MW01096822

Principles and Practice of Phytotherapy

This book is dedicated to Hein Zeylstra, a beloved colleague, and Principal of the College of Phytotherapy in England, who through his enormous energy over 25 years has inspired us both in our work.

About the Authors

Simon Y. Mills

A Cambridge graduate in medical sciences, Simon Mills has also completed the 4-year professional training provided in the UK by the 135 year-old National Institute of Medical Herbalists and has practised as a medical herbalist since 1977. In 1987 he co-founded, and remains the Director of, the Centre for Complementary Health Studies at the University of Exeter, probably the first ever University unit dedicated to studying therapeutic options outside the conventional medical curriculum. Since January 1997, he has been Secretary of the European Scientific Cooperative on Phytotherapy (ESCOP), which is the major European body working to ensure quality, safety and efficacy for herbal medicinal products in collaboration with the European medicines regulators. He also previously co-ordinated the first international research programme on phytomedicines funded by the European Commission entitled *Determining European standards for the safe and effective use of phytomedicines*. He was, for 8 years, President of the National Institute of Medical Herbalists and is currently Chairman of the British Herbal Medicine Association (the primary negotiating body for herbal medicines with the UK regulators) and President of the College of Practitioners of Phytotherapy. He co-produced the 1996 edition of the authoritative *British Herbal Pharmacopoeia* and is the author of several seminal texts on herbal and complementary medicine. As well as his work in the area of herbal medicine, Simon has for many years been in the forefront of developments in the wider development of complementary medicine in the UK. He is currently on the Council of the Foundation for Integrated Medicine, established through the personal instigation of HRH The Prince of Wales.

Kerry Bone

Kerry Bone was an experienced research and industrial chemist before studying herbal medicine in the UK, where he graduated from the full-time course at the School of Phytotherapy. He is currently a practising herbalist of 15 years' experience, Head of Research and Development at MediHerb (Australia's largest manufacturer of high quality herbal extracts) and Principal of the Australian College of Phytotherapy. His research interests include natural insecticide products, and he recently developed a herbal lice control formula that is more effective than synthetic products.

Kerry's technical articles, such as the MediHerb Professional Review, are regularly published in Australia and overseas. His standing as an expert herbalist was acknowledged by his appointment from 1990 to 1997 to the Traditional Medicines Evaluation Committee of the Therapeutic Goods Administration (equivalent to the FDA). He is currently Chair of the Herbal Task Force, a government-industry initiative.

Professional association memberships include; Fellow, National Institute of Medical Herbalists, Fellow, National Herbalists Association of Australia and Member, College of Practitioners of Phytotherapy.

For Churchill Livingstone

Publishing Manager: Inta Ozols
Design Direction: George Ajayi

Principles and Practice of Phytotherapy

Modern Herbal Medicine

Simon Mills MCPP FNIMH MA
Director, Centre for Complementary Health Studies, University of Exeter, Exeter, UK; Chairman, British Herbal Medicine Association; Secretary, European Scientific Cooperative on Phytotherapy (ESCOP)

Kerry Bone MCPP FNHAA FNIMH DipPhyto BSc(Hons)
Head of Research and Development, MediHerb (Pty) Ltd, Warwick, Queensland; Principal, Australian College of Phytotherapy, Australia

Forewords by:

Desmond Corrigan FRSI FLS PhD MA BSc(Pharm)
Senior Lecturer in Pharmacognosy; Director, School of Pharmacy, Trinity College, Dublin; Irish Association of Phytotherapy, Dublin, Eire

James A. Duke
Ethnobotanist, Maryland, USA; formerly US Department of Agriculture

Jonathan V. Wright MD
Medical Director, Tahoma Clinic, Kent, Washington, USA

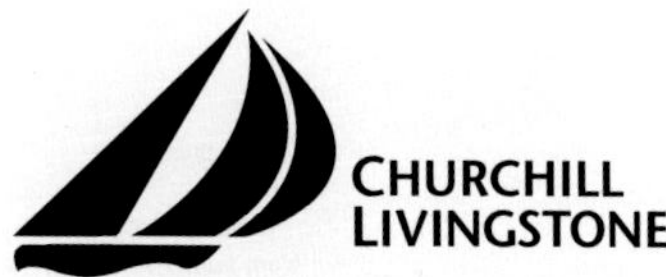

CHURCHILL
LIVINGSTONE

EDINBURGH LONDON NEW YORK PHILADELPHIA ST LOUIS SYDNEY TORONTO 2000

CHURCHILL LIVINGSTONE
An imprint of Harcourt Publishers Limited

First published 2000
Reprinted 2000 (twice)

ISBN 0 443 060169

British Library Cataloguing in Publication Data
A catalogue record for this book is available from the British Library.

Library of Congress Cataloging in Publication Data
A catalog record for this book is available from the Library of Congress.

Note
Medical knowledge is constantly changing. As new information becomes available, changes in treatment, procedures, equipment and the use of drugs become necessary. The editors, contributors and the publishers have, as far as it is possible, taken care to ensure that the information given in this text is accurate and up to date. However, readers are strongly advised to confirm that the information, especially with regard to drug usage, complies with latest legislation and standards of practice.

The publisher's policy is to use **paper manufactured from sustainable forests**

Printed in China

Contents

Forewords

It was not so long ago that much of the material covered by this book would have been considered in the pharmacy curriculum. Departments of pharmacognosy were the rule in schools of pharmacy. Pharmacists would be expected to know how to identify and to prepare and compound plant drugs in their professional work, and to know much about their practical applications. Now pharmacognosy departments are a rarity and only a few of us keep the flame alive in pharmacy education in the English-speaking world. It is somewhat surprising, that a uniquely pharmaceutical science, is nowadays more often taught outside of schools of pharmacy, in new herbal medicine degrees and courses in homeopathy and aromatherapy.

Those of us who have continued to believe in pharmacognosy have been heartened by the increased amount of research on phytochemistry, and on the pharmacology of plant drugs and extracts. It does look as though academic interest in this area is paying off again. There are positive developments elsewhere as well. Our work in developing monographs on the medicinal uses of plant drugs within the European Scientific Cooperative on Phytotherapy (ESCOP) has demonstrated how much expertise there now is, at least in Europe, so that really substantial therapeutic dossiers are now available for many herbal medicinal products. The European Pharmacopoeia is publishing draft quality monographs for plant drugs at an accelerating pace and the WHO series also addresses key quality issues.

However, what we have singularly lacked is the informed insight of clinical practice. There is still too little professional interest among the English-speaking medical profession. Without this it is difficult to fill the information gap between the few clinical research papers published in the medical literature and the vast but often poorly articulated traditional reputation of these remedies. A reliable guide to what works in a modern practice is still hard to find.

In *Principles and Practice of Phytotherapy* we have a serious contribution to filling this gap. The two authors are both grounded in scientific disciplines, one in medical sciences and the other in chemistry. They both have international reputations for setting standards in this field and this is clearly evident in these pages. Most important however, is that they are both in herbal practice, still regularly seeing patients amongst their other duties, and have been doing so for many years. The clinical realities imbue the text. As practitioners, the authors know that clinical judgement is made on the best available rather than the ideal evidence base. As inheritors of a long tradition of herbal practice they know that there are treatments often honed over centuries with well-established reputations for efficacy. When these reputations are rigorously reviewed, as they are here, they may provide a fair basis for prescription in many clinical conditions where confirmed modern drug treatments do not exist. However it is gratifying to see that these authors rarely leave established reputations without comment. Considerable researched material is brought in to qualify or illuminate the material.

Particularly exciting is the pharmacology section, demonstrating with impressive sources how herbal constituents are likely to affect the body. This is especially innovative in including one of the most useful applications of pharmacokinetics to herbal medicine I have ever read. An impressive array of almost 350 references in this section alone is eloquent testimony to the breadth of scholarship brought to bear on this key topic. The herb monographs are also very thorough; clearly differentiating traditional reputation from established or projected activity based on modern evidence.

The clinical recommendations are carefully balanced. Two well-considered chapters on the general issues of efficacy and safety are followed by a large section, Practical Clinical Guides. This starts with very revealing reviews of the current issues of dosage and prescribing that are a major contribution to the debate on these matters. Reviews of the treatment of a wide range of clinical conditions follow. In each case there is a realistic rather than exaggerated range of treatable conditions, and cautions are also given. Helpful treatment plans follow and the remedies to be used clearly identified. Useful case studies add to the relevance of this material and remind us that this information is born of experience rather than theory.

No clinical text on herbal medicine can be entirely a hard-nosed scientific exercise but this at least reassures by its balance and thoroughness. A modern health practitioner interested in the potential of phytotherapy can be encouraged to use this as a practical clinical guide. Students on herbal medicine courses are likely to find this book invaluable as a standard text. For pharmacists and pharmacy students this book provides an excellent opportunity to develop the integration of herbal medicine into the rapidly developing area of pharmaceutical care because of its clinical emphasis. Equally all pharmacy courses could do worse than include the chapters on herbal pharmacology and on optimizing safety (Chapter 5) into the pharmacognosy courses which they should be providing in order that their graduates can truly claim to be society's experts on medicines.

1999 Desmond Corrigan.

Everyone seems to be interested in herbal medicine these days. And the interested parties are hungry for exciting new practical books like this one. Sure, books are surfacing right and left, like never before. But this one, appropriate for the new millennium, is different, an authoritative fact-packed book, reliable and well researched, and written by people who actually *prescribe* real herbal remedies to real people. Herbal medicine has been with us for millennia; synthetic organic poisons less than 200 years.

Therein encapsulated is the reason for modern man's return, his resort, to herbal medicine, safer and gentler, and often as effective. Herbal medicine has always been more empirical than theoretical, never a subject confined to scholarly texts. Herbal medicine has been practised for centuries. Contrary to naive opinions in the first world, herbal medicine is once again in ascendancy, not a dying fossil relic of the past. The 25-year-old herbal renaissance is coming to great fruition, including great new books like this one. Herbal medicine will continue to be used for millennia. Why? Because our genes know many of these phytochemicals, and know how to handle and balance the phytochemicals. Our genes have had little experience with new synthetic drugs.

Mills and Bone pose and answer some fascinating questions: if our foods are chemically complex, then should not our medicines be. (I think that the answer is yes, and that side effects of simple monochemical drugs are what are leading many people to turn to the polychemical herbs). They give good (and fresh) examples of the synergies, which appear to be the rule rather than the exception in herbal medicines. And I love their conclusion to their herbal safety chapter, that possibly the safety record for herbal medicine is better than that for any other widespread human activity, be it eating, drinking, exercise, sleeping, travel, or work.

In this book we are extremely fortunate. These authors, representing respectively the traditions of Great Britain and Australia, have 40 years of clinical practice of herbal medicine between them. They are also both solid scientists; able to apply rigorous scrutiny to the many claims made for their medicines. Every traditional claim offered forth in their book is countered by an exhaustive pharmacological and phytochemical analysis. And excitingly new, the authors have comprehensively covered, and covered well: herbal pharmacodynamics (effect of an active phytochemical at target site(s)) and pharmacokinetics, explaining what actually happens to the phytochemicals in the body when humans consume herbal medicines, and how much of a phytochemical can be concentrated at the site. It is most exciting to read what the authors have to say in this important and understudied area of herbal medicine. These pharmacokinetic observations alone would make the book worthwhile.

The authors rightfully devastate some overextensions of in vitro enzyme assays to real life, where they could not work. This treatise seems to effectively balance authentic traditional use with the latest research priorities. It makes it obvious that laboratory 'in vitro' studies cannot substitute for human 'in vivo' experience. And here we often have centuries of human experience around the world written up in the eyes of phytomedicinal scientists with decades of clinical experiences. Readers will enjoy sharing the erudite observations reported in this fascinating book.

Part Three contains their Materia Medica, a nice selection of almost 50 species. I find it interesting that of these, Andrographis, Angelica (dong-quai), Astragalus, Arctostaphylos, Barosma, Berberis, Bupleurum, Chelidonium, Chrysanthemum (Feverfew), Euphrasia, Hydrastis, Oenothera, Phytolacca, Rehmannia, Tabebuia, and Withania, about a third, were not approved or studied by Commission E. But I have a great respect for these clinicians' experience and will give their selections equal weight with the Commission E selections. I want the best medicine for my family and myself, whether it be African, American, Australian, British, Chinese, German, Japanese or what have you.

What a shame. I didn't have time to devour all the new information in this exciting book, now. I'll have to wait until it's published at which time it will be a must for my coworkers and me, especially when trying to sort out the herbal hyperbole from the herbal truth. Thanks Simon and Kerry. The millennium needed this.

1999 James A. Duke

Our great-great-grandmothers are back. They may be wearing white laboratory smocks and using mainframe computers, but our great-great-grandmothers are indeed back. Perhaps your great-great-grandmother, perhaps mine; very likely great-great-grandmothers (and great-great-grandfathers, too) from the Amazon, China, the Outback, India, and the Congo. They've been trying to tell us for most of the 20th century that the plants of our Earth contain great healing power, but only a few of us have listened. So they've returned to tell us again, making sure to use language our contemporary high priests (scientists) can understand and disseminate to 'the masses'.

For those who don't believe in re-incarnation, I'll state right away: this image is figurative, not literal, but the meaning is the same. Using the most powerful tools and techniques of contemporary science, researchers all over the world are 'proving' that great-great-grandmother (and great-great-grandfather) were right about herbs and health in many, many cases. (Certainly our ancestors weren't infallible, any more than are we, but it's likely they were just as smart and observant as we are.) With the information gained with today's powerful research tools, our scientists can now tell us: 'Take your polysaccharides (including heteroglycans and inulin), flavonoids (including quercitin and rutoside), caffeic acid derivatives (including chicoric acid, chlorogenic acid and cynarin), essential oils (including borneol, and alpha-pinene), polyacetylenes, and alkylamides. They'll boost your immune system and help chase that cold.'

Great-great-grandmother would have put it more simply: 'Take your Echinacea. It'll help that cold.' But chances are she'd also have smiled and agreed with Will Shakespeare who reminded us: 'That which we call a rose by any other name would smell as sweet'.

No matter if we describe Echinacea molecule-by-molecule, it'll do the same job she said it would.

Of course great-great-grandmother wouldn't take all the credit, and we can't take away the achievements of contemporary science. Following the many paths pioneered by our herbalist ancestors, today's researchers into botanicals have (as each succeeding generation should) added another dimension to the accumulating storehouse of information about the preventive and therapeutic uses of the plants of our planet. And very likely to great-great-grandmother's satisfaction ('they're so clever, our great-great-grandchildren') contemporary researchers have found and proven a few uses for herbals not known in the past.

Kerry Bone and Simon Mills are two of these 'great-great-grandparents in spirit'. Using a clear and understandable style, they've woven the latest in-depth research data into the millenia-old herbal tradition. They have written us not only an excellent 'take this herb for that health problem, and here's the science why' volume, but they also take care to put it into the larger context of traditional herbalism. They gently remind us that the 'magic bullet herbal' (they term it 'alternative allopathic') approach is only a part of a much greater herbal healing tradition, a tradition as yet unexplored by contemporary science. (For example, they discuss the traditional herbalists' approaches of cleansing, heating, cooling, and tonification, and how they fit into an over-all health improvement pattern.)

My own medical practice of nearly 30 years (after conventional medical school and 'residency') relies on intensive study of natural approaches, emphasizing diet, vitamins, minerals, allergies and sensitivities, and natural hormones. Over the years, I've added more and more 'herbal tools' (I'm guilty of using the alternative allopathic' approach in most instances), many of which I've learned from Kerry Bone's exceptionally well-done columns in the *Nutrition and Healing* newsletter (edited by myself in the USA). I'm very grateful to Kerry and his colleague Simon Mills for the furthering of my education with the information in this volume, and recommend it as 'top of the list' for contemporary students of herbal medicine.

1999

Jonathan V. Wright

Prefaces

In the 25 years since I started practice as a medical herbalist the profession in Britain has changed dramatically, the challenges that face it growing with it. I was introduced to the profession by one of its great advocates. Fred Fletcher Hyde, who had graduated from the University of London with a first-class degree in Botany in 1923, and almost single-handedly steered the practice of herbal medicine through its darkest days after the 1941 Pharmacy Act and on through its apparent nemesis, with the first draft of the 1968 Medicines Act, to successful legal protection under that Act. I shall be forever grateful for his inspiration, for his vision of herbal medicine as the most noble of healing professions, at least as old as mankind, and able to take on all comers, here always and forever more. He was painfully aware of the labours necessary to survive in a modern world. The National Institute of Medical Herbalists (NIMH), of which he had been president for many years, had in 1964 celebrated its centenary as by far the oldest professional body of medical herbalists in the Western world but with a membership down to double figures and declining. For obvious reasons, therefore, the profession in recent years has been in defensive rather than enterprise mode. The major developments of strategy had been in the previous century and again briefly before the Second World War. Fletcher Hyde was a valiant defender and was concerned most urgently with applying scientific method to support traditional practice. However, there was little opportunity at that time for philosophical innovation. As the profession began to grow in the 1970s and especially with the establishment of the new school under the direction of Hein Zeylstra, herbal practitioners found themselves heir to a miscellany of influences, few clearly articulated.

The original therapeutic core was Anglo-American, the simple but radical system developed by Samuel Thomson out of a blend of settler and Indian practices in early 19th-century North America and later developed by his successors to the physiomedical tradition that briefly flowered in the American Midwest in the late 1800s, taking in all the latest physiological insights of the time, notably the discovery of the autonomic nervous system. Both Thomsonism and physiomedicalism found a welcome reception among new working-class urban herbal associations of the Midlands and northern British Industrial Revolution. The NIMH until the mid-1980s was still describing itself as a professional body of physiomedical practitioners. This was in spite of the fact that apart from published texts by Albert Priest and one or two others, the relevant theoretical material had barely changed since its inception. There was an important kernel of a radical pharmacology in the Thomsonian tradition of 'heating' rather than suppressing fevers but few modern practitioners could embrace the old system in its entirety. North America also provided us with other legacies that have fared rather better. The Eclectic tradition, contemporary with physiomedicalism (and with the new professions of osteopathy and chiropractic in the same setting), crossbred European naturopathy with a vigorous new American materia medica to provide a new professional impetus that currently flourishes in the north-west of North America.

Nevertheless, in setting out a new professional identity, the new NIMH school opted instead for European phytotherapy, from the established herbal medicine of Germany and France, where modern physicians and pharmacists still supply plant medicines and increasingly integrate them with modern medicine. From this tradition, we learnt how to appraise herbs as alternatives to synthetic drugs, attempting to explain their action by reference to the activity of their chemical constituents, and we began the process, still under way, of standardizing quality, safety and efficacy for the requirements of the national and European legislatures. In this, we have begun to have some success and have been considered with some envy by practitioners in other countries where herbal medicine is still dismissed by orthodoxy as a fringe activity. There is a growing body of clinical and pharmacological research to justify the use of individual remedies. However, any radical therapeutic approaches in European phytotherapy emerge only dimly out of the *Mittel*european naturopathic and vitalistic traditions. Very often, it is merely *médicin douce*, a gentle alternative to chemical drugs. Herbs are often provided on the same symptomatic basis as other drugs (from *drogen*, dried herb) but at least in over-the-counter supply, mainly for the 'minor, self-limiting conditions' deemed appropriate for the therapy by legislators.

Our student practitioners are now taught in the European tradition how to apply herbs for more complex conditions in the consulting room context. However, these strategies often have only a fragmentary pharmacological rationale (How far do the herbs recommended for arthritis or peptic ulceration or bowel disease really go to the underlying causes of these conditions?) or continue naturopathic approaches (e.g. eliminating 'acids' in arthritis, giving expectorants in catarrhal conditions, using depuratives in inflammatory disease). That these often appear to help remains the justification for using the treatments but, as we shall see, without a sound pharmacological rationale this is emphatically not a basis for a new professional therapeutic. In any case, the strategies were not sufficient to prevent a widespread outbreak of philosophical drifting by the new generation of medical herbalists.

It has sometimes appeared, unlike almost anywhere else in the world, as though indigenous herbal medicine has been a Cinderella among the new complementary disciplines in Britain. The first big sister has clearly been dietary therapy. The results of a diet change, the elimination of coffee, tea, pork, dairy, even the addition of a dietary supplement, have often obscured the perceived effect of the concurrent herbal treatment, to the latter's disadvantage. There is no doubt, as the following text makes clear, that there are very close links between diet and herbal medicine, with the latter in many ways informing and facilitating the former. However, as shall also be made clear, herbal medicine has many features that distinguish it from diet. Both can probably do things that the other could never achieve. It will be helpful for both to distinguish herbal from dietary treatments.

Then there has been the lure of the Orient. With its sophistication, comprehensiveness, subtleties and insights pertinent to a postmodern era, Chinese medicine especially has been a major success story in the West. Many graduates of herbal medicine have moved smartly to learn the new materia medica, philosophies and diagnostic systems, perhaps reflecting the very lack of systematics in the homegrown version. As we shall hopefully demonstrate, Chinese and Ayurvedic medicine provide us with important insights into the effect of herbal medicines on the human body and it should be possible to transcribe some of these to a modern Western format.

Other practitioners have embraced the physical therapies. Traditionally in Britain, many herbalists were also osteopaths-naturopaths;

now they are as likely to learn aroma-massage, applying essences of plants to a distinctly more immediate and beguiling therapy.

Herbal medicine has always mixed well with other treatments. In modern times, however, it is unique in that it competes for its rationale directly with synthetic chemical pharmacology. This has held it back, for example where other complementary disciplines have gone for state registration or licence. It leaves herbal medicine vulnerable to the benefit:risk ratio applied to evaluating modern drugs, where to the public guardian unproven benefit equates with zero benefit and even a suggestion of risk is enough to cast doubts on its value to the public.

Even to survive in the modern world, let alone to be able to take its place again as the most noble form of healing, herbal medicine needs to develop a more muscular pharmacological and therapeutic case for itself. It needs frankly to take on the phenomenon of the placebo effect, to develop new verifiable models of efficacy that satisfactorily distinguish it from the alternatives. It needs to identify the areas where it can make a valuable contribution and those where it probably has little direct benefit. It can almost certainly withstand the pressure.

Exeter, UK 1999 Simon Y. Mills

In the early 19th century, Samuel Thomson established and promoted a system of herbal medicine that drew heavily from the native Americans. In 1838, a student of Thomson with the unfortunate name of Dr Albert Isaiah Coffin arrived in England to spread the word about Thomsonian medicine. (John Skelton, an English herbalist, teamed with Coffin briefly but later became aligned with another group of practitioners who called themselves the Eclectics.) Nonetheless, professional herbalism had truly arrived in the UK.

In 1864, the British Medical Reform Association was founded, later to become the National Institute of Medical Herbalists (NIMH) which prospers to this day. Meanwhile in the USA, a relatively obscure system known as physiomedicalism evolved from Thomsonian medicine, with key works by Thurston, Cook and Lyle. Although the physiomedicalists were relatively few in the USA compared to the Eclectics, English herbalists aligned themselves with the physiomedicalists in the early 20th century. At around the same time, the National Herbalists Association of Australia (NHAA) was established, with practice along physiomedical/Thomsonian lines. The NHAA remains the prime body for herbalists in Australia.

Thomson was not an intellectual in his approach and developed a simple but sound philosophical basis for his system. In one sense, he was a true naturopath who strongly believed in a vital force, as expressed by the body's innate healing capacity. Since physiomedicalism evolved from Thomsonian medicine, this system also stressed the importance of the vital force. The physiomedicalists promoted an elaborate philosophy and chose their name because their approach to therapy was based on theories emphasizing the known physiology of the time. According to Lyle (1897): 'Physiomedicalism is medication in harmony with true Physiology, recognizing in all conditions the indications of the vital force and hence abstaining from all poisonous medicines'.

While the practice of physiomedicalism died out in the USA, it was perpetuated in England and Australia (with influences also from the Eclectics and local herbal medicine) as the Anglo-American school of herbal medicine. This is arguably the only tradition of Western herbal medicine in which the passage of knowledge from teacher to student has survived unbroken to this day. It retains the elements central to any traditional system of medicine. These are the recognition of a vital force, respect for traditional knowledge, treatment of the patient as a unique individual and a system of comprehending the therapeutic needs of the patient more in terms of physiology than pathology and more in terms of allaying causes than treating symptoms.

The authors of this book are (through our original training in herbal medicine) steeped in the Anglo-American tradition. But we also recognize the importance of the considerable scientific endeavour that has been applied in recent times to the study of medicinal plants. The successful blending of tradition with science is leading to a new robust system of Western herbal medicine, a system best encompassed by the term 'phytotherapy'. As such, phytotherapy defines a new medical paradigm that combines the wisdom of an ancient tradition with the cutting edge of current research. However, scientific rigour must not be compromised. If science is an integral part of phytotherapy, then it should be good science. Too many texts about herbs and herbal medicine contain misleading information because of excessive extrapolation from scientific publications, be they in vitro, animal or clinical studies, or because of vague allusions to traditional use. While it is appropriate to speculate on new uses for herbs, such speculation should be transparent. Hypotheses should not be presented as fact and all sources of information, be they traditional or scientific, should be clearly cited. Anecdotal information that has no traditional basis should be heavily discounted.

A number of approaches have emerged in the modern practice of Western herbal medicine. At one extreme is the model where herbs are viewed as plant-based drugs. As such, they are administered in monopreparations or sometimes simple combinations of two herbs. The approach to prescribing is very simple, being based on symptoms or a particular condition, and medicines are chosen on the basis of proof of efficacy and safety from controlled clinical trials. This model predominates among medical doctors, particularly in Europe. Herbal products are prescribed in the context of a conventional medical consultation and are viewed as an additional therapeutic option when chemical drugs are inappropriate. Preparations are usually in tablet form and often contain standardized extracts. Adherents to this style of herbal medicine will probably be most interested in the monograph section of this book but will hopefully enjoy learning about the practice of phytotherapy in a wider context.

At the other end of the spectrum are traditional Western herbalists, who compound different formulations for each patient on the basis of a detailed consultation, which, while it might resemble a conventional medical consultation, is ultimately seeking different endpoints. Such practitioners generally employ the traditional galenical extracts of herbs, which come in liquid form as either tinctures or fluid extracts. The advantages of these preparations are largely that they represent a minimal processing of the crude herb into a convenient dosage form but, more importantly, that they can be readily compounded into an individual prescription. The attitude of the more traditional practitioners to scientific information about herbs and the new style of products tends to vary. This book is intended to encourage traditional practitioners in what they already do. Its primary objective is to assist them by providing a contemporary rationale for their therapy and perhaps new insights into the management of common health problems, backed up by concise and up-to-date scientific information on the plants they use.

One feature which is generally lacking from books about herbs or herbal medicine is adequate treatment of herbal therapeutics. To be fully effective in herbal therapy, it is not enough simply to know about the herbs themselves. Information must also be sought about how and when to use these herbs in response to the various therapeutic challenges. It is the therapeutic content in this text, complete with actual case histories, which differentiates it from other works and genuinely defines its audience as the student or professional reader.

A form of herbal medicine is practised in every culture and in every country of the world, be it industrialized or not. Something deep within us recognizes that there is healing power in the plant kingdom which, after all, is the nourishment of all animal life. Herbal medicine is not an anachronism practised by ignorant people. It is time to embrace the concept of phytotherapy and further develop its art and science for the benefit of all humanity.

Queensland, Australia 1999 — Kerry Bone

Acknowledgments

It is obviously a large task to comprehensively capture and review at any one time the now extensive literature on major medicinal plants. Several herbalists assisted with Part Three of this text which contains the herbal monographs. The contributions of Mark Walker, Berris Burgoyne, Andrew Pengelly and Michael Thomsen are gratefully recognized. But in particular the diligence and meticulous research and drafting skills of Michelle Morgan, who made a major contribution to Part Three, is acknowledged with thanks and gratitude by the authors.

Secretarial staff who helped throughout the preparation of the book were Jacinta McGahan, Patti Steele, Jan Frousheger and Trish Burt. The input of Sue Radford on both the manuscript and the chemical structures needs to be particularly noted with due appreciation.

Finally our respective wives Rachel and Patricia tolerated much and offered great moral support for this project. We hope that the book meetings in Bali were sufficient compensation.

S.Y.M.

K.B.

Herb terminology

There are three conventions for naming herbal remedies. All are used freely in this book to reflect common parlance among herbal practitioners. Familiarity with all three will be useful for any reader.

The **common name** (here in English and occasionally pinyin Chinese) is the language used with patients and is rendered in this text in ordinary lower case as in 'dandelion'.

The botanical name, the most precise and globally applicable, used to define the plant scientifically and professionally, rendered here in the usual convention of the generic name starting with a capital letter and the specific name in lower case, all in italics, as in *Echinacea angustifolia* or *Taraxacum officinale*.

The abbreviated pharmaceutical name, the common shorthand terminology among practitioners and in the pharmaceutical sector, used especially where the generic name is sufficient (either because only one species is generally used or because the species used is not critical or one understands it to refer to the best species available); in this text the convention is to use an initial capital and no italics, as in 'Echinacea' or 'Taraxacum'.

Introduction

Herbal medicine is a triumph of popular therapeutic diversity. Plants above all other agents have been used for medicines because they have fitted the immediate personal need: they are accessible and inexpensive, they speak to those who have used them in their own language and they are not provided from a remote professional or government apparatus. For these and other reasons, the use of plants for medicines around the world still vastly exceeds the use of modern synthetic drugs. Such activity is not completely dismissed in scientific society either: plants are also appreciated in pharmaceutical research as the major resource for new medicines and a growing body of medical literature supports the clinical efficacy of herbal treatments. Even where traditional use has largely died out in developed countries, there is an increasing yearning for a new deal in healthcare in which the old remedies feature strongly. To meet this demand, there is a growing number of well-educated herbalists and phytotherapists.

Most herbal use has been very parochial and empirical: local reputations have often been disparate; herbal lore has rarely travelled well. However, herbs have also provided the basis for the great medical systems in human history, of Hippocrates and Galen and the great Islamic medical eras, of the Ayurveda of the Indian subcontinent, of waves of Chinese systematizations over two millennia and the many smaller cultural traditions that were often hybrids of the foregoing. All these systems were formed in large part by the peculiar characteristics of their materia medica; plants have clearly demanded and been granted their own therapeutic approach.

The era of grand systems has probably passed but it may be time to develop a new coherent approach to herb use for a scientific age. Apart from a general view that herbs are safer, there has been only a fragmentary rationale for using them as medicines in modern times. Now that there are increasing media attacks on herbal safety, mostly alarmist, there is the risk that even the perceived safety advantage is being whittled away. There is a pressing need to salvage from the wealth of tradition, empirical practices and modern research a new positive, muscular and consistent pharmacological strategy that can meet the valid challenges of medical science, the safety and the placebo issues above all.

Four main sources of information were used in preparing the following text. Traditional use of herbs is both the largest and most difficult resource. The bewildering variety of folk practices around the world, the powerful confounding effect of social context and other non-specific or placebo effects make reliable conclusions from any one tradition difficult. However, evidence will be presented that in general, folk use and pharmacological activity are indeed closely correlated. More usefully, it will be shown that there are recurring themes in indigenous use: persistent therapeutic approaches and consistent use of 'archetypal' chemical groups within plants. These resonances will be identified and will provide the backdrop to discussions of modern use.

There is also the clinical experience of modern practitioners to consider. This has the advantages of being up to date and set in a modern medical context. It still suffers, however, from the confounding effect of non-specific effects of treatment: in many of the conditions for which modern phytotherapy is applied the placebo effect is likely to be high, sometimes very high, and without controlling for this effect the independent activity of the herbs themselves is extremely hard to isolate. Nevertheless, there are ways in which the fog can be cleared and practitioners can often obtain quite reliable insights into the action of their prescriptions; where these accord more widely, they may also add usefully to a growing caseload.

The third data resource is less clinically relevant but is both substantial and scientifically sound. The available published literature on phytochemistry (the chemistry of plants) and preclinical pharmacology of plant extracts grows at an astounding pace. There are several peer-reviewed scientific journals devoted to the subject and there is of course a powerful incentive for such work in the pharmaceutical industry's search for new drugs. Researchers have no doubt that nature is still the preeminent synthetic chemist and that in plants particularly, there are almost infinite reserves of fascinating chemical constituents with actual and potential effects on the human body. As such information accumulates it is sometimes possible better to understand traditional uses of plants. Where such associations can be made they will be posited in the text as leads for further exploration. They will not be used, however, as confirmation of a clinical effect; experience in practice is that the effect of the whole plant is rarely predicted by the effects of its parts. The pharmaceutical industry's own experience is that preclinical activity only occasionally translates into clinically useful benefits.

Finally, there is the evidence that counts most in the court of clinical judgement. There are still too few well-conducted, placebo-controlled, double-blind clinical trials into the effect of herbal drugs. These are expensive to conduct and present awesome methodological and logistical challenges (especially in satisfactorily measuring outcomes in the less pathologically defined conditions for which herbs are most often applied). Without patent protection, industry is less inclined to invest in such studies. However, the evidence is accumulating. A number of meta-analyses of clinical trial data have shown that for the few individual herbs most studied, the clinical evidence is indeed persuasive. In most such cases, the plants concerned are pharmacologically unremarkable; their survival through the most intense scrutiny reassures that other remedies could do the same. More importantly for this book, there are specific lessons that can be applied in judging likely efficacy of a wider range of plants.

No single source above can absolutely confirm that herbs are a rational treatment strategy. It is for this reason that herbs have sometimes been dismissed as the refuge of the romantic and the uncritical. However, when all sources of information are integrated something genuinely exciting emerges: traditionally based coherent treatment policies for a range of conditions are given new relevance in modern practice and resonate with new pharmacological insights into the activity of plant constituents. As most of the strategies developed are unique to herbal medicine and address clinical problems that are notoriously difficult to treat in modern times, they will repay further investigation.

The different data sources above are elaborated in the contents of this book. In Part One, traditional systematic approaches to herbal therapeutics from around the world are outlined first; this section finishes with a brief review of modern insights into the behaviour of dynamic systems, which have lead to the development of chaos and complexity models and which incidentally provide new explanations for healing phenomena. There then follows an introduction to the pharmacological principles emerging from current knowledge of the activity of plant constituents. Many constituents are classified into 'archetypal' chemical groups with well-established pharmacological activities; understanding these activities allows for preliminary assessments of a plant's potential with only minimal information of its taxonomic group and constitution. The presence of prominent archetypal groups can often lead to fertile cross-referencing with traditional reputations to raise fascinating clinical prospects. This section extends to consideration of a radically new explanation for the effects of herbs on the body. It will be pointed out that most herbal constituents start with topical effects (i.e. locally at the site of application) and that they are particularly likely to stimulate the wide range of functions linked to trigger sites on the lining of the digestive tract. Traditional reputations will be linked to modern physiological insights to provide promising new strategies for a wide range of diseases.

There follow a number of sections which elaborate the practical implications of applying herbal remedies compared with other treatments. There is a section on the most persistent herbal therapeutic principles found in the traditional records, updated into modern terminology, and providing a basis for the more detailed discussions later. The most appropriate diagnostic information required for herbal prescription is discussed next, emphasizing the importance of assessing functional performance in the body as much as morbid states; the ancient techniques of pulse and tongue diagnosis used around the world are reviewed in this context. Important discussions of the issues of validation and safety follow; in both areas herbal medicine is subject to challenge but in both reassuring progress is being made.

Part Two looks more closely at the herbal approach to particular clinical conditions. These are divided into two groups: general disease conditions that lead to the most common pathological states afflicting humanity and the more particular functional disturbances of the body's organ systems to which herbal medicine has so often been applied. Functional disturbances can have many causes; pathological processes are the most serious but probably not the most common. Herbal remedies have persistently been viewed as addressing what might be called 'misbehaviours' of body functions, a term that includes the notion of psychosomatic disorders but also all the other ways in which the living body finds it difficult smoothly to coexist with its environment.

No practical guide to using herbal remedies could be complete without a good review of the dosage issue and indeed this opens Part Two. There is much confusion abroad on this with widely varying dose regimes being recommended. The authors explore the relative cases for each approach, taking account of a wide range of sources, and make clear recommendations in all the following sections.

Part Three is devoted to individual remedies. Over 40 plants most widely used in the Western herbal tradition, but including examples from around the world, are reviewed in considerable depth. Clinical imperatives still rule and the information most important to the practitioner opens each monograph – practical guides as to when to use and not to use each plant, cautions and doubts honestly raised as appropriate. However, there also follow comprehensive details of the current scientific information on each herb, fully referenced, so that the best available technical assessments can be made by each reader.

There are a number of reference guides for easy access. As well as a detailed general index, there is an index of symptoms and conditions and one for herb activities. All sections of the book are comprehensively supported with citations so that the reader can pursue further reading in depth.

Any new therapeutic framework needs broad agreement from current practitioners. There are now thousands of highly educated individuals in the developed countries, many of them physicians, who prescribe herbal medicines regularly in their clinical work. Most of these have been bypassed by the vigorous scientific activity currently found at phytomedicine conferences or in the technical literature. They have obviously acquired valuable experience but rarely have the tools with which to separate the effects of the remedy from other clinical phenomena and still lack the institutional support that might underpin their aspirations. Nevertheless, they remain a vital community. Both authors of this book are experienced herbal practitioners and are guided in this work mainly by clinical priorities. They will aim to provide new information for debate among their colleagues, possible new rationales for their practices, even new approaches for difficult clinical problems.

The book should also reassure other healthcare workers, for example doctors, pharmacists, osteopaths and chiropractors, who are tempted to try herbal medicines themselves but want a sound basis first. Although many doctors in Europe prescribe phytomedicines, this is rare in English-speaking countries in which there is more scepticism about using crude historical folk remedies as a serious substitute for scientific medication. Although there is a growing interest in other complementary techniques herbal medicine has not managed to persuade that it has a coherent strategy for treating difficult conditions. That patients increasingly resort to herbs is seen as something separate from medicine, unless a safety issue is perceived. This text will present a substantial and well-documented case for herbs as unique strategies in the treatment of some of the most intractable problems in modern healthcare.

In many developed countries natural healthcare alternatives are provided by a range of naturopathic professional groups. As well as dietary treatment and various complementary disciplines, these practitioners frequently use herbal remedies. Often, the herbal component has only a minor and adjunctive role in the overall treatment strategy. This text will surely persuade that there are many areas where informed application of herbs might transform the prospects of difficult conditions and that, in particular, dietary measures can be powerfully reinforced or amended by the established modulatory effects of herbs on the digestive processes. There is also a trend among complementary practitioners to favour herbal remedies from China and India, accompanied as these are by their own elaborate therapeutic system. This account should allow such practitioners better to understand the underlying principles and may reinstate indigenous remedies in their materia medica.

In the countries of Asia, Africa and South America, a much larger proportion of the population still choose or rely on herbal medicines for their day-to-day healthcare. The World Health Organization and other international agencies have long recognized that traditional health practitioners and their remedies represent a vital resource to be encouraged, to more effectively maintain health in remote regions and better to maintain plant biodiversity and local communities and industries. As these practitioners work to develop their therapeutic approaches and integrate them better with Western delivery systems, they may welcome the insights of those with long experience of coexistence with Western medicine. The remedies will be different but the principles are likely to be the same.

The patient can also learn from this book. Anyone who wishes to be informed about the treatment of their personal condition, who wants to take responsibility for their own health, who is fascinated that there may be effective remedies provided freely in nature and who is able to grasp basic medical concepts will find this a treasure trove. All such readers must be reminded, however, that illness can often be complex and sometimes dangerous. They should never proceed far without expert advice and never stray from adequate supervision of any illness.

What follows is a contribution to a debate among those interested in herbal medicine. It will lay out as effectively as possible a realistic strategy in line with scientific evidence but based also on experience in practice and on the legacy of much longer traditions. It will inevitably be contentious in parts: some cherished beliefs will be challenged but if this stimulates productive debate then nothing should be lost.

Part 1

Background and Strategies

1 Herbal therapeutic systems

A useful way to appreciate the potential of herbal remedies is to review those approaches to using them which have developed in a number of cultures through history. Some common themes emerge in this review, though varied by their background; when these are recast in the light of modern scientific enquiry one may glimpse therapeutic approaches that are radically different from those which underpin conventional medicine.

What also emerges again and again is that, contrary to modern prejudice, writers on medicine from the very earliest eras demonstrate a respect for rigorous observation and humane pragmatism that still may provide a valuable lesson for healthcare today. These sources are not to be dismissed lightly.

FROM THE BEGINNING: POPULAR PRACTICES

As it is now known that animals use plants for medicinal purposes[40,41], it is unlikely there was a time that humans did not use herbal remedies. There is prehistoric evidence of the use of medicinals, from the USA[1] and medicinal plant traces found at Neolithic sites.[2] There are also innumerable accounts of medicinal plant use by small communities around the world, living wholly within the natural world and crafting their survival from the facilities around them[42–44].

Most of what is known about herbal use in recorded history is provided by early texts, often among the earliest of all known books. However, one overwhelming gap in this record is that although in its original mode herbal medicine was most probably practised in local communities, largely by women, this is barely reflected in contemporary accounts.[3] After the demise of organized medicine with the collapse of the Roman empire, healthcare in Europe for most people was again provided at a very local level, probably including a mix of herbs and diet, together with faith and holy relics, as well as astrology, pagan incantation and ritual[4] (the Inquisition permitting – millions of women were killed for practising 'witchcraft' across Europe from the 13th to the 18th centuries).[5] Hildegarde von Bingen, one of the first prominent woman authorities in Europe, achieved particular renown through her medicinal text *Physica*. In it, she became the first woman publicly to discuss plants in relation to their medicinal properties.[6] She was, however, a solitary exception to the prevailing view that women were not in the forefront of academic, professional or literary efforts. Like her, however, most European writers of the time were from the monastic tradition, only moving into the popular arena around Chaucer's time. By then well-organized medicinal gardens and practices were recorded in England by authors such as Henry Daniel, John Arderne, John Bray and Chaucer himself, all reflecting on current medicinal practice across Europe in the 14th century.[7] Where systems were apparent in these texts, they appear to have been derived from the Graeco-Roman tradition with varying amounts of astrology, especially in works by Culpeper and Gerard. It was only with the works of Paracelsus that scholarship began substantially to question the previous deference to Galen and medicine moved into the modern technological age, leaving folk practice way behind.

Such was the enormous variety of folk practices around the world that one must conclude that most rationales were based on a mix of empiricism with local shibboleths and traditions. Nevertheless, there are likely to have been common features. A fascinating account of one remote group in Central America[45] shows significant similarities between their and other humoral approaches around the world. It is also certain that where therapeutic systems did develop, they were based on popular practices.

GRAECO-ROMAN AND ISLAMIC MEDICINE

The systematic development of medical ideas that started with the Hippocratic writings from the Greek island of Kos in the fifth and fourth centuries BC and climaxed in the work of Galen in the second century AD laid the foundations for European medicine until the scientific era and the framework for Islamic medicine until the present time. They were marked by almost modern standards of empiricism, logic and rigour.

The Hippocratic writings,[8] a complex series of treatises from a school rather than from one individual, were an astonishing event. In passages of renaissant illumination, they evidenced an enlightened tradition that invoked dietary, lifestyle, environmental and psychotherapeutic means to encouraging health. The Hippocratic tradition is generally associated with the concept of the natural healing power of life, the *vis medicatrix naturae*. In fact, most of the texts are pragmatic guides to maintaining health and to the practice of medicine, with some passages (e.g. *The Art of Medicine*) as undisguised paeans to the importance of physicians in healthcare.

There were herbs included in the Hippocratic canon, but it was a wider doctrine of whole healthcare that was being formulated. It was left to others to formulate the materia medicae of the day. The Greek Dioscorides in the first century AD rigorously collected information about 500 plants and remedies in tours with the Roman armies and collated them in his seminal *Materia Medica*.[9]

Galen is widely regarded as the pivotal Graeco-Roman authority in medicinal matters. He wrote extensively about his subject, setting out comprehensive principles of sometimes surprising topicality. For example, he proposed a research agenda for establishing the 'powers' of a remedy, based on the observance of eight conditions:

1. the drug must be of good unadulterated quality;
2. the illness must be simple, not complex;
3. the illness must be appropriate to the action of the drug;
4. the drug must be more powerful than the illness;
5. one should make careful note of the course of illness and treatment;
6. one must ensure that the effect of the drug is the same for everybody at every time;
7. one must see that the effect of the drug is specific for human beings (in an animal it can have another effect);
8. one must distinguish the effect of drugs (working by their qualities) from foods (working by their substance).

In further passages (most have never been translated) he shows clear evidence of modern logical thought in setting out a series of experiments to prove that the kidneys were the source of urine into the bladder.[10]

The fundamental principle in Galen's work was that nature was an active dynamic force manifesting phenomena as it expressed its purpose. Treatments engaged these powers, either in the case of drugs through their own dynamic 'qualities' or in the case of foods by the qualities of their substance. In classifying the dynamic qualities of medicines, he refined the widely established view that they had 'temperaments' reflecting well-understood climatic influences. The most prominent were the effects they appeared to have on the mobilization of body heat, especially in relation to fevers. His authoritative definitions of pharmaceutical qualities were widely used throughout medieval Europe:

> All medicines considered in themselves are either hot, cold, moist, dry or temperate.
>
> The qualities of medicines are considered in respect of man, not of themselves; for those simples are called hot which heat our bodies; for those cold which cool them; and those temperate which work no change at all…
>
> Such as are hot in the first degree, are of equal heat with our bodies, and they only add a natural heat to them, if it be cooled by nature or by accident thereby cherishing the natural heat when weak, and restoring it when wanting. Their use is 1. To make the offending humours thin, that they may be expelled by sweat or perspiration. 2. By outward application to abate inflammations and fevers by opening the pores of the skin.
>
> Such as are hot in the second degree, as much exceed the first, as our natural heat exceeds a temperature. Their use is, to open the pores, and take away obstructions, by relaxing tough humours and by their essential force and strength, when nature cannot do it.
>
> Such as are hot in the third degree, are more powerful in heating, because they tend to inflame and cause fevers. Their use is to promote perspiration extremely, and soften tough humours, and therefore all of them resist poison.
>
> Such as are hot in the fourth degree, burn the body, if outwardly applied. Their use is to cause inflammation, raise blisters, and corrode the skin.

> Such as are cold in the first degree, fall as much on the one side of temperate as doth hot on the other. Their use is, 1. To qualify the heat of the stomach and cause digestion. 2. To abate the heat in fevers; and 3. To refresh the spirits being almost suffocated.
>
> Such as are cold in the third degree, are such as have a repercussive force. Their use is 1. To drive back the matter, and stop defluctions. 2. To make the humours thick; and 3. To limit the violence of choler, repress perspiration, and keep the spirits from fainting.
>
> Such as are cold in the fourth degree, are such as to stupefy the senses. They are used, 1. In violent pains; and 2. In extreme watchings, and the like cases, where life is despaired of.

This is a clinically elaborate classification. Heating remedies start as at 'equal heat with our bodies' (i.e. normalizing a healthy body temperature), rising in stages to those that must only be 'outwardly applied' in counterirritation and blistering strategies (see p. 81).

Their primary function is to thin 'offending humours', or toxic accumulations, a process that may have been likened to the effect of warming congealed meat stock, so that they may be expelled by perspiration (in fever). This strategy implied that fevers were a healthy response and that such remedies supported this response 'when nature cannot do it'. As they become stronger they are more forceful, till they actually 'cause fevers' and 'cause inflammations', taking over entirely from a failing constitution.

Cooling remedies are inherently more risky. The ultimate cold is the corpse. Nevertheless, they can be used to contain excessive vital responses such as pain, 'choler' and excessive eliminations ('defluctions'). Intriguingly, at the gentlest such level, the effect is to 'cause digestion'; the bitters (see p. 38) were included in this category, the attraction being that these cooled but did not depress, reducing heat by switching the bias towards increased digestive activity (universally seen as cooling) and thus increased nourishment, a highly attractive tactic in many fevers. Also intriguing is the insight at the other end of the spectrum. Using powerful sedatives when all else fails and death is imminent ('in extreme watchings') is one of the less formally advisable clinical knacks from a more desperate age; it appears that the effect can be to wipe out the clamour of adversity at that stage of crisis so that new life might just flicker back.

The works of the Graeco-Roman writers were most extensively reworked by the medical writers of the Islamic era. Up to 100 authors on pharmaceutics and materia medica are identifiable in the Arabic bibliographies, most copying and adapting directly from Dioscorides and Galen. There were, however, notable developments, including the work of the Persians al-Majusi (Haly Abbas), ar-Rhazi (Rhazes) and Ibn-Sina (Avicenna), the Jew Maimonides and the Christian Hunayn ibn-Ishaq. However, not for the first time in reviews of classic texts (the Chinese canon is another example), there is a sense that much that was written was truly theoretical, with evidence of systematization by rote, showing little regard for likely actual practices.[11]

Nevertheless, it is apparent that in Islamic pharmaceutics considerable respect was paid to the qualities of individual herbs (unlike the Chinese emphasis on formulations, these were seen as reflecting a secondary skill). Physicians were expected to understand intimately the nature of each remedy, its natural habitat, its specific energy pattern, actions, indications, specific relationships to the organs, duration of action, toxicity and contraindications, types of preparation, dosage, administration and antidotes.[12]

The Islamic medical tradition has been maintained in its heartland to the present day and also generated important benefits for the medicine of Europe at its fringes. Montpellier and Salerno were among the first of the new medical centres of Europe. Rather than relying just on ancient texts, a new experimental culture led to reports of the tested effects of substances from identified plants. This advance was fostered by the foundation of universities and greatly aided by the later invention of the printing press, which also allowed wider dissemination of the classical texts.[13] In Salerno, medical training could last for 7 years or more.[14]

CHINESE HERBAL MEDICINE

The traditions of medicine that developed in China from prehistoric times have survived as a major part of healthcare provision to the present day and through this extraordinary continuity, constitute the most comprehensive clinical strategy for the use of herbal medicines anywhere.

This text is not the place for an exhaustive overview of Chinese medicine. There are effective texts available in English, notably the essential work by Unschuld,[13] other classic texts[14–17] and one very accessible introduction[18] (and see also[19] for a brief review in the context of the Western herbalist's perspective). What will be attempted here is the distillation of uniquely herbal strategies and concepts from the vast corpus of Chinese medicine. There is much to choose from. Over the last 2000 years a number of seminal texts and systems have been developed, each incorporating the developments of their predecessors. These were often very intricate systems, reflecting perhaps the priorities of scholarship and portent lore (much theorizing at the early stages was for the Imperial court[14]). At more than one stage, there appears to have been some difficulty in organizing the empirical folk traditions into neat systems[13] and there is always a suspicion that realities may have been squeezed to justify the cosmology.

However, Chinese medicine was certainly not idle theorizing. In one review of the medicine of early China,[20] it has been pointed out that among other 'modern' advances were the use of androgens and oestrogens (in placentas) to treat hypogonadism, the development of forensic medicine, the advocation of hand washing to avoid infection, the association of hardening of the arteries with high salt intake. Qualifying examinations for physicians were conducted by the Chinese state as early as the first century AD and there was an elaborate system of medical ethics.

It is first important to emphasize that the Chinese world view has been fundamentally different from that in the West since the time of Aristotle. In Chinese thought everything moves (the seminal classic, the *I Ching*, is translated as the 'Book of Changes'). Events are automatically described by their transient qualities in relation to other events and are manifestations of energies in ways that the West understood only after Einstein (see also[21]). The generic term for these energies is *qi* but in the case of the living body there are many forms of varying density, from *wei qi* as the most rarefied on the body surface, manifest in acute defensive reactions like fever and colds, through *ying qi*, the nourishing *qi* flowing through the meridians, to *xue* or blood, the most substantial aspect of *qi*, manifest in many somatic events. *Qi* is also manifest in *jing* (essence) and the body fluids. The comparison with modern physics is even more apposite as *qi* is simultaneously energy, movement and fluid (reminiscent of attempts to define light as waves and/or particles).

Transience continues: thus, in what has become known as Traditional Chinese Medicine (TCM – in fact the mainstream tradition in China after the Communist Revolution of 1948 and the one most widely used by Western practitioners), the framework by which diseases are addressed is made up of four sets of polar opposites, the 'eight conditions'.

Each pair denotes a spectrum of qualities onto which any illness can be placed; each implies that the aim of any therapeutic measure is to move extremes back towards a comfortable mean. Although used as a diagnostic framework for acupuncture, it is widely agreed that TCM is primarily based on herbal therapeutics. Thus herbs are ascribed temperaments or tendencies accordingly: they may be *Yin* or *Yang*, tonic or dispersive, cooling or heating, eliminative or constructive. These manifestations are in turn aspects of fundamental properties of the remedies.

Condition	Attributes
Yang	Active, expanding, transforming, dispersive, centrifugal, aggressive, light
Yin	Constructive, sustaining, completing, condensing, centripetal, responsive, dark
Full	Repleted
Empty	Depleted
Hot	Active
Cold	Passive
External	Acute
Internal	Chronic

Herbs gathered in the spring, in the morning or at the waxing moon, made up of rapidly growing tissues, the leaves, green tips and other parts when green, will tend to encourage upward movement. Herbs gathered in midsummer, at noon and at the full moon, made up of the mature parts of the plant, the flowers, fruit and associated structures, would tend to encourage outward movement. One would use such remedies to disperse cold, to assist superficial defences against both cold and heat and to counteract symptoms of excessive sinking in the body (such as prolapse, diarrhoea, excessive menstruation) or excessive penetration (i.e. disease conditions moving past primary defences to establish themselves as chronic pathologies). Rising remedies might include heating remedies, emetics and expectorants, the astringents and the peripheral vasodilators.

Herbs gathered in the autumn, in late afternoon and during the waning moon, with drying plant tissues, stalks, fallen leaves, parts of the plant that have lost their full colour, the rhizomes and tubers that condense nourishment for the following year, will encourage downward movement while those associated with dormancy, latency, hidden potency, with the plant in winter, at night and at the new moon, with quiescent latent tissues, especially seeds, buds and rootstocks, will encourage inward movement. Both tendencies are encouraged by harvesting and storage. They would tend to be used to reduce excessive heat, encourage nourishing and eliminatory activities and counteract symptoms of excessive rising in the body, such as vomiting, coughing, headaches, convulsions, spastic conditions such as asthma and nervous dyspepsia, and neuromuscular tensions. These remedies might include the antispasmodics, sedatives, bitters, antitussives, purgatives and diuretics.

In Chinese medicine there is little regard for anatomy and the main entities upon which pathogenic or therapeutic forces act are essentially functional and physiological. There are six pairs of functions, often confusingly translated in the West as 'organs'. These, like all phenomena in the Chinese world, are ascribed to points on the five-phase cycle that further illuminate their qualities. The five phases (the frequently used term 'five elements' is clearly not appropriate here) are seasonal and cyclical transition states through which all the universe moves. They have a multitude of dynamic relationships with each other and a vast array of more or less consistent qualities. The five phases, their attributes and their relationship with the six pairs of functions are illustrated in tabular form as follows.

Following the strictures of Porkert,[15] words in this text which may be confused with their Western meanings are distinguished typographically (with capitals and italics though not, as he insisted, using completely new words altogether).

THE FIVE TASTES

In days before laboratory investigations, taste was obviously a major arbiter of a plant's quality and it is easily seen how an association with pharmacological activity could be made. In the case of Chinese medicine the taste became a pharmacological force in its own right.

Two of the *Tastes* are primarily *yang* and tend to disperse upwards in the body. They are the pungent

Phase	*Fire*	*Earth*	*Metal*	*Water*	*Wood*
Attributes	Heating, attracting, burning, destructive, ascending, illuminative	Nourishing, stable, restful, central, fertile	Hard, strong but mouldable, cold but responsive to heat, lustrous, protective	Soaking, sinking, cold, still, deep, dark, potent, latent	Growing, spreading outward
Function (*yin*)	*Heart/ pericardium*	*Spleen*	*Lungs*	*Kidney*	*Liver*
Attributes	1) Sovereign, rules *xue*, stores *shen*, maintains individual integrity, seen in face, tongue, pleasure, sweating and laughter 2) Ambassador, origin of pleasure and social skills	Transformation, primary digestive function, in charge of upward movement, stores nourishing *qi*, rules flesh and limbs, seen also in lips, mouth, sympathy, saliva and singing	Prime minister, source of rhythm, directs movement outward (defence) and fluid downward, site of *qi* production, rules *qi*, seen also in nose, skin, sorrow, nasal secretions and crying	Root of life and will, stores *jing* (essence), rules birth, development and reproduction, source of *yin* and *yang*, heat and power, rules bones and marrow, seen also in hair, ears, fear, sputum and moaning	Allocation of resources, spreading, stores *xue*, rules sinews, also seen in nails, eyes, anger, tears, shouting
Function (*yang*)	*Small Intestine /Triple Heater*	*Stomach*	*Large Intestine*	*Bladder*	*Gallbladder*
Attributes	1) Rules separation of pure from impure 2) Smelting, distillation and condensation, regulates movement of fluids	Receives and digests food, in charge of downward movement, starts separation of pure from the impure	Rules elimination, continues separation of pure from impure	Rules fluid eliminations, confluence of fluids	Directs other functions, stores bile
Pharmacological attribute (*Taste*)	Bitter	Sweet	Pungent	Salty	Sour

and sweet *Tastes* (the latter is usually yoked with a sixth non-taste quality, referred to here as the bland *Taste*).

Three *Tastes* are primarily *yin* and tend to flow downwards in the body. They are the sour, bitter and salty *Tastes*.

The *Tastes* were assigned to the five phases and their functional manifestations in the body, as above. In turn, this came to mean that the normal role of each *Function* included being a vehicle for the activity of its own *Taste* and depended on acquiring a quantum, primarily from food but if necessary from medicine.

While a moderate amount of each *Taste* is necessary for its corresponding *Function*, there are also wider effects arising from their consumption. The relationships are expressed in Figure 1.1 (For a review of the implications of the four-phase nature of the relationships and the peculiar position of the *Spleen*, see[22].)

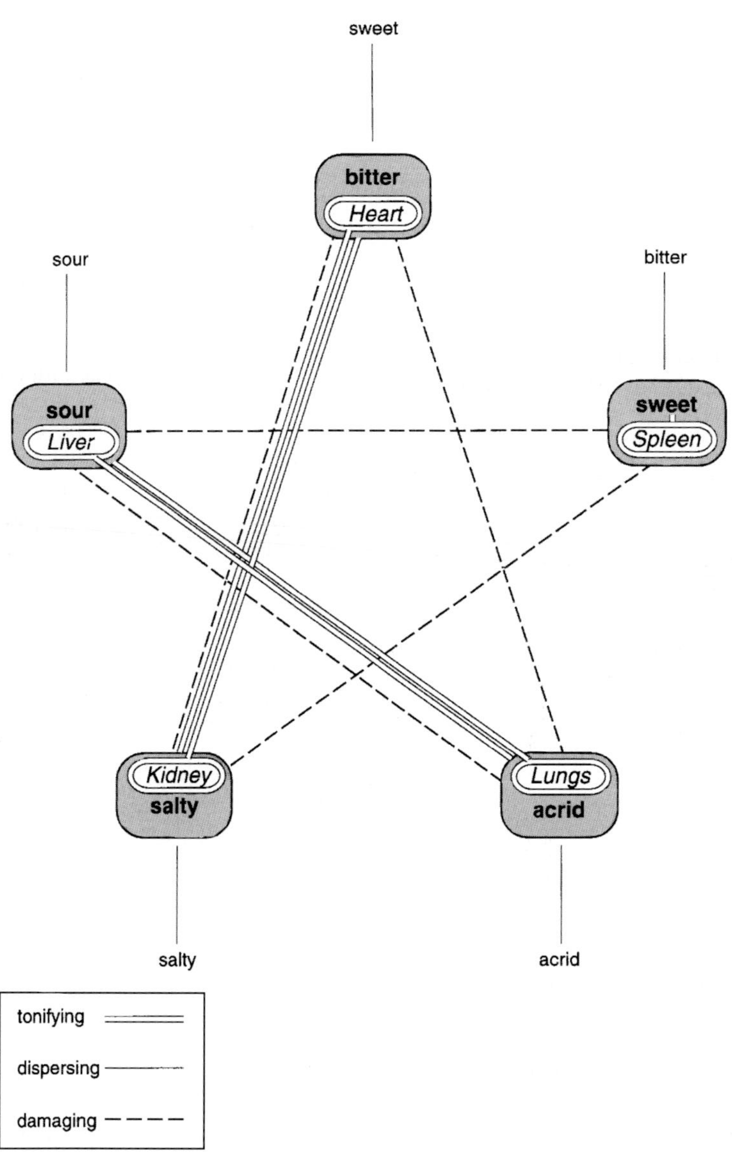

Figure 1.1 The Five *Tastes* and their relationships (reproduced with permission from Penguin Books)

Tonification

As well as being associated with one *Function*, each *Taste* is also seen to tonify, i.e. at moderate levels support, another *Function*.

Dispersing

Extra amounts of each *Taste* disperse excessive activity in the *Function* with which it is linked. This is straightforward except in the case of the *Spleen* which is already tonified by sweet: it appears therefore to do a swap with the *Heart*.

Damaging

The effects of taking excessive amounts of any particular *Taste* follow a conventional destructive *ko* cycle pattern in the five-phase relationship.

A brief review of the properties of each *Taste* is instructive.

Salty

The taste of common salt and seafood but not well represented in the herbal materia medica. However, seaweeds are occasionally used in maritime cultures and in Japan. It is possible to classify the occasional remedy like celery seed in this category. In China, however, the main group of drugs classified as salty are animal remains and tissues and the minerals.

The salty *Taste* is directed by the *Spleen* to the *Kidneys*. It is *yin* and tends to flow downwards in the body and particularly to the bones.

It is said to 'moisten' and 'soften' and salty remedies are used for 'dry, hard' pathologies, such as tumours, fibroses (e.g. liver cirrhosis), constipation and other abdominal swellings.

In moderation, it tonifies the *Heart* but damages it in excess. It is interesting to see how closely ancient observations tie in with current views on the influence of salt and electrolytes on the circulation.

Sour

This arises as the result of the stimulation of the sour taste buds by hydrogen ions. It is the taste of fruit acids, vinegar and tannins.

The sour *Taste* is directed by the *Spleen* to the *Liver*; it is *yin* and tends to move downwards in the body. It moves particularly to the muscle fibres (or 'sinews').

It is said to 'absorb' and 'bind' and is applied to discharges, excessive diuresis, incontinence, perspiration and premature ejaculation. Some of these indications recur in the discussion of the effect of tannins (see p.37).

It disperses excess activity in the *Liver* and tonifies the *Lungs*. Among other roles, the latter is concerned with the maintenance of the body's defences against external pathogens. The role of fruit as protection, particularly against respiratory infections, was thus apparently not a new discovery.

In excess it damages the *Spleen*. Excessive consumption of tannins interferes with assimilation of foods.

Bitter

This taste is mediated by bitter taste buds in the mouth which are stimulated by a number of chemical structures. It is thus a quality recognized by the Chinese, and others, as being intrinsic to herbal remedies.

It is directed by the *Spleen* to the *Heart*; it is *yin* and tends to flow downwards in the body. It moves particularly to *xue* ('blood'). As the most dense of the circulating energies in the body, *xue* is in effect the speculative force behind the more somatic events in the body. Compared to acupuncture, which is seen to primarily affect *qi*, the more rarefied circulating energy, the archetypal bitterness of herbal remedies is strongly associated with treating more substantial deep-seated clinical problems.

It is said to 'sedate', 'dry' and 'harden'. The first reflects bitter's cool temperament while 'drying' refers to bitter's use in 'damp-heat' conditions (e.g. hepatitis); 'harden' may be better translated by the term 'consolidate' to express the effect of improving assimilation and nourishment.

It disperses excess in the *Spleen*. A modern manifestation of such a condition is the excessive consumption of sweet foods with the consequent possible disruptions in blood sugar levels. There is clinical experience of the benefits of bitter herbs in stabilizing such disruptions.

It tonifies the *Kidneys*. As the repository of constitutional reserves, the *Kidneys* provide the greatest tonifying challenge, another example of the universal traditional reverence for bitters.

In excess it damages the *Lungs*. Excessive cooling suppresses vital defences.

Sweet

In a time when sugar was almost unknown, this was a far more subtle taste and was used to refer to the intrinsic sweetness of the rural diet: cereals, pulses, cooked root vegetables and those fruits suitable for drying and storing as winter food such as apricots, figs and prunes. In days when even honey was rare, the taste of extracted sugar would have been considered intrinsically excessive. In herbal remedies the sweet taste is exhibited particularly by the saponins, a chemical group often found in Chinese tonics and adaptogens.

The *Spleen* keeps the sweet *Taste* to itself; it is *yang* and tends to move upwards in the body, particularly to the soft tissues. Sweetness is nourishment: it is the quality of a simple agrarian diet and has its most potent metaphor in mother's milk. It thus manifests in the soft tissues and in overall body shape.

It is said to 'tonify' and to 'balance'. As well as being the obvious tonic influence, a good stable agrarian diet is the most effective way to promote homoeostasis; many saponin-rich adaptogenic remedies have a similar clinical reputation.

It disperses excess in the *Heart*, including symptoms of anxiety and nervous tension.

In excess it damages the *Kidneys*, a terminal effect in Chinese medicine, resulting in premature ageing. The Chinese in effect predicted an enfeeblement of general vitality through excessive sweet consumption.

Pungent

Sometimes also called 'acrid', this is the taste of the hot spices, cayenne, ginger, mustard, the peppers, horseradish, raw onions and garlic (both the latter become sweet when cooked) and generally all the 'heating' herbal remedies. Unlike the other four tastes, the effect is not linked to any special taste bud but simply follows direct irritation of any exposed tissues and sensory nerve fibres. The association with the *Metal* phase may have followed inhaling the fumes given off from smelting.

It is directed by the *Spleen* to the *Lungs*; it is *yang* and tends to move upward, particularly to *qi*. The heating properties of the pungent *Taste* are always its dominant feature.

It is said to 'move *qi*', 'disperse', 'activate the body fluids', 'cause expulsion from the *Lungs*' and 'open the pores'. It tends to be used therefore for superficial, external disease conditions, to counteract external pathogenic influences, especially *Wind* and *Cold*, and to mobilize stagnant body energies.

It disperses excess in the *Lungs*, notably that manifested by congested bronchial inflammations. It tonifies the *Liver*, the *Function* responsible for ensuring a balanced dispersal of all the body's energies and activities, but in excess also damages the *Liver*.

Bland

A substance seen as having no character and without dynamic action in the body. It is not therefore a typical *Taste* and is not recognized in all classical texts. Where it is, it is said to slip through the body without hindrance or interaction. It moves straight through from the *Spleen* to the *Bladder*, i.e. the urinary system, and thus out of the body.

Its only effect, therefore, is that it is a diuretic. Many of the diuretics used in herbal medicine have a characteristic blandness of taste.

AYURVEDIC HERBAL MEDICINE

The written record of the traditional medicine of India is less comprehensive than that for China, with a few texts from India itself (e.g. [23–25]) and a few notable but exceptional texts written in the West (e.g. [26–28]). Nevertheless, it is clear that this tradition includes significant systematizing of medical practices in one of the major cultures in history. Medicines were classified, for example, by their Tastes and therapeutic categories, as in Chinese medicine, and their effects on illnesses linked to constitutional types (*doshas*) and humours.

The *doshas* provide the primary orientation. The word derives from the same root as the English 'dys-' as in 'dysfunction': the *dosha* is essentially a fault in the healthy state of the body. Three *doshas* have survived as fundamental, each being a condensation of pairs of the five elements, waste products produced when the body replenishes its elements. The *doshas* support the body only as long as they continually flow out of it, as proper eliminations of urine, faeces and sweat.

Kapha is a condensation of water and earth (the damp and dry elements of matter) and projects itself into the production of lubricant fluids in the body. It is the stabilizing influence in the body and generally concentrates in the thorax to contain rising *vata*; it is associated with mucus. Illnesses of excessive *kapha* are marked by symptoms of cold, damp and heaviness (e.g. catarrh, oedema, abdominal congestion) and are relieved by warming, drying, stimulating remedies such as the pungent spices, warming diaphoretics and expectorants, emetics, aromatic and bitter digestives and carminatives and, to a lesser extent, perhaps combined with the above, diuretics, laxatives and astringents.

Pitta collects fire and water elements into the production of bile and is associated with digestive juices more generally; it is in charge of transformation and processing and concentrates in the mid-abdomen.

Illnesses of excessive or obstructed *pitta*, are marked by biliary disturbances and may include symptoms of heat, damp and excessive activity (e.g. fever, inflammation, infection, blood toxicities, bleeding); they are relieved as appropriate, and perhaps in combination, by cooling, drying, nutritive or calming remedies such as the bitters, purgatives, sweet tonic remedies, astringents, cooling diaphoretics, alteratives and diuretics.

Vata arises from condensation of air and space and is the (often unstable) windy form of *prana*, linked to the functions of the respiratory system, and is in charge of all movement in the body; it concentrates in the lower abdomen to help lift *kapha*. Illnesses of the *vata* type, marked by cold, dryness and excessive (especially nervous) activity, are of two types. Deficient *vata* (e.g. emaciation and constitutional dehydration) is treated with sweet and nutritive tonics, bulking laxatives, demulcents and salty remedies. Accumulated or obstructed *vata* is a congestive version that may include abdominal distension and gas, constipation and rheumatic and arthritic conditions. This is treated with modest pungent herbs in the short term only, moderate warming diaphoretics, carminatives and antispasmodics and temporary laxatives. All *vata* conditions are indications for traditional Ayurvedic enema therapy.

In a bias that often recurs in herbal medicine texts, the Ayurvedic tradition also sees many conditions as combinations of the *doshas* with toxicity or *ama*. This is a *kapha*-like influence, being generally cold, slimy, heavy and dense, with phlegm and mucus, loss of taste and appetite, indigestion, depression and irritability as common symptoms, and may arise from emotional difficulties as well as physical reasons. It lies at the root of much chronic disease and immune disturbance. Where there is evidence of *ama*, improving eliminations is the first priority of treatment, a universal theme in herbal therapeutics. The prime herbal influences in the elimination of *ama* are the bitter and pungent herbs, often in that sequential order, perhaps after a fast. Sweet, salty and sour herbs can increase *ama*.

The treatment of *ama* is, however, complicated by its combinations with the *doshas* (in which case it has the suffix *sama*). Combined with *kapha* (*kapha sama*), it is marked by severe mucus conditions and is a clear indication for pungent with bitter herbs. *Pitta sama* is the classic Galenic damp-heat condition, with yellow tongue coating, urine and faeces, congestive anorexia, loss of thirst and biliousness. Bitter herbs lead the treatment, with modest amounts of pungent as appropriate. *Vata sama* is associated with constipation, painful abdominal congestion and flatulence, anorexia and bad breath and is treated with pungent herbs, warming aromatic digestives and carminatives combined with laxatives as required.

THE SIX TASTES (*RASAS*)

As with the Chinese view, the effects of foods and the pharmacology of medicines were classified in terms of their immediate impact on the body. *Rasas* are not only subjective impressions but attributes of the body itself in its relationship with its environment: everyone craves the taste most lacking within. The choice of both medicines and foods is thus often determined by such assessments, the distinction between them again being a function of their effects on the body: foods nourish, medicines balance and poisons disturb.

The effects of *rasas* on the body are complex and rarely isolated. For example, the sweet, sour and salty tastes decrease *vata* and increase *kapha* but sour, salty and pungent tastes increase *pitta*. Bitter, pungent and astringent tastes increase *vata* and decrease *kapha*.

THE PRIMACY OF CLEANSING

The Indian traditions of therapeutics concurred with most other older cultures in seeing disease as initially a toxic accumulation. The disease process is seen generally to start with an obstruction to the pathways and an accumulation of one or more of the *doshas* (one recalls that the healthy manifestations of *doshas* are as eliminations from the body) in their respective locales: the stomach for *kapha*, the intestine for *pitta* and the bowel for *vata*. It is easiest to combat diseases at this earliest stage and there are several cleansing routines that people are encouraged to observe to remove accumulations of *doshas* before they lead to the next stages of disease development.

If hygienic and other observances are insufficient to deal with the accumulations, a range of therapeutic measures are indicated. These may include an elaborate structure of procedures called *pancakarma*, designed to purify the body from the accumulations and pacify associated disturbances. Always the physician had to respect the relative strength of the patient and of the disease and adopt only those treatments that did not disturb or debilitate (there was little attraction in the 'healing crisis' of some more recent alternative traditions). Often a treatment would start with fasting, especially to promote removal of any *ama* or in acute outbreaks. Thereafter, there might be variously intense body massages with oils or heating and sweating to soften and loosen the *dosha* accumulations (as in the Galenic tradition referred to earlier).

Herbal or other remedies would be applied at any stage (or as a substitute for a stage of *pancakarma* where this was not indicated), with the most active tactics being those that led to the most vigorous eliminations (emetics for accumulated *vata* and *kapha*, purgatives for *pitta*) but because of the risks of depletion there were many approaches to consider, some being particularly gentle. For every purification treatment successfully completed, there would be a mandatory convalescence to allow recovery, perhaps augmented by appropriate rejuvenating remedies.

AN EMPIRICAL AND ALLOPATHIC TRADITION

Ayurvedic texts provide considerable detail in their therapeutic recommendations. Preparation of herbal remedies, for example, is most elaborate, with a wide range of methods designed to transform the original plant material in a variety of ways to match the typology of the disturbance being treated. The remedies were also applied to the body in many forms and at various times in the treatment according to its development. It was clear, however, that the texts were meant to be enabling rather than prescriptive; they encouraged a respect for diversity and complexity, for the individuality of the patient, rather than formulaic prescription. Ayurvedic medicine is also marked in the clarity of its therapeutic objectives. As admirably expressed in one of the standard texts:

> We nourish the emaciated and starve the corpulent. We treat the man afflicted by heat with cooling measures, and with hot things him who is afflicted by cold. We replenish body elements that have suffered decrease, and deplenish those that have undergone increase. By treating disorders properly with measures which are antagonistic to their causative factors we restore the patient to normal.[29]

Like most ancient herbal traditions, Ayurveda was essentially 'allopathic'.

Empiricism and pragmatism are essential features of any survival strategy but the repeated emphasis in the texts on judging a remedy or tactic by its effects on the body in clinical adversity rather than in theory, and the transparency of the therapeutic tactics, all provide an encouraging antidote to idle acquiescence to the elders.

NINETEENTH-CENTURY NORTH AMERICAN HERBAL MEDICINE

The majority of the early immigrants to North America were Europeans looking for a new chance in the vast spaces of the 'New World'. Although new towns and cities emerged significant numbers lived remotely from any organized services, for example often hundreds of miles from any doctor (who was often poorly qualified). These were hardy self-reliant people who had to find all resources on their doorstep. They had to rediscover their self-sufficiency in health terms as well, combining their (imported) old European home remedies with native North American flora and a considerable amount of Indian lore as well. Their experience provides the reader of the new millennium with a unique precedent: the rediscovery of traditional herbal medicine by a modern population.

A new group of practitioners emerged, sometimes referred to now as 'travelling medicine shows', more often contemporarily as 'white Indian doctors', often peripatetic, exploiting their claimed skills and usually their own patent nostrums. Many were opportunists with little to contribute in a lasting way to the development of healthcare (although one 19th-century herbal tonic was to become, as Coca-Cola, the most massively consumed product of all time). Nevertheless, there were also true pioneers among this group, some passionately keen to develop a self-reliant healthcare system based on what they knew of plant remedies.

One 'white Indian doctor' went into print. Samuel Thomson (1769–1843), was brought up as a shepherd boy in New Hampshire and introduced to herbs by a 'wise woman', Mrs Benton, who was versed in Indian lore. He very quickly became adept, being called upon by neighbours in competition with what may have been particularly poor service from the local doctor.

Thomson was horrified by the remedies used in 'regular physic', these being dominated by toxic minerals based on mercury, arsenic, antimony and sulphur. He also saw that there was a fundamental difference in therapeutic approach. He saw the objective of the doctors as being to stop the disease at all costs. The main conditions of the day were febrile infections and the regular approach was to use mineral products and bloodletting to stifle the symptoms and bring the temperature down (this was before germ theory redefined the objective as eliminating pathogens). Thomson had ministered to patients almost killed by the combination of calomel (mercurous chloride), antimony, bloodletting and fever. In native Indian tradition (as seen in the sweat lodge), Thomson treated fevers in the opposite way, by maintaining and supporting them. He saw the fever as a sign of healthy resistance: it was possible for damage to follow if the fever got out of hand but the main risk was failure of the febrile defence. Thus Thomson used *Capsicum* (cayenne) as a powerful support to the febrile mechanism, along with a range of other remedies including *Lobelia inflata* (lobelia), *Myrica cerifera* (bayberry), *Viburnum opulus* (cramp bark) and *Zanthoxylum* (prickly ash) to modulate and support various aspects of the febrile response.

Thomson was sufficiently enthused by the distinction between his and the regular approaches to learn to read and write so that he could pass on his message. He set out a principle that at once encapsulated this tradition and fired the public imagination. The book in which he propagated his views [30] was a runaway publishing success across the East and Mid West and at the time it was calculated that over half the population of Ohio were adherents of Thomsonism.

Thomson's language was simple, even simplistic, and aimed at a God-fearing readership. However, he seemed to have touched a gut instinct, that life and health are positive virtues, to be protected or recovered through personal self-sufficiency using the medicinal aids provided by the Maker. In one key passage he appears to have adopted some of the language of Graeco-Roman humoral medicine:

> I found that all animal bodies were formed of four elements. The Earth and Water constitute the solid; and the Air and Fire (or heat) are the cause of life and motion; that the cold, or the lessening of the power of heat, is the cause of all disease; that to restore heat to its natural state was the only way health could be produced, and that, after restoring the natural heat, by clearing the system of all obstruction and causing a natural perspiration, the stomach would digest the food taken into it, and the heat (or nature) be enabled to hold her supremacy.

To a readership versed in the Book of Genesis, the fact that earth and water (or clay) were the stuff of life, the dry and wet principles respectively, would have been readily appreciated. For those spending all their lives in the open, Air would have been easily equated with its former meaning, wind, a persistent metaphor for movement. The important vital principle, of course, was Fire or Heat, the obvious difference between a living body and a corpse, the universal metaphor for life.

Thomson's message was simple. Heat is life. Disease (and death) are degrees of cold. Heating thus provides the fundamental principle of healing. Other measures, principally in improving eliminations and digestive performance, are often essential supports to this central measure. Cayenne is literally a life promoter.

In the case of fever this message was particularly appropriate in its radical emphasis. The battle lines between heat and cold are more clearly drawn. Thomson was of course essentially correct in his judgement: fevers are defence mechanisms and the symptoms of pyrexia, anorexia, nausea, vomiting, diarrhoea or convulsions are all side effects of this mobilization, not to be confused with the underlying pathogen. Clinical experience is that a fever well fought, with a clear crisis and lysis, no hyperpyrexia and side effects prevented from causing collateral damage, can leave the body in a stronger position. Effective fever management can be a more helpful strategy than suppression.

The central point, of course, was that Thomson had articulated, with popular success, an essential feature of the herbal tradition: that the primary task was to support the body's own recuperative efforts. Everything else was secondary. He also sounded the essential difference between that tradition and what had already become conventional medicine. The fact that his relationship with the medical establishment was almost entirely acrimonious only served to reinforce his position as a fundamentalist.

Some of his followers were less keen on absolute simplicities. Much to the old man's disgust, several started developing variations on his teachings, recognizing for example that there were conditions that could be diagnosed as excessive heat. There were different emphases on the need to control heat (in fact, circulation) and variations in the mechanisms for keeping the blood 'clean'.

Thomsonism was to develop in the second half of the 19th century to inspire both eclecticism and physiomedicalism, at the same time as osteopathy and chiropractic emerged. Unlike these latter, however, the medicinal therapies did not fare well. The main colleges of physiomedicalism and eclecticism, along with those of homoeopathy, were 'invited' to come within the umbrella of established medical training in talks held with the American Medical Association at the turn of the century. This was an inspired example of the establishment eliminating radicalism by accommodation.

Three figures stand out. TJ Lyle produced a superb herbal materia medica,[31] concentrating on the observed influence of each remedy on the human being rather than listing its symptomatic indications. JM Thurston produced the last authoritative physiomedical text, posing operational definitions of the vital force, health and disease and the distinctions between functional symptoms and those arising from organic ('trophic') origins, and elaborating on the need to use only such remedies as supported vitality. He also, rather prematurely, sought to classify remedies in terms of the newly discovered autonomic nervous system, reasoning that in its vasomotor activity control could be exerted on local circulation and thus on all tissue functions, including digestion, elimination and hormonal and nervous activity.[32]

Of the physiomedical theorists, WH Cook was particularly inspired. Like the others, Cook attempted to link the rapid new discoveries of medical science to traditional approaches. Through his arguments appears to run the theme that the living body is essentially a functional entity and that disease starts as a disturbance of normal functional rhythms, for example:

> Regularity in periods of alternate labor and rest is characteristic of all vital action …
>
> … the earliest departure of the tissues from under the full control of the vital force will be in the lack of ability either to relax or to contract some of the tissues as readily as in the healthy state …[33]

Like other physiomedicalists, Cook started with the principle that the ideal medicine should support recuperative functions but added considerably to the view that thereafter they should have a gentle dynamism, helping to correct distorted functions, either 'relaxing' overstimulated tissues or functions or 'contracting' those that are sluggish.

Thomsonism and physiomedicalism both travelled to Britain to a welcome from the newly urbanized medical herbalists of the Industrial Revolution. Their approaches formed the foundation of the oldest body of medical herbalism in the Western world, the National Institute of Medical Herbalists, established in 1864. Although the vigour of the American pioneers faded in the following century, their ideas at least survived on foreign shores while they singularly failed to do so after the AMA takeover at home.

MIDDLE EUROPEAN HERBAL MEDICINE

Much of Western herbal therapeutics is imbued with the values of a healthcare tradition that arose in central Europe from the 18th century. Built on the philosphical foundations of Goethe and Schiller, a cultural view arose of health as a refinement, a separation of the pure from the greater impure.

The Goethian view achieved practical therapeutic form in Germany in the homeopathy of Samuel Hahnemann, the biochemic tissue salts of Schussler and, in the 20th century, the anthroposophical medicine that arose as one aspect of the holistic world view of Rudolph Steiner (and indirectly in the Flower remedies of Edward Bach in England). It also provided the founding principles of a variety of practices that have been grouped under the heading of naturopathy. The use of dietary changes (and in later years dietary supplements), hydrotherapy and a range of physical therapies in order to allow 'nature cure' has one of its strongest cultural roots in this tradition.

The European naturopathic tradition also developed Galenic concepts of heat and cold and notably (as a northern European phenomenon) that of damp. The concept of 'catarrh' and 'mucus' became a cornerstone of naturopathic treatment. Following the Graeco-Roman lead, many infectious and inflammatory diseases were seen as congestive toxicities to be warmed and dried. When germ theory established the role of bacteria in infections these were seen as 'saprophytes' rather than pathogens; in other words, essentially beneficial cleansing organisms, like forest fungi breaking down dead wood, taking advantage of the catarrhal nutrients to effect extraordinary healing responses like inflammation and fever. As in all other foregoing traditions, herbal remedies were seen as important contributions to detoxifying damp conditions, although these were closely interwoven with dietary techniques in ways that have permeated much herbal practice in the West to this day.

The main impact of the Middle European tradition of herbal medicine was on dosage. Whereas the historical emphasis has always been on large 'heroic' doses of herbs, often single preparations for short-term use in acute diseases, the homoeopathic initiative led to a general move towards smaller doses, often linked to the use of their 'mother tinctures'. Some of today's leading German phytomedicine companies were formed by homoeopaths and have provided plant products over a mixed range of doses and potencies, with the herbal remedies having sometimes tiny material doses. In some European countries, notably The Netherlands, the public perception of herbal or phytomedicine is that it uses homoeopathic remedies. The significance of this is that the German industry makes up the largest single part of the European herbal market and the overwhelming part of the herbal clinical research literature. Much of this literature relates to products supplied in much lower doses than those commonly used elsewhere in the world.

The clinical implications, and possible limitations, of low-dose phytotherapy are reviewed in Chapter 6 on dosage. Whatever the pharmacological doubts, however, one beneficial effect is that it marked the move from primitive drastic shortterm medication for acute conditions to a therapy that could, and did, take its place in the modern mainstream in the treatment of chronic disorders. Remedies changed their role when so transformed (for example, hawthorns moved from a fever management treatment in high doses to a gentle cardiovascular modulator, valerian from an alterative to a mild sedative, garlic from an antiseptic to a treatment for high blood cholesterol). It can be argued that the Western fascination with Chinese and Ayurvedic herbal medicine is for traditions that have yet to be adequately exposed to the clinical realities of illnesses of a modern developed society

COMMON ELEMENTS. READING THE BODY-MIND AS A NATURAL PHENOMENON

Several themes emerge from the foregoing reviews of traditional herbal therapeutic systems.

1. Medicines, most of which were herbal, were seen as correcting internal disharmonies (literally 'diseases') rather than targeting symptoms.
2. In the absence of modern instrumentation, internal disharmonies were understood as *subjective* matters, often described in climatic or emotional metaphors or by metaphysical constructs (*yin/yang*, the *doshas*, the humours) that were widely understood among the general population.
3. From the herbalist's perspective most internal disharmonies involved literal or substantial disruptions in the body, most often involving body fluids or humours (including Chinese Blood/*xue*, *jing* and *qi*): in this sense most herbal medicine has been *humoral* medicine.
4. By definition the humours suffused equally the body and the mind (and often the spirit), so that one internal disharmony could affect all planes of experience. There was *no Cartesian body/mind split*.
5. Herbal remedies were often classified by the internal disharmony they affected; thereafter they were used as allopathic remedies, in the strict sense of that term.

If modern herbal therapeutics is to be true to its traditions then it should be able to postulate modern versions of the above themes.

Unfortunately, there are no such constructs widely understood among the general population. Any postulates at this stage have to remain speculative and theoretical, operational rationales for the practitioner rather than an effective language for the patient.

It will also be difficult to arrive at acceptable modern versions of the humours. It may be that modern systems analysis of body fluid dynamics increasingly supports the prospect for oceanic currents through the tissues rather than the mechanistic pipes and channels of Harvey.[34] Although this provides a possible rationale for meridianal movement this is not really the point. Humours were equally of the body and mind and while there is a Cartesian split in the biological and physical definition of the two, the prospect of a modern 'humour' is bleak.

There may be a much stronger basis for a modern subjective physiology and pathology. Indeed, one of the concerns about the way modern medicine has developed is that its language has long left the patient behind. Doctors have become better and better at differentiating pityriasis alba from seborrhoeic eczema but are not as good at telling the patient what is wrong, especially if there is only superficial treatment available.

Again, there is a long way to go. However, there are few conceptual barriers to a new physiology, one that might become understood by anyone. Much of the theoretical ground has been broken in such disciplines as endocrinology and neuropeptide science, neurophysiology, immunology (and the radical North American hybrid with almost every other human science: psychoneuroimmunology). In embryology and developmental biology, researchers regularly think in four dimensions and models of transience that are rare in the other medical sciences. For some time biology has been taking mathematics, physics and computer sciences into its domain. As will be seen in the next section, the fascinating insights that have followed a better understanding of the behaviour of complex living systems have also begun to affect the biomedical model, at least slightly. All these disciplines are, of course, still highly arcane, barely comprehensible even to other biologists let alone the general public. They are certainly too difficult to enter into here. However, they do offer opportunities to check and amend the postulates of a functional physiology that in turn can be drawn from the insights of much earlier physicians.

The traditional herbal therapeutic systems reviewed in preceding sections were all constructed from empirical insights, honed by generations of observers of the human condition. Without instrumentation, they nevertheless were able to draw meaningful clinical connections between observed body functions in health and disease. As outlined earlier, there was an assumption that a principle applying at one level applied equally across others; there was also much more interest in function than anatomical structure, malfunctions rather than pathologies. Most principles were established with the acquiescence and knowledge of the wider population, using the common language. They were usually workaday and pragmatic, with only occasional efforts to construct elaborate systems from above. The vast number of local cultures means that there is considerable diversity and even contradictions in the detail. Nevertheless, fundamental principles about vital functions were widely agreed.

All living organisms clearly:

- *perceive* and respond to their environment;
- either *accommodate* to or *react* against each environmental stimulus;
- on *ingestion* of environmental influences, either *assimilate* or *reject* them;
- engage in a confusing and largely impenetrable triad of linked functions to *process* and *circulate* assimilated material and *remove* its metabolites;
- *integrate* all these functions with an endogenous vital force that was manifest primarily as vital rhythms but was often also literal and material;
- reproduce themselves, generally using functions analogous to the integrative functions.

Moreover, living organisms manifested these vital functions at every level of body, mind and spirit and in their social groups. In modern parlance, we would say equally at the cell, tissue, organ, body, psyche, society and wider ecosystem levels (the Gaia model develops similar principles).

A diagrammatic relationship between these functions (Fig. 1.2) resonates with clinical insights over several traditional systems and provides a model on which a therapeutic language could be built.[35] For example, Figure 1.3 shows how the archetypal properties of herbal remedies impact upon such a model. Other examples outline what would have been considered key therapeutic issues.

- Disorders of *assimilation*, whether of nutrients like glucose (diabetes), fats (high blood cholesterol and lipids, obesity) or minerals (e.g. iron deficiency anaemia) or of oxygen (anaemia, arteriosclerosis), may constitute part of wider patterns of disharmony, linked in old systems to inadequate nurturing (excessive sweet, fat and alcohol consumption for example being seen as a regression to unfulfilled infantile needs). In herbal medicine aromatic and bitter digestives (and cholagogues) were accorded wider roles than merely improving digestive performance.

- *Reaction, rejection* and *removal* are overlapping defence/eliminatory functions arranged topographically from the outside in. Failure in one burdens the others. Thus it is generally better that external pathogenic influences are headed off as close to the surface as possible (using, first, the primary defences of the skin and upper digestive tract, including the gastric secretions; and second, the secondary defences such as coughing, vomiting, diarrhoea, the phagocytic reticuloendothelial or lymphatic systems, fever and inflammatory responses). Next best is to have effective *removal* functions in the bowel, bile, kidneys, sweat glands and lungs, which themselves may have extra burdens if the principal defences are down. The fall-back mechanism is better not overburdened: the immune system is the most effective surveillance mechanism of all but it also has the greatest potential for long-term harm if persistently perturbed. Coupling it with the *rejection* function is a reminder that its primary role is to screen dietary antigens (most of the body's immune system is in gut-associated lymphatic tissue) and that failure in preliminary screening of that material and, significantly, other malfunctions of *assimilation* are likely to be a major factor in the aetiology of many autoimmune diseases. Herbal strategies are strong in supporting both primary and secondary defences (including gastric activities, fever and inflammation) and especially in mobilizing eliminations; they may thus reduce the burden on immune defences. Particular disturbances in the balance between assimilation and rejection (what the Chinese refer to as *Stomach, Small* and *Large Intestine Functions*) are possibly a modern problem for which the many herbal strategies in the digestive tract are applicable.

- The common features of integration and reproduction (the steroidal hormone link to the Chinese *Kidney Function* for example) emphasize that disturbances in one can be tied to those in the other. Traditional herbal remedies for infertility and impotence were also tonics used for wider conditions (and many have been found to contain significant levels of steroidal precursors). The overlap of course is seen also in the integration of social, relationship, sexual and childrearing activities.

This is an emerging area. There are enough leads, however, to suggest that further mining of traditional herbal strategies and the development of new biomedical models may together build a stronger rationale for the application of herbal remedies.

The impact of modern insights on a new therapeutic approach based on traditional strategies may be greatest in the fascinating work on complex dynamic systems.

A NEW SYNTHESIS. THE BODY AND MIND AS COMPLEX DYNAMIC SYSTEMS

This theory of life's origins is rooted in an unrepentant holism, born not of mysticism, but of mathematical necessity
Stuart Kauffman, *At Home in the Universe*

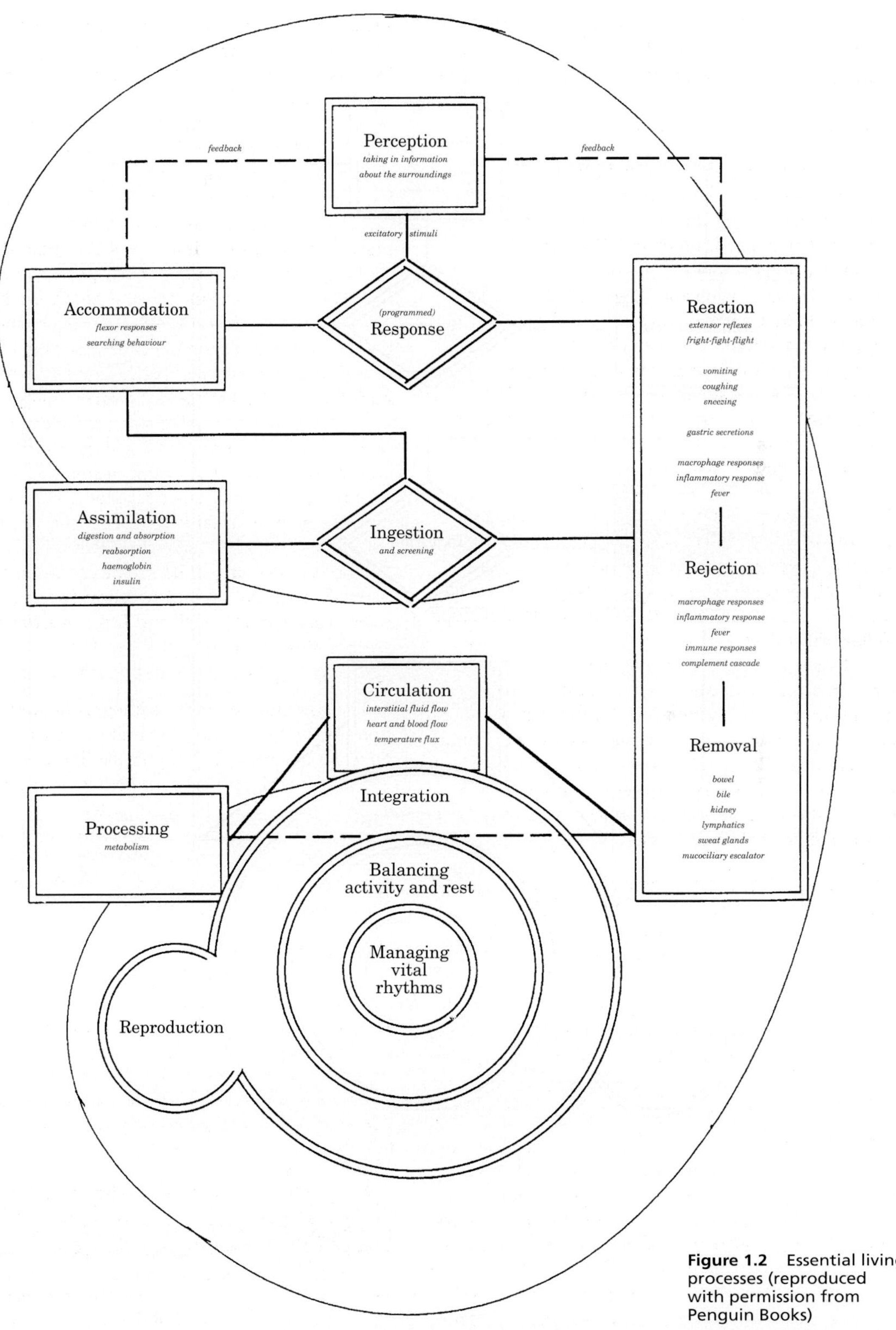

Figure 1.2 Essential living processes (reproduced with permission from Penguin Books)

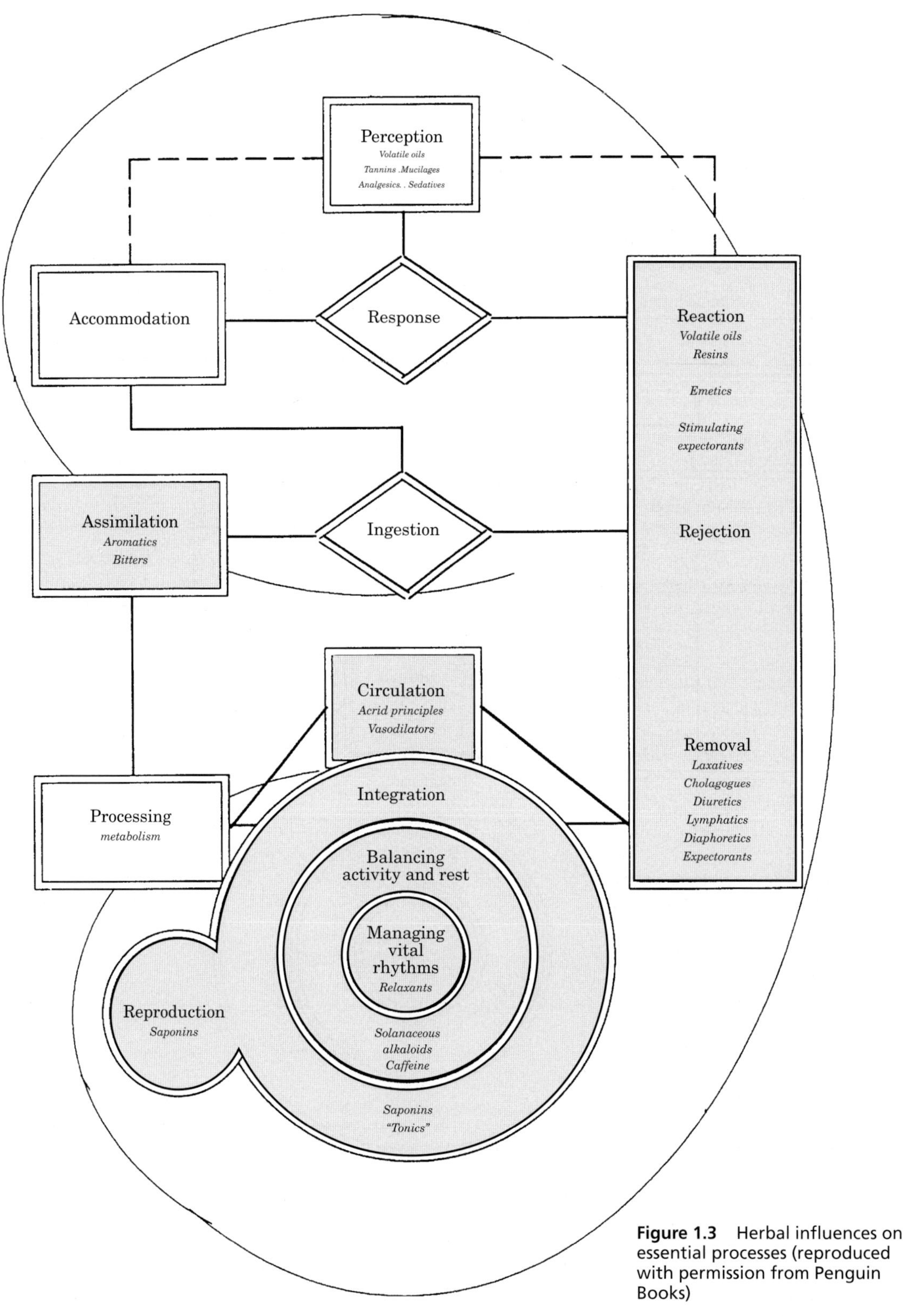

Figure 1.3 Herbal influences on essential processes (reproduced with permission from Penguin Books)

One of the serious drawbacks of the science inspired by Galileo and Newton and honed in the 19th century is that it was never designed to understand wholes. Its strength is in reduction of complexities to their parts. While modern science is therefore unprecedented in understanding the constituents of life and nature and building new edifices and realities with the results, it has been poor in understanding or predicting the behaviour of life and nature itself.

It is difficult to put this right. Scientific tools have not been readily available to understand patterns. Nevertheless, the study of complex systems has been tackled by leading scientific minds since computers provided the tools. Traditionally, the study has been one of high mathematics as the permutations and calculus of relationships between entities are worked through. Latterly, however, computer modelling has provided far more powerful artificial complexities with which to run. Application of often relatively simple mathematical formulae or simple modelling has shown that surprising things can happen in apparently random arrays. Programmed with only two simple instructions, dots on the screen behave spontaneously like flocks of birds, and a simple mathematical formula creates myriad self-similar fractal patterns, the Mandelbrot sets, of astonishing natural beauty. New properties that are genuinely more than the sum of the parts emerge from simple constituents.

The subject of complexity is a vast and often difficult one. It is home to mathematicians, computer programmers, physicists and engineers. Nevertheless, it is a subject that is coming of age. It has enormous implications for those who wish that there was another way rigorously to observe life and health and the reader is strongly recommended to read the excellent introductory texts now available.[36–39]

One of the most stunning proposals in the biological realm is the radical riposte to conventional views of the origin and, by inference, the mechanics of life. So far, the current view is that life formed once upon a time after the fortuitous combination of numbers of organic molecules in a primeval soup, perhaps aided by the odd burst of lightning. The first key stage in reproducible life was the formation of strands of ribonucleic acid, RNA, that could provide the mechanism for protein synthesis and eventually replication. A mathematical review of this scenario shows how astonishingly improbable it is that such events could have happened by chance, even in the billion years or so that were available for this leap. Visions of monkeys producing not one but many Shakespearean texts by random play with a typewriter come to mind.

However, if there were enough organic molecules in the chemical soup, some with the capacity to catalyse transformations between others, enough so that a catalytic loop was closed (i.e. some catalysts were formed by transformations they themselves initiated), then the molecules in that loop could become self-sustaining: they become an 'autocatalytic set'. Their levels will be built up within their locale, they will 'consume' building block molecules and 'excrete' metabolites and they will colonize any other locales into which they spill. This is not only possible, it is inevitable if there is sufficient diversity of organic molecules with catalytic properties in the medium and this seems most likely to have been the case. Self-organization is shown to happen spontaneously, simply out of the mathematical permutations of the events. This is 'order for free', as the leading proponent of this scenario, Stuart Kauffman, puts it.[39] It implies that organized structures arise spontaneously all the time. It supports a much wider view that complex systems tend to self-organization as an essential property of their complexity.

But this order is not fixed. If it were, it could not grow, move or adapt. It would be dead. It is important that there be some adaptability in self-organization. Science and mathematics are now very familiar with the phenomena of chaotic behaviour in natural systems. The patterns of clouds or sand dunes or flames, the flow of water down pipes, the weather, all are manifestations of the behaviour of particles acted upon by natural forces. Chaos in this sense is not random; its patterns are deterministic, not actually predictable overall but made up of elements which at any one point follow a predictable trajectory. Chaotic behaviour also creates moving zones of minimum energy or 'attractors' (a 'point attractor' is reached by a ball dropped into a bowl) which behave in characteristic ways: these are the 'strange attractors'. The trajectories of activity to and from strange attractors mean that a small initial stimulus, if on the appropriate trajectory, could amplify to massive effects: the fabulous 'butterfly wing effect' where in theory a hurricane in the Gulf of Mexico could start with a butterfly flapping in the Amazon ... or not.

Chaos, although sometimes manifest in astonishing patterns, is not consistent with sustainable life and health. What appears to happen, however, in self-organized complex systems is that they spontaneously tend to a state just on the 'edge of chaos', a position where, in information theory terms, there is enough stability to store information, and enough fluidity to send it. It has been described as a 'phase transition' such as exists between the solid and fluid state of substances. Complexity therefore is seen as a state between fixed order and chaos, one to which complex systems seem gravitationally to revert. The cell is a stable focus of high potassium in a dissipative sea of sodium; the heart beats most effectively when it is neither too regular nor too sensitive but somewhere in between (and this behaviour may well be the inevitable dynamic effect of circulatory structures – the heart doesn't beat, it resonates); an ant colony appears automatically to adjust its boundaries so that its density is always at optimum levels for effective ant-to-ant interactions; human civilizations consume chaotic phenomena and construct stable systems from them before eventually decaying through too much order or too much chaos.

Without going through the many fascinating arguments, it really does appear possible that the hovering of complex systems on the edge of order and chaos is itself an attractor, a state of lowest energy for such systems. And this is the punchline: *health itself could be seen as a biological attractor, the state to which living systems revert, effortlessly!*

The interest of the herbalist in a science of wholes, of qualities rather than quantities, is obvious. Unlike conventional pharmaceutical medicine, the herbal practitioner has been unable to hide behind the comfort that at least one part of the therapeutic encounter was narrowly scientific. For the herbalist even the medicine is a complex and unquantifiable thing. The fact that isolated drugs could produce unpredictable side effects because real people were still unfathomably complex has not been philosophically as strong an argument for the herbalist as it could be because the counter argument was that a complex medicine given to a complex person compounded rather than reduced complexity and unpredictability. If someone could come up with an operational model to improve understanding of the behaviour of whole beings then administering complex medicines may also be chartable.

This cannot be a thorough review of the impact of complexity theory on therapeutics; indeed, such a text has not yet been written. However, the subject is beginning to generate vigorous debate in some quarters and taking all the discussions in this chapter together, as well as reviewing the section on the placebo effect (see p. 87), it is possible to make the following tentative therapeutic propositions.

- Health in biological systems emerges out of an essential drive to self-organization. Moves to self-correction are therefore the principal responses to pathogenic forces and the main reason for disease symptoms.
- System failure in adapting to disturbances is more likely to lead to ill health than pathogens as such.
- While a system is capable of adaptive self-organization, including competent resistance to disturbance, selection of inputs from its environment and elimination of metabolites, therapeutic interventions are unnecessary except to steady the recovery (such healthy adaptations include fevers, inflammations and increased eliminations like coughing, vomiting and diarrhoea).
- Therapeutic measures are justified mainly in supporting self-organization if it is failing; the value of any medication can be judged in relation to its effect on these adaptive processes.
- All recovery is self-repair. The placebo effect and spontaneous remission are merely examples of a principle that underpins all therapeutic efficacy – Medicines in themselves do not heal.

Somewhere in this there is the basis of a truly rational therapeutic approach ideally suited to the use of herbal remedies.

References

1. Leach JD Holloway RG Almarez FA. Prehistoric evidence for the use of Chenopodium (Goosefoot) from the Hueco Bolson of west Texas. Texas Journal of Science 1996; 48 (2): 163–165.
2. Litynska-Zajac M. Polish archaeobotanical studies in north Africa: Armant (Egypt). Wiadomosci Botaniczne 1993; 37 (3–4): 171–172.
3. Petrucelli RJ II. Monastic incorporation of classical botanic medicines into the renaissance pharmacopeia. American Journal of Nephrology 1994; 14 (4–6): 259–263.
4. Sabatini S. Women, medicine and life in the Middle Ages (500–1500 AD). American Journal of Nephrology 1994; 14 (4–6): 391–398.
5. Trevor-Roper H. Medicine in the court of Charles I. In: Dickinson CJ. Marks J, ed. Developments in cardiovascular medicine. MTP Press, Lancaster, Eng., 1978: pp 305–317
6. Strehlow W, Hertzka G. Handbuch der Hildegard-Medizin. Verlag Hermann Bauer, Freiburg, 1987.
7. Harvey JH. Gardening in the age of Chaucer. 1994; 46 (4): 564–573.
8. Lloyd GER (ed). Hippocratic writings. Pelican, London, 1978.
9. Scarborough J. Drugs and medicines in the Roman world. Expedition 1996; 38 (2): 38–51.
10. Brock AR (trans). Galen: on the natural faculties. Heinemann, London, 1952.
11. Ullmann M. Islamic medicine. Edinburgh University Press, Edinburgh, 1978, pp 103–106.
12. Khan MS. Islamic medicine. Routledge and Kegan Paul, London, 1986.
13. Unschuld PU. Medicine in China: a history of pharmaceutics. University of California Press, Berkeley, 1986.

14. Needham J. Science and civilisation in China, vol 2: history of scientific thought. University of Cambridge, Cambridge, 1956.
15. Porkert M. The theoretical foundations of Chinese medicine. MIT Press, Massachusetts, 1978.
16. Larre CSJ, Schatz J, Rochat de la Vallee E. Survey of traditional Chinese medicine. Institut Ricci, Paris, 1986.
17. Wiseman N (trans). Fundamentals of Chinese medicine. Paradigm Publications, Brookline, Massachusetts, 1994.
18. Kaptchuk TJ. The web that has no weaver: understanding Chinese medicine. Congdon and Weed, New York, 1983.
19. Mills SY. Out of the earth: the essential book of herbal medicine. Viking, London, 1991, pp 596–632.
20. Chan ELP, Ahmed TM, Wang M, Chan JCM. History of medicine and nephrology in Asia. American Journal of Nephrology 1994; 14 (4–6): 295–301.
21. Capra F. The turning point: science, society, and the rising culture. Wildwood House, London, 1982.
22. Mills SY. *ibid*, pp 166–170.
23. Murthy KR, Srikantha Murthy KR (transl). Vagbhata's Astanga Hrdayam. Krishnadas Academy, Varanasi, 1991.
24. Ray P, Gupta HN. Charaka samhita: a scientific synopsis. National Institute of Sciences of India, New Delhi, 1965.
25. Savnur H. Ayurvedic materia medica. Sri Satguru Publications, New Delhi, 1984.
26. Wujastyk D, Meulenbeld GJ (eds). Studies in Indian medical history. Forsten, Groningen, 1987.
27. Leslie C (ed). Asian medical systems: a comparative study. University of California Press, Berkeley, 1976.
28. Svoboda R. Theory and practice of Ayurvedic medicine.
29. Svoboda R. *ibid*, p 87.
30. Thomson S. New guide to health; or the botanic family physician. Boston, 1835.
31. Lyle TJ. Physio-medical therapeutics, materia medica and pharmacy. Salem, Ohio, 1897.
32. Thurston JM. The philosophy of physiomedicalism. Nicholson, Richmond, Indiana, 1900.
33. Cook WH. The science and practice of medicine. Cincinnati, 1893.
34. Guyton AC. Textbook of medical physiology, 7th edn. WB Saunders, Philadelphia, 1986, pp 230–236.
35. Mills SY. *ibid*, pp 23–131.
36. Waldrop MM. Complexity: the emerging science at the edge of order and chaos Viking, London, 1992.
37. Lewin R. Complexity: life on the edge of chaos. JM Dent, London, 1992
38. Goodwin B. How the leopard changed its spots: the evolution of complexity. Weidenfeld & Nicolson, London, 1994.
39. Kauffman S. At home in the universe: the search for laws of self-organisation and complexity. Viking Penguin, London, 1995.
40. Jisaka M, Ohigashi H, Takegawa K et al. Antitumoral and antimicrobial activities of bitter sesquiterpene lactones of Vernonia amygdalina, a possible medicinal plant used by wild chimpanzees. Biosci Biotechnol Biochem 1993; 57 (5): 833–834
41. Page JE, Balza F, Nishida T, Towers GH Biologically active diterpenes from Aspilia mossambicensis, a chimpanzee medicinal plant. Phytochemistry 1992; 10; 3437–3439
42. Crandon L. Grass roots, herbs, promotors and preventions: a re-evaluation of contemporary international health care planning. The Bolivian case. Soc Sci Med 1983; 17 (17): 1281–1289
43. Ngilisho LA, Mosha HJ, Poulsen S. The role of traditional healers in the treatment of toothache in Tanga Region, Tanzania. Community Dent Health 1994; 11 (4): 240–242
44. Le Grand A, Sri-Ngernyuang L, Streefland PH. Enhancing appropriate drug use: the contribution of herbal medicine promotion. A case study in rural Thailand. Soc Sci Med 1993; 36 (8): 1023–1035
45. Messer E. Systematic and medicinal reasoning in Mitla folk botany. J Ethnopharmacol 1991; 33 (1-2): 107–128

2 Principles of herbal pharmacology

DEFINING OUR GROUND

Pharmacology can be defined as the study of the interaction of biologically active agents with living systems.[1] The study of pharmacology is further divided into two main areas. *Pharmacodynamics* looks at the effects of an agent at active sites in the body. In contrast, *pharmacokinetics* is concerned with the effects the body has on the medicine and specifically the concentrations which can be achieved at active sites. The approach used in this and throughout the therapeutic chapters is to examine the pharmacology of key chemical groups in plants, the 'archetypal plant constituents', as much as individual herbs. (For detailed information on the pharmacology of individual herbs see Part Three).

The chemical nature and classification of these archetypal plant constituents is studied in the discipline known as phytochemistry. Hence any discourse on herbal pharmacology must be founded on a knowledge of phytochemistry. A common misconception about 'why medicinal plants work' occurs in lay and sometimes even professional circles. This is that the various nutrients such as vitamins, minerals and so on are responsible for the pharmacological activity of plants. Almost without exception, this is not the case. In fact, the archetypal plant constituents generally come from the class of plant metabolites known as secondary metabolites. Primary metabolites are necessary to sustain the life of the plant and include enzymes and other proteins, lipids, carbohydrates and chlorophyll. In contrast, secondary metabolites do not appear to be necessary to sustain life. However, they probably do have more subtle functions which increase the survival prospects of the plant in its natural environment. Some of the known functions of secondary metabolites (there are many gaps in this knowledge) are discussed below.

The phytochemistry of secondary metabolites is comprehensively covered in a number of texts. Textbooks on pharmacognosy are especially relevant for the student of herbal medicine. Two pharmacognosy texts have been drawn on for the phytochemistry content of this chapter:

- Bruneton J. Pharmacognosy, phytochemistry, medicinal plants. Lavoisier Publishing, Paris, 1995.
- Evans WC. Trease and Evans' pharmacognosy, 14th edn. WB Saunders, London, 1996.

Why should secondary metabolites have biological activity in animals? One suggestion put forward by Baker is that enzymes in animals can share a common ancestry with enzymes or proteins in plants.[2] This evolutionary kinship, when combined with structural similarities between plant and animal substrates for these enzymes, could explain the hormone-like or hormone-modulating effects of several archetypal plant constituents in humans.

HOW DO HERBS DIFFER FROM CONVENTIONAL DRUGS?

While many conventional drugs or their precursors are derived from plants, there is a fundamental difference between administering a pure chemical and the same chemical in a plant matrix. It is this issue of the advantage of chemical complexity which is both rejected by orthodoxy as having no basis in fact and avoided by most researchers as introducing too many variables for comfortable research. Herein lies the fundamental difference between the phytotherapist, who prefers not just to prescribe chemically complex remedies but often to administer them in complex formulations, and the conventional physician who would rather prescribe a single agent.

Is there any advantage in chemically complex medicines? Life is indeed chemically complex, so much so that science is only beginning to grasp the subtle and varied mechanisms involved in processes such as inflammation and immunity. It does seem logical that, just as our foods are chemically complex, so should our medicines be. But hard proof of this advantage has been difficult to establish. There are, however, several examples from the literature of how an advantage might arise from chemical complexity and some of these are discussed below.

Synergy is an important concept in herbal pharmacology. In the context of chemical complexity, it applies if the action of a chemical mixture is greater than the arithmetical sum of the actions of the mixture's components: the whole is greater than the sum of the individual parts. A well-known example of synergy is exploited in the use of insecticidal pyrethrins. A synergist known as piperonyl butoxide, which has little insecticidal activity of its own, interferes with the insect's ability to break down the pyrethrins, thereby substantially increasing their toxicity. This example emphasizes what is probably an important mechanism behind the synergy observed for medicinal plant components: increased or prolonged levels of key components at the active site. In other words, components of plants which are not active themselves can act to improve the stability, solubility, bioavailability or half-life of the active components. Hence a particular chemical might in pure form have only a fraction of the pharmacological activity that it has in its plant matrix. This important example of synergy therefore has a pharmacokinetic basis.

Chemical complexity leading to enhanced solubility or bioavailability of key components has been the theme of a number of scientific studies. The basic issues were discussed by Eder and Mehnert.[3] The isoflavone glycoside daidzin given in crude extract of *Pueraria lobata* achieves much greater concentrations in plasma than equivalent doses of pure daidzin.[4] Ascorbic acid in a citrus extract was more bioavailable than ascorbic acid alone.[5] Coadministration of procyanidins from *Hypericum perforatum* (St John's wort) significantly increased the in vivo antidepressant effects of hypericin and pseudohypericin. This effect was attributed to the observed enhanced solubility of hypericin and pseudohypericin in the presence of procyanidins and indicates that pure hypericin and pseudohypericin have considerably less antidepressant activity than their equivalent amounts in St John's wort extract.[6]

Synergy can also have a pharmacodynamic basis. One example is the antibacterial activity of major components of lemongrass essential oil. While geranial and neral individually elicit antibacterial action, the third main component myrcene did not show any activity. However, myrcene enhanced activities when mixed with either of the other two main components.[7] Sennoside A and sennoside C from senna have similar laxative activities in mice. However, a mixture of these compounds in the ratio 7:3 (which somewhat reflects the relative levels found in senna leaf) has almost double the laxative activity.[8] Additional examples of synergy in herbal pharmacology are reviewed in Part Three.

THE ROLE OF SECONDARY METABOLITES

Before discussing the pharmacodynamics of the archetypal plant constituents, it is worthwhile to briefly consider some examples of their value to the plant.

The immobility of plants in diverse and changing physical environments, along with the possibility of attack by animals and pathogens, has necessitated the development of numerous chemical mechanisms for protection and offence. In recent years, considerable attention has been paid to the specific ecological roles of secondary metabolites, which were often formerly regarded as waste products.

Alkaloids are thought to play a defensive role in plants against herbivores and pathogens.[9] Glucosinolates have a role in protecting against insect attack.[10] Tannins act to preserve the wood in living trees from microbial decomposition and insects.[11] Several classes of secondary metabolites are induced by infection, wounding or grazing. Variation in the speed and extent of such induction may account, at least in part, for the differences between resistant and susceptible varieties.[12] Both salicylic and jasmonic acids have been implicated as signals in such responses. Toxic chemicals formed in response to damage, especially from fungal attack, are called phytoalexins.[11] In legumes, secondary metabolites are involved in interactions with beneficial microorganisms (flavonoids as inducers of the Rhizobium symbiosis) and in defence against pathogens (isoflavonoid phytoalexins).[13]

Plants have also developed defences against other plants, a phenomenon known as *allelopathy*. Many compounds are implicated, including phenolics[14] and terpenoids.[15] Positive interaction, or facilitation, among plants is also becoming increasingly recognized.[16]

PHARMACODYNAMICS OF THE ARCHETYPAL PLANT CONSTITUENTS

SIMPLE PHENOLS AND GLYCOSIDES

Phenols comprise the largest group of plant secondary metabolites. They range from simple structures with only one benzene ring to larger molecules such as tannins, anthraquinones, flavonoids and coumarins. They are defined as compounds that have at least one hydroxyl group attached to a benzene ring. Phenols differ in their chemical properties from other tertiary alcohols because the presence of the benzene ring stabilizes the phenolate ion; they are therefore more acidic and more reactive.

Glycosides are secondary metabolites that yield one or more sugars on hydrolysis. The most frequently occurring sugar is glucose (a glycoside yielding glucose is called glucoside). The non-sugar component of the molecule, which may be a simple phenol, flavonoid, anthraquinone, triterpenoid or many other structures, is called the *aglycone*. If the glycosidic bond is via an oxygen, the molecule is termed an *O-glycoside*; if it is via a carbon, it is a *C-glycoside*. The glycosidic linkage is usually resistant to human digestive enzymes (being a beta linkage) and glycosides are often poorly absorbed from the digestive tract. Hence their usual fate is to travel to the distal ileum or large bowel where microbial activity forms the aglycone, which is then absorbed into the bloodstream (see Pharmacokinetics below, p.58).

Phenolic acids are a special class of simple phenols which in addition have at least one carboxylic acid group. Phytochemists usually restrict this term to benzoic and cinnamic acid derivatives only, such as gallic acid, salicylic acid, caffeic acid, vanillic acid and ferulic acid. Phenolic acids derived from cinnamic acid are usually found in plants as esters (phenolic acid esters). These include chlorogenic acid and rosmarinic acid. Caffeic acid esters of quinic acid such as chlorogenic acid are also known as caffeoylquinic acids (see the

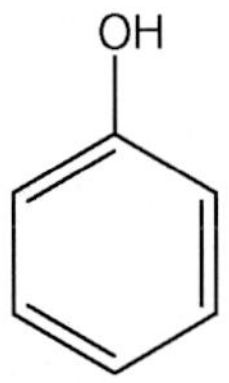

Phenol 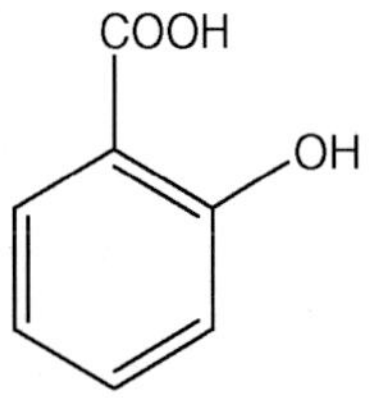 **Salicylic acid**

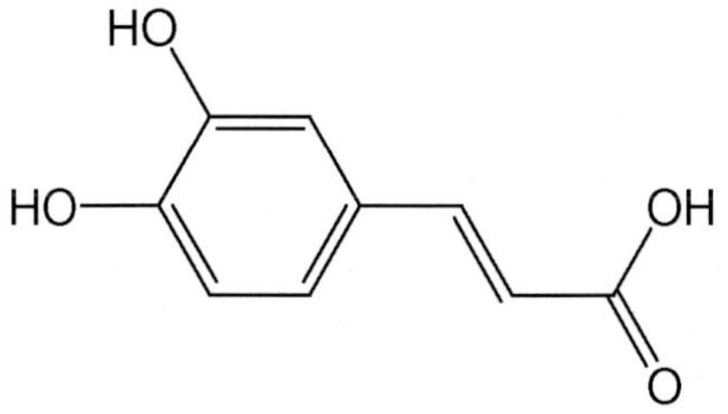

Caffeic acid also known as 3,4-Dihydroxycinnamic acid

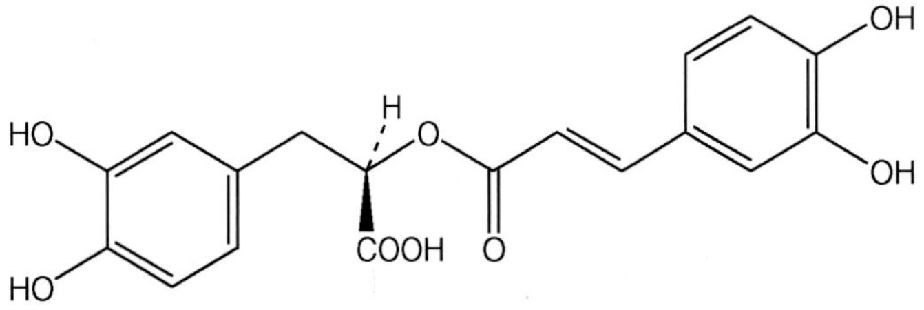

Rosmarinic acid

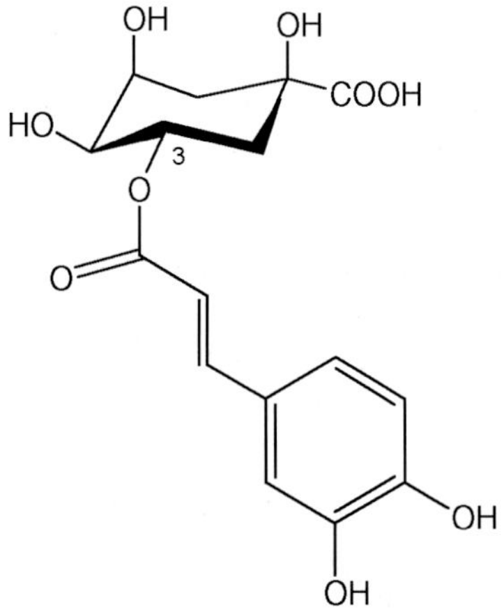

Chlorogenic acid (3-caffeoylquinic acid)

monograph on globe artichoke p.433). Some of these compounds are sometimes called pseudotannins, since they have astringent characteristics but lack all the properties of true tannins.

From a pharmacological perspective, the best known simple phenol is salicylic acid. Its precursors are found in willow (*Salix species*) and poplar barks (*Populus species*) and salicylic acid is subsequently formed on ingestion (see Pharmacokinetics below, p.58). Salicylic acid has recognized antipyretic and antiinflammatory properties which underlie the use of willow bark for arthritis. Acetylsalicylic acid (aspirin) is a synthetic derivative of salicylic acid which in addition has pronounced antiplatelet properties due to the presence of the acetyl group.[17] Salicylic acid lacks this property and consequently willow bark is not suitable as a natural substitute for aspirin in cardiovascular patients. Simple phenols are also powerful antiseptics. Arbutin is a phenolic glycoside which confers bacteriostatic properties on urine (see the monograph on bearberry, p. 280).

Gastrodin, a simple phenol glycoside from the sedative Chinese herb *Gastrodia elata*, antagonized the effects of scopolamine in rats, which suggests it could facilitate learning and memory.[18] The root extract of *Fagara zanthoxyloides* possesses antisickling properties in sickle cell anaemia. The constituents responsible for this activity were identified to be simple phenolic acids such as vanillic acid.[19] Several studies have shown that extracts of many members of the mint family (Lamiaceae) have considerable antioxidant activity due to the presence of phenolic acids such as rosmarinic acid. Highest antioxidant activity was found in *Prunella vulgaris*, which had a rosmarinic acid content of about 5%.[20]

Caffeic acid, as well as its derivatives such as rosmarinic acid and chlorogenic acid, were found to exert antithyroid activity after oxidation. This activity may form the basis of the clinical use of *Lycopus species* for hyperthyroidism.[21] Similar oxidation products of caffeic acid inhibit protein biosynthesis in vitro and these compounds probably account for the clinically established antiviral activity of a topical preparation of *Melissa officinalis*.[22]

CYANOGENIC GLYCOSIDES

Cyanogenic glycosides are capable of generating hydrocyanic acid (prussic acid, cyanide). Structurally they are glycosides of 2-hydroxynitriles which can be hydrolysed by the enzyme beta-glucosidase into cyanohydrin. This is unstable and dissociates to hydrocyanic acid. Common cyanogenic glycosides include amygdalin, which is found in bitter almonds and peach kernels (both used in Chinese medicine), and prunasin which occurs in wild cherry bark (*Prunus serotina*). The small quantities of cyanide generated from this bark are said to be responsible for its antitussive properties, although this has not been confirmed in modern pharmacological experiments. Both amygdalin and prunasin yield benzaldehyde on hydrolysis which accounts for the characteristic almond-like aroma of wild cherry bark.

Although hydrocyanic acid is a violent poison, oral intake of cyanogenic glycosides (which often occurs via food, especially in primitive diets) is not necessarily toxic. Hydrolysis of the glycosides in the digestive tract or by the liver leads to a slow release of hydrocyanic acid which can be readily detoxified by the body. Addition of 10% apricot kernels to the diet of rats for 18 weeks showed only moderate toxic effects.[23] Amygdalin given orally to humans at 500 mg three times a day produced no toxic effects and only moderately raised blood cyanide levels.[24] However, coadministration of beta-glucosidase with amygdalin to rats substantially increased its toxicity.[25]

Considerable interest arose in the 1970s in the use of a synthetic cyanogenic glycoside, patented as laetrile (mandelonitrile beta-glucuronide), as an alternative anticancer compound.[26] However, most of what was subsequently sold as laetrile was in fact amygdalin (which probably had similar properties on injection or ingestion).[27] The theory was that cancer tissues contain beta-glucosidase and that circulating

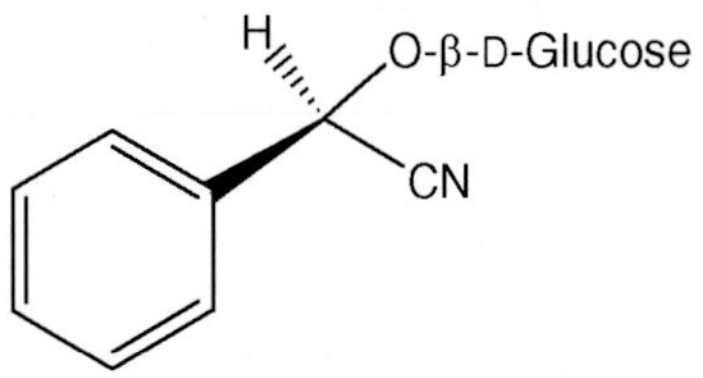

H O-β-D-Glucose CN

Prunasin

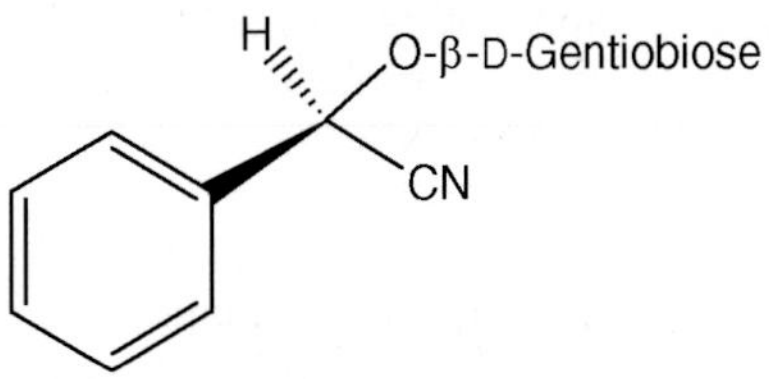

H O-β-D-Gentiobiose CN

Amygdalin

cyanogenic glycosides would therefore act as selective cytotoxic agents. However, amygdalin did not prove to be an effective anticancer agent either in animals[28] or humans,[29] presumably because the beta-glucosidase activity of cancer cells is quite low.[30] In an interesting development of the laetrile theory, beta-glucosidase was conjugated to a tumour-associated antibody. When combined with amygdalin in vitro, the cytotoxicity of amygdalin to tumour cells was increased 36-fold.[31]

MUCILAGES

Although from a phytochemical standpoint mucilages are often considered to be a minor category of the group of large plant polysaccharides (a category which includes gums, the various mannans, hemicelluloses and pectins), they are highly prized by phytotherapists. Strictly speaking, the class of compounds which the phytotherapist considers as 'mucilages' are acidic heterogeneous polysaccharides or the 'acidic mucilages'.

Mucilages are generally not chemically well defined. They are large, highly branched polymeric structures built from many different sugar and uronic acid units (uronic acids are carboxylic acids derived from sugars). They are very hydrophilic (water loving) and are capable of trapping water (and other molecules) in their cage-like structures to form a gel. Consequently, when a mucilage is mixed with water it swells to many times its original volume as it absorbs water. The saccharide linkages are in a beta configuration which means that human digestive enzymes cannot break down mucilages. However, they can at least be partially decomposed by bowel flora into short-chain fatty acids (SCFA). This may explain the traditional use of slippery elm bark (*Ulmus rubra*) as a food for convalescents. Not only would the mucilage soothe a disturbed digestive tract, the SCFA formed in the colon would provide a source of readily absorbed and assimilated nourishment.

Mucilaginous remedies have been primarily used for topical emollient and demulcent properties and their direct, if temporary, benefits in the management of inflammatory conditions of the digestive tract. This antiinflammatory effect is probably more than just mechanical, although the protective benefits of a layer of mucilage on the digestive mucosa are obvious, especially as an extra barrier to gastric acid. The protective effect of mucilage isolated from *Plantago major* leaves against aspirin-induced gastric ulcer has been demonstrated in rats.[32] Similar gastroprotective activity has been demonstrated for guar gum.[33] It has also been shown that guar gum forms a layer closely associated with the intestinal mucosal surface when given to rats, providing a protective barrier.[34]

Mucilages are topically applied for an antiinflammatory (demulcent) effect but also for a drawing and healing effect on wounds and infected skin lesions. This latter application is analogous to the use of hydrocolloid dressings in modern medicine.

Mucilages can also function as bulk laxatives and the most widespread use in this regard is ispaghula or psyllium husks as proprietary products such as Metamucil. However, the traditional uses of mucilages such as linseed (flaxseed) and fenugreek as bulk laxatives often provide a valuable alternative,[35] particularly where psyllium causes the characteristic side effects of bloating, abdominal pain and flatulence.[36] Mucilages can also be used as weight loss agents and presumably act by creating a sensation of fullness.[36] Since they have been known to cause oesophageal obstruction, mucilages should be taken with plenty of water and not prescribed in tablet form.[37]

Mucilages are also used by phytotherapists to effect reflex demulcency, especially to ease irritable and ticklish dry coughs. It is clear that there is no readily recognized pharmacological model for the transfer of demulcent properties directly to the bronchial mucosa: mucilages are too large to be absorbed and transported to this site. The emetic effect in reverse, that is, the reflex effects on the tracheobronchial musculature of a soothing effect on the upper digestive tract, is instead postulated, mediated by the vagus nerve. Similar associations are used to justify the use of mucilages in painful conditions of the urinary tract.

This reflex effect does have experimental support. An extract of marshmallow root (*Althaea officinalis*) and the isolated mucilage demonstrated significant antitussive activity in an animal test. Doses were administered orally and cough from both laryngopharyngeal and tracheobronchial stimulation was depressed[38]. The mucilage was as potent as some non-narcotic antitussive drugs. The reverse phenomenon has also been observed; acid reflux into the distal oesophagus can trigger cough and an association between nocturnal asthma attacks and oesophageal reflux has been demonstrated.

Mucilages are also a class of soluble fibre and in this context the properties of psyllium husks have been well studied. In particular, the mucilage from psyllium is effective at lowering blood cholesterol, as evidenced by a recent review and double-blind crossover clinical trial.[39] Trial results suggest that it must be taken with food to be effective.[40]

Soluble fibre helps to retain glucose in the gut and to reduce blood insulin levels after eating. Psyllium seed was shown to have particular benefits in this regard, with a clear dose-related response on the effects of glucose challenge.[41] Soluble fibre and mucilages in particular also act as a prebiotic, enhancing the population of beneficial organisms in the gut flora. More studies are required to confirm this effect.

Since mucilages are water soluble and relatively insoluble in ethanol, liquid galenical preparations of mucilages are not appropriate (except for their use as reflex demulcents); for demulcent effects in the digestive tract, mucilages are best given as powders or capsules. In any case, an effectively made liquid extract of slippery elm, for example, would be so viscous that it could not be poured.

ESSENTIAL OILS

Phytochemistry

Essential oils (from the word 'essence') are mixtures of fragrant compounds which can be isolated from plants by the process of steam distillation. In this procedure, steam is driven through the plant material and then condensed, with the subsequent oil and water phases separating out. Since they are volatile in steam and usually have pronounced aromas, essential oils are often referred to as volatile oils. However, this term is not accurate since they have boiling points well above 100°C. Often the oil is slightly modified by the steam distillation process, so that it does not exactly reflect what is found in the plant. In some cases, such as chamazulene from German chamomile, steam distillation actually produces substantial quantities of a new chemical.

Other processes are also used to produce essential oils and these include solvent extract using hexane or liquid or supercritical carbon dioxide, enfleurage (oil extraction of delicate essential oils in flowers) and expression (used to produce orange and lemon oils from the peel). Essential oils are important items of commerce, being used for perfumes, food flavourings and personal care and pharmaceutical products. They also comprise the medicines of the therapeutic system known as aromatherapy.

Essential oils are water-insoluble oily liquids which are usually colourless. Despite the fact that they are called oils, they are not chemically related to lipid oils (fixed oils) such as olive oil, corn oil and so on. Although often hydrocarbon in nature, they are unrelated to the hydrocarbon oils from the petrochemical industry. They will slowly evaporate if left in an open container and placing a drop of oil on blotting paper can be used as a simple technique to test for adulteration with a fixed oil. If a fixed oil is present an oily smear will remain on the paper a few days later.

Adulteration is an important issue in the trading of essential oils and many sophisticated techniques have been developed to imitate and extend essential oils. In some cases, such as oil of wintergreen, trade in the synthetic oil has completely supplanted the natural product. A recent survey found a large variability between the biological activities of different samples of oils and groups of oils under the same general name, for example, lavender, eucalyptus or chamomile.[42] This reflected on the blending, rectification and adulteration which occurs with commercial oils. Of course, this issue does not apply for oils prescribed as part of the whole plant extract, as used by phytotherapists.

The synthesis and accumulation of essential oils are generally associated with the presence of specialized structures in the plant which are often located on or near the surface; for example, the delicate glandular trichomes (hairs) of the mint family (Lamiaceae). Essential oil composition can vary quite dramatically within a species and often distinct chemotypes are recognized. This means that the same plant species can produce quite different oils in terms of chemistry, pharmacology and toxicology. From a biosynthetic perspective, the components of essential oils can be classified into two major groups: the terpenoids and the phenylpropanoids. Any given essential oil might contain more than 100 of these components.

When the chemical structures of terpenoids are examined, they can be seen to be theoretically constructed from five-carbon isoprene units. Plants produce terpenoids using the mevalonic acid biosynthetic pathway. The building block is actually isopentenylpyrophosphate, not isoprene, but the final outcome is molecules based on five-carbon units. Naming of terpenoids is based on multiples of 10 carbons (two isoprene units). Hence molecules with 10 carbons are called monoterpenes, those with 15 are called sesquiterpenes (sesqui means one and a half) and so on. Only mono- and sesquiterpenes are found in essential oils. Higher terpenoids are too large and are not volatile in steam. However, diterpenes occur in resins as resin acids and triterpenes are found in saponins. Not even all mono- and sesquiterpenes are volatile in steam – the iridoids which are mentioned in the eyebright monograph are one example. Examples of monoterpenes in essential oils include

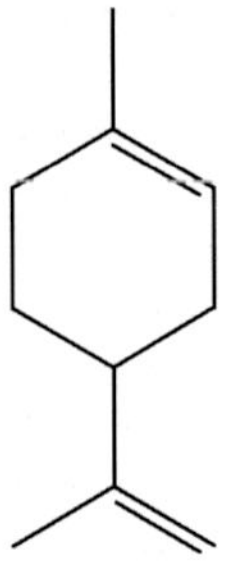

Limonene 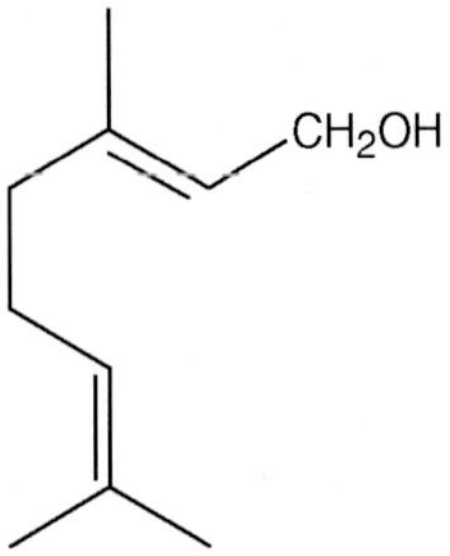 Gerianiol 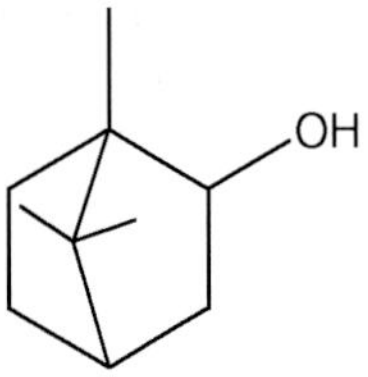 Borneol 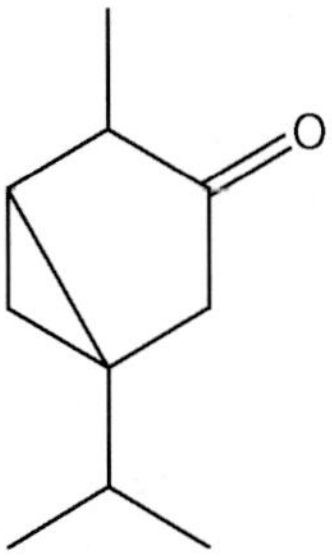 Thujone 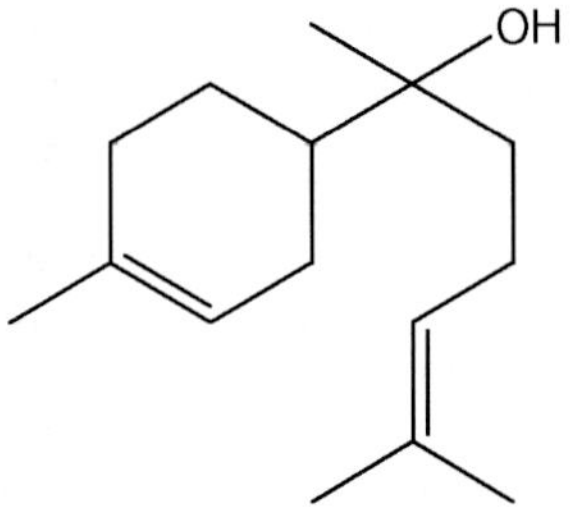 (-)-α-Bisabolol

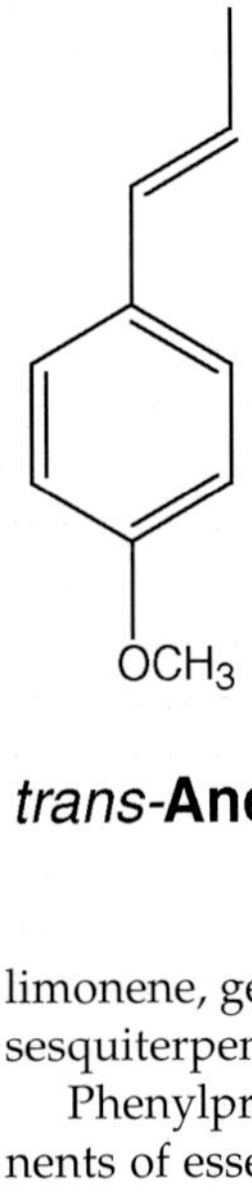

trans-Anethole 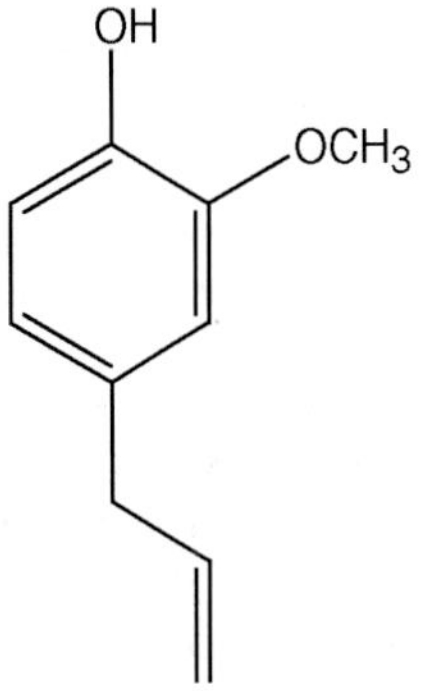 Eugenol

limonene, geraniol, borneol and thujone. Bisabolol is a sesquiterpene.

Phenylpropanoids are far less common as components of essential oils. Their basic chemical skeleton is a three-carbon chain attached to a benzene ring. They are formed by the shikimic acid biosynthetic pathway and examples are anethole and eugenol.

Essential oil components can also be classified according to their functional groups. The most common compounds found in essential oils are hydrocarbons, alcohols, aldehydes, ketones, phenols, oxides and esters. These functional groups play a large part in determining the pharmacology and toxicology of the essential oil component; for example, ketones are more active and toxic than alcohols and alcohols and phenols are more potent as antimicrobial agents, with phenols being more irritant. Essential oil components often exhibit optical isomerism (where the two isomers are mirror images of each other). For example, (+)-carvone isolated from caraway oil has a caraway-like odour and (–)-carvone isolated from spearmint oil has a spearmint-like odour.

Pharmacodynamics

Aromatherapy is a treatment system based on the use of essential oils. The oils may either be inhaled, applied to the skin or orifices, added to baths or ingested. There is no doubt that ingested oils or those applied to the skin or added to baths are absorbed into the bloodstream in significant quantities.[43] However, the use of essential oils by inhalation, mainly to influence mental function, is more controversial. In fact, in the German-speaking world, aromatherapy is defined as the therapeutic use of fragrances only by means of inhalation. Evidence is now accumulating that this form of aromatherapy also has a pharmacological basis and is not placebo, nor is it a manipulation of emotions via the sense of smell.[44]

Given the great chemical diversity of essential oils, it is not surprising that they exhibit a wide variety of pharmacological activities. However, some common themes do emerge, notably antimicrobial and spasmolytic actions.

Most of the evidence for the antimicrobial activity of essential oils comes from in vitro tests, although recently case reports and clinical trials have started to appear in the literature. A review of the published in vitro work between 1976 and 1986 found that results were difficult to compare.[45] Test methods used differed widely and important factors influencing results were frequently neglected. One of these factors was the composition of the essential oil being tested (given the existence of chemotypes and adulteration). This was highlighted in a recent study of commercial essential oils which found a wide variation in the antimicrobial activities of commercial samples of thyme oil, eucalyptus oil and geranium oil, among others.[42]

Of 53 essential oils tested against four organisms, only a few oils exhibited remarkable activity, particularly thyme and origanum which contain phenols.[46] *Pseudomonas aeruginosa* was the least susceptible organism and *Candida albicans* the most susceptible.

All 66 isolates of *Staphylococcus aureus* tested were susceptible to tea tree oil (*Melaleuca alternifolia*) at 0.5% concentration, including antibiotic-resistant strains.[47]

Attempts have been made to identify the mechanisms behind the antimicrobial activity of essential oils and the key components responsible for this activity. Antimicrobial activity was said to parallel cytotoxic activity, which suggests a similar mode of action, most probably exerted by membrane-associated reactions.[48] Concentrations of tea tree oil which inhibit or decrease growth of *Escherichia coli* also inhibit glucose-dependent respiration and stimulate the leakage of intracellular potassium.[49] Of five components tested for antibacterial activity, cinnamic aldehyde was the most active, followed by citral, geraniol, eugenol and menthol.[50] In another study linalool was the most active antibacterial agent and citral and geraniol were the most effective antifungal agents.[51] Essential oils with high monoterpene hydrocarbon levels were very active against bacteria although not against fungi, with the exception of dill.[42] There was a negative correlation between cineole content and antifungal activity. In the case of tea tree oil, terpinen-4-ol was identified as the most important antimicrobial compound[52,53] and cineole detracts from its antifungal activity.[53]

Clinical studies of the antimicrobial activity of essential oils have been published, with a focus on tea tree oil. In a double-blind trial, 10% tea tree oil cream reduced symptoms of tinea pedis but was not effective in achieving eradication of the fungus.[54] However, a 5% tea tree oil gel was as effective as a 5% benzoyl peroxide lotion in the treatment of acne and patients experienced few side effects.[55] An essential oil mouth rinse was more effective at reducing oral plaque than a conventional preparation.[56] Information about topical use is important but phytotherapists also rely on essential oils to achieve antimicrobial effects within the body. In particular, the excretion of essential oils via the lungs or urine might be expected to exert at least mild antimicrobial activity at these sites. This is the basis of the use of juniper for urinary tract infections and one of the reasons for the use of thyme in respiratory infections. However, essential oil components are excreted into the urine in metabolized forms, mainly as glucuronide conjugates and sulphates. Hence any antibacterial activity may not be reflected in the urine. Studies are necessary to further understand this traditional use.

The spasmolytic activity of essential oils has been observed many times on isolated smooth muscle preparations and forms much of the basis of their use in functional gastrointestinal disorders. The effects of essential oils from 22 plants and some of their constituents on tracheal and ileal smooth muscle were investigated.[57] All of the oils had relaxant effects on tracheal smooth muscle, the most potent being angelica root, clove and elecampane root. Sixteen oils inhibited the phasic contractions of the ileal muscle preparation, the most potent being elecampane root, clove, thyme and lemon balm. Two oils (anise and fennel) increased the phasic contractions. Spasmolytic activity has also been confirmed clinically. For example, peppermint oil added to barium sulphate suspension significantly relieved colonic muscle spasm ($p<0.001$) during barium enema examination in a double-blind, placebo-controlled study on 141 patients.[58]

Carminatives relax sphincters and assist in the expulsion of intestinal gas. Their activity is somewhat related to spasmolytic activity. Certain essential oils or essential oil-containing herbs have been traditionally used as carminatives over many years. Oils of peppermint, sage and rosemary all relaxed Oddi's sphincter but peppermint was the most active.[59] The carminative activity of cardamom and dill was confirmed in human studes.[60] However, they were also shown to cause oesophageal reflux and should be used cautiously in susceptible patients.

Some essential oils are traditionally regarded as diuretics because they act as 'kidney irritants'. The infusion and essential oil of juniper berries as well as terpinen-4-ol were tested for diuresis response in rats.[61] On initial dosing, all three test substances exhibited an antidiuretic effect but a significant diuretic effect was established on repeated doses, with the infusion having the strongest effect. The 'irritant' effect of juniper oil on the kidneys was investigated since there are concerns in the literature about its long-term use. No nephrotoxic effects were observed in an animal study and the authors suggested that provided high-quality oil is used (distilled from the ripe berries), concerns about the kidney irritant effects of juniper are unfounded.[62]

Certain essential oils (or the herbs which contain them) are used as expectorants. A proprietary product containing myrtle oil known as Gelomyrtol is popularly prescribed by doctors in Germany as an expectorant and mucolytic for acute and chronic bronchitis and sinusitis. The oil contains limonene, cineole and alpha-pinene. An expectorant activity for this oil was confirmed in a clinical trial on patients with chronic obstructive airways disease.[63] Earlier animal experiments by Boyd suggested an expectorant activity for anise oil.[64]

The sedative activity of essential oils such as lavender is commonly recognized and has been supported

$$R{-}C(=N{-}O{-}SO_3^{\ominus}K^{\oplus})(S{-}glucose) \xrightarrow[\text{steam}]{\text{myrosinase}} R{-}N{=}C{=}S$$

glucosinolate **isothiocyanate**

by animal studies.[65] A proprietary essential oil combination known as Melissengeist exhibited anxiolytic activity in a double-blind, placebo-controlled clinical trial.[66] Myrcene and lemongrass oil exhibited peripheral analgesic activity.[67] Clove oil is a powerful local anaesthetic.

Stimulant activity has been attributed to some essential oils. Inhalation and oral doses of rosemary oil increased locomotor activity in mice.[68] Infusions of essential oil-containing herbs are often taken as diaphoretics especially during acute respiratory infections. In this context, it is interesting to note that a case report describes a patient who exhibited pronounced diaphoresis attributed to up to 10 cups a day of sassafras tea.[69]

For more information about the pharmacology of essential oils and associated antiinflammatory, antiulcer, spasmolytic, oestrogenic, expectorant, antimicrobial and analgesic activities, see the monographs on chamomile, fennel, peppermint and thyme in Part Three.

Toxicology

Essential oils are highly concentrated compared to the original plant and as a result can present specific safety issues when used as such. Their toxicology has already been comprehensively reviewed.[70] Nevertheless, a few issues are worth noting here. Certain toxic essential oils, notably pennyroyal, tansy and parsley, have been used as abortifacients but as early as 1913 it was found that these oils have absolutely no specific or direct stimulating action on the uterine muscle.[71] In fact, consistent with the known pharmacodynamics of essential oils, they were found to inhibit uterine contractions. Their abortifacient action was concluded to be due to general poisoning or gastrointestinal irritation, which makes their use not only uncertain but extremely dangerous.

Thujone is a constituent of commonly used herbs such as wormwood, yarrow, thuja and sage. This compound is neurotoxic and its presence in liqueurs such as absinthe caused widespread toxicity and abuse syndromes in the early 20th century[72]. The first sign of toxicity is a headache. High and prolonged doses of the above herbs should be avoided unless they are low-thujone varieties. It has been suggested that thujone intoxication may have played a part in Van Gogh's style of painting[73]. Safrole, a major component of sassafras oil, is carcinogenic and its use should be avoided.

GLUCOSINOLATES

Phytochemistry

Glucosinolates are sulphur- and nitrogen-containing glycosides which are responsible for the pungent properties of horseradish, nasturtium and mustard. The glucosinolate itself is not pungent. When it comes into contact with the enzyme myrosinase, which is normally stored in another compartment of the cell, the aglycone is formed which usually rearranges into the pungent and corrosive isothiocyanate. Isothiocyanates can also be formed from glucosinolates by steam distillation and so are also called mustard oils. For this reason, they are sometimes classified as essential oils but from a phytochemical perspective this is inappropriate. The structure of a typical glucosinolate is given above. They are ionic in nature and occur in the plant as potassium salts.

Glucosinolates are also found in brassicas such as cabbage, broccoli and Brussels sprouts. As such, they are frequently consumed as a normal part of human diet.

Pharmacodynamics

In traditional herbal medicine and folk medicine, strong skin irritants and inflammatory substances were empirically used to combat inflammatory processes in tissues and organs remote from the site where the irritant was applied. This is the principle of counterirritation. This poorly understood effect is recognized in pharmacology and can often provide misleading antiinflammatory effects for substances which have no pharmacological activity other than being irritants. The mode of action of skin irritants is characterized by an ability to influence deeper regions of the body, probably by reflex effects mediated by the nervous system. The stinging of arthritic joints with nettles and the subsequent reduction in pain and inflammation is one such example. Hyperaemic medicines can be used in the form of ointments, compresses, liniments or plasters. The mustard compress or plaster is still used in Europe today, particularly for bronchial infections and detoxification in chronic diseases. Mustard oil is highly corrosive and if applied for too long will cause blistering and may even permanently scar the skin.

The main component of nasturtium oil (*Tropaeolum majus*) is benzyl isothiocyanate. This has potent antibacterial and antifungal activity and in Europe enteric-coated capsules of the oil are used to treat bronchial and urinary tract infections.[74] Horseradish preparations are used in the treatment of bronchial and sinus conditions. Presumably the sulphur compounds confer a mucolytic effect.

Isothiocyanates and some of their products (such as goitrin) are goitrogenic and interfere with the function of the thyroid gland.[75] Goitrin inhibits iodine incorporation and the formation of thyroxin and its effects cannot be countered by iodine administration. Although this is a potentially toxic effect, it could be exploited in cases of patients with hyperthyroidism.

The bulk of recent research attention on glucosinolates and their various transformation products has focused on their potential to prevent cancer. This phenomenon has been known for more than 20 years. The anticarcinogenicity of these compounds, specifically in relation to brassica vegetables, has been recently reviewed for in vitro assays, animal experiments and various human studies.[76] Alterations in phase I and particularly phase II detoxification enzymes are suggested as possible mechanisms by which these plant constituents might inhibit chemical carcinogenesis. On the other hand, possible mutagenicity and carcinogenicity are also discussed, indicating that caution should be exercised if recommending long-term intake of these compounds at well in excess of optimum dietary levels.

FLAVONOIDS

Phytochemistry

Flavonoids are extremely common and widespread in the plant kingdom. They function as plant pigments, being responsible for the colours of flowers and fruits. Being abundant in plants, flavonoids are commonly consumed in the human diet, especially if it is rich in fruits and vegetables.

The word 'flavonoid' is derived from the Latin word *flavus* meaning yellow and many flavonoids are indeed yellow in colour. However, many others are white and the special flavonoid-related anthocyanidins are red, blue or purple. (For a discussion of the pharmacological properties of anthocyanidins, see the bilberry monograph on p.297.) Flavonoids are also present in leaves where they are said to protect the plant tissue against the damaging effects of ultraviolet radiation.

Flavonoids consist of a single benzene ring joined to a benzo-gamma-pyrone structure. They are formed from three acetate units and a phenylpropane unit (shikimic acid pathway). More than 2000 are known with nearly 500 occurring in the free (aglycone) state and the rest as O-or C-glycosides. Flavonoid glycosides are generally water soluble. There are three main types, classified according to the state of oxygenation at carbon 3. These are flavones, flavonols and flavonones. The properties of isoflavonoids are discussed in the Phytooestrogen section on p.000.

Pharmacodynamics

Most of the studies conducted on flavonoids have used in vitro models, often isolated enzyme systems. The findings of these studies need to be interpreted with caution since it is uncertain that oral doses of flavonoid glycosides or even their aglycones can reach sufficient concentrations in living organisms to reproduce these effects. This reservation applies even more for oral doses of herbs containing flavonoids, since the flavonoid dose will be commensurately lower. The issue was well illustrated by a clinical pharmacology study which found that while quercetin and apigenin inhibited platelet aggregation in vitro, no significant effect was found in human volunteers.[77] For these reasons, such in vitro studies (and those where flavonoids were administered in high doses by injection) have not been reviewed in detail. For a further discussion on the bioavailability of flavonoids, see the Pharmacokinetics section on p.58.

The original pharmacological interest in flavonoids arose during vitamin C research in the 1930s. Studies by Hungarian workers indicated that a number of vegetables and fruits (notably citrus) contained substances capable of correcting certain abnormalities associated with scurvy. In particular, this new factor, designated as vitamin P, corrected the capillary fragility associated with ascorbic acid deficiency. Vitamin P was subsequently found to be a mixture of flavonoids. Additional research disputed that vitamin P was essential to maintain human life and the term was dropped in the 1950s. However, research did confirm the therapeutic value of flavonoids for fragile capillaries (actually fragile connective tissue

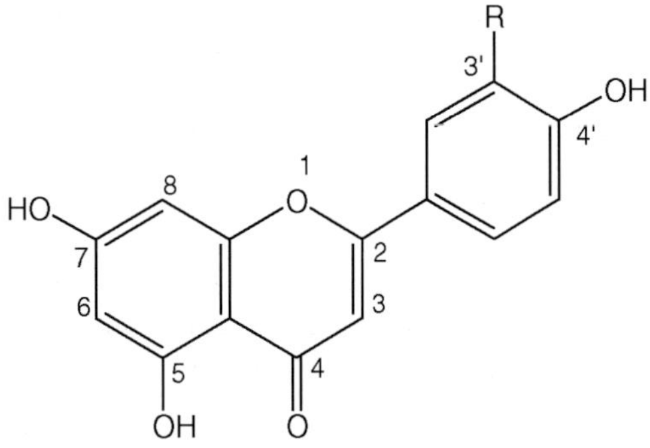

R = H: Apigenin
R = OH: Luteolin

Flavones

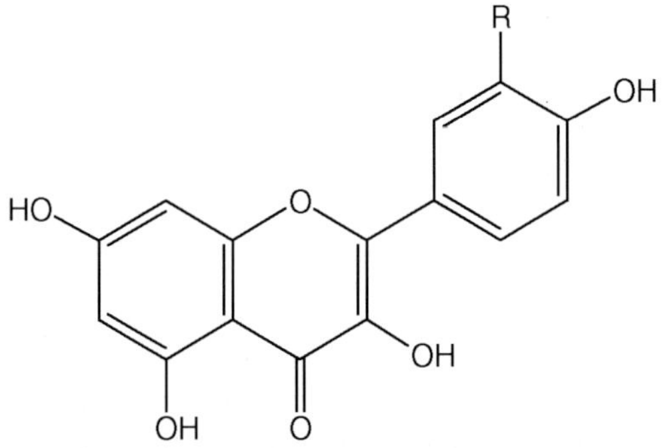

R = H: Kaempferol
R = OH: Quercetin

Flavonols

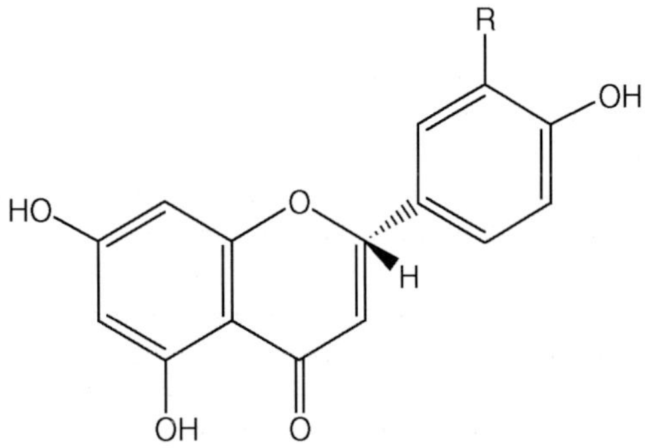

R = H: Naringenin
R = OH: Eriodictyol

Flavonones

surrounding capillaries) and as extenders of vitamin C activity, possibly through improved absorption and protection from oxidation and by partially substituting for some of its biological functions.[78]

Decreased capillary fragility means improved connective tissue tone and a reduced tendency for capillary contents to leak into surrounding tissue. This implies that flavonoids will prevent oedema associated with inflammation and stasis. Such effects from flavonoids are the only benefits which are reasonably well established from clinical trials.

Daflon is a proprietary mixture of micronized flavonoids consisting of 90% diosmin and 10% hesperidin, which is usually administered at a dose of 1000 mg per day. Double-blind, placebo-controlled clinical trials have shown that this flavonoid combination improves venous tone in normal volunteers,[79] enhances microcirculation in patients with venous insufficiency,[80] assists healing of venous ulcers,[81] and relieves symptoms of acute haemorrhoids.[82]

Flavonoids are polyphenolic compounds (they contain several phenolic hydroxyl groups) and some are more so than others. The chemical properties which flow from this feature underlie many of the impressive in vitro pharmacological effects of these compounds. In particular, they are able to complex metal ions, act as antioxidants and bind to proteins such as enzymes and structural proteins (this last feature could also explain the ability of flavonoids to enhance the integrity of connective tissue).

The in vitro antioxidant properties of flavonoids have been the focus of much research in recent years. The ability of flavonoids to complex prooxidant metallic ions such as iron probably augments their antioxidant effects in specific circumstances.[83] Of particular interest is the ability of flavonoids to inhibit macrophage-mediated oxidation of low-density lipoprotein and thereby attenuate atherogenesis.[84] The antioxidant properties of flavonoids could also contribute to observed antiinflammatory and antiplatelet effects[85] and are related not only to their structural characteristics but also to their ability to interact with and penetrate the lipid bilayers of the cell membrane.[86] Flavonoids scavenge the nitric oxide radical,[87] the superoxide anion[88] and singlet oxygen.[89] Like most other antioxidants, flavonoids can also act as prooxidants in particular circumstances.[90]

The following enzyme activities are inhibited to varying degrees by flavonoids in vitro: cyclooxygenase,[91] lipoxygenase,[91] lens aldose reductase,[92] xanthine oxidase,[93] cyclic GMP phosphodiesterase,[94] cyclic AMP phosphodiesterase,[95] angiotensin-converting enzyme,[96] aromatase[97] and thyroid peroxidase.[98] However, more research is needed to determine which of these activities can realistically translate into clinical effects. Since enzyme-inhibiting activity depends on the structure of the flavonoid, some compounds are more likely to be clinically effective than others.

Using isolated cells in vitro, the following activities have been demonstrated for flavonoids: antiviral activity, especially 3-methoxylated flavones,[96] antimicrobial activity,[96] inhibition of histamine release from mast cells,[99] antiplatelet activity,[96] tumour cell cytotoxicity, especially for highly methoxylated flavones,[96] spasmolytic activity[100] and prevention of otosclerosis-like changes in bone.[101] The flavonoid 8-isopentenylnaringenin isolated from the Thai herb *Anaxagorea luzonensis* was found to be an oestrogen agonist with an activity about 10 times greater than genistein.[102] Other flavonoids also bind to oestrogen receptors.[103] Type II oestrogen-binding sites have been identified on normal and tumour cells from various tissues and flavonoids and their metabolites (but not isoflavones) show strong binding to these sites. This has potential for anticancer activity.[104]

Animal experiments (usually using high doses) have demonstrated a number of interesting pharmacological effects for flavonoids. One study found antioxidant effects in vivo for dietary flavonoids (quercetin and catechin) which reduced lipid peroxidation in rats.[105] Flavonoids have also demonstrated hepatoprotective, antiulcer and analgesic activity in vivo.[96] Several flavonoids tested showed antiinflammatory effects in acute and chronic animal models.[106] The favourable effect of quercitrin on experimentally induced diarrhoea was probably related to antiinflammatory effects.[107]

Flavonoids exhibit preventative activity against chemical carcinogens and tumour promotion in animal models.[108,109] Anxiolytic properties have been demonstrated for some flavonoids (chrysin and apigenin) which selectively bind with high affinity to the central benzodiazepine receptor.[110]

The relationship between dietary flavonoid intake and cardiovascular disease has been tested in several epidemiological studies. The Zutphen Study in Holland found that flavonoid intake in elderly men (largely via tea, onions and apples) was significantly inversely associated with mortality and incidence of stroke.[111] A Finnish study also found that people with very low intakes of flavonoids have higher risks of coronary disease[112] but a US study found no significant association.[113]

For more information about the pharmacology of flavonoids, see the monographs on Astragalus (p.273), chamomile (p.319), Ginkgo (p.404), hawthorn (p.439), horsechestnut (p.448) and licorice (p.465). In particular the monographs on Ginkgo and hawthorn extensively review the cardiovascular effects of flavonoids which have not been emphasized in this chapter.

Toxicology

Flavonoid aglycones, but not their glycosides, are mutagenic in various assay systems. Quercetin is probably the most mutagenic (and most widespread) flavonoid. When glycosides are incubated with beta-glucosidase or bacteria possessing this enzyme, they acquire mutagenic properties.[114] The presence of methoxy groups markedly decreases the mutagenicity of the flavonoid.[115] Concerns about the mutagenicity and carcinogenicity of quercetin first arose among Japanese researchers who were searching for the carcinogenic compounds in bracken fern. However, those compounds were later identified to be ptaquilosides. It is therefore interesting to find that both bracken fern and quercetin are co-carcinogens for the oncovirus BPV-4.[116] Dietary quercetin also enhanced pretumorous lesions in a model of rat pancreatic carcinogenesis, indicating promoting and progressing effects,[117] but lacked tumour-promoting effects in a different model.[118] On the other hand flavonoids, including quercetin, have shown antimutagenic effects and are widely considered to be antimutagens.[119,120]

With the initial discovery of the mutagenicity of quercetin and concerns about the carcinogenicity of bracken fern, tests were conducted to determine if quercetin was carcinogenic. While two studies were positive in rats, many other studies (at least nine) in rats, mice and golden hamsters failed to demonstrate carcinogenic activity.[121] This is reassuring since quercetin is the most common flavonoid in human diet. Proposed reasons for the lack of carcinogenicity included poor absorption and rapid microbial degradation (which are in fact the case; see Pharmacokinetics on p.58).

However, the lack of carcinogenicity of massive exposure to quercetin at 10% of diet suggests more active mechanisms might be at work. This has been confirmed by a study which demonstrated the rapid metabolic inactivation of quercetin, catalysed by catechol-O-methyltransferase, to form non-mutagenic methoxy groups on the flavonoid.[121] This could be a major reason for the lack of carcinogenicity of flavonoids in vivo.

TANNINS AND OLIGOMERIC PROCYANIDINS

Tannins are defined as vegetable substances capable of tanning animal hides to produce leather. This is used as a method to preserve the hide and at a molecular level is effected via the crosslinking by the tannins of hide proteins. This definition is prescriptive and powdered hide is still used as a phytochemical test for tannins. Like flavonoids, tannins are polyphenolic compounds which have an affinity for proteins. However, the higher number of phenolic groups and the larger molecular size of tannins mean that they are capable of binding strongly to proteins at several sites and can precipitate them from solution.

The phytochemical classification of tannins can be complex but two main groups are usually recognized: hydrolysable tannins and condensed tannins (procyanidins or proanthocyanidins). Hydrolysable tannins usually consist of a central glucose molecule linked to molecules of gallic acid (gallitannins) or hexahydroxydiphenic acid (ellagitannins). They are readily hydrolysed, hence their name. Ellagitannins are found in cranesbill, oak bark and meadowsweet. Oak bark (*Quercus robur*) also contains condensed tannins.

Unlike hydrolysable tannins, condensed tannins are polymeric flavans which are not readily hydrolysable. They often consist of molecules of catechin and epicatechin joined by carbon-carbon bonds. Hence catechin and epicatechin are referred to as monomers and molecules containing 2–4 monomers are referred to as oligomeric procyanidins (OPC). Protein-binding capacity increases markedly with the degree of polymerization, hence dimers are much less astringent than hexamers. It is, however, difficult to define the point at which OPC end and

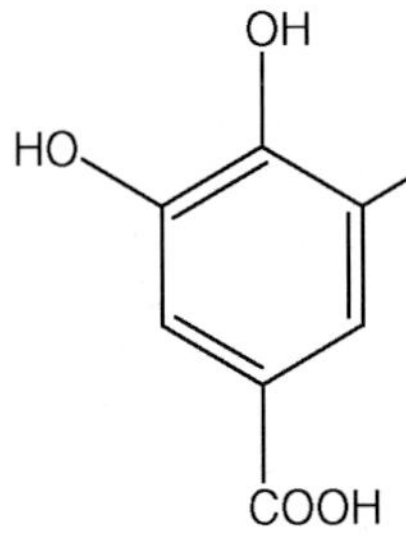

Gallic acid

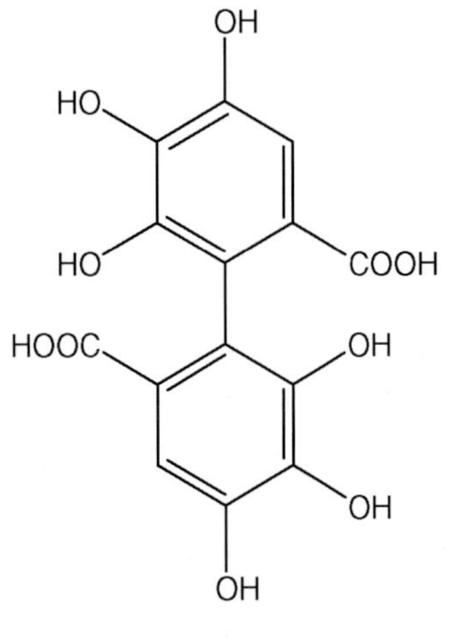

Hexahydroxydiphenic acid

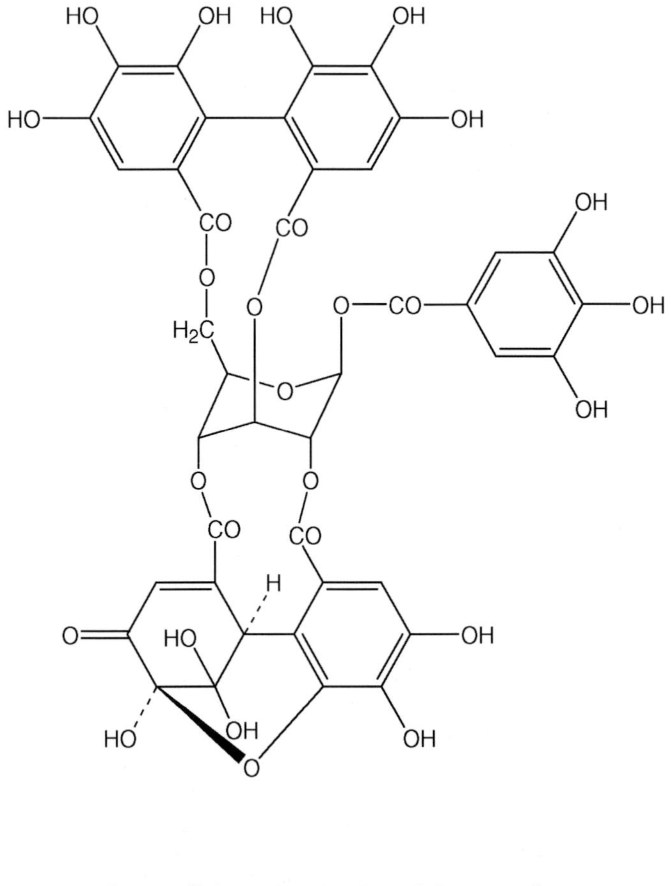

Geraniin - a hydrolysable tannin

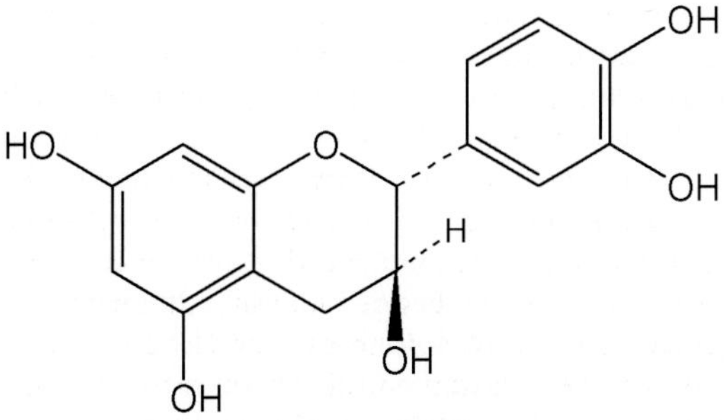

(+)-Catechin

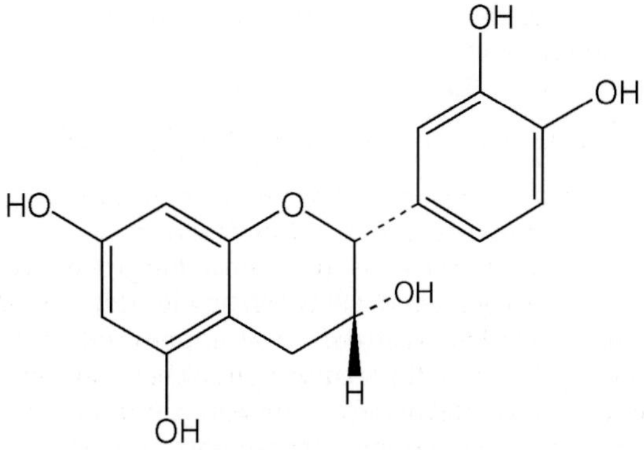

(–)- Epicatechin

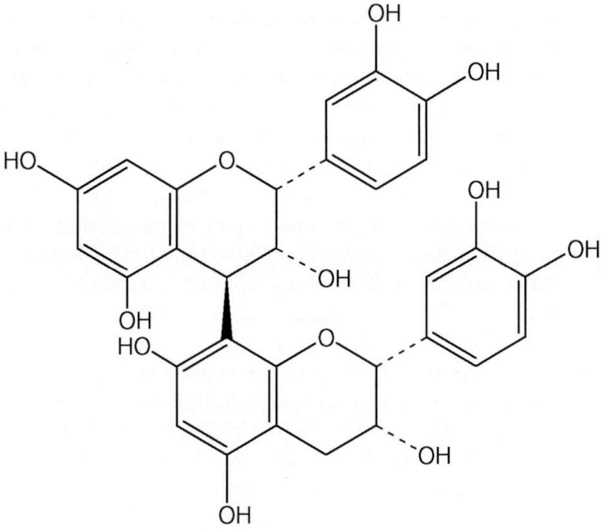

Procyanidin B-2

true tannins start. From a pharmacological perspective, OPC and their monomers behave much like flavonoids (they also resemble them chemically) and they are sometimes classified with them.

Hydrolysable tannins generally decompose slowly when kept in aqueous solution. They may also be hydrolysed by acids or enzymes such as tannase into their component molecules. Condensed tannins are more resistant to decomposition into their monomeric components. However, they are readily oxidized over time as shown by their colour change to purplish pink. These oxidized tannins are responsible for the reddish colour of many barks and roots. Long storage of solutions of condensed tannins (such as tinctures and fluid extracts) induces extensive precipitation of condensate products known as phlobaphenes or phlobatannins. Glycerol was traditionally added to liquid galenicals to decrease this effect. Tannins complex with and precipitate alkaloids and herbal extracts containing tannins should not be mixed with alkaloid-containing extracts.

Pharmacodynamics

When tannins come into contact with mucous membranes, they react with and crosslink proteins in both the mucus and epithelial cells of the mucosa. The mucosa is consequently bound more tightly and rendered less permeable, a process referred to as *astringency*. If this phenomenon is experienced in the mouth, such as when eating an unripe banana, a puckering and drying sensation is experienced. Astringency affords increased protection to the subadjacent layers of the mucosa from microorganisms and irritant chemicals. It also creates an antisecretory effect on the mucous membrane.

Since tannins are large polar molecules, they are poorly absorbed through the skin or gastrointestinal tract. Hence the pharmacological effects of tannins can be largely explained in terms of their local effects on these organs (such as astringency) or effects within the gastrointestinal lumen. However, decomposition products of tannins are absorbed and do exert systemic effects (see Pharmacokinetics section on p.58). The poor bioavailability of tannins is fortunate, since they can be quite toxic if absorbed in large amounts.

One of the most notable effects of tannins in the gut is their dramatic effect on diarrhoea. It can be proposed that the effect of tannins is to produce a protective (if temporary) layer of coagulated protein on the mucosa along the upper levels of the gut wall, so numbing the sensory nerve endings and reducing provocative stimuli to additional peristaltic activity.

Supporting this central astringent activity, tannins will also inhibit the viability of infecting microorganisms, check fluid hypersecretion and neutralize inflammatory proteins. Because of their affinity for free protein, they will concentrate in damaged areas. Condensed tannins were able to bind to and inactivate the hypersecretory activity of cholera toxin.[122]

Tannins in herbs such as meadowsweet were traditionally regarded as beneficial in mild peptic ulceration and inflammation. This application is analogous to the use of the synthetic antiulcer drug known as sulcrafate. Sulcrafate is an astringent aluminium-based compound (aluminium is highly astringent). It is said to selectively bind to exposed proteins at the ulcer base and the barrier thus created protects the ulcer crater from gastric contents. Antiulcer activity has been demonstrated for black tea extract (which is rich in tannins)[123] and for condensed tannins.[124] Ellagic acid suppresses acid secretion.[125]

Tannins also can affect bowel flora composition. For example, tea tannins fed to chicks significantly changed the levels of particular microflora.[126] This may explain why rhubarb and other tannin-containing herbs reduced levels of uraemic toxins in rats with renal failure (perhaps at least in part by inhibition of the bowel flora production of some of these compounds).[127] Whatever the mechanism, tannin-containing containing herbs such as rhubarb are currently used in China to treat renal failure.

Local use of tannins on bleeding surfaces renders a styptic or haemostatic effect due to localized vasoconstriction and possibly an increased rate of coagulation. Since the presence of tannins is widespread in higher plants, this would explain the folk use of so many different plants as 'wound herbs'. An aqueous extract of a tannin-containing herb demonstrated haemostatic activity due to vasoconstriction and the formation of an 'artificial clot' (presumably resulting from a tannin-protein reaction), which tended to produce a mechanical plug to arrest bleeding from small blood vessels.[128] This styptic effect can also be useful for mild internal bleeding.

Topical application of tannins will cause favourable effects on burns, weeping eczema and viral infections. In the early 20th century, tannin sprays were applied to severe burns as preferred therapy. The tannin-protein complex thus formed acted as an artificial semipermeable membrane known as an eschar.[129] This procedure was abandoned because toxic levels of tannic acid (the hydrolysable tannin used) were sometimes absorbed through the damaged skin. Tannic acid damaged epithelial stem cells and caused excessive scar formation. However, the procedure is still practised in China using condensed tannins which are less toxic and kinder to the regenerating epidermis.

One of the notable properties of tannins which has emerged in recent research is their antioxidant effects. This is not surprising, given their polyphenolic nature. Hamamelitannin (from witchhazel) and gallic acid were more active than ascorbic acid in scavenging reactive oxygen species.[130] Oral administration of geraniin was found to lower the level of lipid peroxide in the serum and liver of rats suffering liver injury.[131] Most of the antioxidant research on tannins has focused on green tea polyphenols. As well as impressive in vitro effects, it appears that antioxidant activity can also be achieved in the human body, presumably brought about by absorption of decomposition products (see Pharmacokinetics section on p.58).

As alluded to previously, the many and impressive in vitro effects of tannins may not have clinical relevance because of their poor bioavailability. This is highlighted by a study which postulated that hydrolysable tannins were responsible for the antiprostatic activity of Epilobium species via inhibition of 5-alpha-reductase.[132] Sufficient quantities of almost any tannin will non-specifically inhibit almost any enzyme. Other effects of tannins unlikely to have clinical relevance include antiviral activity (except topically and in the gut lumen),[133] inhibition of elastase,[134] cytotoxic effects,[135] reverse transcriptase inhibition,[131] antimutagenic activity,[131] host-mediated antitumour activity[131] and inhibition of lipoxygenase.[131]

The lower than expected rate of coronary artery disease in France has been termed the French paradox. Several reasons have been proposed for this effect, notably the high consumption of red wine rich in OPC. Independently of this development, a French scientist named Masquelier researched the antioxidant and connective tissue-stabilizing benefits of OPC over many years. This led to the development of two OPC products, one from grape seeds and the other from the bark of the maritime pine (*Pinus pinaster*). These products are prescribed for applications similar to flavonoids and clinical research supports their use for varicose veins, capillary fragility and chronic venous insufficiency.[136] Given the postulated beneficial effects of OPC in heart disease, it should come as no surprise that hawthorn, the most important herb for the heart in modern phytotherapy, is rich in these substances (for more details on the cardiovascular pharmacology of OPC, see the hawthorn monograph on p.439).

Important tannin-containing herbs not already mentioned include agrimony (*Agrimonia eupatorium*), tormentil (*Potentilla erecta*) and bistort (*Polygonum bistorta*). There is also a monograph on witchhazel on p. 590).

Adverse reactions and toxicology

Tannins are found to some extent in many plant medicines. The following comments about adverse reactions refer only to those with significant quantities applied in relatively high doses. It is unlikely that incidental exposure to tannins at low levels has any significant impact. In fact, condensed tannins are found in several commonly consumed foods. In contrast, hydrolysable tannins are rare in foods and this suggests that the long-term therapeutic intake of this group of tannins should be avoided.

High doses of tannins lead to excessive astringency on mucous membranes which has an irritating effect. This probably led to the practice of adding milk to tea whereby the tannins preferentially bind to proteins in the milk rather than the gut wall. However, even adding milk does not prevent the constipation which results from chronic intake of high levels of tannins. For these reasons, high doses of strongly astringent herbs should be used cautiously in highly inflamed or ulcerated conditions of the gastrointestinal tract.

Chronic intake of tannins inhibits digestive enzymes, especially the membrane-bound enzymes of the small intestinal mucosa.[137] Tannins complex metal ions and inhibit their absorption. One study found that as long as tea and iron are consumed separately, iron absorption is not affected.[138] This iron-complexing property of tannins could be exploited in male patients with haemochromatosis, which is now recognized to be a relatively common disorder. Tannins can also react with thiamine and decrease its absorption.[139]

Addition of tannic acid, a hydrolysable tannin, to the barium sulphate mixture used in barium enemas increases the yield and accuracy of the examination. The colonic mucosa stands out clearly and tumour visualization is improved. However, the practice was banned in 1964 by the US FDA.[140] Several deaths caused by acute hepatotoxicity, the majority in children, were attributed to this practice.[141] In these cases quantities of tannic acid sufficient to cause massive liver damage were absorbed directly into the bloodstream from the colon. This effect is highly unlikely to follow from use of tannin-containing herbs. Nonetheless, some unexplained cases of herbal hepatotoxicity have been recorded. It is therefore prudent to avoid the use of high doses of highly astringent herbs in patients with damaged gastrointestinal tracts, other than in the circumstances outlined above.

Tannins are carcinogenic when injected subcutaneously[142] and herbal teas containing tannins have been implicated in the possible development of oesophageal cancers.[143] While these associations probably have little relevance to phytotherapy, they do suggest caution with the long-term oral and topical use (on damaged skin) of tannin-containing herbs.

RESINS

Resins are sticky, water-insoluble substances often exuded by the plant. The term is used in several contexts. When certain plants are damaged, either by incision or naturally due to the action of animals or the environment, they secrete a viscous fluid which soon hardens. This probably serves as protection. The resultant exudate is an amorphous, complex mixture of chemicals which softens on heating. Such resins are often associated with essential oils (oleoresins), with gums (gum resins) or with oil and gum (oleo-gum resins). Their resin components, which mainly comprise diterpenes known as resin acids, resin alcohols and resin phenols, are soluble in alcohol and ether but are insoluble in water and hexane.

In another context, the term 'resin' (or occasionally 'resinoid') means that part of the plant which is soluble in ether or alcohol, as in kava resin, guaiacum resin (also prepared by burning the heartwood) and jalap. These resins are chemically diverse and can contain resin acids, pyrones, lignans, esters and glycosides among others. On microscopic examination of the tissues of these plants, secretion cells with resinous contents are sometimes visible.

Myrrh (*Commiphora molmol*) is an oleo-gum resin with astringent and antimicrobial properties. The former quality is probably entirely due to the resin and the latter is a combined effect from the resin and the essential oil. Tincture of myrrh is a potent antiseptic in the mouth and throat. There is a modern tradition that one of its effects is to provoke a local leucocytosis, to effectively stimulate defensive white blood cell responses and so involve the body in eliminating local infections. Clinical experience of long-standing improvement in recurrent throat and gum disease, for example, lends support to this view.

Resins have also been applied to inflammatory conditions of the upper digestive tract with some benefit. This probably reflects on their astringent property. The oleoresin mastic (*Pistacia lentiscus* var. chia) is traditionally used for the relief of dyspepsia and peptic ulcers.[144] Mastic demonstrated a duodenal ulcer

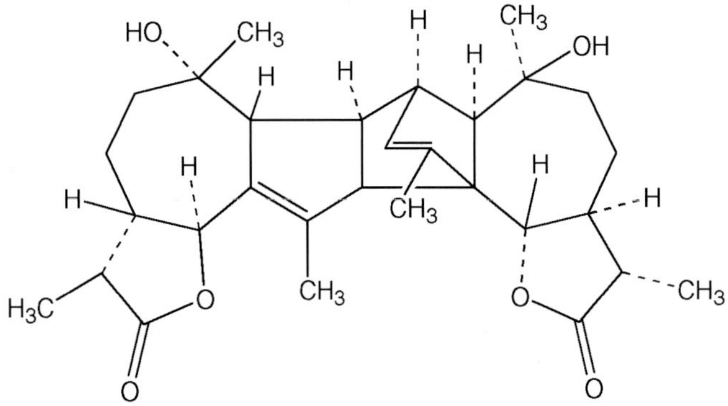

Absinthin

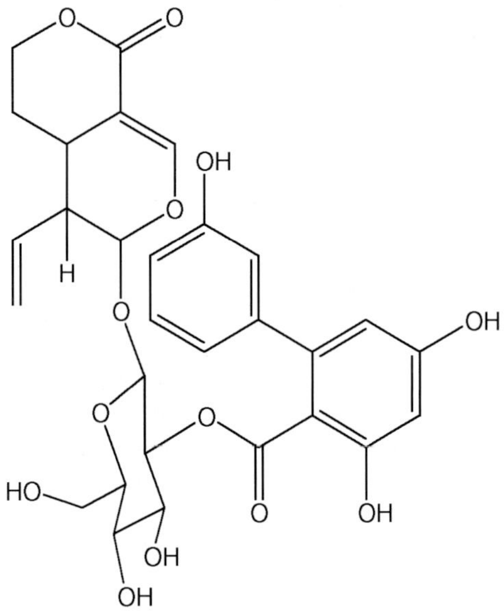

Amarogentin

healing effect at 1 g per day in a double-blind, placebo-controlled clinical trial.[144] Cytoprotective and mild antisecretory effects were demonstrated in a rat model of ulceration, consistent with astringent activity.[145]

Important resin-containing herbs not already mentioned include propolis (not actually a herb but collected by bees from resinous plants), Grindelia, Calendula, guggul, Boswellia, juniper and the various balsams.

Resins are contact allergens which can cause oral ulceration and contact dermatitis.[146]

BITTERS

Bitters are substances capable of strongly stimulating the bitter receptors in the taste buds at the back of the tongue. The taste stimulus is triggered by an intramolecular bonding with these receptors. Each taste bud contains approximately 20–30 sensory cells whose microvilli extend to the bud opening. The taste receptors lie in the membrane of these microvilli and consist of glycoproteins.

Given that bitters are defined physiologically, it might be expected that bitter compounds come from a number of different phytochemical classes. This is certainly the case; monoterpenes, sesquiterpenes, diterpenes, flavonoids and triterpenes can exhibit bitter properties. However, the most notable bitter compounds are the monoterpene secoiridoid glycosides of gentian (particularly amarogentin), centaury and bogbean, and the sesquiterpene lactone dimers (such as absinthin) of wormwood. These compounds are among the most bitter substances known.

Many cultures recognize the value of bitter substances in promoting digestive function and general health. In Holland, older people would celebrate the bitter hour in the early evening when they would partake of bitter food and drink to support their fading digestive powers. In India, it is said that those with liver problems seek bitter-tasting substances. In Africa the medicinal value of bitter herbs, particularly as digestive stimulants, is commonly recognized in traditional medical systems.[147] Bitter drinks taken before meals are still called aperitifs.

In the early 20th century it was still widely accepted in medical and scientific circles that bitters promoted digestion. Even Pavlov was said to have acknowledged this connection.[148] However, this was a time when such assumptions were being subjected to scientific scrutiny. In 1915 the American physiologist Carlson and co-workers published a study entitled 'The Supposed Action of the Bitter Tonics on the Secretion of Gastric Juice in Man and Dog'.[148] The group found that bitters, applied either to the mouth or directly to the stomach, produced no change in the acidity and pepsin concentration of the gastric juice produced prior to food actually being in contact with the stomach. Despite the fact that this study had a number of methodological flaws, notably that gastric secretions were not tested under the stimulus of actual contact with food, it was largely interpreted as discrediting the concept of bitters as digestive stimulants.

However, work published also in 1915 by Moorhead, a colleague of Carlson, demonstrated a radically different activity profile for bitters.[149] Moorhead found that a tincture of the herb gentian (*Gentiana lutea*) given by mouth or directly in the stomach of cachectic dogs caused a marked increase in appetite. Also, only when gentian was given by mouth (i.e. tasted) did it cause a marked increase in gastric secretion and its acid and pepsin content. This effect only occurred after normal feeding. All the above effects were absent in normal animals.[149]

The conclusions which could be drawn from this early research are several.

- Bitters increase appetite only if a cachectic, malnourished or debilitated state exists in the body.
- Similarly, bitters increase digestive power mainly when it is below optimum, as in a state of cachexia.
- Experiments with bitters should involve actual feeding, that is, the presence of food in the stomach is important for their activity.
- At normal doses, bitters act in the mouth, that is, they must be tasted.

From this research the mode of action of bitters can be postulated. Bitters applied to the mouth (tasted) before a meal have a priming effect on upper digestive function. This effect is most marked in states where digestion is below optimum, where a positive effect on appetite is also observed. This increase in upper digestive function is probably mediated by a nerve reflex from the bitter taste buds and involves an increase in vagal stimulation. From physiology we know that vagal stimulation causes:

- an increase in gastric acid secretion;
- a transient rise in gastrin;
- an increase in pepsin secretion;
- a slight increase in gallbladder motility;
- a priming of the pancreas.

Therefore bitters could have a promoting effect on all components of upper digestive function, namely the stomach, liver and pancreas. Why does this reflex exist? It may have developed as a protective mechanism since many poisonous substances taste bitter.

Modern research supports this activity profile for bitters. Oral doses of liquid preparations of gentian and wormwood (*Artemisia absinthium*) were tested in human subjects 5 minutes before a meal.[150] Both bitter tonics stimulated gastric secretion. Gentian also stimulated bile release from the gallbladder and both herbs increased bile production by the liver. Another study found that oral doses of liquid wormwood caused a dramatic increase in duodenal levels of pancreatic enzymes and bile.[151] Studies have also shown that bitters increase the secretion of saliva. A lemon wedge saturated with Angostura bitters was also found to cure hiccups in 88% of subjects in an open trial.[152]

Some bitter herbs may also have a direct effect on the stomach. Wolf and Mack carried out an excellent study on the action of various bitters on the stomach of their famous patient, Tom, who had an occluded oesophagus and a gastric fistula.[153] Bitters were administered by mouth and swallowed into the blind oesophagus; the resulting salivary volume and gastric secretion were compared with direct administration into the stomach. In the 96 experiments conducted it was found that there was considerable variation in the effect of the bitters. Golden seal (*Hydrastis canadensis*) was the most active herb and gentian was virtually inactive at the levels tested. The increase in salivation when given orally was usually comparable with the increase in gastric secretion after direct introduction into the stomach. The alcoholic content of the bitters was shown to evoke no response. It was concluded that bitters had a direct effect on the stomach, since no significant effect was observed in the stomach following oral administration. These results therefore contrast with the work of Moorhead but Tom's digestion function was probably normal (despite his injury) and the experimental design did not include a test meal, a common flaw in some of the early research.

A recent publication also suggests that bitters exert a direct effect in the stomach.[154] When isolated stomach cells were exposed to different levels of an extract of gentian root, a concentration-dependent rise in gastric acid production was observed. No stimulatory effect was exerted by globe artichoke extract (*Cynara scolymus*). Significant effects for gentian extract were observed at concentrations of 10–100 μg/ml. This concentration range can be readily achieved by normal doses of gentian. The author suggests that his results can explain why encapsulated gentian extracts also show therapeutic effects and he downplays the importance of the reflex effect to one of 'supportive importance only'. However, the above findings must be verified in clinical studies before such a reappraisal of the activity of bitters.

Some preliminary support for this idea comes from a recent multicentre uncontrolled study of gentian capsules involving 205 patients.[155] Patients took on average about five capsules per day containing 120 mg of a 5:1 dry extract of gentian root to achieve rapid and dramatic relief of symptoms which included constipation, flatulence, appetite loss, vomiting, heartburn, abdominal pain and nausea.

Healthy upper digestive function is important for maintaining health and preventing disease. Gastric secretion declines with age[156] and a significant percentage of people aged 65 years or older have abnormally low gastric acidity.[157] Low acidity can lead to poor nutrient absorption and abnormal bowel flora. Patients with reduced gastric secretion are more susceptible to bacterial and parasitic enteric infections.[158] The contribution of poor upper digestive function to the chronicity of intestinal dysbiosis is often overlooked by therapists.

Early studies associated low gastric acidity with a number of chronic diseases such as rosacea, gallbladder disease, eczema and asthma and this has been reflected in recent writings.[159] The experimental method used in these early studies usually measured gastric pH following a test meal. This is now considered to be an invalid way to investigate a pathological hydrochloric acid deficiency (hypochlorhydria). Instead, a potent gastric cell stimulus such as pentagastrin is currently preferred to establish the diagnosis of hypochlorhydria.

The early studies were probably measuring the physiological response of the stomach to food rather than a pathological absence or deficiency of the secretory apparatus. If this is the case, then the observation is still valid that a poor physiological response to food may be associated with certain chronic diseases. The use of bitters is particularly relevant in this context, since they could act via a vagal reflex, which is the normal physiological way that the upper digestive tract is primed for food.

As early as 1698 Floyer in his Treatise of the Asthma reflected that:

> Some writers, as Sylvius and Etmuller, have observed the hypochondriac symptoms in the stomach, and conclude the asthma is a hypochondriacal flatus, and wants digestives … It is commonly observed that fulness of diet, and all debauches render the fits most severe, and a temperate diet makes the fits more easy … This defect of digestion and mucilaginous slime in the stomach are very obvious and observed by writers, and were supposed the immediate cause of the asthma.

A modern study found that allergic asthma was associated with a reduction in histamine-stimulated peak acid output from the gastric mucosa (about 60% of normal). There is therefore a depression of gastric H_2-histamine receptor function in asthma.[160]

Diabetics respond well to bitters and some herbalists believe they can assist in normalizing blood sugar levels in both reactive hypoglycaemia and diabetes. A lack of insulin could impair the vagal stimulation of gastric acid secretion[161] and oral doses of a bitter herb lowered blood sugar in healthy rats.[162] Long-standing diabetics may have impaired upper digestive function secondary to vagal neuropathy.[163]

It has even been found that in some cases patients' responses to herbal medicines depend on their upper digestive function.[164] A Japanese study found that the antioxidant properties of a herbal product could be increased by fermentation. It was found that the brewing process degraded high molecular weight polymers to smaller molecules which were more active. The unfermented herbal product was tried on patients with autoimmune diseases. Some responded to the product, others did not. Those who responded had a greater capacity to produce the small antioxidant molecules in their gastric secretions, which was correlated with their acid and pepsin secretion. It was concluded that one of the factors determining the patients' response was the ability of their digestive system to produce low molecular weight compounds from the natural polymers.

Herbalists consider that bitters have a tonic effect on the body and the term 'bitter tonic' is often used. In addition to their use for poor upper digestive function, low appetite and hypochlorhydria and its consequences, bitters are used to treat anaemia. Bitters are valuable for food allergies, since poorly digested proteins and other compounds probably contribute to this condition. Herbalists also believe that bitters stimulate immune function and a patient who is pale, lethargic and prone to infections is a prime candidate for bitters.

The famous herbalist Dr Weiss stressed that the action of bitters was most pronounced after continued use (probably because it is a conditioned reflex).[165] He described how a physician in Vienna noted that dyspeptic patients liked wormwood tea and kept asking for it, despite the taste. Another Viennese paediatrician considered bitters to be an excellent remedy for anorexic children. Weiss claimed that bitters neutralize the negative influence of higher mental functions on digestion, which usually results from chronic stress. He claimed that bitters had a toning effect on the colon when applied over a long period.

Bitters are contraindicated in states of hyperacidity, especially duodenal ulcers. Tasted bitters may actually be beneficial in gastric ulcers, since this condition is often associated with atrophic gastritis. Tasted bitters may also help oesophageal reflux because they could improve the tone of the oesophageal sphincter. However, they should be used with caution here.

The main bitter herbs used in Western herbal medicine are gentian and wormwood. For a reflex effect, bitters do not usually have to be given in high doses. Enough to promote a strong taste of bitterness is usually sufficient. This is typically 5–10 drops of the 1:5 tinctures of the above herbs in about 20 ml of water. (Bitters are one exception where drop doses are appropriate.) Since bitters have a priming effect on upper digestive function and work by a visceral reflex (which is slow) they are best taken about 15 minutes before meals. Also bitters work best if they are sipped slowly, to prolong the stimulation of the reflex. This can be difficult for some people but will give optimum results.

For a direct effect on the gastric mucosa, higher doses need to be used. About 300–600 mg of gentian root before meals would be an appropriate dose. Be careful of such high doses of gentian taken in liquid form, since they can cause nausea in some people.

One question which has vexed herbalists is whether the taste of bitters given in liquid form can be masked and yet their reflex activity still be preserved. This is probably the case, since masking agents will change the conscious perception of bitterness but the bitter taste buds will still be stimulated.

A number of papers have been published on the subject of supertasters.[166] Supertasters perceive the greatest bitterness and sweetness from many stimuli as well as the greatest oral burn from alcohol and capsaicin (from Capsicum species). This is an inherited ability produced by a dominant allele. Women are more likely than men to be supertasters. This phenomenon needs to be kept in mind because some patients may be very sensitive to the taste (and possibly effects) of bitter and other strong-tasting herbs. These patients are also more likely to experience nausea if the dose of bitters used is too high.

PUNGENT CONSTITUENTS

Like bitters, pungency is a physiological classification rather than a phytochemical one. The three most commonly used hot spices are the cayenne pepper (capsicum), the black pepper and ginger and whilst their pungent components (respectively capsaicin, piperine and the gingerols) are chemically distinct, it has been suggested that they act upon a common group of nerve cell receptors: the postulated vanilloid receptors.[167] Capsaicin and piperine are alkaloids based on homovanillic acid (hence vanilloid receptor), whereas the gingerols are substituted alkylphenols.

Pharmacodynamics

Capsaicin has been the most commonly studied of the pungent compounds. C-fibre sensory neurons, which release inflammatory neuropeptides such as substance P, mediate a wide variety of responses including neurogenic inflammation, thermoregulation and chemical-initiated pain. Capsaicin functions to activate and then, at higher doses and over time, desensitize this class of neurons. This latter response, by a process known as *tachyphylaxis*, provides the basis for the current therapeutic interest in capsaicin. Capsaicin is postulated to stimulate C-fibres by interacting with vanilloid receptors.[168] The intense sensation of pain and heat which is experienced after eating a hot curry is testimony to this C-fibre activation. But as experienced curry eaters will testify, they can tolerate hotter and hotter food over time due to tachyphylaxis.

Although the pain and burning from consumption of cayenne or capsaicin can be disturbing, no actual harm results from its consumption. In effect, the specific action on nervous system receptors creates an illusion of pain and burning. Tissue damage is not concurrent with these sensations. This contrasts strongly with the mustard oils, which are highly corrosive and produce sensations of pain and burning in association with actual tissue damage. On the other hand, capsaicin is a pronounced irritant, as evidenced by the incapacitating effect of capsicum sprays. Sometimes ingestion of cayenne does seem to produce lingering sensations of discomfort and this probably highlights the role of substance P in neurogenic (nervous system-mediated) inflammation. Once the process of neurogenic inflammation has been triggered, it can become self-perpetuating. Neurogenic inflammation has been implicated in a number of chronic functional disorders of uncertain aetiology such as interstitial cystitis and irritable bowel syndrome.

The desensitization of C-fibres has value for pain relief in a number of chronically painful disorders. Controlled clinical trials of topical use of capsaicin cream has demonstrated symptom relief in osteoarthritis,[169] neuropathy[170] and postherpetic neuralgia.[171] Topical capsaicin is effective for painful skin disorders such as psoriasis and pruritis and may be useful for neural dysfunction in the form of cluster headaches and phantom limb pain.[172,173] Vasomotor rhinitis may also be susceptible to topical capsaicin.[174]

The higher fibrinolytic activity observed in Thai people has been attributed to daily intake of cayenne pepper.[175] Capsicum also increases gastric acid output.[176] Since gastric acid is a natural defence against gastrointestinal pathogens, it can be speculated that

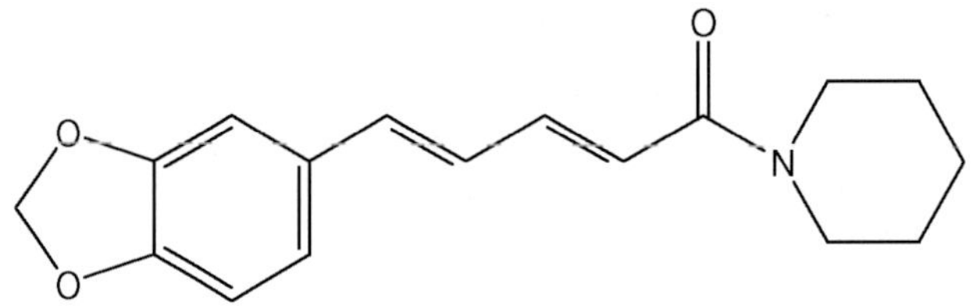

Piperine

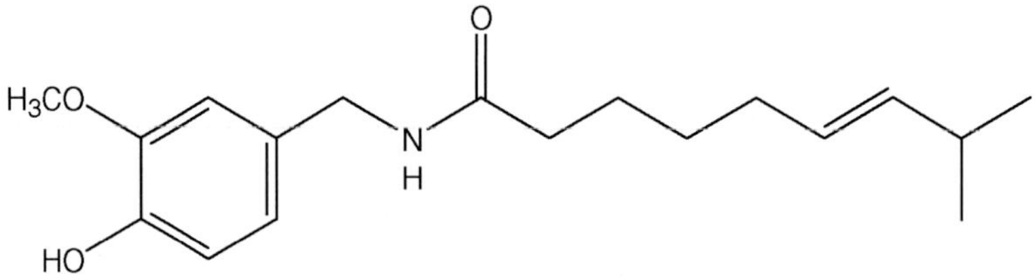

***trans*-Capsaicin**

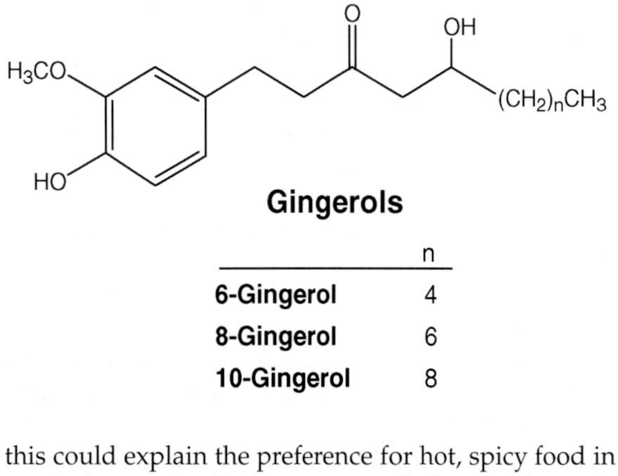

H_3CO, HO, O, OH, $(CH_2)_nCH_3$

Gingerols

	n
6-Gingerol	4
8-Gingerol	6
10-Gingerol	8

this could explain the preference for hot, spicy food in tropical countries. In the rat stomach there is clear evidence that capsaicin-sensitive sensory nerves are involved in a local defence mechanism against gastric ulcer. However, excessive capsaicin exposure caused tachyphylaxis and impaired this defensive mechanism.[177] Perhaps the maxim of 'too much of a good thing' applies here.

Like capsaicin, piperine has attracted research interest but for quite different reasons. Attention has focused on the capacity of piperine to enhance the bioavailability of other agents. These include aflatoxin B1 in rats[178] and propanol, theophylline,[179] curcumin,[180] vasicine and spartenine in humans.[181] While there is good evidence that piperine inhibits drug metabolism by the intestine and liver,[182] other possibilities include increased permeability of intestinal cells[183] and even complexation with drugs.[184]

In traditional Chinese medicine, a mixture of radish and pepper is used to treat epilepsy. Piperine and some synthetic derivatives have been shown to be anticonvulsant agents that antagonize convulsions induced by physical and chemical methods.[185] Antiepilepsirine, one of the derivatives of piperine, is widely used as an antiepileptic drug in China.

Hot spices are used around the world for their general warming effects on the body, in modern terms stimulating circulatory activity. A mechanism for this universal experience is suggested. In a study that compared the effects of various pungent agents, an increase in catecholamine secretion, especially adrenaline, from the adrenal medulla was observed. Capsaicin was most active but piperine and zingerone (from ginger) also showed activity, although allylisothiocyanate (from mustard) and diallyldisulphide (from garlic) did not have this effect. The effective principles were readily transported from the gut around the body.[186] Capsaicin is known to increase energy expenditure in the body and boost basal metabolic rate, which has implications for its use in weight control.[187]

The above findings hark back to the use of cayenne promoted by Samuel Thomson, who regarded it as a life-promoting heating herb and a general metabolic stimulant. The physiomedicalists extended this concept and proposed that cayenne administered in conjunction with another herb would augment the particular stimulatory activity of that herb. Given what we now know about the bioavailability effects of piperine (and therefore possibly capsaicin), this apparently arcane dictum may have a rational basis.

A discussion of the pharmacology of the gingerols is included in the ginger monograph (see p.394).

Toxicology

Numerous investigations have been conducted to determine the potential mutagenic and carcinogenic activity of capsaicin and cayenne but findings are contradictory.[188] Results from recent studies indicate that capsaicin also demonstrates chemoprotective activity against some chemical carcinogens and mutagens.[189] Piperine appears to lack mutagenic activity.[190]

SAPONINS

Phytochemistry

Saponins are phytochemicals which produce a foam when dissolved in water. Their name derives from the same root as the word soap (Latin *sapo* = soap). Like soaps or detergents, saponins are large molecules which contain a water-loving (*hydrophilic*) part at one end, separated from a fat-loving (*lipophilic* or *hydrophobic*) part at the other. In aqueous solution, the saponin molecules align themselves vertically on the surface with their hydrophobic ends oriented away from the water. This has the effect of reducing the surface tension of the water, causing it to foam. For this reason saponins are classified as surface-active agents. Similar to other surface-active agents, saponin molecules can align to form a spherical configuration in water, creating a micelle. Micelles have a lipophilic centre and this creation of a fat-loving compartment explains why detergents can dissolve grease and oils.

Saponins are glycosides (the sugar part comprises the hydrophilic end). Two classes are recognized, based on the structure of their aglycone or sapogenin: steroidal saponins, which contain the characteristic four-ringed steroid nucleus, and triterpenoid saponins, which have a five-ringed structure. Both of these have a glycosidal linkage usually at carbon 3 and have a common biosynthetic origin via the mevalonic acid pathway. Steroidal saponins are mainly found in the monocotyledons and triterpenoid saponins are by far the most common. There are some unusual classifications; for example, the ginsenosides in ginseng are grouped with the triterpenoid saponins, even though they exhibit a steroidal structure. Steroidal saponins typically contain extra furan and pyran heterocyclic rings, which is not a feature of ginsenosides. (Furans and pyrans are respectively five- and six-membered rings containing oxygen.)

Saponins are consumed in many common foods and beverages including oats, spinach, asparagus, soya beans and other legumes, peanuts, tea and beer.

Pharmacodynamics

The pharmacological events which follow the ingestion of saponins can be broadly classified into two categories: the general actions which follow from their detergent-like properties and are determined by the interaction of intact saponins, and those specific actions which follow after the saponin (or more usually the sapogenin) is absorbed into the bloodstream. This discussion will concentrate on the general pharmacodynamic actions of saponins but will also provide a context for their specific activities. The antiinflammatory, tonic, adaptogenic, aldosterone-like and mucoprotective properties (among others) of specific saponins are examined in detail in the monographs on Astragalus (p.273), black cohosh (p.303), Bupleurum (p.313), ginseng (p.418), Horsechestnut (p.448), licorice (p.465), poke root (p.515) and Withania (p.595).

Saponins are capable of destroying red blood cells (RBCs) by dissolving their membranes, a process known as *haemolysis*, releasing free haemoglobin into the bloodstream. Red blood cells are particularly susceptible to this form of chemical attack because they have no nucleus and therefore cannot effect membrane repair. Haemolysis explains why saponins are much more toxic when given by injection than when they are administered orally. The toxic dose of an injected saponin occurs when sufficient haemoglobin is released to cause renal failure (haemoglobin is damaging to the delicate membranes of the glomerulus). After oral intake much of the saponin is not absorbed or is slowly and partially absorbed as the aglycone. The kidneys are thereby spared the sudden influx of haemoglobin. For a long time this feature of saponin toxicity was interpreted by many pharmacologists as an indication that saponins were largely inert after oral doses. While it is true that saponins and even their sapogenins are generally not well absorbed from the gut, there can be no doubt that they can exert significant pharmacological activity after ingestion (for example, licorice side effects).

A common misconception is that the haemolytic activity of saponins is related to their detergent-like characteristics. However, as early as the 1960s this was shown to be false. The mechanism of saponin-induced haemolysis was investigated by extracting the active haemolysing factor from ghost cells of

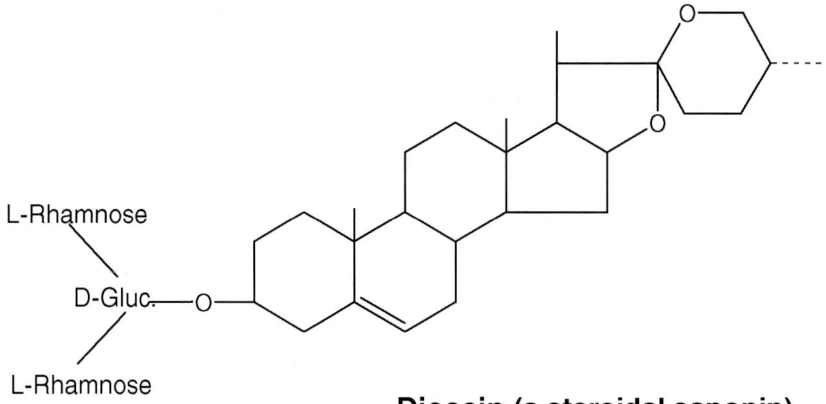

Dioscin (a steroidal saponin)

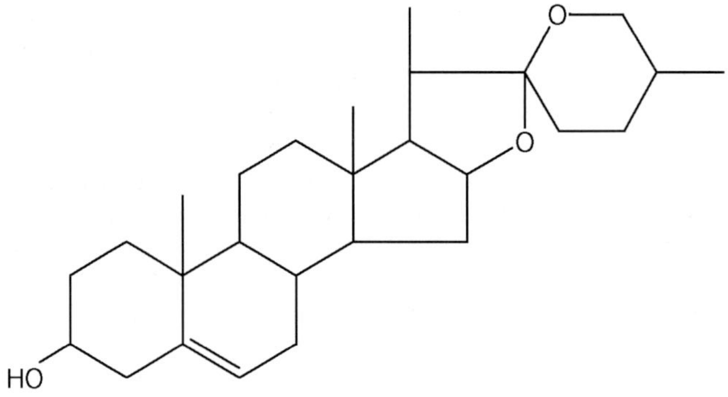

Diosgenin (a steroidal sapogenin)

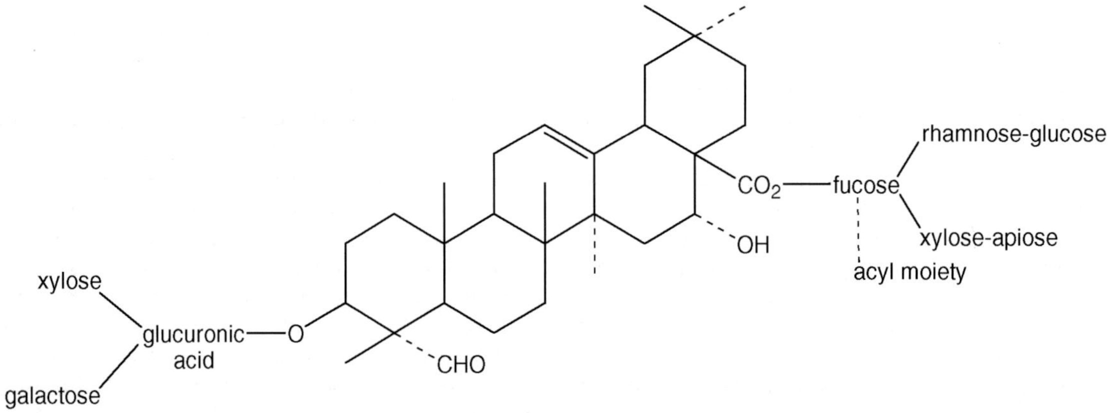

Component of quillaia saponin (a triterpenoid saponin)

saponin-haemolysed blood. The fact that only the corresponding aglycones could be extracted shows that hydrolysis of the glycosidic bond precedes haemolysis (red blood cell membranes possess a beta-glucosidase). The lack of haemolytic activity of a saponin was either due to the fact that it could not be hydrolysed by the beta-glucosidase or that it could not adsorb onto the RBC membrane.[191] This is further supported by the observation that some sapogenins are also quite haemolytic (for example, glycyrrhetinic acid is actually more haemolytic than glycyrrhizin)[191] and that haemolysis by saponins is inhibited by aldonolactones, which are glycosidase inhibitors.[192]

Saponins are more or less irritant to gastrointestinal mucous membranes (whether this is related to their detergent or haemolytic properties is not understood). This irritant property creates an acrid sensation in the throat when a saponin-containing herb is chewed. One effect, like the emetics, may be by upper gastrointestinal irritation to induce a reflex expectoration. Certainly many of the traditional expectorant herbs such as soap bark, senega, primrose root and ivy leaf are rich in acrid saponins. This reflex expectorant effect, and its relationship to emesis, has been demonstrated in animal models.[193] Presumably it is mediated via the vagus nerve.

The detergent effect of saponins helps to increase the solubility of lipophilic molecules via micelle formation. One example which illustrates this phenomenon is the kava lactones. These compounds are quite insoluble in water, yet water can readily extract a percentage of lactones from kava root, which also contains a significant amount of saponins. Moreover, the bioavailability of kavain from a kava matrix is much greater than for the pure compound (see the kava monograph on p.456).

Early research suggested that the incorporation of saponins into the cell membrane probably forms a structure that is more permeable than the original membrane.[194] Saponins readily increase the permeability of the mammalian small intestine in vitro, leading to the increased uptake of otherwise poorly permeable substances and a loss of normal function.[195] The disruptive effect of saponins on the architecture of the cell membrane could lead to impaired absorption of smaller nutrient molecules which are otherwise rapidly absorbed. This appears to be the case for glucose and ethanol, based on in vitro models.[196,197] Tablets containing an extract of the Ayurvedic herb *Gymnema sylvestre* are sold in Japan as a weight loss agent, which is attributed to reduced glucose absorption.

Sapogenins, both steroidal and triterpenoid, resemble cholesterol in their structure and may have a profound effect on cholesterol metabolism in the liver. Diosgenin is well studied in this regard. It interferes with the absorption of cholesterol of both dietary and endogenous origin; such interference is accompanied by increased rates of hepatic and intestinal cholesterol synthesis. Diosgenin also markedly enhanced cholesterol secretion into bile which, in conjunction with the unabsorbed cholesterol, resulted in increased faecal excretion of cholesterol (neutral sterols) without affecting excretion of bile acids.[198] Higher levels of ingestion of saponins or sapogenins leads to cholestasis and jaundice associated with the presence of cholesterol-like crystals in hepatocytes. In grazing animals this can result in photosensitivity due to the photosensitizing effect of high plasma levels of chlorophyll metabolites (see Toxicology on p. 46).

It is well established that saponin intake lowers plasma cholesterol levels in animal models.[199] Various mechanisms have been put forward such as increased faecal excretion of bile salts[199] and loss of cholesterol via exfoliated mucosal cells[195] but the mechanism suggested by the above research on diosgenin seems most likely.[198] In this context it is pertinent to note that diosgenin (a sapogenin) inhibits cholesterol absorption, suggesting that the mechanism behind this phenomenon might have more to do with the haemolytic or steroid-like nature of the saponins rather than their detergent properties. As an interesting footnote, it has been suggested that the Masai, who consume 2000 mg of cholesterol per day yet maintain very low blood levels, might achieve this feat by their high consumption of saponins from both foods and medicines.[200]

Saponins may have beneficial effects on bowel flora; yucca saponins are added to commercial piggery feeds to suppress ammonia production. As testimony to the fact that a percentage of saponins pass through the digestive tract unabsorbed, the product brochures maintain that the faecal material is easier to hose down because of the detergent action of the saponins.

Saponins are very gentle detergents which can be used to wash the hair and skin in conditions such as acne without causing a rebound increase in sebum production. Decoctions of soapwort have been used to wash and restore ancient fabrics in stately homes; modern soaps are too harsh and disintegrate the fabrics.

One of the most interesting effects of saponins (or sapogenins) which follows from their ingestion is their capacity to interact with and influence steroid hormone metabolism. Much of this is covered in the monographs but some of the principles behind this are worth highlighting here. It is only in the last few years that the role of enzymes that metabolize steroids in regulating the actions of these hormones has been appreciated. For example, 11-beta-hydroxysteroid dehydrogenase regulates glucocorticoid action by catalysing the interconversion of hydrocortisone (cortisol) and cortisone, an inactive steroid. In the kidney, hydrocortisone is oxidized to cortisone by this enzyme, a reaction that prevents circulating hydrocortisone from occupying kidney mineralocorticoid receptors and stimulating a mineralocorticoid response. Aldosterone is inert to 11-beta-hydroxysteroid dehydrogenase and can regulate mineralocorticoid responsive genes in the kidney. Inhibition of the enzyme in the kidney allows hydrocortisone to exert an additional aldosterone-like effect. This is exactly what licorice does.[2]

An important consequence of this mechanism for regulating hormone action is that compounds that inhibit these enzymes will appear to be acting as hormones (or antihormones). Thus the active sapogenin from licorice appears to behave like aldosterone, even though it has no affinity at all for mineralocorticoid receptors. Similar examples need to be better understood. For example, the antiinflammatory effect of escin from horsechestnut is abolished in the absence of steroid hormones (see p.451).

The influence of steroidal saponins on oestrogen metabolism may follow similar lines but perhaps with some noteworthy differences. This is illustrated by research on *Tribulus terrestris*. Saponins from Tribulus appear to increase FSH in women, which in turn increases levels of oestradiol.[201] They may do this by binding with, but only weakly stimulating, hypothalamic oestrogen receptors, which are part of the negative feedback mechanism of oestrogen control. The weak stimulus (as opposed to oestrogen) leads the body to interpret that oestrogen levels are lower than they really are and it subsequently increases production. In the postmenopausal woman, herbs such as tribulus, wild yam (*Dioscorea villosa*) and false unicorn (*Chamaelirium luteum*) appear to alleviate symptoms of oestrogen withdrawal. It is possible that a binding of plant steroids to vacant receptors in the hypothalamus (in this low-oestrogen situation) is sufficient to convince the body that more oestrogen is present in the bloodstream than actually is.

Claims have arisen in the popular literature that the female body can manufacture progesterone from diosgenin, particularly if a wild yam cream is applied to the skin. This is despite the fact that wild yam contains dioscin, not diosgenin, and there is no information about the dermal absorption of these compounds. Furthermore, no evidence exists for mammalian enzymes which are capable of effecting what is a difficult chemical conversion. The evidence that does exist strongly disputes the possibility of this conversion.[202] The above discussion should demonstrate that the interaction of saponins with steroid hormones is far more subtle than this. In fact, diosgenin appears to have oestrogenic properties in mice and lacks progesteronic effects.[203]

In addition to this already impressive array of diverse activities for saponins, further effects have been demonstrated using in vitro models. However, the results of these studies need to be interpreted with caution since in the majority of cases saponins will not be absorbed in sufficient quantities to manifest these effects systemically (and the sapogenins do not appear to share these properties). These findings may have relevance to the topical activity of saponins and effects in the gut lumen. They include antiviral activity,[204] antifungal activity[205] and cytotoxicity.[206]

Adverse reactions and toxicology

Saponins are gastrointestinal irritants. In milder examples this can lead to oesophageal reflux in sensitive or overweight patients which can be remedied by using enteric-coated preparations or by taking the saponin-containing herbs during a meal. In more severe examples, such as with poke root, this irritation can lead to acute vomiting and diarrhoea. If the irritation is sufficiently prolonged, erosion of the gastrointestinal mucosa can occur, resulting in substantial absorption of saponins into the bloodstream with the expected toxic sequelae. This is probably the mechanism via which acute oral doses of saponins cause death in humans.

Saponins are toxic to fish and other cold-blooded animals and have been used to kill snails which harbour the bilharzia parasite.[207] However, normal intake of the majority of saponins is not toxic to humans, as evidenced by the fact that saponin intake by vegetarians is in the range of 100–200 mg per day.[199] Saponins are permitted as food additives in many countries (for example, to give a satisfactory head to beer), although there are inconsistencies.[208] Long-term feeding of saponins to animals did not demonstrate any signs of toxicity.[208]

As noted previously, grazing animals which consume large amounts of saponins can develop cholestatic liver damage. In South Africa, consumption of Tribulus by sheep contributes to a bilirubin-induced disorder known as geeldikkop.[209] While it is unlikely that normal human doses would cause cholestasis, this phenomenon should be considered in unexplained cases of this disorder in patients taking herbs. More importantly, saponin-containing herbs are best kept to a minimum in patients with preexisting cholestasis.

CARDIAC GLYCOSIDES

Phytochemistry

These compounds, also known as cardioactive glycosides, are steroidal glycosides which are similar to, but essentially different from, steroidal saponins. They constitute a well-defined and highly homogeneous group from both a structural and a pharmacological perspective. They (or the plants which contain them) have been used as conventional medical drugs for 200 years and are still widely used today, despite their potential toxicity and the current controversy over their clinical value. There are two main types, which either have a steroidal aglycone with 23 carbons (the cardenolide glycosides) or 24 carbons (the bufadienolide glycosides). The sugar part usually consists of 2–4 sugars joined together (an oligosaccharide).

Pharmacodynamics

The properties of cardiac glycosides are very well documented. They inhibit the sodium-potassium cellular pump leading to a rise in intracellular calcium levels which increases the contractile force and speed of the heart muscle (*positive inotropy*). In patients with compromised cardiac function, this positive isotropic effect translates into increased cardiac output and associated events which flow from this central effect. Heart rate is decreased (*negative chronotropy*) via the autonomic nervous system. Digitalis glycosides in particular also cause electrophysiological changes in the heart: conduction velocity at the atrioventricular node is slowed, together with an increase in its refractory period (*negative dromotropy*). This last feature underlies the use of digitalis glycosides in subventricular rhythm abnormalities such as atrial fibrillation.

It is beyond the scope of this chapter to discuss the pros and cons of digitalis therapy or the various adverse reactions and toxicity considerations associated with its use. Phytotherapists find digitalis to be too powerful for comfort and prefer to see it used, if necessary, under appropriate specialist care (generally the legal restrictions on its use render it available only on a medical prescription).

In some countries, herbalists and physicians practising phytotherapy find value in the use of milder herbs containing cardiac glycosides, in particular lily of the valley (*Convallaria majalis*). Its properties are similar to those of digitalis, but much less cumulative. The principal glycoside is convallatoxin, but the plant contains many minor cardenolides. Convallatoxin is poorly absorbed as a pure compound but the other components in the herb are said to aid its absorption.[210] It is unsuitable for manifest congestive heart failure but combines well with hawthorn in the management of milder forms of this condition, for digitalis hypersensitivity or for heart failure associated with a low pulse rate.[210] All the usual cautions governing the use of cardiac glycosides should be observed.

As an interesting footnote, an ouabain-like compound has been identified in humans (ouabain is a

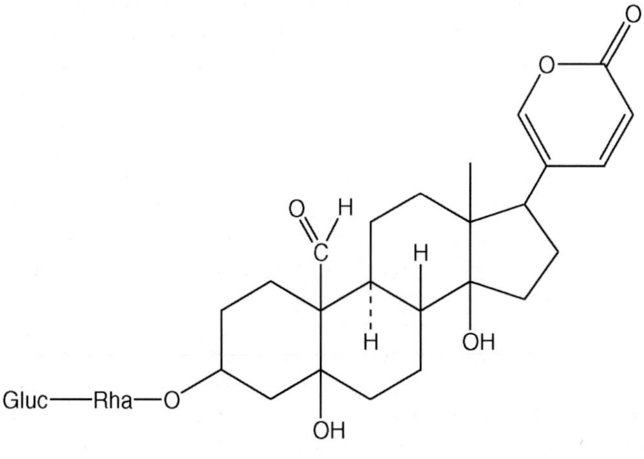

Gluc—Rha—O, OH, H, OH, O, H, C, H, O, O

Hellebrin - a bufadienolide glycoside

R_2O, OH, R_1, O, O

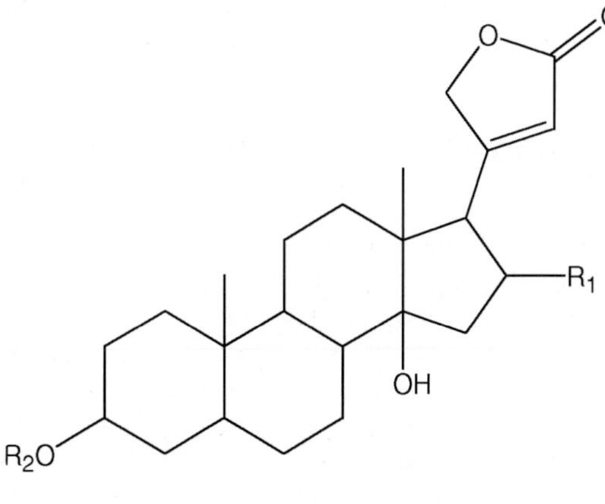

The cardenolide aglycone

cardenolide). This endogenous mammalian cardiotonic factor may be involved in renal function and in the pathogenesis of hypertension.[211]

ANTHRAQUINONES

Phytochemistry

Anthraquinones, as the name implies, are phytochemicals based on anthracene (three benzene rings joined together). At each apex of the central ring is a carbonyl group (carbon double-bonded to oxygen), which is the quinone part. Not all anthraquinones are strictly quinones; for example, the sennosides are dianthrones which consist of two anthrone units, each bearing only one carbonyl group. Anthraquinones usually occur in plants as glycosides; for example the sennosides from senna (*Cassia species*) are O-glycosides and the aloins from aloe are C-glycosides. The cascarosides from cascara (*Rhamnus purshiana*) are unusual molecules in that they are C,O-glycosides, having one glucose linked to a central anthrone via a carbon atom and a second glucose linked via oxygen. If aglycones do occur in dried herbs, they are always anthraquinones; anthrones are too unstable in the free state. Dianthrone glycosides such as the sennosides are not found in the living plant, being formed on harvesting and drying from monomeric anthrone glycosides.

Pharmacodynamics

Plants like rhubarb, senna and cascara have been used for their laxative effects from prehistory. Given their widespread contemporary use, it should not be surprising that their pharmacology is relatively well studied. Of particular interest is the pharmacokinetics of the anthraquinone glycosides. This topic will be more extensively discussed in the pharmacokinetics section (p.58) but briefly put, these agents travel to the large bowel where bacterial action forms anthrone aglycones, which are the true active forms.

The laxative effect on the gut is largely a local one; systemic absorption is limited. Two distinct mechanisms are in force: a modification of intestinal

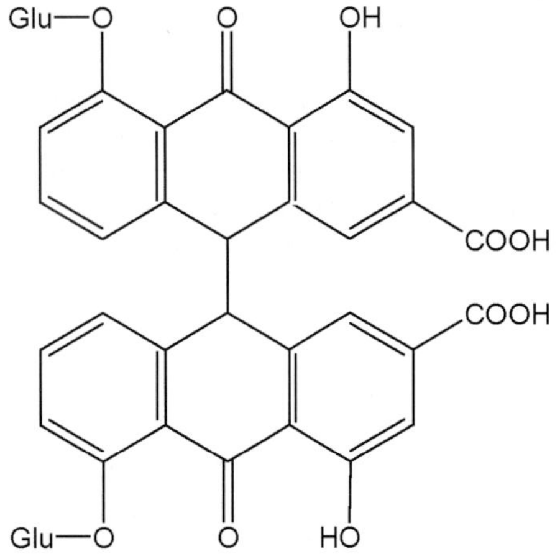

Sennosides A, B (stereoisomers)

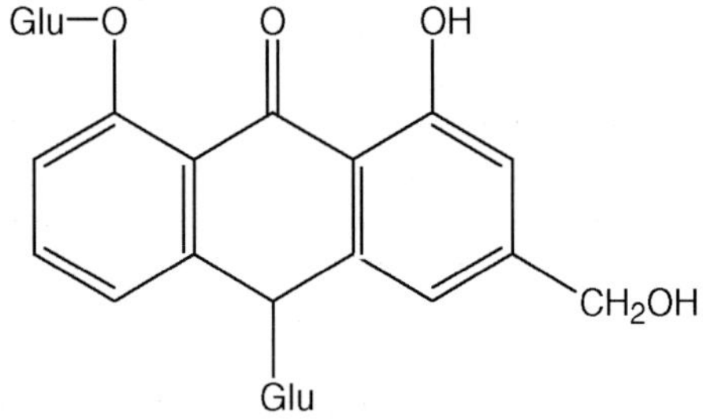

Cascarosides A, B (stereoisomers)

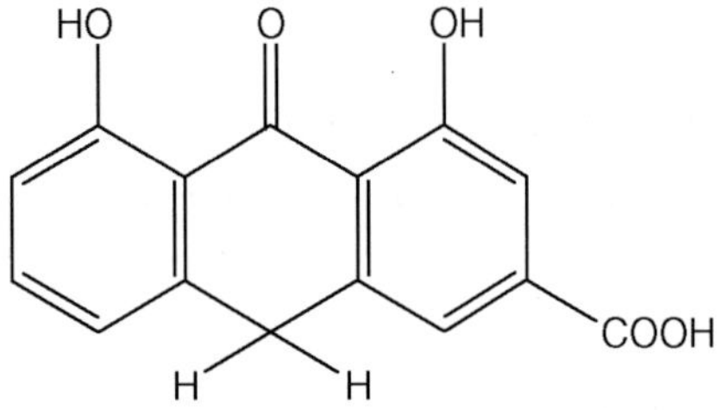

Rheinanthrone

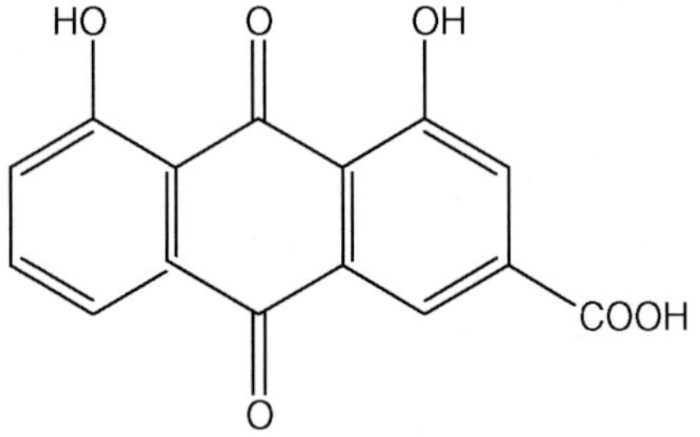

Rhein

motility and an accumulation of fluid in the intestinal lumen.[212] Experiments in animals and humans have shown that the introduction of anthrones into the colon quickly induces vigorous peristaltic movements.[212] Such a fast response is certainly not a secondary effect resulting from increased faecal water. This effect on motility is at least in part due to the release of prostaglandins, since its action is abolished by indomethacin and other cyclooxygenase inhibitors.[213] However, other research shows that inhibition of intestinal tone and segmentation (and therefore reduced colonic transit time) could be the primary motility effect.[212]

Accumulation of fluid in the colonic lumen can also lead to laxative effects. While it has been suggested that this could be due to the inhibitory effect of anthrones on the sodium pump,[212] these agents have instead been shown to stimulate active chloride secretion into the lumen, which is balanced by an increase in sodium and water flow.[214] Prostaglandins may be involved in this process[215] but not platelet-activating factor.[216] Alteration of calcium transport may also play a role.[212]

The dual action of anthraquinones highlights an important aspect of their safe and effective usage. In lower laxative doses that produce a normal motion, the effects on motility are apparent, but in higher doses, electrolyte secretion and diarrhoea will predominate. Habituation and adverse effects are more likely to follow the electrolyte loss associated with the use of high doses. Chronic abuse of laxatives raises aldosterone levels in response to electrolyte loss, which diminishes their effectiveness. Higher doses empty a larger portion of the colon. The resulting natural absence of defaecation over the next day or so leads to reuse, perhaps of an even higher dose, and the cycle of use is perpetuated.

Natural anthraquinones in the form of chrysarobin have also been used topically in the treatment of psoriasis. Chrysarobin, a mixture of substances including chrysophanol, is obtained from araroba or goa powder. Araroba is extracted from cavities in the trunk of the South American tree *Andira araroba*.[217] Dithranol (or anthralin), a cheaper synthetic analogue of chrysarobin, has been the focus of the most studies. Chrysarobin is an effective topical agent for psoriasis, as was demonstrated in an open comparative study with coal tar and ultraviolet radiation.[218] However, it has a number of drawbacks: it is only stable in a greasy base and it irritates and stains the skin.

The antiproliferative mode of action of dithranol, and presumably chrysarobin, is thought to be either through its effect on DNA, probably mitochondrial DNA, which reduces cell turnover or through its effects on various vital enzyme systems.[219] A possible relationship with reduction-oxidation potential has recently been observed.[220] Most recent research on chrysarobin has been concerned with its tumour-promoting activity.[221] Not surprisingly, this finding has further reduced its use in therapy.

Hypericin and pseudohypericin are dianthrones (structurally related to anthraquinones) with antiviral activity. Several anthraquinone aglycones including rhein, alizarin and emodin also demonstrated antiviral activity against human cytomegalovirus.[222] This may explain the traditional use of applying leaves of *Cassia species* to viral skin conditions.[217] It is unlikely that systemic antiviral effects would follow from the ingestion of these compounds, due to their low bioavailability.

Rhein is an anthraquinone aglycone found in rhubarb which inhibits the activity of cytokines in models of osteoarthritis.[223] This observation led to the development of diacetylrhein, a synthetic derivative with better bioavailability. Clinical studies of oral diacetylrhein at 100 mg per day improved symptoms in patients with osteoarthritis.[223] Diarrhoea was a common side effect.

Madder root (*Rubia tinctorum*) contains a characteristic spectrum of intensely coloured anthraquinone glycosides such as glycosides of lucidin and alizarin. As well as being used as a vegetable dye and natural food colouring, madder has traditionally been employed for the prevention and treatment of kidney stones. The anthraquinones in madder can function as chelating agents with some metal ions such as calcium and magnesium. With oral doses of glycosides and aglycones, a pronounced calcium complexing effect and a significant reduction in the growth rate of kidney stones was observed in an animal model.[217] A therapeutic oral dose of madder root will colour the urine slightly pink, which indicates that significant quantities of anthraquinones are excreted in the urine. Its regular use is said to slowly dissolve kidney stones. Perhaps madder might also have value as an oral chelation therapy in patients with atherosclerotic lesions.

Adverse reactions and toxicology

Madder has been withdrawn from the German market due to concerns over its mutagenicity and potential carcinogenicity. In particular, rats metabolize alizarin glycosides to alizarin and 1-hydroxyanthraquinone, a known rodent carcinogen.[224] However, long-term feeding of madder root to mice failed to produce neoplastic lesions.[225]

Anthraquinone laxatives may cause mild abdominal complaints such as cramps and abdominal pains and should be used cautiously in patients with these symptoms. Other side effects include discoloration of the urine and haemorrhoid congestion. Overdosage can result in diarrhoea and, coupled with prolonged use, can result in excessive loss of electrolytes, particularly potassium.[212]

Abuse of anthraquinone laxatives has been stated to cause damage to the myenteric plexus. However, results from animal studies and a controlled study in humans have challenged this finding.[226] Habituation can occur with laxative abuse, due to hyperaldosteronism. The evidence is that anthraquinone laxatives, used sensibly, are unlikely to cause habituation. In fact, in several studies senna has been claimed to have a reeducative function and helped to restore normal bowel function.[227] For example, out of 210 patients in a psychiatric hospital, 44% were taking laxatives at the outset, but 3 months' treatment with senna lowered this to 8%.[228]

Cathartic colon coupled with hypokalaemia (low serum potassium) is a characteristic finding associated with chronic laxative abuse (not just anthraquinones). The cathartic colon is characterized by the existence of a segment of intestine (typically the ascending colon) which has become largely non-functioning. Cathartic colon presents as chronic diarrhoea resistant to therapy. This is probably a rare disorder and is often associated with psychological abnormalities.[229] Cathartic colon can be reversed; a case has been described of a 78-year-old woman with cathartic colon who, after treatment was switched to psyllium, demonstrated complete reversal of the condition after 4 months.[230]

Contraindications for anthraquinone laxatives include ileus from whatever cause. Use in pregnancy and lactation is controversial. In traditional Chinese medicine they are contraindicated in pregnancy because they promote a downward movement of energy. Apart from this consideration, they are unlikely to cause adverse effects since their effects in the gut are largely topical: systemic absorption is limited (see Pharmacokinetics, p.58). Results from several clinical studies on senna indicate that its normal use does not involve any increased risk for the pregnancy or the foetus.[231] Moreover, clinical observations of infants and analytical studies of breast milk both lead to the conclusion that the treatment of lactating mothers with senna does not carry a risk of producing a laxative effect in the infant.[232]

Long-term use of anthraquinone laxatives leads to a condition known as melanosis (or pseudomelanosis) coli. This is a brown discoloration of the intestinal mucosa which begins at the ileocolonic junction and may extend to the rectum. This harmless pigmentation is not staining by the anthraquinones but is due to a lipofuscin-like substance within macrophages of the colonic mucosa.[212] (Lipofuscin is a pigmented, peroxidized fatty acid residue which is found in many organs with advancing age.) However, the intrinsic colour of anthraquinones may play some part in the development of this pigment. It is generally accepted that melanosis is a benign, reversible condition.[233]

The mutagenicity of isolated anthraquinones has been extensively studied and established in several models, particularly microbial assays such as the Ames test.[234] On the other hand, some recent studies involving both in vitro and in vivo models found an absence of mutagenicity for senna, sennosides and rhein.[235] The same research group recently concluded that senna does not represent a genotoxic risk to humans when used periodically at therapeutic doses.[236]

Nonetheless, their putative mutagenicity has led to investigation of carcinogenic effects associated with the use of anthraquinone laxatives. One review examined the relationship between anthraquinone laxatives and colorectal cancer.[237] Danthrone (two studies) and 1-hydroxyanthraquinone (one study) were carcinogenic in rodent models. Three clinical studies did not show an association of colorectal cancer with laxative abuse but these studies also included bulk laxatives. When melanosis coli was taken as an indicator of anthraquinone laxative use, a retrospective study of 3049 patients undergoing endoscopic diagnosis for suspected colorectal cancer found an association between anthraquinone use and colorectal adenomas.[237] A prospective study by the same research group found that 18.6% of patients with colorectal carcinoma had evidence of anthraquinone use.[237] From their data they suggested that a relative risk of 3.04 could be calculated for colorectal cancer due to anthraquinone laxative abuse. These studies did not differentiate between natural and synthetic (danthrone) laxative use. This is significant because relatively higher doses of danthrone are required for laxative effects and, since it is not a glycoside, its systemic absorption is greater. It has recently been asserted that epidemiological studies do not give conclusive evidence for any association with colorectal cancer.[212]

Given the above concerns, whatever their basis in fact, most regulatory authorities now require that anthraquinone laxatives are to be labelled as a short-term treatment for constipation. Since the goal of the phytotherapist is to effect change (reeducate the bowel) rather than compensate for a deranged physiology, this approach is consistent with good herbal medicine.

COUMARINS

Phytochemistry

Coumarins owe their name to 'coumarin' which was the common name for the tonka bean (*Dipteryx odorata*) from which the simple compound coumarin was first isolated in 1820. Coumarins are benzo-alpha-pyrones (lactones of o-hydroxycinnamic acid) formed via the shikimic acid pathway. Except for a few rare cases, including coumarin itself which is unsubstituted, all plant coumarins contain a hydroxyl or methoxy group in position 7. These substituted simple coumarins such as scopoletin, aesculetin and umbelliferone are common and widespread in higher plants and often occur as glycosides.

Simple coumarin has a pleasant vanilla-like odour. It is probably not present in the intact plant but is rather formed by enzymatic activity from a glycoside of o-hydroxycinnamic acid (such as melilotoside) after harvesting and drying. This accounts for the odour of new-mown hay, which is not present in the undamaged plant. Coumarin is used to perfume pipe tobacco and can be sometimes found as an adulterant in commercial vanilla flavouring.[238]

The furanocoumarins are closely related furano derivatives of coumarin (furan is a five-membered heterocyclic ring containing oxygen) which are commonly found in the Rutaceae (rue family) and Umbelliferae (Apiaceae, celery family). Linear furanocoumarins are often called psoralens and act as photosensitizing agents (see below).

The furanochromones such as khellin from *Ammi visnaga* are structural derivatives of benzo-gamma-pyrone (furanobenzo-gamma-pyrones) and therefore are as much related to flavonoids as coumarins. In other words, the carbonyl group is opposite the oxygen rather than adjacent to it. However, they are usually classified as coumarins and will be considered in this section. *Ammi visnaga* also contains visnadin, a pyranocoumarin.

The widespread nature of coumarins means that they are consumed in human diet, for example, carrots, celery and parsnip.[239] Coumarins are fluorescent compounds and this property is widely utilized in a number of biochemical techniques. Simple substituted coumarins are also used as pigments in sunscreens.

Pharmacodynamics

Dicoumarol is a potent anticoagulant compound formed from coumarin by bacterial action in spoiled sweet clover hay (*Melilotus species*). Its discovery led to the development of modern anticoagulant drugs. Dicoumarol and related anticoagulants are hydroxylated in the 4 position. This is deemed to be an essential requirement (among others) for powerful anticoagulant activity. All of the common plant coumarins are not substituted at this position and therefore lack significant clinical anticoagulant activity, although many do possess measurable activity when given to animals in high doses.[240] Coumarin has antioedema, antiinflammatory, immune-enhancing and anticancer activities which are more fully described in the Melilotus monograph (p.483).

Simple substituted coumarins such as scopoletin and umbelliferone have exhibited a diverse range of pharmacological activities. The spasmolytic activity of scopoletin is probably a major reason behind the use of *Viburnum species* such as cramp bark and black haw for hypertension and dysmenorrhoea. Scopoletin and aesculetin were identified in black haw as having significant spasmolytic action on guinea pig small intestine.[241] Another research team working at the same

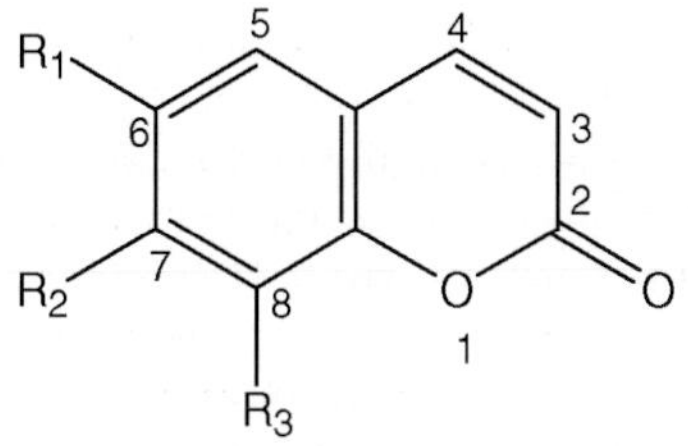

R_1	R_2	R_3	
H	H	H	Coumarin
H	OH	H	Umbelliferone
H	OCH_3	H	Herniarin
H	OH	OH	Daphnetin
OH	OH	H	Aesculetin
OCH_3	OH	H	Scopoletin

Simple coumarins

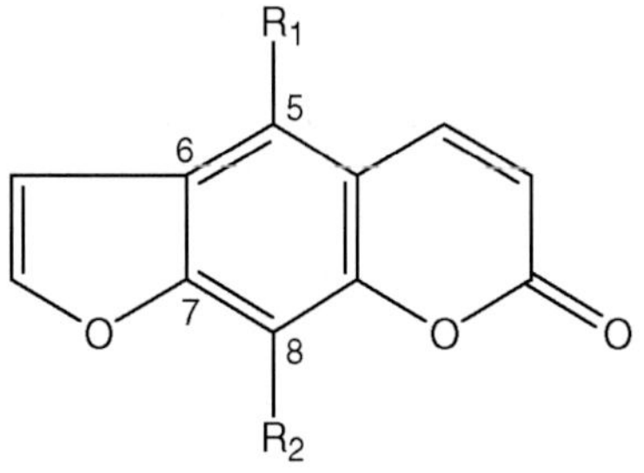

R_1	R_2	
H	H	Psoralen
H	OCH_3	Xanthotoxin
H	OH	Xanthotoxol
OCH_3	H	Bergapten
OH	H	Bergaptol

Linear furanocoumarins

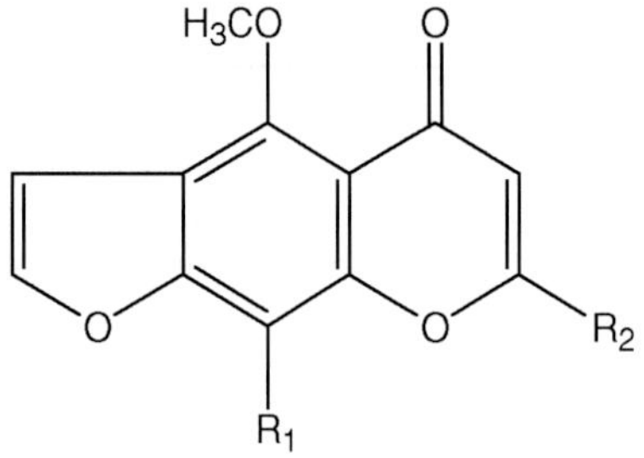

R_1	R_2	
H	CH_3	Visnagin
OCH_3	CH_3	Khellin
OH	CH_2OH	Khellol

Furanochromones

Visnadin

time also identified scopoletin as a component of the Viburnums which exhibited uterine spasmolytic activity.[242] It has been suggested that the spasmolytic activity of scopoletin might be due to a blockade of autonomic neurotransmitters.[243]

Further studies are required to establish if scopoletin, umbelliferone and related compounds possess clinically relevant antiinflammatory and analgesic activities but such activities have been established in animal studies.[244] Inhibition of cyclooxygenase and 5-lipoxygenase may play a role.[245] Aesculetin and umbelliferone are also strong xanthine oxidase inhibitors in vitro.[246]

Like coumarin, substituted coumarins may have a role to play in cancer prevention and treatment. Umbelliferone and scopoletin are antimutagenic[247,248] but were much less protective than coumarin in one model of chemical carcinogenesis.[249] Aesculetin exhibited considerably higher cytotoxic activity than coumarin in vitro on two tumour cell lines but scopoletin was inactive.[250] Umbelliferone has similar cytotoxic activity to coumarin.[251]

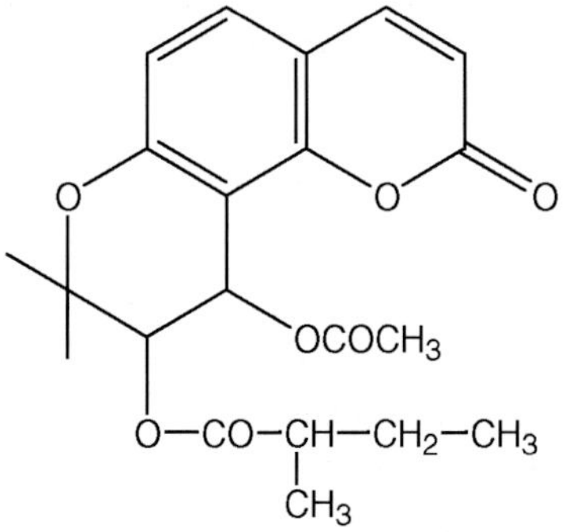

Furanocoumarins have a long history of therapeutic use in humans. More than 3000 years ago it was recorded in both Egyptian and Ayurvedic medicine that the ingestion of herbs containing psoralens followed by exposure to sunlight could assist in the treatment of vitiligo, a skin condition characterized by loss of pigmentation.[252] This traditional knowledge was developed into a modern therapy in the 1940s when xanthotoxin (8-methoxypsoralen, 8-MOP) plus sunlight exposure was introduced as a therapy for vitiligo.[253] The treatment was not very successful, mainly due to phototoxic side effects, and it was only when ultraviolet A light sources (UVA) became available that significant advances were made. UVA radiation is less energetic and therefore less damaging than ultraviolet B (UVB) radiation. It was demonstrated that oral 8-MOP and UVA were highly effective in the control of psoriasis and the malignant skin condition mycosis fungoides.[253] The treatment was called PUVA (psoralen plus UVA) and the new field of photochemotherapy was initiated.

More recently, it has been realized that bergapten (5-methoxypsoralen, 5-MOP) is a psoralen with superior therapeutic characteristics in PUVA. Furanocoumarins in conjunction with ultraviolet radiation stimulate melanogenesis (tanning) and cause antiproliferative effects but also initiate phototoxic erythema (inflammation). For 8-MOP, the therapeutic dose is similar to the dose that causes erythema. With the use of oral 5-MOP it is possible to obtain melanogenic doses of drug-UVA or drug-sunlight combinations without the development of phototoxicity. This provides a wider margin of safety and permits the induction of a tan (known as a PUVA tan) which is more effective than a normal tan in attenuating the damaging effects of UV exposure. Psoralens are now the basis of yet another new field of therapy: photochemoprotection.[253]

The use of 5-MOP has provided a more effective treatment for vitiligo and gives fewer side effects in PUVA therapy of psoriasis.[254] As a further development of photochemoprotection, studies have shown that this furanocoumarin, in conjunction with UVB sunscreens, provides a faster tan (without burning) which is more protective against the harmful effects of ultraviolet radiation[255] and even chemical irritation.[256] It should be noted that certain citrus oils are rich sources of bergapten (5-MOP) and are used in these tanning products in preference to the synthetic chemical.

Furanocoumarins in conjunction with UV light kill bacteria and inactivate viruses.[257,258] In addition, they may be responsible for the enhanced bioavailability which grapefruit juice affords to several pharmaceuticals (see Pharmacokinetics section, p.58).

The decoction of the fruits of *Ammi visnaga* has been used since ancient times in Egypt as a spasmolytic for kidney stones and in the treatment of angina pectoris. The pyranocoumarin visnadin was isolated which exhibited positive inotropic and marked coronary vasodilatory activities. Visnadin is still used as a treatment for angina and possibly acts as a calcium channel blocker.[259] *Ammi visnaga* also contains the spasmolytic furanochromone khellin, which was adopted for the treatment of angina and asthma. Its use was discontinued because of side effects such as drowsiness, headache and nausea.

As further evidence that the archetypal plant constituents still provide much of the inspiration for the development of modern drugs, sodium cromoglycate (Intal) was developed in an attempt to find a derivative of khellin which was devoid of its side effects. Unlike khellin, the antiasthmatic activity of Intal is believed to result from increased stability of mast cells.

Toxicology

The toxicology of coumarin is reviewed in the Melilotus monograph (p.483). It is hepatotoxic in the rat and also less commonly in humans. Coumarins are structurally related to fungal aflatoxins, which are potent hepatotoxins, but it appears that the substituted coumarins do not share this property (see the Melilotus monograph). Although a case of increased haemorrhagic tendency was attributed to coumarin intake from tonka beans, sweet clover and woodruff, intake was excessive and there were a number of confounding factors.[260]

Furanocoumarins are potent photosensitizing agents. Chance exposure to these compounds in the field can lead to severe photodermatitis with blistering. The giant hogweed is one example of a plant which consistently causes this problem. Celery pickers can develop photodermatitis after handling celery infected with fungus, which induces celery to produce high levels of psoralens.[261]

Furanocoumarins are powerful mutagens in the presence of UVA and psoralens are light-activated carcinogens.[261] In the presence of UV light, psoralens are capable of binding to and cross linking DNA, which causes genetic damage and mutations. Only linear furanocoumarins (psoralens) are able to bind to two DNA bases to cause crosslinks. Non-linear furanocoumarins (isopsoralens) can only bind to one base to form monoadducts. Although concerns were expressed that the development of isopsoralens as photochemotherapeutic agents may increase carcinogenic risk because monoadducts are subject to error-prone DNA repair mechanisms,[261] this does not appear to be the case.[262]

Use of UV filters decreases the photomutagenic and photocarcinogenic effects of psoralens but the employment of 5-MOP in suntanning lotions remains controversial.[263,264] Given the advantages of a PUVA tan, it is likely that the benefits will outweigh risks provided that UV exposure is carefully controlled. This may only occur under clinical supervision.

Use of PUVA therapy in psoriasis is postulated to be associated with an increased risk of skin cancer, particularly squamous cell carcinoma.[265] Risk of developing skin cancer was claimed to be proportional to the number of treatments and the degree of exposure to UVA.[265] However, these associations have been disputed by at least one study, which proposed that prior exposure to arsenic treatments or X-rays largely explained the higher incidence of skin cancer in PUVA-treated psoriasis patients.[266] Significant exposure of the unprotected human eyes to PUVA may accelerate cataract formation but this is readily alleviated by protective eyeglasses.[265]

PHYTOOESTROGENS

Phytooestrogens are phytochemicals which have oestrogenic activity. Compounds belonging to several phytochemical classes interact with oestrogen receptors but research has focused on isoflavones and lignans. Oestrogenic isoflavones, which include genistein, daidzein and their glycosides, are mainly found in members of the Leguminosae (pea family) such as soya beans and red clover. Linseed (flaxseed) is the richest source of the oestrogenic lignans enterodiol and enterolactone, which are formed by bacterial action on the precursor secoisolariciresinol diglucoside, found in the seed.

Pharmacodynamics

Interest in the oestrogenic effects of plants first arose in the scientific world when clover disease was identified in Australia in the 1940s. It was observed that infertility in sheep developed after grazing on various species of clover (Trifolium species). Research interest at the time focused on understanding the factors that caused clover disease, which were identified as isoflavone glycosides. It was several decades later, when results from epidemiological studies suggested that the dietary consumption of soya products might have a protective role in breast cancer, that interest in the oestrogenic properties of isoflavones was rekindled.

Studies using various animal tissues demonstrated that, while isoflavones compete strongly with oestradiol at oestrogen receptors, their stimulation of these receptors is much weaker than oestradiol.[267] In other words, they are partial oestrogen agonists which can function as oestrogen agonists or antagonists depending on the hormonal milieu. In a high-oestrogen environment (such as in the premenopausal woman), their displacement of endogenous oestrogens is postulated to have an antioestrogenic effect. In

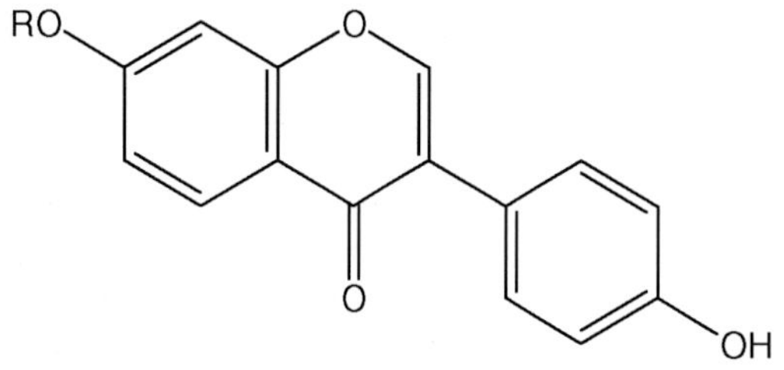

Daidzein R = H
Daidzin R = Glucose

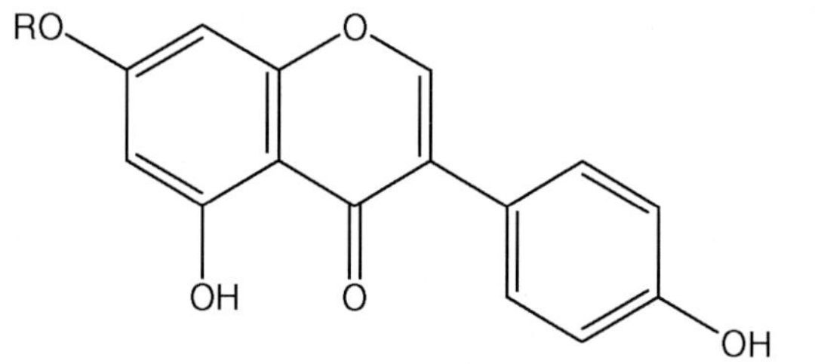

Genistein R = H
Genistin R = Glucose

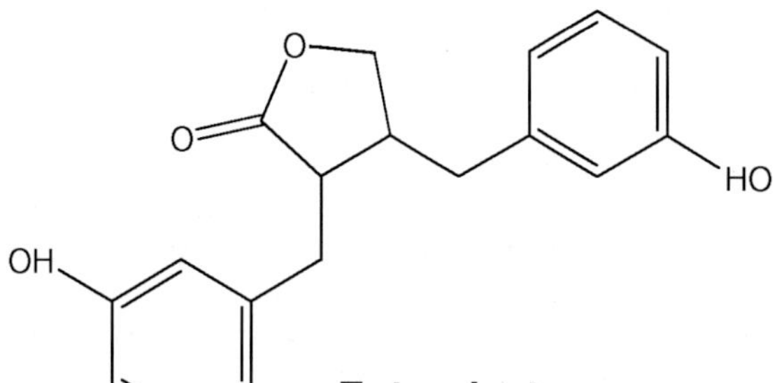

Enterolactone

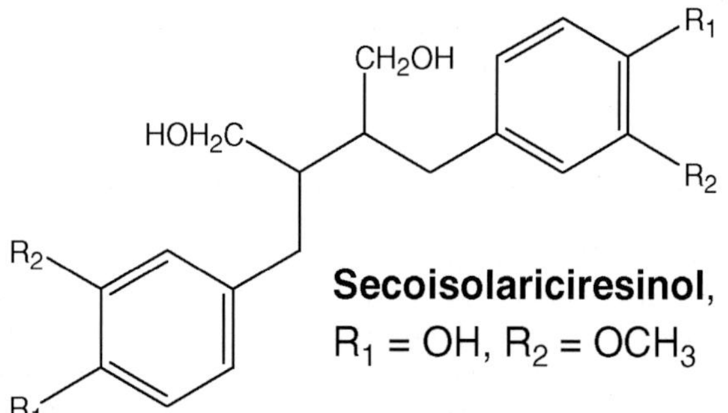

Secoisolariciresinol, $R_1 = OH, R_2 = OCH_3$

Enterodiol, $R_1 = H, R_2 = OH$

contrast, in a lower oestrogen environment, as in the postmenopausal woman, they are expected to provide a net oestrogenic effect.

Animal studies have shown that isoflavones influence many aspects of the mammalian reproductive process via effects on the development and physiology of female reproductive organs and alteration of sexual behaviour.[268] It is now recognized that the rat, mouse and human oestrogen receptor exists as two subtypes, alpha and beta. The alpha receptors predominate in the kidney, pituitary and reproductive tract while beta receptors are found in bone, prostate, brain and reproductive organs. Whereas environmental oestrogens (xenooestrogens) such as pesticides bind to both subtypes with a similar preference and degree, isoflavone phytooestrogens compete more strongly with oestradiol for binding to beta-oestrogen receptors.[269]

Phytooestrogens also appear to influence sex hormone metabolism. Lignans and isoflavones are postulated to increase levels of sex hormone-binding globulin (SHBG), which is deemed to be a favourable effect for protection against breast cancer and coronary heart disease in women.[270] They also inhibit aromatase in vitro, which converts androgens in adipose tissue into oestrogen.[271]

A study in six premenopausal women indicated that intake of soya protein (60 g per day for one month containing 45 mg of isoflavones) significantly ($p<0.01$) increased follicular phase length or delayed menstruation.[272] Midcycle surges of LH and FSH were significantly suppressed and plasma oestradiol concentrations increased in the follicular phase. Tamoxifen causes similar changes, which are considered to indicate a reduced breast cancer risk.

The incidence of hot flushes is said to be lower in menopausal women in Asian countries where soya intake is high.[273] Dietary supplementation with soya flour significantly reduced hot flushes in a randomized double-blind trial.[274] In another double-blind, placebo-controlled study involving 104 menopausal women, 60 g of soya protein per day caused a significant reduction in the frequency of hot flushes.[275] These findings in pre- and postmenopausal women are clinical confirmation of the partial oestrogen agonist effects of soya isoflavones.

Studies are in progress to determine if isoflavones share other putative effects of hormone replacement therapy in postmenopausal women, notably reduced loss in bone density and favourable cardiovascular activity. Positive effects have been noted on bone metabolism in vitro[276] and in vivo[277] and ipriflavone, a synthetic isoflavone, has been demonstrated to maintain or increase bone density in postmenopausal women.[273] Nonetheless, more studies are required to define the influence of isoflavone consumption on bone density in postmenopausal women. Dietary soya protein intake appears to be antiatherogenic in animal models and lowers cholesterol in humans.[273] Whether these effects are due to the isoflavones remains in question. In this context, it is interesting to note that removal of the phytochemicals (including the isoflavones) from soya protein eliminates the antiatherosclerotic effects observed with untreated soya.[278]

Most of the recent interest in isoflavones has focused on their potential to prevent and possibly treat cancer, especially hormone-dependent cancers such as breast and prostate cancer. These effects can be categorized as following from either the hormonal activity of isoflavones or from their inhibition of a number of aspects of tumour cell function. Epidemiological studies have shown that in populations at low risk from breast cancer, urinary and plasma levels of isoflavones and their metabolites are usually higher.[279] Isoflavonoids are competitive with regard to the binding of oestradiol to its receptors in breast cancer cells and genistein and daidzein were shown to be antiproliferative in cultures of breast cancer cells in the presence of oestrogen.[279] Isoflavones inhibited the proliferative effects of xenooestrogens on human breast cancer cells.[280] However, the oestrogenic function of genistein means it can also induce proliferation of human breast cancer cells in vitro in the absence of oestradiol.[281]

Isoflavone intake may prevent the development of prostate cancer. The mortality from prostate cancer is low in countries such as Japan where soya intake is high[279] and genistein inhibits the growth of human prostatic cancer cells in vitro.[282] A 66-year-old man took 160 mg of isoflavones from red clover daily for 1 week before radical prostatectomy for a moderately high-grade adenocarcinoma. The resected specimen showed prominent apoptosis, typical of response to high-dose oestrogen therapy and suggestive of tumour regression.[283]

Isoflavones, particularly genistein, exhibit anticancer potential which is independent of their hormonal effects and appear to inhibit several aspects of tumour cell growth regulation. Two particular enzymes that play key roles in cell proliferation and differentiation are the protein tyrosine kinases (PTK) and the DNA topoisomerases. Genistein specifically inhibits most PTK and, together with other flavonoids, inhibits DNA topoisomerases.[279,284]

Genistein specifically inhibited the growth of several tumour and non-tumour cell lines in vitro, including those which were not oestrogen responsive.[284] In rat models of breast cancer genistein, like oestradiol, has the most protective effect when administered early in the life of the animal.[285] In ovariectomized mice, dietary genistein increases breast cancer proliferation. This oestrogen-like effect is not observed in non-ovariectomized rats.[285] Genistein has also shown an anticarcinogenic effect in many other animal models of carcinogenesis involving a range of inducing agents.[286] An important aspect of the anticancer activity of genistein may be its marked capacity to inhibit endothelial cell proliferation and in vitro angiogenesis.[287] Unregulated angiogenesis is associated with several diseases and the formation of new blood vessels is critical for the growth of tumours.

In contrast to the isoflavones, research on the oestrogenic lignans enterolactone and enterodiol has not been as extensive. Initial interest in these compounds resulted from the observation in the early 1980s that their urinary levels in menstruating women exhibited a cyclic pattern during the menstrual cycle, with maximum excretion in the luteal phase.[288] The relatively high concentrations of these new lignans in urine, their cyclic pattern of excretion and their increased excretion in early pregnancy suggested that they were a new class of human hormone. It transpired that what had been found was a plant chemical which had been modified by bacteria in the human digestive tract.[288] Selective antibiotic administration to humans suppressed oestrogenic lignan formation.[288]

Enterolactone, like isoflavones, inhibited oestradiol stimulated breast cancer cell growth in vitro.[289] Increased lignan ingestion has been associated with increased concentrations of SHBG, but this was not confirmed in a clinical study.[289] Linseed intake by normal premenopausal women was consistently associated with longer luteal phase (LP) lengths and higher ratios of LP progesterone to oestradiol.[289] These findings may reflect favourably on breast cancer risk. An earlier animal study found that linseed supplementation reduced early risk markers for breast cancer.[290] Dietary studies and assays of urinary lignans in postmenopausal women showed that lignan excretion is significantly lower in the urine of women with breast cancer.[291]

Adverse reactions and toxicology

Epidemiological studies have not found adverse effects from dietary consumption of isoflavones or lignans. However, if quantities well above dietary exposure are used in a therapeutic context, adverse events might well ensue. The phytooestrogens are partial oestrogen agonists similar to the drug tamoxifen. Research has shown that while tamoxifen has potential for preventing both breast cancer and cardiovascular disease, its use increases the risk of developing endometrial cancer. Moreover, concurrent intake of phytooestrogens and tamoxifen may reduce the therapeutic effects of the drug in breast cancer. For this reason, and also because of the observation that phytooestrogens can stimulate the growth of oestrogen-dependent tumours in some circumstances, intake of these phytochemicals should be limited to dietary levels in women with oestrogen-sensitive breast cancers until clinical studies suggest otherwise.

Controversy has arisen over the possible adverse effects of soya-based infant milk formulas. A recent study found that infant exposure to isoflavones from these products was relatively much greater than levels shown to alter reproductive hormones in adults.[292] It was suggested that further studies of possible developmental effects are highly desirable.

ALKALOIDS

Phytochemistry

Because they are a vast and diverse group of archetypal plant constituents, it is consequently difficult to arrive at a consistent definition of alkaloids. The word derives from the term 'vegetable alkali' which refers to the alkaline nature of these compounds, a property which results from the fact that they always contain nitrogen. The following definition is concise and descriptive: alkaloids are alkaline (basic) nitrogen-containing heterocyclic compounds derived from higher plants and often exhibiting marked pharmacological activity. However, there are several exceptions to this definition. For example, the nitrogen in ephedrine is not part of a ring, so it is not heterocyclic. For this reason it is sometimes referred to as a protoalkaloid. Berberine is not alkaline and some alkaloids are derived from animals and microorganisms. Generally alkaloids are white but some are highly coloured; for example, berberine is yellow and sanguinarine is red. (By now it should be apparent that names of alkaloids end with the letters *–ine*.)

Alkaloids were the first chemical drugs to be derived from plants; a mixture of morphine and narcotine was isolated from opium in 1803. They have maintained an important role in conventional drug therapy since then; names such as codeine, morphine, atropine, quinine, pilocarpine, theophylline, colchicine, pseudoephedrine and vincristine are a familiar part of modern drug medicine. These drugs are potent pharmacological agents and their properties are well described in conventional pharmacology texts. A high risk of adverse reactions ensues from their use. In contrast, while phytotherapists do rely on plants containing alkaloids, their activity is at the milder end of the pharmacological spectrum. Alkaloids as a group are not nearly as important to the phytotherapist as they are to the conventional doctor.

Accordingly, this section will not include a broad and detailed treatment of various classes and subclasses of alkaloids but will instead focus on a few examples which are important to phytotherapy. Nevertheless, it is worthwhile to consider the basic structures of the important classes of alkaloids and these are provided in the diagram below.

Examples of each class named are: pyrrolidine – hygrines; piperidine – lobeline; pyridine – nicotine; indole – strychnine; quinoline – quinine; isoquinoline – morphine; pyrrolizidine – seneciphylline; tropane – hyoscyamine; purine (xanthine) – caffeine; imidazole – pilocarpine; quinolizidine (norlupinane) – sparteine.

Most alkaloids are synthesized by the plant from amino acids. If they are not, they are called pseudoalkaloids. Most of the known examples of pseudoalkaloids are isoprenoids and are referred to as terpenoid alkaloids. Aconitine from various species of aconite is an example of a diterpene alkaloid and is one of the most toxic substances known. Steroidal alkaloids are also found in plants. Some are combined as glycosides; for example, solanine from potato shoots.

Despite being the most important archetypal plant constituents from an orthodox perspective, little is known about the function of alkaloids in plants. They may have a defensive role but many other theories are still suggested in texts, including that they are a byproduct of primary metabolism.

Pharmacodynamics

Alkaloids have two key properties which determine much of their pharmacology: an ability to cross the blood–brain barrier and exert depressant or stimulant effects on the central nervous system, and an ability to interact with various neurotransmitter receptors.

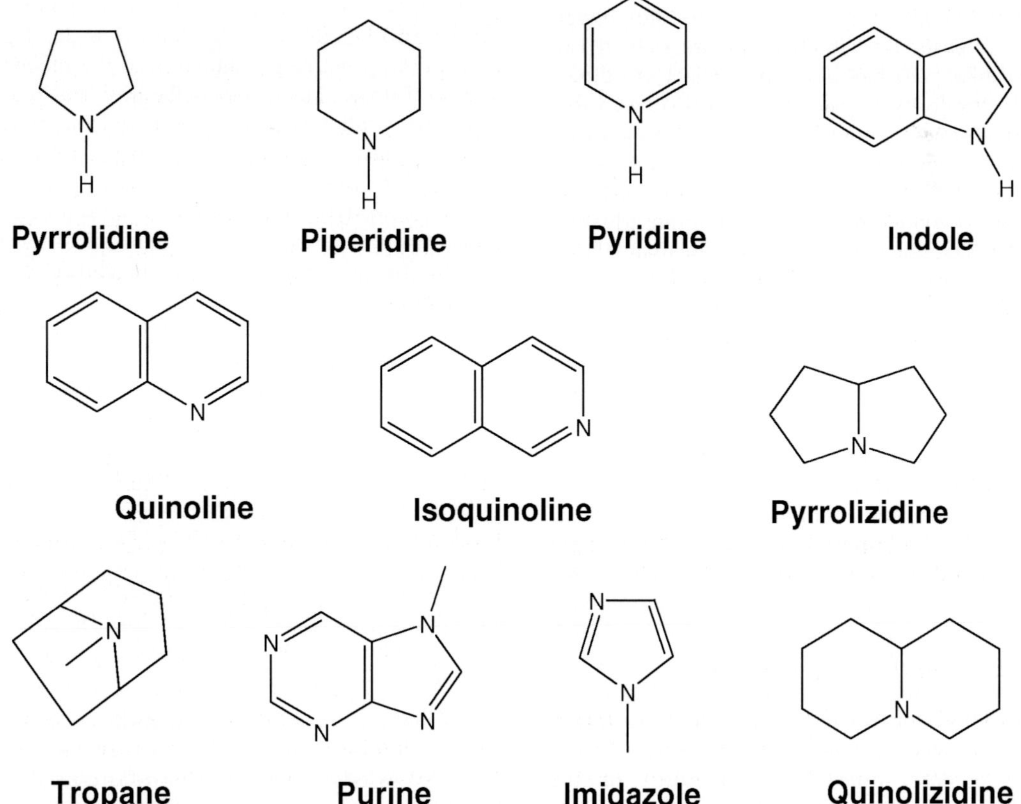

Examples include CNS depressants such as morphine and codeine, CNS stimulants such as caffeine and cocaine and sympathetic nervous system stimulants such as ephedrine.

Alkaloids are important to phytotherapy but their role is less significant than other archetypal plant constituents, as demonstrated by the fact that only three alkaloid-containing herbs are covered by monographs in this text, namely chelidonium, barberry and golden seal. Some additional examples of important alkaloid-containing herbs and their pharmacodynamic properties are discussed below.

Lobelia (*Lobelia inflata*) and ipecacuanha root (*Cephaelis ipecacuanha*) contain emetic alkaloids (lobeline and emetine respectively) which act as reflex expectorants at subemetic doses (similar to the expectorant saponins). Oral preparations of lobelia are also used as an aid to stop smoking, since lobeline is very similar to nicotine in its pharmacodynamic actions.

Several alkaloid-containing herbs are used as mild analgesics and anxiolytics. Californian poppy (*Eschscholtzia californica*) is a traditional medicine used by the rural population of California for its analgesic and sedative properties. Animal studies verified these actions and demonstrated low toxicity.[293] A proprietary formula consisting of 80% Californian poppy and 20% *Corydalis cava* (both herbs are rich in isoquinoline alkaloids) has been the subject of clinical studies.[294] Results from two clinical trials showed that disturbed sleeping behaviour could be normalized by the combination, without evidence of carry-over effects or addiction.[294] In vitro studies suggest that the two herbs cooperate in establishing an advantageous catecholamine status necessary for maintaining sedative and antidepressant effects.[295]

Various species of Ephedra contain the protoalkaloids ephedrine and pseudoephedrine.[296] Ephedra is a commonly used Chinese herb which possesses diaphoretic, antipyretic, antiallergic and antiasthmatic effects. It is also favoured in phytotherapy, particularly for the latter two activities. Ephedrine has been used as a conventional treatment for asthma.

Broom tops (*Cytisus scoparius*) contains the alkaloid sparteine and is an important herb for the treatment of cardiac arrhythmias.[297] Sparteine acts as a potassium channel antagonist[298] and delays systolic depolarization. Normal sinus frequency is slightly reduced, the refractory period is prolonged and the threshold raised, reducing the risk of fibrillation and extrasystoles. Indications for broom tops include sinus tachycardia, ventricular extrasystoles and arrhythmias following a heart attack.[297] High doses of the herb are necessary to achieve therapeutic levels of sparteine and related alkaloids. Sparteine was once widely used as an oxytocic drug, but it fell out of favour because of the uterine spasm which occurred in women who were unable to metabolize it effectively. About 5% of male and female subjects studied were unable to metabolize sparteine by N-oxidation[299] and this defect appears to have a genetic basis.[300]

PHARMACOKINETICS IN HERBAL MEDICINE

Pharmacokinetics can be defined as the study of the absorption, distribution, metabolism and elimination of pharmacologically active agents in the body. This discussion is not intended to be a primer on the principles of pharmacokinetics (there are appropriate texts for this purpose[301]); however, certain basic issues will be discussed where there is particular relevance to plant chemicals.

One important issue which should underlie much of the study of herbal pharmacokinetics is that herbs are not usually directly introduced into the bloodstream by injection or other means but rather the traditional oral or topical routes of administration are preferred. This renders the study of bioavailability of paramount importance for active constituents in plants. Bioavailability can be defined as the degree of absorption of active substances into the bloodstream after oral doses. Hence bioavailability is also a factor of the preparation which is used to deliver the dose of active substance. Conventional drugs intended for oral use are designed to have good bioavailability. In contrast, phytochemicals are of natural origin and may exhibit unusual or poor bioavailability, which may be further compounded by the choice of dosage preparation.

In this discussion, the issue of the bioavailability of some of the archetypal plant constituents will be emphasized. For pharmacokinetic details on individual herbs, see the monograph section of this book (or a recent review).[302]

Some practitioners and students of herbal medicine question the value of studying herbal pharmacokinetics. The following premises should be considered.

- If it is accepted that medicinal plants act at a chemical level in the body (as well as probably other levels of activity), then knowledge of herbal pharmacokinetics is vital.
- Given that, with a few exceptions in some countries, oral and topical doses are used for herbal medicines, a better knowledge of bioavailability is critical to meet the challenge of future health problems.

In particular, the information derived from the detailed study of herbal pharmacokinetics will confer certain advantages. These would include:

- information to further assess the traditional and anecdotal uses of a medicinal plant;
- better information on which to base rational dosages;
- a better interpretation of scientific information, particularly in vitro research or in vivo studies where the active compounds are administered by injection. There is an abundance of misinformation in the herbal literature related to excessive extrapolation from such studies, with no consideration of bioavailability;
- a better appreciation of the safety and toxicity of a plant;
- anticipation of potential herb-drug interactions;
- supporting evidence for the synergistic nature of herbal medicine;
- ways to optimize the bioavailability and hence efficacy of herbal medicines.

The study of herbal pharmacokinetics is a unique field which is extraordinarily complex. This is due to the following reasons:

- the chemical complexity of plant medicines and thus potential interactions between constituents
- the different bioavailability of different compounds
- the active components are often not known, so the components in the plant which should be studied cannot be identified
- herbal medicines are not designed for predictable pharmacokinetic characteristics and in particular, natural compounds are often metabolized in the digestive tract; that is, they are prodrugs; this feature is emphasized in this chapter
- often large polar molecules are involved, which might be expected to have poor and unpredictable bioavailability.

But this does not mean to imply that existing information is without value. On the contrary, there are now many studies which can lead to a far better understanding of this topic than previously.

Before particular examples of the pharmacokinetics of plant constituents are discussed, it is worthwhile examining some of the key issues pertaining to bioavailability. The bioavailability of a molecule depends on several factors which determine how the molecule traverses the barrier of the gastrointestinal tract and survives into the bloodstream. These include:

Table 2.1 Effect of lipid solubility on bioavailability[303]

Cardiac glycoside	P	B%
g-Strophanthin	0.01	6.6
Convallatoxin	0.33	13.6
Digoxin	18.2	26.4
Digitoxin	70	74.9
Oleandrin	338	86.0

P = partition between water and octanol, an indication of fat solubility
B = bioavailability

- the pharmaceutical preparation;
- the size of the molecule – very large molecules still have some bioavailability (about 1% or less) which may be due to pinocytosis;
- the fat (lipid) solubility of the molecule – the more fat-soluble, the better the bioavailability (see Table 2.1 for examples of how fat solubility influences bioavailability for cardioactive glycosides);
- the water solubility of the molecule on a molecule is both water and fat soluble, it will exhibit very good bioavailability because it will dissolve in the digestive juices and then cross lipid membranes; otherwise, purely water-soluble molecules can be expected to have poor bioavailability. Ionization of the molecule usually means poor bioavailability;
- specific factors related to crossing the gut wall, e.g. active transport;
- factors within the gut – interaction with food, stability in the gut, gastric emptying;
- metabolism in the gut and first-pass metabolism by the liver;
- individual factors in the patient, including the influence of pathological factors.

Food is known to affect the bioavailability of conventional drugs (see Table 2.2 and 2.3 for examples). The presence or absence of food may also influence the absorption and bioavailability of plant constituents.

Grapefruit juice is a plant substance which can have a marked effect on bioavailability. For example, it increases the bioavailability of oral 17-beta-oestradiol and its metabolite oestrone.[305] Grapefruit juice also substantially increases the bioavailability of the following drugs: felopidine,[306] caffeine,[307] nifedipine and similar drugs,[308] cyclosporine[309] and triazolam[310] and similar drugs. The major interaction seems to be in the gut wall with enzymes belonging to various cytochrome P-450 subfamilies.[311] It also appears to inhibit renal 11-beta-hydroxysteroid dehydrogenase in humans and could therefore potentiate side effects from licorice.[312] Although the flavonoids naringin

Table 2.2 Drugs with absorption enhanced by food[304]

Drug	Mechanism
Carbamazepine	Increased bile production; enhanced dissolution and absorption
Diazepam	Food enhances enterohepatic recycling; increased dissolution secondary to gastric acid secretion
Griseofulvin	Drug is lipid soluble; enhanced absorption
Metoprolol	Food may reduce first-pass extraction and metabolism
Phenytoin	Delayed gastric emptying and increased bile production improve dissolution and absorption

Table 2.3 Drugs with absorption decreased by food[304]

Drug	Mechanism
Isoniazid	Food raises gastric pH preventing dissolution and absorption; also delayed gastric emptying
Captopril	Mechanism unknown
Chlorpromazine	Drug undergoes first-pass metabolism in gut; delayed gastric emptying affects bioavailability
Tetracyclines	Bind with calcium ions or iron salts forming insoluble chelates

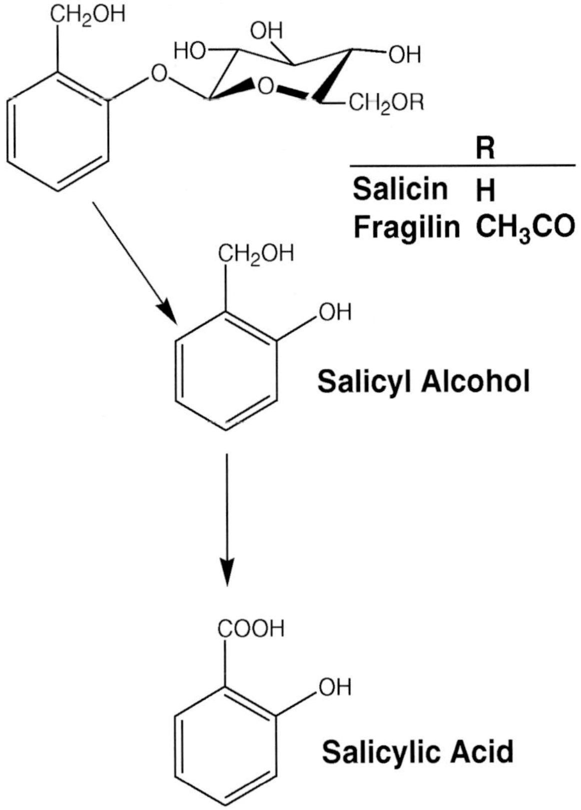

Figure 2.1 Salicin and its conversion products

and naringenin were at first implicated, they are probably not the only active components.[313,314] In fact, the furanocoumarin bergamottin and related compounds appear to be largely responsible for this activity.[315] This ability of plant furanocoumarins to inhibit drug-metabolizing enzymes was first noted by Korean researchers in 1983.[316] This phenomenon raises the question of how other plants and their phytochemicals may influence the bioavailability of both drugs and herbal constituents.

Bioavailability is also affected by the preparation used to deliver the dose of the medicine. This is an area of study which has largely been neglected for herbal medicines. However, some general statements about aqueous preparations such as infusions and decoctions can be proposed. Infusions and decoctions extract water-soluble compounds from plants. Many of these will have poor bioavailability. One important exception is plants containing essential oils and taken by infusion. Here the hot water acts almost as a distillation medium and the oil will collect on the surface of the water. However, the addition of saponin-containing herbs to the mixture will increase the solubility of compounds that are not as water-soluble, which may then have better bioavailability. This is often done in traditional Chinese medicine which relies heavily on aqueous preparations. Changes in water-soluble compounds in the digestive tract, most significantly the conversion of glycosides to aglycones in the caecum and large bowel, will render them more lipid soluble and they will be bioavailable as the aglycone. In general, however, bioavailability and solubility considerations suggest that infusions and decoctions are inferior preparations for extraction and delivery of herbal actives except where those actives are largely water soluble anyway such as some saponins, tannins, polysaccharides and proteins. However, only small quantities of these relatively large molecules will be absorbed as such (see later).

A good starting point in the study of herbal pharmacokinetics is those archetypal plant constituents which have been relatively well studied. The phenolic glycoside salicin and the anthraquinone glycosides are two such examples.

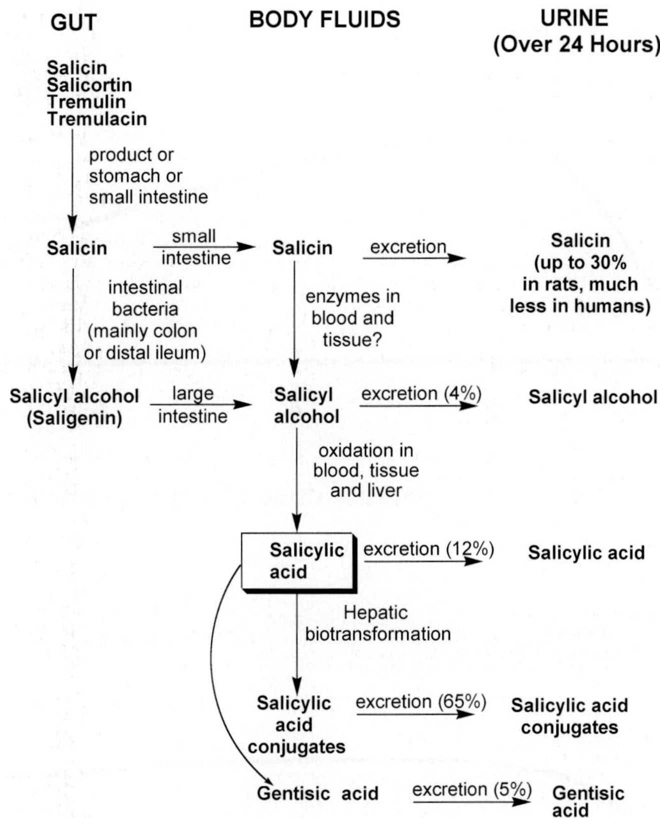

Figure 2.2 Pharmacokinetics of salicin and its derivatives[317,318]

SALICIN

Salicin and its conversion products are illustrated in Figure 2.1 and a schematic diagram of the pharmacokinetics of salicin is provided in Figure 2.2. As shown in Figure 2.2, salicin derivatives are first converted into salicin in the stomach or small intestine. The salicin may then be absorbed in the small intestine but in humans it is mainly carried to the distal ileum or colon where gut flora convert this glycoside into its aglycone, known as salicyl alcohol. The salicyl alcohol is absorbed and oxidized in the blood, tissue and liver to give salicylic acid, which is the main active form. The excretion of these various products is also outlined in Figure 2.2.

Despite the elaborate route by which salicin (and indeed willow bark) delivers salicylic acid into the bloodstream, the relative bioavailabilites of sodium salicylate and salicin are remarkably similar (Fig. 2.3). The curve for salicin is slightly lower and flatter, indicating a greater half-life. The rapid absorption of salicin as salicylic acid additionally implies that its conversion is also rapid, which suggests the distal ileum or caecum as the site of conversion rather than the large intestine (orocaecal transit time is about 1 hour).

At this point it is worth reflecting upon the traditional use of willow bark and the history of the development of aspirin. When scientists in the 19th century began to investigate the antipyretic and antiinflammatory effects of willow bark, their crude extraction techniques isolated salicylic acid, not salicin, from the bark. Salicylic acid was adopted into mainstream therapy but had the drawback of being a strong irritant to the stomach. This led to the development of aspirin, a derivative of salicylic acid, in an attempt to minimize this gastric irritation. (Unfortunately aspirin was still a gastric irritant, but it was vastly more active than salicylic acid as an analgesic and antiplatelet agent). Had the early scientists studied salicin instead, they might have recognized that nature had already designed a derivative of salicylic acid which gave a

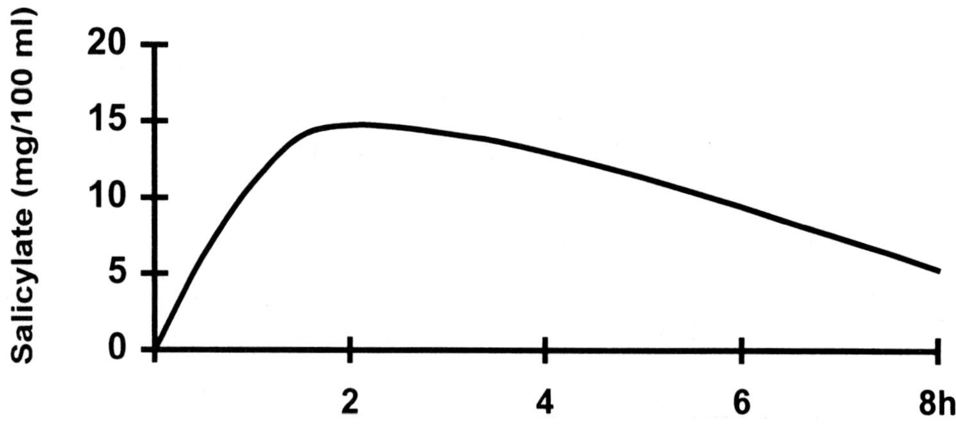

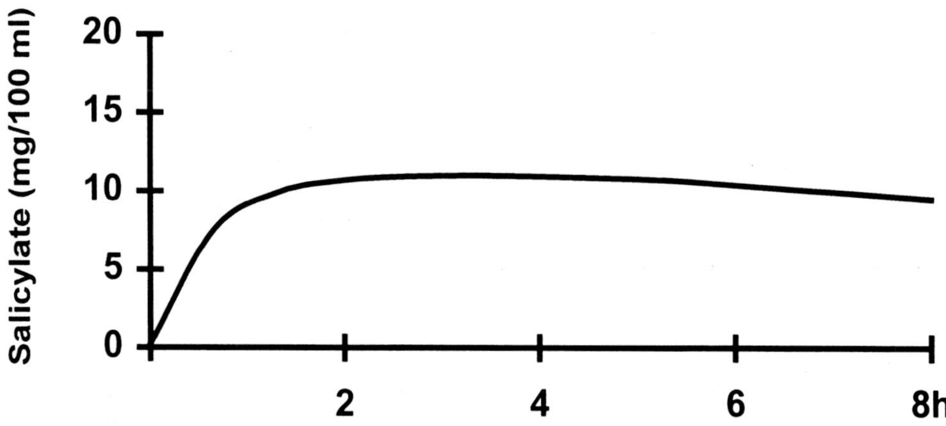

Figure 2.3 Relative bioavailabilities of salicin and salicylic acid (doses are approximately equivalent)[317]

good yield of bioavailable salicylic acid and was also kind to the stomach.

ANTHRAQUINONE GLYCOSIDES

Early research on the laxative properties of anthraquinones and their glycosides baffled researchers. When equivalent doses were used, only the glycosides were active orally, not their aglycones. However, when equivalent doses were administered by injection, the reverse situation applied: the aglycones were more active. Equally baffling was the observation that oral doses of the anthraquinone glycosides took 6–8 hours to exert their laxative effect and that the effective dose for laxation often varied dramatically from person to person.

Modern understanding of the pharmacokinetics of anthraquinone glycosides provides a simple explanation for these paradoxical observations. This is illustrated schematically in Figure 2.4.

As anthraquinone glycosides pass through the digestive tract, a significant proportion undergoes polymerization to inactive polymers. Any remaining glycoside is unchanged and unabsorbed until it

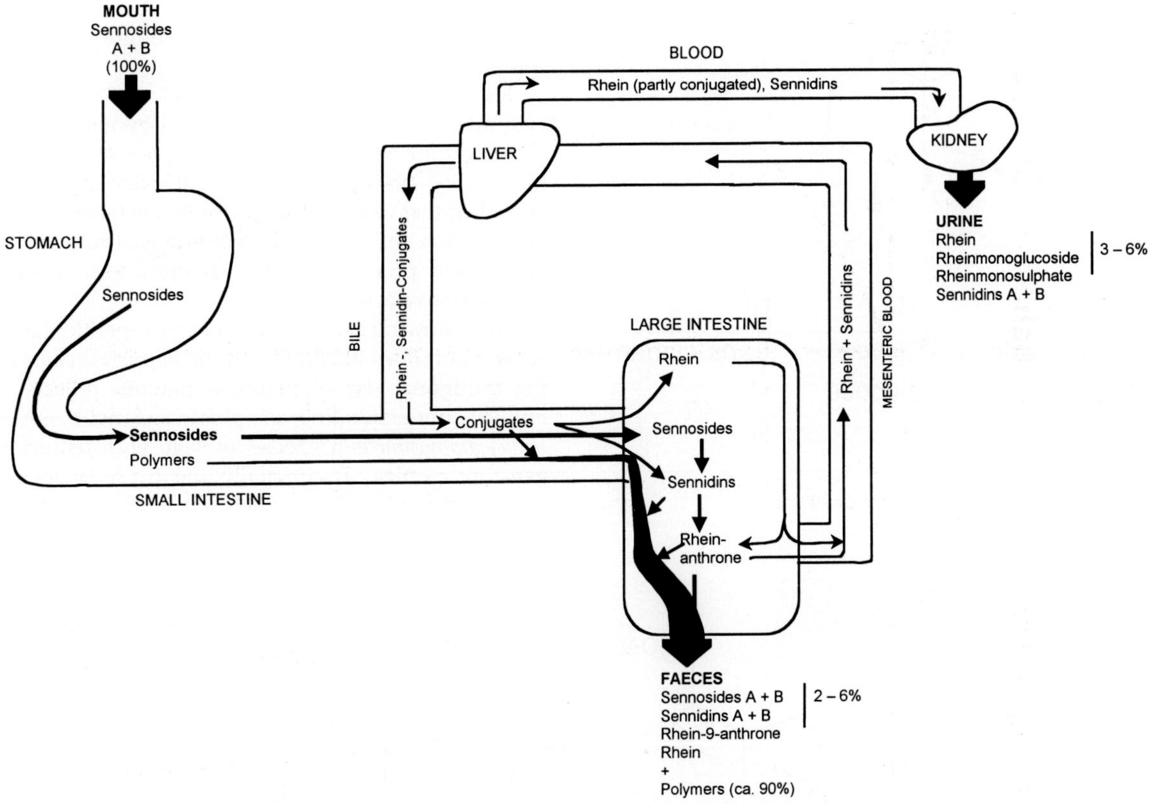

Figure 2.4 Pharmacokinetics of sennosides[319]

reaches the large intestine. There the action of certain bowel flora convert the glycosides into their anthrone aglycones and it is these active aglycones which then exert a laxative action in situ in the colon.[319]

Hence, the anthraquinone glycoside given by injection exerts less activity, because this is not the active form. On the other hand, the aglycone given orally also exerts little activity because it is broken down or absorbed before it reaches the colon. (Some modern laxative drugs are anthrone aglycones but they are administered orally in quite high doses). The 6–8 hour lag-time for activity reflects the time it takes for ingested anthraquinone glycosides to reach the appropriate part of the colon for conversion to aglycones.

We can only wonder at this elegant and, when one considers the quantities of liberated anthrone aglycone involved, exquisitely sensitive mechanism designed by nature. One inference from this example is that the composition of an individual's bowel flora is highly relevant to the pharmacokinetic equation and hence to the final pharmacological effect.[319] This is a common theme for several of the archetypal plant constituents and emphasizes the herbalist's obsession with the health of the gut, not just as the central focus for restoring robust health but also for delivering effective therapy.

GLYCOSIDES AND GASTRIC MODIFICATION

A number of plant glycosides are modified by the action of gastric acid or the alkaline conditions of the duodenum. The following examples and their implications serve to illustrate this phenomenon.

Harpagoside from devil's claw (*Harpagophytum procumbens*) has oral antiinflammatory activity (Fig. 2.5). However, when it is incubated with gastric acid, which generates harpagogenin from harpagoside, it loses this activity in oral dose models.[320] While harpagoside may not be the final bioavailable form, this research suggests that the action of gastric acid is detrimental to the antiinflammatory activity of devil's claw. Preparations of this herb should be

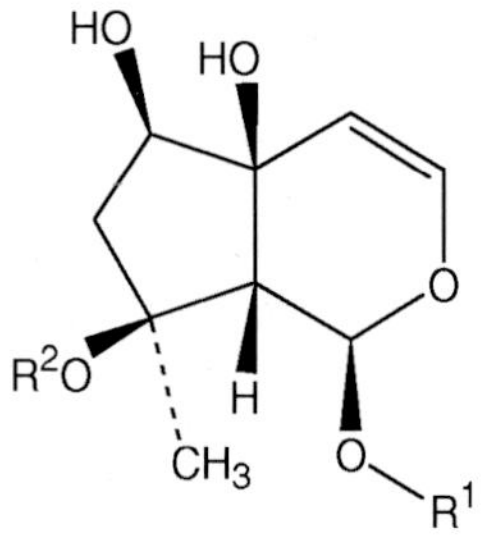

	R	R^2
Harpagoside	glucose	trans-cinnamoyl
Harpagide	glucose	H
Harpagogenin	H	H

Figure 2.5 Harpagoside from devil's claw.

enterically coated or at least taken between meals to optimize the bioavailability of antiinflammatory components.

The valepotriates (Fig. 2.6) of valcrian havc cytotoxic activity when administered by injection but do not exhibit this effect after oral doses. This initially raised concerns about the safety of valerian but it is now clear that valepotriates are quite unstable in aqueous solution and are decomposed by gastric acid. The breakdown products of the valepotriates still have some sedative activity.[321]

The following example is not of therapeutic significance but it does illustrate that the empirical basis for the traditional use of plants sometimes reflects an implicit understanding of pharmacokinetic issues. *Salvia divinorum* is a species of sage with hallucinogenic properties. Traditionally the fresh leaves are chewed for this effect, which led to the belief that

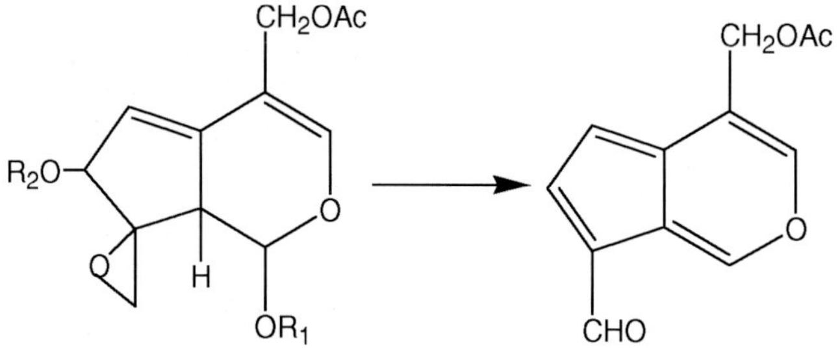

R_1	R_2	
Aiv	Iv	1-Acevaltrate
Iv	Iv	Valtrate

Baldrinal

Ac	CH_3CO-	Acetyl
Iv	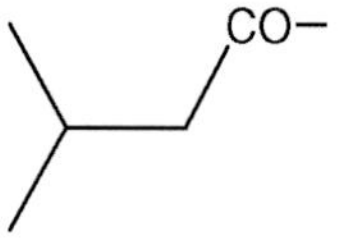	Isovaleryl
Aiv	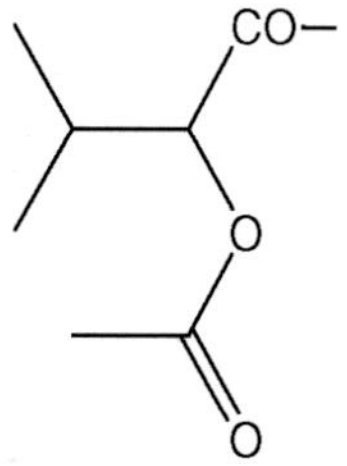	Acetoxyisovaleryl

Figure 2.6 Valepotriates from valerian

the hallucinogenic component(s) were inactivated by drying the herb. Recent research has revealed that this is not the case. The active hallucinogenic component in *Salvia divinorum* is salvinorin A (Fig. 2.7).[322] This is converted by gastric acid into salvinorin B which is inactive. Hence the chewing of leaves by the shamans was in fact a delivery mechanism for salvinorin A which bypassed decomposition in the stomach. That hallucinogenic quantities of salvinorin A can be absorbed through the oral mucosa underlines the potent activity of this compound.

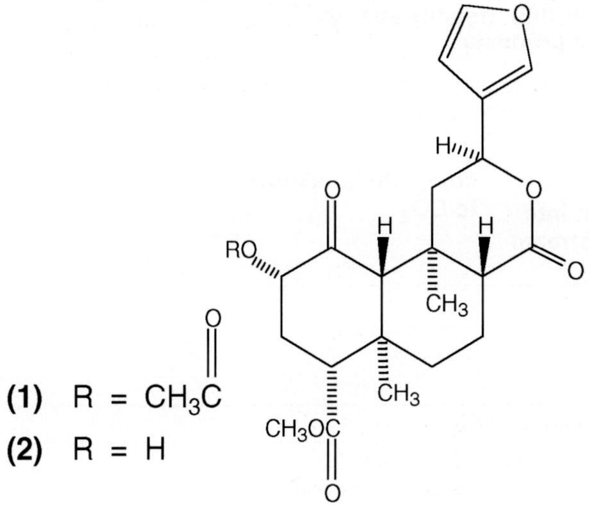

(1) R = CH_3C(=O)

(2) R = H

Figure 2.7 Salvinorins A (1) and B (2) isolated from *S. divinorum*

FLAVONOID GLYCOSIDES AND ENTERIC MODIFICATION

Flavonoid glycosides are a common component of many plants and are a significant class of archetypal plant constituents with pharmacological activity. However, in vitro models dominate the pharmacodynamic research on flavonoids and their glycosides. This is of concern because an understanding has existed for some time (and has been recently confirmed) that flavonoids often have poor bioavailability as such because they are largely decomposed by bowel flora.

Studies have shown that flavonoid-O-glycosides are converted into the aglycone by bowel flora. But the decomposition can extend further than this; the aglycones undergo further breakdown by a process known as C-ring fission (the C-ring is the central ring in the flavonoid structure) to give two different phenolic products. An example of C-ring fission is illustrated in Figure 2.8. The ring fission products for several common flavonoids, flavonoid glycosides and related products are summarized in Table 2.4 and a general scheme for the pharmacokinetics of flavonoid glycosides is outlined in Figure 2.9.

Studies have also shown the following.

- Oral doses of flavonoid aglycones are less bioavailable (as the flavonoid) than their glycosides because they are more susceptible to ring fission.
- Levels of a flavonoid aglycone in the bloodstream will vary according to:

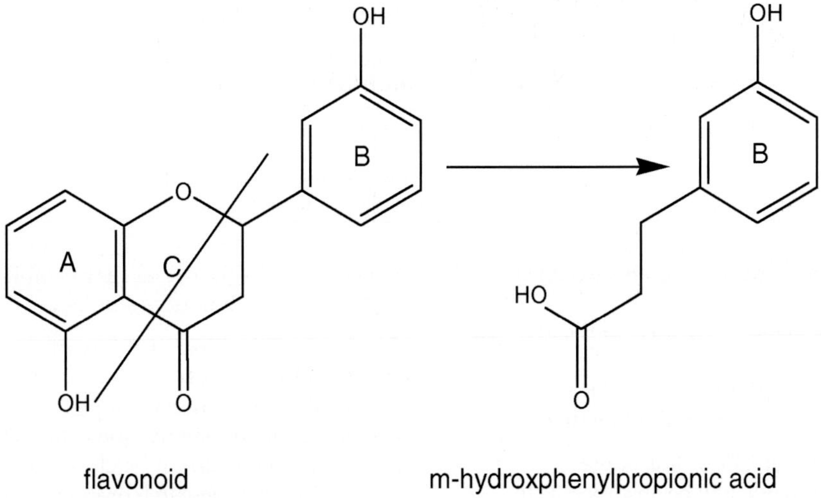

flavonoid → m-hydroxphenylpropionic acid

Figure 2.8 An example of C-ring fission.

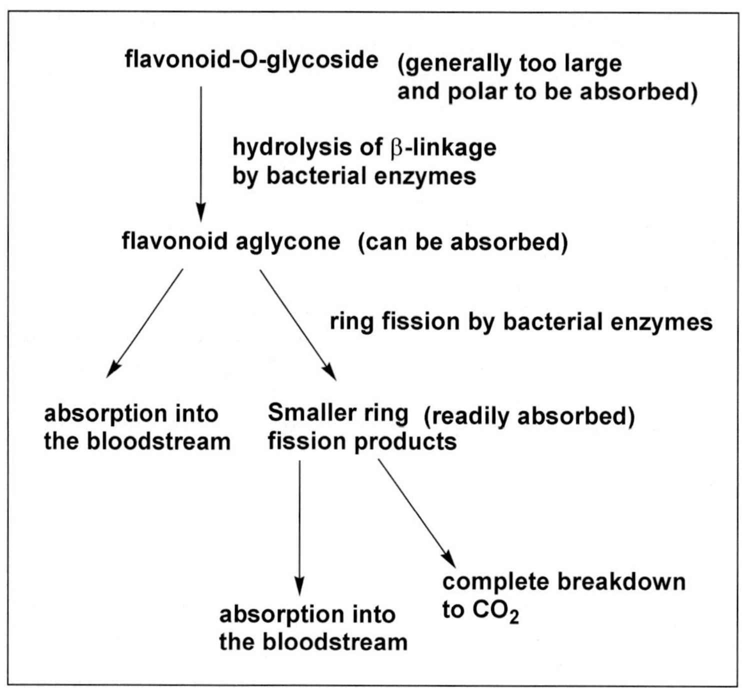

Figure 2.9 Pharmacokinetics of flavonoid glycosides

Table 2.4 Flavonoid ring fission metabolites[323]

Flavonoid administered	Ring fission products
Quercetin, rutin	3,4-dihydroxyphenylacetic acid, 3-methoxy-4-hydroxyphenylacetic acid, *m*-hydroxyphenylacetic acid
Hesperidin, diosmin, eriodictyol, homoeriodictyol	*m*-hydroxyphenylpropionic acid, *m*-coumaric acid (rat), 3-hydroxy-4-methoxyphenyl-hydracrylic acid (human)
(+)-Catechin	delta-(hydroxyphenyl)-gamma-valerolactones *m*-hydroxyphenylpropionic acid, *m*-hydroxybenzoic acid, *m*-hydroxyhippuric acid
Kaempferol	delta-(*p*-hydroxyphenyl)-gamma-valerolactone *p*-hydroxyphenylacetic acid
Myricetin, myricitrin	3,5-dihydroxyphenylacetic acid, *m*-hydroxyphenylacetic acid
Tricetin, tricin	3,5-dihydroxyphenylpropionic acid, *m*-hydroxyphenylpropionic acid

1. whether it is administered as an aglycone or glycoside;
2. if given as a glycoside, the form of the glycosidic prodrug;
3. the nature of the individual bowel flora, which is partly dependent on the individual diet.

- Generally only about 20% or less of the administered glycoside will be absorbed as the intact aglycone.
- Flavonoid C-glycosides may exhibit similar mechanisms, but more studies are needed.

The issue of the bioavailability of the flavonoid aglycone quercetin serves to illustrate many of these issues. Many nutritional supplement companies market products containing quercetin. The rationale for including quercetin in such products is generally based on in vitro research or in vivo models following dosage by injection. However, the general consensus of studies is that the bioavailability of quercetin (as quercetin) is poor. This is due to its propensity to rapidly undergo C-ring fission. Following the Zutphen Elderly Study and the Netherlands Cohort Study, both conducted in The Netherlands, where flavonol and flavone dietary intake were inversely associated with mortality from coronary heart disease and risk of stroke, Dutch researchers have once again studied quercetin bioavailability.[324] Conclusions from their first study on ileostomy patients were uncertain because they did not measure quercetin in the bloodstream.[325] It was assumed that because of the ileostomy, any unrecovered quercetin was absorbed. But significant microbial degradation could also have occurred. This is supported by the minimal level of quercetin (0.5% of original dose) found in subjects' urine. Their second study on onions (a source of quercetin glycosides) did measure plasma quercetin concentrations.[326] Following intake of the equivalent of 215 g raw yellow onions in two subjects, a mean peak plasma concentration of 196 ng/ml (approx. 0.6 μM) was reached after 2.9 hours. The elimination half-life was slow at about 17 hours, suggesting possible enterohepatic recirculation. This concentration probably only represents a small proportion, say 5% or less, of the administered dose.

A recent study on C-ring fission products of quercetin found that 3,4-dihydroxyphenylacetic acid possessed significant antioxidant activity.[327] Future pharmacodynamic research on flavonoids should include more studies on C-ring fission products, which in many instances are probably the true bioavailable and active form of this important group of archetypal plant constituents.

ISOFLAVONES

The isoflavones are a group of archetypal plant constituents attracting increasing attention because of their affinity for oestrogen receptors. The principal isoflavones are the glycosides genistin and daidzin and their aglycones genistein and daidzein, from the soya plant, and the aglycones formononetin and biochanin A from red clover (*Trifolium pratense*) (see Fig. 2.10). Formononetin can be converted to daidzein which in turn can be metabolized to equol by bowel flora. This is a significant reaction pathway from a pharmacodynamic perspective, because equol has substantially more oestrogenic activity than its precursors. However, equol appears to be produced to different degrees in different people. Table 2.5 illustrates that individuals can be grouped into high and low equol producers. The high equol producers are likely to experience significantly greater oestrogenic effects from the consumption of soya or red clover.

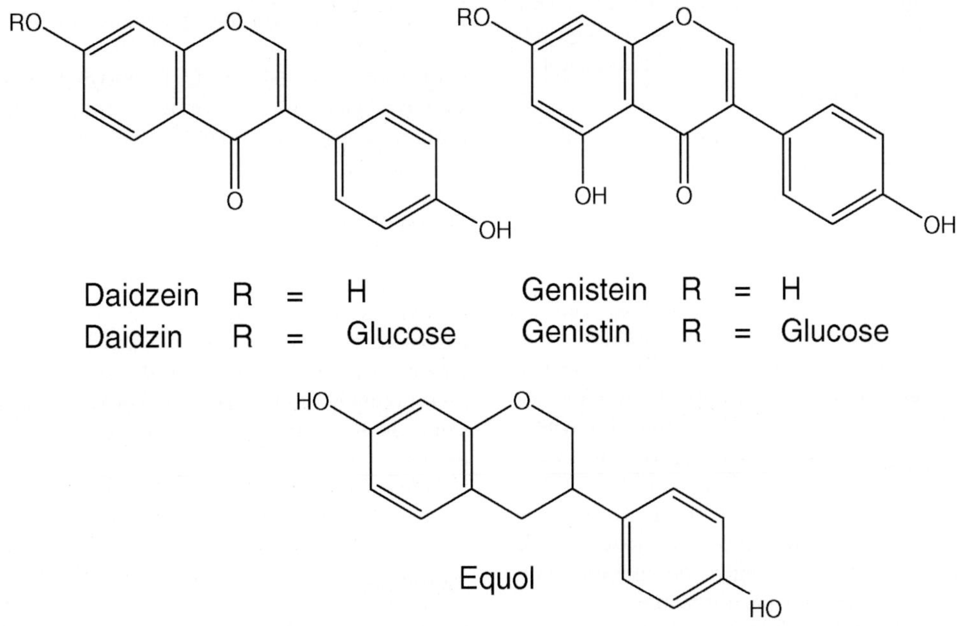

Daidzein R = H
Daidzin R = Glucose

Genistein R = H
Genistin R = Glucose

Equol

Figure 2.10 Major isoflavones and equol

Table 2.5 Comparison of the urinary excretion rates of daidzein and two daidzein[328] metabolites in individuals over a 3-day period following soya challenge[a]

Metabolite	Mean (SD) excretion (μmol) per 3 days	
	<8 μmol equol (n = 8)	>25 μmol equol (n = 4)
Daidzein	23.05 (12.43)	14.95 (6.69)
Equol	1.53 (2.60)	64.89 (59.23)
O-Dma	21.72 (17.93)	6.97 (6.47)

[a]*Individuals are grouped as either low equol producers (less than 8 μmol in 3 days) or high equol producers (over 25 μmol in 3 days)*
Note: Equol is substantially more oestrogenic than daidzein or O-Dma

Other studies have found the following.

- Soya isoflavones are 85% degraded in the intestine.[329]
- Differences in faecal flora account for the differing metabolism of soya isoflavones.[330]
- Faecal flora could completely degrade genistein and daidzein.[330]
- Differences in faecal excretion of isoflavones profoundly altered isoflavone bioavailability: higher faecal excretion is correlated with higher bioavailability. Such subjects may have fewer bacteria which degrade isoflavones, leaving more intact for absorption.[327] Bioavailability varied from 13% to 35% depending on the individual gut microflora.[330]
- Soya protein (containing isoflavone glycosides) increased follicular phase length in women, while miso (containing isoflavone aglycones) did not.[331] This suggests that the glycosidic group delays the degradation of isoflavones, resulting in higher bioavailability of their aglycones or equol.

These studies again serve to emphasize the importance of bowel flora in determining bioavailability and hence pharmacodynamic activity.

SAPONINS

If saponins have good fat solubility they can be absorbed unchanged in significant quantities in the small intestine. This is the case for many cardiac glycosides, a related chemical group. If saponins are not absorbed they will pass to the large intestine where gut flora will convert them to the sapogenin (aglycone). The aglycone usually has better lipid solubility and will be absorbed to some extent. Hence in these cases saponin is a prodrug. Since the bioactivity of saponins may be due to their aglycone, extrapolation of in vitro results for saponins is unreliable.

Glycyrrhizin (GL) is a triterpenoid saponin which has hepatoprotective activity in vitro and by injection. It also has antiviral activity, even against HIV-1. This has led to suggestions that oral doses of licorice can be used as a systemic antiviral treatment or for hepatoprotective activity. Pharmacokinetic experiments with licorice or GL have shown that the aglycone glycyrrhetinic acid (GA) is the predominant form absorbed into the bloodstream after oral doses.[332,333] GL is converted to GA by human intestinal flora.[334] Some GL may be absorbed, although this could be recycled GA-glucuronide being misread as GL on chromatograms.[332,335] So licorice may possess antiviral activity after oral doses but as the GA-glucuronide. Ironically GA has recently been shown to be more hepatoprotective than GL,[336] so licorice may also prove to be a valuable hepatoprotective herb (this awaits clinical confirmation for oral doses). Other triterpenoid saponins appear to follow a similar pathway, for example the ginsenosides.[337]

Some studies on the bioavailability of steroidal saponins have also been published. Ruscus extract (1 g) containing 60 mg degluconeoruscin and other steroidal saponins was orally administered to three human volunteers.[338] Plasma analysis showed significant absorption: degluconeoruscin concentrations peaked at about 2 mg/ml after about 90 minutes. Some steroidal saponins may therefore show good bioavailability (this work does need to be repeated). However, others probably follow the same pattern as glycyrrhizin; the aglycone is the absorbed form. This is supported by extensive historical work on cardioactive glycosides which shows that some glycosides such as digitoxin are quantitatively absorbed (the oral dose of digitoxin is the same as the intravenous dose) and that digoxin is excreted largely unchanged in the urine. In contrast, ouabain (from Strophanthus) has poor and erratic oral absorption and is now only given by injection.

TANNINS

Because of their large size, their high affinity to bond with proteins and poor lipid solubility, tannins have

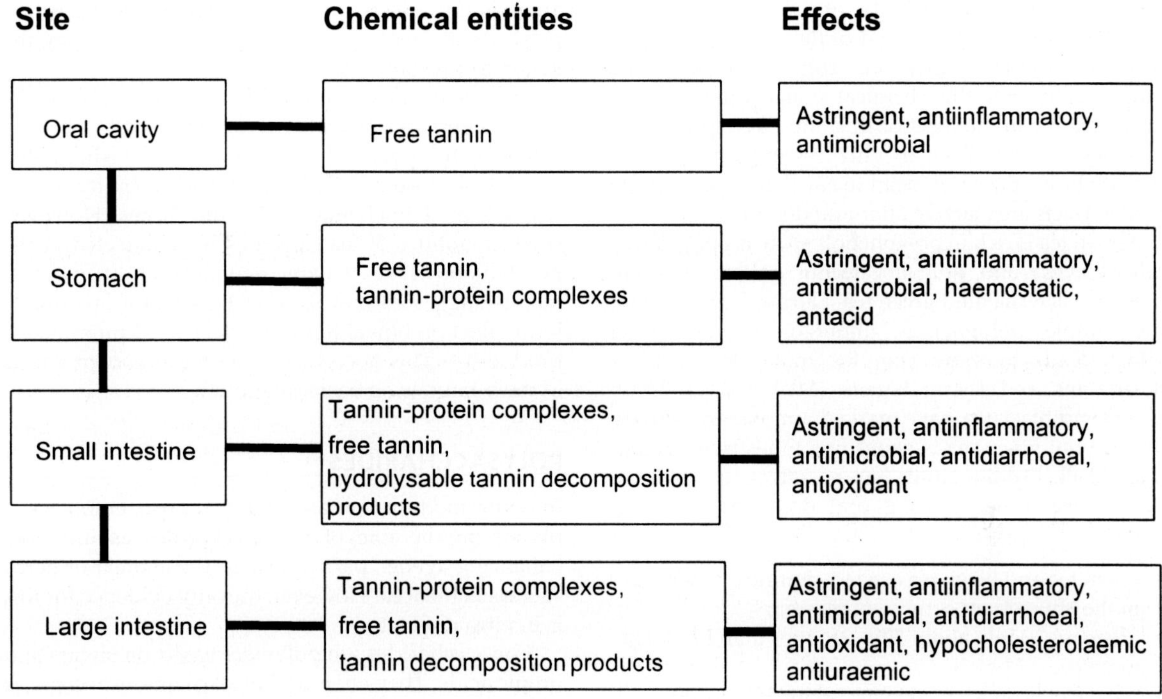

Figure 2.11 The 'lifecycle' of a tannin through the gut.

negligible bioavailability as such. Hence the activity of tannins (and the herbs which contain them) should be explained in terms of local effects. This poor bioavailability of intact tannins is important, since hydrolysable tannins absorbed into the bloodstream cause hepatotoxicity. Many common herbs would be poisonous if tannins were highly bioavailable. Also tannins injected subcutaneously cause cancers, so it is also fortunate that they do not penetrate the skin. Breakdown products of tannins which are produced in the large bowel by bowel flora (and perhaps spontaneously in the small intestine in the case of hydrolysable tannins) are absorbed and probably explain many of the modern uses of tannin and oligomeric procyanidin (OPC)-containing herbs, e.g. as antioxidants.

In vitro experiments found that ellagic acid was liberated from condensed tannins at pH 7–8 (not at pH 2) and also by microflora when in contact with caecum contents (ellagic acid has antioxidant and anticancer properties).[339] About 95% of orally administered tannic acid is decomposed (as assessed by faecal excretion).[340] Tannic acid is a hydrolysable tannin which probably releases gallic acid and other compounds on decomposition. Condensed tannins and green tea polyphenols show more complex decomposition patterns but microflora again produce smaller bioavailable phenolic compounds.[341]

The probable behaviour of tannins as they pass through the digestive tract is summarized in Figure 2.11. Apart from antioxidant activity, which can be a systemic effect mainly from the decomposition products of tannins, all the other possible effects are due to local activity at the designated site. Remote astringency and antihaemorrhagic properties sometimes attributed to tannin-containing herbs must be in doubt (in other words, tannins given orally will not, for example, astringe lung tissue or staunch uterine bleeding).

As stated earlier, OPC are a part of the archetypal group known as condensed tannins. Products high in OPC such as pine bark and grape seed extract, sometimes known as pycnogenol, have enjoyed enormous popularity recently as antioxidants and even cure-alls. Much of this popularity is based on the work of the French scientist Masquelier and one feature of this work is the reputed high bioavailability of OPC which are even said to cross the blood–brain barrier.

Masquelier conducted pharmacokinetic studies on OPC using radioactively labelled compounds. On the basis of these studies, he concluded that OPC have good bioavailability and cross the blood–brain barrier.

However, the bioavailability of OPC observed by Masquelier was probably that of their smaller decomposition products, since his study only measured radioactivity, not the chemical entity carrying that radioactivity. In the light of this, the many properties assigned to OPC from in vitro research need to be revisited (this does not mean to say that pine or grape seed extracts are inactive after oral doses).

Green tea is rich in polyphenols such as epigallocatechin (EGC) and epigallocatechin gallate (EGCG). Black tea is fermented green tea. During fermentation, the simple polyphenols undergo polymerization which leads to more complex molecules such as theaflavins and therarubigens (MW 500 to 3000). Green and black tea have marked antioxidant activity in vitro but green tea is about five times more potent than black. Adding milk has no effect. In contrast, human experiments using oral doses have shown that:[342]

- green tea and black tea cause a significant increase in the antioxidant activity of plasma;
- green tea is only about 50% stronger than black tea in vivo;
- the effect is rapid, peaking at about 30 minutes after consumption for green tea and 50 minutes for black tea;
- adding milk completely destroys this effect.

One possible explanation is that the tea polyphenols undergo spontaneous decomposition in the gut and the smaller antioxidant molecules are then absorbed. This would explain the similar activities of green and black tea in vivo. Adding milk causes protein binding which would inhibit this decomposition. This implies that only tea without milk will render significant antioxidant activity in the bloodstream. However, this study did not monitor plasma antioxidant activity after more than a few hours. It is possible that the tannin-protein complexes formed after milk is added are decomposed further down in the gut and bacterial action on the liberated tannins (or just spontaneous breakdown) leads to absorption of antioxidant phenolics from the colon into the bloodstream.

Another possible explanation is that the observed antioxidant effects in plasma were due to absorption of unchanged tea phenolics. Both EGC and EGCG were detected in the plasma of healthy human volunteers 90 minutes after they consumed capsules containing green tea extract.[343] However, as might be expected for such large polar molecules, levels detected corresponded to only 0.2–2.0% of the ingested amount. It still remains to be established if these amounts are sufficient to confer significant antioxidant effects or whether the decomposition products of green tea polyphenolics instead play the major antioxidant role.

Studies on EGCG found that it was stable in the upper digestive tract but was decomposed to a certain extent by bacteria in the large intestine.[344] About 40% of a 50 mg dose of EGCG administered orally to rats was excreted unchanged with the faeces. However, small quantities of tea catechins were detected in the portal blood of rats.[345] Other animal and human experiments suggested that tea catechins had a favourable local effect on bowel flora and decreased putrefactive products.[344] This is consistent with the known effects of these tannins on bacterial growth.

POLYSACCHARIDES

In some modern herbal literature, great emphasis is placed on the role of polysaccharides as immune-enhancing agents, particularly in the context of herbs such as Echinacea. However, the only evidence for this is in vitro research.

Polysaccharides are polymers based on sugars and uronic acids. They are found in all plants, especially as a component of the cell wall. However, some plants particularly accumulate polysaccharides. Any herbal extract prepared in 50% ethanol or stronger will not contain significant quantities of polysaccharides because of their insolubility in ethanol. Since they are large water-soluble molecules, which may even carry an ionic charge, polysaccharides will have low (but not zero) bioavailability. Pharmacokinetic considerations therefore dictate that if a herb is to be used as a source of polysaccharides it must be rich in these compounds, be prepared in a way to preserve or extract the polysaccharides and be administered in sufficient doses to compensate for the poor bioavailability. Such considerations will only apply in special cases and probably do not apply for oral doses of any Echinacea preparation. Unabsorbed polysaccharides pass into the large intestine where they are broken down by bowel flora (and may have an effect on flora balance).

Whole-leaf *Aloe vera* preparations appear to be one good source of active polysaccharides, provided they are prepared to contain high levels of acemannan (about 1%). Acemannan is a polysaccharide found under the skin in *Aloe vera* leaves and is often not present in aloe gel or juice preparations because the outer leaf is not incorporated or enzymes used during manufacture have destroyed the acemannan. Doses of 50–100 ml per day of this concentrate can provide significant doses of acemannan. In a little-known, open, uncontrolled clinical study, 29 AIDS patients received *Aloe vera* whole-leaf juice, essential fatty acids and nutrients.[346] The aloe dose was the equivalent of 1200 mg per day of acemannan. Karnofsky scores improved in 100% of these patients after 180 days. Although this study had many design flaws, it does suggest that this type of preparation as a source of polysaccharides is worthy of further study. Other potentially rich sources of polysaccharides include the various mushroom species such as Ganoderma and Lentinus.

OPTIMIZING EFFICACY

It should be clear from the above discussion that a knowledge of factors influencing bioavailability can lead to the more effective use of herbal medicines. In particular, the bowel flora characteristics which can optimize the efficacy of many herbal treatments need to be better understood. This bowel factor probably underlines the importance of a wholesome diet and adequate fibre intake, which will lead to healthy bowel flora. Other issues which should be considered in the context of optimizing efficacy include the following.

- Relationship to meals:
  1. polyphenolics should be taken away from meals because of their interaction with protein;
  2. components relying on gastric acid hydrolysis should be taken with meals;
  3. components damaged by gastric acid should be taken away from meals.
- Saponins can be used to improve absorption and/or solubilization.
- Some foods can be used to inhibit gut biotransformation, e.g. grapefruit juice.
- The frequency of dosage should be based on bioavailability and metabolism.

References

1. Munson PL, Muller RA, Beese GR. Principles of pharmacology. Basic concepts and clinical applications. Chapman and Hall, New York, 1995, pp 1–5.
2. Baker ME. Endocrine activity of plant-derived compounds: an evolutionary perspective. Proceedings of the Society for Experimental Biology and Medicine 1995; 208: 131–138.
3. Eder M, Mehnert W. Bedeutung pflanzlicher Begleitstoffe in Extrakten. Pharmazie 1998; 53 (5): 285–293.
4. Keung W, Lazo O, Kunze L et al. Potentiation of the bioavailability of daidzin by an extract of Radix puerariae. Proceedings of the National Academy of Science USA 1996; 93: 4284–4288.
5. Vinson JA, Bose PB. Comparative bioavailability to humans of ascorbic acid alone or in a citrus extract. American Journal of Clinical Nutrition 1988; 48: 601–604.
6. Butterweck V, Petereit F, Winterhoff H et al. Solubilized hypericin and pseudohypericin from Hypericum perforatum exert antidepressant activity in the forced swimming test. Planta Medica 1998; 64: 291–294.
7. Onawunmi GO, Yisak W, Ogunlana EO. Antibacterial constituents in the essential oil of Cymbopogon citratus (DC.) Stapf. Journal of Ethnopharmacology 1984; 12: 279–286.
8. Kisa K, Sasaki K, Yamauchi K et al. Potentiating effect of sennoside C on purgative activity of sennoside A in mice. Planta Medica 1981; 42: 302–312.
9. Castells E, Penuelas J. Towards a global theory of chemical defense: the case of alkaloids (French). Orsis 1997; 12: 141–161.
10. Oleszek W. Glucosinolates: occurrence and ecological significance (Polish). Wiadomosci Botaniczne 1995; 39 (1–2): 49–58.
11. Laks PE. Wood preservation as trees do it. Scottish Forestry 1991; 45 (4): 275–284.
12. Bennett RN, Wallsgrove RM. Tansley review no 72: secondary metabolites in plant defence mechanisms. New Phytologist 1994; 127 (4): 617–633.
13. Dixon RA, Lamb CJ, Masoud S et al. Metabolic engineering: prospects for crop improvement through the genetic manipulation of phenylpropanoid biosynthesis and defense responses: a review. Gene 1996; 179 (1): 61–71.
14. Inderijt. Plant phenolics in allelopathy. Botanical Review 1996; 62 (2): 186–202.
15. Langenheim HJ. Higher plant terpenoids: a phytocentric overview of their ecological roles. Journal of Chemical Ecology 1994; 20 (6): 1223–1280.
16. Callaway R. Positive interactions among plants. Botanical Review 1995; 61 (4): 306–349.
17. Patroni C. Aspirin as an antiplatelet drug. New England Journal of Medicine 1994; 330 (18): 1287–1294.
18. Wu C, Hsieh M, Huang S et al. Effects of Gastrodia elata and its active constituents on scopolamine-induced amnesia in rats. Planta Medica 1996; 62: 317–321.
19. Lamba S, Buch K, Lewis H III. Potential antisickling agents: activated ester derivatives of hydroxybenzoic acid. Planta Medica 1990; 56: 681
20. Lamaison JL, Petitjean-Freyet C, Carnat A. Lamiacées médicinales à propriétés antioxydantes, sources potentielles d'acide rosmarinique. Pharmaceutica Acta Helvetica 1991; 66 (7): 185–188.
21. Auf'mkolk M, Amir SM, Kubota K et al. The active principles of plant extracts with antithyrotropic activity: oxidation products of derivatives of 3, 4-dihydroxycinnamic acid. Endocrinology 1985; 116 (5): 1677.
22. Chlabicz J, Galasinski W. The components of Melissa officinalis L. that influence protein biosynthesis in-vitro. Journal of Pharmacy and Pharmacology 1986; 38 (11): 791–794.
23. Miller KW, Anderson JL, Stoewsand GS. Amygdalin metabolism and effect on reproduction of rats fed apricot kernels. Journal of Toxicology and Environmental Health 1981; 7 (3–4): 457–467.
24. Moertel CG, Ames MM, Kovach JS et al. A pharmacologic and toxicological study of amygdalin. Journal of the American Medical Association 1981; 245 (6): 591–594.
25. Adewusi SR, Oke OL. On the metabolism of amygdalin. 1. The LD50 and biochemical changes in rats. Canadian Journal of Physiology and Pharmacology 1985; 63 (9): 1080–1083.
26. Fenselau C, Pallante S, Batzinger RP et al. Mandelonitrile beta-glucuronide: synthesis and characterization. Science 1977; 198 (4317): 625–627.
27. Dorr RT, Paxinos J. The current status of laetrile. Annals of Internal Medicine 1978; 89 (3): 389–397.
28. Hill GJ 2nd, Shine TE, Hill HZ et al. Failure of amygdalin to arrest B16 melanoma and BW5147 AKR leukemia. Cancer Research 1976; 36 (6): 2102–2107.

29. Moertel CG, Fleming TR, Rubin J et al. A clinical trial of amygdalin (Laetrile) in the treatment of human cancer. New England Journal of Medicine 1982; 306 (4): 201–206.
30. Hill HZ, Backer R, Hill GJ 2nd. Blood cyanide levels in mice after administration of amygdalin. Biopharmaceutics and Drug Disposition 1980; 1 (4): 211–220.
31. Syrigos KN, Rowlinson-Busza G, Epenetos AA. In vitro cytotoxicity following specific activation of amygdalin by beta-glucosidase conjugated to a bladder cancer-associated monoclonal antibody. International Journal of Cancer 1998; 78 (6): 712–719.
32. Obolentseva GV, Khadzhai YaI, Vidyukova AI et al. Effect of some natural substances on ulceration of the rat stomach caused by acetylsalicylic acid. Bulletin of Experimental Biology and Medicine 1974; 77: 256–257.
33. Rafatullah S, Al-Yahya MA, Al-Said MS et al. Gastric anti-ulcer and cytoprotective effects of Cyamopsis tetragonolaba ('Guar') in rats. International Journal of Pharmacognosy 1994; 32 (2): 163–170.
34. Blackburn NA, Johnson IT. The influence of guar gum on the movements of insulin, glucose and fluid in rat intestine during perfusion in vivo. Pflügers Archiv 1983; 397: 144–148.
35. Morcos SR, El-Baradie AA. Fenugreek mucilage and its relation to the reputed laxative action of this seed. Egyptian Journal of Chemistry 1959; 2 (1): 163–168.
36. Stevens J, Levitsky DA, Van Soest PJ et al. Effect of psyllium gum and wheat bran on spontaneous energy intake. American Journal of Clinical Nutrition 1987; 46: 812–817.
37. Voinchet O, Mouchet A. Obstruction de l'oesophage par mucilage. La Nouvelle Presse Médicale 1974; 3 (19): 1223–1225.
38. Nosalova G, Strapkova A, Kardosova A et al. Antitussive Wirkung des Extraktes und der Polysaccharide aus Eibisch (Althaea officinalis L., var. robusta). Pharmazie 1992; 47: 224–226.
39. Roberts DCK, Truswell AS, Bencke A et al. The cholesterol-lowering effect of a breakfast cereal containing psyllium fibre. Medical Journal of Australia 1994; 161: 660–664.
40. Leeds AR. Psyllium – a superior source of soluble dietary fibre. Food Australia 1995; 47 (2) (supp): S2–S4.
41. Frati-Munari AC, Flores-Garduno MA, Ariza-Andraca R et al. Effect of different doses of Plantago psyllium mucilage on the glucose tolerance test. Archives of Investigative Medicine (Mexico) 1989; 20 (2): 147–152.
42. Lis-Balchin M, Deans SG, Eaglesham E. Relationship between bioactivity and chemical composition of commercial essential oils. Flavour and Fragrance Journal 1998; 13: 98–104.
43. Römmelt H, Zuber A, Dirnagl K et al. Zur Resorption von Terpenen aus Badezusätzen. Munchener Medizinische Wochenschrift 1974; 116 (11): 537–540.
44. Bone K. Report on the 24th International Symposium on Essential Oils, Berlin 1993. MediHerb Monitor 1993; 7: 1–4.
45. Janssen AM, Scheffer JJC, Baerheim Svendsen A. Antimicrobial activity of essential oils: a 1976–1986 literature review. Aspects of the test methods. Planta Medica 1987; 53: 395–398.
46. Janssen AM, Chin NLJ, Scheffer JJC et al. Screening for antimicrobial activity of some essential oils by the agar overlay technique. Pharmaceutisch Weekblad Scientific Edition 1986; 8: 289–292.
47. Carson CF, Cookson BD, Farrelly HD et al. Susceptibility of methicillin-resistant Staphylococcus to the essential oil of Melaleuca alternifolia. Journal of Antimicrobial Chemotherapy 1995; 35 (3): 421–424.
48. Soderberg TA, Johansson A, Gref R. Toxic effects of some conifer resin acids and tea tree oil on human epithelial and fibroblast cells. Toxicology 1996; 107 (2): 99–109.
49. Cox SD, Gustafson JE, Mann CM et al. Tea tree oil causes K+ leakage and inhibits respiration in Escherichia coli. Letters in Applied Microbiology 1998; 26 (5): 355–358.
50. Moleyar V, Narasimham P. Antibacterial activity of essential oil components. International Journal of Food Microbiology 1992; 16 (4): 337–342.
51. Pattnaik S, Subramanyam VR, Bapaji M et al. Antibacterial and antifungal activity of aromatic constituents of essential oils. Microbios 1997; 89 (358): 39–46.
52. Carson CF, Riley TV. Antimicrobial activity of the major components of the essential oil of Melaleuca alternifolia. Journal of Applied Bacteriology 1995; 78 (3): 264–269.
53. Williams LR, Home VN. Factors determining the quality of tea tree oil in formulations for clinical use. Cosmetics, Aerosols and Toiletries in Australia 1995; 9 (2): 14–18.
54. Tong MM, Altman PM, Barnetson RS. Tea tree oil in the treatment of tinea pedis. Australasian Journal of Dermatology 1992; 33 (3): 145–149.
55. Bassett IB, Pannowitz DL, Barnetson RS. A comparative study of tea-tree oil versus benzoylperoxide in the treatment of acne. Medical Journal of Australia 1990; 153 (8): 455–458.
56. Moran J, Addy M, Newcombe R. A 4-day plaque regrowth study comparing an essential oil mouthrinse with a triclosan mouthrinse. Journal of Clinical Periodontology 1997; 24 (9 Pt 1): 636–639.
57. Reiter M, Brandt W. Relaxant effects on tracheal and ileal smooth muscles of the guinea pig. Arzneimittel-Forschung 1985; 35 (1A): 408–414.
58. Sparks MJ, O'Sullivan P, Herrington AA et al. Does peppermint oil relieve spasm during barium enema? British Journal of Radiology 1995; 68 (812): 841–843.
59. Giachetti D, Taddei E, Taddei I. Pharmacological activity of essential oils on Oddi's sphincter. Planta Medica 1988; 54: 389–392.
60. Creamer B. Oesophageal reflux and the action of carminatives. Lancet 1955; 1: 590–592.
61. Stanic G, Samarzija I, Blazevic N. Time-dependent diuretic response in rats treated with juniper berry preparations. Phytotherapy Research 1998; 12: 494–497.
62. Schilcher H, Leuschner F. Studies of potential nephrotoxic effects of essential juniper oil (German). Arzneimittel-Forschung 1997; 47 (7): 855–858.
63. Dorow P, Weiss TH, Felix R et al. Effect of a secretolytic and a combination of pinene, limonene and cineole on mucociliary clearance in patients with chronic pulmonary obstruction. Arzneimittel-Forschung 1987; 37 (12): 1378–1381.
64. Boyd EM. Expectorants and respiratory tract fluid. Pharmaceutical Reviews 1954; 6: 521–542.
65. Guillemain J, Rousseau A, Delaveau P. Effets neurodépresseurs de l'huile essentielle de Lavandula angustifolia Mill. Annales de Pharmaceutiques Françaises 1989; 47 (6): 337–343.
66. Büchner KH, Hellings H, Huber M et al. Double blind study as evidence of the therapeutic effect of Melissengeist on psycho-vegetative syndromes. Medizinische Klinik 1974; 69: 1032–1036.
67. Lorenzetti BB, Souza GE, Sarti SJ et al. Myrcene mimics the peripheral analgesic activity of lemongrass tea. Journal of Ethnopharmacology 1991; 34 (1): 43–48.
68. Kovar KA, Gropper D, Friess D et al. Blood levels of 1,8-cineole and locomotor activity of mice after inhalation and oral administration of rosemary oil. Planta Medica 1987; 53: 315–318.
69. Haines DJ Jr. Sassafras tea and diaphoresis. Postgraduate Medicine 1991; 90 (4): 75–76.
70. Tisserand R, Balacs T. Essential oil safety: a guide for health care professionals. Churchill Livingstone, Edinburgh, 1995
71. Macht DI. The action of the so-called emmenagogue oils on the isolated uterine strip. Journal of Pharmacology and Experimental Therapeutics 1912; 4: 547–552.
72. Arnold WN. Absinthe. Scientific American 1989; 260: 86–91.
73. Albert-Puleo M. Van Gogh's vision: thujone intoxication. Journal of the American Medical Association 1981; 246 (1) : 42.
74. Pulverer G. Benzylsenföl: ein Breitbandantibiotikum aus der Kapuzinerkresse. Deutsche Medizinische Wochenschrift 1968; 93: 1642–1649.
75. Langer P, Štolc V. Goitrogenic activity of allylisothiocyanate – a widespread natural mustard oil. Endocrinology 1965; 76: 151–155.

76. Verhoeven DTH, Verhoeven H, Goldbohm RA et al. A review of mechanisms underlying anticarcinogenicity by brassica vegetables. Chemico-Biological Interactions 1997; 103: 79–129.
77. Janssen K, Mensink RP, Cox FJ et al. Effects of the flavonoids quercetin and apigenin on hemostasis in healthy volunteers: results from an in vitro and a dietary supplement study. American Journal of Clinical Nutrition 1998; 67 (2): 255–262.
78. Hughes RE, Wilson HK. Flavonoids: some physiological and nutritional considerations. Progress in Medicinal Chemistry 1977; 14: 285–301.
79. Amiel M, Barbe R. Study of the pharmacodynamic activity of daflon 500 mg. Annales de Cardiologie et Angiologie 1998; 47 (3): 185–188.
80. Le Devehat C, Khodabandehlou T, Vimeux M et al. Evaluation of haemorheological and microcirculatory disturbances in chronic venous insufficiency: activity of Daflon 500 mg. International Journal of Microcirculation: Clinical and Experimental 1997; 17 (supp 1): 27–33.
81. Guilhou JJ, Fevrier F, Debure C et al. Benefit of a 2-month treatment with a micronized, purified flavonoidic fraction on venous ulcer healing. A randomized, double-blind, controlled versus placebo trial. International Journal of Microcirculation: Clinical and Experimental 1997; 17 (supp 1): 21–26.
82. Cospite M. Double-blind, placebo-controlled evaluation of clinical activity and safety of Daflon 500 mg in the treatment of acute hemorrhoids. Angiology 1994; 45 (6 pt 2): 566–573.
83. Ferrali M, Signorini C, Caciotti B et al. Protection against oxidative damage of erythrocyte membrane by the flavonoid quercetin and its relation to iron chelating activity. FEBS Letters 1997; 416 (2): 123–129.
84. Aviram M, Fuhrman B. Polyphenolic flavonoids inhibit macrophage-mediated oxidation of LDL and attenuate atherogenesis. Atherosclerosis 1998; 137 (supp): S45–50.
85. Robak J, Gryglewski RJ. Bioactivity of flavonoids. Polish Journal of Pharmacology 1996; 48 (6): 555–564.
86. Saiija A, Scalese M, Lanza M et al. Flavonoids as antioxidant agents: importance of their interaction with biomembranes. Free Radical Biology and Medicine 1995; 19 (4): 481–486.
87. Van Acker SA, Tromp MN, Haenen GR et al. Flavonoids as scavengers of nitric oxide radical. Biochemical and Biophysical Research Communications 1995; 214 (3): 755–759.
88. Hu JP, Calomme M, Lasure A et al. Structure-activity relationship of flavonoids with superoxide scavenging activity. Biological Trace Element Research 1995; 47 (1–3): 327–331.
89. Tournaire C, Croux S, Maurette MT et al. Antioxidant activity of flavonoids: efficiency of singlet oxygen (1 delta g) quenching. Journal of Photochemistry and Photobiology B – Biology 1993; 19 (3): 205–215.
90. Cao G, Sofic E, Prior RL. Antioxidant and prooxidant behaviour of flavonoids: structure-activity relationships. Free Radical Biology and Medicine 1997; 22 (5): 749–760.
91. Alcaraz MJ, Ferrandiz ML. Modifications of arachidonic metabolism by flavonoids. Journal of Ethnopharmacology 1987; 21: 209–229.
92. Okuda J, Miwa I, Inagaki K et al. Inhibition of aldose reductases from rat and bovine lenses by flavonoids. Biochemical Pharmacology 1982; 31 (23): 3807–3822.
93. Chang WS, Lee YJ, Chiang HC. Inhibitory effects of flavonoids on xanthine oxidase. Anticancer Research 1993; 13 (6A): 2165–2170.
94. Ruckstuhl M, Beretz A, Anton R et al. Flavonoids are selective cyclic GMP phosphodiesterase inhibitors. Biochemical Pharmacology 1979; 28: 535–538.
95. Petkov E, Nikolov N, Uzunov P. Inhibitory effect of some flavonoids and flavonoid mixtures on cyclic AMP phosphodiesterase activity of rat heart. Planta Medica 1981; 43: 183–186.
96. Pathak D, Pathak K, Singla AK. Flavonoids as medicinal agents – recent advances. Fitoterapia 1991; 62 (5): 1991.
97. Pelissero C, Lenczowski MJ, Chinzi D et al. Effects of flavonoids on aromatase activity, an in vitro study. Journal of Steroid Biochemistry and Molecular Biology 1996; 57 (3–4): 215–223.
98. Divi RL, Doerge DR. Inhibition of thyroid peroxidase by dietary flavonoids. Chemical Research in Toxicology 1996; 9 (1): 16–23.
99. Amella M, Bronner C, Briancon F et al. Inhibition of mast cell histamine release by flavonoids and biflavonoids. Planta Medica 1985; 51: 16–20.
100. Hammad HM, Abdalla SS. Pharmacological effects of selected flavonoids on rat isolated ileum: structure-activity relationship. General Pharmacology 1997; 28 (5): 767–771.
101. Sziklai I, Ribari O. Flavonoids alter bone-remodelling in auditory ossicle organ cultures. Acta Oto-Laryngologica 1995; 115 (2): 296–299.
102. Kitaoka M, Kadokawa H, Sugano M et al. Prenylflavonoids: a new class of non-steroidal phytooestrogen (Part 1). Isolation of 8-isopentenylnaringenin and an initial study on its structure-activity relationship. Planta Medica 1998; 64 (6): 511–515.
103. Miksicek RJ. Estrogenic flavonoids: structural requirements for biological activity. Proceedings of the Society for Experimental Biology and Medicine 1995; 208 (1): 44–50.
104. Ferrandina G, Almadori G, Maggiano N et al. Growth-inhibitory effect of tamoxifen and quercetin and presence of type II estrogen binding sites in human laryngeal cancer cell lines and primary laryngeal tumors. International Journal of Cancer 1998; 77 (5): 747–754.
105. Fremont L, Gozzelino MT, Franchi MP et al. Dietary flavonoids reduce lipid peroxidation in rats fed polyunsaturated or monounsaturated fat diets. Journal of Nutrition 1998; 128 (9): 1495–1502.
106. Pelzer LE, Guardia T, Osvaldo JA et al. Acute and chronic antiinflammatory effects of plant flavonoids. Farmaco 1998; 53 (6): 421–424.
107. Galvez J, Zarzuelo A, Crespo ME et al. Antidiarrhoeic activity of Euphorbia hirta extract and isolation of an active flavonoid constituent. Planta Medica 1993; 59: 333–336.
108. Elangovan V, Sekar N, Govindasamy S. Chemopreventive potential of dietary bioflavonoids against 20-methylcholanthrene-induced tumorigenesis. Cancer Letters 1994; 87: 107–113.
109. Yasukawa K, Takido M, Takeuchi M et al. Inhibitory effects of flavonol glycosides on 12-O-tetradecanoylphorbol-13-acetate-induced tumor promotion. Chemical and Pharmaceutical Bulletin 1990; 38 (3): 774–776.
110. Salgueiro JB, Ardenghi P, Dias M et al. Anxiolytic natural and synthetic flavonoid ligands of the central benzodiazepine receptor have no effect on memory tasks in rats. Pharmacology, Biochemistry and Behavior 1997; 58 (4): 887–891.
111. Keli SO, Hertog MG, Feskens EJ. Dietary flavonoids, antioxidant vitamins, and incidence of stroke: the Zutphen Study. Archives of Internal Medicine 1996; 156 (6): 637–642.
112. Knekt P, Jarvinen R, Reunanen A et al. Flavonoid intake and coronary mortality in Finland: a cohort study. British Medical Journal 1996; 312 (7029): 478–481.
113. Rimm EB, Katan MB, Ascherio A et al. Relation between intake of flavonoids and risk for coronary heart disease in male health professionals. Annals of Internal Medicine 1996; 125 (5): 384–389.
114. Nagao M, Naokata M, Yahagi T et al. Mutagenicities of 61 flavonoids and 11 related compounds. Environmental Mutagenesis 1981; 3: 401–419.
115. Czeczot H, Tudek B, Kusztelak J et al. Isolation and studies of the mutagenic activity in the Ames test of flavonoids naturally occurring in medical herbs. Mutation Research 1990; 240 (3): 209–216.
116. Connolly JA, Morgan IM, Jackson ME et al. The BPV-4 co-carcinogen quercetin induces cell cycle arrest and up-regulates transcription from the LCR of BPV-4. Oncogene 1998; 16 (21): 2739–2746.
117. Barotto NN, Lopez CB, Enyard AR et al. Quercetin enhances pretumorous lesions in the NMU model of rat pancreatic carcinogenesis. Cancer Letters 1998; 129 (1): 1–6.
118. Chaumontet C, Suschetet M, Honikman-Leban E et al. Lack of tumor-promoting effects of flavonoids: studies on rat liver preneoplastic foci and on in vivo and in vitro gap junctional intercellular communication. Nutrition and Cancer 1996; 26 (3): 251–263.

119. Wall ME, Wani MC, Manikumar G et al. Plant antimutagenic agents, 2. Flavonoids. Journal of Natural Products 1988; 51 (6): 1084–1091.
120. Duthie SJ, Collins AR, Duthie GG et al. Quercetin and myricetin protect against hydrogen peroxide-induced DNA damage (strand breaks and oxidised pyrimidines) in human lymphocytes. Mutation Research 1997; 393 (3): 223–231.
121. Zhu BT, Ezell EL, Leihr JG. Catechol-O-methyltransferase-catalyzed rapid O-methylation of mutagenic flavonoids. Journal of Biological Chemistry 1994; 269 (1): 292–299.
122. Hör M, Rimpler H, Heinrich M. Inhibition of intestinal chloride secretion by proanthocyanidins from Guazuma ulmifolia. Planta Medica 1995; 61: 208–212.
123. Maity S, Vedasiromoni JR, Ganguly DK. Anti-ulcer effect of the hot water extract of black tea (Camellia sinensis). Journal of Ethnopharmacology 1995; 46: 167–174.
124. Ezaki N, Kato M, Takizawa N et al. Pharmacological studies on Linderae umbellatae Ramus, IV. Effects of condensed tannin related compounds on peptic activity and stress-induced gastric lesions in mice. Planta Medica 1985; 51: 34–38.
125. Murakami S, Isobe Y, Kijima H et al. Inhibition of gastric H+, K+-ATPase and acid secretion by ellagic acid. Planta Medica 1991; 57: 305–308.
126. Terada A, Hara H, Nakajyo S et al. Effect of supplements of tea polyphenols on the caecal flora and caecal metabolites of chicks. Microbial Ecology in Health and Disease 1993; 6: 3–9.
127. Yokozawa T, Fujioka, Oura H et al. Confirmation that tannin-containing crude drugs have a uraemic toxin-decreasing action. Phytotherapy Research 1995; 9: 1–5.
128. Akah PA. Haemostatic activity of aqueous leaf extract of Ageratum conyzoides L. International Journal of Crude Drug Research 1988; 26 (2): 97–101.
129. Root-Bernstein RS. Tannic acid, semipermeable membranes and burn treatment. Lancet 1982; 2: 1168.
130. Haslam E. Natural polyphenols (vegetable tannins) as drugs: possible modes of action. Journal of Natural Products 1996; 59: 205–215.
131. Okuda T, Yoshida T, Hatano T. Chemistry and biological activity of tannins in medicinal plants. In: Wagner N, Farnsworth NR (eds) Economic and medicinal plant research, volume 5. Academic Press, London, 1991, pp 130–165.
132. Ducrey B, Marston A, Göhring S et al. Inhibition of 5a-reductase and aromatase by the ellagitannins oenothein A and oenothein B from Epilobium species. Planta Medica 1997; 63: 111–114.
133. Mizuno T, Uchino K, Toukairin T et al. Inhibitory effect of tannic acid sulfate and related sulfates on infectivity, cytopathic effect, and giant cell formation of human immunodeficiency virus. Planta Medica 1992; 58: 535–539.
134. Lamaison JL, Carnat A, Petitjean-Freytet C. Teneur en tanins et activité inhibitrice de l'élastase chez les Rosaceae. Annales de Pharmaceutiques Francaises 1990; 48 (6): 335–340.
135. Kashiwada Y, Nonaka G, Nishioka I et al. Antitumor agents, 129. Tannins and related compounds as selective cytotoxic agents. Journal of Natural Products 1992; 55 (8): 1033–1043.
136. Schwitters B, Masquelier J. OPC in practice, 2nd edition. Alfa Omega Editrice, Rome, 1995.
137. Ahmed AE, Smithard R, Ellis M. Activities of enzymes of the pancreas, and the lumen and mucosa of the small intestine in growing broiler cockerels fed on tannin-containing diets. British Journal of Nutrition 1991; 65: 189–197.
138. South PK, House WA, Miller DD. Tea consumption does not affect iron absorption in rats unless tea and iron are consumed together. Nutrition Research 1997; 17 (8): 1303–1310.
139. Ruenwongsa P, Pattanavibag S. Effect of tea consumption on the levels of alpha-ketoglutarate and pyruvate dehydrogenase in rat brain. Experientia 1982; 38: 787–788.
140. Eshchar J, Friedman G. Acute hepatotoxicity of tannic acid added to barium enemas. Digestive Diseases 1974; 19 (9): 825–829.
141. Paton A. Tannic acid in barium enemas. Lancet 1964; 1: 934.
142. Kapadia GJ, Chung EB, Ghosh B et al. Carcinogenicity of some folk medicinal herbs in rats. Journal of the National Cancer Institute 1978; 60 (3): 683–686.
143. Morton JF. Further associations of plant tannins and human cancer. Quarterly Journal of Crude Drug Research 1972; 12: 1829–1841.
144. Al-Habbal MJ, Al-Habbal Z, Huwezi FU. A double-blind controlled clinical trial of mastic and placebo in the treatment of duodenal ulcer. Clinical and Experimental Pharmacology and Physiology 1984; 11: 541–544.
145. Al-Said MA, Ageel AM, Parmar NS et al. Evaluation of mastic a crude drug obtained from Pistacia lentiscus for gastric and duodenal anti-ulcer activity. Journal of Ethnopharmacology 1986; 15: 271–278.
146. Lee TY, Lam TH. Allergic contact dermatitis due to a Chinese orthopaedic solution tieh ta yao gin. Contact Dermatitis 1993; 28 (2): 89–90.
147. Ogeto JO, Maitai CK. The scientific basis for the use of Strychnos henningsii (Gilg) plant material to stimulate appetite. East African Medical Journal 1983; 60: 603–607.
148. Carlson AJ, Torchiani B, Hallock R. Contributions to the physiology of the stomach. XXI The supposed actions of the bitter tonic on the secretion of gastric juice in man and dog. Journal of the American Medical Association 1915; 64 (1): 15–17.
149. Moorhead LD. Contributions to the physiology of the stomach. XXVIII Further studies on the action of the bitter tonic on the secretion of gastric juice. Journal of Pharmacology and Experimental Therapeutics 1915; 7: 577–589.
150. Glatzel H, Hackenberg K. Röntgenologische Untersuchungen der Wirkungen von Bittermitteln auf die Verdauungsorgane. Planta Medica 1967; 3: 223–232.
151. Baumann IC, Glatzel H, Muth HW. Untersuchungen der Wirkungen von Wermut (Artemisia absinthium L.) auf die Gallen-und Pankreassaft-Sekretion des Menschen. Zeitschrift fur Allgemeinmedizin 1975; 51 (17): 784–791.
152. Herman JH, Nolan DS. A bitter cure. New England Journal of Medicine 1981; 305: 1654.
153. Wolf S, Mack M. Experimental study of the action of bitters on the stomach of a fistulous human subject. Drug Standards 1956; 24 (3): 98–101.
154. Gebhardt R. Stimulation of acid secretion by extracts of Gentiana lutea L. in cultured cells from rat gastric mucosa. Pharmaceutical and Pharmacological Letters 1997; 7 (2–3): 106–108.
155. Wegener T. Anwendung eines Trockenextraktes Augentianae luteae radix bei dyspeptischem Symptomkomplex. Zeitschrift für Phytotherapie 1998; 19: 163–164.
156. Krentz K, Jablonowski H. In: Hellemans J, Vantrappen G (eds) Gastrointestinal tract disorders in the elderly. Churchill Livingstone, Edinburgh, 1984; pp 62–69.
157. Hurwutz A, Brady DA, Schaal SE et al. Gastric acidity in older adults. Journal of the American Medical Association 1997; 278 (8): 659–662.
158. Ralph A, Giannella MD, Selwyn A et al. Influence of gastric acidity on bacterial and parasitic enteric infections. Annals of Internal Medicine 1973; 78 (2): 271–276.
159. Werbach MR. Nutritional influences on illness: a sourcebook of clinical research. Third Line Press, California, 1987.
160. Gonzalez H, Ahmed T. Suppression of gastric H2-receptor mediated function in patients with bronchial asthma and ragweed allergy. Chest 1986; 89 (4): 491–496.
161. Kemp DR, Herrera F, Isaza J et al. On the critical nature of blood sugar levels in the vagal stimulation of gastric acid secretion in normal and diabetic dogs. Surgery 1968; 64 (5): 958–966.
162. Mukherjee B, Mukherjee SK. Blood sugar lowering activity of Swertia chirata (Buch-Ham) extract. International Journal of Crude Drug Research 1987; 25 (2): 97–102.
163. Saltzman MB, McCallum RW. Diabetes and the stomach. Yale Journal of Biology and Medicine 1983; 56: 179–187.
164. Niwa Y, Miyachi Y, Ishimoto K et al. Why are natural plant medicinal products effective in some patients and not in others with the same disease? Planta Medica 1991; 57 (4): 299–304.
165. Weiss RF. Amara in current therapy (German). Planta Medica 1966; 14 (supp): 128–132.
166. Bartoshuk LM, Duffy VB, Reed D et al. Supertasting, earaches and head injury: genetics and pathology alter our taste worlds. Neuroscience and Behavioural Reviews 1996; 20 (1): 79–87.

167. Eldershaw TP, Colquhour EQ, Bennett KL et al. Resiniferatoxin and piperine: capsaicin-like stimulators of oxygen uptake in the perfused rat hindlimb. Life Sciences 1994; 55 (5): 389–397.
168. Biro T, Acs G, Acs P et al. Recent advances in understanding of vanilloid receptors: a therapeutic target for treatment of pain and inflammation in skin. Journal of Investigative Dermatology Symposium Proceedings 1997; 2 (1): 56–60.
169. Towheen TE, Hochberg MC. A systematic review of randomized controlled trials of pharmacological therapy in osteoarthritis of the knee, with an emphasis on trial methodology. Seminars in Arthritis and Rheumatism 1997; 26 (5): 755–770.
170. Kingery WS. A critical review of controlled clinical trials for peripheral neuropathic pain and complex regional pain syndromes. Pain 1997; 73 (2): 123–139.
171. Rains C, Bryson HM. Topical capsaicin. A review of its pharmacological properties and therapeutic potential in post-herpetic neuralgia, diabetic neuropathy and osteoarthritis. Drugs and Aging 1995; 7 (4): 317–328.
172. Hautkappe M, Roizen MF, Toledano A et al. Review of the effectiveness of capsaicin for painful cutaneous disorders and neural dysfunction. Clinical Journal of Pain 1998; 14 (2): 97–106.
173. Baron R, Wasner G, Lindner V. Optimal treatment of phantom limb pain in the elderly. Drugs and Aging 1998; 12 (5): 361–376.
174. Sanico A, Togias A. Noninfectious, nonallergic rhinitis (NINAR): considerations on possible mechanisms. American Journal of Rhinology 1998; 12 (1): 65–72.
175. Visudhiphan S, Poolsuppasit S, Piboonnukarintr O et al. The relationship between high fibrinolytic activity and daily capsicum ingestion in Thais. American Journal of Clinical Nutrition 1982; 35: 1452–1458.
176. Desai HG, Venugopalan K, Philipose M et al. Effect of red chilli powder on gastric mucosal barrier and acid secretion. Indian Journal of Medical Research 1977; 66 (3): 440–448.
177. Abdel-Salam OM, Szolcsanyi J, Mozsik G. Capsaicin and the stomach. A review of experimental and clinical data. Journal of Physiology Paris 1997; 91 (3–5): 151–171.
178. Allameh A, Sexena M, Biswas G et al. Piperine, a plant alkaloid of the piper species, enhances the bioavailability of aflatoxin B1 in rat tissues. Cancer Letters 1992; 61 (3): 195–199.
179. Bano G, Raina RK, Zutshi U et al. Effect of piperine on bioavailability and pharmacokinetics of propranolol and theophylline in healthy volunteers. European Journal of Clinical Pharmacology 1991; 41 (6): 615–617.
180. Shoba G, Joy D, Joseph T et al. Influence of piperine on the pharmacokinetics of curcumin in animals and human volunteers. Planta Medica 1998; 64 (4): 353–356.
181. Atal CK, Zutshi U, Rao PG. Scientific evidence on the role of Ayurvedic herbals on bioavailability of drugs. Journal of Ethnopharmacology 1981; 4 (2): 229–232.
182. Atal CK, Dubey RK, Singh J. Biochemical basis of enhanced drug bioavailability by piperine: evidence that piperine is a potent inhibitor of drug metabolism. Journal of Pharmacology and Experimental Therapeutics 1985; 232 (1): 258–262.
183. Johri RK, Thusi N, Khajuria A et al. Piperine-mediated changes in the permeability of rat intestinal epithelial cells. The status of gamma-glutamyl transpeptidase activity, uptake of amino acids and lipid peroxidation. Biochemical Pharmacology 1992; 43 (7): 1401–1407.
184. Khajuria A, Zutshi U, Bendi KL. Permeability characteristics of piperine on oral absorption – an active alkaloid from peppers and a bioavailability enhancer. Indian Journal of Experimental Biology 1998; 36 (1): 46–50.
185. Pei YQ. A review of pharmacology and clinical use of piperine and its derivatives. Epilepsia 1983; 24 (2): 177–182.
186. Kawada T, Sakabe S, Watanabe T et al. Some pungent principles of spices cause the adrenal medulla to secrete catecholamine in anesthetized rats. Proceedings of the Society for Experimental Biology and Medicine 1988; 188 (2): 229–233.
187. Doucet E, Tremblay A. Food intake, energy balance and body weight control. European Journal of Clinical Nutrition 1997; 51 (12): 846–855.
188. Surh YJ, Lee SS. Capsaicin in hot chili pepper: carcinogen, co-carcinogen or anticarcinogen? Food and Chemical Toxicology 1996; 34 (3): 313–316.
189. Surh YJ, Lee SS. Capsaicin, a double-edged sword: toxicity, metabolism, and chemopreventive potential. Life Sciences 1995; 56 (22): 1845–1855.
190. Karekar VR, Mujumdar AM, Joshi SS et al. Assessment of genotoxic effect of piperine using Salmonella typhimurium and somatic and germ cells of Swiss albino mice. Arzneimittel-Forschung 1996; 46 (10): 972–975.
191. Segal R, Shatkovsky P, Milo-Goldzweig I. On the mechanisms of saponin hemolysis-I. Hydrolysis of the glycosidic bond. Biochemical Pharmacology 1974; 23: 973–981.
192. Segal R, Milo-Goldzweig I. On the mechanism of saponin hemolysis-II. Inhibition of hemolysis by aldonolactones. Biochemical Pharmacology 1975; 24: 77–81.
193. Boyd EM, Palmer ME. The effect of quillaia, senega, squill, grindelia, sanguinaria, chionanthus and dioscorea upon the output of respiratory tract fluid. Acta Pharmacologica 1946; 2: 235–246.
194. Bangham AD, Horne RW. Action of saponin on biological cell membranes. Nature 1962; 196: 952–953.
195. Gee JM, Johnson IT. Interactions between hemolytic saponins, bile salts and small intestinal mucosa in the rat. Journal of Nutrition 1988; 118: 1391–1397.
196. Yamasaki K. Effect of some saponins on glucose transport system. In: Waller GR, Yamasaki K (eds) Saponins used in traditional and modern medicine. Plenum Press, New York, 1996; pp 195–206.
197. Yoshikawa M, Yamahara J. Inhibitory effect of oleanene-type triterpene oligoglycosides on ethanol absorption: the structure-activity relationships. In: Waller GR, Yamasaki K (eds) Saponins used in traditional and modern medicine. Plenum Press, New York, 1996, pp 207–218.
198. Cayen MN, Dvornik D. Effect of diosgenin on lipid metabolism in rats. Journal of Lipid Research 1979; 20 (2): 162–174.
199. Oakenfull D, Sidhu GS. Could saponins be a useful treatment for hypercholesterolaemia? European Journal of Clinical Nutrition 1990; 44: 79–88.
200. Sears C. How to survive the world's worst diet. New Scientist 1995; 18 February: 10.
201. Milanov S, Maleeva E, Taskov M. Tribestan: effect on the concentration of some hormones in the serum of healthy volunteers. Medicobiologic Information 1985; 4: 27–29.
202. Zava DT, Dollbaum CM, Blen M. Estrogen and progestin bioactivity of foods, herbs and spices. Proceedings of the Society for Experimental Biology and Medicine 1998; 217: 369–378.
203 Aradhana, Rao AR, Kale RK. Diosgenin – a growth stimulator of mammary gland of ovariectomized mouse. Indian Journal of Experimental Biology 1992; 30(5): 367–370.
204. Fukushima Y, Bastom KF, Ohba T et al. Antiviral activity of dammarane saponins against herpes simplex virus I. International Journal of Pharmacognosy 1995; 33 (1): 2–6.
205. Favel A, Steinmetz MD, Regli P et al. In vitro antifungal activity of triterpenoid saponins. Planta Medica 1994; 60: 50–53.
206. Hasegawa H, Matsumiya S, Uchiyama M et al. Inhibitory effect of some triterpenoid saponins on glucose transport in tumour cells and its application to in vitro cytotoxic and antiviral activities. Planta Medica 1994; 60: 240–243.
207. Marston A, Hostettmann K. Plant molluscicides. Phytochemistry 1985; 24 (4): 639–652.
208. Oakenfull D. Saponins in food – a review. Food Chemistry 1981; 6: 19–40.
209. Van Tonder EM, Basson PA, Van Rensburg IBJ. Geeldikkop: experimental induction by feeding the plant Tribulus terrestris L (Zygophyllaceae). Journal of the South African Veterinary Association 1972; 43 (4): 363–375.
210. Weiss RF. Herbal medicine. Beaconsfield Publishers, Beaconsfield, 1988.
211. Nakanishi K, Berova N, Lo LC et al. Search for an endogenous mammalian cardiotonic factor. In: Waller GR, Yamasaki K (eds) Saponins used in traditional and modern medicine. Plenum Press, New York, 1996, pp 219–224.

212. Mascolo N, Capasso R, Capasso F. Senna. A safe and effective drug. Phytotherapy Research 1998; 12: S143–S145.
213. Nijs G, De Witte P, Geboes K et al. In vitro demonstration of a positive effect of rhein anthrone on peristaltic reflex of guinea pig ileum. Pharmacology 1993; 47 (supp 1): 40–48.
214. Leng-Peschlow E. Sennoside-induced secretion is not caused by changes in mucosal permeability or Na(+), K(+)-ATPase activity. Journal of Pharmacy and Pharmacology 1993; 45 (11): 951–954.
215. Yagi T, Miyawaki Y, Nishikawa A et al. Suppression of the purgative action of rhein anthrone, the active metabolite of sennosides A and B, by indomethacin in rats. Journal of Pharmacy and Pharmacology 1991; 43 (5): 307–310.
216. Capasso F, Izzo AA, Mascolo N et al. Effect of senna is not mediated by platelet-activating factor. Pharmacology 1993; 47 (supp 1): 58–63.
217. Anton R, Haag-Berrurier M. Therapeutic use of natural anthraquinone for other than laxative actions. Pharmacology 1980; 20 (supp 1): 104–112.
218. Rossi-Soffar G. Psoriasis. Dermatologica 1965; 130: 53–79.
219. Ashton RE, Andre P, Lowe NJ et al. Anthralin: historical and current perspectives. Journal of the American Academy of Dermatology 1983; 9 (2): 173–192.
220. Muller K, Leukel P, Ziereis K et al. Antipsoriatic anthrones with modulated redox properties. 2. Novel derivatives of chrysarobin and isochrysarobin-antiproliferative activity and 5-lipoxygenase. Journal of Medicinal Chemistry 1994; 37 (11): 1660–1669.
221. Wang XJ, Warren BS, Rupp T et al. Loss of mouse epidermal protein kinase C isozyme activities following treatment with phorbol ester and non-phorbol ester tumor promotors. Carcinogenesis 1994; 15 (12): 2795–2803.
222. Barnard DL, Huffman JH, Morris JL et al. Evaluation of the antiviral activity of anthraquinones, anthrones and anthraquinone derivatives against human cytomegalovirus. Antiviral Research 1992; 17 (1): 63–77.
223. Spencer CM, Wilde MI. Diacerein. Drugs 1997; 53 (1): 98–106.
224. Blomeke B, Poginsky B, Schmutte C et al. Formation of genotoxic metabolites from anthraquinone glycosides present in Rubia tinctorum L. Mutation Research 1992; 265 (2): 263–272.
225. Ino N, Tanaka T, Okumura A et al. Acute and subacute toxicity tests of madder root, natural colorant extracted from madder (Rubia tinctorum), in (C57BL/6 X C3H)F1 in mice. Toxicology and Industrial Health 1995; 11 (4): 449–458.
226. Leng-Peschlow E. Senna and its rational use. Pharmacology 1992; 44 (supp 1): 26–29.
227. Leng-Peschlow E. Senna and its rational use. Pharmacology 1992; 44 (supp 1): 30–32.
228. Howard LRC, Hughes-Roberts HE. The treatment of constipation in mental hospitals. Gut 1962; 3: 89–90.
229. Leng-Peschlow E. Senna and its rational use. Pharmacology 1992; 44 (supp 1): 36–40.
230. Campbell WL. Cathartic colon: reversibility of roentgen changes. Diseases of Colon and Rectum 1983; 26: 445–448.
231. Leng-Peschlow E. Senna and its rational use. Pharmacology 1992; 44 (supp 1): 20–22.
232. Leng-Peschlow E. Senna and its rational use. Pharmacology 1992; 44 (supp 1): 23–25.
233. Leng-Peschlow E. Senna and its rational use. Pharmacology 1992; 44 (supp 1): 33–35.
234. Brown JP. A review of the genetic effects of naturally occurring flavonoids, anthraquinones and related compounds. Mutation Research 1980; 75: 243–277.
235. Heidemann A, Miltenburger HG, Mengs U. The genotoxicity status of senna. Pharmacology 1993; 47 (supp): 178–186.
236. Brusick D, Mengs U. Assessment of the genotoxic risk from laxative senna products. Environmental and Molecular Mutagenesis 1997; 29: 1–19.
237. Siegers CP. Anthranoid laxatives and colorectal cancer. Trends in Pharmacological Science 1992; 13: 229–231.
238. Marles RJ, Compadre CM, Farnsworth NR. Coumarin in vanilla extracts: its detection and significance. Economic Botany 1987; 41 (1): 41–47.
239. Stohr H, Herrmann K. On the phenolic acids of vegetables. III Hydroxycinnamic acids and hydroxybenzoic acids of root vegetables (German). Zeitschrift für Lebensmittel-Untersuchung und-Forschung 1975; 159 (4): 218–224.
240. Arora RB, Mathur CN. Relationship between structure and anticoagulant activity of coumarin derivatives. British Journal of Pharmacology 1963; 20: 29–35.
241. Hörhammer L, Wagner H, Reinhardt H. On new constituents from the barks of Viburnum prunifolium L. (American Snowball) and Virbunum opulus (Common Snowball). Zeitschrift für Naturforschung 1967; 22b: 768–776.
242. Jarboe CH, Zirvi KA, Nicholson JA et al. Scopoletin, an antispasmodic component of Viburnum opulus and prunifolium. Journal of Medicinal Chemistry 1967; 10: 488–489.
243. Ojewole JAO, Adesina SK. Mechanism of the hypotensive effect of scopoletin isolated from fruit of Tetrapleura tetraptera. Planta Medica 1983; 49: 45–50.
244. Chen YF, Tsai HY, Wu TS. Anti-inflammatory and analgesic activities from roots of Angelica pubescens. Planta Medica 1995; 61 (1): 2–8.
245. Kimura Y, Okuda H, Arichi S et al. Inhibition of the formation of 5-hydroxy-6, 8,11,14-eicosatetraenoic acid from arachidonic acid in polymorphonuclear leukocytes by various coumarins. Biochemica et Biophysica Acta 1985; 834 (2): 224–229.
246. Chang WS, Chiang HC. Structure-activity relationship of coumarins in xanthine oxidase inhibition. Anticancer Research 1995; 15 (5B): 1969–1973.
247. Ohta T, Watanabe K, Moriya M et al. Anti-mutagenic effects of coumarin and umbelliferone on mutagenesis induced by 4-nitroquinoline 1-oxide or UV irradiation in E. coli. Mutation Research 1983; 117: 135–138.
248. Romert L, Jansson T, Curvall M et al. Screening for agents inhibiting the mutagenicity of extracts and constituents of tobacco products. Mutation Research 1994; 322 (2): 97–110.
249. Wattenberg LW, Lam LKT, Fladmoe AV. Inhibition of chemical carcinogen-induced neoplasia by coumarins and α-angelicalactone. Cancer Research 1979; 39: 1651–1654.
250. Kolodziej H, Kayser O, Woerdenbag HJ et al. Structure–cytotoxicity relationships of a series of natural and semi-synthetic simple coumarins as assessed in two human tumour cell lines. Zeitschrift für Naturforschung 1997; 52 (3/4): 240–244.
251. Weber US, Steffen B, Siegers CP. Antitumor-activities of coumarin, 7-hydroxy-coumarin and its glucuronide in several human tumor cell lines. Research Communications in Molecular Pathology and Pharmacology 1998; 99 (2): 193–206.
252. Pathak MA, Carbonare MD. Melanogenic potential of various furocoumarins in normal and vitiliginous skin. In: Fitzpatrick TB, Forlot P, Pathak MA et al (eds) Psoralens: past, present and future of photochemoprotection and other biological activities. John Libbey Eurotext, Paris, 1989, pp 87–101.
253. Fitzpatrick TB. The psoralen story: photochemotherapy and photochemoprotection. In: Fitzpatrick TB, Forlot P, Pathak MA et al (eds) Psoralens: past, present and future of photochemoprotection and other biological activities. John Libbey Eurotext, Paris, 1989, pp 5–10.
254. Kalis B, Sayag S, Forlot P. Photochemotherapy (PUVA) of psoriasis: a double-blind comparative study of 5- and 8-methoxypsoralen. In: Fitzpatrick TB, Forlot P, Pathak MA et al (eds) Psoralens: past, present and future of photochemoprotection and other biological activities. John Libbey Eurotext, Paris, 1989, pp 277–282.
255. Forlot P. Psoralen induced pigmentation in human skin: overview of clinical evidence, mechanisms of induction and future research. In: Fitzpatrick TB, Forlot P, Pathak MA et al (eds) Psoralens: past, present and future of photochemoprotection and other biological activities. John Libbey Eurotext, Paris, 1989, pp 63–71.
256. Kligman AM, Forlot P. Comparative photoprotection in humans by tans induced either by solar stimulating radiation or after a psoralen-containing sunscreen. In: Fitzpatrick TB, Forlot P, Pathak MA et al (eds) Psoralens, past, present and future of photochemoprotection and other biological activities. John Libbey Eurotext, Paris, 1989, pp 407–420.

257. Musajo L, Rodighiero G, Colombo G et al. Photosensitizing furocoumarins: interaction with DNA and photoinactivation of DNA containing viruses. Experientia 1965; 21: 22.
258. Oginsky EL, Green GS, Griffith DG et al. Lethal photosensitization of bacteria with 8-methoxy-psoralen to long wave length ultra-violet radiation. Journal of Bacteriology 1959; 78: 821.
259. Rauwald HW, Brehm O, Odenthal KP. The involvement of Ca^{2+} channel blocking mode of action in the pharmacology of Ammi visnaga fruits. Planta Medica 1994; 60: 101–105.
260. Hogan RP. Hemorrhagic diathesis caused by drinking an herbal tea. Journal of the American Medical Association 1983; 249 (19): 2679–2680.
261. Ivie GW. The chemistry of plant furanocoumarins and their medical, toxicological, environmental, and coevolutionary significance. Revista Latinoamericana De Quimic 1987; 18 (1): 1–5.
262. Cassier-Chauvat C, Averbeck D. Photomutagenic effects induced by psoralen derivatives in the yeast Saccharomyces cerevisiae. In: Fitzpatrick TB, Forlot P, Pathak MA et al (eds) Psoralens: past, present and future of photochemoprotection and other biological activities. John Libbey Eurotext, Paris, 1989, pp 329–335.
263. Marzin D, Olivier P. Study of the protective activity against photomutagenicity of 5-MOP. In: Fitzpatrick TB, Forlot P, Pathak MA et al (eds) Psoralens: past, present and future of photochemoprotection and other biological activities. John Libbey Eurotext, Paris, 1989, pp 337–343.
264. Young AR, Walker SL. Experimental photocarcinogenesis of psoralens. In: Fitzpatrick TB, Forlot P, Pathak MA et al (eds) Psoralens: past, present and future of photochemoprotection and other biological activities. John Libbey Eurotext, Paris, 1989, pp 357–366.
265. Stern RS. PUVA: its status in the United States, 1988. In: Fitzpatrick TB, Forlot P, Pathak MA et al (eds) Psoralens: past, present and future of photochemoprotection and other biological activities. John Libbey Eurotext, Paris, 1989, pp 367–376.
266. Henseler T. Risk of non melanoma skin tumors in patients treated with long-term-photochemotherapy (PUVA). In: Fitzpatrick TB, Forlot P, Pathak MA et al (eds) Psoralens: past, present and future of photochemoprotection and other biological activities. John Libbey Eurotext, Paris, 1989, pp 377–386.
267. Molteni A, Brizio-Molteni L, Persky V. In vitro hormonal effects of soybean isoflavones. Journal of Nutrition 1995; 125: 751S–756S.
268. Kaldas RS, Hughes CL. Reproductive and general metabolic effects of phytoestrogens in mammals. Reproductive Toxicology 1989; 3: 81–89.
269. Kuiper GG, Lemmen JG, Carlsson B et al. Interaction of estrogenic chemicals and phytoestrogens with estrogen receptor beta. Endocrinology 1998; 139 (10): 4252–4263.
270. Adlercreutz H. Western diet and western diseases: some hormonal and biochemical mechanisms and associations. Scandinavian Journal of Clinical and Laboratory Investigations 1990; 50 (201): 3–23.
271. Adlercreutz H, Bannwart C, Wahala K et al. Inhibition of human aromatase by mammalian lignans and isoflavonoid phytoestrogens. Journal of Steroid Biochemistry and Molecular Biology 1993; 44: 147–153.
272. Cassidy A, Bingham S, Setchell KDR. Biological effects of a diet of soy protein rich in isoflavones on the menstrual cycle of premenopausal women. American Journal of Clinical Nutrition 1994; 60: 333–340.
273. Knight DC, Eden JA. Phytoestrogens – a short review. Maturitas 1995; 22: 167–175.
274. Murkies AL, Lombard C, Strauss BJG et al. Dietary flour supplementation decreases post-menopausal hot flushes: effect of soy and wheat. Maturitas 1995; 21: 189–195.
275. Albertazzi P. Effect of dietary soy supplementation on hot flushes. Obstetrics and Gynecology 1998; 91: 6–11.
276. Yamaguchi M, Gao YH. Anabolic effect of genistein and genistin on bone metabolism in the femoral-metaphyseal tissues of elderly rats: the genistein effect is enhanced by zinc. Molecular and Cellular Biochemistry 1998; 178 (1–2): 377–382.
277. Fanti P, Monier-Faugere FC, Geng Z et al. The phytoestrogen genistein reduces bone loss in short-term ovariectomized rats. Osteoporosis International 1998; 8 (3): 274–281.
278. Clarkson TB, Anthony MS, Williams JK et al. The potential of soybean phytoestrogens for postmenopausal hormone replacement therapy. Proceedings of the Society for Experimental Biology and Medicine 1998; 217: 365–368.
279. Herman C, Adlercreutz T, Goldin BR et al. Soybean phytoestrogen intake and cancer risk. Journal of Nutrition 1995; 125: 757S–770S.
280. Verma SP, Goldin BR. Effect of soy-derived isoflavonoids on the induced growth of MCF-7 cells by estrogenic environmental chemicals. Nutrition and Cancer 1998; 30 (3): 232–239.
281. Hsieh CY, Santell RC, Haslam SZ et al. Estrogenic effects of genistein on the growth of estrogen receptor-positive human breast cancer (MCF-7) cells in vitro and in vivo. Cancer Research 1998; 58 (17): 3833–3838.
282. Onozawa M, Fukuda K, Ohtani M et al. Effects of soybean isoflavones on cell growth and apoptosis of the human prostatic cancer cell line LNCaP. Japanese Journal of Clinical Oncology 1998; 28 (6): 360–363.
283. Stephens F. Phytoestrogens and prostate cancer: possible preventive role. Medical Journal of Australia 1997; 167: 138–140.
284. Peterson G. Evaluation of the biochemical targets of genistein in tumor cells. Journal of Nutrition 1995; 125: 784S–789S.
285. Barnes S. The chemopreventive properties of soy isoflavonoids in animal models of breast cancer. Breast Cancer Research and Treatment 1997; 46: 169–179.
286. Barnes S. Effect of genistein on in vitro and in vivo models of cancer. Journal of Nutrition 1995; 125: 777S–783S.
287. Fotsis T, Pepper M, Adlercreutz H et al. Genistein, a dietary ingested isoflavonoid, inhibits cell proliferation and in vitro angiogenesis. Journal of Nutrition 1995; 125: 790S–797S.
288. Setchell KDR, Lawson AM, Borriello SP et al. Lignan formation in man – microbial involvement and possible roles in relation to cancer. Lancet 1981; 2: 4–7.
289. Phipps WR, Martini MC, Lampe JW et al. Effect of flax seed ingestion on the menstrual cycle. Journal of Clinical Endocrinology and Metabolism 1993; 77 (5): 1215–1219.
290. Serraino M, Thompson LU. The effect of flaxseed supplementation on early risk markers for mammary carcinogenesis. Cancer Letters 1991; 60: 135–142.
291. Adlercreutz H, Fotsis T, Heikkinen R et al. Excretion of the lignans enterolactone and enterodiol and of equol in omnivorous and vegetarian postmenopausal women and in women with breast cancer. Lancet 1982; 2: 1295–1299.
292. Irvine CHG, Fitzpatrick MG, Alexander SL. Phytoestrogens in soy-based infant foods: concentrations, daily intake, and possible biological effects. Proceedings of the Society for Experimental Biology and Medicine 1998; 217: 247–253.
293. Rolland A, Fleurentin J, Lanahers MC et al. Behavioural effects of the American traditional plant Eschscholzia californica: sedative and anxiolytic properties. Planta Medica 1991; 57: 212–216.
294. Schäfer HL, Schäfer H, Schneider W et al. Sedative action of extract combinations of Eschscholtzia californica and Corydalis cava. Arzneimittel-Forschung 1995; 45 (1): 124–126.
295. Kleber E, Schneider W, Schäfer HL et al. Modulation of key reactions of the catecholamine metabolism by extracts from Eschscholtzia californica and Corydalis cava. Arzneimittel-Forschung 1995; 45 (1): 127–131.
296. Lui LM, Sheu SJ, Chiou SH et al. A comparative study on commercial samples of Ephedrae herba. Planta Medica 1993; 59: 376–378.
297. Thies PW. Spartium und spartein. Pharmazie in unserer Zeit 1986; 6: 172–176.
298. Northover BJ. Effect of pre-treating rat atria with potassium channel blocking drugs on the electrical and mechanical responses to phenylephrine. Biochemical Pharmacology 1994; 47 (12): 2163–2169.

299. Eichelbaum M, Spannbrucker N, Steincke B et al. Defective N-oxidation of sparteine in man: a new pharmacogenetic defect. European Journal of Clinical Pharmacology 1979; 16: 183–187.
300. Vinks A, Inaba T, Otton SV et al. Sparteine metabolism in Canadian Caucasians. Clinical Pharmacology and Therapeutics 1982; 31 (1): 23–29.
301. Munson PL, Mueller RA, Breese GR. Principles of pharmacology. Basic concepts and clinical applications. Chapman and Hall, New York, 1995, pp 39–74.
302. De Smet PAGM, Brouwers JRB. Pharmacokinetic evaluation of herbal remedies. Basic introduction, applicability, current status and regulatory needs. Clinical Pharmacokinetics 1997; 32 (6): 427–436.
303. Hempelmann FW, Heinz N, Flasch H. Lipophilicity-protein binding relationship in cardenolides. Arzneimittel-Forschung 1978; 28 (12): 2182–2185.
304. Tschanz C, Stargel WW, Thomas JA. Interactions between drugs and nutrients. Advances in Pharmacology 1996; 35: 1–26.
305. Schubert W, Culberg G, Edgar B et al. Inhibition of 17 beta-estradiol by grapefruit juice in ovariectomized women. Maturitas 1995; 20: 155–163.
306. Bailey DG, Arnold JM, Spence JD. Grapefruit juice and drugs. How significant is the interaction? Clinical Pharmacokinetics 1994; 26 (2): 91–98.
307. Fuhr U, Klittich K, Staib AH. Inhibitory effect of grapefruit juice and its bitter principle, naringenin, on CYP1A2 dependent metabolism of caffeine in man. British Journal of Clinical Pharmacology 1993; 35 (4): 431–436.
308. Miniscalco A, Lundahl J, Regardh CG et al. Inhibition of dihydropyridine metabolism in rat and human liver microsomes by flavonoids found in grapefruit juice. Journal of Pharmacology and Experimental Therapeutics 1992; 261 (3): 1195–1199.
309. Min DI, Ku YM, Perry PJ et al. Effect of grapefruit juice on cyclosporine pharmacokinetics in renal transplant patients. Transplantation 1996; 62 (1): 123–125.
310. Hukkinen SK, Varhe A, Olkkola KT et al. Plasma concentrations of triazolam are increased by concomitant ingestion of grapefruit juice. Clinical Pharmacology and Therapeutics 1995; 58 (2): 127–131.
311. Lundahl JUE, Regårdh CG, Edgar B et al. The interaction effect of grapefruit juice is maximal after the first glass. European Journal of Clinical Pharmacology 1998; 54: 75–81.
312. Lee YS, Lorenzo BJ, Koufis T et al. Grapefruit juice and its flavonoids inhibit 11 beta-hydroxysteroid dehydrogenase. Clinical Pharmacology and Therapeutics 1996; 59 (1): 62–71.
313. Edwards DJ, Bernier SM. Naringin and naringenin are not the primary CYP3A inhibitors in grapefruit juice. Life Sciences 1996; 59 (13): 1025–1030.
314. Runkel M, Bourian M, Tegtmeier M et al. The character of inhibition of the metabolism of 1,2-benzopyrone (coumarin) by grapefruit juice in humans. European Journal of Clinical Pharmacology 1997; 53: 265–269.
315. He K, Iyer KR, Hayes RN et al. Inactivation of cytochrome P450 3A4 by bergamottin, a component of grapefruit juice. Chemical Research in Toxicology 1998; 11 (4): 252–259.
316. Woo WS, Shin KH, Lee CK. Effect of naturally occurring coumarins on the activity of drug metabolizing enzymes. Biochemical Pharmacology 1983; 32 (11): 1800–1803.
317. Steinegger E, Hövel H. Analytic and biologic studies on Salicaceae substances, especially on salicin. II. Biological study. Pharmaceutica Acta Helvetiae 1972; 47: 222–234.
318. Fotsch G, Pfeifer S, Bartoszek M et al. Biotransformation of phenolglycosides leiocarposide and salicin. Pharmazie 1989; 44 (8): 555–558.
319. Leng-Peschlow E. Senna and its rational use. Pharmacology 1992; 44 (suppl): 10–15.
320. Soulimani R, Younos C, Mortier F et al. The role of stomachal digestion on the pharmacological activity of plant extracts, using as an example extracts of Harpagophytum procumbens. Canadian Journal of Physiology and Pharmacology 1994; 72: 1532–1536.
321. Wagner H, Jurcic K, Schaette R. Comparative studies on the sedative action of Valeriana extracts, valepotriates and their degradation products. Planta Medica 1980; 39: 358–365.
322. Valdes LJ III. Salvia divinorum and the unique diterpene hallucinogen Salvinorin (Divinorin) A. Journal of Psychoactive Drugs 1994; 26 (3): 277–283.
323. Griffiths LA, Barlow A. The fate of orally and parenterally administered flavonoids in the mammal. The significance of biliary excretion. Angiology 1972; 9 (3–6): 162–174.
324. Hertog MGL, Hollman PCH. Potential health effects of the dietary flavonol quercetin. European Journal of Clinical Nutrition 1996; 50 (2): 63–71.
325. Hollman PC, De Vries JH, Van Leeuwen SD et al. Absorption of dietary quercetin glycosides and quercetin in healthy ileostomy volunteers. American Journal of Clinical Nutrition 1995; 62 (6): 1276–1282.
326. Hollman PC, Van Der Gaag M, Mengelers MJ et al. Absorption and disposition kinetics of the dietary antioxidant quercetin in man. Free Radical Biology and Medicine 1996; 21 (5): 703–707.
327. Merfort I, Heilmann J, Weiss M et al. Radical scavenger activity of three flavonoid metabolites studied by inhibition of chemiluminescence in human PMNs. Planta Medica 1996; 62 (4): 289–292.
328. Kelly GE, Joannou GE, Reeder AY et al. The variable metabolic response to dietary isoflavones in humans. Proceedings of the Society for Experimental Biology and Medicine 1995; 208 (1): 40–43.
329. Xu X, Wang HJ, Murphy PA et al. Daidzein is a more bioavailable soymilk isoflavone than is genistein in adult women. Journal of Nutrition 1994; 124 (6): 825–832.
330. Xu X, Harris KS, Wang HJ et al. Bioavailability of soybean isoflavones depends upon gut microflora in women. Journal of Nutrition 1995; 125 (9): 2307–2315.
331. Cassidy A, Bingham S, Setchell K. Biological effects of isoflavones in young women: importance of the chemical composition of soyabean products. British Journal of Nutrition 1995; 74 (4): 587–601.
332. Wang Z, Kurosaki Y, Nakayama T et al. Mechanism of gastrointestinal absorption of glycyrrhizin in rats. Biological and Pharmaceutical Bulletin 1994; 17 (10): 1399–1403.
333. Krahenbuhl S, Hasler F, Krapf R. Analysis and pharmacokinetics of glycyrrhizic acid and glycyrrhetinic acid in humans and experimental animals. Steroids 1994; 59 (2): 121–126.
334. Hattori M, Sakamoto T, Kobashi K et al. Metabolism of glycyrrhizin by human intestinal flora. Planta Medica 1983; 48 (1): 38–42.
335. Sakiya Y, Akada Y, Kawano S et al. Rapid estimation of glycyrrhizin and glycyrrhetinic acid in plasma by high-speed liquid chromatography. Chemical and Pharmaceutical Bulletin 1979; 27 (5): 1125–1129.
336. Nose M, Ito M, Kamimura K et al. A comparison of the antihepatotoxic activity between glycyrrhizin and glycyrrhetinic acid. Planta Medica 1994; 60 (2): 136–139.
337. Hasegawa H, Sung JH, Matsumiya S et al. Main ginseng saponin metabolites formed by intestinal bacteria. Planta Medica 1996; 62 (5): 453–457.
338. Rauwald HW, Grunwild J. Ruscus aculeatus extract: unambiguous proof of the absorption of spirostanol glycosides in human plasma after oral administration. Planta Medica 1991; 57 (supp 2): A75–A76.
339. Daniel EM, Ratnayake S, Kinstle T et al. The effects of pH and rat intestinal contents on the liberation of ellagic acid from purified and crude ellagitannins. Journal of Natural Products 1991; 54 (4): 946–952.
340. Bravo L, Abia R, Eastwood MA et al. Degradation of polyphenols (catechin and tannic acid) in the rat intestinal tract. Effect on colonic fermentation and faecal output. British Journal of Nutrition 1994; 71 (6): 933–946.
341. Groenewoud G, Hundt HKL. The microbial metabolism of condensed (+)-catechins by rat-caecal microflora. Xenobiotica 1986; 16 (2): 99–107.

342. Serafini M, Ghiselli A, Ferro-Luzzi A. In vivo antioxidant effect of green and black tea in man. European Journal of Clinical Nutrition 1996; 50 (1): 28–32.
343. Nakagawa K, Okuda S, Miyazawa T. Dose-dependent incorporation of tea catechins, (-)-epigallocatechin-3-gallate and (-)-epigallocatechin, into human plasma. Bioscience, Biotechnology and Biochemistry 1997; 61 (12): 1981–1985.
344. Hara Y. Influence of tea catechins on the digestive tract. Journal of Cellular Biochemistry 1997; 27 (supp): 52–58.
345. Okushio K, Matsumoto N, Kohri T et al. Absorption of tea catechins into rat portal vein. Biological and Pharmaceutical Bulletin 1996; 19 (2): 326–329.
346. Pulse TL, Uhlig E. A significant improvement in a clinical pilot study utilizing nutritional supplements, essential fatty acids and stabilized aloe vera juice in 29 HIV seropositive ARC and AIDS patients. Journal of Advancement in Medicine 1990; 3 (4): 209–230.

3 Principles of herbal treatment

FIRST PRINCIPLES OF TRADITIONAL HERBAL TREATMENT

The history of herbal treatments is marked by the enormous diversity of local traditions, with much more variety than consistency. However, themes are apparent. These emerge most clearly where local folk practices were systematized in the great written traditions in history, reviewed in Chapter 1. When these are distilled further and then translated into modern terminology, it is possible to identify a few features that recur consistently. These appear to encapsulate essential characteristics of the material, universal archetypes of the effects plants have on humans. They reflect also the therapeutic priorities of earlier ages and, at the least, need adaptation to be incorporated into a phytotherapy appropriate to modern needs. They are valuable, however, because they probably represent the roots of herbal therapeutics, those characteristics of the remedies that are the most potent. They also draw stark contrasts with the approaches that have emerged with the development of modern technological medicine. They are antidotes to the modern tendency to view herbs solely as milder versions of modern drugs. In essence, they should underpin any rational phytotherapy.

CLEANSING: DETOXIFICATION AND ELIMINATION

In almost all traditional practice there was an explicit or implicit assumption that before healing could take place, noxious influences need to be removed. In the earliest animistic traditions, pathogens could be literally demons and shamanistic practices emerged to drive them out. However, there was also a consistent, more mundane view of toxins and poisons: these needed to be removed by the body's eliminatory functions. Disease was widely seen as a failure of elimination and the vomiting, diarrhoea, coughing, diaphoresis and diuresis of most acute diseases as evidence that the body was being driven to extraordinary eliminative measures. In Chinese medicine the development of chronic disease was a clear indication that acute eliminatory responses had failed in their primary task of keeping pathogens out and that penetration into the interior had occurred[1].

The task of the physician was equally clear: to support eliminatory functions as vigorously as possible compatible with the body's vital reserves (eliminatory functions were mostly seen as taxing the body's energies). In practice this meant robust heroic treatments in acute disease, notably involving emetics, purgatives, powerful expectorants and diaphoretics in fever management. In chronic and debilitated conditions the aim was to use gentler treatments, peeling away toxic accumulations like the layers of an onion, always making sure that eliminatory measures, laxatives, diuretics, choleretics, expectorants and the more systemic lymphatics and alteratives were supported by adequate sustenance for the vital functions: rest, nourishment and the use of tonic remedies (see below).

Typically in traditional therapeutics, eliminatory measures were the first stage of treatment, to be followed increasingly by more adjustive and sustaining treatments, as outlined next.

HEATING: MOVING THE CIRCULATION

It was apparent to all humans that heat equated to vitality. The extreme absence of heat was the striking coldness of the corpse. When Samuel Thomson in North America built his therapeutics around the principle that disease was essentially a cold intrusion and that before all else remedies should heat the struggling body, he was only highlighting an almost universal instinct. In every tradition there is frequent use of heating remedies; the hot spices, or 'pungent' remedies, were the strongest for internal use but there was always a raft of gentler warming remedies as well. Some were applied as aromatic digestives to failing 'cold' digestion, others as warming expectorants or mucolytics in treating the effects of cold and damp on the chest and respiratory system. There were warming tonics (*yang* tonics in traditional Chinese medicine) and a variety of remedies that brought heat to the head, reproductive system or kidneys.

All the above could be used, along with hot packs, hot baths, 'sweat lodges' or hot drinks, in the major indication for supportive heating: the fever. In modern terms heating remedies used in fever management are called 'diaphoretics' as their main effect is to increase perspiration. Sweat was understood not only as a cooling agent but also as the prime eliminatory route in febrile disease; in this context, therefore, heating was an obvious cleansing strategy, as above.

Indications for the use of heating agents apart from fevers were easily understood. If the patient felt cold, as a whole or in the diseased part, or favoured hot food, hot drinks, hot packs or hot baths; if there was diminished vitality; if there was pallor (the nail beds or quicks were particularly sensitive guides) or signs of cumulative cold-damp conditions like catarrh or gravity-dependent oedema, then heating remedies were indicated. The fact that a headache or arthritic joint or abdominal swelling was relieved by a hot pack was more important in choosing the course of treatment than determining what pathological factor was involved.

When the focus of cold was clearly demarcated then extreme heating, in the form of powerful counterirritation, cayenne or mustard plasters, blistering croton oil or formic acid or stinging nettles, might be applied topically, with sometimes dramatic beneficial effects.

Heat in modern terms equates also to circulation and a rationale that speaks of improved tissue perfusion, oxygenation and metabolite removal could easily be made. A modern phytotherapist might avoid the more drastic topical heating agents and may have less need to manage fevers but could nevertheless consider the role of heating agents in a prescription if these appeared to be indicated.

The major caveat in modern circumstances is that many patients are also debilitated, at least from the perspective of earlier, more robust times. Heating agents do not heat directly but instead stimulate increased thermogenesis and circulatory activity. They thus require reserves of energy in the body. Someone weakened by chronic ill health may suffer if stimulated in this way too much. An assessment of vital reserves is essential in such treatment.

COOLING: STIMULATING DIGESTION

Whereas heating was clearly 'on the side of the angels' in traditional healthcare, cooling was altogether a more serious matter. It is, after all, perfectly possible to have hot spicy foods at every mealtime (especially in the tropics where they prompt gastric defences against enteric infections) but with a few notable exceptions, cooling was confined to therapeutics. Cooling meant reducing vitality. The ultimate cold was death. In their simple restatement of fundamental principles, Samuel Thomson and his followers denied any prospect of cooling in heathcare and even saw something diabolical in it. Nevertheless, more considered views have throughout history recognized that one can have too much, or inappropriate, heat. The obvious examples were hyperpyrexia in fevers, inflammatory diseases, hypersensitivity or allergic reactions, nervous agitation and, above all, pain. The respective treatments, febrifuges, antiinflammatories, antiallergic remedies, sedatives, hypnotics (and narcotics) and analgesics, would all be classified as cooling in these terms. Indeed, some of the eliminatory treatments often applied for these purposes, especially the laxatives and cholagogues, were also seen as cooling. Reference to the Galenic classification (see p.4) will put all this into context.

The classification of sedatives is illuminating. In former times neurosis and anxiety, irritability and tension were aspects of heat. Children were hotter than adults and there was progressive constitutional cooling with age. Psychological explanations were not considered and no one was told 'it is all in the mind'. The Cartesian body-mind split had not occurred.

Clearly, each of the above types of remedy involved a particular therapeutic decision. There was more likely to be care in prescription of cooling remedies. Although many popular treatments existed, it was probable that professional expertise would be called for, especially in the treatment of severe pains and inflammations. Almost everything now prescribed by modern doctors would have been classified as cooling.

There was one striking exception to the cautions linking cooling to reduced vitality. As referred to in the Galenic classification, the most gentle category of cooling remedy (those 'cold in the first degree') did 'qualify the heat of the stomach and cause digestion'. Digestion was widely seen as a cooling activity, marked of course by a shift of blood flow from the periphery to the core (so that excessive exercise after a big meal can lead to cramps).

The archetypal cooling digestive stimulants were the bitters. Of all the herbal strategies in history, these are probably the most respected (the Chinese even gave them the awesome role in their five-phase classification of tonifying the *Kidneys* – the source of constitutional energies in their system). Bitters are universally used before and after eating as appetite stimulants ('aperitifs') and digestives. They were the first resort in digestive difficulties, especially when associated with heat and hepatobiliary ('damp-heat') disorders (bitters are also the most commonly used choleretics). Critically, they were also favourite febrifuges, apparently lowering body temperature in fever. They appeared to correct an apparent design inconsistency in the febrile response, wherein digestion is shut down, leaving undigested material as a source of new toxicity and even the original source of infection in the case of gastroenteritis. Bitters appeared to switch on digestive defences as well as to bring the fever down. Unlike other cooling agents which counteracted vital functions, bitters appeared to transcend these limitations, to convert heat and vitality into nourishment. This was sometimes regarded as magical.

The modern phytotherapist in effect competes in cooling remedies with modern orthodox medicine. Technology has produced the most powerful analgesics, sedatives and antiinflammatory and antiallergic drugs yet (although many are still derived from natural sources). Phytotherapy may score in two ways: first, by producing a more gentle and sustained and perhaps even a longer lasting alternative (treating an inflammatory disease with cleansing remedies, for example) and second, by having recourse to the cooling digestives to transform a hot condition in the most constructive way. The phytotherapist might also be sensitive to the risks of excessive cooling, especially when vital reserves are low (there is a particular risk of provoking latent kidney inflammations).

Bitters and other cooling herbs and other strategies (such as cooling drinks, baths and cold packs) could be considered by the phytotherapist when the patient, whatever the diagnosis, favours cool applications or is thirsty, abhors heat, has a reddened complexion, is excessively animated or distressed, has a dry and possibly red tongue and/or coloured tongue coating, Any sign of liver difficulties (particularly with fatty food or alcohol) or a history of hepatobiliary problems or digestive troubles strongly indicates bitter remedies. When so appropriate, they are one of the best tactics available.

TONIFICATION: SUPPORTING NOURISHMENT AND REPAIR

So far all the foregoing strategies make demands on the patient's reserves. In more robust times (i.e. when not being robust seriously compromised one's chances of survival) and in the treatment of acute disease, this was not a major issue. However, it quickly becomes one when there is diminished vitality. It can be argued that traditional practitioners would see most clinical conditions in modern times as marked by degrees of debility. The low-grade viral or fungal infections, the persistent catarrhal state, recurrent headaches or migraines, allergies, skin and arthritic disease and other chronic inflammatory diseases, stress problems and anxiety neuroses and cancer are all marked by a failure to cope or adequately to defend. One perspective on this development is that modern medicine has so effectively neutered the acute battle, especially in the too frequent use of antibiotics and antiinflammatories, that most people in developed countries have never had to muster their defences. Life is also much easier in these societies and there is less rigorous testing of physiological functions generally.

Whatever the reason, the modern phytotherapist will need much more than the traditional practitioner to ensure that there are adequate vital supports in their prescriptions. In large part this involves mobilizing the principles of convalescence – rest, exercises and diet (see below) – but in herbal terms the remedies involved are the 'tonics'.

Tonics have been poorly defined, with different meanings in different contexts. In this text they are taken to refer to remedies with substantially supportive reputations. Some are also classified as adaptogens, i.e. they appear to encourage the body to better adaptability under stress (so reflecting the concept elaborated by Hans Selye as the general adaptation syndrome, as a marker of health and vitality in the face of stresses. At one extreme remedies used as tonics overlap wholly with foods: different parts of the oat, wheat, barley, rye, asparagus and artichoke, for example, have been used as both foods and medicines. In modern times dietary supplements like evening primrose oil and grape seed have further blurred the distinction. Other tonics are more dynamic, notably some of those used in Chinese medicine, particularly the *yang* tonics like Trigonella (fenugreek) and Eucommia and the *qi* tonics like *Panax ginseng* (asiatic ginseng): these move beyond the simply sustaining towards their own contraindications in the very debilitated.

Within this spectrum there is a vast range of remedies which are used in modern phytotherapy because they appear to support some aspect or other of body function: Silybum (St Mary's thistle) and Taraxacum (dandelion root) for the liver and hepatobiliary functions, Crataegus (hawthorn) for the cardiovascular system, *Plantago lanceolata* (ribwort) for the upper respiratory system, Verbascum (mullein) and Inula (elecampane) for the chest, Hypericum (St John's wort), Withania and Turnera (damiana) for nervous with hormonal symptoms, Foeniculum (sweet fennel), Cardamomum (cardamon) for the digestion, Linum (linseed), *Plantago psyllium* (psyllium seed) and Mentha (peppermint) for the bowel, Echinacea, Picrorrhiza and Astragalus for the immune defences, *Vitex agnus-castus* for the female reproductive system, *Serenoa serrulata* (saw palmetto) for the prostate, and many more in this and other herbal traditions. In earlier times tonification was often the final stage of a course of herbal treatment. The phytotherapist most often has to start a prescription with at least some tonic element.

APPROACHES TO USING HERBS

AS INSTANT TREATMENTS: TRIGGER-POINT PHYTOTHERAPY

Herbal medicine has developed the reputation in modern times of being an innocuous alternative to conventional drug treatment. It is often thought that if the remedies work at all, it can only be after weeks or months. The French term *médicin douce* sums up a modern European view of herbal medicine; that it is 'soft' and above all safe, free from the side effects of modern chemical drugs.

This is not how herbal medicines were developed. Before ambulances and hospital casualty wards men and women had to turn to the remedies they had available, sometimes for life-and-death emergencies. Until a few hundred years ago there were practically no other options than to use plant products. These were often administered in heroic doses and judged on their ability to produce dramatic results. In most people's daily lives there was little room for sentiment or for the modern romantic view of natural medicine maintaining holistic health and balance. The imperative was simple and urgent: 'Will this measure work, and work soon? If not, I do not want to waste time in trying it'.

All this should not be surprising. The notion that people used somehow to be less interested in efficacy or had less wit in seeking out and recommending the best strategies available would be more extraordinary. There is no doubt that the measures actually adopted in the past, often by ordinary people, did work dramatically when needed.

It is of course unlikely that while modern emergency facilities are available anyone would choose to adopt the traditional alternatives, which were often uncomfortable, crude and imprecise. What may be more interesting is to consider the many ways in which these traditional herbal techniques were applied to lesser problems. In having to learn how to survive illnesses, early practitioners appear to have gained considerable insight into the way the body behaves.

One of the tactics adopted was the use of remedies for provocation. The heroic techniques of emesis and catharsis were merely the most dramatic of the approaches used and which are still applied: the bitter digestives and cholagogues, circulatory stimulants and topical rubefacients and expectorants are examples of remedies that gently nudge the body towards hopefully useful activity. All these effects are short term, even immediate, as are the measures adopted for symptom relief: the demulcents, carminatives and spasmolytics. These categories of activity link closely to categories of plant constituents (see Chapter 2) and recur again and again in human history. They make a persuasive case for a modern herbal therapeutics still.

FOR LONG-TERM REPAIR

In modern times herbal medicine has come to be seen as gentle, almost inocuous, most suitable for long-term therapy. Patients often expect herbs to take a long time to work. As has been discussed so far, this perspective says more for the conditions being treated than for the herbs themselves. Chronic diseases cannot be corrected quickly. An informal rule of thumb used by some practitioners is to allow 3 months' treatment for a problem of a year's standing and a month for every further year (or a week's treatment for every month in problems of shorter duration). Such formulae can of course only be approximate but at least they provide guidelines to aim for. They also imply that real correction of chronic disease is possible. This may be unattainable in conditions that are too far established but there are many pleasant surprises in herbal practice and most patients may gain some long-term benefits.

In general, herbal treatment for chronic conditions uses relatively smaller doses, less robust remedies and more tonics.

AS ALTERNATIVE ALLOPATHICS

Herbal remedies perhaps too easily lend themselve to being characterized as natural drugs, gentler versions of conventional medicines. Indeed, the majority of Western European use is as substitutes for conventional prescriptions or over-the-counter (OTC) medicinal products. Almost all herbal research is predicated on the same assumption. European regulators treat herbs as individual medicinal products in the same legislative framework as other medicines and similar assumptions are found elsewhere in the world.

It is also the case that in developed Western countries the human consumption of herbal remedies as natural alternatives to synthetic drugs far outstrips any other use. We have sought to argue that there is much more to herbal medicine than this, that it becomes more powerful when used in a more considered way. A literally allopathic character has been accepted in the review of herbal therapeutic systems but this was in relation to a humoral approach which is much more integrative. However, if a conventional use cannot be denied it is a consolation at least that there is likely to be some benefit in using gentler, more broad-based remedies if they are suitable. There are also undeniable advantages in using herbs individually, for whatever rationale, in learning more about their effects on the human body: it is an approach that can sometimes be recommended to first-time practitioners.

The great majority of 'gentle drug' herbal use relates to the production of OTC goods by herbal manufacturers. These may have legally- permitted labelled claims but these are highly conservative and most often the patient makes a personal choice, based on recommendations or articles in the popular health press. Practitioners may make their own recommendations, especially if they do not hold the herb concerned in stock. They may even prescribe or recommend a product themselves, as do a high proportion of physicians in Europe.

Dosages of simple herbal products are often determined on the label. They are sometimes at smaller doses than used by a herbal practitioner. Production costs and selling prices effectively discourage heroic dosing and this is in any case inappropriate without trained practitioner supervision.

PHYTOTHERAPY AS A COMPONENT OF OTHER HEALING STRATEGIES

CONVALESCENCE

It is ironic that at the very time that healthcare has to deal with so much chronic and debilitated disease it has abandoned the best strategic approach inherited from tradition. In the past it was taken for granted that any illness would require a decent period of recovery after it had passed, a period of recuperation, of convalescence, without which recurrence was possible or likely. For the really debilitating diseases convalescent care was the primary treatment, reaching its apogee in the many European sanatoria for tuberculosis patients.

Convalescence fell out of favour as powerful modern drugs emerged. It appeared that penicillin and the steroid antiinflammatories produced so dramatic a resolution of the old killer diseases, including tuberculosis, that all the time spent convalescing was no longer necessary. Then, as healthcare provision became generally more effective and public expectations increased, pressure on hospital facilities led to shorter stays, whilst the increasing angst of the modern working rhythm has conspired to ensure that most people now could not consider time off to convalesce after a bout of flu. That this means they are more likely to get another bout the next year, is a second, crueller, irony.

A good convalescence is a marvellous thing. It rounds off an illness and gives it meaning; it makes the sufferer stronger for having had it. In a way no vaccination could do, it arms and strengthens the immune defences and provides real protection against recurrence, possibly forever. It is probably the only strategy that will allow real recovery from debilitating disease, fatigue syndromes, recurrent infections and states of compromised immunity. It is the therapeutic recognition that healing, like the growth of children, is almost inevitable but that it needs to be allowed to proceed. Convalescence needs time, one of the hardest commodities to find now.

There are four essential features of convalescence, in general agreed through history, though with many cultural embellishments.

Rest

This is by far the most important element. It should include maximum sleep, as physiologically this is the body's time for repair. In the early stages of vigorous convalescence almost constant sleep should be encouraged (as in the former 'sleep clinics'). Thereafter it should be promoted as much as possible. Rest also means less activity: if work has to be done it should be in brief bouts, switching frequently between different activities ('change is as good as a rest'). Patients should be encouraged to pace themselves, to go to bed early, sleep late and not to volunteer for any work that is not absolutely necessary.

Exercise

The flipside and necessary adjunct to rest, the equivalent to 'turning the engine over', to prevent congestion and stagnation. Essentially the body needs to be taken to aerobic exercise (defined for these purposes as any activity producing a pulse rate of between approximately 60–80% of 220 minus one's age, e.g. 108–144 for a 40-year-old) at least briefly each day. Using the pulse rate to set exercise levels has the advantage of being self-adjusting: the very debilitated will reach high pulse rates with minimal activity. Nevertheless, caution is required. The debilitated will have very little stamina and even a minute may be too long. If exercise is followed by more fatigue, it is too much. Rather, one should build up to being able to undertake aerobic activity for up to 15 minutes each day. The main benefit of the aerobic mode is that it quickly dissipates adrenaline, the enemy of convalescence which is constantly generated during the day in response to perceived stressors. Timing one's exercise for the evening will encourage better sleep that night.

Diet

The principle of the convalescent diet is that it should simply nourish. It should not stimulate or impose demands. Subject to individual dispositions, a convalescent diet is based on vegetables, especially root vegetables, cereals and pulses (if tolerated), fish and eggs, as the most easily assimilated protein sources, and chicken and other fowl if acceptable (chicken stock and soup remain one of the most universal and puzzling convalescent recommendations of history!). There should be no stimulants, caffeine, nicotine, alcohol or sugar, little dairy food and a minimum of convenience foods and food additives. Patients should thus be encouraged to take a simple peasant diet, sharing also with the peasant a simple respect for the food, taking time over it, building their daily rhythm around it.

Medication

It is obviously important to maintain treatment during convalescence, herbal or conventional. However, there is also a key contribution to the measures above in herbal traditions. It was accepted that rest, exercise and diet alone might not be sufficient to bring about recovery. A range of herbal remedies have been directed to facilitating the process, to drive recovery. Many of these are the tonics listed earlier. If recovery is from febrile disease, sustaining warming remedies like achillea (yarrow), *Angelica archangelica* (common angelica), *Cinnamonum zeylanicum* (Ceylon cinnamon), Cardamomum (cardamon) or Foeniculum (sweet fennel) might be indicated. Recovery from low-grade assault on the immune system, chronic viral or fungal infections, conditions marked by swollen lymph glands, persistent sore throats or catarrhal states would need Echinacea, Picrorrhiza or *Baptisia tinctoria* (wild indigo). Digestion is often in need of support, whether from cooling bitters or warming aromatic digestives. Cleansing should be managed, above all, by gentle eliminatives.

For the phytotherapist convalescence is often the main strategy in making headway in chronic debilitated conditions such as a fatigue syndrome or persistent low-grade infections. Often these problems start with an infection early in life – a glandular fever or infectious mononucleosis, perhaps. The phytotherapist might suggest to the patient that the task was to go back and complete the convalescence from the original illness. The remedies available are probably uniquely appropriate to the job.

NUTRITION: HELPING TO CONVERT FOODS INTO NOURISHMENT

The revival in holistic and traditional healthcare rightly highlights the importance of good diet. It can also be argued that in an age of processed foods and widespread adulteration of the environment, additional foods and food supplements are sometimes essential. Most phytotherapists will attend to these matters as an intrinsic part of their treatment. This text is not the place to rehearse this complex matter but it is the place to explore the phytotherapist's particular perspective on dietary therapy.

One could start with a principle, literally a fundamental principle. New-wave dietetics has been associated with the dictum that 'You are what you eat'. This pop simplicity might be derided but it reflects much of what inspires nutritional therapy. A phytotherapist, on the other hand, grounded in the affairs and rude robustness of the digestive tract and liver, might respond: 'No, you are what you assimilate'. To almost every popular dietary measure it is possible to add a functional modifier or a caveat.

Is there any real point giving extra vitamins, minerals or other food supplements if they are not being well absorbed or utilized, or are being excessively metabolized? What is the point of eliminating potential dietary allergens if the gut is in hypersensitivity mode (when one simultaneously reduces vital dietary variety and creates new allergens)? If there is abdominal bloating or flatulence after eating a food, improving digestive performance might be better than removing the food. Correcting bowel environment by attending to biliary or gastric functions may be more useful in containing Candida outbreaks than drastic eliminations of starches and yeasts.

The phytotherapist would want to answer such questions satisfactorily before embarking on extra dietary measures. Referral to the sections on treating digestive, bowel and liver problems and the section on acupharmacology (p.166) should provide a rich range of tactics to modify digestive performance and modulate dietary measures. Appropriate use of eliminative or heating remedies may provide additional influence on dietary metabolism. Phytotherapy provides unique opportunities to convert food into useful nourishment. It gives dietary therapy much added value.

References

1. Porkert M. The essentials of Chinese diagnosis. Acta Medicinae Sinensis, Zurich; 1983: 39–44.

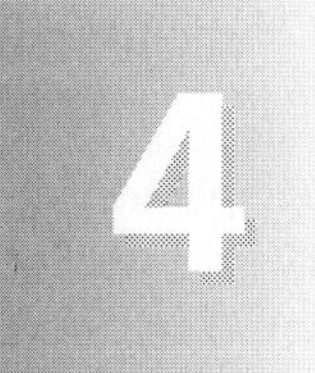

Validating herbal therapeutics

BUT DO HERBS ACTUALLY WORK?

This book is constructed largely on the foundation of published scientific literature. It is clear that there is now a sufficient case to construct a rational therapeutic system for remedies that have previously been poorly articulated. However, in spite of this and the presence in medicinal plants of many pharmacologically active constituents, the most persistent doubt expressed by the medical world is whether whole herbs actually work in practice.

Although there is indeed considerable published research, much reviewed in this text, there is still a relative paucity of top-quality controlled clinical studies of the whole herb that clearly separate its effect from placebo, and most good clinical studies show only a modest additional effect. Where relevant debates have been held (e.g. Office of Alternative Medicine/Food and Drug Administration Joint Conference on Botanicals in Medicine, Washington, 1994), critics also point out that pharmacological constituents in most herbs are at relatively low levels in a final therapeutic dose, that the complexity of constituents is at least as likely to reduce as to potentiate activities and that traditional reputation is often clouded by plagiarism and inappropriate transmission.

On the other hand, most herbal practitioners will attest to consistent therapeutic performance and will also have accounts of dramatic responses from their patients, where genuinely powerful pharmacological effects have followed consumption of herbal prescriptions. They will also point to the essential 'neutering down' of clinical trials data as denying precisely that which they value most about their therapy – the individulization of treatment and response (for example, experimental data consistently deny the possibility of appreciable diuretics among plant remedies yet substantial diuresis in individual patients, often not to traditional 'diuretics', is one of the most familiar treatment reactions in practice). This is enough to convince most practitioners that herbal medicine is a serious alternative to conventional drug treatment with few of the adverse effects.

Any move in the stand-off between the sceptics and the believers is, however, likely to include a full discussion of the placebo effect.

THE PLACEBO EFFECT

It is likely that most benefits seen in taking any therapy are not produced directly by the treatments themselves. This is the main conclusion reached after taking the substantial literature about placebo effects into account.

The term 'placebo effect' is not wholly appropriate for this discussion. It originally derived from observations in double-blind clinical studies where the treatment was compared with a dummy pill made to look as close as possible to the treatment, with neither the patient nor the practitioner aware of which was which. Early observations were that a significant proportion of subjects in such studies who were taking the dummy nevertheless got better. Initial impressions in the 1940s and 1950s, when such rigorous studies became more common, were that figures varied from trial to trial but it appeared that about a third of subjects were likely to be 'placebo responders'. This behaviour was put down, in the psychosomatic model emerging at the same time, as reflecting a particular suggestibility on the part of that proportion of the population. As a result the placebo response has been seen to be a non-serious event, not something to be confused with real medicine and at worst a confounding nuisance in establishing therapeutic efficacy for treatments.

Many doctors and other practitioners became used to thinking that about a third of their patients would get better whatever they were given and many thought they knew who they were! After discounting this element they were pleased to feel that any further improvement in their patient population was a result of therapeutic efficacy and skill. Herbal practitioners have therefore been able to confirm to themselves that there must be much more to account for the evidence before their eyes.

Both practitioners and sceptics must review their opinion about the placebo effect in the light of overwhelming later evidence. The last 50 years have completely overturned early prejudices. In brief, it is now possible, after analysis of the clinical trial literature, to confirm that:

- placebo benefits can occur in any proportion of a treatment group, from zero to almost 100%,[1] depending on the condition and circumstances;[2]
- there are no particular 'placebo responders' as such;[3]
- placebos have time-effect curves and peak, cumulative and carryover effects similar to those of active medications;[2] they can also generate significant levels of adverse effects[4] (see also the discussion of the 'nocebo effect' on p.101);
- placebo responses can involve real cures over the long term [5] – they are not, as often thought, transient, imaginary events;[6]
- placebo response can lead to long-term benefit even in difficult conditions such as multiple sclerosis,[7] ulcerative colitis,[8] benign prostatic hyperplasia[6] and schizophrenia.[9]

The first real shock to the herbal practitioner is that those 'conditions and circumstances' where placebo responses have been recorded as particularly high include many of those covered by herbal and other complementary treatments. There is support for the cynic's case that the success of herbal tradition over centuries, especially that drawn from close-knit early societies (where placebo responses were likely to be particularly high because of stronger peer pressures and belief systems), could be due to benefits other than the treatment itself.

The shock also applies, however, to conventional medicine and especially surgery where placebo responses, as evidenced by examining data from non-controlled clinical studies of surgical interventions which were later found to be valueless, are among the highest recorded.[2] The simple instruction from a doctor carries enormous 'placebo' impact[19]. In whole industries, such as those promoting antidepressant drugs, the impact of placebo relative to treatment response has probably been systematically understated.[10]

Among both conventional and complementary healthcare practitioners there is an understandable feeling that cures that have nothing to do with the treatment so skilfully provided are something of an embarrassment and even a challenge to one's choice of vocation. Thus the placebo effect is one of the least discussed phenomena in clinical medicine. Yet it is by far the most powerful factor of all.

The way out of this potential difficulty is to reconsider what the placebo response means.

NON-SPECIFIC SUPPORTS FOR SELF-REPAIR: A DIFFERENT THERAPEUTIC STRATEGY?

When a moderate cut is sustained, one assumes it will heal itself. A cold or bout of influenza will generally get better on its own. The only treatment for serious trauma like broken bones or operation wounds is to put the tissues back together and leave them for natural healing to occur.

No one doubts that self-repair is a vital phenomenon. Nevertheless, medicine has moved away from the classic principle that all healing is self-healing, that the *vis medicatrix naturae*, the healing power of life, is the only healer and that the physician should do no more than help it on its way. Exasperation at the slow and uncertain pace of natural healing, the realization that one can save lives and health by stepping in with something direct and powerful has led man to find his own healing bullets. The modern success in this venture has allowed medicine to forget the fundamental principle that ultimately no drug or surgery actually heals: its value is in reducing pain and distress, returning an acceptable function and at best enabling spontaneous repair to occur when it had previously been prevented.

There is no problem with the modern strategy in many clinical cases; it is certain that it can save lives and protect health in ways inconceivable to prescientific medicine. Nevertheless, there is another strategy that may be more appropriate in many other clinical conditions, a therapeutic approach with the primary objective of supporting self-repair. This could be most appropriate in facing the challenge of chronic diseases, the broad range of indeterminate syndromes, along with the numerous minor self-limiting symptoms that make up the vast majority of the family practitioner's caseload.

What researchers have labelled as the placebo effect in their clinical trials is of course an improvement in self-repair. That it was merely the effect of being recruited into the clinical study and being given a dummy treatment (actually the main feature of most clinical trials is the increased attention that subjects receive for their condition) is surely evidence of how little it can take to mobilize this self-repair. Dismissing placebo healing as just suggestibility is to miss the point; as shown above, placebo healing can occur in any subject when the circumstances are right.

Indeed, some medical practitioners have got the point. There is a long unspoken tradition of non-specific prescribing, with vitamins, laxatives, aspirin and, unfortunately, antibiotics, to keep the patient happy (*placebo* means 'I please'), although actual prescription of placebos as such usually breaches ethical and legislative codes.

Many researchers prefer to use the term 'non-specific effects' to describe contributions to improvements in clinical studies that are not caused by the treatment in isolation. As well as the placebo effect itself, they include the natural course of the illness ('getting better anyway' is something 'control groups' of non-treated patients are supposed to quantify in the better organized clinical trials but even here confusion reigns about hidden placebo effects[11]), 'spontaneous remission' (generally used to describe recovery that cannot otherwise be explained), a trend for improvement ('regression to the mean') due to the fact that people tend to get recruited to studies (and come to obtain treatment) when they are at their worst. All these phenomena are of course aspects of self-repair. A shift in terminology so that the generally prejudicial 'placebo effect' becomes 'non-specific effects' will be welcome.

HERBAL REMEDIES AND PLACEBOS

In reflecting on practice experience with the full impact of the placebo literature in mind, one could easily become dismayed at the difficulty in separating possible treatment effects from non-specific effects. Nevertheless, one is quickly reminded of the peculiar properties of herbal remedies; time and again one sees in practice changes that are characteristic of the remedies rather than fitting any preconceived notion of a placebo response. Changes in physiological functions, in digestion, bowel performance, expectoration, diuresis and many others can often be invoked in a herbal strategy crafted to reach the symptom goal indirectly. There is enough evidence to support the view that many herbal remedies have appreciable effects on various organ and tissue functions, much of which is considered throughout this book.

If the objectives of treatment are to better mobilize self-repair functions, then herbal remedies really appear to have unique prospects for this job. If non-specific responses are manifestations of such mobilization then, to put it simply, the role of the herbal practitioner is to improve such responses.

No one needs to feel their vocation is challenged if they acknowledge the large contribution of non-specific factors in their professional performance. It may even be possible to develop research questions that test the hypothesis that herbal remedies have unique prospects for mobilizing the self-repair functions.

Whatever the argument for or against the benefits of herbal medicine, it is clear that this is driven more by prejudice on both sides rather than the evidence. It is time to review the status of research so far and pose new, more appropriate methods for the future.

THE DIFFICULTY OF ENQUIRY

Judging by the substantial markets for herbal products in the developed world, let alone the vast use in traditional cultures, a great many people have already found herbal medicines useful. Compared with the experience of most modern drugs, the human use and approval of most herbal remedies is awesome. The requirement by the medical and scientific establishment for research to 'prove' that herbs are effective is not found among the population at large. It is apparent that most ordinary people are content to rely on their impressions of the world to get by in it.

However, the public do want to be assured that someone is looking after them. They therefore assume the questions are being asked by those who ought to do it. The physician and the regulators are charged with the job of making sure that medicine is safe and effective.

Knowledge within traditional medicine, however, has generally been in the form of received wisdom moulded to the individual needs and prowess of each practitioner. Such means of acquiring healing skills seem temperamentally suited to most practitioners, herbal and conventional, even today. Their interest in inquiry for its own sake, with secure truths up for constant possible refutation, is understandably secondary to their concern to survive in practice. In the case of herbal medicine, adherents understandably tend to give it the benefit of doubt. The view that 'What worked for our grandparents is good enough for me, and at least it is natural' probably sustains a considerable casualness about research. It is also possible to question the validity of the research forum and only to play it as far as absolutely necessary (so that the rights to supply herbs are not restricted by law). Nevertheless, simple pride in the therapy should encourage an enthusiasm for research along the lines of the challenge: 'If what you say is so valuable and powerful then it should be able to stand up for itself in any forum'.

There are, however, three practical problems in pursuing good clinical research in herbal medicine.

1. To produce results carrying sufficient statistical weight is expensive and laborious (each trial has to be costed in research salaries plus logistical expenses). Herbal medicine in the West can boast no teaching hospitals or research institutes, nor funding by government or a wealthy industrial sector. The necessary infrastructure is lacking. Neither can the costs of undertaking research studies easily be justified commercially. It is difficult to patent herbs and the size of the market for any individual product is not comparable to that for any patentable conventional drug.

2. Herbs are complex medicines, occupying an unusual position in being medicines with many of the characteristics of foods. Being a complex of pharmacologically active chemicals, the whole package will have different properties from that of any single constituent acting alone. The action of the latter will not predict the effect of the former, particularly if the experimental evidence is based on work done on laboratory animals.

3. The application of herbs and their effect on the body are not always the same as usually understood for conventional medicines. As has been suggested above, herbal medicines may be used more to evoke healing responses in the body than to attack symptoms; this generates a different research question.

CONVENTIONAL CLINICAL TRIALS

Even with these difficulties, conventional double-blind randomized clinical trials can sometimes be completed. The monographs in this text include well-conducted clinical trials, notably for garlic, ginkgo, St John's wort, valerian, feverfew and ginger. These studies show that the conventional methodology is very powerful and can be suited to understanding herbal remedies in some contexts at least. They also show that even such unremarkable plants, when researched thoroughly, can demonstrate efficacy beyond the placebo.

The benefits of well-conducted controlled clinical trials are that effects separate from the non-specific can be quantified in a way no other study can permit and that this is still the only currency accepted as evidence of efficacy by those medicine regulators who determine what is legally available for the public. They are also very flexible devices. It is possible, for example, to use the double-blind placebo-controlled methodology to test the efficacy of individual prescribing (random assignment of the tailored prescription or placebo is done by a third person in the dispensary); it does not test an individual remedy but could establish whether the prescribing skill was any better than placebo. Such trials will remain the gold standard research method for the foreseeable future.

The limitations of the controlled clinical study include the homogenization of the patient population so that only an average effect is confirmed. The fact that people react differently to the same treatment and that a good practitioner will work with this individualized approach means that clinical trial data will help with but still do not answer the basic question 'Is this drug going to be good for this patient?' It is also likely that genuinely important benefits for a minority of the population will be overlooked.

Some herbal practitioners have resisted the controlled study as inherently unethical, in denying a proportion of subjects the most useful treatment. This argument is easily challenged, however. In the first place, one goes into a controlled clinical study professionally neutral to the outcome. Second, no study in a developed country could proceed without painstaking adherence to the principle of informed consent and to other reassurances that the interests of the subject are paramount. The ethics committees that legally review all orthodox study protocols are charged to represent the interests of the subjects (and this includes rejecting studies that are not sufficiently well designed to actually answer the question). Indeed, medical researchers may point out in their terms that administering a remedy that has not been proved by good quality research is itself unethical. This may not be an argument for herbal practitioners to pursue too far!

However, for the reasons outlined, the conventional trial approach is not always possible or appropriate in actual clinical practice. It would be helpful to develop other techniques to explore how herbs affect human beings.

There have fortunately been some considerable efforts in constructing appropriate methodologies of sufficient weight.[12] These include looking at different outcome measures, applying rigorous observational studies and monitoring individual case studies.

THE MEASUREMENT OF TRANSIENT CLINICAL EFFECTS: THE FUNCTIONAL ASSAY

In the review earlier in this chapter, the tendency to use herbs to support individual self-repair rather than simply to target disturbances was raised as prompting different research questions.

Traditional views of herbal remedies emphasize their primary influence on transient body functions, e.g. they are classed as diaphoretics, expectorants, circulatory stimulants, diuretics, digestive stimulants, laxatives and so on. These effects, contrary to common beliefs about the effect of herbal remedies, can occur very quickly after treatment. The requirement is to devise a process by which such properties can be substantiated.

By working with both healthy individuals or, more appropriately, cohorts of patients, it should be possible to monitor functional changes after administering herbal remedies, although this will be more straightforward in some areas than others. Monitoring urine or bowel production is simple enough in theory but demanding in practice; most internal functions are beyond simple measure. On the other hand, recent advances in electronic biochemical monitors provide the possibility of following changes in liver function and blood levels of various markers very simply. Moreover, monitoring changes in blood flow to various organs with thermal imaging or cutaneous thermocouples is a most elegant way of pursuing one of the persistent traditional claims for herbal medicines, that they affect the circulation to (heat or cool) various tissues, organs or functions.

Such outcomes could be explored in as double-blind controlled studies. Although involving physiological changes rather than symptom relief, they could in some cases be translated into the labelled claims that are the main motivation for industrial sponsorship of clinical research. However, the main justification for the practitioner in examining functional changes is that they may provide the currency for a wholly appropriate herbal clinical science.

Given that herbs do not have isolated pharmacological actions and that their effects are upon complex living beings (for example, there is the impression that herbal remedies are more interactive with the patient than conventional drugs, i.e. their actual effect varies with the nature of the disturbance treated), it may be better to chart several changes within individuals, using such parameters as are relevant, useful and non-invasive. Emphasis would shift to the simultaneous recording of several parameters of change. Synchronous events mutually influence each other rather than act as causes or effects of each other; they are thus all equally related to each other and to the outcome of their use. It is precisely this interdependence, this inductive relationship, that leads to their exclusion from conventional trials as distracting variables. Acceptance of these variables as important data is a key feature of such work and must therefore profoundly change the nature of the information gathered.

Instead of trying to eliminate all variables that might cloud the specific issue in question ('Is it drug A that reduces inflammation in this organ or other factors?', for example), the aim of the 'functional assay', as it might be called,[13] is ideally to define all factors which determine the medicinal substance's influence on the course of disease ('What, in fact, is drug A likely to do in this individual?'). The task would in some ways resemble homoeopathic 'proving'; in other ways it might take advantage of modern computerized and multilevel diagnostic techniques known as 'metabolic profiles'.

Any conclusions drawn from such complex information would be qualitative rather than quantitative: relationships induced rather than causes analysed. The process may resemble anthropological rather than conventional medical research. It could, of course, augment the collation of exhaustive case stories as described below.

The demonstration of transient effects would not always lead to predictable changes in pathologies, representing as these do the somatic accumulation of various, previous functional disorders. However, many clinical presentations are wholly functional (e.g. acute inflammations, asthma, migraine, digestive disorders and the whole range of psychosomatic disorders). Even in the worst case, knowing the functional impact of a herbal remedy would be a most useful guide to its use in clinical practice.

Thus, it might be more valid to say that a herb, in certain individuals at least, changed the constitution of phlegm or urine or altered circulatory activity to one or other tissues or over the body as a whole, for example, rather than that it is statistically likely to be effective against bronchitis, urinary stones or other disease state.

These latter multiple measurements lead the discussion onto the role of observational studies as a whole in assessing the impact of herbal remedies.

OBSERVATIONAL STUDIES

There are many ways in which rigorous, though uncontrolled observations can illuminate therapeutic events. Although it is difficult to establish cause and effect in observational or field studies or specifically to separate specific from non-specific treatment effects, there are a number of particular ways that observational studies could productively be used in herbal research.

Performance and effectiveness of a therapy overall can be measured with various outcome measures, including the whole range of clinical or biochemical measures, patient questionnaires or analysis of records. This information can inform those determining health policy or the allocation of resources (a good observational study could demonstrate that herbal medicine was a sufficiently cost-effective strategy in the management of interstitial cystitis, for example, to enable a clinical group to bid for public health funding for treatment of the condition). Of course, only limited evidence of efficacy can be obtained; however, if a herb were to be given to one group of patients with a condition while another group with the same condition was observed as a matching control, then any clear improvement in the first group will suggest follow-up research.

Whereas such studies have a second-best feel to them, there is at least one way in which observational studies are a highly appropriate method for herbal medicine. Following the earlier discussion about self-repair and the supportive role of the practitioner of herbal medicine, as well as the review of the self-organization found in living complex systems in Chapter 1 and the therapeutic principles that arise (see p.20), then it is apparent that different research methodologies are required. These should:

- have regard to global behaviour of the system rather than particular variables in isolation;
- aim to measure quantifiable components of health, rather than of morbidity, mortality or other indicators of disease;
- involve minimal intervention.

This suggests observational rather than controlled studies. Non-invasive monitoring of physiological functions, as in the 'functional assay' above, may be applied, perhaps coupled with patient self-rated questionnaires, clinical observations of overall behaviour and epidemiological methods, to establish as far as possible what actually happens to living patients when they do or do not seek treatments.

One source of data on self-organization in humans, for example, is remission from disease. The normal remission rate may be obtained from medical texts and the clinical research literature; levels of the more unusual 'spontaneous remissions' can be obtained from the Remission Project of the Institute of Noetic Sciences.[14] Having benchmarks for the natural course of disease is generally helpful in research but they also allow assessment of treatment effectiveness in determining how far perceived recovery rates in any study differed from that expected.

Routine collection of patient and clinical data at a teaching clinic, for example, including self-rating questionnaires for general health and target conditions, perhaps combined with a number of other non-invasive observations, compared with general remission rates, is feasible. Modern database technology and touch-screen inputs facilitate routine data collection and can allow meaningful collation, retrieval and analysis. Such a programme is under way at a leading student herbal clinic in London; over several years such data will provide very useful therapeutic information about the use of herbal remedies.

WHERE N=1: THE SINGLE-CASE STUDY

The main charge against single-case studies is that they cannot credibly select out real effects from confusing variables, specific from non-specific treatment effects and so on. The following scenario for such research, however, shows both that it can have more credibility than might be supposed and that it is not a soft option.

The criteria for validity of such trials have been well reviewed by Reason and Rowan:[15] they are challenging, even daunting. They include ensuring that the perceptive faculties of the researchers are constantly and clearly sharpened, providing as many points of view as possible, clarifying these perspectives and recycling observed data around the researchers (including the patient as co-researcher) for checking and possible refutation. At stake is the need to ensure that, while accepting the difficulty of a truly objective view, researchers do not confine themselves to the subjective, aiming instead to create a perspective which transcends the two.

In an ideal study design, data about a particular treatment could be drawn from:

- the patient, acting as co-researcher and with a uniquely intimate though slanted view of the internal landscape;
- the practitioner, with sufficient competence and clinical experience to provide both an informed and empathic account of the encounter;
- a third person acting as coordinator and observer.

The account of each participant could be assembled individually and then crosschecked and combined at a case conference editorial discussion so as to produce a final consensus report of the treatment. Each such report can be examined by the coordinating researcher or assistant, applying a form of grounded inquiry similar to that originally proposed by Diesing in the social sciences.[16] In other words, themes of disturbance and incapacity are elicited by formal contents analysis of the original material, then used to construct the working case story, both steps being subjected to reevaluation by all co-researchers. As each case is thus graphically characterized, it can be used for comparative purposes with other cases to see whether a pattern occurs and can be sustained.

Inherent validity in even rigorous consensual research is, of course, no greater than when a number of people agree among themselves that 'all swans are white' (to use Popper's image) but it can still be argued that this is a fair basis on which to base practical predictions and applications (it would be considered very sound intelligence in the business world). It has the advantage that all conclusions are based on real experiences and can more thoroughly be applied to meaningful clinical application.

It is also possible to conduct double-blind, placebo-controlled studies in a series of such individual case studies with each patient being his or her own control. Standard sequences of treatment, placebo and/or control can be conducted, described as ABAB, ACABCBCB, complex patterns that, say in the case of dietary exclusion and challenge, are nevertheless attainable in everyday clinical practice.[17]

Such rigorous exercises are best conducted in the environment of a training clinic, where there is likely to be a more overt climate of inquiry and debate and extra administrative labour. It could allow for a useful database of reliable case histories to be assembled over the years as both an educational and research exercise.

FUNDAMENTAL RESEARCH

Any rationale for herbal medicine is likely to be based on the activity of many plant chemical constituents. There are fundamental technical questions raised in building a rational case for herbal therapeutics. The following might usefully form the basis of pharmacological research questions.

- In what ways are plant constituents likely to interact, in the context of the gut and body tissues, to affect bioavailability and activity (obvious interactions are between tannins/alkaloids/saponins/minerals /complex carbohydrates)?
- What is known of hepatic action on plant constituents, both in terms of the results of the 'first-pass effect', as plant constituents move into the tissues from the digestive tract, and the impact of enterohepatic recycling (see p.184)?
- Following from both the above, what plant-derived constituents are likely to reach the systemic circulation (an answer to this question is an essential requisite for meaningful tissue culture experiments – see below)?
- How do changes in pharmaceutical preparation affect the bioavailability and activity of plant constituents? For example, do alcoholic extracts have significantly different actions from the aqueous extracts generally dominant in traditional practice?

With new biochemical monitoring technology it is feasible that some of these answers could be obtained non-invasively in healthy human subjects. However, such topics would have been addressed traditionally with animal and organ culture experiments.

ANIMAL EXPERIMENTS

There can be no doubt of the problems of using animals to support research into herbal remedies. Apart from the difficulty of applying findings to the human situation, there are extremely strong ethical objections from almost all those who support the use of herbal medicines, especially in the English-speaking developed world.

Nevertheless, the subject cannot be dismissed entirely. In the first place much phytotherapeutic research in Europe has involved animal experimentation and the findings have entered everyday debate about the action of herbal remedies. Second, it is quite possible to devise trials that involve no pain or discomfort to the animals involved, as is the obvious practice in gerontological research (animals live longest when well treated). It is recalled that herbal therapy aims to support vital functions (in China the worth of any therapeutic practice is determined by how successfully its use appears to encourage a long and healthy life). If the intention of a trial was to assess the effects of herbal medication applied in approximately therapeutic doses adjusted for body weight and metabolism, there could be little complaint that the animals would be harmed and they are likely to actually benefit. Advice is that authorities responsible for licensing animal experiments are likely to consider such studies as indistinguishable from keeping animals as pets.

Feasible trials might include monitoring the effects of posited 'adaptogens' on life expectancy, stamina and reproductive capacity, the effects of antimicrobial remedies on normal resistance to disease among large populations and observing changes in digestive and urinary performance (as judged by changes in excretion, appetite and weight). As the common laboratory animal with a metabolism closest to the human being, the humble rat would probably be the creature of choice.

It might also be valuable to have the results of careful observations of the use of herbs in veterinary practice, where many of the limitations attending patient-practitioner interaction can be minimized.

Nevertheless, in modern times political sensitivities to any animal research are so great that few herbal researchers are likely to consider the modest net contribution of such trials to a useful understanding of the effects of herbal remedies on human beings as justifying the effort.

CELL, TISSUE AND ORGAN CULTURES

As part of the modern move to find alternatives to animal experimentation, increasing attention is being paid to techniques for assessing the effects of drugs on cultures of cells, tissues and organs in vitro. Conventional drug research is switching in this direction for preliminary screening in drug discovery programmes and there is a lesser move for at least initial toxicological testing.

The advantages are in the opportunity for the direct observation of the action of an agent on target cells, with reduced ethical difficulties (although the sacrifice of animals is often necessary to supply short-lived organ and tissue samples).

The problems are the limited application of such observations to the in vivo situation and the need to confirm any in vitro findings anyway. From the point of view of herbal research there is the additional problem that it is impossible at this stage to reproduce that balance of plant constituents that will actually reach internal tissues (after digestion, absorption and the 'first-pass' hepatic effect). Difficulties are increased by the desirability of using tissues most closely mimicking the real situation, i.e. mammalian organ cultures (rather than the easier to culture amphibian tissues or the less sophisticated cell lines).

Nevertheless, in vitro techniques could provide valuable supplementary information to other research, as in the following suggested projects.

- The influence of herbal extracts on epithelial tissue cultures (e.g. gastric, enteric and tracheal tissues; unfortunately the former two decline rapidly in culture). This represents a point of genuine tissue interaction with herbal remedies and might add much to pharmacokinetic research.
- Observations on the biotransformation of plant constituents using liver cultures (again short-lived and a technically difficult operation but one that is well established in conventional pharmacological research).
- Alteration in the migratory behaviour and internal metabolism of macrophages as a result of exposure to herbal extracts (herbal medicine claims to improve resistance to infections by a general enhancement of defensive mechanisms; looking directly at macrophage response is an established screening technique).
- The influence of herbal preparations on microbiological cultures (direct antiseptic action for some plant constituents has been established but many questions remain unanswered).
- Non-specific observations (as in gerontological research) on cell migrations, length of interphase, longevity and other pointers to in vitro cell health.

CONCLUSION

In reviewing the prospects for validating herbal medicine in a sceptical age, the first conclusion is that the job is overwhelming. The large number of medicines in use, the complexity of their pharmacology and the low financial gearing of the industry rule out an early overhaul by scientific scrutiny. The public will have to rely largely on the precedent of tradition in choosing to use herbal remedies for some time yet.

But choose herbs they will: modern demand continues to grow. The suppliers of herbal medicines and the legislators overseeing the supply have a common interest in working together to improve the level of knowledge available as best they can. The industry and profession may thus consider adopting an integrated, moderate-cost but rigorous and validatable research programme that reflects the special character of the material. The projects should be able to be conducted in small clinics and laboratory facilities and without prohibitive capital investment. To screen out the time-wasting project, protocol design and project oversight should be performed by university specialists.

In return for such endeavours, the herbal industry and profession could expect cooperation from regulatory authories. They should have clear encouragement for investigation that is not necessarily identical to that appropriate to the proving of new synthetic drugs and a declared willingness to include expert testimony from within the industry and profession in deliberations on the fate of herbal medicines. An undertaking of this nature will provide a strong incentive for the suppliers to invest time and finance in the necessary infrastructure for research activity.

However, by far the best reason for doing research is that it provides the best educational deal possible, for herbal students and practitioners alike. Many of the project ideas are feasible for student clinics associated with undergraduate degree training programmes and are even being piloted. Being trained to ask questions of their working environment is the best way to produce effective practitioners, able to adapt to different circumstances and avoid formulaic and lazy practice.

At its heart research is a process by which it is possible to develop the professional ideal of critical acumen, to select, sort and clarify the information available about a healing technique, to answer the fundamental question: 'Is this treatment likely to make the patient well or is it not?' As Carl Rogers put it:

> Scientific methodology needs to be seen for what it truly is: a way of preventing me from deceiving myself in regard to my creatively formed subjective hunches which have developed out of the relationship between me and my material.[18]

or as Oliver Cromwell is said to have cried: 'By the bowels of Christ, I beseech ye, bethink yourselves that ye may be mistaken'.

References

1. McQuay H, Carroll D, Moore A. Variation in the placebo effect in randomised controlled trials of analgesics: all is as blind as it seems. Pain 1996; 64 (2): 331–335.
2. Turner JA, Deyo R A, Loeser J D, Von Korff M, Fordyce W E. The importance of placebo effects in pain treatment and research. Journal of the American Medical Association 1994: 271 (20): 1609–1614.
3. Wilcox CS, Cohn JB, Linden RD et al. Predictors of placebo response: a retrospective analysis. Psychopharmacology Bulletin 1992; 28 (2): 157–162.
4. Rosenzweig P, Brochier S, Zipfel A. The placebo effect in healthy volunteers: influence of experimental conditions on the adverse events profile during phase I studies. Clinical Pharmacology and Therapeutics 1993; 54 (5): 578–583.
5. Hansen BJ, Meyhoff HH, Nordling J, Mensink HJA, Mogensen P, Larsen EH. Placebo effects in the pharmacological treatment of uncomplicated benign prostatic hyperplasia. Scandinavian Journal of Urology and Nephrology 1996; 30 (5): 373–377.
6. Fine PG, Roberts WJ, Gillette RG, Child TR. Slowly developing placebo responses confound tests of intravenous phentolamine to determine mechanisms underlying idiopathic chronic low back pain. Pain 1994; 56 (2): 235–242.
7. La Mantia L, Eoli M, Salmaggi A, Milanese C. Does a placebo-effect exist in clinical trials on multiple sclerosis? Review of the literature. Italian Journal of Neurological Sciences 1996; 17 (2): 135–139.
8. Ilnyckyj A, Shanahan F, Anton PA et al. Quantification of the placebo response in ulcerative colitis. Gastroenterology 1997; 112 (6): 1854–1858.
9. Lewander T. Placebo response in schizophrenia. European Psychiatry 1994; 9 (3): 119–120.
10. Brown WA. Placebo as a treatment for depression. Neuropsychopharmacology 1994; 4: 265–269.
11. Hrobjartsson A. The uncontrollable placebo effect. European Journal of Clinical Pharmacology 1996; 50 (5): 345–348.
12. Lewith GT, Aldridge D (eds). Clinical research methodology for complementary therapies. Hodder and Stoughton, London, 1993.
13. After Professor Manfred Porkert at the University of Munich
14. O'Regan B, Hirshberg C. Spontaneous remission: an annotated bibliography. Institute of Noetic Sciences, Sausalito, CA, 1993.
15. Reason P, Rowan J. Human inquiry: a sourcebook of new paradigm research. John Wiley, Chichester, 1981.
16. Diesing P. Patterns of discovery in the social sciences. Routledge and Kegan Paul, London, 1972
17. Aldridge D. Single case research designs. In Lewith GT, Aldridge D (eds) Clinical research methodology for complementary herapies. Hodder and Stoughton, London, 1993, pp 136–168.
18. Rogers CR. On becoming a person: a therapist's view of psychotherapy. Constable, London, 1961.
19 Laskin DM, Greene CS. Influence of the doctor-patient relationship on placebo therapy for patients with myofascial pain-dysfunction (MPD) syndrome. J Am Dent Assoc 1972; 85(4): 892–894

5 Optimizing safety

INTRODUCTION

Medical opinion generally has been that it is impossible for any medicine to have effects without side effects, that if herbs are claimed to be free from side effects they are probably not effective either.

This is a rational view, within its own terms. Any intervention at one site is always likely to lead to reactions at other sites, either because of functional or structural connection or because of similarity in sensitivity.

On the other hand, there is a persistent popular belief that herbs are safe. Probably the main reason why patients first turn to herbs is they assume they are free from side effects, 'not like drugs'. Many herbalists emphasize the same point. They refer to the uninterrupted use of the most established remedies by millions of people since prehistory. They also talk of herbs being used for different reasons than conventional drugs, promoting healing responses rather than targeting pathology or symptoms, of the whole herb being a complex package around the active constituents.

How can these discrepancies be resolved? The answer is not clear or satisfactory. The evidence shows that toxic effects of herbal remedies are rarely recorded, although there are a few cases that prompt concern. The main problem is a serious information vacuum into which adherents can project safety and critics hidden dangers. Most significantly, government regulators, in the interests of public safety, can exercise due diligence and reduce access to any herb over which even theoretical doubt may arise.

For all concerned, what is needed is more information on safety.

THE CASE FOR CONCERN

ADVERSE REPORTS

There have been a number of cases reported in the medical literature indicating a link between herbal consumption and adverse effects.

During the early 1990s several patients with renal failure were admitted to hospitals in Brussels with progressive interstitial fibrosis and tubular atrophy that was linked to a herbal slimming preparation. At least 30 individuals were found to have sustained terminal renal failure from the incident, making it perhaps the single most serious adverse event linked to herbal consumption in modern times. The Chinese herb *Aristolochia fangchi* was found to be an ingredient of the formulation instead of the intended *Stephania tetrandra*. The consequent presence of aristolochic acid, a known toxin, was put forward as a hypothesis for the aetiology of the nephropathies in the literature. However, the case prompted the Association Pharmaceutique Belge at the Service du Contrôle des Médicaments to probe the matter further.[1] They pointed to the idiosyncratic nature of the reactions and the presence of other powerful synthetic drugs in the mixture as suggesting a more complex story. They considered that the cocktail of sometimes powerful preparations adopted by some observing slimming regimes might have significantly lowered the threshold for renal damage. It is important to note that Aristolochia is still used in traditional medicine and that cases of toxicity are not recorded. It is more likely, therefore, that this tragic case is one of a herb-drug interaction than a simple herb toxicity. Nevertheless, in their report the Belgian authorities voiced wider concerns about the way in which

Chinese herbs were available in their country with few clear quality standards and without even observance of traditional preparation techniques and declared themselves unable to make any statement about their safe use.

During the early 1990s liver units in France began to report a number of cases of liver disease. The hepatotoxicity of germander (*Teucrium chamaedrys*) was confirmed in isolated rat hepatocytes, particularly a crude fraction containing the diverse furanoditerpenoids. It was concluded that they are activated by cytochrome P-450 3A into electrophilic metabolites that deplete glutathione and protein thiols and form plasma membrane blebs.[2] On the other hand, the ethanolic extract of another species of Teucrium has been found to have substantial hepatoprotective activity in the case of paracetemol-induced hepatic damage in mice.[3]

From January 1991 to December 1993, the Medical Toxicology Unit (formerly Poisons Unit) at Guy's and St Thomas's Hospital in London received reports of 11 cases of liver damage following the use of Chinese herbal medicine for skin conditions. There was strong evidence of an association in two cases in which recovery after withdrawal and recurrence of hepatitis after rechallenge were observed. The time-course relationship, recovery after ceasing Chinese herbal medicine and absence of alternative causes of liver damage suggested an association in two further symptomatic cases following a single period of exposure. Herbal material was available for analysis in seven cases. The plant mixtures varied so no single ingredient could account for liver injury. Effects did not appear dose related and it was concluded they were probably idiosyncratic.[4] Two patients were additionally described who suffered an acute hepatic illness related to taking traditional Chinese herbs for skin disease. Both recovered fully. The mixtures that they took included two plant components also contained within the mixture taken by a previously reported patient who suffered fatal hepatic necrosis.[5]

Animal exposure to pyrrolizidine alkaloids (PAs), found in several medicinal plants, has led to a dose-dependent swelling of hepatocytes and haemorrhagic necrosis of perivenular cells of the liver, with concomitant loss of sinusoidal lining cells with sinusoids filled with cellular debris, hepatocyte organelles and red blood cells. These are all features of venoocclusive disease.[6] LD_{50} for a pyrrolizidine-rich extract of Senecio was found to be 160 mg/kg.[7] Despite their similarity in structure, PAs vary in their individual LD_{50} and in the organs in which toxicity is expressed. In one study of four PAs the proportion of the PA removed by liver cultures varied considerably due to variation in the production of reactive metabolites (dehydroalkaloids), which appear to be largely responsible for the toxicity of PAs, and in their conversion to a safer form (GSDHP).[8] Among pyrrolizidine-containing plants, heliotrope[9] and *Senecio*[10] have been found to be responsible for venoocclusive disease in humans. Clinical manifestations of poisoning in humans include abdominal pain, ascites, hepatomegaly and raised serum transaminase levels. Prognosis is often poor with death rates of 20–30% being reported.[11] In vivo studies of coltsfoot, containing senkirkine, have shown some evidence of toxicity.[12] The main reported case turned out to be a substitution problem. Tea containing peppermint and what the mother thought was coltsfoot (*Tussilago farfara*) was associated with venoocclusive liver disease in an 18-month-old boy. Pharmacological analysis of the tea compounds revealed high amounts of PAs, mainly seneciphylline and the corresponding N-oxide. It was calculated that the child had consumed at least 60 μg/kg body weight per day of the toxic pyrrolizidine alkaloid mixture over 15 months. Macroscopic and microscopic analysis of the leaf material indicated that *Adenostyles allariae* had been erroneously gathered by the parents in place of coltsfoot. The child was given conservative treatment only and recovered completely within 2 months.[13]

A report from Denver in the USA described the cases of three children and three adults in whom severe toxic effects developed after ingestion of a Chinese herbal medication, jin bu huan, sold as a natural anodyne. A single, acute ingestion in children rapidly produced life-threatening neurologic and cardiovascular manifestations, while long-term jin bu huan use in adults was associated with hepatitis. Jin bu huan was found to contain levo-tetrahydropalmatine, a constituent with neuroactive activity.[14]

A case of acute hepatitis associated with the use of ma huang was reported from the USA. Ma huang, *Ephedra sinica et spp*, is advertised as being useful for causing weight loss and enhancing energy levels. Given the lack of reports in the literature of hepatotoxicity with ma huang and ephedrine, the authors speculated that the ma huang product concerned contained some other ingredient or contaminant or was misidentified. Nevertheless, the obvious adrenergic effect of ephedrine has led the USA Food and Drug Administration to restrict the sale of Ephedra products containing more than 8 mg of ephedrine per dose. This move was regretted by practitioners who use Ephedra for a range of beneficial effects in lung problems, febrile disease and allergic conditions.[15]

A review of 18 case reports of pennyroyal ingestion documented moderate to severe toxicity in patients who had been exposed to at least 10 ml of pennyroyal oil. In one fatal case, postmortem examination of a serum sample, which had been obtained 72 hours after the acute ingestion, identified 18 ng of pulegone per ml and 1 ng of menthofuran per ml.[16]

Traditional intoxication with the Chinese remedy *Atractylis gummifera* usually occurs in the spring and is related to chewing the roots of these plants. Severe hepatocellular lysis may occur less than 24 hours after ingestion.[17] One case reported was in a 7-year-old boy who drank an extract made from the plant's root for medicinal purposes. He was admitted to hospital 2 days after ingestion, in coma, with epigastric pain, vomiting and general anxiety. Laboratory findings showed severe hepatocellular damage and acute renal failure. In spite of all treatment and therapeutic efforts, the boy died 8 days after admission. A postmortem histopathological study of the liver confirmed the panlobular hepatic necrosis and allowed the differential diagnosis of the intoxication from Reye's syndrome.[18]

PLANTS AS POISONS

It is accepted by all involved that not all plants are safe to use as remedies. The incidence of these clearly varies from country to country. In Britain, for example, a Ministry of Agriculture, Fisheries and Food publication reviewed the published literature on the toxicology of plants in that country.[19] Adverse effects after their consumption by animals or humans are reported for a high proportion of natural flora. Nevertheless, most reports concern damage to livestock after undue or excessive grazing and clear harm to humans is seldom reported. In very few cases are plants seen to be poisonous in low doses. The authors concluded that while many plants in Britain are known to be poisonous, few are dangerously so and cases of severe poisoning in animals or man are relatively rare.[19] They went on to point out, however, that the full effects of toxic constituents of plants are difficult to assess and left open the possibility that many plants, including ordinary foodstuffs, might have low-level toxicity that would be difficult to isolate.

Some plants historically used by herbalists are generally understood as potentially poisonous. Under the terms of the UK Medicines Act 1968 herbal practitioners are permitted to use some of these plants for internal use (marked below with their maximum permitted dosage) or externally (marked *) but they are not permitted for general sale (although some marked † are available for external use only). Others are available only on doctor's prescription.[20] Most are, in any case, only used rarely.

*Aconitum spp**
Adonis vernalis (100 mg tds)
Arnica montana †
Areca catechu
Atropa belladonna (herba 50 mg; radix 30 mg tds)
Bryonia alba
Chelidonium majus (2 g tds)
Chenopodium ambroisioides
Cinchona spp. (250 mg tds)
Colchicum autumnale (100 mg tds)
*Conium maculatum**
Convallaria majalis (150 mg tds)
Corynanthe yohimbi
Crotalaria spp
Cucurbita maxima
Datura stramonium (50 mg tds)
Digitalis spp
Duboisia spp
Ephedra sinica (600 mg tds)
Gelsemium sempervirens (25 mg tds)
Hagenia abyssinica
Heliotropium europaeum
Hyoscyamus niger (100 mg tds)
Juniperus sabina
Mallotus philippinensis
Mandragora officinarum
Papaver somniferum
*Pilocarpus microphyllus**
Podophyllum peltatum
Rauwolfia spp
*Rhus toxicodendron**
*Senecio jacobaea**
Strychnos spp

PLANTS PROMOTING CANCER?

Several herbal constituents have been shown to have in vivo carcinogenic activity. These include the alkenylbenzenes safrole, estragole and methyleugenol. However, others in the same chemical group such as anethole, myristicine, parsleyapiol, dill-apiol, elemicin, eugenol and isosafrole have been shown to have little or no such activity in vivo.[21]

On the other hand, plant material, including fruit and vegetables, has demonstrated sometimes substantial antimutagenic activity in a number of studies[22–25] (see also p.158).

PHOTOTOXICITY

Plants of the family Umbelliferae cause a dermatitis due to a phototoxic reaction caused by furanocoumarins (psoralens) and simultaneous exposure to sunlight. In one report four patients were found with partial skin thickness burns, induced by this phototoxic reaction. One occurred after contact with parsley (*Petroselinum crispum)* and three others after contact with giant hogweed (*Heracleum mantegazzianum*) and simultaneous exposure to sunlight.[26]

Cattle grazing heavy quantities of St John's wort have also suffered photodermatitis[26a].

Except for skin contact with hogweed, which is notoriously irritant, there is no serious suggestion that normal consumption of any of these plants leads to any risk.

HYPERSENSITIVITY REACTIONS

The literature refers to a number of cases where acute hypersensitivity reactions have occurred to herbal remedies. The Umbelliferae[27] and spice plants[28] have been most often implicated with reactions to chamomile and feverfew also listed.

It is possible that a proportion of adverse effects otherwise cited in this chapter may be due to idiosyncratic reactions rather than to overt toxicity. The classic features of idiosyncratic reactions are that they are not predictable, i.e. there is no obviously toxic element identifiable. They are also usually rare. Although they may sometimes be serious it is difficult, on the basis of occasional idiosyncratic reactions, to justify the withdrawal of a product from general use.

HEROIC REMEDIES

A number of remedies are often referred to as toxic because they provoke vomiting or catharsis or eliminate worms (which necessitates some toxicity). In the past, however, when survival imperatives outweighed comfort, powerful drugs were highly prized in acute gut infections. Most of the following examples are limited in the UK and elsewhere.

Aspidosperma quebracho-blanco (50 mg tds)
Euonymus atropurpureus
Euonymus europaeus
Dryopteris filix-mas
Ipomoea jalapa
Ipomoea purpurea
Lobelia inflata (200 mg tds)
Sanguinaria canadensis

Of these, only lobelia and sanguinaria find current use among herbal practitioners, the former for its relaxant rather than its emetic properties.

PREGNANCY AND LACTATION

It is a general principle that one should refrain from giving medicines to a pregnant woman unless clearly necessary. Although some herbs have been used safely by women when pregnant and may thus be seen to have a degree of positive vetting, they should be prescribed particularly carefully in the crucial first trimester when foetal organ development is under way. Although there are very few accounts that link any pregnancy problems to herb consumption, too little is known for any sweeping recommendation. Particular caution should be exercised for plants with alkaloidal principles, strong volatile constituents (notably including pure essential oils and plants with high levels of thujone) and anthraquinone laxatives and in cases where there is a history of miscarriage or where low back or abdominal pains occur.

There are a number of herbs which should be particularly avoided in pregnancy. In many popular herb books, the term 'emmenagogue' is used to refer to a gynaecological remedy. Probably the most frequent indication for such remedies in earlier times was to bring on delayed menstruation; in other words, many 'emmenagogues' were used for birth control, as abortifacients. This was likely to be one of the specialist skills of 'wise women' and theoretically remedies affecting the gravid uterus are as likely to harm foetal growth as to abort pregnancy. The following should be included in such a list.

Artemisia absinthium et spp
Berberis vulgaris
Caulophyllum thalictroides
Chelidonium majus
Cimicifuga racemosa
Cinchona spp
Crocus sativa
Dryopteris filix-mas
Gossypium herbaceum
Hydrastis canadensis
Juniperus communis
Mentha pulegium
Origanum vulgare

Phytolacca decandra
Rosmarinus officinalis
Ruta graveolens
Salvia officinalis
Sanguisorba canadensis
Tanacetum vulgare
Thuja occidentalis

In regulatory terms the caution referred to above in the case of pregnancy is also extended to the stage of lactation. Although critical organ development is not threatened there remains doubt about how secondary plant metabolites, many of which pass easily and even preferentially into breast milk, affect the baby. Practitioners should therefore maintain a degree of caution in attending to clinical problems affecting mother and suckling baby.

CASES OF CONTENTION

FALSE ALARMS?

There has been increasing concern among herb users about recent initiatives by regulators around the world. Lists of 'dangerous herbs' have sometimes included plants for which evidence of any realistic toxicity in normal human usage is very poor. The European Commission Committee for Proprietary Medicinal Products in 1992 circulated a list of herbal remedies that it considered should be withdrawn (at least for over-the-counter sale) for safety reasons. As well as many undoubtedly powerful and toxic plants, they include many remedies still widely used and indeed popular among practitioners and the wider public, such as the following examples.

Angelica archangelica (angelica seed and herb)
Berberis vulgaris (barberry bark and root)
Borago officinalis (borage herb and flowers)
Juglans regia (walnut fruit shell)
Petroselinum crispum (parsley seed)
Pulsatilla vulgaris (pasqueflower herb)
Ruta graveolens (rue herb and leaf)
Tanacetum vulgare (tansy flower and herb)
Vinca minor (lesser periwinkle herb and leaf)

There was no consultation with practitioner representatives before this list was produced and its appearance caused a shock to the profession. The fact that the list has had little impact on availability in practice has not reduced the disquiet that representation of herbal expertise on controlling bodies is inadequate and that it is too easy for legislative diktat to constrict herb availability.

A climate of restriction may be created by reports of potential adverse effects in the medical literature. On the other hand, these are not always as conclusive as they may seem. In one paper in 1989[29] the authors implicated British over-the-counter herbal sedative products in four cases of liver damage. However, on closer examination there was no indication whether the herbal remedies were primarily or secondarily involved, no evidence that might implicate either a constituent or an adulterant, hypersensitivity or interaction with other events, and no mechanism for hepatotoxicity. Although the authors freely admitted that they had no firm evidence to suspect any individual constituents, the fact that both products concerned had at certain times contained valerian and skullcap led to these herbs being suspected. However, given the lack of comparable reports in a country where use of these herbs is popular and the other poorly charted predisposing factors, it was difficult to see how the implications of direct hepatotoxicity could be substantiated. On further follow-up, the evidence was found not to be overwhelming and the British Medicines Control Agency were not moved to act against either the constituents or the products themselves. Nevertheless, a shadow was cast over both herbs and indeed on herbal products in general, spurring frequent articles and letters in the leading British journals on the the hidden dangers of herbal use.

It may be easier to publish reports in medical journals on the risks of herbal remedies than it is to prepare a publishable account of their efficacy. In the first case anecdotal evidence is the norm, in the latter case it would be dismissed out of hand. It is therefore incumbent on authors who rely on anecdote (and editors who review the results) to be assiduous in their presentation of the evidence (to get the botanical details correct, for example), to look for other possible factors in the pathogenesis and consistently to insert caveats about their inability to generalize from their evidence.

At the end of the day, risk assessment is more a political than scientific discipline. The BSE crisis in Europe led to a marked increase in sensitivity to risk, with food policy measures being made in that case on the basis of risks less than one in many millions. It is inconceivable that truly dangerous activities like driving and smoking would ever be banned, although each may be curtailed to some extent. Unfortunately, for the same reason, herbal medicine is vulnerable; although its political weight is apparent when there have been serious threats to its future (in Britain, Germany and the USA, for example), it is less able to muster strong political reasons to save its outlying positions. A question of definition arises in these discussions. What does toxicity actually mean in real life?

POISONOUS FOOD

Many ordinary foods naturally contain poisonous constituents.

- Wheat, rye, barley and oats contain a protein gluten that is hydrolysed in the digestive system to yield the peptide alpha-gliadin, a well-established and occasionally dangerous intestinal irritant that has caused many thousands of deaths around the world through coeliac disease and sprue.
- Apple seeds and the kernels of apricots, plums and other stone fruits, as well as bitter almonds, contain significant quantities of glycosides that yield cyanide on hydrolysis in the digestive tract.
- The cabbage family contain glucosinalates that yield toxic nitriles and goitrogenic thiocyanates.
- The oil from rapeseed, widely grown in temperate climates as a cheap vegetable oil, contains erucic acid, which is known to cause heart damage in experimental animals.[30]
- Potatoes are members of the deadly nightshade family; when the tuber turns green under the influence of light it produces the same poisonous alkaloids.
- Many common household pulses, including soya bean, red kidney bean and haricot bean (as in baked beans), contain toxic lectins called phytohaemagglutinins as well as trypsin inhibitors, that can only reliably be neutralized by boiling for at least 30 minutes.

The foods listed above are considered safe to eat, most in unlimited quantities. They do, however, demonstrate how difficult it is to predict the toxicity of a plant from the presence of toxic constituents alone. The action of the whole plant and the way in which it is normally consumed clearly in these cases count for more than any individual constituent list. It is at least possible that medicinal plants impugned for their inclusion of toxic constituents are in the same position. In the absence of clear reports of adverse side effects, it can be argued that the burden of proof falls on those who would restrict access to popular remedies.

THE NOCEBO EFFECT

The potency of the placebo effect as a contributor to clinical efficacy is discussed elsewhere (p.87). Although the scale of the impact may be surprising, the fact of placebo or non-specific activity is generally accepted.

What is much less debated are negative placebo effects. In reports on most double-blind clinical trials there are accounts of adverse effects among the placebo group. The symptoms listed cover a wide range and are not necessarily short-term and transient. In one report of studies of 1228 healthy volunteers the overall incidence of adverse events during placebo administration was 19%. Complaints were more frequent after repeated dosing (28%) and in elderly subjects (26%). Overall, the most frequent adverse events were headache (7%), drowsiness (5%) and asthenia (4%), with some variation depending on study design and populations.[31] Pain can certainly be induced by placebo[32] and placebo can also interact negatively with other medications.[33]

The nocebo effect raises an intriguing prospect. It is quite likely that some adverse effects ascribed to a remedy are as non-specific as placebo-induced efficacy. Most of these nocebo effects are likely to be clinically insignificant but there are real possibilities that more serious adverse effects could also have nothing directly to do with the remedy itself.

Unfortunately, placebo-controlled safety studies are not feasible but it will be helpful in assessing overall herbal safety to have some better understanding of the potential of the nocebo effect to confound the picture.

HERBAL SAFETY: THE ARGUMENTS

A MATTER OF DEBATE

With the paucity of hard facts, the issue of herbal safety is a matter of contention. The following are the arguments marshalled by the doubters, particularly those who feel that their duty to public safety is to assume the worst-case scenarios.

The doubts

- Herbal remedies are complex mixtures of chemicals, about whose effects on the body little is known even in their isolated state, let alone when mixed in infinitely variable ways.
- Chemical complexity can work in both directions, buffering against and towards potentiation of adverse effects.
- Traditional use is likely to have spotted only acute and relatively frequent adverse reactions; chronic, delayed or infrequent reactions would probably not have been associated with the herb.

• Traditional reputations are in any case highly unreliable in their transmission.

• It is possible to exceed modern standards of risk, say 1:1000, and still statistically mean that very few working practitioners will see the adverse events in their lifetimes (although this argument does not apply to consumer branded products selling in millions of units per annum).

• There are particularly heavy biases in the way of reporting adverse effects of herbal remedies at the present time (see below); therefore the current state of information is almost certainly understating the risk.

The reassurances

• The remedies used in herbal medicine represent only a tiny proportion of available plant species around the world. It is likely that humans through history moved inexorably to using those plants that were effective with a minimum of toxic or other adverse consequences.

• Even allowing for underreporting of adverse events, the levels in the database are remarkably low and certainly do not compare with the levels of iatrogenic problems in conventional medicine.

• Some benign qualities may arise from the very complexity of the plants for which they are dismissed by conventional pharmacologists. The existence of tannins, mucilages, saponins or other constituents is likely to buffer or modulate the effect of more active constituents, which are often in any case present in only low levels.

• Most of the serious adverse events reported involve problems of product quality and adulteration. Attendance to pharmaceutical standards of quality assurance and quality control (as is the norm for European herbal medicinal products) and insisting on minimal training standards for those who prescribe herbal remedies will reduce risk.

• Most importantly, the thrust of treatment in herbal medicine is often different from that of conventional pharmacology. The herbs may better be understood as promoting healing responses in the body rather than directly targeting symptoms or pathology; this allows for a more elliptical, nutritional tilt at the body with consequent reduced negative impact. Certain herbs may be contraindicated in certain cases, not because they can cause side effects or threaten danger but because they may simply be inappropriate for the job.

CONDITIONAL CONCLUSIONS

None of the arguments presented above are mutually contradictory. An honourable position is possible on either side.

Given the low profile of adverse effects compared with other human activities, however, it could be argued strongly that herbal use be given the benefit of the many doubts that remain. The burden of proof should lie with the regulator rather than with the herbal sector; that theoretical reasons for impugning safety (such as the presence of constituents with toxic potential in isolation) are not sufficient in themselves for banning herbal remedies. Nevertheless, the herbal sector has a professional responsibility to assiduously and continuously monitor the situation and to react responsibly if genuine concerns arise.

INTERACTIONS WITH CONVENTIONAL DRUGS

There is a major deficit of useful information about the interactions between herbal and synthetic remedies.

Interactions between herbs and synthetic drugs can be classified as either pharmacodynamic or pharmacokinetic. Pharmacodynamic interactions, that is those of pharmacological activities, are at least predictable in theory and much of this section will be focused on these. On the other hand, pharmacokinetic interactions, whereby ingestion of a herb modifies the absorption, distribution, metabolism or excretion of a drug or vice versa, are far less predictable. It is this latter type of interaction which generates the major uncertainties in the use of synthetic drugs with herbal remedies. More information is urgently required about herb-drug interactions which have a pharmacokinetic basis.

It is not surprising that most suggestions for pharmacodynamic interactions involve herbal remedies that contain conventionally researched active constituents, many of which are not widely used by herbal practitioners and even fewer are generally available over the counter in health shops. To what extent the lack of information on the greater proportion of the herbal materia medica reflects genuine lack of interaction or simply inadequate research is an open question. It is most unlikely that incidences of interaction have been clarified when there is so little use of herbal remedies within the usual conventional system. On the other hand, most herbal remedies, especially those bought by the users directly, are likely to be of only moderate pharmacological impact.

Even where there is a pharmacological case it very rarely reflects actual clinical experience. The following adverse reactions are in most cases theoretical risks only and may be even less likely where the constituents concerned occur in the context of crude herbal preparations because:

- the concentration of each active is usually relatively low compared with synthetic counterparts or experimental experience;
- interactions within herbal remedies often involve neutralizing and buffering of actives by modifying constituents such as mucilages, tannins and resins.

For such reasons it is also unlikely that all the expected generic interactions involving classes of conventional agents such as diuretics, antihypertensives or sedatives apply to their herbal counterparts where activity is significantly milder and where pharmacological mechanisms are different (e.g. osmotic diuresis and antispasmodic and vasodilating antihypertensives).

Areas where hidden interactions may occur include the following.

- Phenolic constituents such as flavonoids and tannins may share some of the cautions attending salicylates, although the lack of interactions noted for conventional rutosides, and for the anthraquinone laxatives, is a reassurance.
- Resins, tannins and mucilaginous constituents are likely to interact with absorption of many substances, most often, but not always, reducing their availability and plasma concentrations.
- Hot spices are likely to increase absorption rates of many pharmacological agents[34] and may also accelerate the metabolism of some, but there is no information as to whether bitter digestives have any comparable effect or whether stimulation of digestive secretions in other ways interacts with the availability of drugs.

There are areas where the information deficit is particularly obvious. The potential effects of herbal constituents on blood sugar levels in insulin-dependent diabetes are almost unknown. In practice, caution has always dictated that herbal treatment concurrent with insulin needs to be done under close expert supervision. Similar cautions apply to the use of herbs along with prescribed warfarin, heparin and other anticoagulants, as well as digoxin, although interactions in these cases are better described.

However, all these uncertainties should be placed in the context of the normal consumption of plant and other organic material in the diet. Any substantial consumption of tea, coffee, alcohol or tobacco will have more effects on drug activity than most herbal prescriptions. The interactions between medicines and foodstuffs is a question for a much larger proportion of prescriptions. The deficit of information in these cases is even more glaring.

The lack of information on interactions benefits no-one. Those in the forefront of herbal medicine have all agreed that it is important that clinical experiences of interactions be reported. Where access to conventional reporting schemes is available, it should be used. In other cases, there is a dedicated reporting mechanism available on the PhytoNET website at http://ex.ac.uk/phytonet/

Table 5.1 reflects the best current assessment of possible interactions, balancing theoretical possibilities (mostly drawn from standard dispensary texts) with experience of the likely impact in clinical reality. It is an incomplete dossier. Suspected herb-drug interactions are also provided in the herbal monograph section.

It is of course possible for the skilled practitioner to use some of the following interactions to therapeutic advantage, either by reinforcing a desired effect or by reducing (in cooperation with the prescribing physician) the amount of synthetic medication required.

It must also be emphasized that the interactions listed are rarely established as such. The great majority of cases are only theoretical. The reason for listing them is to encourage practitioners to be alert to the possibilities rather than to predict likely outcomes.

However, prudence and good practice suggest that the following combinations be considered with caution. Particular care should be taken in cases highlighted in bold text where possible reactions are especially serious.

THE ISSUE OF QUALITY

APPRECIATING QUALITY

Medicinal herbs are sourced from nature and hence, unlike conventional chemical drugs, vary from batch to batch. This can be readily understood by comparison with another plant product – wine. In technical terms, wine is the fermented juice of the fruit of *Vitis vinifera*. However, factors such as the grape variety, climatic conditions, soil type, time of harvest and fermentation conditions can all determine whether a batch of wine will be either poor or good quality

Table 5.1 Herb-drug interactions

Herbal remedy or class	Possible conventional drug interactions	*Possible* reactions
Antimuscarinics (e.g. belladonna, datura, henbane)	Analgesics	Increased antimuscarinic effects
	Antiarrhythmic agents	Increased antimuscarinic effects; delayed absorption of antiarrhythmics
	Anticholinergic drugs	Additive effects
	Antidepressants: monoamine oxidase inhibitors (MAOIs) and tricyclics	Increased antimuscarinic effects
	Antiemetics	Antagonism of metoclopramide and domperidone
	Antifungals	Reduced absorption of ketoconazole
	Antihistamines	Increased antimuscarinic side effects
	Cisapride (GI motility stimulant)	Antagonism
	Dopaminergics	Increased antimuscarinic side effects
	Nitrates	Reduced sublingual absorption (due to dry mouth)
	Parasympathomimetics	Antagonism
Cardioactive glycosides (e.g. foxglove, lily-of-the-valley)	ACE inhibitors	Potentiation of cardiac glycosides
	Antiarrhythmic agents	Plasma concentration of cardioactive glycosides increased
	Anthranoid laxatives	Potassium depletion leading to adverse cardiovascular effects
	Antibiotics	Effect of cardioactive glycosides enhanced by erythromycin and other macrolides; digitoxin metabolism increased by rifampicins
	Antiepileptics	Metabolism of digitoxin accelerated by carbamazepine
	Antifungals	Plasma concentration increased by itraconazole; **increased cardioactive glycoside plasma concentration with amphotericin**
	Antimalarials	**Plasma concentration of cardioactive glycosides raised by quinine and possibly chloroquine**; possible bradycardia
	Barbiturates	Metabolism of digitoxin accelerated
	Beta-blockers	Increased AV block, bradycardia
	Calcium channel blockers	AV block, bradycardia, increased plasma concentration of digoxin reported
	Digoxin	Potentiation, increased risk of adverse effects
	Diuretics	**Increased toxicity if hypokalaemia occurs; effects of cardioactive glycosides enhanced by spironolactone**
	Muscle relaxants	Arrhythmias
	Non-steroidal antiinflammatory drugs (NSAIDs)	Increased plasma concentrations of cardioactive glycosides; heart failure exacerbated by NSAIDs
	Steroids	Hypokalaemia
	Ulcer-healing drugs	Plasma concentration of cardioactive glycosides possibly increased by proton pump inhibitors; increased toxicity if hypokalaemia occurs with carbenoxolone

Herbal remedy or class	Possible conventional drug interactions	*Possible* reactions
Gammalinoleic acid (GLA)-rich remedies (e.g. evening primrose, borage,	Antiepileptics	Increased risk of seizure (equivocal evidence)
Grapefruit juice	Antihistamines	Increased plasma concentration of terfenadine
	Calcium channel blockers	Increased plasma concentration of dihydropyridines
	Immunosuppressants	Increased plasma concentration of cyclosporin; also many other enhancing effects on bioavailability of drugs
Potatoes, tomatoes, eggplants and other nightshades (containing solanaceous alkaloids)	Anaesthetics and muscle relaxants	Increased plasma half-life of anesthetics and muscle relaxants
Garlic, artichoke, fenugreek	Cholesterol-lowering agents	Additive effects
Ginseng	MAOI antidepressants	Interaction with phenelzine suspected
Guar gum (and other bulking agents?)	Antibiotics	Absorption of phenoxymethylpenicillin reduced
Herbal sedatives (e.g. valerian, hops, wild lettuce)	Alpha-blockers	Enhanced sedative effects
	Anaesthetics	Enhanced sedative effects
	Analgesics	Enhanced sedative effects
	Tricyclic antidepressants	Enhanced sedative effects
	Antiemetics	Potentiation of sedative side effects
	Antiepileptics	Potentiation of sedative side effects
	Beta-blockers	Enhanced sedative effects
	Hypnotics	Additive effects
Anthranoid laxatives	Antidiarrhoeals	Antagonism
	Cardioactive glycosides	Potassium depletion leading to adverse cardiovascular effects
Licorice	Antihypertensives	Antagonism
	Cardioactive glycosides	Potassium depletion leading to adverse cardiovascular effects
	Diuretics	Potassium depletion with adverse effects especially likely when combined with cardiovascular glycosides as above
Opioid plants (e.g. Californian poppy)	Antidepressants, MAOIs	CNS excitation, hyper- or hypotension
	Antipsychotics	Increased sedative effect
	Anxiolytics	Increased sedative effect
	Dopaminergics	CNS excitation, hyperpyrexia
	Ulcer-healing drugs	Cimetidine inhibits opioid metabolism, increases plasma concentration
Cinchona bark (containing quinine)	Antiarrhythmics	Plasma concentration of flecainide increased
	Antihistamines	Ventricular arrhythmias with astemizole and terfenadine

contd. ....

Table 5.1 Herb-drug interactions.....Contd

Herbal remedy or class	Possible conventional drug interactions	*Possible* reactions
	Cardioactive glycosides	**Plasma concentration of digoxin increased (reduce digoxin dose)**
	Ulcer-healing drugs	Metabolism inhibited by cimetidine (i.e. increased plasma concentration)
Pungent (hot) remedies (e.g. cayenne, ginger, horseradish, mustards)	Antacids	Antagonism, increased mucosal irritation
	General medication	Increased absorption from gut wall and other mucosal surfaces generally likely; also possible increased metabolism, i.e. increased rises in plasma concentration, possibly shorter half-life
Remedies interacting with platelet function (e.g. ginger, garlic, clove, feverfew)	Anticoagulants	Potentiation of bleeding
Remedies alkalinizing urine (e.g. celery)	Aspirin	Aspirin excretion increased
Salicylate-rich remedies (e.g. willow bark, poplar bark) NB: most natural salicylates have less activity than aspirin so cautions are less necessary	Abortifacients	**Avoid with mifepristine and for 12 days after**
	Anticoagulants	**Potentiation**
	Antiemetics	Metoclopramide enhances effect of salicylates
	Antiepileptics	Transient enhancement of effects of phenytoin and valproate
	Cytotoxics	**Reduced excretion (increased toxicity) of methotrexate**
	Diuretics	Antagonism of spironolactone; reduced excretion (increased toxicity) of acetazolamide
	NSAIDs	Increased side effects
	Uricosuric drugs	Effect of probenecid and sulphinpyrazone reduced
Sympathomimetics (e.g. ephedrine and pseudoephedrine, myristicin from ma huang, nutmeg respectively)	ACE inhibitors	**Severe hypertension**
	Anaesthetics	Arrhythmia
	Antidepressants	Hypertensive crises with MAOIs; hypertension, arrhythmias with tricyclics
	Antihypertensives	Antagonism
	Antipsychotics	Antagonize pressor action
	Beta-blockers	**Hypertension (possibly severe)**
	Bronchodilators	Potentiation
	Diuretics	Increased risk of hypokalaemia
	Dopaminergics	Increased risk of toxicity with bromocriptine
	Muscle relaxants	Potentiation
	Sympathomimetics	Potentiation and hypertension
	Vasoconstrictor sympathomimetics	Increased vasopressor effects
Vasoconstrictors (e.g. broom)	Antihypertensives	Antagonism
	Sympathomimetics	Hypertension
Vasodilators (e.g. hawthorn)	Antihypertensives	Additive effects

Herbal remedy or class	Possible conventional drug interactions	*Possible* reactions
Vitamins	Anticoagulants	Vitamin K antagonizes
	Antiepileptics	Folic acid occasionally reduces plasma concentration; vitamin D requirements increased
	Diuretics	Hypercalcaemia with thiazides and vitamin D supplementation
	Dopaminergics	Levodopa antagonized with pyridoxine
Xanthine-rich remedies (e.g. cola, maté)	Antidepressants, selective serotonin reuptake inhibitors (SSRIs)	Plasma concentration of xanthines increased
	Antihypertensives	Antagonism

(which is subsequently reflected in the price of the wine).

In the case of wine, factors such as the texture, colour, aroma and taste determine if the product is of good quality or otherwise. For medicinal plants, the situation is much more complex. Most of the chemical components of herbs which are important for therapeutic activity are secondary metabolites. Secondary metabolites are defined as those not likely to be important for normal growth and survival of the plant, although they are sometimes produced in higher levels in response to infection, insect attack and adverse growing conditions. One consequence of this is that even though they may give an impression of its quality, the appearance and colour of a herb are not necessarily indicators of its therapeutic benefit or safety. Indeed, plants grown under adverse conditions may sometimes have a poor appearance but higher levels of secondary metabolites. One corollary of this is that while herb batches which have a good appearance and a pleasant taste might be suitable for a herbal tea, they may not be optimum for use as medicines. For example, in chamomile, matricine is considered to be an important active component and varieties of chamomile have been bred which have higher levels of this compound. Since matricine imparts a bitter taste to the flowers, these high medicinal grade varieties are not suitable for a culinary herbal tea.

MARKERS OF QUALITY?

One approach adopted by the various pharmacopoeias and used by manufacturers is to set minimum levels of marker chemical compounds for a herbal raw material. These are seen to give an indication of activity and hence quality. This approach is fraught with difficulties. Even where the marker compound is known to contribute to the therapeutic activity of the herb (and this is not always the case), herbalists stress that the chemical complexity of the plant confers the sum total of its activity. However, until there is better understanding of how individual herbs work in their chemical totality, setting markers is a good starting point. The uncertainties can be lessened by choosing phytochemical classes of marker compounds (flavonoids, essential oil, oligomeric procyanidins, etc.) rather than just individual chemical constituents. In addition, testing for different marker compounds (or groups of marker compounds) in the one plant can lead to a better assessment of activity. However, none of this should occur at the expense of the chemical totality of the plant's extractable material.

GMP

In a number of countries, including those in Europe as well as Japan and Australia, all herbal medicines must, by law, be made according to the code of pharmaceutical GMP (Good Manufacturing Practice). This is a fail-safe system of quality assurance and quality control which defines a number of procedures and observances including:

- validation of equipment and processes;
- documented standard operating procedures covering every aspect of manufacture;
- documented cleaning and calibration logs for equipment;
- control of the manufacturing environment, air and water;
- quarantining and unique identification and testing of raw materials, labels and packaging;
- discrete batch identification;
- comprehensive batch record documentation;

Box 5.1 Herbal raw material testing

- Identity and quality with thin layer chromatography (TLC)
- Microscopic analysis
- Macroscopic analysis and organoleptic assessment
- Pesticide residues
- Microbial levels
- Aflatoxins
- Heavy metals
- Foreign material
- Infestation
- Radiation levels
- Active or marker compounds (quantitative)

Box 5.2 Thin Layer Chromatography

- An extract of a herb is spotted at the bottom of a thin layer of silica gel on a glass plate.
- The plate is dipped in a solvent mixture.
- The solvent draws up the layer and carries the components in the herb for different distances.
- Sprays and/or ultraviolet light are used to view the components, giving a characteristic pattern of spots.
- Each spot corresponds to a component in the herb.
- Different solvent systems draw out different classes of components in the herb.

Box 5.3 Quality considerations for finished liquid herbal products

- Extraction efficiency
- Identity
  a) organoleptic assessment
  b) TLC or HPLC fingerprint
- Active or marker components
- Microbial testing
  a) total count
  b) pathogens
  c) yeast and mould
- Pesticides

Box 5.4 Quality considerations for finished tablet herbal products

- Identity
  a) organoleptic assessment
  b) TLC
- Microbial testing
  a) total count
  b) pathogens
  c) yeasts and mould
- Hardness and friability
- Disintegration time
- Weight
- Active or marker components

- reconciliation of raw materials, product, packaging and labels;
- quarantining and testing of finished products;
- documented release-for-sale procedures;
- testing of stability of finished product;
- documentation of customer complaints and recall procedures.

In the USA, large herbal medicine manufacturers comply with full pharmaceutical GMP; however, the recently proposed legal requirement is that less than full GMP (the smaller GMPs) must be adhered to.

In practice, herbal manufacturing under GMP is more complex than conventional drugs. This is because a herb is biologically rather than chemically defined and:

- may be incorrectly identified;
- may vary in chemical content and hence efficacy;
- carries with it 'a history', i.e. it may be contaminated with unwanted substances;
- processing of herbs may enhance or impair their safety and efficacy;
- stability may be difficult to define and measure.

Nevertheless, all the considerations above point strongly to the importance of herbal product manufacture under appropriate GMP.

As part of GMP, herbal raw materials are subjected to a battery of tests to ensure their quality and purity. These tests are outlined in Box 5.1. A useful guide to the British and European standards in these areas is provided by the *British Herbal Pharmacopoeia*.[35]

Thin layer chromatography (TLC) is a particularly useful technique for the identification of plant material. It can also be used to quantify plant constituents. The process of performing TLC is outlined in Box 5.2

Finished herbal products also need to undergo testing before their release. Boxes 5.3 and 5.4 provide examples of possible testing protocols for finished products.

MICROBIAL CONTAMINATION

Since plants come from nature, herbal raw materials carry a microbial burden which needs to be reduced during processing.

The *European Pharmacopoeia* sets limits for microbial contamination for herbal remedies in Category 4 under Part 1, VIII.15 Microbial Quality of Pharmaceutical Preparations (1995) as follows.

A. Herbal remedies to which boiling water has been added before use

- Total viable aerobic count. Not more than 10^7 aerobic bacteria and not more than 10^5 fungi per gram or per millilitre.
- Not more than 10^2 *Escherichia coli* per gram or per millilitre.

B. Other herbal remedies

- Total viable aerobic count. Not more than 10^5 aerobic bacteria and not more than 10^4 fungi per gram or per millilitre.
- Not more than 10^3 enterobacteria and certain other Gram-negative bacteria per gram or per millilitre.
- Absence of *Escherichia coli* (1.0 g or 1.0 ml).
- Absence of salmonella (1.0 g or 1.0 ml).

These levels are incidentally much tighter than those applied to food supply industries where absolute levels are often absent.

SUBSTITUTION PROBLEMS IN HERBAL MEDICINE

Substitution of one herbal raw material with another can pose a considerable problem in herbal manufacture. Substitution can occur at several different levels:

- within a species of a less active chemical race or subspecies;
- of the wrong or less active plant part;
- within a genus of a related plant;
- of a completely different genus.

Many problems associated with herbal quality have been caused by substitution. This particularly threatens remedies that have suddenly become wildly popular so that demand exceeds supply, e.g. the substitution of Echinacea with *Parthenium integrifolium* and the replacement of *Hypericum perforatum* (St John's wort) with other Hypericum species. It is particularly serious where safety is compromised, e.g. the substitution of *Teucrium species* (germander) for *Scutellaria lateriflora* (skullcap).

Some substitution practices avoid detection at manufacture, even under GMP, and can occasionally be detected in over-the-counter products in some countries. Despite the substitution of Stephania by Aristolochia being implicated in renal disease (see p.96), this practice still commonly occurs.

CONTAMINATION ISSUES IN HERBAL MEDICINE

Herbal products can sometimes be contaminated with other agents and a few isolated instances have raised public health concerns. These include:

- products made in China and India contaminated with heavy metals (sometimes added intentionally) or microbial contaminants;
- products made in China contaminated with conventional drugs;
- contamination of a safe herb with a toxic herb, e.g. Digitalis (foxglove leaves) found among Symphytum (comfrey leaves).

The practice of GMP in a well-regulated environment should eliminate the possibility of these types of contamination.

RESOLVING THE SAFETY ISSUE: PHARMACOVIGILANCE INITIATIVES

POSTMARKETING SURVEILLANCE

Given that so few plant drugs have ever been submitted to preclinical studies, toxicological information about herbal remedies is generally poor. In European legislation the principle has been accepted that drugs already widely used in the population need not go back to the laboratory for new toxicological studies. Instead, those supplying such remedies are under increasing burden to establish safety on an ongoing basis; postmarketing surveillance or *pharmacovigilance* are terms generally used to describe this monitoring process. There is an overwhelming mathematical case for systematizing observations of adverse reactions. Statisticians have calculated that if, for example, an adverse event occurred in as many as 1 in 1000 cases, one would need to see 3000 cases to have a 95% probability of spotting one.[36] This 'law of three' makes the individual practitioner of little use in identifying even substantial risks.

All modern medicine legislatures have drug monitoring administrations and encourage physicians to report adverse events they encounter. In some countries reporting to the authority is mandatory and various forms are produced for the purpose. There is thus in most countries a database of adverse drug reports

(ADRs) which contribute to the warnings added to drug labels and datasheets. A very small number of ADRs relate to herbal remedies but for a number of reasons (see below) these have been poorly evaluated.

In the cases where analysis of the data has been done, reports of adverse effects from human consumption of herbs appear to be relatively infrequent, making up around 1% of spontaneous reporting[37]. There is a widespread concern among the regulatory authorities, however, that these cases represent only a small proportion of such incidents. Spontaneous reporting is for even conventional prescribed drugs an inefficient mechanism, with reporting rates among physicians as low as a few percent of actual cases.[38] In the case of herbal remedies, so many of which are self-prescribed or are prescribed by non-doctors, there is much less opportunity for doctors to become aware of this factor in adverse events. Reporting mechanisms for non-doctors are rarely in place and even pharmacists have only variable opportunities or tradition for notifying adverse events. Even where reporting is possible there are other reasons why spontaneous notification is likely to be particularly ineffective for herbal remedies (Box 5.5).

On the other hand the herbal sector can claim that uncontrolled observations of adverse events are likely to be misleading for the case of herbal safety and even the regulators accept that there are particular problems (Box 5.6)

All this has contributed to a situation where the herbal sector is sometimes accused by the regulators of ignoring a potential safety problem and the regulators are often seen by the herbal sector as intrinsically unable to understand the issue. Attempts have been made to reduce the prospect of such adversarial positions. From 1994 to 1996 a network of researchers, clinicians and manufacturers linked to ESCOP (the European Scientific Cooperative on Phytotherapy) received funding from the Biomedical and Health Research Programme of the European Community for a series of Concerted Action projects under the title 'Determining European standards for the safe and effective use of phytomedicines'. Faced with the Commission's own acknowledgement that pharmacovigilance schemes in general needed improvement,[39] the projects included a number of exercises to improve marketing surveillance of the safety of herbal remedies.

The BIOMED project identified and evaluated the different potential sources of ADRs from herbs:

- published papers
- hospital consultants
- general practitioners
- pharmacists
- phytotherapists and medical herbalists
- healthfood retailers
- manufacturers
- patients and users

Box 5.5 Problems affecting the reporting of ADRs involving herbal remedies

There may be fewer ADRs for herbal remedies due to the following.

- Lethargy (general reporting rates for all drugs are very poor)
- Physicians are usually unaware of natural product consumption
- Physicians do not routinely ask about non-prescribed medications
- Common bias against associating adverse effects with natural medicines
- Ignorance of reporting mechanisms by potential non-physician notifiers
- Users reluctant to talk to professionals if self-prescribed treatment goes wrong
- Potential notifier's reluctance to get involved in 'the system'
- Potential notifier's reluctance to risk losing a favourite remedy
- Uncertainty of connections in multiple ingredient prescriptions

Box 5.6 Perceived problems in applying ADRs to assessing the safety of herbal remedies

ADR reporting is not sensitive to herbal use; it does not easily:

- detect adverse reactions that are:
  subtle
  infrequent
  delayed;
- pick out causative agents from multiple ingredients;
- disentangle multiple/multicausal pathologies most often seen in chronic diseases.

There is a wider lack of context in which to place herbal ADRs, in particular concerning:

- market availability/consumption;
- pharmacotoxicology;
- drug interactions.

and sought ways to maximize the effectiveness of each. In particular, it has set up:

- a long-term (low-maintenance) on-line reporting mechanism (PhytoNET) to parallel and augment orthodox reporting schemes (this can be found on http://ex.ac.uk/phytonet/)
- a network of specialists and a panel of toxicologists from across Europe to actively pursue and evaluate safety data in this area.

ESCOP has also been involved in other initiatives to reduce risks in the consumption of herbal remedies, notably the production of ESCOP monographs to standard drug dossier formats including the best consensus on likely adverse effects, effects of overdosage and constraints on use[40].

ESCOP's UK member, the British Herbal Medicine Association, has set up voluntary codes, supported by the British regulators, which as a condition of membership oblige manufacturers to institute medicinal level GMP and pharmacopoeial standards for the production of unlicensed herbal remedies. This reflects the opinion that most safety problems with herbs are likely to arise from poor quality standards in their production.

In general, the ESCOP effort has led to the advice to all herbal users that attendance to adverse effects is not a threat but both a responsibility and an opportunity, that there are no two sides to the truth and not to let uncertainty about the cause of adverse effects deter reporting.

CONCLUSION

There is no absolute safety in life. Every human activity is risky and accidents will happen, even to herbalists. Some plants are likely to be dangerous when consumed; as material medicines, herbs are bound to interact with the body in ways that are not always convenient. So little is known about the long-term consequences of herbal intake that it would make good practical sense to discourage patients from taking the same prescriptions for long periods.

It is surprising, however, how few problems have been laid at the door of herbal medicine. Considering the vast usage around the world of plants as medicines, it is remarkable that there is so little epidemiological or clinical evidence that this is a harmful activity. It is possible that the safety record for herbalism is better than for any other widespread human activity, including eating, drinking, sleeping (a particularly dangerous activity), taking exercise, working or travelling.

The problem with legislators, medical professionals and public guardians is that they inevitably find themselves balancing risk with benefit. If they can see a public benefit as well as a demand for an activity they will feel able to cover themselves against public and media attack if something ever went wrong. Unfortunately, the case for the efficacy of herbal remedies is making only little more headway with the legislators than the case for their safety.

References

1. Violon C. Belgian (Chinese herb) nephropathy: why? Journal Pharmaceutique Belge 1997; 52(1): 7–27
2. Lekehal M, Pessayre D, Lereau JM et al. Hepatotoxicity of the herbal medicine germander: metabolic activation of its furano diterpenoids by cytochrome P450 3A depletes cytoskeleton-associated protein thiols and forms plasma membrance blebs in rat hepatocytes. Hepatology 1996; 24(1): 212–218
3. Rasheed RA, Ali BH, Bashir AK. Effect of Teucrium stocksianum on paracetamol-induced hepatotoxicity in mice. General Pharmacology 1995; 26(2): 297–301
4. Perharic L, Shaw D, Leon C et al. Possible association of liver damage with the use of Chinese herbal medicine for skin disease. Veterinary and Human Toxicology 1995; 37(6): 562–566
5. Kane JA, Kane SP, Jain S. Hepatitis induced by traditional Chinese herbs; possible toxic components. Gut 1995; 36(1): 146–147
6. Yeong ML, Clark SP, Waring JM et al. The effects of comfrey derived pyrrolizidine alkaloids on rat liver. Pathology 1991; 23(1): 35–38
7. White RD, Swick RA, Cheeke PR. Effects of microsomal enzyme induction on the toxicity of pyrrolizidine (senecio) alkaloids. Journal of Toxicology and Environmental Health 1983; 12(4): 633–640
8. Yan CC, Cooper RA, Huxtable RJ. The comparative metabolism of the four pyrrolizidine alkaloids, seneciphylline, retrorsine, monocrotaline, and trichodesmine in the isolated, perfused rat liver. Toxicology and Applied Pharmacology 1995; 133(2): 277–284
9. Datta DV, Khuroo MS, Mattocks AR et al. Herbal medicines and veno-occlusive disease in India. Postgraduate Medical Journal 1978; 54(634): 511–515
10. Ortiz Cansado A, Crespo Valadés E, Morales Blanco P et al. Veno-occlusive liver disease due to intake of Senecio vulgaris tea. Gastroenterology and Hepatology 1995; 18(8): 413–416
11. Mokhobo KP. Herb use and necrodegenerative hepatitis. South African Medical Journal 1976; 50(28): 1096–1099
12. Hirono I, Mori H, Culvenor CC. Carcinogenic activity of coltsfoot, Tussilago farfara 1. Gann 1976; 67(1): 125–129
13. Sperl W, Stuppner H, Gassner I et al. Reversible hepatic veno-occlusive disease in an infant after consumption of pyrrolizidine-containing herbal tea. European Journal of Pediatrics 1995; 154(2): 112–116
14. Horowitz RS, Feldhaus K, Dart RC et al. The clinical spectrum of jin bu huan toxicity. Archives of Internal Medicine 1996; 156(8): 899–903
15. Nadir A, Agrawal S, King PD, Marshall JB. Acute hepatitis associated with the use of a Chinese herbal product, Ma-huang. American Journal of Gastroenterology 1996; 91(7): 1436–1438
16. Anderson IB, Mullen WH, Meeker JE et al. Pennyroyal toxicity: measurement of toxic metabolite levels in two cases and

review of the literature. Annals of Internal Medicine 1996; 124(8): 726–734
17. Larrey D. Liver involvement in the course of phytotherapy (editorial). Presse Medicale 1994; 23(15): 691–693
18. Georgiou M, Sianidou L, Hatzis T et al. Hepatotoxicity due to *Atractylis gummifera* L. Journal of Toxicology. Clinical Toxicology 1988; 26(7): 487–493
19. Cooper MR, Johnson AW. Poisonous plants in Britain and their effects on animals and man. Ministry of Agriculture Fisheries and Food, Reference Book 161. HMSO, London, 1984
20. Fletcher Hyde F. Herbal practitioners guide to the Medicines Act. National Institute of Medical Herbalists, Tunbridge Wells, 1978
21. Randerath K, Haglund RE, Phillips DH, Reddy MV. 32P-post-labelling analysis of DNA adducts formed in the livers of animals treated with safrole, estragole and other naturally-occurring alkenylbenzenes. I. Adult female CD-1 mice. Carcinogenesis 1984; 5(12): 1613–1622
22. Edenharder R, John K, Ivo Boor H. Antimutagenic activity of vegetable and fruit extracts against in-vitro benzo(a)pyrene). Zeitschrift für die gesamte Hygiene und ihre Grenzgebiete 1990; 36(3): 144–147
23. Ebata J, Inoue T. Antimutagenic activity of vegetables harvested in different growing conditions. Mutation Research 1989; 216: 359
24. Shinohara K, Kuroki S, Miwa M, Hosoda H. Antimutagenicity of dialyzates of vegetables and fruits. Agricultural and Biological Chemistry 1988; 52: 1369–1375
25. Ito Y, Maeda S, Sugiyama T. Suppression of 7,12-dimethylbenz(a)anthracene-induced chromosome aberrations in rat bone marrow cells by vegetable juices. Mutation Research 1986; 172: 55–60
26. Lagey K, Duinslaeger L, Vanderkelen A. Burns induced by plants. Burns 1995; 21(7): 542–543
26a Araya OS, Ford EJH. An investigation of the type of photosensitisation caused by the ingestion of St. John's Wort (Hypericum perforatum) by calves. J Comp Pathol. 1981; 91: 135–141.
27. De Maat Bleeker F. Etiology of hypersensitivity reactions following Chinese or Indonesian meals. Nederlands Tijdschrift voor Geneeskunde 1992; 136(5): 229–232
28. Zuskin E, Kanceljak B, Skuric Z et al. Immunological and respiratory findings in spice-factory workers. Environmental Research 1988; 47(1): 95–108
29. Macgregor FB, Abernethy VE, Dahabra S, Cobden I, Hayes PC, Hepatotoxicity of herbal remedies. British Medical Journal 1989; 299(6708): 1156–1157
30. Van Vleet JF, Ferrans VJ. Myocardial diseases of animals. American Journal of Pathology 1986; 124(1): 98–178
31. Rosenzweig P, Brohier S, Zipfel A. The placebo effect in healthy volunteers: influence of experimental conditions on the adverse events profile during phase I studies. Clinical Pharmacology and Therapeutics 1993; 54(5): 578–583
32. Benedetti F, Amanzio M. The neurobiology of placebo analgesia: from endogenous opioids to cholecystokinin. Progress in Neurobiology 1997; 52(2): 109–125
33. Kleijnen J, De Craen AJM, Van Everdingen J, Krol L. Placebo effect in double-blind clinical trials: a review of interactions with medications. Lancet 1994; 344: 1347–1349
34 Atal CK, Zutshi U, Rao PG. Scientific evidence on the role of Ayurvedic herbals on bioavailability of drugs. Journal of Ethnopharmacology 1981; 4(2): 229–232
35. British Herbal Medicine Association. British herbal pharmacopoeia BHMA, Christchurch, 1996; 14–16
36. De Smet PAGM. An introduction to herbal pharmacoepidemiology. Journal of Ethnopharmacology 1993; 38: 197–208
37. Report to 9th Meeting of Working Group for International Program on Chemical Safety (IPOS) INTOX Project 2-6th Sept 1996
38. Leiper JM, Lawson DH. Why do doctors not report adverse drug reactions? Netherlands Journal of Medicine 1985; 28: 546–550
39. Fracchia GN. Euro-ADR: pharmacovigilance and research. Biomedical and Health Newsletter 1992; 3(3): 5–6
40. The European Scientific Cooperative on Phytotherapy. Monographs on the medicinal use of plant drugs. ESCOP, Exeter, England 1996–1998

Part 2

Practical Clinical Guides

Introduction

In Part Two the strategic options in clinical phytotherapy are reviewed. Practical issues of dosage and prescribing are followed by individual chapters on the phytotherapeutic approach to pathological states and to system dysfunctions.

As far as possible the commentary in this section is based on material that is both subjected to modern research and supported by the most persistent therapeutic traditions distilled from the long human battle with illness. If there is a choice between the two sources of information, the text is biased in favour of traditional use; in general, only when there is such use will scientific pointers to plant activity be cited. This is particularly so in the great majority of cases where experimental data are restricted to in vitro or animal or other non-clinical models. Until the modern research effort becomes much more substantial this bias will remain the only appropriate option.

This is not a book on general medicine; not every infirmity encountered in the clinic is covered in depth or even mentioned. Nor is there any attempt to review the wider natural approaches to healthcare; there is little on dietary or other naturopathic strategies. The aim is to highlight the strengths of herbal medicine and to commend the unique approaches to many difficult clinical conditions that are possible. The authors believe that phytotherapy can provide a major resource for future healthcare. The groundwork is set out in these pages.

The work is not complete. The sections vary in substance, size, detail and authority. The support provided by modern research is particularly patchy. In some areas, notably the digestive system, the liver, the urinary and nervous systems, there is a great deal of underpinning at a theoretical level but little clinical evidence. In most areas there are some strong therapeutic commendations to make but less pathophysiological or pharmacological rationale or research evidence. Only in the circulatory system is there a reasonable mix of theoretical and clinical research support. The work continues for future editions.

In all sections summary indications and contraindications are included at the beginning. In some sections, summary materia medica for therapeutic group or chemical subgroup is appropriate. A few case histories are included for illumination.

In general, the authors have stayed with the European and North American tradition they practise. Nevertheless, readers who would rather use herbs from other traditions should still find the mechanisms and rationales discussed here appropriate.

6 Dosage and dosage forms in herbal medicine

The subject of appropriate dose is probably the most controversial aspect of contemporary Western herbal medicine. Among Western herbal practitioners, many different dosage approaches are found from country to country and within countries. Underlying these different approaches are different philosophies about the therapeutic action of medicinal plants.

At one extreme is the assumption that the therapeutic effect relies on a specific dose of the active chemicals contained in each particular plant. At the other extreme, emphasis is often placed on the assumption that a herbal medicine, being derived from a living organism, carries a certain energy or vital force. The quality of this energy confers the therapeutic effect and hence the amount of actual herb is not as important, as long as some is present. Others perhaps feel that the active components act as catalysts to restore health and do not need to be present in pharmacological quantities.

The low dosage approach should not be confused with homoeopathy, although it has been influenced by this system. One important difference from homoeopathy is that the therapeutic indications are not derived from the principle of similars and mainly come from traditional indications. Like homoeopathy, this approach probably relies on a high degree of patient susceptibility to the medication.

Both the high and low dosage approaches have their adherents who maintain that their respective systems give good results in the clinic. While it is inappropriate to label one approach as correct and the other incorrect (indeed, even high doses of herbs possibly also act in part through an energetic factor), it is useful to review and contrast current and historical dosage approaches. By doing this, one can arrive at an appropriate dosage system for modern phytotherapy in that it is consistent with:

- dosage ranges used in other important herbal traditions, e.g. China and India;
- dosages used by important historical movements in Western herbal medicine, e.g. the Eclectics;
- dosages currently recommended in pharmacopoeias;
- dosages established from pharmacological and clinical research.

In any discussion of herbal doses, the influence of dosage form and quality of preparations must also be considered, as should the mechanics of formulation and prescription writing.

REVIEW OF DOSAGE APPROACHES

TRADITIONAL CHINESE MEDICINE

The daily dose for individual non-toxic herbs in traditional Chinese medicine is usually in the range of 3–10 g, given as a decoction or in pill or powder form.[1] Often higher doses are prescribed by decoction than for pills, as might be expected since not all active components readily dissolve in hot water.[2] (Pills generally consist of the powdered herb incorporated into a suitable base.) Herbs are invariably prescribed in formulations. Doses for such formulations are about 3–9 g taken three times daily but can be higher in the case of decoctions.

For each individual herb a wide dosage range is usually given in texts. This applies for all herbal systems. One reason for this is that if a herb is used by itself or with just a few other herbs, a larger dose is used than when it is combined with many other herbs.[2] Dose also varies according to the weight and age of patients and the severity or acuteness of their condition.

Recently, a more processed form of dosage has become popular among practitioners of Chinese

Table 6.1 Comparison of dosages used in Chinese and Western herbal medicine

Herb	Chinese dosage[1] g/day	Western dosage[3,4] g/day
Ephedra sinica	3–9	3–12 (decoction) 3–9 (extract)
Zingiber officinale	3–9	0.75–3 (decoction) 0.38–0.75 (tincture)
Taraxacum mongolicum	9–30	6–24 (decoction) 3–6 (tincture)
Glycyrrhiza uralensis	3–12	3–12 (decoction) 6–12 (extract)
Rheum palmatum	3–6	2.3–4.5 (decoction) 1.8–6 (extract)

Note: For dosages of tinctures and extracts given three times daily, the corresponding amount of dried herb per day has been calculated

Table 6.2 Comparison of dosages used by the Eclectics and modern dosages

Herb	Eclectic dosage[7,8] g/day	Current dosage[3,4] g/day
Euphorbia hirta	1.8–10.8	0.36–0.9
Echinacea angustifolia	0.9–5.4	0.75–3.0
Hydrastis canadensis	0.9–10.8	0.9–3.0
Passiflora incarnata	1.8–10.8	1.5–3.0
Valeriana officinalis	2.1–6.0	0.9–3.0
Rumex crispus	1.8–10.8	6.0–12.0
Viburnum opulus	3.6–10.8	6.0–12.0
Sabal serrulata	2.7–10.8	1.8–4.5

Note: The corresponding amount of dried herb per day has been calculated from recommended dosages for fluid extracts

medicine. This involves the prescription of formulas in a granulated form. The granules are prepared by drying or freeze-drying decoctions, that is aqueous extracts, of herbal formulas. Usually 2 g of granules is prescribed three times daily, which corresponds to about 6–10 g of original dried herbs per dose.

Some herbs, or closely related species, are used in both Chinese and Western herbal medicine. Table 6.1 compares dosages for a few of these herbs.

In general, the similarity in the dosage range between the different systems is striking. Discrepancies do exist for Zingiber and Taraxacum, which in the case of Zingiber can be explained by a higher content of the active components in the alcoholic tincture compared to the decoction, and in the case of Taraxacum may be a reflection on the different species used.

AYURVEDA

Ayurveda often involves complex formulations which are prepared over several days and can contain many herbal and mineral components. Consequently, there is more dosage diversity than for Chinese medicine. Dosage ranges for individual non-toxic herbs are generally in the range of 1–6 g per day as powders or tinctures, with higher doses often recommended for decoctions.[5]

ECLECTIC MEDICINE

Eclectic medicine was a largely empirical school of medicine which developed in America during the 19th century.[6] The movement was most prominent for a brief period from the late 19th to the early 20th centuries, when there were several teaching universities and many eminent scholars in the USA. Although the Eclectics used simple chemical medicines such as phosphoric acid, they mainly prescribed herbal medicines. Their knowledge of materia medica was their greatest contribution to Western herbal medicine; for example, herbs such as Echinacea and golden seal were made popular by them after observation of their use by the native Americans.

The Eclectics tended to use higher doses than those recommended in current texts and pharmacopoeias, although the ranges tend to overlap. Table 6.2 compares dosages currently used[3,4] with those found in Eclectic texts[7,8] for alcoholic extracts of herbs.

THE BRITISH HERBAL PHARMACOPOEIA

The *British Herbal Pharmacopoeia* 1983 (BHP) carries extensive dosage information for individual herbs and is generally regarded as an important reference

Table 6.3 Comparison of extract and tincture dosages in the BHP 1983

Herb	Dose range 1:1 extract[3]	Dose range 1:5 tincture[3]	Expected dose range for 1:5 tincture
Agrimonia eupatoria	1–3 ml	2–4 ml	5–15 ml
Achillea millefolium	2–4 ml	2–4 ml	10–20 ml
Eupatorium purpureum	2–4 ml	1–2 ml	10–20 ml
Menyanthes trifoliata	1–2 ml	1–3 ml	5–10 ml

Note: The expected dose range for the 1:5 tincture is calculated by multiplying the dose range for the 1:1 extract by 5

on this subject for Western herbal practitioners. Dosages given in the BHP were derived from earlier texts such as the *British Pharmacopoeia* (BP) and the *British Pharmaceutical Codex* (BPC) but also resulted from a survey of herbal practitioners. More recently, the *British Herbal Compendium* (BHC) has been published with dosage information for the practitioner.

The doses given by the BHP contain some inconsistencies. The main problem is that doses for tinctures often do not correlate to corresponding doses for liquid extracts. For a 1:1 extract and a 1:5 tincture of a particular herb to correlate in terms of dose, the dose range for the tincture should be five times that of the extract, since it is five times weaker. This problem contrasts with other pharmacopoeias such as the BPC 1934 where the correlation is generally, but not exactly, observed. Some examples which highlight this problem are provided in Table 6.3.

The poor correlation demonstrated in Table 6.3, where in the case of *Eupatorium purpureum* the tincture dose is actually *less* than the extract dose, probably arises for two reasons.

1. As stated above, the BHP doses were in part derived from a survey of herbal practitioners. It is probable that there were different dosage philosophies between practitioners using extracts compared to those using tinctures. Hence a correlation should not be expected.

2. Tinctures are manufactured using different techniques to 1:1 fluid extracts. This aspect is particularly important. Fluid extracts are now often prepared by reconstituting more concentrated extracts, rather than the traditional method of reserved percolation. In either case, the heat or vacuum used in concentration can rob the preparation of important active chemicals. Tinctures better preserve the activity of the whole plant because they are made without heat or a concentration procedure. Fluid extracts are also often manufactured using lower alcohol strengths than tinctures and important active components may therefore not be extracted from the starting plant material. The result of these factors is that a 1:1 fluid extract can have an activity which is much less than five times that of a 1:5 tincture. This will be dealt with in more detail in the part of this chapter which discusses liquid preparations.

Since tinctures better preserve the chemical profile of the dried herb, more credibility should be given to the tincture doses when using the dosage ranges in the BHP.

COMMISSION E MONOGRAPHS

Under the direction of the German Health Department, the Commission E prepared a series of monographs on commonly used medicinal herbs during the 80s. The Commission E is an expert committee consisting of doctors, pharmacologists, pharmacognocists and toxicologists from both academia and industry. If a herb did not receive a positive monograph from the Commission E, it could not be registered as a medicine in Germany. In the preparation of a monograph, the Commission E took into account relevant traditional use as well as scientific research.

A positive monograph for a herb also included dosage information. Many of the monograph doses are for infusions or decoctions since this reflects the common use in the German marketplace.[9] Such daily doses are usually in the range of 2–10 g. Occasionally a monograph will specify a dose for a herb in terms of major active constituents; e.g. for Ephedra the daily dose is 45–90 mg of alkaloids (about 4–8 g of herb which is similar to the range in Table 6.1). Occasionally, where tincture and extract doses are given by the Commission E, there is not always a good correlation. For example, the single dose for valerian tincture is 1–3 ml and yet the single dose for a fluid extract is 2–3 ml. The reasons for this may be the same as those discussed above for the BHP.

CLINICAL TRIALS

The clinical trial is arguably the best way to determine the effective dose of either a single herb or a herbal formulation. This will not always be applicable to traditional medicine, however, since prescriptions are usually prepared on an individual basis. Also, a clinical trial does not necessarily determine the optimum dose. It does, however, confer a relative certainty to the clinical results. That is, at a given dose of a given preparation a certain percentage of patients are likely to respond; e.g. *Ginkgo biloba* standardized extract at 120 mg per day (which corresponds to about 6 g per day of dry leaves), given for 2 months, will improve intermittent claudication in 60% of patients.[10]

Sometimes the clinical trial has used a standardized extract of the herb which can then be correlated to the whole herb; e.g. silymarin in liver disorders at 240 mg per day corresponds to 8–24 g per day of *Silybum marianum* seeds.[11]

THE LOW DOSAGE APPROACH

Currently in the United States, New Zealand, parts of Europe (especially among homoeopaths) and to some extent Australia, there are practitioners who prefer to prescribe drop doses of 1:5 or even more dilute tinctures. It is useful to examine the possible origins of this approach.

In Europe, homoeopaths often use combinations of herbal mother tinctures in drop dosage, for example 'drainage'. This approach is sometimes incorrectly labelled as 'phytotherapy'.

In the United States a more direct influence comes, ironically, from a development of Eclectic medicine. In 1869, the Eclectic physician John Scudder proposed the concept of 'specific medication'.[7] With this concept, medicines were matched specifically to the symptom picture of the patient and then given in the minimum dose required. Although this system may seem similar to homoeopathy, there were important differences.[12] Material doses were always used, albeit lower than those prescribed by other Eclectics, and the prescription was not based on the law of similars. However, there was a tendency to use only one medicine at a time, similar to classical homoeopathy.

Scudder initially proposed that 'specific medicines' should be tinctures prepared from the fresh plant.[12] A fresh plant tincture is sometimes still called a 'specific tincture'. Hence the approach of using drop doses of tinctures, especially fresh plant tinctures, also comes from Scudder.

Although Scudder's system of specific medication was seen as an important development in Eclectic medicine, it was considerably modified by Lloyd.[13] Lloyd felt that drop doses of tinctures were too low and described the preparations proposed by Scudder as 'superficial'.[13] Lloyd proceeded to develop elaborate herbal preparations which were concentrated, semi-purified liquids. He also called these 'specific medicines' and they were widely adopted by Eclectic practitioners. However, in the early 20th century, English herbalists aligned themselves with the American physiomedicalists because specific medicines proved too costly to import from America.

Lloyd sometimes used solvents other than ethanol and water in the preparation of his specific medicines.[13] His methods were kept secret and even today are not widely known. Lloyd writes: 'The aim has been to exclude colouring matters ... and inert extractive substances also from these preparations ...'. In this sense he was tending towards the concept of orthodox drugs. However, his preparations were still chemically complex and 'very characteristic' of the original herb.[13] According to Felter, the specific medicines developed by Lloyd were at least eight times stronger than 1:5 tinctures.[7] It is these highly concentrated preparations which were generally used by Eclectic physicians in drop doses and even then, doses could be quite high – up to 60 drops (3 ml) three times daily.[7]

In conclusion, the use of drop doses of tinctures, especially fresh plant tinctures, was an early development of specific medication and was not representative of the general practice of Eclectic medicine.

THE CURRENT SYSTEM IN THE UK

In the UK in the past herbalists used fluid extracts, usually prepared using heat or from concentrates. However, among newer practitioners there was a disenchantment with these preparations because of their inconsistent quality. These practitioners have instead adopted the use of 1:5 tinctures. Usually, formulations of tinctures are prescribed at doses of 2.5–5 ml three times daily. However, BHP doses for tinctures can only be achieved by this approach if the formulation contains one to three herbs (see Table 6.3 for examples). Unfortunately, this restriction is usually not followed and it can be concluded that the move to tinctures has resulted in the use of lower doses.

A RATIONAL SYSTEM FOR MODERN PHYTOTHERAPY

The dosages used by the traditional systems of India and China, by most of the Eclectics and those established by clinical trials or recommended by expert committees or in pharmaceutical texts all tend towards the higher end of the dosage spectrum. Such an agreement should not be ignored if there is to be consistency in modern phytotherapy.

If liquid preparations are to be used, then the BHP 1983 is an appropriate guide. However, as discussed above, more credibility should be given to the tincture doses. The difficulty in using 1:5 tinctures is the large volumes which are required to achieve BHP doses for multiherb formulations. One way to overcome this problem is to make a more concentrated preparation but without the use of heat or vacuum. Such a preparation would be more akin to a 1:5 tincture than a fluid extract, since it would better reflect the chemical characteristics of the starting herb. The most concentrated preparation which can be achieved from a dried herb without using heat or vacuum concentration, and yet achieving a high extraction efficiency, is a 1:2. A process of cold percolation is necessary to achieve a 1:2 extract. Dosages for 1:2 extracts can be calculated as 0.4 of the dose for 1:5 tinctures, since they are 2.5 times stronger.

This approach enables the use of multiherb formulations consistent with BHP and BHC dosage guidelines. For special preparations, such as herbal extracts standardized for active components, dosages established by clinical trials should be followed.

ORAL DOSAGE FORMS IN HERBAL MEDICINE

It is worth examining the relative advantages and disadvantages of the various oral dosage forms used by practitioners of Western herbal medicine.

LIQUIDS

Liquid preparations are widely used because of their considerable advantages. The main advantage is the easy preparation of formulations for each individual patient (extemporaneous dispensing). The other considerable advantage of liquids is that, if properly prepared, they involve minimal processing and truly reflect the chemical characteristics of the herb in a compact, convenient form. They also confer considerable dosage flexibility which is especially relevant when prescribing low doses for small children. Liquids are readily absorbed and are convenient to take.

The main disadvantage of liquids is taste, although in the case of bitters, the taste is an essential part of the therapy. The taste problem is somewhat exaggerated by some patients. Most patients get used to the taste of their mixture and some even grow to like it. If taste becomes a problem, there are flavouring preparations available and these are particularly useful for children. Another disadvantage of liquids which applies in a few cases is the alcohol content. This is either because the patient is allergic to alcohol or is an ex-alcoholic who does not wish to take alcohol in any form. Strict Muslims will also not take alcohol.

Only a very small minority of patients are genuinely sensitive to alcohol. In others, a presumed sensitivity is only an exaggerated reflex response to the medicine. This can usually be alleviated by lower doses at greater frequency, taken with copious water or food. Usually the small quantities of alcohol involved will not affect a mildly damaged liver – a 5 ml dose contains as much alcohol as about one-sixth of a glass of beer or wine. The alcohol content of liquids is not a problem for children since correspondingly lower amounts of liquids, and hence alcohol, are prescribed.

Use of alcohol in herbal liquid preparations is important since it is a good solvent for herbal active components and also an excellent preservative. This is discussed in more detail later in this chapter.

TABLETS

Herbal tablets are a convenient dosage form and no problems with taste or alcohol are associated with their use. However, tablets contain fixed formulations which cannot be adapted to the needs of the individual patient. Therefore, it is critical that the herbs contained in a tablet are carefully chosen for the disorder they are intended to treat. Even then, the degree of treatment flexibility is limited.

A major potential problem with tablets is the degree of processing required. Processing is minimal for tablets containing the powdered herb but the amount of herb which can be incorporated into such tablets is limited (without making them excessively large). Tablets are therefore usually made from extracts which are more concentrated than the original dried herb. In order to achieve this, the herb is first extracted with a solvent. Often water is used to keep costs down. The resultant liquid is then dried to either a soft or powdered concentrate using processes such as vacuum concentration or spray drying. Heat-sensitive or volatile components can be damaged or lost by this process. Heat is also sometimes used in the tablet-making process via a granulation step: the tablet mixture may be wetted and then dried in an oven before the final pressing. This risks further damage to the active components. Hence when manufacturing tablets, quality may be sacrificed for the sake of quantity. One way to compensate for this problem with concentrates is to standardize each herbal ingredient for key active components. However, the components chosen for standardization must be meaningful in terms of the desired activity of the herb. In other words, they must be meaningful indicators of quality.

Another problem with tablets is that, despite the use of concentrates, they are sometimes formulated to contain low amounts of herbs. Many tablets contain herbs in equivalent dried herb doses of 1–50 mg (i.e. the herb is there as a concentrate and the equivalent amount of dried herb is calculated from the known strength of the concentrate). It is difficult to see how therapeutic doses can be achieved from such small quantities.

POWDERS

Sometimes the best way to prescribe a herb is as a powder. This particularly applies to mucilage-containing herbs. When these herbs are mixed with water, the mucilage reacts with the water to form a gel and the wet herb swells to many times its original volume. Mucilage is not very soluble in alcohol-water mixtures, hence it is difficult to use mucilaginous herbs effectively as liquids. In any case, if fluid extracts of, say, slippery elm and marshmallow were properly made, they would be so gelatinous that they could not be poured.

When giving mucilaginous herbs as powders it is best to advise the patient to mix them quickly with water and to take the mixture without delay before it swells. Otherwise, the patient often experiences difficulty negotiating the gelatinous mass which results. A copious amount of water should then be consumed to allow swelling in the stomach. Other herbs given as powders are also best taken slurried with water and rinsed down by additional water.

Tannin-containing herbs for the treatment of colon problems should also be given as powders. This is because the tannins are only slowly dissolved from the herb matrix and are therefore still being released in an active form when the powdered herb reaches the colon.

A big advantage of powders is that the total constituents of a herb are presented to the patient's digestive tract, rather than those constituents which only dissolve in alcohol or water. Where the fat-soluble components are an important part of the activity of a herb, the powder should be followed by a dose of vegetable oil or lecithin to assist absorption.

CAPSULES

Capsules are a convenient way to give powdered herbs because they conceal unpleasant tastes or textures. A drawback is that even large capsules can only hold 300–600 mg of powdered herb, which means that sometimes many capsules need to be taken to achieve adequate doses. Capsules containing herbal formulations are subject to the same limitation of flexibility as tablet formulations. Single herbs in capsules do confer prescription flexibility, since one merely prescribes each of the required herbs in capsule form. The disadvantage is that the patient may need to take a large number of capsules in order to achieve adequate doses for several herbs.

Concentrated extracts can be used in capsules instead of the powdered herb. In this instance, the same disadvantages discussed above for tablets apply. In other words, quality may be sacrificed for quantity.

INFUSIONS AND DECOCTIONS

Infusions and decoctions are time-honoured methods for delivering oral doses of herbs. In modern phytotherapy, they are mainly used where the active components of the herb are water soluble, e.g. for herbs containing polysaccharides, tannins or mucilage or some glycosides. They also can be advantageous for the treatment of urinary tract problems and for the administration of alterative herbs. Diaphoretics should be given hot to maximize their effectiveness, hence they are often administered as infusions or decoctions.

The major disadvantage of infusions or decoctions is that water is not a good solvent for many of the active components in herbs. This problem is compounded by the relatively short extraction time used in their preparation (usually 5–10 minutes). In addition, the large volume of hot liquid usually means that exposure to any unpleasant taste is considerably prolonged.

THE PREPARATION OF LIQUIDS

It is useful to consider in detail some of the factors involved in the preparation of herbal liquids.

THE STRENGTH OR RATIO

The strength of a liquid preparation is usually expressed as a ratio. For example, 1:5 means that 5 ml of the final preparation is equivalent to 1 g of the dried herb from which the preparation was made. Liquid preparations weaker than 1:2 are usually called 'tinctures' whereas 1:1 and 1:2 preparations are called 'extracts'. Tinctures are usually made by a soaking process known as maceration, whereas extracts are best made using percolation. However, tinctures can also be adequately manufactured by a percolation process. These days, 1:1 liquid extracts are often made by reconstituting soft or powdered concentrates.

It has been argued that 1:2 extracts are relatively new, are not mentioned in the BHP or other

Table 6.4 Essential oil and phenol content of various pharmaceutical preparations of thyme[16]

	Essential oil content %	Phenol content %	Equivalent content in the dried herb Essential oil %	Phenol %
Dried herb	2.81	0.59	2.81	0.59
1:1 extract	–	0.13	–	0.13
1:2 extract	–	0.11	–	0.22
Soft extract (13:1)	0.88	0.51	0.07	0.04
Powdered extract (16:1)	3.54	1.84	0.22	0.12

pharmacopoeias and therefore should not be used. In fact, 1:2 extracts are mentioned in 19th century texts[12,14] and are described in the *German Pharmacopoeia* (DAB).[13] The seventh edition of the DAB actually defines a liquid extract as a 1:2 extract.[15]

The dominant historical use of 1:1 extracts may not have been the wisest choice because of the extra processing required. In 1953, a Dutch PhD student studied the impact of pharmaceutical processing on some active components of thyme (*Thymus vulgaris*).[16] The components tested were the phenols (thymol and carvacrol), which are responsible for the antiseptic activity of thyme. Thymol and carvacrol are found in the essential (volatile) oil of thyme and could conceivably be lost under conditions of vacuum or heat. The following preparations were made.

1. A 1:1 liquid extract in 50% ethanol by the method of reserved percolation which is described in most pharmacopoeias.
2. A 1:2 liquid extract in 50% ethanol by cold percolation.
3. A soft extract (13:1) by evaporating some of the liquid described in (2) under vacuum.
4. A powdered extract (16:1) by drying some of the liquid described in (2) in a spray dryer.

The phenol content in all four preparations and in the original herb was measured and the results are summarized in Table 6.4. The table also provides the essential oil content of some of the preparations.

As can be seen from Table 6.4, the 1:2 extract contains only marginally less phenol content than the 1:1. This is presumably because the phenols were largely lost during the heating of the second percolate which occurs in reserved percolation. Hence, on the basis of the active components tested, the 1:2 is almost as strong as the 1:1. It should be noted from Table 6.4 that neither the 1:1 nor the 1:2 quantitatively extracted all the phenols from the dried herb, presumably because these components were not completely soluble at the ethanol percentage chosen. The 1:2 contained 37% of the original phenol content in the dried herb, compared to 22% for the 1:1.

The results for the soft and powdered extracts are disturbing. For the soft extract, 82% of the phenols were lost in processing and for the powdered extract, the loss was 48%. Compared to spray drying, conditions of vacuum therefore seem more likely to cause the loss of essential oil components, although the losses in both cases are considerable. A Swiss study found that concentration of a chamomile extract under vacuum caused the loss of about half of the essential oil.[17]

The content of essential oil and phenols in the corresponding amount of dried herb are also provided for the various preparations in the right-hand columns of Table 6.4. As can be seen from the table, the soft and powdered extracts only contain a fraction of the essential oil and phenol content of the dried herb. Hence for this example, the use of these concentrates in the manufacture of liquids, tablets or capsules would clearly represent a substantial sacrifice of quality for the sake of an increase in quantity. If the soft extract was reconstituted to a 1:1 which is a common practice, it would contain about 30% of the phenol content of the 1:2 (0.04% versus 0.11%).

THE ETHANOL PERCENTAGE

Ethanol (or alcohol) has been used for hundreds of years to prepare liquid herbal preparations and indeed ethanol-water mixtures do appear to be quite efficient for the extraction of a wide variety of compounds found in medicinal plants.

A number of studies have highlighted the importance of the correct choice of the ethanol percentage in terms of maximizing the quality of liquid preparations. The Swiss study mentioned above found that 55% ethanol was the optimum percentage for the extraction of the essential oil from chamomile (*Matricaria chamomilla*).[17] Higher percentages of ethanol did not extract any additional oil and there was a decrease in the solids content of the extract, which indicates that other components were being less efficiently extracted. More recently, Meier found that 40–60% ethanol was the optimum range for achieving the highest extraction efficiency for the active components of a variety of herbs.[18] For example, at 25% ethanol none of the saponins in ivy leaves (*Hedera helix*) were extracted but at 60% ethanol they were maximally extracted.

Higher ethanol percentages do not always confer higher activity. French researchers found that *Viburnum prunifolium* bark extracted at 30% ethanol was five times more spasmolytic than a 60% extract.[19]

The basic guidelines for the choice of the ethanol percentage to optimize the activity of the final liquid are as follows.

25%	Water-soluble constituents such as mucilage, tannins, and some glycosides (including some flavonoids and a few saponins)
45–60%	Essential oils, alkaloids, most saponins and some glycosides
90%	Resins and oleoresins

Glycetracts or glycerites are liquid preparations made using glycerol and water instead of ethanol and water. They are useful preparations where the active components are water soluble, for example marshmallow root (*Althaea officinalis*), since they do not contain alcohol and the sweetness of the glycerol gives them a better taste. However, their importance should not be overrated. Glycerol is a poor solvent for many of the active components found in herbs and glycetracts are less stable than alcoholic extracts. Moreover, because of the viscosity of glycerol, concentrated preparations are difficult to make by percolation. The manufacture of 1:1 or 1:2 glycetracts therefore invariably requires the use of a concentration step involving heat or vacuum.

QUALITY VERSUS QUANTITY

Essentially this problem arises because herbs are chemically complex biological drugs which need to be processed in some way and losses of activity can occur during this processing. Few of these kinds of problems arise when using pure chemicals.

But even if the problems of processing the herb are ignored, there still remains the problem of the quality of the herb itself. A herb is biologically defined and even if this biological definition is adhered to (and sometimes unfortunately it is not), there is an element of chemical uncertainty. The active components of a particular dried herb can vary considerably. This is due to factors such as climate, soil conditions, genetic characteristics, time of harvest, methods of harvest and drying techniques.

One way to partially solve this problem is to use 'organic' and 'wildcrafted' herbs. By definition, these are herbs which not only have been organically grown or harvested from the wild under ideal growing conditions but have also been subjected to maximum care at all stages of harvesting and drying to ensure that quality is optimized.

A more certain way to overcome the problem of the chemical variation of herbs and herbal preparations is to quantify them for indicator chemicals. In other words, the content of a particular component or group of components should always be greater than a minimum level. These components may not be solely responsible for the complete spectrum of the therapeutic effects of the herb but rather will act as indicators of consistent quality. However, they should be meaningful indicators of quality. Although more research is needed in this direction, many common herbal medicines can now be quantified for active components and the appropriate dosage range can be set accordingly.

STANDARDIZED EXTRACTS

The use of standardized extracts, where chemical components are set to a consistent level in a herbal extract, has become widespread. There are basically four types of standardized extracts currently on the world market.

1. Extracts which have been produced using defined conditions of processing and extraction. Standardization is used to ensure batch-to-batch consistency, which then allows the extensive clinical testing of these extracts, and their clinical efficacy and safety is thereby well established. Examples of this type of standardized extract include those of *Ginkgo biloba, Hypericum perforatum* and *Serenoa repens.* It is the extract as a whole which has been clinically proven. The standardization serves to define this clinically proven extract. Any issues pertaining to safety would be documented in the various clinical trials.

2. Extracts, which may or may not have been proven effective in clinical trials, for which the level of standardization gives some indication of the potency of the whole extract. This can only apply where there is clear evidence of a relationship between the compounds chosen for standardization and the pharmacological activity of the plant. Examples of this type of extract include *Coleus forskohlii* and forskolin, *Matricaria chamomilla* and essential oil and Salix species and salicylate derivatives.

3. Extracts for which the chemical chosen for standardization merely guarantees the identity and batch-to-batch consistency of the product. The extract as a whole has not been extensively studied clinically and the marker compound does not have relevant pharmacological activity. An example here would be *Echinacea angustifolia* and echinacoside.

4. Adulterated herbal products which contain isolated chemicals added to an inert or herbal matrix and sold as a 'standardized extract'. One example is the addition of caffeine, which is cheap and readily available, to extracts of guarana and kola nut.

The concern that there may be manipulation of the key components of the herb to achieve standardization requires clarification. Apart from the fourth example above, there is little evidence of how and where this might have occurred. Manufacturers will naturally select and extract herbal raw materials according to various quality criteria, including marker compounds. Such quality criteria are defined in the various pharmacopoeias including the *European Pharmacopoeia*; e.g. horsechestnut (Aesculus) as a raw material must contain a minimum level of escin to have pharmaceutical quality.

There is the case that if the chemical component of a plant is purified to a high degree, efficacy and safety concerns may arise. Such pure chemicals would not indeed be herbal substances. Such cases need to be evaluated on an individual basis. Here the issue is not really one of 'standardization' but rather one of isolation and purification. It is therefore incorrect to include this type of issue under the heading of 'herbal standardization', even though it may be represented as such in the marketplace.

From the perspective of the herbalist, these practitioners have long maintained that a herb's action is an expression of the sum total of known and unknown chemical constituents. There is a strong belief that the relationship between the constituents may be as important as the actual constituents themselves. Hence, the majority of herbal preparations used in practice are galenicals, that is, extracts based on whole herbs prepared in a manner which best extracts the balance of constituents. However, the use of well-chosen chemical components as markers of quality is not necessarily inconsistent with this approach.

A MECHANISM FOR FORMULATING LIQUIDS

There are a number of mechanisms for writing liquid prescriptions but a simple system widely used in the UK is worth describing. This is the system of formulating in terms of weekly doses.

If the dose for a herb is 1–2 ml three times daily, then the weekly dose is 21 times this or 21–42 ml per week, which is usually rounded down to 20–40 ml. Prescriptions for patients are then written in terms of weekly doses.

Assuming the patient is to take 5 ml of a liquid formulation three times daily, this amounts to 105 ml per week which can be rounded down to 100 ml. Hence the weekly dosages of the individual herbs in a formulation should total 100 ml. If the total amount of herbs in a formula is less than 100 ml, water or aqueous-ethanol can be added to bring the volume to 100 ml. Using this system the patient then automatically receives the correct amount of each herb in each dose, provided they take 5 ml tds (three times a day).

An example prescription for 1 week might be as follows.

Sambucus nigra	1:2	20 ml
Echinacea angustifolia	1:2	25 ml
Glycyrrhiza glabra	1:1	20 ml
Mentha piperita	1:2	25 ml
Zingiber officinale	1:2	10 ml
	Total	100 ml

The dosage is 5 ml of the mixture three times daily with water.

When dispensing for more than 1 week, the weekly doses are simply multiplied by the number of required weeks. This system confers considerable flexibility and ease in prescription writing and dispensing.

Even using 1:1 and 1:2 extracts, formulations based on 100 ml for 1 week should not contain more than about 6–7 herbs. Otherwise therapeutic doses will not be achieved. If more than this number of herbs is required then the week's formulation should be based on 150 ml. The single dose becomes 7.5 ml (which can be rounded up to 8 ml) three times daily.

COMPARING DOSES

Often it is difficult for practitioners to compare doses between liquid and/or solid preparations made with various types of extracts. The concept of 'dried herb equivalent' is a useful way of comparing doses between different strengths of liquids or between liquids and tablets. Using the product ratio, the dried herb equivalent of a given amount of product can be calculated. The product ratio expresses the weight of original dried herb starting material to the volume or weight of finished product (in that order), e.g. 5:1, 1:4, 1:1, etc. For example, a dried herb equivalent of 1 g might be:

2 ml of a 1:2 liquid
1 ml of 1:1 liquid
250 mg of 4:1 soft extract
200 mg of a 5:1 spray-dried powder

References

1. Bensky D, Gamble A. Chinese herbal medicine materia medica. Eastland Press, Seattle, 1986
2. Yanchi L. The essential book of traditional chinese medicine, volume 2: clinical practice. Columbia University Press, New York, 1988
3. British herbal pharmacopoeia. British Herbal Medicine Association, Bournemouth, 1983
4. British Pharmaceutical Codex. Pharmaceutical Press, London, 1934
5. Nadkarni KM, Nadkarni AK. Indian materia medica. Popular Prakashan Private Ltd, Bombay, 1976
6. Griggs B. Green pharmacy. Jill Norman and Hobhouse, London, 1981
7. Felter HW. The eclectic materia medica, pharmacology and therapeutics, First published Cincinnati, Ohio, 1922. Reprinted by Eclectic Medical Publications, Portland, 1983
8. Felter HW, Lloyd JU. King's American dispensatory, 18th edn. Reprinted by Eclectic Medical Publications, Portland, 1983
9. Eberwein E, Vogel G. Arzneipflanzen in der Phytotherapie. Kooperation Phytopharmaka, Bonn, 1990
10. De Feudis FV. Ginkgo biloba extract (EGb 761): pharmacological activities and clinical applications. Elsevier, Paris, 1991
11. Ravanelli OV, Haase W. Zur Wirksamkeit von Silymarin bei Leberkrankheiten. Zeitschrift für Praktische Anasthesie und Wiederbelebung 1976; 30(355): 1592–1612
12. Scudder JM. Specific medication and specific medicines. Scudder Bros Co, Cincinnati, 1913
13. Ellingwood F. American materia medica, therapeutics and pharmacognosy. Reprinted by Eclectic Medical Publications, Portland, 1983
14. Lyle TJ. Physio-medical therapeutics, materia medica and pharmacy. Originally published Ohio, 1897. Reprinted by the National Association of Medical Herbalists, London, 1932
15. Deutsches Arzneibuch der BRD – 7 Ausgabe 1968
16. Van Es MJ. Some applications of the spray-dryer in galenical pharmacy. PhD thesis, Utrecht University, 1953
17. Munzel K, Huber K. Extraction procedures in the preparation of chamomile fluid extract. Pharmaceutica Acta Helvetica 1961; 36: 194–204
18. Meier B. The extraction strength of ethanol/water mixtures commonly used for the processing of herbal drugs. Planta Medica 1991; 57(supp 2): A26
19. Balansard G, Chausse D, Boukef K et al. Selection criteria for a Viburnum extract, Viburnum prunifolium L., as a function of its veino-tonic and spasmolytic action. Plantes Médicinales et Phytothérapie 1983; 17(3): 123–132

7 A systematic approach to herbal prescribing

INTRODUCTION

In order to appreciate the approach behind Western herbal therapeutics, we must make the assumption that the normally functioning human body is free from disease and capable of resisting disease. Therefore a true understanding of the cause and treatment of disease should come from a consideration of physiology, the normal functioning of the body, as well as pathology and pathophysiology. An excessive focus on pathology will lead to a medical system which is interventionist and directed towards compensating for the physiological deficiencies and imbalances which arise in disease, without seeking a greater understanding of how they arose in the first place. The basic strategy will be superficial and short term. This is increasingly the orthodox medical system which we have today. While it is a very useful system for advanced pathologies and life-threatening states, it is incomplete and especially inadequate for the treatment of chronic diseases.

In contrast, most traditional medical systems, systems which are partially or completely based on herbal medicine, concern themselves more with the underlying physiological imbalances which led to and sustain the disease. As such, they are more focused on physiology than pathology. The treatment is aimed at physiological support or correction, rather than just compensating for the chemical deficiencies or excesses resulting from an abnormal physiology. The orthodox approach of physiological compensation often requires the constant presence of the medicine to achieve the desired effect whereas physiological support can, in time, lead to a permanent correction of an abnormal body chemistry.

One group of herbalists in the 19th century recognized these considerations and, in an attempt to translate traditional herbal thinking into more modern concepts, named their discipline 'physiomedicalism'. Obviously, other traditional herbal practitioners did not and could not express their understanding of physiology in modern scientific theories but this does not detract from the value or elegance of their comprehension of the functioning of the human body.

An example of physiological support versus physiological compensation can be seen in the treatment of bacterial infections. The traditional herbal approach is to support immunity and to fine tune the normal physiological responses to infection such as fever. In contrast, the orthodox approach is to suppress the fever and kill the bacteria with antibiotics, thereby compensating for weakened or overloaded bodily defences. The latter approach has life-saving value but will not prevent infections from recurring. The traditional herbal approach may see a higher rate of failure in acute situations, although this is debatable, but will lead to improved immunity and a reduced rate of recurrent infections. Clearly an important complementary role for traditional herbal medicine can be argued from this and other examples.

Western herbal medicine is also not opposed to employing physiological compensation when needed, although the approach is far less interventionist than that possible with modern drugs. It recognizes that a disease process can often create a vicious cycle and that only direct intervention to break that cycle can restore health in some instances. At a pragmatic level, interventionist treatment gives quicker relief of symptoms which encourages the patient to persist with the treatment. Sometimes the very concepts treated might require an interventionist approach because they are orthodox concepts, e.g. hypertension and high serum cholesterol. This is not to say that a more traditional herbal approach cannot be of assistance as well.

THERAPEUTIC STRATEGY

The treatment strategy in modern Western herbal medicine therefore arises from a consideration of both physiological enhancement and physiological compensation.

PHYSIOLOGICAL ENHANCEMENT

General strategy

In general terms, the goal of physiological enhancement is to create a state of active, robust health. This is more than just the absence of overt disease, although such a positive state of body and mind would be free of disease and capable of resisting disease. It is the optimum state of body chemistry and body energy. The term 'energy' in this context is more than just physical or chemical energy. All traditional health systems without exception assert the existence of a vital energy which integrates the normal physiological functioning of the body and maintains homoeostasis. This controversial concept, 'vitality', represents a fundamental difference between traditional and orthodox medical systems.

The treatment goals of physiological enhancement can be elaborated as follows.

- Optimize body chemistry by improving nutrition and enhancing detoxification. This applies not just to the body as a whole but to every cell, organ and system within the body.

- Optimize body energy by raising vitality. Improved vitality automatically follows from optimized body chemistry. But it can also be specifically encouraged using tonics, which make more energy available, and adaptogens, which optimize the capacity to cope with stressors of all kinds, thereby helping to conserve vitality.

Specific strategies

With the exception of 'whole-body' medicines such as the tonics and adaptogens, the general goals of physiological enhancement are achieved by enhancing the function of individual systems, organs or even tissues and cells. Enhancement often involves the correction of imbalances. Deficient function in one physiological compartment can lead to overstimulated function in another which in turn can create a deficiency elsewhere. For this reason the specific treatment is sometimes not aimed at the problem site: for example, in constipation caused by deficient liver function, liver function would be enhanced instead of, or in conjunction with, enhancing bowel function. In another example, an excess of female hormones causing a menstrual problem may again be treated by enhancing liver function, since the liver is the organ which breaks down these hormones. But it may also be treated by regulating the pituitary, which controls ovarian function. However, direct regulation of ovarian function may not be used.

From the brief examples above it becomes apparent that fundamental to the specific strategy of physiological enhancement is the individualization of the patient. If the concept of a vital force is the first pillar of traditional herbal medicine, the treatment of the patient as an individual is the second. This is in direct contrast to current medical science, since double-blind, placebo-controlled clinical trials only examine the effect of a medicine in a group of patients (the more the better, for statistical power) rather than individuals.

Where appropriate, specific physiological enhancement might involve the regulation or boosting of digestive function, immunity, circulation, respiratory function and hormone output. It may also involve the enhancement of specific organs such as the liver, kidneys, ovaries and so on. Specific tissues may also be targeted, e.g. the exocrine cells of the pancreas. Specific functions of organs may also be targeted, e.g. the bile secretion from the liver or the detoxification enzyme systems in the liver. In all cases this must be assessed on an individual basis and periodically reviewed.

An important general goal of physiological enhancement is the stimulation of detoxification. This is particularly required for problems where toxin overload is significant, as may be the case in chronic fatigue syndrome, autoimmune disease and cancer, for example. Detoxification can be achieved by both stimulating detoxification processes with depuratives, immunostimulants and liver herbs and stimulating elimination with diaphoretics, diuretics, lymphatics, laxatives and expectorants.

PHYSIOLOGICAL COMPENSATION

Sometimes an overstimulated function needs to be directly controlled or deficiencies need to be compensated because the pathological process has gone too far. In other cases, a vicious cycle needs to be broken or the patient needs relief from uncomfortable or debilitating symptoms. These are circumstances where physiological compensation is appropriate. Actions which begin with 'anti' usually denote a role in physiological compensation, e.g. antiinflammatory, antiviral, antispasmodic, antiseptic, antiallergic and so on. Sedative and hypnotic actions also involve compensatory mechanisms and there are many other examples. Many of the 'specific' herbs come into this category. Experience has shown that these herbs work well for particular disease states, e.g. *Tanacetum parthenium* and migraine, Arnica and bruises etc. Their mechanism of action is not necessarily known but probably involves compensatory effects, although more fundamental mechanisms may also apply. Knowledge about 'specifics' often originates from folk medicine, where often just one herb is used at a time.

TREATING THE PERCEIVED CAUSES

The question which must be asked at the outset and through all stages of treatment is: 'What is the cause of disease in this individual?' Depending on the perceived cause, treatment involving physiological enhancement and/or compensation will be directed at that cause. Using the word 'cause' can lead to a metaphysical debate, therefore the adjective 'perceived' is an important qualification. As perception and understanding of the patient's problem improve, so one gets closer to the 'real' cause. Often there is a chain of causal events and the traditional herbal approach is usually to treat as many of the links in the chain as are amenable to treatment and are active at the time of treatment. Perception of the cause should always be linked to a correct medical diagnosis, although this diagnosis need not be as specific as that required by orthodox medicine.

Factors involved in disease causation can be divided into predisposing, excitatory and sustaining causes. A *predisposing* cause is any factor which renders the body more liable to disease. Such predisposing causes include stress, lowered vitality, poor diet, inherited defects and so on. *Excitatory* causes are the direct provoking causes of a disease, such as infection and trauma. *Sustaining* causes usually come into play as a result of the initiation of a disease process and hinder the resolution of the disease. In this context, inflammation can be a sustaining cause. In general, orthodox medical treatment is aimed only at excitatory and sustaining causes, at best.

As much as is possible, predisposing causes should be removed through physiological enhancement. Neutralization of excitatory causes usually requires only compensatory mechanisms. Similarly, treatment of sustaining causes usually only needs physiological compensation to break the sustaining cycle.

An example of treating the links in a causal chain can be illustrated by the following sequence of events:

1. stress → 2. insomnia → 3. lowered vitality → 4. weakened immunity → 5. viral infection → 6. catarrhal state of mucous membranes → 7. cough

Table 7.1 Example of a treatment approach for a causal chain

Link in chain	Treatment	Physiological enhancement (E) or compensation (C)
1	Adaptogens	E
2	Sedatives	C
	Hypnotics	C
3	Tonics (choosing those which will not aggravate insomnia)	E
4	Immunostimulants	E
5	Antivirals	C
6	Anticatarrhals	C
7	Expectorants	E
	Antitussives	C

In the context of the above causal sequence, 1–4 are predisposing causes, 5 is the excitatory cause, 6 is a sustaining cause and 7 is the symptomatic expression of the disease.

The treatment approach is set out in Table 7.1

While all this may not be achievable in one prescription, over time all the links in a chain might be addressed. By choosing herbs which cover several of the required actions, it may be possible to treat many or most links in the one prescription e.g. Hypericum is antiviral and a mild hypnotic, Echinacea is immunostimulant and lymphatic. Other actions might also be required if the body retraces the links in order to resolve the problem, e.g. the catarrhal state may be resolved by an acute infection and this would require stimulants (in the herbal sense) and diaphoretics in addition to some of the above. If the catarrhal state were found to be more than just a sustaining cause then it would require deeper treatment using lymphatic and expectorant herbs.

Sometimes, where there is a good understanding of the main predisposing cause and a very effective treatment, only this cause needs to be treated. For example, Ross River virus infection, which is endemic in Australia, can lead to a chronic condition with joint pain, lethargy and night sweats due to the persistence of the immune imbalance caused by the virus. Treatment with just *Echinacea angustifolia* in sufficient doses usually resolves the condition in 6–10 weeks.

Some causes are not treatable by herbal medicine; e.g. if insomnia is caused by a traumatic experience, then herbs can compensate but cannot treat or remove the cause. Causes amenable to herbal treatment are listed in Box 7.1.

Some of the causes which cannot be removed but can be compensated for by herbal treatment are listed in Box 7.2

Box 7.1 Causes amenable to herbal treatment

Lowered vitality	Weakened immunity
Toxicity	Allergy
Tumour	Infection – chronic, subclinical or acute
Emotional imbalance	Stress
Organ malfunction	Catarrhal state of mucous membranes
Organ damage	Autoimmunity
Inflammation	Unhealthy bowel flora
Hormonal imbalance	

Box 7.2 Causes which can only be compensated for by herbal treatment

Attitudes to life
Emotional or physical trauma
Heredity
Climate
Age
Lifestyle
Diet

Often, as part of arriving at an individual treatment framework based on the above considerations, it is also necessary to take into account the current medical understanding of the patient's condition. This orthodox understanding needs to be carefully interpreted but nonetheless the current scientific literature is yielding very useful information. For example, potential causative factors which have been identified in autoimmune disease include chronic bacterial and/or viral infections, abnormal bowel flora, dietary allergies and chemical sensitivities. Factors identified in gastric ulceration include bacterial infection, defective sphincter function and poor mucosal resistance.

THE CRITICAL ROLE OF CASE TAKING

The major aim of case taking is to establish the treatment goals or treatment protocols for that individual. Even for the same medical disorder, this can vary greatly from patient to patient; e.g. a patient with eczema with a history of insecticide exposure when young will be treated differently to a patient with eczema which developed after her first child. The following is a basic outline for a consultation which seeks to obtain the information needed to arrive at the treatment framework. Particular emphasis should be given to:

- the historical factors behind the development of the presenting complaint;
- factors which modify the presenting complaint;
- current and previous medication;
- information about the patient's constitution and current condition;
- diet;
- social history;
- past serious disorders or health problems and disorders related to the presenting complaint, as these can lead to information about underlying causes.

THE TREATMENT FRAMEWORK

The treatment framework or protocol sets out the aims or goals of treatment. This is mainly derived from an understanding of the perceived causes of the condition together with an assessment of the need for physiological enhancement or compensation.

Information used to arrive at the treatment framework for a particular disorder is drawn from the following sources.

- The traditional herbal understanding of the disorder.
- The clinical experiences of the practitioner in the treatment of the disorder.
- A general understanding of the type of the disorder, e.g. if it is an infection, what usually leads to this, or if it is an autoimmune disease, what factors usually precipitate and sustain an autoimmune process.
- A scientific understanding of the causes involved in the particular disorder, e.g. ankylosing spondylitis. This information might be derived from clinical and epidemiological studies which have revealed factors which precipitate and sustain the disease process.
- A knowledge of scientific studies which have defined the underlying pathological process for that particular disorder.
- The individual case history. In a sense, the individual case history acts as a filter for all the above information. An obvious example is lung cancer. Smoking is known to cause lung cancer but if a patient has never smoked then this consideration is irrelevant to that particular patient. In other words, only those known or suspected causative factors which apply to the particular patient should be incorporated into his or her treatment framework.

• The need for symptomatic treatment; again, this relies largely on the individual case history.

For many disorders, development of the treatment framework is a relatively simple process. However, in some instances this process may become quite complex, especially in the case of chronic disorders.

THE ACTIONS

The concepts which link the treatment goals or treatment framework to the choice of herbs are the actions. These are traditional herbal concepts but scientific research also yields information about the actions of a herb. The stepwise process in linking treatment goals to choice of herbs for prescription is then as follows.

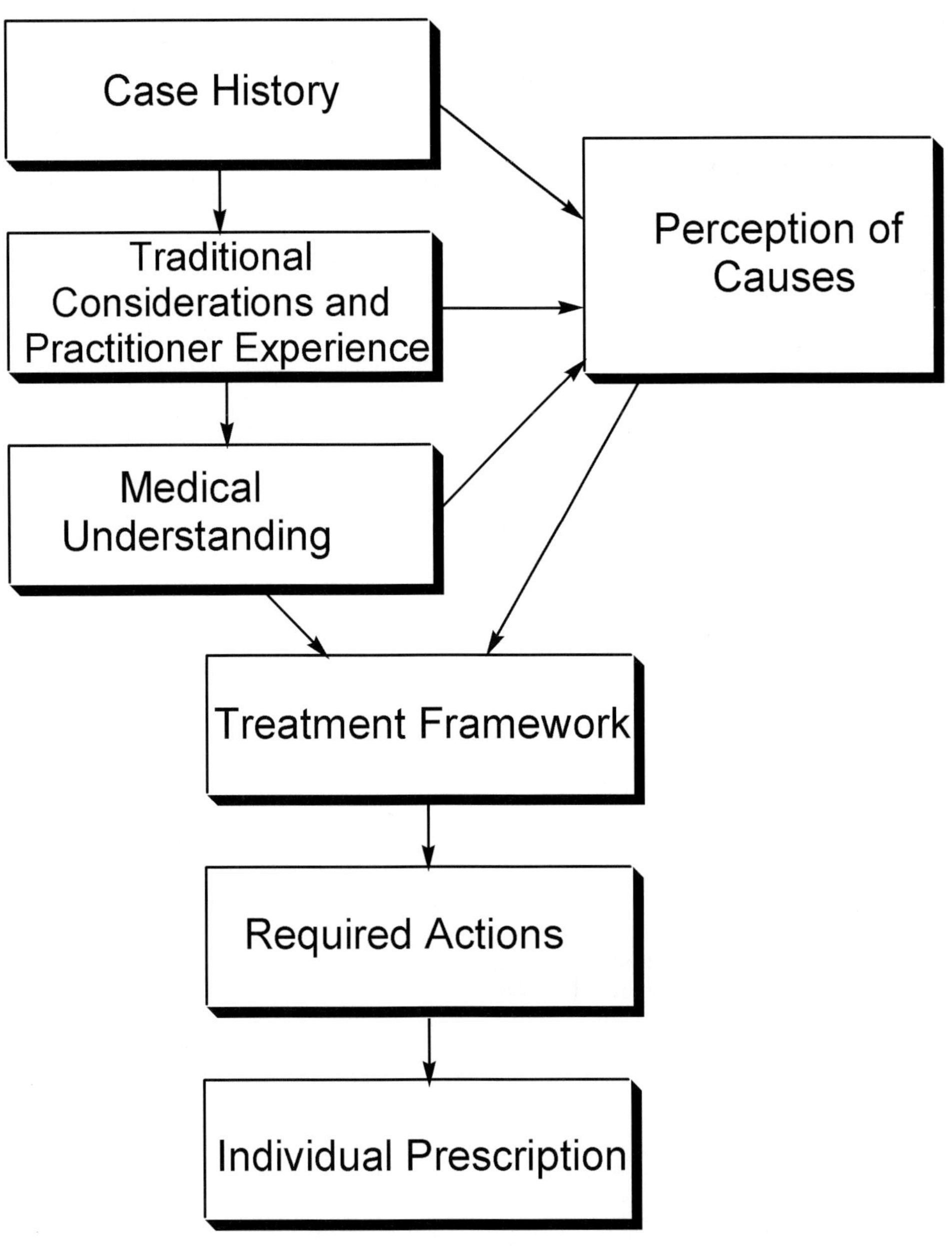

Figure 7.1 A summary of the event sequence in Western herbal therapeutics

1. Decide the treatment goals based on traditional herbal concepts, the orthodox medical understanding of the disorder and the patient's case.

2. Ensure that the goals are individualized to the requirements of the individual case.

3. Decide upon the immediate priorities of treatment.

4. On the basis of the immediate treatment goals, decide what actions are required.

5. Choose reliable herbs which have these actions, with as much overlap as possible. For example, if anti-inflammatory and antispasmodic actions are required for the gut, Matricaria can effectively cover both these requirements. Make sure that these herbs are matched to the patient's constitution and general condition according to the considerations outlined in Chapter 3.

6. If a particular action needs to be reinforced, do this by choosing more than one herb with this action or by using a very effective herb in a higher dose.

7. Combine the herbs in a formula with appropriate doses (this is usually done as a mixture of fluid extracts or tinctures). Do not choose too many herbs as this will compromise their individual doses in the formula and may lead to undefined interactions.

To facilitate this process, the practitioner needs a clear understanding of herbs in terms of their reliable, well-established actions. Reference lists of herbs classified under each action and ranked in order of priority from the most reliable herb to the least reliable are a useful tool. For example, under the heading of immune stimulants, one might list the following herbs in this order:

Echinacea angustifolia
Echinacea purpurea
Astragalus membranaceus
Andrographis panniculata
Picrorrhiza kurroa
down to *Allium sativum* and *Baptisia tinctoria* which are less proven.

This list could be annotated, e.g. Echinacea species, best at increasing phagocytic activity and early aspects of immune recognition, Picrorrhiza best at stimulating all aspects of immune function and Astragalus, best in chronic states of impaired immunity and contraindicated in acute infections, and so on. (There will be a considerable element of subjectivity in the compilation of such lists!) The interactive preparation of these lists by a group of practitioners can be a useful learning experience.

The event sequence in Western herbal therapeutics is summarized in Figure 7.1.

Herbal approaches to pathological states

TOPICAL APPLICATIONS

SCOPE

Apart from their use to provide non-specific support for recuperation and repair, specific phytotherapeutic strategies include the following.

Treatment of:

- minor wounds and lesions;
- sprains and bruises;
- seborrhoeic inflammations;
- cutaneous infections and infestations;
- minor inflammations of mouth, throat, anus and nasal and vaginal mucosa;
- certain inflammatory conditions affecting the surface of the eye.

Management and relief of:

- pruritic symptoms;
- cutaneous eruptions from skin and systemic inflammatory diseases;
- inflammations affecting joints, muscles and other subcutaneous tissues;
- varicose ulceration and pressure sores.

Because of its use of secondary plant products, particular caution is necessary in applying phytotherapy in cases of:

- broken skin;
- individuals with certain contact sensitivities.

ORIENTATION

Background

Plants contain many constituents with local physical impact on body tissues. The topical use of herbal remedies is among the first emphases in the earliest and simplest traditions of healthcare. Wound healing was an obvious primal indication for which plant remedies appeared especially suitable.

From a modern perspective direct effects on tissues are readily testable in research. Most antiseptic, antiinflammatory and antitumour effects in the research literature relate to in vitro observations, of little direct application to anticipating the effects of oral consumption but quite relevant to the prediction of topical activity.

Referral to Chapteı 2 will provide much of the detail for this review. The following topical properties, however, can be highlighted.

Demulcents

Plant material often contains apparently soothing effects on physical contact and plant remedies must have been a very early instinctive application to wounds. Plants with high mucilage content form the basis of poultices and creams. Linum (linseed, flaxseed) is one of the most impressive poultices where the skin (or subdermal tissue in even unbroken skin) is painfully inflamed. *Ulmus fulva* (slippery elm bark) when powdered is one of the most obviously mucilaginous plant materials available for poultices. Stellaria (chickweed) in a cream base provides effective relief for many itchy conditions. Althaea (marshmallow root) and *Trigonella foenum-graecum* (fenugreek) have notably soothing reputations. Above all, Symphytum (comfrey root) cream, applied only to unbroken skin, combines an unparalleled local demulcent action with an active promoter of repair, allantoin, which is known to be very rapidly absorbed into the subdermal tissue.[1] The expressed juice of *Aloe vera* also has impressive topical demulcent properties when applied directly to broken or unbroken skin.[2,3,4]

Astringents

Tannins and related polyphenols are very common plant constituents with the simple property of curdling protein molecules into which they come in contact. The principle of tanning animal skins to make leather, most often using oak galls or oak bark, follows from this property. Simple washes with strong decoctions of high-tannin preparations (like broadleaved tree bark) are well-established country first-aid treatments for open wounds and burns and the technique was formally revived among 'barefoot doctors' in China after the Cultural Revolution in the 1960s. The aim here was to produce a sealing eschar over the exposed tissues formed from coagulated protein on the surface. In modern clinical application, suspensions of decoctions of high-tannin herbs in gum tragacanth or gum arabic can produce impressive healing effects in open wounds or skin lesions. The antioxidant effects of such preparations have also drawn attention.[5,6,7] Plants to be considered for this role include decoctions of Hamamelis (witchhazel bark), *Potentilla tormentilla* (tormentil root), Quercus (oak bark), Krameria (rhatany) and *Geranium maculatum* (American cranesbill root).

Antiinflammatories

A number of plant constituents appear to possess topical antiinflammatory effects, frequently in addition to their demulcent and astringent properties. They might be considered as alternatives to conventional steroidal and other antiinflammatory prescriptions. Calendula (marigold),[8] at least when extracted in high-strength alcohol, and *Matricaria recutita* (German chamomile),[9] both included in creams, have useful benefits in soothing inflamed skin lesions.[10] *Berberis aquifolium* has demonstrated efficacy in the treatment of psoriatic lesions.[11] Echinacea applied topically appears to have local antiinflammatory effects on minor wounds.[12] Hypericum (St John's wort) extracted in oil as a red pigment is a long-standing remedy for the relief of burns and skin pain, as is oil of lavender applied over unbroken skin. Other traditional remedies used topically for antiinflammatory effects include *Curcuma longa* (turmeric), juniperus (juniper oil) and *Angelica archangelica* (angelica oil). Bruising is traditionally treated with external applications of *Aesculus hippocastanum*[13] and *Arnica montana* (arnica).

Antiseptics

The topical effects of herbal remedies can include some antiseptic effects in vitro, although only a few whole preparations have significant clinical prospects. For a review of antimicrobial effects of herbal remedies see p.140.

FORMULATIONS

Many types of topical formulation have evolved for the application of plant materials on body surfaces. A brief summary of their characteristics well reflects the diversity of possible approaches.

Liquids

Liniments (and embrocations)

Semiliquid preparations prepared in oily or alcoholic solution respectively, with rubefacient or analgesic intentions, are rubbed into unbroken skin. Examples include liniments of mustard and Capsicum, used to stimulate circulation, and liniment of Arnica for healing.

Lotions

These are non-oily liquids applied externally and generally not rubbed in. They are applied to the body surface or any external orifice. Sometimes a lotion will be a herbal tincture used, for example, as topical treatments for skin or nail fungal infections.

Eardrops

The external ear canal can be treated with oil or alcohol/water-based preparations to help clear obstructions, to treat inflammation or infection of the canal or ear drum or to influence the middle ear by diffusion across the ear drum. Warm olive oil is a popular treatment for waxy obstructions and may be augmented by garlic and Verbascum (mullein flowers) steeped in the oil. However, bacterial contamination of such products is a concern and non-industrially produced preparations are often not to be recommended.

Eyebaths

Aqueous solutions are the usual basis for irrigation of the eye in blepharitis, conjunctival and corneal affections. Bacterial contamination of the eye tissues is particularly hazardous in any home-produced eyebath and these should be discouraged. Great care must be taken to ensure sterility of the fluid which must be boiled for at least 15 minutes in its final container (or added to a sterilized container after boiling). Any water added to the preparation must also be boiled or sterilized. Preparations must be used immediately or stored in sterile frozen blocks. Decoctions of Euphrasia (eyebright), Foeniculum (fennel seed), Agrimonia (agrimony), Glycyrrhiza (licorice root), made at 30 g per 500 ml and then diluted 1:1 with water for application, may be used to reduce inflammatory symptoms.

Gargles

These are preparations in water or alcohol/water solution to be used for throat problems. They may be antiseptic, soothing and/or healing. Herbal gargles may also be swallowed to obtain a secondary, systemic effect. Effective gargles can be made with tinctures of Salvia (sage), Commiphora (myrrh), Calendula and Echinacea, these ideally combined with fluid extract of Glycyrrhiza (licorice) or mucilaginous ingredients. Honey is another effective ingredient.

Inhalants (or vapours)

Volatile components may be inhaled either from a pad applied to the nose and mouth or from liniments or ointments applied to the skin under the nose or on the chest or, most effectively, with steam from hot water. They allow deep and accurate penetration of medicinal agents throughout the whole respiratory system, including the sinuses and middle ear. They will clear catarrhal congestion, soothe irritable mucous membranes and reduce some hypersensitivity reactions. The simplest steaming herb is Matricaria (chamomile) strewn onto the surface of recently boiled water. Recommended oils include pine, aniseed, eucalyptus and, to a limited extent, peppermint.

Baths

Adding herbs or volatile oils to baths has been a traditional technique, with the particular benefit of allowing inhalation of the volatile components in the steam. One common non-volatile application is the mustard bath, used to bathe feet or hands affected by arthritic trouble or as a means of stimulating circulation generally throughout the system. Mustard powder is added at up to 1% by weight to hand-hot water and the part bathed in it till cool.

Douches

Aqueous solutions may be directed against the body or into a body cavity to cleanse or disinfect. The vaginal douche is the most frequently used: infusions or decoctions of astringent or antiseptic herbs may be prepared and applied deep into the vagina with a bulb syringe or similar applicator whilst the patient is lying supine, for vaginal and cervical infections and inflammations. Douches can also be used for the nasal cavity although this is rarely done nowadays.

Solids

Creams

These are emulsions of oil in water or water in oil designed to be well absorbed by the skin. They may have various remedies dissolved in either the oil or water fraction. Creams are generally softer than ointments and are more complex in their formulation. For this reason, they were not common in pharmacies of the past but with technical advances are very prominent today, especially in the cosmetics industry. Where available, preparations with Stellaria (chickweed), Calendula, Echinacea and Symphytum (comfrey) are suitable for the treatment of pruritic or inflammatory skin conditions.

Ointments (or unguents)

These are semisolid solutions of various preparations in non-aqueous bases that are not absorbed easily into the skin and are therefore used to provide a protective or remedial film over the skin. Being immiscible with water or skin secretions, ointments effectively form an occlusive layer over the skin, preventing evaporation by transpiration or sweating and allowing the skin to become hydrated. This permits easier absorption of any water-soluble materials in the ointment.

Jellies (or gels)

Suspensions or colloids made from gums, pectin or gelatin allow non-oily applications to be applied to mucous membranes (like the vagina and rectum) and to open or discharging wounds or lesions. They are the most effective way of applying an astringent treatment, especially if gum tragacanth is used as the gelling/suspending agent. Infusions, juices or tinctures may be used for the fluid part. Soothing astringent preparations made, for example, with witchhazel are ideal for irritated wounds, slow-healing leg ulcers or haemorrhoids. Without preservatives, gels should be made and used freshly or from frozen samples.

Plasters

Unlike the modern item, traditional plasters were impregnated dressings applied over the skin where a long-term and concentrated medication was required. The plaster mass was a waxy, rubber, resinous or other base incorporating medical agents, spread on to fabric. It was often designed to convey rubefacient, analgesic or protective effects. Cayenne plasters are notable applications for arthritic disease.

Poultices

The oldest traditional application was a mass of material soaked in hot water in a fabric bag and applied to the skin while still hot. Poultices have particular ability to draw wounds and infections and to soothe, heal and astringe. Linseed, comfrey, marshmallow and cabbage leaf are frequently used in poultice form in traditional practice.

Suppositories and pessaries

Solid preparations suitable for rectal and vaginal insertion respectively, generally consisting of a solution or suspension of active agents in a solid base designed to melt at body temperature (and thus needing to be stored at cool temperatures). Two main types of base are cocoa butter and gelatin-glycerin mixes. The former is most immediately applicable where dry herbal preparations are to be added. Gelatin-glycerin bases are better able to hold fluid; nevertheless, their use may lead to drying of the mucosal membranes and this may provoke inflammation if used frequently.

References

1. Sznitowska M, Janicki S. The effect of vehicle on allantoin penetration into human skin from an ointment for improving scar elasticity. Pharmazie 1988; 43: 218
2. Chithra P, Sajithlal GB, Chandrakasan G. Influence of aloe vera on the healing of dermal wounds in diabetic rats. Journal of Ethnopharmacology 1998; 59(3): 195–201
3. Strickland FM, Pelley RP, Kripke ML. Prevention of ultraviolet radiation-induced suppression of contact and delayed hypersensitivity by Aloe barbadensis gel extract. Journal of Investigative Dermatology 1994; 102(2): 197–204
4. Visuthikosol V, Chowchuen B, Sukwanarat Y, Sriurairatana S, Boonpucknavig V. Effect of aloe vera gel to healing of burn wound a clinical and histologic study. Journal of the Medical Association of Thailand 1995; 78(8): 403–409
5. Masaki H, Sakaki S, Atsumi T, Sakurai H. Active-oxygen scavenging activity of plant extracts. Biological and Pharmaceutical Bulletin 1995; 18(1): 162–166
6. Sawabe Y, Yamasaki K, Iwagami S, Kajimura K, Nakagomi K. Inhibitory effects of natural medicines on the enzymes related to the skin. Yakugaku Zasshi 1998; 118(9): 423–429
7. Mrowietz U, Ternowitz T, Wiedow O. Selective inactivation of human neutrophil elastase by synthetic tannin. Journal of Investigative Dermatology 1991; 97(3): 529–533
8. Klouchek-Popova E, Popov A, Pavlova N, Krsteva S. Influence of the physiological regeneration and epithelialization using fractions isolated from Calendula officinalis. Acta Physiologica et Pharmacologica Bulgarica 1982; 8(4): 63–67
9. Glowania HJ, Raulin C, Swoboda M. Effect of chamomile on wound healing – a clinical double-blind study. Zeitschrift für Hautkrankheiten 1987; 62(17): 1262, 1267–1271
10. Shipochliev T, Dimitrov A, Aleksandrova E. Antiinflammatory action of a group of plant extracts. Veterinarno-Meditsinski Nauki 1981; 18(6): 87–94
11. Wiesenauer M, Lüdtke R. Mahonia aquifolium in patients with Psoriasis vulgaris – an intraindividual study. Phytomedicine 1996; 3(3): 231–235
12. Kinkel JH, Plate M, Töllner HU. Verificable effect of Echinacin ointment on wound healing. Medizinische Klinik 1984; 79: 580–583
13. Bombardelli E, Morazzoni P. Aesculus hippocastanum L. Fitoterapia 1996; 67(6): 483–510

FEVER

SCOPE

Apart from their use to provide non-specific support for recuperation and repair, specific phytotherapeutic strategies include the following.

Treatment of:

- uncomplicated and moderate fevers from infectious causes.

Management and relief of:

- febrile symptoms of non-infectious origin.

Particular **caution** is necessary in applying phytotherapy in cases of:

- severe, rampant fever with hyperpyrexia and/or when due to virulent causes.

ORIENTATION

Introduction

Fever is most often associated with viral and bacterial infectious illnesses of varying degrees of severity, such as 'flu', measles, rubella, rheumatic fever, pneumonia, malaria, scarlet fever, polio, tuberculosis and meningitis. It can also accompany a wider range of problems such as cardiovascular and autoimmune diseases, drug reactions and some cancers. Many cases, especially in children, remain mysterious.[1]

It is therefore vital that the onset of any fever is diagnosed as accurately as possible, especially in the very young and elderly, pregnant women, among overseas travellers and those with immune disorders. Orthodox drug therapy and even hospitalization may be essential.

The fever as friend?

Perhaps because of the associations above, the fever process has come to be seen as a problem to be treated in its own right ('We must bring the fever down'). The serious risks from hyperpyrexia (overheating) are well understood and the accompanying unpleasant symptoms are reason enough to regard fever with suspicion. However, if it is clear that fever is not part of a serious condition there are also good reasons for not suppressing the process unnecessarily. This view is gaining support in conventional medicine,[2,3] particularly in reaction to the fashion for using paracetamol, and previously aspirin, to treat common childhood fevers.[4]

Such modern reassessment of fever treatment echoes the older traditional view that fever was not the disease itself but the body's extraordinary efforts to resist disease. It was therefore something to be supported, or at least managed, rather than unduly suppressed. In this view, a 'good fever', one which went through its natural course satisfactorily, would not only lead to better resolution of the immediate crisis but would actually rearm the body's defences and increase its resistance to future onslaughts. Indeed, it was on this issue above all others that the revivalist practices of Samuel Thomson in the 19th century were based (see p.12). It was common practice among 'regular' physicians to suppress fevers with mineral drugs based on mercury, arsenic and antimony. Thomson was moved by Indian practices, especially the sweat lodge, to vehemently challenge such principles and insist instead on the view that fever was a sign of healthy defences (the 'natural heat' of the body resisting 'cold' intrusion) and should be supported in its efforts rather than suppressed. To this end, he recommended the use of heating remedies, including cayenne, and other measures to support the body through the episode, managing excesses of the febrile condition along the way. Although Thomson's message was simple (reflecting the predominance of fevers as the main clinical priority of the times), he identified a fundamental difference between traditional practices and the new direction of orthodox medicine – supporting body defences versus attacking disease processes.

Other traditional approaches to fever management were similar. Because fever was so common, the universal classification of remedies as heating or cooling was made very largely on the basis of their observed effects in this condition. Heating herbs would be used to support a flagging fever and, by promoting perspiration, were additionally seen as aiding elimination through the sweat glands (sweat glands do resemble primitive nephrons and can stand in for kidney function to some extent); cooling remedies would be used to temper excessive pyrexia. Herbs with subtle heating or cooling (e.g. the Galenic 'hot in the first degree') were seen as exerting a normalizing effect, helping to steady body temperature. Other remedies were classified for their ability to reduce the impact of febrile convulsions, diarrhoea, vomiting and distress.

There is modern support for the traditional view. The body's febrile response is accompanied by the arousal of powerful, unpleasant and debilitating defensive measures, the release of inflammatory chemicals, temperature-stimulated activity in the circulation and in various blood cells, including the scavenger white blood cells, and associated alterations in a wide range of other functions.[5,6] In many ways it is like inflammation, for which an analogous traditional view applies (see p.145): it generally proceeds in defined stages, tends to be self-limiting and is directed to mobilizing defensive resources to the rapid elimination of an intrusion into the tissues. Both inflammation and fever are accompanied by what may be regarded as guarding symptoms, in the case of fever often by nausea (leading to reduced eating and unnecessary digestive, eliminative and metabolic burdens), thirst (increasing fluid consumption and compensating for fever-induced dehydration), lassitude and exhaustion (ensuring adequate rest during the process) and photophobia (encouraging withdrawal to a darkened place so as to reduce visual and other stimulation).

In contrast to our forebears, modern practitioners can now accept the far superior diagnostic and treatment prospects that medicine can bring and be grateful that the killer fevers are largely in the past. Nevertheless, there is real value in revisiting some fundamental fever management approaches in the majority of feverish illnesses that do not present serious threat. There is a real concern that suppressive measures like aspirin and paracetamol and preemptive (and often unsuitable) antibiotic treatments are aborting an important natural healing process. Earlier observers predicted that unresolved fevers would lead to recurrent low-grade problems thereafter. The current frequency of chronic catarrhal problems, sore throats, cervical lymphadenopathy (swollen glands), sinusitis and otitis media (glue ear), especially among children, reminds many modern practitioners of such a syndrome.

It is possible to retrieve some of the early measures as part of a new strategy of fever management, taking advantage of insights and technology unavailable to our forebears.

Practical fever management

Fevers present serious challenges for any practitioner more used to dealing with modern chronic and low-grade conditions. **Fevers can be dangerous. They can change rapidly and initial diagnoses can be wrong. It would be professionally negligent to take responsibility for managing a fever without the necessary personal medical qualifications and experience unless supported by an effective health team. The following suggestions can only be applied in such circumstances.**

After best available medical diagnosis has determined that dangerous disease is unlikely, the phytotherapeutic approach to fever is to see the condition as something to be managed, even nurtured, to allow the body temperature to stay at acceptable febrile levels (usually the range 100–102°F or 37.8–38.9°C) until the fever breaks, then to switch to recuperative measures as required. During the fever the practitioner watches for dangerous symptoms (and ensures ongoing medical supervision as necessary), works with herbal and other measures to prevent body temperature rising too high and provides relief for ancillary symptoms like nausea, vomiting, diarrhoea, coughing, convulsions and general malaise and discomforts.

Many fever-causing bacteria and viruses either produce as metabolites or present as surface antigens trigger chemicals, referred to as *exogenous pyrogens*, that stimulate the temperature control mechanism in the hypothalamus – in effect, they 'set the thermostat higher'. The result is a stimulus to the heat-generating and heat-conserving mechanisms of the body so that body temperature can rise to match the new setting in the hypothalamus. Such mechanisms include shutting down the blood flow to the surface (pallor), shivering and seeking warmth. In short, **when the temperature is rising the patient feels cold**.

This is the 'chill' phase of fever. When the body temperature rises to the level set by the hypothalamus, a new stability with balance of heat gain and loss returns. The symptoms of chill recede and a less uncomfortable phase commences.

With the rise in body temperature, blood flow through the tissues and the activity of the phagocytes increase. The body's defenses are alerted and mobilized. The intruder's prospects are reduced, as eventually is its production of exogenous pyrogens. The upward stimulus on the hypothalamus is reduced and the thermostat setting falls. The outward sign of this change could be predicted from knowing that the body temperature will now be higher than that set in the thermostat so heat has to be lost. The circulation to the periphery opens up again, the sweat glands operate, clothing and coverings are thrown off. **The temperature falls and for that reason the patient feels hot**. In traditional terms, the fever has 'broken', 'crisis' has been reached and 'lysis' or resolution intervenes. With luck, the infection has been successfully rejected and recovery can commence.

This is a very simple account. There can be complicating factors. For example, there are a range of peptides, such as interleukin-1-beta, produced by the body itself and known as *endogenous pyrogens* which, possibly interacting with prostaglandins, can induce relapsing and other complex fever patterns with no clear cause.[7,8] Yet this account provides an acceptable basis for a policy of fever management, in which basic principles of nursing can be augmented by herbal remedies.

The first requirement is for some means of monitoring the situation. A clinical thermometer is obviously central but its usefulness is greatly enhanced by knowing how to interpret its findings. Referring to the account of fever above will explain the following points.

1. Feeling cold, pale cyanosed skin and shivering mean that the body temperature is lower than that set in the hypothalamus and is most likely to be *still rising*.
2. Feeling hot, flushed skin and sweating mean that the body temperature is higher than the thermostat setting and is most likely to be *coming down*.
3. Having no dominant feeling of being hot or cold suggests relative equilibrium between thermostat and body temperature.

With these clues and a thermometer, it is generally possible to assess progress through the fever. If, for example, the temperature was 104°F (40°C), its importance would depend on whether the patient was feeling hot or cold. In the former case, one would expect the temperature to fall; in the latter case, some quick treatment would be called for.

Apart from the usual techniques for bringing temperature down, such as cold wet face flannels or tepid baths, there is conventional aspirin. This, however, simply turns the thermostat controls down without attending to any other aspects of the fever; there is the risk of an unresolved problem with symptoms lasting for years. Its use in children has in any case been discontinued in recent years because of the incidence of serious side effects.[9,10] Paracetamol is still used for similar purposes in spite of growing concerns about its dangers.[11,12] Herbal remedies, by contrast, appear to interact more constructively and there are a number of peripheral antipyretic mechanisms associated with plant remedies.[13,14,15]

Herbal treatments during fevers are best provided in the form of aqueous infusions or decoctions (see p.121), either hot or warm depending on the wider context.

As a steadying influence, the peripheral vasodilators or diaphoretics are appropriate, including remedies such as Achillea (yarrow,) Sambucus (elderflower,) Matricaria (chamomile), Tilia (limeflowers), *Nepeta cataria* (catmint) and *Eupatorium perfoliatum* (boneset). Their effect in hot infusion, seen only in a febrile state, is subjectively to reduce chill and encourage cooling perspiration; they also have a variety of other useful benefits for the digestion, mucous membranes and neuromuscular system. They may be combined with peppermint tea for a more accelerated cooling effect.

For gentle but stronger reduction in febrile temperature, the cooling bitters, like Taraxacum (dandelion root), Gentiana (gentian root) and Cichorium (chicory root) and Erythraea (centaury), are favoured. They have the additional advantage of stimulating the otherwise dormant digestive system, thus helping to counter fermentation or infection arising from the gut. Throughout history some plants were particularly favoured for their fever-reducing properties; most were notable bitters as well as having a range of antipathogenic and antiinflammatory properties. They are, however, inherently more powerful and should be applied with more caution and under closer supervision. They include Cinchona (Peruvian bark that later yielded quinine) various members of the Artemisia or wormwood family, Jateorhiza (calumba), *Berberis vulgaris* (barberry bark) and Hydrastis (golden seal).

Apart from body temperature, there are other symptoms of fever that need to be watched. Many, such as nausea, vomiting, diarrhoea, headaches, coughing, pains and spasms, can usually be controlled by the appropriate herbal remedy, covered elsewhere in this book. Accepting the potential value of the febrile reaction does not mean consigning the patient to unnecessary discomfort. There are of course danger signs as well (a pulse that does not rise with temperature as expected might herald meningitis; convulsions, although common enough in children, can disguise and exacerbate polio; a dry cough of measles can resemble that of pneumonia, which can also be heralded by rapid breathing rates; malaria remains impossible to diagnose without blood tests).[16] The untrained must not attempt to take full responsibility for any such treatment.

Raising fever

In addition to containing excessive body temperature, there may be a need to encourage it to rise. If it is clear that the fever is not adequately materializing and that there is no serious infection or underlying pathology, warming remedies might be chosen. This is a common scenario in affluent societies. Here, fevers are rare after childhood but unresolved low-grade chronic infections are not. In a case of persistent catarrh, for example, it is often useful to take advantage of a partial attempt by the body to raise the stakes, a cold or sore throat perhaps, and set a 'therapeutic fever' in train.

The patient should be advised to prepare properly. Bed rest, a minimal fresh diet and plenty of fluid are basic requirements. It is then possible to take one of the many circulatory stimulants, such as *Cinnamomum zeylanicum* (cinnamon,) *Angelica archangelica* (angelica), Zingiber (ginger), Allium (raw garlic) or even Capsicum (cayenne). A modest febrile process can then be nudged into existence, often to considerable advantage. Echinacea, being both warming and stimulating to mucosal immune defences, may be particularly useful here.

Aftermath

As important as any other part of the treatment is adequate convalescence (see p.84) after it is all over. There are a range of remedies traditionally used for postfever recuperation. These include some of the warming and cooling remedies above, those with additional tonic reputations, like *Inula helenium* (Elecampane), Cardamomum (cardamon seed), Echinacea, Taraxacum (dandelion root) and Gentiana (Gentian root).

References

1. McCarthy PL, Klig JE, Shapiro ED, Baron MA. Fever without apparent source on clinical examination, lower respiratory infections in children, other infectious diseases, and acute gastroenteritis and diarrhea of infancy and early childhood. Curr Opin Pediatr 1996; 8(1): 75–93
2. Kluger MJ, Kozak W, Conn CA et al. The adaptive value of fever. Infect Dis Clin North Am 1996; 10(1): 1–20
3. Klein NC, Cunha BA. Treatment of fever. Infect Dis Clin North Am 1996; 10(1): 211–216
4. Adam D, Stankov G. Treatment of fever in childhood. Eur J Pediatr 1994; 153(6): 394–402
5. Norman DC, Castle S, Yamamura RH, Yoshikawa TT. Interrelationship of fever, immune response and aging in mice. Mech Ageing Dev 1995; 80(1): 53–67
6. Muzyka BC. Host factors affecting disease transmission. Dent Clin North Am 1996; 40(2): 263–275
7. Sakata T, Kang M, Kurokawa M, Yoshimatsu H. Hypothalamic neuronal histamine modulates adaptive behavior and thermogenesis in response to endogenous pyrogen. Obes Res 1995; 3(Suppl 5): 707–712
8. Derijk RH, Van Kampen M, Van Rooijen N, Berkenbosch F. Hypothermia to endotoxin involves reduced thermogenesis, macrophage-dependent mechanisms, and prostaglandins. Am J Physiol 1994; 266(1 Pt 2): 1–8
9. Chalasani N, Roman J, Jurado RL. Systemic inflammatory response syndrome caused by chronic salicylate intoxication. South Med J 1996; 89(5): 479–482
10. Whelton A. Renal effects of over-the-counter analgesics. J Clin Pharmacol 1995; 35(5): 454–463
11. Czerwionka-Szaflarska M, Sobkowiak E. Acute gastrointestinal hemorrhage in a 12-month-old child following treatment with panadol. Pediatr Pol 1996; 71(5): 471–472
12. Stamm D. Paracetamol and other antipyretic analgesics: optimal doses in pediatrics. Arch Pediatr 1994; 1(2): 193–201
13. Tsai TH, Lee TF, Chen CF, Wang LC. Thermoregulatory effects of alkaloids isolated from Wu-chu-yu in afebrile and febrile rats. Pharmacol Biochem Behav 1995; 50(2): 293–298
14. Backhouse N, Delporte C, Givernau M et al. Anti-inflammatory and antipyretic effects of boldine. Agents Actions 1994; 42(3–4): 114–117
15. Lalé A, Herbert JM. Polyunsaturated fatty acids reduce pyrogen-induced tissue factor expression in human monocytes. Biochem Pharmacol 1994; 48(2): 429–431
16. Svenson JE, Gyorkos TW, MacLean JD. Diagnosis of malaria in the febrile traveler. Am J Trop Med Hyg 1995; 53(5): 518–521

INFECTIOUS DISEASES

SCOPE

Apart from their use in providing non-specific support for recuperation and repair, specific phytotherapeutic strategies include the following.

Treatment of:

- minor to moderate acute infections of the respiratory, urinary and gastrointestinal mucosa;
- minor to moderate systemic infections especially when accompanied by lymphadenopathy;
- topical bacterial and fungal infections;
- minor to moderate febrile infections;
- minor to moderate chronic viral, bacterial and fungal infections.

Management of:

- refractory cases of chronic viral, bacterial and fungal infections especially accompanied by lowered immune resistance.

Because of its use of secondary plant products, particular **caution** is necessary in applying phytotherapy in cases of infections of the kidney parenchyma.

Note: In most developed countries there are usually legal constraints on non-physicians treating or claiming to treat notifiable infections, for example, contagious infections, tuberculosis and venereal infections. Severe acute infections, especially involving vital organs, should in general be approached with extreme care and never without full medical supervision unless this is clearly not available.

ORIENTATION

Background

A modern observer might presume that one area where traditional herbal medicine could not be claimed as a useful model is in the area of infections. It is generally accepted that until Pasteur's germ theory of disease and the isolation of effective antimicrobials, humanity had seriously missed the plot. The history of pestilences and plagues, the decimation caused by the killer infections such as smallpox, cholera, typhoid and scarlet fever, the waking medieval nightmares of tuberculosis and syphilis, the Russian roulette that every mother and infant played with perinatal mortality, along with the near universal ignorance of the dangers of living in filth and squalor along with dark mutterings about 'contagions' and 'toxins' in lieu of simple hygienic measures; all this looks rather bad for traditional medicine.

Much of this is undeniable. There is no doubt that healthcare shifted beyond recognition with public hygiene measures like clean water and separate sewage systems from the 19th century and the discovery of penicillin in the early decades of the 20th. Herbal practitioners can admit this gracefully and be grateful they no longer have to attempt to thwart life-threatening infectious diseases.

Nevertheless, the herbal cupboard is not entirely bare. Most of the horrors referred to above were features of life in cities and towns, of crowded squalid conditions, far from sources of fresh food (and with no refrigerated delivery) and clean water. The historical and archaeological evidence available suggests that life was more equable in traditional rural communities, that, leaving perinatal mortality aside, average lifespans in the ancient world differed little from those reached until the middle of the 20th century[1,2,3] and that longevity was not uncommon where land was fertile.[4] In such circumstances, the case against the traditional remedies used by country people is harder to sustain.

Furthermore, if the killer diseases are taken out of the picture and more ordinary everyday infections are considered, the balance shifts in favour of historical treatment. There are a number of traditional remedies that appear to support the body in its battle against infections. From an exhaustive review of traditional cooking practices and recipes and correlation with exposure to infections, it has been concluded that the pungent spices were adopted as flavourings, consciously or unconsciously, at least in part because of their protective effect against enteric infections, with the hottest used where there is greatest exposure.[5] There are other indications that chillies in particular are antimicrobial in moderate doses.[6,7]

As another example of a dietary antimicrobial, various publications indicate that garlic extract also has broad-spectrum antimicrobial activity against many genera of bacteria and fungi. This activity, particularly in respect of Gram-negative bacteria, seems to be stronger than that of other members of the onion family.[8,9] Allicin was the early candidate as the most active constituent in garlic.[10] However, more recent research has demonstrated that ajoene, the prominent metabolite of allicin, conveys particular antimicrobial activity, including against such Gram-negative bacteria as *Escherichia coli* and *Klebsiella pneumoniae*. The disulphide bond in ajoene appeared to be necessary for this activity, since reduction by cysteine, which reacts with these bonds, abolished its antimicrobial activity.[11] This activity is, however, significantly exceeded by another metabolite, 10-devinylajoene, marked by substitution of the allyl group in ajoene by a methyl group and sulfinyl group.[12]

The incidence of stomach cancer is lower in individuals and populations with high allium vegetable intakes. To investigate this further, an aqueous extract of garlic cloves was standardized for its thiosulfinate concentration and tested for its antimicrobial activity on *Helicobacter pylori*. Minimum inhibitory concentration was 40 µg thiosulfinate per millilitre. This study may have detected a particular sensitivity of *H. pylori* to garlic constituents as *Staphylococcus aureus* tested under the same conditions was not susceptible to garlic extract up to the maximum thiosulfinate concentration tested (160 µg/ml).[13] Systemic antifungal activity has been supported in a study where commercial garlic extract was given intravenously to two patients with cryptococcal meningitis and three patients with other types of meningitis. Plasma titres of anti-*Cryptococcus neoformans* activity rose twofold over preinfusion titres.[14]

The position with other plant constituents is less clear. Essential oils have demonstrated antimicrobial effects in vitro (e.g.[15,16,17]). In one study, for example, the antimicrobial effects of some essential oils on oral bacteria were surveyed. Tea tree oil, peppermint oil and sage oil proved to be the most potent essential oils, whereas thymol and eugenol were potent essential oil components.[18] Tea tree oil has demonstrated a number of antimicrobial effects, even against methicillin-resistant *Staphylococcus aureus*,[19] and in a rare clinical study apparently against the bacteria of acne.[20] In other tea tree studies, the monoterpenes terpinen-4-ol, linalool and alpha-terpineol were found to be particularly active.[21] In research on antifungal effects, those of phenolics such as iso-eugenol, cinnamaldehyde, carvacrol, eugenol and thymol were linked to the presence of a free hydroxyl group linked to an alkyl substituent.[22] Camphor and camphene have been shown to be bacteriostatic and fungistatic constituents in another study.[23] However, all these studies generally refer to isolated oils rather than to the whole plant and it is difficult to infer from these that traditional treatments had much antimicrobial efficacy.

On the other hand, ethnobotanical reviews of traditional plants (often reported in the excellent *Journal of Ethnopharmacology*) have shown in vitro efficacy of whole-plant preparations (e.g.[24–27] and in one study a high correlation was demonstrated between traditional use and in vitro antisepsis among plants in North America.[28] It is possible that modest antimicrobial effects may lie in other plant constituents: tannins (especially tannic acid and propyl gallate) have demonstrated such properties. This activity is suggested as being associated with the hydrolysis of ester linkage between gallic acid and polyols hydrolysed after ripening of many edible fruits. Tannins in these fruits thus may serve as a natural defence mechanism against microbial infections.[29]

There were other particular remedies, generally at least a few in each tradition, whose role was directly to help the body resist infections. Raw garlic in Europe, Echinacea and Baptisia (wild indigo) in North America and *centella asiatica* (hydrocotle) and Picrorrhiza in Asia and Andrographis in China were all accorded great respect in their respective cultures. Some were mobilized in managing the fevers that often resulted (see p.137), others were used to support recovery and the hopefully increased defensive strength of the well-managed convalescence. There is little evidence that any of these are antibiotics in the modern sense: most were understood as supporting some defensive function or other. This list would also contain other supporters of host resistance.

- The powerful bitters – *Artemisia absinthaium* (wormwood), Columbo, Marsdenia (condurango), Cinchona (quinine bark), Swertia, *Berberis vulgaris* (barberry bark) and *Hydrastis canadensis* (golden seal bark) – that were likely to have been effective protectors against enteric and hepatic infections.
- The hot pungent spices – Capsicum spp (chillies), Zingiber (ginger) – that complement this role in enteric infections and, with Cinnamomum (cinnamon), that still today provide effective treatments in respiratory infections.
- Remedies like Juniperus (juniper berries), *Arctostaphylos uva-ursi* (bearberry), *Barosma betulina* (buchu), *Piper cubeba* (cubeb) in the treatment of urinary infections.

For the many non-serious infections in everyday life the deathbed recantation attributed to Pasteur is increasingly relevant. No seed can develop without *le terrain*, the soil to nourish it, no infections can establish without the body, by deficit, enabling a sympathetic environment for colonization to occur. There are very few genuinely aggressive pathogens; there are always some people, usually the majority, unaffected in even the most notorious epidemics. The normal environment, food, air, skin, mouth and gut lining, is full of theoretically pathogenic bacteria (legally allowable counts in many foods are still in the millions of bacteria per milligram). In the absence of supporting immune defences, it is likely that the drive to kill pathogens has gone too far. While antibiotics have changed the prospects for bacterial infections beyond traditional recognition, and antifungals, antiprotozoals and antiviral medicines have played important parts in the management of other infections, it is also clear that infectious diseases remain major clinical problems in even the most modern societies. In particular, there is concern about the increasing resistance of many pathogens to new drugs. Antibiotic resistance is causing particular worries, with the spectre of 'super-bugs' now occupying the attention of the popular press. In Britain the government instructed doctors in September 1998 to avoid prescribing antibiotics in minor self-limiting infectious conditions such as colds and sore throats or when infections are likely to be viral in origin.

The role for phytotherapy in infectious diseases is likely to increase rather than diminish.

PHYTOTHERAPEUTICS

General approach to infections

It is worthwhile reviewing the considerations for the herbal management of infections. These are as follows:

- Immune-enhancing herbs like *Echinacea angustifolia* or *E. purpurea* or Baptisia (wild indigo root) are an effective core element in the treatment of any infection, acute or chronic (see below for a treatment protocol for Echinacea).
- Warming circulatory stimulants will act to promote defensive immune activities in many cases of acute infections. Zingiber (ginger) is particularly helpful in these circumstances; Capsicum (cayenne) and Cinnamomum (cinnamon) are respectively stronger and milder substitutes or accompaniments.
- If the infection is located in a particular organ, herbs are prescribed to support that organ or its defensive functions: strong bitters in the case of enteric infections; Silybum (milk thistle) for liver infections; expectorants for lung infections; Juniperus for the urinary system; Sabal (saw palmetto) for prostate infections.
- Hypericum (St John's wort) may be applied in the long-term treatment of infections with enveloped viruses; Thuja (arbor-vitae) more widely for viral infections.
- For topical treatment of accessible surfaces a different range of products can be used. Melaleuca (tea tree oil) can be applied directly to some skin infections and, in suitable carriers, for vaginitis, in either case of both bacterial or fungal origin. Melissa (lemon balm) and Glycyrrhiza (licorice) have topical antiviral activity and can be applied to herpes and similar outbreaks. Thuja and Calendula tinctures are effective for fungal infections of the skin and nails. For the mouth and throat mouthwashes and gargles can be made with *Echinacea angustifolia* root, high-strength alcoholic tinctures of Commiphora (myrrh), Calendula, *Populus gileadensis* (balm of Gilead) or propolis, all best combined with fluid extract of Glycyrrhiza.

Poor immunity and recurrent infections

Patients with poor immunity and/or recurrent infections should receive treatment selected from the following groups:

- Immune-enhancing herbs: Echinacea, Astragalus, Picrorrhiza, Andrographis, Phytolacca. Astragalus should not be prescribed during acute episodes and Picrorrhiza and Andrographis should not be prescribed if the patient is constitutionally cold.
- Tonic and adaptogenic herbs: Panax, Eleutherococcus, Withania. Panax and Eleutherococcus should not be prescribed during an acute infection.
- Bitter herbs: Gentiana, *Artemisia absinthium* especially where the patient appears anaemic or undernourished. Exercise caution if the patient is also constitutionally cold or counter the cooling effect with heating herbs.

Echinacea protocol

Echinacea alone, either the root of *E. angustifolia* or *E. purpurea*, has helped countless patients with poor immunity in doses equivalent to 2.5–7.5 g per day (5–15 ml of a 1:2 preparation). The treatment protocol is as follows:

1. Take a 5 ml dose each day (2.5 g) as a maintenance dose (take twice this dose for maintenance if immunity is very poor).
2. If infection threatens, double or triple the daily maintenance dose until the threat passes.
3. If infection takes hold, maintain the higher dose until the infection is completely gone and then return to the normal daily dose.

References

1. Montagu JD. Length of life in the ancient world: a controlled study. Journal of the Royal Society of Medicine 1994; 87(1): 25–26
2. O'Rourke DA. Three score and ten. Medical Journal of Australia 1976; 131(11): 356
3. Jarcho S. The longevity of the ancient Greeks. Bulletin of the New York Academy of Medicine 1967; 43(10): 941–943
4. Kottek SS. Old age in Biblical and Talmudic lore. Israeli Journal of Medical Science 1996; 32(8): 702–703
5. Billing J, Sherman PW. Antimicrobial functions of spices: why some like it hot. Quarterly Review of Biology 1998; 73(1): 3–49
6. Cichewicz RH, Thorpe PA. The antimicrobial properties of chile peppers (Capsicum species) and their uses in Mayan medicine. Journal of Ethnopharmacology 1996; 52(2): 61–70
7. Caceres A, Alvarez AV, Ovando AE, Samayoa BE. Plants used in Guatemala for the treatment of respiratory diseases 1. Screening of 68 plants against gram-positive bacteria. Journal of Ethnopharmacology 1991; 31: 193–208
8. Elnima EI, Ahmed SA, Mekkawi AG, Mossa JS. The antimicrobial activity of garlic and onion extracts. Pharmazie 1983; 38(11): 747–748
9. Dankert J, Tromp TF, De Vries H, Klasen HJ Antimicrobial activity of crude juices of Allium ascalonicum, Allium cepa and Allium sativum. Zentralblatt für Bakteriologie [Orig A] 1979; 245(1–2): 229–239
10. Adetumbi MA, Lau BH. Allium sativum (garlic) – a natural antibiotic. Medical Hypotheses 1983; 12(3): 227–237
11. Naganawa R, Iwata N, Ishikawa K, Fukuda H, Fujino T, Suzuki A. Inhibition of microbial growth by ajoene, a sulfur-containing compound derived from garlic. Applied and Environmental Microbiology 1996; 62(11): 4238–4242
12. Yoshida H, Iwata N, Katsuzaki H et al. Antimicrobial activity of a compound isolated from an oil-macerated garlic extract. Bioscience, Biotechnology and Biochemistry 1998; 62(5): 1014–1017
13. Sivam GP, Lampe JW, Ulness B, Swanzy SR, Potter JD. Helicobacter pylori – in vitro susceptibility to garlic (Allium sativum) extract. Nutrition and Cancer 1997; 27(2): 118–121
14. Davis LE, Shen JK, Cai Y. Antifungal activity in human cerebrospinal fluid and plasma after intravenous administration of Allium sativum. Antimicrobial Agents and Chemotherapy 1990; 34(4): 651–653
15. Kartnig T, Still F, Reinthaler F. Antimicrobial activity of the essential oil of young pine shoots (Picea abies L.). Journal of Ethnopharmacology 1991; 35(2): 155–157
16. Kalodera Z, Pepeljnjak S, Blaevi N, Petrak T. Chemical composition and antimicrobial activity of Tanacetum parthenium essential oil. Pharmazie 1997; 52(11): 885–886
17. Briozzo J, Núñez L, Chirife J, Herszage L, D'Aquino M. Antimicrobial activity of clove oil dispersed in a concentrated sugar solution. Journal of Applied Bacteriology 1989; 66(1): 69–75
18. Shapiro S, Meier A, Guggenheim B. The antimicrobial activity of essential oils and essential oil components towards oral bacteria. Oral Microbiology and Immunology 1994; 9(4): 202–208
19. Carson CF, Cookson BD, Farrelly HD, Riley TV. Susceptibility of methicillin-resistant Staphylococcus aureus to the essential oil of Melaleuca alternifolia. Journal of Antimicrobial Chemotherapy 1995; 35(3): 421–424
20. Bassett IB, Pannowitz DL, Barnetson RS. A comparative study of tea-tree oil versus benzoylperoxide in the treatment of acne. Med J Aust 1990; 153(8): 455–458
21. Carson CF, Riley TV. Antimicrobial activity of the major components of the essential oil of Melaleuca alternifolia. Journal of Applied Bacteriology 1995; 78(3): 264–269
22. Pauli A, Knobloch K. Inhibitory effects of essential oil components on growth of food-contaminating fungi. Zeitschrift für Lebensmittel-Untersuchung and Forschung 1987; 185(1): 10–13
23. Tirillini B, Velasquez ER, Pellegrino R. Chemical composition and antimicrobial activity of essential oil of Piper angustifolium. Planta Medica 1996; 62(4): 372–373
24. Ritch-Krc EM, Turner NJ, Towers GH. Carrier herbal medicine: an evaluation of the antimicrobial and anticancer activity in some frequently used remedies. Journal of Ethnopharmacology 1996; 52(3): 151–156
25. Cáceres A, Girón LM, Alvarado SR, Torres MF. Screening of antimicrobial activity of plants popularly used in Guatemala for the treatment of dermatomucosal diseases. Journal of Ethnopharmacology 1987; 20(3): 223–237
26. Taylor RS, Manandhar NP, Towers GH. Screening of selected medicinal plants of Nepal for antimicrobial activities. Journal of Ethnopharmacology 1995; 46(3): 153–159
27. Desta B. Ethiopian traditional herbal drugs. Part II: Antimicrobial activity of 63 medicinal plants. Journal of Ethnopharmacology 1993; 39(2): 129–139
28. McCutcheon AR, Towers GHN. Ethnopharmacology of North American Plants. Lecture at the 2nd International Congress on Phytomedicine, Sept 11–14 1996, Institute of Pharmaceutical Biology, D-80333 Munich, Germany
29. Chung KT, Wong TY, Wei CI et al. Tannins and human health: a review. Critical Reviews in Food Science and Nutrition 1998; 38(6): 421–464

AUTOIMMUNE DISEASES

SCOPE

Apart from their use in providing non-specific support for recuperation and repair, specific phytotherapeutic strategies include the following.

Treatment of:

- acute inflammations of muscles, joints and connective tissues.

Management of:

- rheumatoid arthritis, ankylosing spondylitis and other chronic inflammatory joint diseases;
- psoriasis, scleroderma and other persisting skin diseases.

Because of the use of secondary plant products, particular **caution** is necessary in applying phytotherapy in cases of:

- inflammatory disease complicated by glomerulonephritis or other kidney disease.

ORIENTATION

Unresolved inflammations

Apart from trauma and wear and tear, the skeletal and connective tissues of the body are susceptible to few functional disorders. By far their most frequent problems involve disturbances of the inflammatory and immunological mechanisms. Inflammations of the skin (dermatitis, including eczema and psoriasis) and joints (arthritis) are among the most familiar chronic inflammatory diseases. Those of other connective tissues, chronic arteritis, cellulitis, chondritis, meningitis, osteitis, pericarditis, phlebitis, pleurisy and vasculitis, can be at least as puzzling. (Although involving different types of tissue, chronic inflammations of glandular tissue, epididymitis, oophoritis, pancreatitis, prostatitis and thyroiditis, as well as endodermal tissue, Crohn's disease, gastritis and ulcerative colitis, share many of the therapeutic challenges and features and may also be considered in this context.)

The modern approach to most of these inflammations is to apply antiinflammatory drugs, either steroids or the non-steroidal antiinflammatories (NSAIDs), or coal-tar products in the case of topical applications to the skin. Traditional herbal practice approached these conditions in radically different ways. The reputation of efficacy for almost universal approaches is sufficiently wide ranging across many cultures and traditions to justify a rational review. Nevertheless, perhaps because these indications demand particularly individual therapy, there is very little direct clinical evidence of efficacy under controlled clinical conditions. Happily, however, some of the traditional insights concur with the latest research findings about the aetiology of inflammatory diseases and it is thus possible to substantiate clinical experience that the use of herbal approaches can be beneficial.

It is, however, obvious that chronic inflammatory diseases are among the most demanding indications. It is likely that only individual treatments have been truly effective in the past and apart from the undoubted power of the placebo effect, these are not very amenable to simple recipes or over-the-counter treatments (fish oils in arthritic disease are perhaps the main exception). Thus when steroidal drugs based on cortisone became widely available in the early 1950s, the transformation these made to the prognosis for arthritic, skin and other connective tissue diseases was dramatic. For two decades, any challenge to these drugs would have been derided. However, it then became apparent that both steroids and their non-steroidal counterparts based on aspirin were associated with a range of side effects that now lead physicians to limit their prescription much more than in the past. There is again a demand for other approaches, especially in the case of those sufferers otherwise condemned to a lifetime of powerful and potentially dangerous drugs.

Nevertheless, the success of the modern drugs in controlling inflammatory diseases has tended to lock medical research and thought into antiinflammatory tramlines. Thus, although new insights into the cause of these diseases are emerging, these have not yet led to new treatments, much less therapeutic approaches or popular advice. The new ideas do, however, have major implications for the herbal treatment of such conditions.

The traditional understanding of inflammatory diseases notably involved ideas of 'toxicity' and, particularly but not exclusively, in Chinese herbal therapeutics, metereological concepts of 'damp', 'wind', 'heat' and 'cold' (see also pp.147). These apparently quaint medieval notions are metaphors for clinical insights into the way the body appears to behave in such illnesses that can indeed inform a modern review. It is this that will now be attempted.

Modern research into the causes of inflammatory diseases has uncovered in particular disturbed reactions to infections and significant events in the digestive tract.

Infectious agents

At the turn of the 20th century the rheumatoid-like condition ankylosing spondylitis was regarded as a venereal disease, though 20 years later the wider association with urinary infection had been made. This, however, was lost by the time steroids transformed the prospects for the condition.

An interesting later brush with ancient notions by modern medical research was seen in an issue of *The British Medical Journal*.[1] It was reported that patients with rheumatoid arthritis had a significantly higher incidence or history of pulmonary disease than the wider population. It was pointed out that the lungs remain subclinically infected, almost indefinitely in many cases, after the incidence of pneumonia, bronchitis and pleurisy and this persistence is obvious in conditions like emphysema and bronchiectasis. The findings were dramatic and led a linked editorial to speculate, probably reluctantly, that 'toxins' in the infected lung base might provoke the inflammatory changes in the rheumatoid joints.

Modern rheumatology has now taken such notions into orthodoxy, although gratefully abandoning any primitive imagery. Rather than 'toxic' influences, the role of 'immunological crossreactivity' has emerged as a leading factor in the aetiology of rheumatic diseases. In this view, the autoimmune nature of these diseases is reinforced; it had long been understood that the body's own immune defences were the main cause of many connective tissue inflammations (the term 'collagen diseases' was used to embrace a wide range of such conditions). In immunological crossreactivity, the immune system is provoked and then confused by the similarity between bacterial, viral or other antigens and those of its own tissues and attacks both.

Infectious agents are now regarded as the major environmental factors that may cause arthritic inflammation in genetically susceptible hosts. Retroviruses, urinary and pulmonary and especially enteric bacteria are the provocateurs most often discussed.[2–5]

'Molecular mimicry' has been found between a white blood cell protein, HLA-B27, and two molecules, nitrogenase and pullulinase D, in the anaerobic gut bacterium *Klebsiella pneumoniae* among ankylosing spondylitis patients[6] and between HLA-DR1/DR4 and the haemolysin molecule in another gut anaerobe, *Proteus mirabilis*, among rheumatoid arthritis patients.[7] Both bacteria can be found as secondary infections elsewhere in the body and prospects for future control of rheumatoid diseases by antibiotic therapy have been raised.[8]

Intestinal wall damage

There is increasing evidence of damage to the gut wall in a range of rheumatoid diseases. One category of diseases, classified as spondylarthropathies, involve inflammatory damage of the joints and the skeleton, the eyes, gut, urogenital tract, skin and sometimes the heart.[9,10] In a series of investigations, histological signs of gut inflammation were found in a high proportion of patients with spondylarthropathies. Most of these patients did not present any clinical intestinal manifestations. Remission of the joint inflammation was always connected with a disappearance of the gastrointestinal inflammation. Persistence of locomotor inflammation was mostly associated with the persistence of gastrointestinal inflammation. It was proposed that some patients with a spondylarthropathy had a form of subclinical Crohn's disease in which the locomotor inflammation was the only clinical expression.[11]

This hypothesis was supported in prospective long-term studies in which the ileocolonoscopied patients were reviewed over periods of up to 9 years. About 6% of spondylarthropathy patients who did not present any sign of Crohn's disease at first investigation (but did show gut inflammation on biopsy) developed full-blown Crohn's disease within 9 years. Electron microscopy of these lesions demonstrated an increase in the number of membranous (M) cells in inflamed mucosa. Necrosis and rupture of these M-cells, with lymphocytes entering the gut lumen, was observed. Such evidence of damage to the gut mucosa could be responsible for an increase in local antigenic stimulation and could readily lead to secondary systemic immunological disorders.[12]

Hormonal factors

Hormonal factors in rheumatoid disease are well accepted. Risk factors include reduced childbearing and breastfeeding; these apparently contradictory influences are both associated with high prolactin levels.[13]

On the other hand, preeclampsia and breast cancer have a negative association with rheumatic and other autoimmune diseases.[14]

Such links are confusing and even contradictory but a defective response of the neuroendocrine system to inflammatory stimuli has been proposed as a feature of rheumatoid arthritis.[15]

TRADITIONAL APPROACHES TO INFLAMMATORY DISEASES

Antiinflammatory remedies

The use of willow bark for rheumatism in traditional medicine is a reminder that where remedies clearly provided symptomatic relief, they were used. More recently, there has been a huge research effort to find new antiinflammatory activities in the plant world. Many chemical subgroups from plants have shown promising experimental activity, including terpenoids and steroids, phenolics and flavonoids, fatty acids, polysaccharides and alkaloids.[16] Platelet-activating factor (PAF) antagonism has been demonstrated by tetrahydrofuran ring structure from plants used traditionally in inflammatory diseases: prehispanolone, from *Leonurus heterophyllus*,[17] kadsurenone from the bulb of *Piper futokadsura*[18] and several compounds from *Biota orientalis*.[19] The effect of the Chinese herbal formulation found effective in the treatment of atopic eczema has been shown to be associated with changes in a number of immunological functions, such as decreasing the higher levels of circulating IgE complexes and interleukin-2 receptors and vascular cell adhesion molecules in atopic eczema patients.[20] The immunological effects of *Tripterygium wilfordii*, for example in the traditional treatment of rheumatoid arthritis, were found to be associated with an in vitro suppression of antigen-stimulated T-cell production, immunoglobulin production by B-cells[21] and reduction of interleukin-2 production and activity.[22]

Counterirritation

The most common application of counterirritation was to inflamed arthritic joints and the technique is discussed further in the appropriate chapter (see p.248). Nevertheless, the approach was also used for other subdermal inflammations, notably in pleurisy and other chest infections, mastitis and other cellulitis conditions. (A traditional treatment of mastitis and pleurisy involved making poultices with cabbage leaves, a close relative of mustard.) Heating inflammations was not always considered appropriate however. As discussed below, some inflammatory diseases are excessively 'hot' and can react violently to additional help. Some rheumatic joints can behave in this way.

Diet

One of the persistent dietary notions in European tradition in the case of degenerative diseases, particularly arthritis, has been the distinction between 'acid' and 'alkaline' foods. The view is that as metabolites tend to be acidic, as acid-buffering agents are a major constituent of the body fluids and as eliminatory channels (lungs, kidney, bile and bowel) pass mainly acidic materials, inflammatory diseases may be marked by, and even result from, greater acidosis. Overt metabolic acidosis is well characterized in medicine and may follow excessive alcohol consumption, laxative abuse, excessive vitamin D and NSAIDs (most often prescribed in arthritis) and salicylate use, among other drugs.[23] The case for a more subtle effect is considered further in the section on joint disease (see p.248). In addition to the prospects for therapy that could, for example, include diuretic herbal remedies, there are associated dietary observations which reinforce the potential for benefit in some chronic inflammatory diseases. There was, for example, a widespread traditional instinct in many inflammatory diseases to reduce animal protein, although chicken and other fowl were a common exception.

There is modern support for this approach in rheumatic diseases. A combination of fasting and vegetarian diets has been shown to reduce the ability of the urine to support the growth of *Proteus mirabilis* and *Escherichia coli*.[24] A substantial placebo-controlled trial has confirmed that gamma-linolenic acid (GLA), a component mainly of plant-based foods, has antirheumatic activity.[25] The possibility of crossreaction between dietary collagen found in animal products and the sufferer's connective tissue has also been postulated.[26,27] The effects of a low-starch diet in reducing the gut levels of anaerobic bacteria such as *Klebsiella* and serum IgA antibody levels in both normal subjects and those suffering ankylosing spondylitis, and in benefiting symptoms in the latter, have been supported by clinical evidence.[28]

PHYTOTHERAPEUTICS

The treatment of chronic inflammatory diseases is complex. Traditional strategies rely on the assessment of prevailing conditions within the body and generally incorporate the idea of change and adaptability in ongoing prescription.

In most traditions inflammatory diseases of the joints, skin and other body tissues were viewed as compounded and deep-seated toxic conditions. It might have been explained that whereas fevers, acute inflammations and infections were examples of noxious intrusions to which the body mounted a frank and usually successful defence (what modern medicine refers to as the 'self-limiting' condition), chronic problems indicated that the body had not 'repelled boarders' at first attack, had primary defences breached (like the digestive tract, skin and lymphatics: the 'reticuloendothelial' phagocytic wing of the immune response) and had allowed toxic pathogenic influences to penetrate and disturb deeper functions. Treatment often therefore involved characterizing the toxicity and constructing the best strategy to help the body better eliminate it. There were many strategies and in the best practice these were tailored to individual circumstances but certain remedies were more popular for joint and skin diseases than others. These are listed below.

In certain traditions diagnosis might include assessing the extent of the following characteristics of the disease process, in most cases more than one of which being likely to occur. These are based very much on insights from traditional Chinese medicine and particular Chinese remedies can be readily allocated to each category or blend of categories. Western herbal medicine is much less systematized and no such classification of treatments can reliably be made. However, it is most likely that in practice intuitive assessments would resemble what follows.

Damp (the presence of tissue congestion or chronic infection)

Damp was the universal metaphor for toxic congestion, recalling the notions of stagnation, brackishness and mould. As expected, it tended to occur in conditions of poor circulation, most often associated with cold but with a hot 'humid' variant as well. Damp is exacerbated and to some extent caused by external climatic dampness (as the Romans noted, a feature of Britain and the Britons). Associated with cold, it tends to gravitate to the lower regions of the body and can be associated with sluggish digestion and congested abdomen. Associated with heat, it involves the liver, with intolerance to fats, rich food and alcohol and perhaps a history of jaundice/hepatitis. Naturally it would need treatment with 'drying' remedies: warming aromatics for cold-damp, and bitters for hot-damp conditions.

Wind (the degree of fluctuation)

The tendency of rheumatic and some skin problems to fluctuate and move rapidly around the body was obvious. Chinese medicine in particular invoked the universal metaphor of change, wind, to characterize this phenomenon. Wind of course occurs with the juxtaposition of hot and cold and implied that there was similar imbalance within the body. Apart from the fluctuation of symptoms, signs of wind might include, when deep seated (a common occurrence in rheumatic disease) wandering, sudden pains in joints. In Chinese medicine there were a number of remedies specifically reputed to calm the wind but the deeper view might be that attendance to the underlying imbalances of hot and cold would be the more lasting strategy.

Heat (the violence of the inflammatory reaction and extent of immunological hypersensitivities)

As the obvious vital sign, heat was seen as a mark of vigorous defence (as in fever and inflammation) and in its place was even encouraged. When stuck, however, or marked by destructive symptoms like allergic reactions or eczema, it signified blocked poisons which needed clearing, perhaps with local cooling as well. When coupled with dryness, there would be respiratory symptoms like asthma, allergic rhinitis or hayfever, dry eczema and/or constipation; when coupled with damp, the liver and digestion would be involved as above. It might also be localized to an organ like the lungs or kidneys or to some other part of the body. Heat was often diagnosed on the basis of simple palpation or by the presence of flushing, a preference for cool drinks, cool weather or cold applications. The tongue might be more red in colour, with less sal-iva (if associated with dryness) or with a coloured coating (if associated with damp). A range of cooling remedies were used to help clear such hot spots and help with a wider strategy to improve circulation.

Cold (the degree of circulatory, immune and other debility)

Cold is the symptom of diminished vitality and death and marks a condition where the metabolic furnace has faltered, either generally or locally. The patient would prefer heat, in food and drink or as hot applications, abhor cold and might be listless, pale and withdrawn. The tongue might be pale and wet and (if associated with damp) the coating would be white. As long as debility was not too extreme, heating remedies like the spices were indicated either systemically or as hot topical applications.

The modern concepts of immunological diseases as disturbed responses to infection or disrupted gut barriers entirely accord with the intuitive and systematized traditional focus on toxicities. In the particular remedies below, their relevant properties are also listed. Not all plants are ascribed temperaments like warming or drying: some, like diuretics and astringents, were considered to have neutral temperaments; in other cases some Western herbs have no consistent tradition that would allow these qualities to be safely ascribed.

Plants with antiinfective properties

- *Allium sativum* (garlic): heating, disinfectant, especially in lungs and gut.

- *Berberis vulgaris* (barberry): cooling and drying.
- *Echinacea spp* (echinacea): warming and promoting defences, particularly of throat and upper gut wall.
- *Hypericum perforatum* (St John's wort): restorative tonic with potential antiviral support.
- *Lavandula spp* (lavender): topically warming and antiseptic.
- *Thuja occidentalis* (arbor-vitae): warming and stimulating.

Plants with eliminative properties

- *Apium graveolens* (celery): diuretic and eliminating acidic metabolites through the kidneys, particularly used in arthritic disease.
- *Arctium lappa* (burdock): general eliminative particularly popular in skin disease.
- *Arctostaphylos uva-ursi* (bearberry): diuretic and urinary antiseptic, most likely to be applied in arthritic disease (often to be recommended in ankylosing spondylitis).
- *Betula spp* (birch): diuretic, particularly used in arthritic disease.
- *Berberis aquifolium* (Oregon grape): cooling and drying, cholagogue and popular in treating skin disease.
- *Fumaria officinalis* (common fumitory): cholagogue, popular in treating skin diseae.[29]
- *Galium aparine* (cleavers): diuretic and lymphatic and used particularly in skin disease.
- *Gaultheria procumbens* (wintergreen): topically warming and used over inflammations.
- *Inula helenium* (elecampane): warming and aiding elimination (expectoration) from the lungs.
- *Juglans nigra* (walnut bark): general alterative and laxative remedy.
- *Rumex crispus* (yellow dock): cooling and drying with mild aperient properties for helping bile and bowel elimination.
- *Scophularia nodosa* (figwort): warming and generally eliminative, traditionally for aggressive skin disease.
- *Solidago spp* (goldenrod): traditional diuretic, used for skin conditions, with some anti-inflammatory properties.[30]
- *Taraxacum officinale* (dandelion root): cooling and drying with cholagogue and diuretic properties, popularly combined with Apium for arthritic disease and as a remedy in skin disease.
- *Trifolium pratense* (red clover): lymphatic and expectorant, used in skin and joint disease.
- *Urtica dioica* (nettle leaf): warming and nutritive taken internally, popular in skin disease.

Plants with digestive antiinflammatory properties

A large number of remedies are effective for intestinal wall problems (see p.145). The following are immediately obvious options in arthritic, skin and other chronic inflammatory diseases.

- *Aloe vera* (aloe juice): reducing digestive wall inflammation.
- *Calendula officinalis* (marigold): lymphatic and reducing inflammation in the throat and stomach.
- *Dioscorea villosa* (wild yam): antispasmodic and antiinflammatory on lower gut wall, possibly steroidal effect systemically.
- *Filipendula ulmaria* (meadowsweet): demulcent and astringent effect on stomach wall overwhelming low levels of salicylates.
- *Hamamelis virginiana* (witchhazel): astringent throughout the digestive tract.
- *Matricaria recutita* and *Chamaemelum nobile* (wild and Roman chamomiles[31]): cooling and reducing inflammatory damage in the upper digestive tract.
- *Myrica cerifera* (bayberry): warming and astringent, traditionally used in fever management associated with diarrhoea and dysentery.
- *Symphytum officinale* (comfrey leaf): potent healing effects on gut wall, to be used only in the short term.
- *Ulmus rubra* (slippery elm): mucilaginous and healing on the upper digestive tract, best used as an early stage of, and preparatory to, wider treatment.

Plants with hormonal properties

Many herbs are rich in stigmasterol and other potentially antiinflammatory phytosterols. Some also have reputations for hormone balancing and all those below also have a traditional reputation in the treatment of inflammatory diseases.

- *Caulophyllum thalictroides* (blue cohosh)
- *Cimicifuga racemosa* (black cohosh)
- *Pfaffia paniculata* (Brasilian ginseng)
- *Smilax spp* (sarsaparilla)

Plants with general antiinflammatory properties

The traditional herbal approach includes antiinflammatories in the modern medical sense. These remedies are, however, less powerful than modern drugs and are most useful as adjuncts to the therapeutic measures listed above.

- *Fraxinus excelsior* (ash): moderate antiinflammatory containing coumarins that inhibit T-cells and prostaglandin biosynthesis.[32]
- *Harpagophytum procumbens* (devil's claw): mild anti inflammatory effects (see monograph).
- *Guaiacum spp* (lignum vitae): traditional reputation in arthritic diseases.
- *Menyanthes trifoliata* (bogbean): a bitter and hepatic remedy applied to rheumatic conditions where such effects are useful.
- *Populus spp* (poplar bark): containing salicylates with established antiinflammatory properties.[32]
- *Salix spp* (willow bark): the original source of salicylates and with a strong traditional reputation as an antirheumatic.
- *Tanacetum parthenium* (feverfew): potential antiinflammatory properties (see monograph)

Contraindications for antiinflammatory remedies

The use of antiinflammatory remedies is inappropriate when there is already prescription of strong antiinflammatory medication.

Traditional therapeutic insights into the use of treatments for inflammatory diseases

Faced with a highly complex condition like a chronic inflammatory disease, the traditional practitioner might of course proceed entirely intuitively to clear the obstacles, using remedies such as the above in their own favoured ways. However, where strategies are systematized, notably in the Chinese tradition, a consistent pattern emerges. There is an almost geological approach. Pathogenic influences are envisaged as penetrating to different strata of the body, becoming more disturbed, disruptive and persistent the deeper they go. In chronic inflammations, by definition, the pathologies are deeply rooted and very mixed up. Looking for a way to disentangle the complexity, the traditional approach was often compared with peeling the layers of an onion, starting from the outside. Any opportunity to use effective 'superficial' eliminative measures would be taken up.

- A cold or fever, provided it could be managed within the patient's often diminished reserves, could lead to an effective clearing of burdens by mobilizing the phagocytic defences. The occurrence of any such event would lead the practitioner to switch treatment rapidly and deal with the acute indications intensively until resolved (see also p. 137).
- Primary eliminatory routes would be an early therapeutic focus; diuretics, aperients and cholagogues are especially likely to be used, as indicated in the individual's story. These might be step-like interventions, each pursued briefly for particular medium-term goals.
- The gut wall was always a priority zone. Dietary approaches would usually be combined with treatments to enhance the digestive process, like bitters or warming aromatic digestives as required, or remedies with antiinflammatory or healing effects on the wall itself. For example, one strategy might be to start or rotate a course of treatment with a demulcent remedy like slippery elm or comfrey.

Chronic inflammatory diseases are often, almost by definition, accompanied by compromised defences and reduced vigour and there may be hotspots of relatively violent inflammations, for example rheumatic joints or skin eruptions. It is thus possible that treatments may be unduly provocative and exacerbations may occur. Contrary to some popular opinion ('Things must get worse before they get better'), these 'healing crises' are rarely a good idea; indeed, they may worsen the condition in the long term. (Therapeutic exacerbations may be justified under carefully controlled conditions to expedite a blocked inflammation or fever but only when the patient is in a sufficiently robust state and the inflammation concerned is relatively simple.) Thus a good practitioner will peel the onion layers with care, only proceeding at a pace the body can stand, avoiding unnecessary exacerbation (for example with remedies that are too heating or cooling or with too strong an eliminative effect) and using remedies that calm and soothe. The practitioner will often take especial care to apply strategies that aid recuperation and restoration of a robust and balanced immune system. This may mean, for example, adopting convalescent dietary principles (see p. 85) and combining these with appropriate digestive or hepatic remedies.

Application

Antiinflammatory remedies are best taken before, or if there is any stomach irritation, after meals.

Long-term therapy with antiinflammatory remedies is usually acceptable although this should be kept under review.

Although the conditions involved are sometimes very complex there should still be early endpoints to aim for. The obvious is relief of the symptoms but there may be stages along the way as well.

References

1. Anonymous. Respiratory complications of rheumatoid disease [editorial]. British Medical Journal 1978; 6125; 1437–1438
2. Krause A, Kamradt T, Burmester GR. Potential infectious agents in the induction of arthritides. Current Opinion in Rheumatology 1996; 8(3): 203–209
3. Aoki S, Yoshikawa K, Yokoyama T et al. Role of enteric bacteria in the pathogenesis of rheumatoid arthritis: evidence for antibodies to enterobacterial common antigens in rheumatoid sera and synovial fluids. Annals of Rheumatic Diseases 1996; 55(6): 363–369
4. Eerola E, Mottonen T, Hannonen P et al. Intestinal flora in early rheumatoid arthritis. British Journal of Rheumatology 1994; 33(11): 1030–1038
5. Melief MJ, Hoijer MA, Van Paassen HC, Hazenberg MP. Presence of bacterial flora-derived antigen in synovial tissue macrophages and dendritic cells. British Journal of Rheumatology 1995; 34(12): 1112–1116
6. Ebringer A, Ahmadi K, Fielder M et al. Molecular mimicry: the geographical distribution of immune responses to Klebsiella in ankylosing spondylitis and its relevance to therapy. Clinical Rheumatology 1996; 15(supp 1): 57–61
7. Tiwana H, Wilson C, Cunningham P et al. Antibodies to four gram-negative bacteria in rheumatoid arthritis which share sequences with the rheumatoid arthritis susceptibility motif. British Journal of Rheumatology 1996; 35(6): 592–594
8. Albani S, Carson DA. A multistep molecular mimicry hypothesis for the pathogenesis of rheumatoid arthritis. Immunology Today 1996; 17(10): 466–470
9. Mielants H, Veys EM. Significance of intestinal inflammation in the pathogenesis of spondylarthropathies. Verhandelingen–Koninkhijke Academie voor Geneeskunde van Belgie 1996; 58(2): 93–116
10. Mielants H, Veys EM, De Vos M et al. The evolution of spondyloarthropathies in relation to gut histology. I. Clinical aspects. Journal of Rheumatology 1995; 22(12): 2266–2272
11. Altomonte L, Zoli A, Veneziani A et al. Clinically silent inflammatory gut lesions in undifferentiated spondyloarthropathies. Clinical Rheumatology 1994; 13(4): 565–570
12. Nissila M, Lahesmaa R, Leirisalo-Repo M et al. Antibodies to Klebsiella pneumoniae, Escherichia coli, and Proteus mirabilis in ankylosing spondylitis: effect of sulfasalazine treatment. Journal of Rheumatology 1994; 21(11): 2082–2087
13. Brennan P, Ollier B, Worthington J et al. Are both genetic and reproductive associations with rheumatoid arthritis linked to prolactin? Lancet 1996; 348(9020): 106–109
14. Polednak AP. Pre-eclampsia, autoimmune disease and breast cancer etiology. Medical Hypotheses 1995; 44(5): 414–418
15. Panayi GS. Hormonal control of rheumatoid inflammation. British Medical Bulletin 1995; 51(2): 462–471
16. Bingol F, Sener B. A review of terrestrial plants and marine organisms having antiinflammatory activity. International Journal of Pharmacognosy 1995; 33(2): 81–97
17. Lee CM, Jiang LM, Shang HS et al. Prehispanolone, a novel platelet activating factor receptor antagonist from Leonurus heterophyllus. British Journal of Pharmacology 1991; 103(3): 1719–1724
18. Shen TY, Hwang SB, Chang MN et al. The isolation and characterization of kadsurenone from haifenteng (Piper futokadsura) as an orally active specific receptor antagonist of platelet-activating factor. International Journal of Tissue Reactions 1985; 7(5): 339–343
19. Yang HO, Suh DY, Han BH. Isolation and characterization of platelet-activating factor receptor binding antagonists from Biota orientalis. Planta Medica 1995; 61(1): 37–40
20. Latchman Y, Banerjee P, Poulter LW et al. Association of immunological changes with clinical efficacy in atopic eczema patients treated with traditional Chinese herbal therapy (Zemaphyte). International Archives of Allergy and Immunology 1996; 109(3): 243–249
21. Tao X, Davis LS, Lipsky PE. Effect of an extract of the Chinese herbal remedy Tripterygium wilfordii Hook F on human immune responsiveness. Arthritis and Rheumatism 1991; 34(10): 1274–1281
22. Li XW, Weir MR. Radix Tripterygium wilfordii – a Chinese herbal medicine with potent immunosuppressive properties. Transplantation 1990; 50(1): 82–86
23. Fukuhara Y, Kaneko T, Orita Y. Drug-induced acid-base disorders. Nippon Rinsho 1992; 50(9): 2231–2236
24. Kjeldsen-Kragh J, Kvaavik E, Bottolfs M, Lingaas E. Inhibition of growth of Proteus mirabilis and Escherichia coli in urine in response to fasting and vegetarian diet. APMIS 1995; 103(11): 818–822
25. Zurier RB, Rosetti EW, Jacobsen DM et al. Gamma-linolenic acid treatment of rheumatoid arthritis: a randomised placebo-controlled trial. Arthritis and Rheumatism 1996; 39(11): 1808–1817
26. Terato K, DeArmey DA, Ye XJ et al. The mechanism of autoantibody formation to cartilage in rheumatoid arthritis: possible cross-reaction of antibodies to dietary collagens with autologous type II collagen. Clinical Immunology and Immunopathology 1996; 79(2): 142–154
27. Mitchison A, Sieper J. Immunological basis of oral tolerance. Zeitschrift für Rheumatologie 54(3): 141–144
28. Ebringer A, Wilson C. The use of a low starch diet in the treatment of patients suffering from ankylosing spondylitis. Clinical Rheumatology 1996; 15(supp 1): 62–66
29. Hentschel C, Dressler S, Hahn EG. Fumaria officinalis (fumitory) – clinical applications. Fortschritte der Medizin 1995; 113(19): 291–292
30. Leuschner J. Anti-inflammatory, spasmolytic and diuretic effects of a commercially available Solidago gigantea herb extract. Arzneimittel-Forschung 1995; 45(2): 165–168
31. Rossi T, Melegari M, Bianchi A et al. Sedative, anti-inflammatory and anti-diuretic effects induced in rats by essential oils of varieties of Anthemis nobilis: a comparative study. Pharmacology Research Communications 1988; 20(supp 5): 71–74
32. Von Kruedener S, Schneider W, Elstner EF. A combination of Populus tremula, Solidago virgaurea and Fraxinus excelsior as an anti-inflammatory and antirheumatic drug. A short review. Arzneimittel-Forschung 1995; 45(2): 169–171

DEBILITY

SCOPE

Apart from their use to provide non-specific support for recuperation and repair, specific phytotherapeutic strategies include the following.

Treatment of:

- chronic fatigue syndrome;
- fatigue and debility after illness, injury or trauma (convalescence).

Management of:

- fatigue linked to clinical depression;
- fatigue due to untreatable or terminal illness.

Because of the use of secondary plant products, **caution** is necessary in applying phytotherapy in cases of:

- severe digestive depletion;
- renal or hepatic failure.

ORIENTATION

A debilitating symptom

Phytotherapists increasingly find that a major indication for treatment is a degenerative or debilitating illness. Unlike their forebears, for whom acute diseases were the norm and recuperative support of debility was usually convalescent aftercare, the modern practitioner will be less often involved in first-line treatment. Patients will more often report for help after years of ill health or when conventional medicine has run out of options.

There are many diseases that can lead to such signs of debility as tiredness, inability to rest, weakness, depression, wasting and anorexia. Indeed, any illness of sufficient duration or severity can lead to such symptoms; chronic low-grade infections, especially viral infections, are particular precursors in modern times. In some cases severe or traumatic diseases from the distant past can lead to a legacy of weaknesses of this type. A few are constitutionally enfeebled and are prone to debilitating responses to a range of stressors. A good practitioner will obviously seek to address current problems as far as possible. However, one of the prominent elements of a debilitating condition is that the weakness imposes its own limitations on any treatment. It is often impractical to embark upon the usual treatment strategy while the patient is at a low ebb as even the gentlest remedies can provoke uncomfortable responses.

Finding a regime of treatment that simply addresses the debility, with little consideration of the causes or background factors, might be the only strategy feasible if the condition is especially severe. The principles involved in such approaches can best be reviewed for a classic modern syndrome of debility – chronic fatigue syndrome.

Chronic fatigue syndrome

Although the name might be new, chronic fatigue syndrome (CFS) is not a new disorder. While the affliction described as 'neurasthenia' in Victorian times does not necessarily represent an early forerunner, the 'bed cases' or 'sofa cases' reported among middle-class women in the period from 1860 to 1910 probably were CFS and by the time of World War I, a syndrome resembling CFS was a common complaint in Europe and North America.[1] CFS is also known as postviral fatigue syndrome or myalgic encephalomyelitis (ME). Although the orthodox medical profession was reluctant at first to recognize CFS as a physical disorder rather than a variant of depression or neurosis, this opinion is changing. Nonetheless, treatment of CFS as a psychiatric problem is still relatively widespread.

CFS was formally defined in 1988 as disabling fatigue of at least 6 months' duration of uncertain aetiology. Additional symptoms can include mild fever, sore throat, painful lymph nodes, weight gain, exertional malaise, muscle weakness, muscle and joint pain, headaches, depression, light-headedness, anxiety, visual and cognitive impairment and disturbed sleep patterns. It usually has a relatively definite onset which resembles influenza. Six of these additional symptoms must be present, plus two or more of the following signs: low-grade fever, non-exudative pharyngitis and palpable or tender lymph nodes.[2]

Currently there is no accepted biochemical test for the condition. Another problem is that the definition is somewhat restrictive. Many patients with chronic, unexplained fatigue and typical symptoms of CFS may not exactly fulfil the above definition.

Possible causes of chronic fatigue syndrome

Viruses

The fact that CFS can occur in epidemics has always pointed to an infectious origin. However, despite the fact that various researchers have implicated a number of viruses, a clear association with a single viral infection has not been established. Originally, Epstein–Barr virus was thought to be the cause, since CFS can follow glandular fever. However, clear links with viral agents remain elusive. Either a number of viruses are capable of triggering CFS, in which case CFS is not an infection in the strict meaning of the term, or CFS may involve the reactivation of the immune response to previous viral infections.

Immunologic abnormalities

The immune abnormalities which occur in CFS are also inconsistent, perhaps because different viral triggers may cause different malfunctions. One important study found no difference between CFS patients and controls for any white blood cell counts, save the CD8 T-lymphocytes.[3] These cells were activated as in a viral infection and the cytotoxic cell subset was increased. These differences were significant (p=0.01) in patients with major symptoms of CFS. The study was noteworthy because of the large number of patients involved and also because the degree of these changes corresponded to the severity of the CFS. The authors concluded that immune activation in CFS leads to increased secretion of cytokines which causes the observed symptoms. Their findings were consistent with chronic stimulation of the immune system, perhaps by a virus. If this is correct, the feeling of malaise experienced in the early stages of influenza, when cytokine output is increased, is similar to the way CFS sufferers feel most of the time. Cancer patients treated with the cytokine interleukin-2 to boost immunity experience side effects remarkably similar to CFS. Serum levels of some cytokines are often raised in CFS. For example, levels of interleukin-1-alpha,[4] tumour necrosis factor (TNF)-alpha and TNF-beta[5] were significantly more often increased in CFS patients.

An increased occurrence of autoantibodies such as rheumatoid factor, thyroid antibodies and antinuclear antibodies (ANA) has been found in CFS patients.[6,7] This, together with an observed high incidence of circulating immune complexes, led a German research team to conclude that CFS is associated with or is the beginning of manifest autoimmune disease.[6] These findings were supported by a large study on 579 patients from Boston and Seattle which found that levels of immune complexes were abnormal in 35% of CFS patients compared to 2% of controls (p=0.0001) and ANA was abnormally high in 15% of CFS patients compared to 0% of controls (p=0.003).[8] The same study found that serum cholesterol and IgG levels were also significantly raised in CFS.

Circulatory abnormalities

A study of 24 CFS patients who were 50 years or younger found that 100% had slightly abnormal ECG readings, compared to only 22.4% of controls (p<0.01).[9] Other research has found that subjects complaining of chronic fatigue were more likely to have abnormally shaped (non-discocytic) red blood cells. The authors concluded that this association with impaired muscle function could indicate a cause-and-effect relationship, which would be in agreement with the physiological concept of fatigue as resulting from inadequate oxygen delivery.[10] The authors suggested the use of evening primrose oil and fish oil to decrease non-discocytes.

Regional cerebral blood flows to the cortex and basal ganglia were significantly reduced in a majority of CFS patients.[11] This finding is supported by a recent study in older patients which found that the abnormal blood flow in CFS was different from that observed in depression.[12] Given the favourable influence of *Ginkgo biloba* on both on red blood cell fragility and blood rheology, it might be indicated for such disturbances.

Brain abnormalities

Magnetic resonance imaging (MRI) scans of the brains of CFS sufferers found a high incidence of inflammation (oedema and demyelination) in association with serological evidence of active human herpes virus-6 infection.[13] This controversial finding of brain abnormalities in CFS has been somewhat supported by a study which observed that CFS patients had significantly more abnormal scans than controls: 27% vs 2%.[14] However, the authors felt that this might instead indicate that some patients labelled with CFS could actually be suffering from other medical conditions. Abnormal MRI and single-photon emission computed topography (SPECT) scans were found with far greater frequency in CFS patients compared to normal controls.[15]

Pituitary and hypothalamic abnormalities

Patients with CFS have a mild central adrenal insufficiency secondary to either a deficiency of corticotropin-releasing hormone (CRH) or some other central stimulus to the pituitary-adrenal axis.[16] This leads to a decreased response of the adrenal cortex. Abnormalities in the regulation of the hypothalamic-pituitary-adrenal (HPA) axis are also a well-recognized feature of endogenous depression. It has been suggested that, since cytokines potently influence the HPA axis, their activation may underlie many of the features found in CFS and depression.[17]

Biochemical abnormalities

It has been hypothesized that the imbalances in immune function, the HPA axis and the sympathetic nervous system in CFS can be explained by changes in essential fatty acid (EFA) metabolism. Dietary EFA modulation afforded substantial improvement in a majority of cases.[18] A Japanese study did find that serum concentrations of EFAs were depleted in CFS sufferers[19] and a controlled clinical trial of evening primrose oil and fish oil demonstrated significant symptom reduction.[20]

Clinical trials

Despite the large number of published studies on CFS, there have been very few clinical trials. In particular, the evening primrose oil study cited above has not been repeated. A Japanese herbal formula was used to successfully treat CFS in an open clinical trial.[19] This complex tonifying formula included Panax, Rehmannia, licorice, cinnamon, Astragalus, dong quai and Schisandra.

PHYTOTHERAPEUTICS

Clinical impressions of fatigue

Chronic fatigue syndrome appears to involve a complex interaction between emotional, infectious and environmental stressors leading to subtle immune dysfunctions. The extreme debility sometimes encountered has the unfortunate effect of blocking many treatment approaches: rest may be disrupted, exercise may be debilitating and even the simplest foods may seem to be too demanding. Many otherwise useful remedies may be too stimulating or unsettling.

Fatigue may take different forms and arise from different stresses. There may be a deficiency condition, there may be an obstruction to normal functions (such as the effects of clinical depression) or fatigue may follow excessive activity, perhaps marked by anxiety and nervous stress. The therapeutic approach in each case will be different. In the first instance, nutritional and supportive therapies will dominate. In the second, there may be the need to embark upon substantial constitutional and metabolic strategies. Where tension is the predominant factor then repair will be difficult if there is not some relaxant or even sedative relief.

Sometimes benefits will follow a focus on what could be exacerbating or even causative factors. These might include:

- intestinal dysbiosis, endotoxaemia or similar syndromes;
- allergies or food intolerances;
- toxins, e.g. dental amalgam, hair dyes, pesticides;
- recurrent fungal, viral or bacterial infection.

Above all else, it is important to ensure that sleep and rest are adequate and much useful treatment effort can be directed to this end as a first priority. Whatever the initiating disturbance, the treatment of fatigue must be marked by extreme gentleness and patience.

Convalescence

With any fatigue syndrome the fundamental principle of treatment is to set up an appropriate recuperative regime. Remedies should be set against a wider programme of convalescence. Convalescence as a strategy is outlined in Chapter 3. Extensive rest is essential and may need to be supported by appropriate treatment: exercise, even if minimal, will help engage adrenosympathetic disturbances; the diet should be based on the most easily assimilable foods possible. Only when such a regime is in place can herbal treatment have a chance of facilitating further improvements.

Herbal remedies useful in chronic fatigue syndrome include the following.

Tonic and adaptogenic herbs

Tonics help revitalize the patient and adaptogens improve the response to stress. Tonics can also correct immune function. Although the immune-boosting function of these herbs might seem unwise, they do help fatigue syndrome, often dramatically.

Major herbs in this group are:

- *Panax ginseng*: tonic, adaptogenic, stimulates hypothalamic output and ACTH and hence adrenal cortex function, increases stamina, spares muscle use of carbohydrate.
- *Eleutherococcus senticosus*: adaptogenic, stimulates T-lymphocyte function.
- *Astragalus membranaceus*: tonic and immune enhancing.
- *Withania somnifera*: a tonic herb which is not stimulating.

Adrenal supportive herbs

The main herbs for this purpose are Glycyrrhiza (licorice) and *Rehmannia glutinosa*. A case study from Japan observed that a chronic fatigue patient went into remission when she developed hyperaldosteronism due to an adrenal tumour. When the adrenal tumour was removed the fatigue returned.[21] Licorice in high doses can cause pseudoaldosteronism due to its aldosterone-like action but obviously should not be used to this level. A high-potassium, low-sodium diet, as in the Gerson therapy, can also raise plasma aldosterone.

Immune-enhancing herbs

Although these may seem contraindicated, immune-enhancing herbs are often needed to help prevent the recurrent viral infections which can plague patients with chronic fatigue syndrome. In cases of infection, treatment with tonic herbs may need to be discontinued so that defensive measures can be applied. *Echinacea angustifolia* and *E. purpurea* are safe to use since, on current knowledge, they mainly enhance phagocytic activity. This can improve antigen recognition which leads to better immune responsiveness. *Picrorrhiza kurroa* should be used with caution as it is a potent promoter of all aspects of immune function, but it may be indicated for patients who have frequent viral infections.

Antiviral herbs

Although the viral association is not always clear, these herbs can be useful in many cases. *Hypericum perforatum* (St John's wort) may contribute to antiviral and antidepressant activity. *Thuja occidentalis* is also active against enveloped viruses as well as naked viruses such as the wart virus and enteroviruses.

Others

Ginkgo biloba, Salvia miltiorrhiza and Zanthoxylum (prickly ash) will improve blood flow. Ginkgo decreases erythrocyte fragility and improves blood rheology and short-term memory. Valeriana (valerian), *Passiflora incarnata* (passionflower), *Piper methysticum* (kava) and other such herbs will help the disordered sleep pattern. Crataegus (hawthorn) may help any cardiac and circulatory abnormalities. EFA therapy with evening primrose oil and fish oil is recommended.

Case histories

'Kylie', aged 17, had glandular fever 6 years previously. Suffered from fatigue ever since, but after beginning Year 12 at school, fatigue was particularly severe. Often catching colds and influenza, her attendance was less than 50%. Even on 'well' days, she often did not have the energy to attend school. Herbal treatment consisted of the following basic formula (written for 1 week).

Astragalus membranaceus	1:2	30 ml
Panax ginseng	1:2	15 ml
Ginkgo biloba (standardized for flavonoids)		20 ml
Echinacea angustifolia	1:2	35 ml
	Total	100 ml

Dose 5 mL tds

In addition, Withania 1:2 5 ml once a day was prescribed.

If a cold came on, the above treatment was stopped for 3–4 days and the following formula was taken.

Zingiber officinale	1:2	10 ml
Echinacea angustifolia	1:2	40 ml
Euphrasia officinalis	1:2	20 ml
Achillea millefolium	1:2	30 ml
	Total	100 ml

Dose 5 ml with warm water up to five times a day.

Initially, 'Kylie' had difficulty taking the herbal formula because it was too stimulating. So the dose was reduced to half and gradually increased. There was only slight improvement in her condition for 3 months but then gradual and steady progress was made. While she received herbal treatment from time to time, she was free of CFS for more than 2 years.

'John' was 35 and had not worked for 3 years. By the time he sought herbal treatment he complained that he was getting sicker and sicker. He had constant headaches and had had chronic sinusitis for about 10 years. His history showed a previous high exposure to insecticides and years of overwork due to family pressures. His wife could not cope with his not working and his marriage was strained. Various formulas were given but the treatment settled at the following (for 1 week).

Panax ginseng	1:2	15 ml
Astragalus membranaceus	1:2	30 ml
Crataegus spp fol.	1:2	20 ml
Ginkgo biloba (standardized)		20 ml
Picrorrhiza kurroa	1:2	15 ml
Glycyrrhiza glabra	1:1	20 ml
Scutellaria baicalensis	1:2	30 ml
	Total	150 ml

Dose 8 ml tds

In addition, *Echinacea angustifolia* 1:2 5 ml once a day was prescribed from time to time. Also an 'acute formula' similar to the one for 'Kylie' was taken during colds and influenza instead of the basic formula. The Crataegus was for the headaches and circulation and the Baical skullcap for the sinusitis. 'John' actually worsened in the first 3 months of treatment, probably because of the natural progression of the disorder. However, after 5 months he thanked the friend who recommended herbal treatment because it was 'the best thing I could have done'. He gradually improved over a period of several more months.

TONICS

Plant remedies traditionally used as tonics

- *Avena sativa* (oatstraw),
- *Cetraria islandica* (Iceland moss),
- *Glycyrrhiza glabra* (licorice),
- *Hypericum perforatum* (St John's wort),
- *Medicago sativa* (alfalfa),
- *Serenoa serrulata* (saw palmetto),
- *Swertia chirata* (chiretta),
- *Trigonella foenum-graecum* (fenugreek),
- *Turnera aphrodisiaca* (damiana),
- *Verbena officinalis* (vervain),
- *Withania somnifera*.

Indications for tonics

- Convalescence
- Debilitating conditions with or without anorexia
- Chronic fatigue syndrome

Cautions in the use of tonics

The use of tonic herbs may be difficult in the following circumstances.

- Very severe debility especially if associated with immune or digestive collapse.
- Renal or hepatic failure.
- Rampant cancer or strong regimes of chemotherapy.

Application

The state of digestion is the main determinant of dosage times. Tonics may be best taken with or after meals if the stomach and digestive system are weakened; in severe cases, they may need to be taken with fluid nourishment. Dosage should be rather more than less frequent: 'little and often' might be a useful axiom.

Long-term therapy with tonics is generally indicated and often advisable.

CHINESE TONICS

In Chinese medicine, tonic remedies are generally divided into four groups, depending on whether they are seen to particularly support *qi*, *yang*, *xue* or *yin*. The first two groups tend to be warming, the last two cooling. They are often more dynamic than the tonics listed above and may thus be more likely to generate adverse reactions. It is more important, therefore, to be careful in their prescription and to take close account of the interpretation of debilitated conditions that Chinese practitioners use. However, they reflect a perspective on debility and its treatment that is not well articulated in the Western traditions.

In the following review, Chinese terms will therefore be used. They are briefly introduced in the summary of Chinese herbal medicine in this text (see p.5) but any practitioner wishing to apply them should be well trained in that tradition. Nevertheless, there is some overlap with Western remedies and some useful insights are possible for a Western phytotherapist.

Qi tonics

These support active energies; they are used for depletion of *qi*, particularly in the *Spleen* and *Lungs*.

In the first case, possibly as a result of prolonged illness or constitutional weakness, debility may affect the functions of assimilation and distribution and be associated with such symptoms as fatigue and depression with depressed digestion, diarrhoea, abdominal pain or tension, visceral prolapse, pale yellow complexion with a tinge of red or purple, pale tongue with white coating and/or languid, frail or indistinct pulses. This may lead in turn to a 'damp' condition developing.

In the second case, extreme or prolonged stress or disease, or chronic pulmonary disease, leads to depletion or cold in the *Lungs*, with easy fatigue and prostration associated with disturbances of regulation, shortness of breath or shallow breathing, rapid, slow or little speech, spontaneous perspiration, pallid complexion, dry skin, pale tongue with thin white coating, weak and depleted pulses.

Plant remedies traditionally used as qi tonics

- *Panax ginseng* (Asiatic ginseng – ren shen)
- *Codonopsis pilulosa* (dang shen)
- *Astragalus membranaceus* (huang qi)
- *Atractylodes macrocephela* (bai zhu)
- *Zizyphus jujuba* (Jujube – da zao)
- *Glycyrrhiza uralensis* (Chinese liquorice – gan cao)

Yang tonics

These remedies support the active energies, particularly those of the *Kidneys* (but also *Heart* and *Spleen*).

Deficient *Kidney yang* leads to listlessness with a feeling of cold and cold extremities, back and loins; there may be weak legs, poor reproductive function, frequency of micturition, nocturia, diarrhoea (especially early in the morning), pale complexion and submerged weak pulses.

Deficiency affecting the *Heart* involves poor performance and coordination associated with profuse cold sweating, asthmatic states, thoracic or anginal pain on exertion, palpitations and fear attacks, cyanosis, white tongue coating and/or diminished, hesitant or intermittent pulses.

Plant remedies traditionally used as yang tonics

- *Trigonella foenum-graecum* (fenugreek – hu lu ba)
- *Morinda officinalis* (ba ji)
- *Juglans regia* (walnut – hu tao ren)
- *Eucommia ulmoides* (du zhong)

Xue tonics

These are remedies that support more substantial energies, those manifesting in substantial disturbances or pathologies. By definition, such disturbances are serious and profound and treatment will need to be prolonged. Symptoms of depletion of *xue* may include cyanosis, pallor, vertigo or tinnitus, palpitations, loss of memory, insomnia or menstrual problems.

There is considerable overlap with *yin* tonics.

Plant remedies traditionally used as *xue* tonics

- *Angelica sinensis* (dang gui)
- *Rehmannia glutinosa* (sheng di huang – fresh – and shu di huang – prepared)
- *Paeonia lactiflora* (paeony root – bai shao)
- *Mori alba* (mulberry fruit – sang shen)

Yin tonics

Remedies for replenishing the body fluids and essence, supplying condensed energies and nourishment, for the most depleted conditions. Areas in most need of support are the *Kidneys, Liver, Lungs* and *Stomach.*

Deficient *Kidney yin* often follows very serious debilitating disease or, alternatively, extended sexual or alcoholic abuse or overwhelming nervous stress. It may manifest as a deficient Fire condition, marked by a pale complexion with red cheeks, red lips, dry mouth, dry but deeply red tongue, dry throat, hot palms and soles, palpitations, vertigo or tinnitus, pains in the loins, night sweats, nocturnal emissions, nightmares, urinary retention, constipation, accelerated though weak pulses.

Deficient *Liver yin*, usually following the above, is often associated with dry eyes, poor vision and vertigo or tinnitus, deafness, muscle twitching, sleeplessness, hot flushed face with red cheeks, red dry tongue with little coating, diminished, stringy and accelerated pulses.

Deficient *Stomach yin* is marked by anorexia, regurgitation, thirst, abdominal rumbling, red lips and red tongue with no coating.

Deficient *Lung yin*, often following prolonged exposure to dryness or chronic pulmonary disease, is marked by dry cough, haemoptysis, hoarseness and loss of voice, strong thirst and/or restlessness and insomnia.

Plant remedies traditionally used as *yin* tonics

- *Asparagus cochinchinensis* (tian men dong)
- *Lycium chinensis* (gou qi zi)
- *Panax quinquefolium* (American ginseng)
- *Ophiopogon japonicus* (mai men dong)
- *Ligustrum lucidum* (nu zhen zi)
- *Sesamum indicum* (sesame seeds – hei zhi ma)

References

1. Shorter E. Chronic fatigue in historical perspective. Ciba Found Symp 1993; 173: 6–16
2. Holmes GP, Kaplan JE, Gantz NM et al. Chronic fatigue syndrome: a working case definition. Ann Intern Med 1988; 108(3): 387–389
3. Landay AL, Jessop C, Lennette ET, Levy JA. Chronic fatigue syndrome: clinical condition associated with immune activation. Lancet 1991; 338 (8769): 707–712
4. Linde A, Andersson B, Svenson SB et al. Serum levels of lymphokines and soluble cellular receptors in primary Epstein-Barr virus infection and in patients with chronic fatigue syndrome. J Infect Dis 1992; 165(6): 994–1000.
5. Patarca R, Klimas NG, Lugtendorf S et al. Dysregulated expression of tumor necrosis factor in chronic fatigue syndrome: interrelations with cellular sources and patterns of soluble immune mediator expression. Clin Infect Dis 1994; 18(Suppl 1): 147–153
6. Hilgers A, Frank J. Chronic fatigue syndrome: immune dysfunction, role of pathogens and toxic agents and neurological and cardial changes. Wiener Medizinische Wochenschrift 1994; 144(16): 399–406
7. Hashimoto N, Kuraishi Y, Yokose T et al. Chronic fatigue syndrome—51 cases in the Jikei University School of Medicine. Nippon Rinsho 1992; 50(11): 2653–2664
8. Bates DW, Buchwald D, Lee J et al. Clinical laboratory test findings in patients with chronic fatigue syndrome. Arch Intern Med 1995; 155(1): 97–103
9. Lerner AM, Lawrie C, Dworkin HS. Repetitively negative changing T waves at 24-h electrocardiographic monitors in patients with the chronic fatigue syndrome. Left ventricular dysfunction in a cohort. Chest 1993; 104(5): 1417–1421
10. Simpson LO, Murdoch JC, Herbison GP. Red cell shape changes following trigger finger fatigue in subjects with chronic tiredness and healthy controls. NZ Med J 1993; 106(952): 104–107
11. Ichise M, Salit IE, Abbey SE et al. Assessment of regional cerebral perfusion by 99T cm–HMPAO SECT in chronic fatigue syndrome. Nucl Med Commun 1992; 10: 767–772
12. Goldstein JA, Mena I, Jouanne E, Lesser I. 1995 The Assessment of Vascular Abnormalities in Late Life Chronic Fatigue Syndrome by Brain SPECT: Comparison with Late Life Major Depressive Disorder. Journal of Chronic Fatigue Syndrome 1(1): 55–79
13. Buchwald D et al: Ann Inter Med 116: 130(1992)
14. Natelson BH, Cohen JM, Brassloff I, Lee HJ. A controlled study of brain magnetic resonance imaging in patients with the chronic fatigue syndrome. J Neurol Sci 1993: 120(2): 213–217.
15. Schwartz RB, Garada BM, Komaroff AL et al. Detection of intracranial abnormalities in patients with chronic fatigue syndrome: comparison of MR imaging and SPECT. AJR Am J Roentgenol 1994; 162(4): 935–941
16. Demitrack MA, Dale JK, Straus SE et al. Evidence for impaired activation of the hypothalamic-pituitary-adrenal axis in patients with chronic fatigue syndrome. J Clin Endocrinol Metab 1991; 73(6): 1224–1234
17. Ur E, White PD, Grossman A. Hypothesis: cytokines may be activated to cause depressive illness and chronic fatigue syndrome. Eur Arch Psychiatry Clin Neurosci 1992; 241(5): 317–322
18. Gray JB, Martinovic AM, Horrobin D. Eicosanoids and essential fatty acid modulation in chronic disease and the chronic fatigue syndrome. Med Hypotheses 1994; 43(1): 31–42
19. Ogawa R, Toyama S, Matsumoto H. Chronic fatigue syndrome—Cases in the Kanebo Memorial Hospital. Nippon Rinsho 1992; 50(11): 2648–2652
20. Behan PO, Behan WM, Horrobin D. Effect of high doses of essential fatty acids on the postviral fatigue syndrome. Acta Neurol Scand 1990; 82(3): 209–216
21. Kato Y, Kamijima S, Kashiwagi A, Oguri T. Chronic fatigue syndrome, a case of high anti-HHV-6 antibody titer and one associated with primary hyperaldosteronism Nippon Rinsho 1992; 50(11): 2673–267

MALIGNANT DISEASES

SCOPE

Apart from their use in providing non-specific support for recuperation and repair, specific phytotherapeutic strategies include the following.

Adjunctive treatment of:

- most cancers.

Management of:

- symptoms of cancer treatment, such as nausea/vomiting of chemotherapy;
- recuperation from chemotherapy and radiotherapy.

Because of its use of secondary plant products, particular **caution** is necessary in applying phytotherapy in cases of cancers of the stomach, liver and kidneys.

ORIENTATION

Background

Whatever their capabilities, herbal practitioners are often asked to provide treatment for cancer patients. This is most often as a complement to conventional treatments. However, in a few cases they are asked to construct completely alternative treatment strategies. In the latter case especially, the practitioner can be put in a most difficult position. Cancer is undoubtedly one of the most serious and also one of the most complex and diverse diagnoses to receive. Modern oncology has confirmed that finding and attacking malignant targets remains most difficult and that different forms of cancer present very different prospects. Modern treatments have, moreover, been powerful, indeed dangerous, assaults on cells that may be more vigorous than their normal neighbours. The efficacy and safety of these treatments depend on being able to focus on their target most selectively. Alternative approaches are usually derided by orthodox authorities because they apparently lack such potency.

Herbal practitioners respond that they are trying a different approach: mobilizing the body's own powerful defences against the proliferation of malignant cells by providing appropriate supportive therapies. They point out that endogenous anticancer defences are formidable in even modest health. It is statistically likely that a tiny fraction of the body's cells (but this could mean thousands of cells) slip out of normal tissue constraints and become malignant each day; through quiet surveillance, the body's defences normally clean up such vagaries without further harm. Against that background, the actual development of a tumour must represent a failure in an impressive protective mechanism. In theory, it may be possible to reactivate these defences, at least in conditions that are not too advanced or debilitating. In practice, there is only a little evidence to guide a practitioner who aimed to work in this direction.

On the positive side, the cases of spontaneous remissions from cancer and unexpected delays in deterioration that all healthcare practitioners encounter are evidence that there are powerful defensive forces to be had. To be set against this, however, is the paucity of evidence for any strategy that could steer a practitioner towards mobilizing these forces. However, there are some pointers, at least to the possibility of improving protection against cancer development before it happens and, by implication (but only by implication), to guide supportive or adjunctive measures to improve the prospects of spontaneous recovery after the event.

Plants and cancer prevention

After a $20 million research campaign over many years and on the basis of in vitro and in vivo studies as well as epidemiological evidence, the American National Cancer Institute (NCI) has identified a range of foods with cancer preventive potential in three categories.[1]

1. Highest anticancer activity is found in garlic, soybeans, ginger, licorice and the umbelliferous vegetables (e.g. carrots, celery, parsley and parsnips).

2. Moderate anticancer activity is found in onions, linseed (flaxseed), citrus, turmeric, cruciferous vegetables (e.g. broccoli, Brussels sprouts, cabbage and cauliflower), solanaceous vegetables (tomatoes and peppers), brown rice and whole wheat.
3. Modest anticancer activity has been demonstrated in oats and barley, cucumber and the kitchen herbs such as the mints, rosemary, thyme, oregano, sage and basil.

The chemical groups suggested by the NCI as conveying some of this activity include allyl sulfides in garlic and onions, phytates in grains and legumes, lycopene, limonoids, glucarates and related terpenes, carotenes and flavonoids in citrus, lignans in linseed[2] and soya, isoflavones in soya, saponins in legumes, indoles, isothiacyanates and dithiolthione in cruciferous vegetables, ellagic acid in grapes and other fruit, phthalides and polyacetylenes in umbelliferous vegetables. Most of these are relatively robust to food preparation and are likely to reach target tissues in the body after oral consumption. Interaction with hormone receptors and other metabolic pathways leading to tumour generation is implicated as a mechanism.

On the other hand, the disappointing outcomes from the large study on the effects of beta-carotene as a food supplement are a reminder that it is not certain that these constituents will turn out to be any improvement on consumption of the whole plant.[3] Epidemiological evidence is so far wholly in this direction. For example, a study in Finland, following a cohort of 9959 cancer-free individuals (from a population of 62 440) for 24 years from 1967, found an inverse relationship between the development of lung and other cancers and the consumption of flavonoid-rich fruits and vegetables.[4] In a study in The Netherlands on a randomly selected cohort of 3123 subjects (from a total study size of 120 852), researchers found an inverse relationship between onion consumption and the development of stomach cancers over 3 years.[5] A review of this and other studies concluded that onions, garlic and other allium vegetables were likely to convey protective effects against cancer development, especially in the gastrointestinal tract.[6]

Antiinflammatory activity, e.g. by aspirin and indomethacin, has been shown to have tumour-inhibitory effects in some models (and aspirin consumption has been linked to reduced human colorectal incidence). Cyclooxygenase inhibition by a polyphenol, resveratrol, has been cited as a mechanism for a range of in vitro and in vivo tumour inhibitory effects of red grapeskin products like red wine. However, the poor bioavailability of this particular substance casts doubt on the benefits of oral consumption.[7]

Plants and cancer treatment

The potential of plant remedies directly to correct established malignancies is apparently limited. In its intensive programme from 1955, screening plant extracts for anticancer activity, the NCI found less than four extracts in every thousand tested containing compounds that demonstrated efficacy. Of the approximately 114 000 extracts studied, 11 000 exhibited antitumour activity in the P338 prescreen but of these only 500 demonstrated such activity in panel testing and only 26 proceeded to secondary testing. Of the plant isolates that reached this stage, most were alkaloids or terpenoids, with a few from plants used in traditional medicine (e.g. a triterpene from *Withania spp*, a diterpene from *Brucea spp*, a lignan from *Podophyllum spp*, a quinone from *Tabebuia spp*, an alcohol from *Aristolochia spp* and alkaloids from *Camptotheca acuminata, Fagara macrophylla, Ficus spp, Heliotropium indicum, Ochorisia moorei* and *Zanthoxylum nitidum*). Only the diterpene taxol from *Taxus brevifolia* eventually received marketing approval from the Food and Drug Administration.[8]

More recently, the NCI has studied the tamoxifen-like properties of the monoterpene perillyl alcohol, a naturally occurring analogue of limonene in citrus fruits and extracted from oil of lavender.[9]

The anticancer benefits of the alkaloids vinblastine and vincristine from the Madagascar periwinkle, *Catharantheus roseus*, were identified separately from the NCI programme. Other plant isolates from traditional remedies have been identified as having antitumour effects in vitro and in vivo in other research programmes.[10] These include:

- the anthraquinones rhein and emodin from *Cassia spp* (the sennas), *Rhamnus spp* (cascara sagrada and alder buckthorn) and *Rumex crispus* (yellow dock);
- the furanocoumarin psoralen from *Angelica spp* and other umbelliferous remedies;
- the alkaloid berberine from *Berberis spp* (barberry and Oregon grape), *Hydrastis canadensis* (golden seal) and the Chinese remedy *Coptis chinensis;*
- the alkaloids matrine and oxymatrine from the Chinese remedies *Sophora spp.*

There have been a few studies that suggest that plant preparations may have anticancer effects in experimental conditions. An extract of garlic was shown to have effects against bladder cancer in mice.[11] A pectin fraction from citrus demonstrated inhibitory effects on metastasis also in mice.[12] In addition to a number of studies demonstrating antitumour effects of extracts of *Camellia sinensis* (green tea), there have also been epidemiological studies supporting its protective effect in humans and there are early studies under way to investigate its benefits in cancer patients.[13]

PHYTOTHERAPEUTICS

All the above evidence suggests that in sufferers from cancer it would generally be wise to start supportive treatment with dietary measures to increase fruits, especially citrus fruits and grapes, and vegetables, particularly of the onion, cabbage, umbelliferous and nightshade families. Supplementation with garlic and green tea seems generally to be advisable. Particularly if there is a tendency to constipation (itself a strong naturopathic focus for correction in cancer patients), the use of linseed as a bulking agent for the bowel seems indicated.

So far, so good. However, all generalities are just that, statistical guides for the population as a whole. None of the above can take account of individual differences. Herbal treatment is most consistently predicated on the uniqueness of each patient and his or her story of illness. It is always possible that there will be some for whom the above advice will not be helpful. It is even more difficult to steer more active treatments, especially without rigorous observations for guidance.

Apart from such general supports, therefore, treatment will concentrate in the first place on supporting what are often depleted resources (see the section on Chronic fatigue syndrome, p.151, for general principles), with perhaps a special resort to Echinacea. Only once everything has been done to bolster endogenous defences can gentle active remedies be considered, using only the mildest remedies until or unless the practitioner can be confident that the patient is strong enough to take anything more vigorous. Without any clear clinical evidence for this next step, the practitioner can only be guided by precedent.

The overwhelming instinct through history is to see cancer as an indication for cleansing. Manifestations of this have included strict dietary eliminations (raw food, grain and fruit only, even grape-only diets have been applied). In the nature cure clinics of *mittel* Europe, often alpine establishments dedicated originally to the treatment of tuberculosis but switching increasingly to cancer management as the former condition diminished, the emphasis was on strict diets, invigorating hydrotherapy treatments and alterative herbal formulations. The latter might include, depending on other indications:

Arctium lappa (burdock)
Calendula officinalis (marigold)
Galium aparine (cleavers)
Phytolacca decandra (poke root)
Rumex acetosella (sheep's sorrel)
Rumex crispus (yellow dock root)
Taraxacum officinale (dandelion)
Thuja occidentalis (arbor vitae)
Trifolium pratense (red clover flowers)
Urtica dioica (nettle)
Viola odorata (sweet violet)
Viola tricolor (heartsease)

Laxatives and cholagogues were often applied where indicated. The relatively toxic laxatives *Podophyllum peltatum* (American mandrake) and *P. emodi* from India were specifically used and have been found to have notable cytotoxic constituents that have featured in conventional chemotherapy; however, these are not part of the conservative strategy being discussed here. The full panoply of phytotherapy would additionally be directed at other factors seen to be contributing to the problem. The inclusion of Zingiber (ginger) in cases judged to be in need of circulatory stimulation seems to be supported by its status in the NCI rankings. The use of Glycyrrhiza (licorice) to modulate a prescription is similarly justified. European medicine also features the specific use of an extract of mistletoe extract (notably a product Iscador) as a non-toxic stimulant of endogenous defences. There are many published studies on this treatment but no substantial controlled clinical trials; nevertheless, it is very widely used as an adjunct to other therapy and has strong professional support.

There were comparable strategies applied in traditional Chinese medicine, although diagnostic differentiation here is consistently more specific and application of such signs as pulse type and tongue appearance might lead to very individual treatments, particularly in replenishing deficient energies.[14] Nevertheless, cleansing or clearing (of toxins, damp-heat *phlegm* or stagnant *qi*, for example) featured highly. The impression from other cultural traditions is that remedies generally considered as eliminatory are those most often used for cancer.

In a major review of traditional treatments for 'tumours', under the aforementioned NCI programme, researchers at the University of Illinois listed several thousand remedies from around the world.[15,16,17] Allowing for semantic confusion about what 'tumours' may have meant in early societies (widely encountered 'tumours' for example, are likely to have included faecal impaction, the result of other digestive obstructions or simple lymphadenopathies), it is still notable how many of the remedies listed could be classified as eliminatives.

In North America the theme has been extended into a number of popular approaches to cancer treatment. The controversial Harry Hoxsey treatments (derived from the formulations of a veterinary practitioner), the Essiac formula (based on sheep's sorrel and burdock and supported by more commendations and professional and political support than other natural approaches) and many other examples usually emphasize the same or comparable remedies and themes. They usually support their theory with dramatic case reports – encouraging but not entirely persuasive. Whatever the doubts about efficacy, these strategies are at least generally consistent with historical approaches. What is less desirable is the occasional promotion of treatments based on whimsical rationale. The claims for apricot kernels and their constituent 'laetrile' or vitamin B_{17} obscured the fact that this active is a cyanogenic glycoside for which the rationale was in effect a selective toxicity against tumour cells. Apart from the fact that the claim was never adequately tested, it sat uneasily in the alternative culture by competing directly with conventional chemotherapy.

The laetrile incident reminds practitioners that cancer patients are notably vulnerable to marketing hype. Claims for treating cancer are for that reason proscribed for over-the-counter medications in the European Union and have been the subject of proscriptive court judgments. A practitioner faced with a request to help an individual patient through cancer will approach the task with humility and a recognition that in most cases the the treatment course will be set without a compass or a map. The most responsible practitioner will privately dread the burden.

References

1. Craig WJ. Phytochemicals: guardians of our health. Journal of the American Dietetic Association 1997; 97 (2): S199–204
2. Jenab M, Thompson L. The influence of flaxseed and lignans on colon carcinogenesis and B-glucuronidase activity. Carcinogenesis 1996; 17 (6): 1343–1348
3. Blumberg JB. Considerations of the scientific substantiation for antioxidant vitamins and beta-carotene in disease prevention. American Journal of Clinical Nutrition 1995; 62: S1521–1526
4. Knekt P, Järvinen R, Sappänen R et al. Dietary flavonoids and the risk of lung cancer and other malignant neoplasms. American Journal of Epidemiology 1997; 146 (3): 223–230
5. Dorant E, van den Brandt PA, Goldbohm RA, Sturmans F. Consumption of onions and reduced risk of stomach carcinoma. Gastroenterology 1996; 110: 12–20
6. Ernst E. Can Allium vegetables prevent cancer? Phytomedicine 1997; 4 (1): 79–83
7. Meishiang J, Cai L, Udeani G et al. Cancer chemopreventative activity of resveratrol, a natural product derived from grapes. Science 1997; 275: 218–220
8. Boik J. Cancer and natural medicine: a textbook of basic science and clinical research. Oregon Medical Press Princeton, Minnesota, 1995, pp 110–111
9. Zeigler J. Raloxifene, retinoids, and lavender: 'Me too' tamoxifen alternatives under study. Journal of the National Cancer Institute 1996; 88 (16): 1100–1101
10. Boik J. ibid, 112–120
11. Riggs DR, DeHaven JI, Lamm DL. Allium sativum (garlic) treatment for murine transitional cell carcinoma. Cancer 1997; 79 (10):1987–1994
12. Briggs S. Modified citrus pectin may halt metastasis. Nutrition Science News 1997; 2 (5): 216–218
13. Muir M. (Green) Tea time: does it help prevent cancer? Alternative and Complementary Therapies 1998; Feb: 43–47
14. Boik J. ibid, 90–104
15. Hartwell JL. Plants used against cancer. A survey. Lloydia 1970; 33 (3): 288–392
16. Hartwell JL. Plants used against cancer. A survey. Lloydia 1971; 34 (1): 103–160
17. Hartwell JL. Plants used against cancer. A survey. Lloydia 1971; 34 (4): 386–425

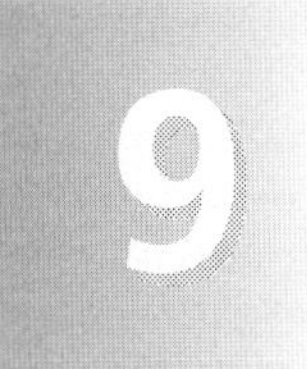

9 Herbal approaches to system dysfunctions

DIGESTIVE SYSTEM AND BOWEL

SCOPE

Apart from their use to provide non-specific support for recuperation and repair, specific phytotherapeutic strategies include the following.

Treatment of:

- functional disorders such as dyspepsia, gastrooesophageal reflux, irritable bowel syndrome;
- inflammatory conditions of the upper tract, such as mouth ulcers, oesophagitis, gastritis;
- chronic gastrointestinal infections and dysbiosis;
- constipation.

Management of:

- digestive deficiency and anorexia;
- food intolerances and allergies;
- peptic ulceration;
- inflammatory diseases of the gut such as Crohn's disease and ulcerative colitis;
- diverticulitis.

Modern research provides support for traditional herbal approaches in treating the gastrointestinal tract as **strategic therapy** in cases of:

- allergic conditions and inflammatory diseases of the skin, joints and connective tissues;
- oedematous and fluid retention problems;
- migraine.

Caution is necessary in applying herbal remedies to:

- severe malabsorption and malnutrition states;
- gastric cancer;
- biliary obstruction and bile duct cancer.

ORIENTATION

A self-correcting assembly line in reverse

The gut is a long passage designed to break down and process food, absorb nutrients and reject waste. Like an assembly line in reverse, it will only work efficiently if the delivery of material to the next stage is coordinated closely with the optimum rate of process at that stage. This subtle coordination is achieved by a robust and remarkably reliable network of control systems, orchestrated by a range of neurochemical and endocrine responses reacting to the material in the gut and managed by the complex circuitry and programmes of the enteric nervous system. This network of nerves, ganglia and neurohormones within the abdomen and the intestinal wall is complex enough to merit the description 'intelligent'. Yet this is a decentralized system, not controlled entirely by the autonomic or higher nervous systems, and most 'decisions' are made at a very local level rather than relying on central controls.[1–3]

Thus when functions are disturbed, treatments at local level may have significant impact. Plant constituents have a unique range of topical effects on the gut. The case will be made that because of the fundamental linkages between gut and other body functions, these effects can account for not only a valuable contribution to the therapeutics of the digestive system but for a very wide range of systemic activity as well (see also p.166).

In phytotherapy there is a traditional emphasis on normalizing the functions of the digestive system. This accords well with its dynamics: like other complex dynamic systems in nature, the digestive system is essentially self-correcting. A gentle trigger stimulation of an appropriate reflex response or the temporary dampening of an inappropriate response may be all that is required to prompt or allow the digestive system to revert to normal patterns of behaviour. Plant constituents seem well suited to such tasks. The following text will review some of the areas of the gut where they may work.

Law of the gut

Normal peristalsis is a simple example of the self-correcting and automatous nature of the digestive system. Gut activity is coordinated by a vast complex of nerve fibres, *intrinsic* fibres within the digestive tract linking to networks of *extrinsic* fibres, these in turn linked to *ganglia* within the abdominal cavity. Ascending intrinsic pathways are excitatory on the gut musculature and descending pathways inhibitory but both are activated by distension. Peristalsis follows the activation, by a bolus of food, of ascending excitatory pathways proximal to each point along the intestine and the simultaneous inactivation of the descending inhibitory pathways distal to the contraction. The propagation of the circular muscle contraction stops when there is no longer a sufficient distension stimulus ahead.[4] The result of this arrangement is known as the 'law of the gut'. Any bolus of food material in the gut, simply by being there, is normally propelled in one direction, towards the lower bowel;[5] the absence of such a bolus leads to quiescence.

Relationship between absorption, secretion and motility

As well as provoking muscular activity, or motility, the presence of food in the gut also stimulates *secretomotor* reflexes via submucous neurons and causes a proportion of water and electrolytes that are absorbed with nutrients such as glucose to be returned to the lumen.

This is a major issue: the balance of absorption and secretion of water and electrolytes in the gut involves levels of fluid and electrolytes much larger than that dealt with by the kidneys. The implications are reviewed below.

The critical control necessary is effected by a balance between activation from the gut wall (as well as mechanical distension by food, stimulants including bile acids, mucosal inflammation and toxic irritation) and inhibitory inputs from other sources (mainly humoral, as discussed below). The whole coordinated response to the presence of food is referred to as the *migrating motor complex*.

Observations in healthy volunteers point to innate rhythms of absorption, secretion and motility in the small intestine and biliary tract during fasting, these marked by variations in plasma levels of gastrointestinal hormones. Current evidence indicates that this fasting periodicity is generated within the intrinsic innervation,[6] i.e. probably by local environmental factors. After ingestion of food, the early part of the migrating motor complex cycle is characterized by low motor activity, low release of bile and pancreatic juice and a little fluid absorption ('absorptive mode'), followed by an increase in motor activity ('motility mode') and pancreaticobiliary secretions and a shift in net fluid transport in the secretory direction ('secretory mode'). There is a significant correlation between motility and secretory modes, so that they are often coupled as the 'secretomotor' mode. As elaborated below, cholinergic neurons seem to mediate the shift in their direction from the absorptive mode.[7]

Carminative herbal remedies, such as the warming spices, reduce motility[8] (and thus possibly secretory activity and, at least in the case of ginger, increase absorptive activity (see p.103). Increases in secretory activity and motility may be seen after the prescription of bitters, cholagogues and stimulating laxatives. However, these responses are not always predictable (in the case of bitters and cholagogues they may even be the opposite reaction in some cases) and it is also observed that reactive bowel looseness may follow a much wider variety of treatments. It appears that increases in gut activity are programmed as a response to any potentially perturbating influence, presumably as a simple defence mechanism.

If there is gut infection or food intolerance, luminal antigens or bacterial products may be detected by the immune system. This may trigger a cascade of events associated with the release of inflammatory mediators. These mediators lead to increased motility and secretory patterns that are characterized by strong muscular contractions, copious secretion and diarrhoea.[9]

The gut and fluid balance

Diarrhoea is an extreme pattern of fluid and electrolyte loss which, as a consequence of enteric infections and malnutrition, is still the most common immediate cause of death around the world. In developed societies it is rarely as dangerous as it is in impoverished regions, where rehydration with fluids and electrolytes is a critical life-saving measure (as seen in the sugar and salt solution widely used by aid agencies around the world for the purpose). Nevertheless, diarrhoea is relatively common, reflecting a wide variety of events in the gut, from food poisoning and enteric infection through hepatobiliary activity (bile being a prominent potential irritant of the gut wall), food intolerance, to irritable bowel behaviour. Often diarrhoea is of short duration and is not explained. It is even seen as a benign transient cleansing event in some healing strategies ('better out than in').

Any looseness of the bowel involves the loss of considerable amounts of fluid and electrolytes which, with the certainty of the excretion of a wide range of other materials, means that the gut can dwarf the function of the kidneys. Even modest fluctuation in bowel consistency and frequency can have significant impact on fluid balance in the body.

Some herbal traditions use remedies that loosen or bulk the bowel contents to reduce fluid accumulation and retention and even in some circumstances reduce weight. Cathartic remedies were included among those with drastic diuretic effects in the Chinese tradition and stimulating anthraquinone laxatives clearly lead to fluid and electrolyte loss. In the French tradition, even bulk laxatives and fibre are used to reduce weight associated with fluid retention.

By contrast, there are also a range of approaches to reducing bowel looseness if this is seen as harmful. These include the temporary use of astringent tannins that reduce reflex irritation of the bowel from the higher reaches of the gut in the case of gastroen teritis (see p.34), the aromatic digestives and volatile antispasmodics (see p.29) and the use of demulcent and topically antiinflammatory remedies like Althaea (marshmallow), Filipendula (meadowsweet), Glycyrrhiza (licorice), Calendula (marigold) and, for short-term use, Symphytum (comfrey).

Stomach activity

The stomach's functions are closely coordinated with the rest of the digestive tract. It stores masticated food as a hopper, delivering its acidic contents into the alkalinized duodenum only at a rate that can be alkalinized: too fast and it damages the duodenal wall, too slow and it leads to discomfort and inhibits digestion of the following meal.

Regulation of gastric emptying represents one of the most important protections of small intestinal structure and function. For example, in humans, gastric emptying is slowed in proportion to the energy density of the meal, which will level out the rate of energy delivery to the duodenum.[10]

The stomach is also the first significant point of contact with most herbal remedies. Many have immediate effects on its function, increasing secretions of acid, pepsin and mucus (bitters and pungent constituents), calming activity (mucilaginous, astringent and some aromatic and antispasmodic remedies) or stimulating motility (saponins and emetic alkaloids). It is often highly sensitive to even minor doses of herbal remedies.

Healthy upper digestive function is important for maintaining health and preventing disease. Gastric secretion declines with age[11] and a significant percentage of people aged 65 years or older have abnormally low gastric acidity.[12] Low acidity can lead to poor nutrient absorption and abnormal bowel flora. Patients with reduced gastric secretion are more susceptible to bacterial and parasitic enteric infections.[13] The contribution of poor upper digestive function to the chronicity of intestinal dysbiosis is often overlooked by therapists: the herbal practitioner has bitters and pungent principles to employ.

The chemical mediators of digestive activity

The coordination of these and digestive processes is mediated in the first instance by batteries of neurohumoral agents, chemicals that range from familiar endocrine hormones, standard neurotransmitters and chemical mediators, found also in the central nervous system and other body tissues, to gut-specific chemical agents. Each may be elicited by several receptor types in the gut wall and thus may be sensitive to different secreted, metabolized, dietary or pharmacological agents. These interactions, although highly complex and multilayered, are all integrated into a whole control mechanism for digestive activity.[14] Many constituents of herbal remedies are likely to interact with chemical mediators and this may provide some mechanisms for their effect on gut function. When these interactions are combined with similar examples in the nervous, endocrine, immunological and reproductive systems it appears that herbal medicine might genuinely provide a unique 'psychoneuroimmunological' strategy for the widest body disharmonies. To centre this range of activity around gut function would simply restate an intuition that has pervaded much traditional medicine.

A vital part of the coordination of gastric emptying referred to above is the control of gastric acid secretion. Serotonin or 5-HT receptors have been shown to mediate the emetic reflex[15] and antagonists of the main receptor concerned, type 5-HT_3, have been developed to reduce emesis of cancer chemotherapy. (These are also found to have anxiolytic effects, confirming the overlap in enteric and higher nervous mediators.[16]) There is evidence, referred to in its monograph later in this book, that ginger also acts on this receptor. 5-HT is also a likely mediator in the lower bowel of both sennoside activity and the diarrhoeal response.[17] It is possibly implicated in the action of the emetic plant remedies.

One common phytotherapeutic constituent has already established a number of contrasting effects on several neurohumoral mechanisms. Capsaicin, from *Capsicum spp*, at quite low concentrations blocks the release of calcitonin gene-related peptide, a peptide found in enteric ganglia and known to be elicited directly by local mucosal irritation leading to increased peristaltic and secretomotor activity. Capsaicin thus results in a concentration-dependent decrease in peristaltic activity following mucosal stimulation.[18] Capsaicin also blocks an alternative stimulant to intestinal contraction, vasoactive intestinal peptide: VIP mediates the effects of noradrenaline and local stressors (like acute hypoxia in vitro) which both depress cholinergic transmission and stimulate non-cholinergic contractions.[19,20] On the other hand, capsaicin is also known to induce intestinal contractions as a stimulant of sensory substance P-containing neurons[21] which are also activated by various luminal stimuli such as the presence of food metabolites and simple physical distension to stimulate intestinal contractions. Incidentally, this is probably the direct mechanism for the hyperperistalsis induced by cholera toxin – perhaps capsicum is contraindicated in cholera. The consumption of hot spices has long been a feature of traditional herbal therapeutics (see also the discussion of 'acupharmacology' below) and the effects of Capsicum on the wider physiology have been confirmed in studies of cutaneous blood flow after ingestion of chillis; variable increases in blood flow have been observed, most consistently in the abdominal area.[22]

One of the most important hormonal regulators of the digestive process is cholecystokinin. This hormone is concentrated in the wall of the upper small intestine and is secreted into the blood on the ingestion of proteins and fats and has also been implicated in the action of bitters. The physiological actions of cholecystokinin include stimulation of pancreatic secretion and gallbladder contraction and regulation of gastric emptying.[23] It is produced particularly by carbohydrate foods and appears to promote a feeling of fullness.[24,25] In humans it has been found that foods that lead to high levels of both cholecystokinin and satiety (e.g. bran) are associated with lower postprandial blood sugar and insulin levels, compared with refined carbohydrate.[26] This may be due to the physical characteristics of the carbohydrate but may also suggest that cholecystokinin helps to suppress hyperinsulinaemia. Cholecystokinin has also been observed to suppress feeding of strongly tasting foods in animals, in direct relation to the strength of the taste.[27] There are suggestions that an increase in cholecystokinin production with age may contribute to the relative anorexia in the elderly.[28]

Gastrin is a polypeptide hormone which is secreted following vagal nerve activity and by the bulk presence of food in the stomach. Some food extractives, including partially digested proteins, alcohol and caffeine have an additional effect and some of the more stimulating plant constituents like resins, spice ingredients and some saponins are likely to compound this activity. Gastrin stimulates gastric acid and pepsin secretion. It extends and indeed multiplies the short-term effect of vagal stimulation on gastric secretions.

When gastric hydrochloric acid spills over into the intestine it lowers intestinal pH and stimulates the secretion of secretin. This acts to stimulate Brunner's glands and bicarbonate-rich bile and pancreatic secretions so as to alkalinize the intestinal contents. Secretin is also a potential mediator of the antiulcer actions of mucosal protective agents; it appears that secretin inhibits gastric acid secretion via endogenous prostaglandins.[29] Glycyrrhiza (licorice) stimulates the release of secretin in humans.[30]

There are a number of herbal constituents shown to have effects on neurosynaptic mediators. These effects are also likely to impinge on gut function as many mediators have been found common to both. Gamma-amino butyric acid (GABA), probably affected by a number of plant constituents, is produced in the myenteric plexus in the gut wall and acts via GABA receptors to both stimulate cholinergic and relax VIP motor neurons contributing to both components of the peristaltic reflex.[31,32]

Disturbed intestinal permeability

The role of the gut wall is to allow for selective absorption of nutrients while providing vital protection against intrusion into the body tissues of harmful substances from the lumen. NSAID treatment has adverse effects on enterocyte mitochondria which may predispose the mucosa to absorption of bacterial and other large molecules that provoke a local inflammatory response. A similar mechanism may operate in patients with untreated Crohn's disease, who show abnormally high permeability. Remission of Crohn's induced by treatment with elemental diets coincides with a reduction in permeability. Significant correlations have been seen between permeability and plasma IgA concentrates in kidney disease and between permeability and the passage of neutrophil chemotactic agents.[33]

It is likely that some plant constituents could reduce excessive intestinal permeability. Tannins are likely to have a limited short-term effect at least in the upper reaches of the tract and healing plants like *Matricaria recutita* (chamomile), Filipendula (meadowsweet), *Ulmus spp* (slippery elm),[34] Glycyrrhiza (licorice), Calendula and Symphytum (comfrey) have long been applied with this effect in mind. In theory local antiinflammatory activity might effectively reduce some types of increased permeability. However, the most promising effect on intestinal permeability is likely to lie in changing biliary constituents, using hepatics and choleretics (see p.183).

Intestinal flora

The balance of flora populations in the gut is highly complex but, in steady-state health and dietary conditions, probably reasonably stable. In humans, for example, there seems to be a moderately predictable sequence of colonization after birth and through to adulthood with fluctuations in the relative numbers of aerobic and anaerobic bacteria in newborns up to a total of 10^{10}/g wet weight, reaching in adulthood between 10^5 and 10^7/g wet weight of aerobic and between 10^{10} and 10^{11}/g wet weight of anaerobic bacteria.[35]

The benefits of a healthy bacterial population in the gut are clear. Anaerobic bacteria in particular are shown to be responsible for considerable secondary digestion and to decrease intestinal transit time.[36] Normal bacteria like *Escherichia coli, Enterococcus faecalis* and *Bacteroides distasonis* have been shown to help protect the gut from pathogenic infiltration and there are a number of other non-specific defences known.[37] Mechanisms are likely to include modification of bile acids, stimulation of peristalsis, induction of immunological responses, competition for substrates and possible elaboration of various bacteriostatic substances.[38] The intestinal flora also contributes to non-specific defences against immunological challenge from dietary antigens by helping to reduce their uptake across the mucosal barrier.[39]

The populations of bacteria and other organisms are, however, obviously dependent on their food supply, i.e. dietary material and its metabolites, reaching the lower intestine. Variation in, for example, lactose and protein levels in infant foods[40] and sugar intake in adults[41] has been shown to have dramatic effects. Probably the most widespread impact on bacterial populations in the gut in modern times, however, is the use of antibiotics. It has long been established that this has an adverse effect on normal gut flora[42,43] especially if the antibiotics are poorly absorbed from the gut[44] and particularly if they are active against anaerobes.[45]

There are potentially negative influences of the bacterial flora in some circumstances. In immunocompromised patients even normal bacteria can cause life-threatening infections.[45] Bacterial hydrolysis of pharmacological agents, including those from plants, as well as other substances left in the intestine may be helpful but may also lead to the possibility of increased gut exposure to carcinogens.[46,47,48]

The relationship of bile products with intestinal flora is complex and works in two directions (see also p.184). Bile salt metabolites variably stimulate growth in bacterial populations,[49] while anaerobic bacteria act on bile products to produce volatile fatty acids that control other pathogenic bacteria.[50] A particularly revealing insight into the relationship is seen in the case of bowel cancer. There are three known endogenous components that affect development of colorectal cancer – colonic bacteria, the mucus layer and bile acids. The major effects of the bacteria are deconjugation and reduction of bile acids, activation of mutagen precursors, fermentation and production of volatile fatty acids, formation of endogenous mutagens and physical adsorption of hydrophobic chemicals. The mucus layer covering the surface acts as a barrier and its composition changes in premalignant and malignant colon tissue. The secretion of protective mucus is elevated by plant cell wall components in the diet. Mucus has some hydrophobic properties and its presence may alter the effect of bile components and bacterial metabolites on the gut wall.

Bowel bacteria have been linked to another cancer. In looking for reasons to explain the epidemiological link between high-fibre diets and lower risks of breast cancer, it was found that both raising fibre content in the diet and suppressing microflora with antibiotics led to reduced intestinal reabsorption of oestrogens and lower levels circulating in the blood. It was concluded that intestinal microflora raise oestrogen levels by deconjugating bound oestrogens that appear in the bile, thereby permitting the free hormones to be reabsorbed.[51] The beneficial levels of a high-fibre diet are likely to be the dominant factor in women susceptible to breast cancer, especially as there is evidence that bacterial flora actually enhance some of its wider benefits.[52]

Correction of disturbed or damaging bowel flora remains a matter of some contention. There seems, after all, little value in the administration of therapeutic cultures such as lactobacillus and yoghurt in disturbances associated with disrupted gut flora.[45] The value of a high bulk diet with reduced simple sugars intake is, however, more accepted. The phytotherapist might combine the benefits of such dietary moves with attendance to hepatic and biliary function and with bitter or aromatic digestive insurance that food matter is well rendered in the upper digestive tract. The value of direct agents like *Artemisia absinthium* (wormwood), Marsdenia (condurango) and *Allium sativum* (garlic) on disruptive bowel flora is likely to be upheld.

Plant fructooligosaccharides have recently been claimed to have 'prebiotic' properties, i.e. to promote the colonization of the bowel with beneficial flora,[53] and to be useful in dysbiotic conditions like candidiasis. They are a mixture of oligosaccharides consisting of glucose linked to fructose units. They are widely distributed in plants such as onions, asparagus and wheat and in herbal remedies such as Cynara (artichoke leaf) and Urginea (squill).[54] They are not hydrolysed by human digestive enzymes but are utilized by intestinal bacteria such as Bifidobacteria, *Bacteroides fragilis* group, Peptostreptococci and Klebsiellae. In clinical studies, improvement of faecal microflora was observed on oral administration of fructooligosaccharides at 8 g[55] and 12.5 g[56] per day; the population of Bifidobacteria in faeces increased substantially compared with before the administration.

It is likely that other animals metabolize fructooligosaccharides differently but they point to other possible effects. Significant beneficial reduction in small intestinal overgrowth has been seen when dogs' diets were supplemented by fructooligosaccharides.[57] Experiments with mice demonstrate that dietary short-chain fructooligosaccharides, unlike wheat bran, counteracted advanced stages of colon carcinogenesis, possibly, the authors suggest, via stimulation of antitumour immunity by modulation of the colonic ecosystem.[58]

Acupharmacology – a pharmacological basis for herbal therapeutics?

Modern insights into the fate of much plant material in the digestive tract support a view that a herbal remedy mostly affects the gut and its immediate surroundings. Adding what is known of the interrelationships between digestive activity and the wider body's physiology allows the modern phytotherapist to develop a rationale for the effect of herbal medicines on the body that is both unique to these remedies and provides potentially very powerful therapeutic strategies.

The body presents two distinct surfaces to the outside world.

The skin is the body's obvious interface. It is also a sensitive template from which it is possible to trigger a wide range of reflex responses elsewhere in the body. When one touches a very hot object, for example, the response is both complex and predictable. As well as the obvious avoidance responses, however, there is the potential for more constructive effects. The benefits of touch, caressing and massage are increasingly well understood. There are a number of established mechanisms by which cutaneous stimulation can have an impact on both specific internal functions and on general well-being: for example, via dermatomes and spinal afferents, stretch sensor stimulation and somatopsychological connections. These have been used to explain the potential benefits of hands-on therapies.

There are other less well-established mechanisms, possibly involving neurohormonal reflexes, that have been suggested as underpinning acupuncture, acupressure and shiatsu and possibly reflexology – the claim that stimulating particular points on the body surface can effect substantial benefits elsewhere. Such possible mechanisms are not the subject of this text except in that they extend the view that the skin is a sensitive organ that allows quite crude stimulation of what in effect are triggerpoints to effect complex reflex responses elsewhere in the system. If stimulation of acupoints leads to changes in neurohormones like enkephalin, then the fact that the stimulant was a steel, stone or gold needle, a warming moxa or finger pressure seems less important than the point that was stimulated. It appears more likely that such reflexes are programmed, even wired, into the system, as part of the marvellous complexity that is the living body.

If the skin has the potential for mediating complex effects within the body then the second of the body's surfaces has much greater potential. The lining of the gastrointestinal tract is a much greater surface than the skin and, with the finest villous foldings, makes up an area covering several playing fields. It is also a dramatically more complex surface structure. Unlike the skin, which has primarily a protective function, the gut surface has a literally intimate engagement with the outer world. It provides by far the largest exposure of the body's immune system and other defences to the outside world (and is thus associated with the largest concentrations of white blood cells). It has to render whatever diverse material is presented to it to a safe and assimilable form, then selectively absorb some of it and excrete the remainder. It has to coordinate the processes of secretion and absorption with the agitation and movement of material down a tube of over

7 metres. It supports a complex population of microflora to augment its digestive processess. The coordination necessary for all these activities is mediated by a vast network of nerve fibres and ganglia, the enteric nervous system, and neurohormones of such complexity that has all the characteristics of an intelligent system.

The main inputs into the decision-making processes involved in digestion are a vast array of receptors and sensory tissues along the gut wall. Each of these provides signals for some effector function elsewhere in the gut or indeed elsewhere in the body. The effects of the following archetypal plant constituents discussed in this chapter and in Chapter 2 can clearly be seen to work primarily on the digestive tract.

Archetypal plant constituents with primary impact on the gut

Mucilages
Tannins
Bitters
Pungent constituents
Anthraquinone glycosides
Resins
Essential oils

The gut is a sensate entity; it functions on the basis of information it receives itself from its environment. As the rest of the body relies on the digestive system to function, this sensory being is literally fundamental.

There are several general ways by which stimulation along the digestive tract can influence wider body functions, some of which were reviewed earlier.

As a source of enteric reflexes

Through neural links forged during embryonic development, stimulation of neural receptors in the gut wall is theoretically able to effect responses in other areas. Vagal modulation can lead to wider adjustment of autonomic activity in the body and particularly in bronchial muscle activity and cardiovascular control signals originating in the thorax. Pungent principles (hot spices) increase blood flow in other areas after ingestion.[59]

As an endocrine organ

The gut is responsible directly or indirectly for the secretion of insulin, glucagon, somatostatin, gastrin, cholecystokinin and a range of other hormones and transmitters with wide effects on body functions.

Through common neurohormonal mechanisms

The gut wall contains many regulatory neurosecretory cells that produce agents with receptors elsewhere in the body. One obvious example of the neurohormonal and endocrine links is the close relationship between digestive status and emotion.

As the body's largest concentration of immunological activity

The body has by far its greatest exposure to immunological challenge in the digestive system.

As a potential route of access for pathogenic materials

Damage to the digestive defences, the digestive secretions or the intestinal wall can permit the absorption of dangerous materials. As well as the extra strain this may put on the immune system referred to above, there are other potential problems that can arise for which digestive treatments may prove beneficial.

As a determinant of blood sugar levels

The awesome effects on behaviour, the functions of the central nervous system and on the major body hormones of undue fluctuations in levels of blood glucose is a reflection of the importance not only of good carbohydrate intake but of coordinated secretion of enteric hormones like gastrin and cholecystokinin.

Via the enterohepatic circulation

The absorption of materials from the gut in the portal bloodstream to the liver presents the latter with its main metabolic load. Hepatic processing of this and other circulating material from elsewhere in the body may include excretion of metabolites into the bile. Depending on the extent of secondary breakdown of these metabolites in the gut, particularly with the activity of gut microflora, these products may to varying extents be reabsorbed for recirculation around the body's general circulation. Levels of many physiological and pharmacological agents in the body can therefore be significantly affected by changes in digestive activity.

As the body's major eliminatory organ

The bowel is the obvious outlet not only of digestive residues but also of bowel microflora detritus and bile products. Any change in eliminatory functions is likely to have significant effects in the body; different traditions around the world have linked catarrhal states, susceptibility to infections, skin and joint diseases, mood disturbances and menstrual problems to disturbed bowel eliminations. The almost universal use in early times of drastic emetics and purgatives, both involving dramatic increase in bile eliminations for the treatment of acute diseases, reflects a widespread human instinct that these eliminatory functions were important.

As the home for the major populations of symbiotic and parasitic organisms in the body

The activity of the gut microflora has an impact on the levels of many nutrients, hormones and drugs in the body.

As the source of all physical and much emotional nourishment and replenishment

The most obvious truism yet provides the herbalist with a potent mechanism for effecting better health. Remedies that could be shown to improve digestive performance would be important elements in convalescence and recuperation.

The main advantage of considering herbal therapeutics as acupharmacology is that it provides a basis for rapid responses, a therapeutics based on intervention and review of early results on an iterative process towards recovery. In this approach to treatment, feedback is almost immediate and a muscular strategy of repair can be constructed.

PHYTOTHERAPEUTIC PRINCIPLES

Archetypal digestive remedies

Following Chapter 2, the approach adopted in this and the following chapters is to look at key chemical groups in plants, the 'archetypal plant constituents', rather than at individual remedies. The fragmentary nature of research support for herbal therapeutics is always a major limitation but fortunately in the area of the digestive tract there is a more than usually reliable experience of efficacy; the digestive tract is one of the most accessible organs in the body and most traditional treatments relied on immediate clinical effects.

Dosage and other prescription practicalities

Most experience of the impact of herbal remedies on the digestion was associated with the use of heroic doses applied to acute indications. Emetics and cathartics were often the first resort of treatment, and dysentery, life-threatening gastrointestinal infections and hepatitis the most common indications. Even with more robust constitutions the occasionally dramatic effects of eating unrefrigerated food were very familiar. The remedies outlined above were favoured because they had rapid effect.

The gastrointestinal tract provides a large surface area and the processes of digestion quickly denature and dilute remedies. For most of the effects referred to, therefore, relatively large doses of plant need to be taken (and the preparation needs to contain the relevant constituent – it is no good having a convenient extract of plant without its mucky mucilage, resin or tannin if those are the constituents one needs!). Many modern prescriptions based on quantities measured in drops or milligrams would be unlikely to have much impact on this system. The main exceptions are the bitters and hot spices or other cases where the target receptors are close to the point of entry or the agent is particularly powerful.

It is also likely that for many effects long-term treatment is inappropriate. The cases of tannins and anthraquinones are examples of when this may even be hazardous. In practice, one finds that for most gut-mediated mechanisms the effect is strongest in the earliest days of treatment and often wears off quite quickly.

It is much better to work on short-term prescriptions of relatively strong doses, constantly monitoring for immediate feedback and adjusting accordingly. In any long-term strategy it is generally wise to treat intermittently, maintaining the option of frequent prescription changes according to results.

BULK LAXATIVES

Plant remedies traditionally used as bulk laxatives
Linum (linseed), *Plantago ovata* (ispaghula), *Plantago psyllium* (psyllium seed and husk).

Indications for bulk laxatives

- Constipation
- Inflammatory bowel disease
- Blood sugar disturbances, including the dietary management of diabetes
- Some dyspeptic and gastric inflammatory conditions

Other traditional indications for bulk laxatives

- Fluid retention
- Obesity

Contraindications for bulk laxatives

There are few contraindications for the use of fibre and the bulk laxatives. However, their supplementation should be kept under review in cases of:

- iron deficiency anaemia;
- osteoporosis;
- chronic malnutrition.

Traditional therapeutic insights into the use of bulk laxatives

Some of the bulk laxatives were also used for their obvious mucilaginous properties (see below) in reducing inflammatory problems in the upper sections of the digestive tract.

Application

Bulk laxatives need to be taken whole as powdered material, most conveniently in capsule form, with food.

Long-term therapy with extra supplementation of soluble fibre is not always advisable and both soluble and insoluble fibre intake should be reviewed where absorption of mineral nutrients is a critical issue.

Advanced phytotherapeutics

Bulk laxatives may also be usefully applied in some cases (depending on other factors) of hypertension.

EMETICS

Plant remedies traditionally used as emetics

Cephaelis (ipecacuanha), Urginea (squill).

Indications for emetics

- Ingestion of poisons

NB. Emesis has been demonstrated as an inefficient way to remove poison material, with appreciable amounts being forced into the small bowel,[60] and activated charcoal as a non-emetic treatment for poisoning is likely to be superior,[61] for example in paracetemol poisoning.[62]

Other traditional indications for emetics

- Any acute toxic and infective condition
- Bronchitis

Contraindications for emetics

The use of emetics is contraindicated in the following.

- Poisoning associated with coma, convulsions
- Poisoning with petroleum products or corrosive substances
- Any debilitated condition or constitutional weakness

Traditional therapeutic insights into the use of emetics

Emetics were used as a first line of treatment especially for enteric and bronchitic infections and for any evidence of biliary toxicity. It was always understood that their use was essentially debilitating so a robust constitution was an essential prerequisite.

Application

For poisoning emergencies use, for example, 15 ml of ipecac syrup for children and adults,[63] repeating the dose in 15–30 minutes if necessary. If Ipecac is unavailable soapy water or detergent with water may be used or manual stimulation of the gag reflex with finger or blunt instrument may be tried.

MUCILAGES

Plant remedies traditionally used as mucilages

Althaea (marshmallow), Ulmus (slippery elm), *Plantago major* (plantain), *Plantago lanceolata* (ribwort), Symphytum (comfrey), Tussilago (coltsfoot), Chondrus (Irish moss), Lobaria (lungwort), Verbascum (mullein).

Indications for mucilages

- Dyspeptic conditions especially with hyperacidity
- Inflammatory diseases of the digestive tract, e.g. reflux oesophagitis, gastritis, peptic ulceration, enteritis, ileitis and colitis
- Non-productive, irritable cough
- Topically: inflamed lesions, pruritus

Other traditional indications for mucilages

- Dysuria

Contraindications for mucilages

The use of mucilages is either contraindicated or at least inappropriate in the following.

- Congestive bronchial and catarrhal conditions
- As a substitute for curative treatments where these are available

Further traditional therapeutic insights into the use of mucilages

Mucilaginous plants were associated in Chinese medicine with a diuretic effect and were also seen as valuable tonics in debilitated conditions, especially with chronic wasting dry lung diseases, such as tuberculosis.

Application

Mucilages should be taken in a formulation that preserves their physical characteristics. Encapsulation is probably the most effective way of administering the whole material (subject to the contents being adequately sterilized) but cold aqueous infusion is the most efficient extraction process, using alcohol later for preservative purposes. Depending on the indication, they may be taken before meals (for digestive problems of the stomach and small intestine), during (for some stomach problems) or after meals (in the case of reflux oesophagitis/hiatus hernia). As mucilaginous expectorants, they may be taken at any time and as frequently as required.

Long-term therapy with mucilages presents few problems but as they are essentially management treatments, such use may disguise the need for more substantial treatments.

SAPONINS

Plant remedies traditionally used for saponin effects

Primula (cowslip), Glycyrrhiza (licorice), Cephaelis (ipecacuanha), Quillaia (quillaia), Senega (snakeroot), Trigonella (fenugreek).

Indications for saponin-containing remedies

- Bronchial congestion
- Digestive difficulties

Other traditional indications for saponin-containing remedies

- As tonics for debilitating conditions
- As hormonal modulators

Contraindications for saponins

The use of saponins is either contraindicated or at least inappropriate in the following.

- Topically to open wounds
- Coeliac disease, fat malabsorption and vitamins A, D, E, and K deficiency
- In some upper digestive irritations

Traditional therapeutic insights into the use of saponins

Saponins are common constituents in plants used in Chinese and Asian medicine as tonics and harmonizing treatments. Modern pharmacological interest in the effects of ginseng has raised speculation that as steroidal molecules, some saponins may modulate steroid hormone control mechanisms in the body (see also p.43).

APPLICATION

Saponin-rich plants may be taken before meals or if there is a sensitive stomach immediately after eating.

Long-term therapy with saponin-rich plants should be avoided unless dosage levels are small or clear benefits are apparent which diminish if treatment is stopped. The impact of saponins on digestion and absorption is insufficiently clear.

TANNINS

Plant remedies traditionally used for tannin constituents

Hamamelis (witchhazel), *Potentilla tormentilla* (tormentil), Quercus (oak), Agrimonia (agrimony), Geum (avens), Krameria (rhatany), Geranium (cranesbill), *Carduus benedicta* (blessed thistle), *Acacia catechu* (catechu), Bidens (bur-marigold), Alchemilla (ladies mantle), Polygonum (bistort), Sanguisorba (burnet).

Indications for tannins

- Inflammation of the upper digestive tract
- Diarrhoea following gastrointestinal inflammation
- Topically: open, discharging lesions, wounds, hemorrhoids and third-degree burns

Contraindications for tannins

The use of tannins is either contraindicated or at least inappropriate in the following.

- Constipation
- Iron deficiency anaemia
- Malnutrition

Traditional therapeutic insights into the use of tannins

Tannins were used throughout history for forming leather from animal tissues and as effective cauterizing agents for burns and other open wounds. The astringent sensation on tasting was a simple guide to efficacy in staunching diarrhoea and other discharges.

Application

Tannins should be taken after food in most cases. For some lesions of the upper digestive tract, short-term use between meals or before food is justifiable.

Long-term therapy with high doses of tannins is to be avoided.

PUNGENT CONSTITUENTS

Plant remedies traditionally used for warming effects

Capsicum (cayenne), Zingiber (ginger), Armoracea (horseradish), Curcuma (turmeric).

Indications for pungent constituents

- Congestive dyspepsia
- Some cases of nausea, emesis, colic, diarrhoea and other hyperperistaltic conditions
- Bronchial congestion
- Poor peripheral circulation
- Topically: for joint and muscle pain, subdermal inflammations

Other traditional indications for heating remedies

- Any effect of cold on body systems

Contraindications for pungent constituents

The contraindications for heating remedies are constitutional rather than symptomatic. The same symptoms in two individuals may provide contrasting indications for this group of remedies. The use of hot spices may be contraindicated or inappropriate in the following.

- Concurrently with powerful drug regimes where dosage levels are critical
- Hyperacidity conditions and gastrooesophageal reflux
- Hepatitis
- Some enteric and bowel inflammatory states with diarrhoea
- Some cases of chronic nephritis

Traditional therapeutic insights into the use of pungent constituents

Early insights into the impact of 'heating' the body have become very developed in some traditions. Most early physicians would have been familiar with the issues that determined how far to 'heat' or 'cool' a prescription (see p.4)

Application

Hot spices can feature in prescriptions taken at various times of the day. When taken primarily for their impact on digestion, they may be taken before meals if there are no local inflammatory conditions in the upper digestive tract, with or after meals if the gut wall proves to be sensitive or there is a tendency to hyperacidity.

Long-term therapy with pungent remedies is acceptable if the individual is comfortable with the regime. It should be discontinued if there are any digestive discomforts.

AROMATICS

Plant remedies traditionally used as aromatics

Elettaria (cardamom), Angelica, Carum (caraway), Pimpinella (aniseed), Foeniculum (fennel), *Cinnamomum spp* (cinnamon), Anethum (dill), Alpinia (galangal), Levisticum (lovage), Myristica (nutmeg).

Indications for aromatics

- Colic and flatulence
- Irritable bowel disease
- Congestive dyspepsia
- Catarrh and bronchial congestion

Other traditional indications for aromatics

- Sluggish digestion and metabolism
- Congestive chronic infections and inflammatory conditions

Contraindications for aromatics

The use of aromatics may be contraindicated or inappropriate in gastrooesophageal reflux.

Traditional therapeutic insights into the use of aromatics

In Chinese medicine aromatics are used for 'damp' conditions affecting the assimilative functions (represented by the *Spleen* in Chinese medicine). Symptoms include abdominal and thoracic congestion (sometimes associated with cough and breathlessness), loss of appetite and loose stools.

Application

Aromatics are best taken immediately before meals. Their impact on the digestion is often increased if taken in hot aqueous infusions.

Long-term therapy with aromatics is often well tolerated.

VOLATILE ANTISPASMODICS

Plant remedies traditionally used as antispasmodics

Matricaria (chamomile), Mentha (peppermint), Melissa (lemon balm), Achillea (yarrow), *Nepeta cataria* (catmint), Petroselinum (parsley root), *Thymus spp (thyme)*.

Indications for antispasmodics

- Nervous dyspepsia
- Colic and flatulence
- Irritable bowel disease
- Gastritis

Other traditional indications for antispasmodics

- As components of fever management strategies
- General nervous, irritable and anxiety syndromes

Contraindications for antispasmodics

The use of antispasmodics may be contraindicated or inappropriate in gastric and enteric poisoning incidents.

Traditional therapeutic insights into the use of antispasmodics

These remedies overlap with the aromatics in their effect on the digestive tract but are more appropriate in hot and febrile conditions. However, in many cases predicting efficacy is difficult and patients may be encouraged to try a number of these or aromatic remedies to see which suits best. In all cases effects are very quick.

Application

Antispasmodics are best taken immediately before meals. Their impact on the digestion is often increased if taken in hot aqueous infusions.

Long-term therapy with antispasmodics is often well tolerated.

RESINS

Plant remedies traditionally used as resins

Calendula (marigold), Commiphora (myrrh), Ferula (asafoetida), Dorema (ammoniacum), Myrica (bayberry).

Indications for resin-containing remedies

- Inflammatory conditions of the mouth, throat and upper digestive tract
- Lymphadenopathies and recurrent infections

Application

Resins will only dissolve in alcohol so resin-rich remedies need to be taken as tinctures with as little water as possible.

Long-term therapy with resins is inadvisable.

ANTHRAQUINONE LAXATIVES

Plant remedies traditionally used as anthraquinone laxatives

Aloe, Cassia (senna), *Rhamnus purshiana* (cascara), *Rhamnus frangula* (frangula), Rheum (rhubarb), *Rumex crispus* (yellow dock).

Indications for anthraquinone laxatives

- Atonic constipation

Other traditional indications for anthraquinone laxatives

- Fluid retention
- Obesity

Contraindications for anthraquinone laxatives

The use of anthraquinone laxatives is either contraindicated or at least inappropriate in the following.

- Constipation associated with bowel irritability
- Bowel disease
- Diarrhoea

Application

Anthraquinones may be taken in laxative doses with the evening meal. Lower doses may be taken with other meals as part of a strategy to increase general bowel activity over the medium term.

Long-term therapy with anthraquinones is formally contraindicated.

Advanced phytotherapeutics

Anthraquinone laxatives may also be usefully applied in some cases (depending on other factors) of detoxifying regimes.

BITTERS

Plant remedies traditionally used as bitters

Gentiana (gentian), Centaurium (centaury), *Artemisia absinthium* (wormwood), Taraxacum (dandelion), Aletris (unicorn root), Marsdenia (condurango), Menyanthes (bogbean), Picrasma (quassia), Swertia (chiretta), Veronicastrum (black root).

Indications for bitters

- Poor appetite and digestion
- Liver and bile disturbances (as choleretics, see p. 190)
- Blood sugar disturbances, including the dietary management of diabetes
- Chronic gastritis and gastric ulceration
- Food intolerances and allergies
- Debilitated conditions associated with any of the above

Other traditional indications for bitters

- Fever management
- Jaundice

Contraindications for bitters

The use of bitters is either contraindicated or at least inappropriate in the following.

- Duodenal ulceration
- Conditions classed as 'cold-dry' in early medicine, involving for example ready shivering with dry cough and notably including some kidney diseases

Traditional therapeutic insights into the use of bitters

Bitters were univerally classified as cooling in early approaches to medicine (see p.5). This insight is likely to have followed observations that administering bitters helped to contain excesses of temperature in fevers and has been associated in Chinese medicine, for example, with the view that increased digestive activity is intrinsically a cooling phenomenon. In supporting the latter, bitters were seen not only to support nourishment but to reduce the symptoms of excessive heat in some pathologies, including some headaches and migraines, skin and other inflammatory diseases and allergic or hypersensitivity conditions.

Application

Since bitters act by reflex, they do not usually have to be given in high doses. Enough to promote a strong taste of bitterness is usually sufficient. This will typically be seen if 5–10% of tinctures are bitters like Gentiana or *Artemisia absinthium* (wormwood).

Long-term therapy with bitters is possible in those individuals where its effect is beneficial. However, it is always valuable to work to a position where the bitters are taken only when necessary and useful.

Advanced phytotherapeutics

Bitters may also be usefully applied in some cases (depending on other factors) of:

- headaches and migraines;
- skin and other inflammatory diseases;
- allergic and hypersensitivity conditions.

PHYTOTHERAPY FOR DIGESTIVE CONDITIONS

Mouth ulcers (aphthous ulceration)

Aphthous ulceration is a common recurrent condition characterized by superficial ulceration in the mouth. Ulcers are often multiple and may recur. The cause is unknown but possible factors include emotional stress, poor immunity, imbalanced oral flora and dentures. In some women ulcers tend to follow a cyclic pattern and occur premenstrually. The presence of serious diseases such as Crohn's disease, ulcerative colitis, coeliac or Behçet's disease should always be excluded.

Glycyrrhiza (licorice)	Antiinflammatory and soothing
Echinacea	Immune enhancing, stimulates saliva, antiinflammatory
Myrrh	Strong antiseptic and antiinflammatory
Propolis	Vulnerary, antiinflammatory, antiseptic, local anaesthetic
Piper methysticum (kava)	Strong local anaesthetic for symptom relief in severe cases
Calendula	Antiseptic, antiinflammatory, vulnerary
Rheum palmatum (rhubarb root)	Antiseptic, antiinflammatory, astringent, possible vulnerary with activity against mouth ulcers confirmed by clinical trials[64]

Treatment

The approach of herbal treatment is to accelerate the healing of the ulcers and to correct any underlying imbalances. Other aspects of treatment include the minimization of stress, attention to a wholesome diet with plenty of fruit and vegetables and attention to oral hygiene.

Case history

A female patient aged 42 had suffered from mouth ulcers almost continuously for 30 years. All her teeth had been removed when she was 15 because they were 'chalky'. She was a worrier and found it difficult to relax.
Initial treatment was as follows (based on 1 week).

Glycyrrhiza glabra (high in glycyrrhizin)	1:1	20 ml
Echinacea angustifolia	1:2	25 ml
Propolis	1:10	25 ml
Valeriana officinalis	1:2	20 ml
	Total	100 ml

Dose 5 ml with water three times a day.

The following mixture was to be applied directly to the ulcers.

Propolis	1:10	50 ml
Calendula	1:2	50 ml
	Total	100 ml

She was also advised to rinse her mouth regularly with a mixture of acidophilus yoghurt and water.
After 4 weeks she had only experienced three ulcers, all in the first week of treatment. In the following 4 weeks there was only one ulcer. One year later she was still taking the herbal treatment at a reduced frequency (one or two doses a day) and was relatively free from mouth ulcers.

Herbs which are prescribed for the treatment of mouth ulcers, and their relevant properties, are as listed above. Most of these herbs are beneficial when applied topically as well as when taken internally.

Topical application of a high alcoholic tincture or extract of calendula, myrrh, kava or propolis is particularly beneficial. This is because such preparations are quite resinous. When they are painted on to the ulcer the alcohol dries and the resin fixes the active components so that they are not readily washed away by saliva. It is also possible that they promote a local leucocytosis (i.e. attract white blood cells).

Dyspepsia and gastrooesophageal reflux (GOR)

Approaches to the herbal treatment of both GOR and functional dyspepsia are similar, although different aspects of treatment are emphasized in each disorder and for individual cases.

Main aspects of treatment include the following.

- *Glycyrrhiza* (licorice) and mucilaginous herbs such as *Ulmus* (slippery elm) and Althaea (marshmallow root) to assist mucoprotection. These are best taken after meals and before bed.
- Bitter herbs at low doses can increase oesophageal sphincter tone and improve gastric emptying. However, they also increase gastric acidity and therefore should be used cautiously.
- Carminative herbs and essential oils in high doses will aggravate GOR by reducing sphincter tone but they can be indicated for functional dyspepsia. Also, in lower doses, they can improve gastrointestinal motility.
- Antiinflammatory herbs relieve symptoms and improve healing and include Filipendula (meadowsweet), Stellaria (chickweed) and Matricaria (chamomile), especially those chemotypes of Matricaria rich in bisabolol. Filipendula is also traditionally thought to reduce excess acidity and Matricaria is also spasmolytic. They are indicated in both functional dyspepsia and GOR.

• GOR and functional dyspepsia may be linked to stress, especially if associated with irritable bowel syndrome. Sedative herbs, e.g. Valeriana, and nervine tonic herbs, e.g. Scutellaria (skullcap), are indicated if this association is evident.

Case history

A female patient aged 58 had suffered irregularly from heartburn for 10–15 years. Over the years she had learnt to avoid alcohol, smoking, wheat, yeast and rice. She was already taking slippery elm powder and had taken antacids in the past. She sought treatment because she was experiencing frequent attacks of heartburn in the past few months. She hated licorice, so it was not included in her formula.
Treatment consisted of (based on 1 week):

Passiflora incarnata	1:2	25 ml
Matricaria chamomilla	1:2	25 ml
Filipendula ulmaria	1:2	25 ml
Stellaria media	*stabilized succus*	25 ml
	Total	100 ml

Dose 5 ml three times a day.
In the 4 weeks following she experienced only one attack of heartburn and in the following 4 weeks had no problems with heartburn, despite being unwell with influenza.

Poor upper digestive function/anorexia

Poor upper digestive function can be a consequence of prolonged or serious illness or can occur with convalescence. Digestive function also deteriorates with age, particularly gastric acid and pancreatic output. It is also reflected in children by their failure to thrive, anaemia and susceptibility to infections. Symptoms include anorexia, a prolonged sensation of fullness or stagnation after eating, undigested food in stools, belching or flatulence, intolerance of fatty foods and nausea. However, poor upper digestive function may be largely asymptomatic in itself but may contribute to other conditions such as food intolerance or allergies, intestinal dysbiosis (abnormal bowel flora), constipation, nutrient deficiencies and migraine headaches. Herbal practitioners believe that many chronic diseases originally begin with poor digestive function and good upper digestive function is a prerequisite for a healthy digestive system.

Herbs which improve upper digestive function can be divided into five major groups.

- Simple bitters such as *Gentiana lutea* which improve most aspects of upper digestive function.
- Aromatic digestives such as *Angelica archangelica*, Cinnamomum (cinnamon) and *Coleus forskohlii* which improve gastric acid secretions. Coleus also improves exocrine pancreatic function.
- Pungent herbs such as Zingiber (ginger) and Capsicum (cayenne) which are potent stimulators of gastric acid.
- Choleretic herbs such as *Berberis vulgaris* (barberry), Silybum (St Mary's thistle) and Taraxacum (dandelion root) which improve bile production by the liver.
- Cholagogue herbs such *Mentha piperita* (peppermint) which improve gallbladder function.

An example formula for improving upper digestive function is:

Gentiana lutea	1:5	10 ml
Coleus forskohlii	1:1	65 ml
Zingiber officinale	1:2	25 ml
	Total	100 ml

Dose 20 drops (about 0.7 ml) with water 20 minutes before meals.

If there is evidence of liver weakness, e.g. previous pesticide exposure, history of hepatitis or symptoms such as nausea after rich or fatty food, the above treatment may need to be supplemented with the choleretic herbs mentioned above. If the patient notices excessive irritability after using any of the above herbs, reduce the dose or delete any bitter herbs, including Berberis.

Nausea

Nausea is a symptom rather than a disease state. A a number of herbs can be used effectively to give relief. If nausea is trace- able to poor liver function, then the treatment approach outlined above should be followed. Other herbs which can provide symptomatic relief in cases of nausea include Zingiber (ginger), *Mentha piperita* (peppermint), Matricaria (chamomile), *Ballota nigra* (black horehound) and Filipendula (meadowsweet). If herbs are used to prevent motion sickness, they should be taken about 1 hour before travel. Ginger is particularly effective for all forms of motion sickness and also for morning sickness. Herbs should not be administered orally to a person who is vomiting.

Peptic ulcer

The herbal approach to the treatment of peptic ulcer disease should take into account all the causative and sustaining factors which are relevant to the individual patients. Rather than being concerned with inhibiting gastric acid, the herbal approach stresses the support of factors which protect the mucosa and improve the capacity of the body to heal the ulcer.

Main aspects of treatment include the following.

- Glycyrrhiza (licorice) and mucilaginous herbs to enhance mucoprotection. These are best taken before meals and, in the case of duodenal ulceration, should be taken at least half an hour before eating. Glycyrrhiza also improves pancreatic bicarbonate secretion.

- Whilst bitter herbs such as Gentiana are contraindicated in duodenal ulcers, they may be valuable in gastric ulcers because of their trophic effect on the gastric mucous membrane.

- *Hydrastis canadensis* (golden seal) is traditionally restorative to mucous membranes and also antibacterial.

- Also other antiseptic treatments such as propolis and raw crushed garlic will help to resolve *Helicobacter pylori* infection, although many ulcer patients find raw garlic difficult to take. Propolis also improves healing.

- Immune-enhancing herbs such as Echinacea will also help resolve *Helicobacter pylori* presence and improve repair mechanisms. They were traditionally used in peptic ulcer disease long before the importance of *H. pylori* was recognized.

- Gently astringent herbs will assist ulcer healing and boost mucoprotection in the vicinity of the ulcer. Good examples are Agrimonia and Filipendula (meadowsweet). Strongly astringent herbs such as *Geranium maculatum* (cranesbill) will aggravate a gastric ulcer but may be suitable for duodenal ulcer treatment.

- Antiinflammatory herbs such as Stellaria (chickweed) and bisabolol-rich Matricaria (chamomile) and vulneraries such as Calendula and Stellaria will help break the vicious cycle of ulceration and accelerate the healing process.

- Spasmolytic and carminative herbs will improve gastrointestinal motility. Carminative herbs, e.g. Foeniculum (fennel) should be administered only in low doses. Good gastrointestinal spasmolytics include Matricaria and *Viburnum opulus* (cramp bark).

- Filipendula is considered by some herbalists to be a normalizer of the acidity of the stomach.[65] It does appear to decrease the negative effects of acid and pepsin on the mucosa but is probably not a true antacid. This positive effect on the mucosa is paradoxical since it contains salicylates.

- Some patients with peptic ulcer disease may experience irritation from herbal treatment and one approach with more severe or chronic cases is to start with a low dose and gradually increase over several weeks.

Example treatments

Gastric ulcer

Foeniculum vulgare	1:2	3 ml
Filipendula ulmaria	1:2	25 ml
Glycyrrhiza glabra (high in glycyrrhizin)	1:1	15 ml
Matricaria chamomilla	1:2	20 ml
Gentiana lutea	1:5	2 ml
Echinacea angustifolia	1:2	20 ml
Calendula officinalis	1:2	15 ml
	Total	100 ml

Dose 5 ml with water three times a day before meals. Also slippery elm powder, one heaped teaspoon with water before meals, and one Hydrastis 500 mg tablet after meals. (Hydrastis contains alkaloids and is incompatible with the tannins in Filipendula.)
If irritation occurs, reduce the dose of liquid herbs to half and stop the Hydrastis.

Duodenal ulcer

Filipendula ulmaria	1:2	20 ml
Glycyrrhiza glabra	1:1	15 ml
Matricaria chamomilla	1:2	25 ml
Propolis	1:10	15 ml
Echinacea angustifolia	1:2	25 ml
	Total	100 ml

Dose 5 ml with water three times a day half hour before meals.
Also slippery elm powder and Hydrastis tablets as above.

Food intolerance and allergies

Food intolerance can have a number of causes such as enzyme defects (e.g. alactasia), pharmacological activity (e.g. salicylates) and immunological reactions (allergy, coeliac disease). There are also a number of less well-defined and less specific, often idiosyncratic, reactions. Food intolerance can follow hepatitis or gastrointestinal infection. In these instances the reaction to some or many foods can continue long after the actual infection has passed.

In the case of immunological reactions, which represent true food allergy, the best approach to treatment is to avoid the offending foods, if they can be identified, and if exclusion is not impractical. In other instances of food intolerance, herbal treatment may prove beneficial by correcting any physiological defects or deficiencies which are contributing to the reaction to foods and by dampening any underlying gastrointestinal inflammation.

The herbal approach to the treatment of food intolerance or allergy is as follows.

- Bitter, aromatic, pungent, choleretic and cholagogue herbs to improve upper digestive function.
- Hepatotrophorestoratives and stimulants of hepatic metabolism, such as Silybum and Schisandra, to improve hepatic screening and detoxification.
- Depurative and lymphatic herbs, e.g. Arctium (burdock) and Calendula, to assist detoxification mechanisms.
- Herbs with healing and protective effects on the gut wall such as Filipendula (meadowsweet), Calendula, Matricaria (chamomile) and Althaea (marshmallow) root.
- Immune-enhancing herbs such as Echinacea which enhances phagocytic activity. Picrorrhiza is both bitter and immune enhancing.
- Hydrastis (golden seal) as a restorative to the mucous membranes of the gut wall and a potential modifier of gut flora. Hydrastis is also bitter.
- Other treatments to restore normal gut flora. This is covered in detail on p.165. See also antimicrobial herbs listed on p.140.
- Antiallergic herbs such as Albizzia and *Scutellaria baicalensis* (Baical skullcap) and antiinflammatory herbs such as Matricaria.

Appropriate herbs should be selected from the above treatment approach on the basis of the individual case.

Case history

A female patient aged 35 had been overseas and developed an acute gastrointestinal infection with pain and diarrhoea. The infection passed but on returning home she experienced bloating and diarrhoea often after eating. Stool culture did not demonstrate the presence of an infection. Symptoms could be controlled by restricting her diet to a very simple one, e.g. rice and vegetables. Treatment consisted of:

Echinacea angustifolia	1:2	30 ml
Picrorrhiza kurroa	1:2	10 ml
Silybum marianum	1:2	20 ml
Matricaria chamomilla	1:2	20 ml
Filipendula ulmaria	1:2	20 ml
	Total	100 ml

Dose 5 ml with water three times a day before meals.
Golden seal tablets 500 mg, one tablet with each meal.
After 4 weeks of treatment, symptoms had improved and she could often be more adventurous with her diet without causing problems. However, symptoms were still occurring on many days.
During the next 4 weeks her condition continued to improve with herbal treatment. After another 4 weeks she could eat normally and the herbs were discontinued without adverse effect.

Gastrointestinal infections and diarrhoea

The most common causes of acute diarrhoea are infectious agents. Acute diarrhoea may also be caused by drugs or toxins. Chronic diarrhoea is also most likely to be caused by infectious agents. However, other common causes include inflammatory bowel diseases, malabsorption, irritable bowel syndrome (idiopathic diarrhoea), medications and food additives. In all cases the source of the diarrhoea should be ascertained and appropriate treatment should then follow.

Acute gastrointestinal diarrhoea with vomiting is generally not suited to herbal therapy. This is because the patient will invariably vomit back the herbal treatment and may consequently develop an aversion to taking herbs.

Acute infectious diarrhoea in the absence of vomiting can be approached in the following way.

- Boost immunity with immune-enhancing herbs, particularly Echinacea and Picrorrhiza.
- Control fever with diaphoretic herbs such as *Mentha piperita* (peppermint) and Achillea (yarrow).
- If the infection does not involve a virus, Hydrastis (golden seal) or *Berberis vulgaris* (barberry) is indicated because of the antimicrobial activity of the berberine they contain. Berberine also inhibits the activity of enterotoxins. Citrus seed extract (*Citrus spp*) is also a highly active antimicrobial.

• If cytotoxins or mucosal invasion are part of the pathogenic process, antiinflammatory herbs such as Matricaria (chamomile) and mucilage-containing herbs, e.g. *Ulmus rubra* (slippery elm) are indicated.

• Tannin-containing herbs, e.g. *Geranium maculatum* (cranesbill), which act as astringents will also gently control diarrhoea without risk of aggravating the infection by reducing intestinal motility. They also reduce mucosal damage.

• Antiprotozoal agents include propolis, *Artemisia annua*, berberine-containing herbs and Euphorbia. Garlic can also be helpful as a gastrointestinal antiseptic.

• Normal conservative measures such as adequate fluid and electrolyte intake should also be implemented.

Chronic infectious diarrhoea is treated in a similar manner to acute infectious diarrhoea. However, particular emphasis should also be given to factors involved in host resistance.

• Gastrointestinal antiseptics, (e.g. Citrus seed, Hydrastis) especially when used (but not concurrently) with agents which encourage growth of normal flora (see Treatment of autoimmune diseases on p.144), will help to restore the protective activity of intestinal flora.

• Herbs to improve gastric acidity to prevent reinfection may also need emphasis. These include Coleus, Angelica, Zingiber (ginger), Capsicum (cayenne) and bitters such as Gentiana.

Case history

A female patient aged 35 presented with chronic infection with the protozoan Giardia which had persisted for more than 3 months. She was prescribed the following treatment (based on 1 week).

Echinacea angustifolia	1:2	35 ml
Picrorrhiza kurroa	1:2	10 ml
Angelica archangelica	1:2	15 ml
Propolis	1:10	20 ml
Zingiber officinale	1:2	5 ml
Matricaria chamomilla	1:2	15 ml
	Total	100 ml

Dose 5 ml with water three times a day.
Hydrastis (golden seal) 500 mg tablets at four per day were also prescribed and regular intake of a Lactobacillus culture at separate times was recommended.
After 4 weeks, symptoms were about the same. There was even a 1-week period when the patient felt that the herbs were aggravating her condition. After another 4 weeks there was considerable improvement and the condition was resolved by a further 8 weeks' treatment. Note that Picrorrhiza in the formula doubled as a bitter to increase gastric acid and as an immune-enhancing agent.

Diverticular disease

The main aim of herbal treatment in uncomplicated diverticular disease is to reduce stagnation and further degeneration of the bowel wall. Aspects of treatment include the following.

• Appropriate dietary measures to increase fibre intake (but excluding seeds and nuts) and supplementation with mucilaginous herbs such as Ulmus (slippery elm). This will also help to maintain healthy bowel flora.

• Gastrointestinal spasmolytics to decrease intracolonic pressure, e.g. *Viburnum opulus* (cramp bark), Dioscorea (wild yam) and Matricaria (chamomile).

• Herbs to improve connective tissue strength such as antioxidant herbs containing flavonoids oligomeric procyanidins (OPC) e.g. Vitis (grape seed extract) and Crataegus (hawthorn). *Polygonum multiflorum* is also thought to improve connective tissue and is also a gentle laxative.

• Gentle treatment of any associated constipation (see below).

Painful or symptomatic diverticular disease can also occur in the absence of diverticulitis. In medical thinking this is considered to be a variant of irritable bowel syndrome. However, it could result from a low-grade 'diverticulosis'. Depending on the assessment of the patient, this problem should either be treated as irritable bowel syndrome or the treatment approach described below to prevent recurrence of acute diverticulitis should otherwise be followed.

Acute diverticulitis usually requires hospitalization. Herbal treatment is more suited to prevention of its recurrence. As well as incorporating the aspects of treatment of uncomplicated diverticular disease described above, the approach to prevention of acute diverticulitis should additionally include:

- immune-enhancing herbs such as Echinacea to reduce pathogenic bacteria;
- gastrointestinal antiseptic herbs (see Gastrointestinal infections above);
- antiinflammatory gastrointestinal herbs such as Filipendula (meadowsweet) and Matricaria (chamomile).

Case history

A male patient aged 72 suffered an attack of acute diverticulitis and was concerned to prevent another episode.
Treatment consisted of the following prescription (based on 1 week).

Echinacea angustifolia	1:2	25 ml
Hydrastis canadensis	1:3	20 ml
Viburnum opulus	1:2	20 ml
Matricaria chamomilla	1:2	20 ml
Propolis	1:10	15 ml
	Total	100 ml

Dose 5 ml with water three times a day.
Slippery elm powder, one heaped teaspoon with water before each meal, was also prescribed.
The patient was also advised to have more fibre in his diet, particularly more fruit. Fresh garlic, one to two cloves a day, was also recommended for 3 days of every week. After 6 months the herbal treatment was discontinued but the fresh garlic (for 1–2 days a week), slippery elm and dietary changes were still observed. Several years later, the patient has not experienced any recurrence of acute diverticulitis.

Constipation

Constipation is medically defined as a bowel frequency of less than three times a week or the need to strain more than 25% of the time during defaecation. However, it is probably less than optimum for health to defaecate less than once a day. Herbalists certainly believe that regular bowel movements are necessary for the maintenance of good health. Constipation may be associated with diseases such as hypothyroidism and Parkinson's disease and these should always be excluded.

Use of the well-known and much maligned anthraquinone-containing herbal laxatives is widespread. On balance, the evidence is that these herbs are safe and effective when used in the short term. However, they are best used as a last resort since their effect is only symptomatic. Their tendency to cause wind and griping can aggravate the pain associated with irritable bowel syndrome and they are not at all suitable for constipation associated with bowel tension, spasm or irritability (see below). Also, the anthraquinone laxatives may become habit forming.

The herbal treatment of constipation can be approached in the following way.

• Improve liver function with choleretic and cholagogue herbs, e.g. Chionanthus (fringe tree), Taraxacum (dandelion root) and Silybum.

• Increase stool bulk through diet and with bulking herbs such as ulmus (slippery elm) and *Plantago ovata* (ispaghula).

• Improve motor function with gastrointestinal spasmolytics such as Matricaria (chamomile) or *Viburnum opulus* (cramp bark).

• Improve gastrointestinal lubrication. Linseeds are particularly suitable because of their oil and mucilage content.

• Judicious use of laxative herbs beginning with gentle agents such as *Juglans cinerea* (butternut), Rumex (yellow dock) Glycyrrhiza (licorice) and Rehmannia. Otherwise a minimum quantity of Cassia (senna) or *Rhamnus purshiana* (cascara) can be introduced.

Irritable bowel syndrome

Irritable bowel syndrome (IBS) can be a difficult disorder to comprehend and treat. One reason for this is that the diagnosis is only conclusively arrived at after exclusion of other known disorders. Hence, it is likely that IBS includes a number of different disorders lumped together under the one label. This can be seen in the fact that patients with IBS have at least three distinct symptom patterns. A more definitive approach towards diagnosis and classification will lead to a better understanding and management. For example, it is unreasonable to assume that IBS characterized by diarrhoea would necessarily respond to the same treatment as IBS in which constipation predominates, yet many clinical trials make no attempt to evaluate therapy in terms of initial symptoms.

IBS is the most common but yet least understood gastrointestinal disorder. There are three basic types:

- Functional diarrhoea, often without pain
- Chronic abdominal pain and constipation (spastic colitis)
- Abdominal pain with disturbed and variable bowel habit, i.e. constipation alternating with diarrhoea

The dated term 'mucous colitis' refers to the excessive amount of mucus which can be passed with stools.

The exact nature of the herbal treatment should depend on the factors identified in the individual case.

• An appropriate exclusion diet should be conducted.

• Spasmolytic herbs including Matricaria (chamomile), *Viburnum opulus* (cramp bark), *Mentha piperita* (peppermint). Matricaria is also a mild sedative.

• Sedative and nervine tonic herbs, particularly *Scutellaria lateriflora* (skullcap) and Valeriana (valerian).

• Hepatorestorative and choleretic herbs to improve liver function such as Silybum (St Mary's thistle), chionanthus (fringe tree) and Schisandra.

• Mucilage-containing herbs such as Ulmus (slippery elm), especially if there is constipation.

• Gastrointestinal antiseptics to restore normal bowel flora such as Hydrastis (golden seal), propolis and citrus seed extract. IBS patients may be intolerant of garlic.

• The presence of mucus implies irritation, and gastrointestinal antiinflammatories such as Filipendula (meadowsweet) and Matricaria (chamomile) are indicated.

• Constipation should be treated with only gentle herbs such as *Rumex crispus* (yellow dock), *Juglans cinerea* (butternut) and Taraxacum (dandelion root).

Case history

A female patient aged 42 complained of chronic episodes of discomfort and distension in the right lower abdomen. This could be quite sharp at times and was associated with a feeling of malaise. She was intolerant of fatty foods and had what she described as a 'sluggish bowel' although her motions were always 'loose'. Past medical history revealed that she had lived on the Solomon Islands for an extended period during which time she had amoebic dysentery and malaria. A number of recent medical tests, including colonoscopy, could not find any abnormalities. She also had a history of heart damage of undefined origin. For this reason Crataegus (hawthorn) was included in her treatment (the Chinese use Crataegus as a digestive herb).
The following treatment was prescribed.

Crataegus spp leaves	1:2	20 ml
Filipendula ulmaria	1:2	20 ml
Chionanthus virginicus	1:2	15 ml
Silybum marianum	1:1	15 ml
Matricaria chamomilla	1:2	20 ml
Viburnum opulus	1:2	20 ml
	Total	110 ml

Dose 5 ml with water three times daily.
Slippery elm, one heaped teaspoon with water three times a day, was also recommended.
After 4 weeks she reported a stunning transformation. In the whole month she had only experienced one bad day. She was feeling very well, eating better and had more energy. The patient will remain on her herbal treatment for some time. This was a patient who had spent many years and thousands of dollars on conventional medical treatment and yet had remained unwell.

Haemorrhoids

Haemorrhoids are aggravated by pelvic congestion (e.g. constipation and pregnancy) and prostatic enlargement. Some degree of loss of elasticity of the anal sphincter may play a role. Lifting heavy weights may aggravate the condition. Treatment could include the following.

• Increase dietary fibre, both soluble and insoluble.

• Mucilage-containing herbs such as Ulmus (slippery elm) and psyllium to keep the stool soft.

• Any associated constipation should be treated (see above).

• Oral treatment using herbs to improve venous and connective tissue tone. These include Aesculus (horsechestnut), Ruscus (butcher's broom) and *Polygonum multiflorum*. Flavonoid-containing herbs, e.g. Crataegus, also have this property. Melilotus (sweet clover) helps to relieve tissue congestion.

• Topical treatment with healing and astringent herbs such as Hamamelis (witchhazel), Symphytum (comfrey) and Calendula. Aesculus also works well topically, especially in gel formulations, but should not be applied if the piles are bleeding.

• If liver congestion exists, which will exacerbate pelvic congestion, treatment with choleretic and hepatoprotective herbs should be applied.

Case history

A male patient aged 35 had suffered from haemorrhoids for 8 years. He had been treated with rubber ligation but was still suffering problems such as irritation and occasional bleeding. He was not suffering from constipation but felt tense in the lower abdomen and was generally an anxious person. Other symptoms included indigestion, abdominal bloating and reflux. Treatment consisted of (based on 1 week):

Artemisia absinthium	1:5	10 ml
Aesculus hippocastanum	1:2	25ml
Melilotus officinale	1:2	20ml
Ruscus aculeatus	1:2	25ml
Valeriana officinalis	1:2	20ml
	Total	100ml

Dose 5 ml with water three times daily.

Slippery elm powder, one heaped teaspoon twice a day was also prescribed, together with comfrey ointment. Over the course of the next 16 weeks, the condition improved and he was free of any symptoms related to the haemorrhoids. He also reported feeling more relaxed.

References

1. Furness JB, Johnson PJ, Pompolo S, Bornstein JC. Evidence that enteric motility reflexes can be initiated through entirely intrinsic mechanisms in the guinea-pig small intestine. Neurogastroenterology and Motility 1995; 7 (2): 89–96
2. Barry MK, Aloisi JD, Yeo CJ Neural mechanisms in basal and meal-stimulated ideal absorption. Journal of Surgical Research 1995; 58 (4): 425–431
3. Kummer W. Neuronal specificity and plasticity in the autonomic nervous system. Anatomischer Anzeiger 1992; 174 (5): 409–417
4. Waterman SA, Tonini M, Costa M. The role of ascending excitatory and descending inhibitory pathways in peristalsis in the isolated guinea-pig small intestine. Journal of Physiology (Lond) 1994; 481 (pt 1): 223–232
5. De Ponti F, Cosentino M, Lecchini S et al. Physiopharmacology of the peristaltic reflex: an update. Italian Journal of Gastroenterology 1991; 23 (5): 264–269
6. Wingate DL. The effect of diet on small intestinal and biliary tract function. American Journal of Clinical Nutrition 1985; 42 (5 supp): 1020–1024
7. Mellander A, Abrahamsson H, Sjovall H. The migrating motor complex – the motor component of a cholinergic enteric secretomotor programme? Acta Physiologica Scandinavica 1995; 154 (3): 329–341
8. May B, Kuntz H, Kieser M, Koler S. Efficacy of a fixed peppermint oil/caraway oil combination in non-ulcer dyspepsia. Arzneimittel-Forschung 1996; 46 (II): 1149–1153
9. Cooke HJ. Neuroimmune signaling in regulation of intestinal ion transport. American Journal of Physiology 1994; 266 (2 pt 1): 167–178
10. Wisen O, Hellstrom PM. Gastrointestinal motility in obesity. Journal of Internal Medicine 1995; 237 (4): 411–418
11. Krentz K, Jablonowski H. In: Hellemans J, Vantrappen G (eds) Gastrointestinal tract disorders in the elderly. Churchill Livingstone, Edinburgh, 1984; pp 62–69
12. Hurwutz A, Brady DA, Schaal SE et al. Gastric acidity in older adults. JAMA 1997; 278 (8): 659–662
13. Ralph A, Giannella MD, Selwyn A et al. Influence of gastric acidity on bacterial and parasitic enteric infections. Annals of Internal Medicine 1973; 78 (2): 271–276
14. Torsoli A, Severi C. The neuroendocrine control of gastrointestinal motor activity. Journal of Physiology Paris 1993; 87 (6): 367–374
15. Minton NA. Volunteer models for predicting antiemetic activity of 5-HT3-receptor antagonists. British Journal of Clinical Pharmacology 1994; 37 (6): 525–530
16. Costall B, Naylor RJ. Neuropharmacology of emesis in relation to clinical response. British Journal of Cancer 1992; 19: 2–7
17. Beubler E, Schirgi-Degen A. Serotonin antagonists inhibit sennoside-induced fluid secretion and diarrhea. Pharmacology 1993; 47 (supp): 64–69
18. Grider JR. CGRP as a transmitter in the sensory pathway mediating peristaltic reflex. American Journal of Physiology 1994; 266 (6 pt 1): 1139–1145
19. Serdiuk SE, Komissarov IV, Gmiro VE. The role of the chemosensory systems in the inhibitory regulation of cholinergic transmission in the small intestine. Fiziologiche Zhurnal 1993; 39 (1): 54–61
20. Furness JB, Costa M. Projections of intestinal neurons showing immunoreactivity for vasoactive intestinal polypeptide are consistent with these neurons being the enteric inhibitory neurons. Neuroscience Letters 1979; 15 (2–3): 199–204
21. Donnerer J, Bartho L, Holzer P, Lembeck F. Intestinal peristalsis associated with release of immunoreactive substance P. Neuroscience 1984; 11 (4): 913–918.
22. Glatzel H, Rüberg-Schweer M. Regional influence on cutaneous blood flow effected by oral spice intake. Nutr. Dieta 1968; 10: 194–214
23. Liddle RA. Regulation of cholecystokinin secretion by intraluminal releasing factors. American Journal of Physiology 1995; 269 (3 pt 1): 319–327
24. Eckel LA, Ossenkopp KP. Cholecystokinin reduces sucrose palatability in rats: evidence in support of a satiety effect. American Journal of Physiology 1994; 267 (6 pt 2): R1496–1502
25. Blundell JE, King NA. Overconsumption as a cause of weight gain: behavioural-physiological interactions in the control of food intake (appetite). Ciba Foundation Symposium 1996; 201: 138–154 154–8, 188–93
26. Holt S, Brand J, Soveny C, Hansky J. Relationship of satiety to postprandial glycaemic, insulin and cholecystokinin responses. Appetite 1992; 18 (2): 129–141
27. Bartness TJ, Waldbillig RJ. Cholecystokinin-induced suppression of feeding: an evaluation of the generality of gustatory-cholecystokinin interactions. Physiology and Behaviour 1984; 32 (3): 409–415
28. Morley JE, Silver AJ. Anorexia in the elderly. Neurobiology and Aging 1988; 9 (1): 9–16
29. Takeuchi T, Shiratori K, Watanabe S et al. Secretin as a potential mediator of antiulcer actions of mucosal protective agents. Journal of Clinical Gastroenterology 1991; 13 (supp): S83–87
30. Shiratori K, Watanabe S, Takeuchi T. Effect of licorice extract (Fm100) on release of secretin and exocrine pancreatic secretion in humans. Pancreas 1986; 1 (6): 483–487
31. Grider JR, Makhlouf GM. Enteric GABA: mode of action and role in the regulation of the peristaltic reflex. Am J Physiol 1992; 262 (4 pt 1): 690–694
32. Krantis A, Costa M, Furness JB, Orbach J. Gamma-aminobutyric acid stimulates intrinsic inhibitory and excitatory nerves in the guinea-pig intestine. European Journal of Pharmacology 1980; 67 (4): 461–468
33. Bjarnason I. Intestinal permeability. Gut 1994; 35 (1 supp): 18–22
34. Lee EB, Kim OK, Jung CS, Jung KH. The influence of methanol extract of Ulmus davidiana var. Japonica cortex on gastric erosion and ulcer and paw edema in rats. Yakhak Hoeji 1995; 39 (6): 671–675
35. Hoogkamp-Korstanje JA, Lindner JG, Marcelis JH et al. Composition and ecology of the human intestinal flora. Antonie Van Leeuwenhoek 1979; 45 (1): 35–40
36. Van Eldere J, Robben J, Caenepeel P, Eyssen H. Influence of a cecal volume-reducing intestinal microflora on the excretion and entero-hepatic circulation of steroids and bile acids. Journal of Steroid Biochemistry 1988; 29 (1): 33–39
37. Ozawa A, Ohnishi N, Tazume S et al. Intestinal bacterial flora and host defense mechanisms. Tokai Journal of Experimental and Clinical Medicine 1986; 11 (supp): 65–79
38. Rolfe RD. Interactions among microorganisms of the indigenous intestinal flora and their influence on the host. Reviews of Infectious Diseases 1984; 6 (supp 1): 73–79

39. Walker WA, Bloch KJ. Gastrointestinal transport of macromolecules in the pathogenesis of food allergy. Annals of Allergy 1983; 51 (2 pt 2): 240–245
40. Heine W, Zunft HJ, Muller-Beuthow W, Grutte FK. Lactose and protein absorption from breast milk and cow's milk preparations and its influence on the intestinal flora. Acta Paediatrica Scandinavica 1977; 66 (6): 699–703
41. Kruis W, Forstmaier G, Scheurlen C, Stellaard F. Effect of diets low and high in refined sugars on gut transit, bile acid metabolism, and bacterial fermentation. Gut 1991; 32 (4): 367–371
42. Bjorneklett A, Midtvedt T. Influence of three antimicrobial agents – penicillin, metronidazole, and doxycyclin – on the intestinal microflora of healthy humans. Scandinavian Journal of Gastroenterology 1981; 16 (4): 473–480
43. Hooker KD, DiPiro JT. Effect of antimicrobial therapy on bowel flora. Clinical Pharmacology 1988; 7 (12): 878–888
44. Grossman RF. The relationship of absorption characteristics and gastrointestinal side effects of oral antimicrobial agents. Clinical Therapeutics 1991; 13 (1): 189–193
45. Graninger W. Disorders of intestinal flora in intensive care patients. Leber, Magen, Darm 1985; 15 (5): 192–197
46. Goldin BR. Intestinal microflora: metabolism of drugs and carcinogens. Annals of Medicine 1990; 22 (1): 43–48
47. Rowland IR. Interactions of the gut microflora and the host in toxicology. Toxicologic Pathology 1988; 16 (2): 147–153
48. Kanazawa K, Konishi F, Mitsuoka T. Factors influencing the development of sigmoid colon cancer. Bacteriologic and biochemical studies. Cancer 1996; 77 (8 supp): 1701–1706
49. Parsonnet J. Bacterial infection as a cause of cancer. Environmental Health Perspectives 1995; 103 (supp 8): 263–268
50. Tazume S, Ozawa A, Yamamoto T et al. Ecological study on the intestinal bacteria flora of patients with diarrhea. Clinical Infectious Diseases 1993; 16 (supp 2): 77–82
51. Gorbach SL. Estrogens, breast cancer, and intestinal flora. Reviews of Infectious Diseases 1984; 6 (supp 1): 85–90.
52. Sacquet E, Leprince C, Riottot M, Raibaud P. Dietary fiber and cholesterol and bile acid metabolism in axenic (germfree) and holoxenic (conventional) rats. III. Effect of nonsterilized pectin. Reproduction, Nutrition, Development 1985; 25 (1A): 93–100
53. Hidaka H, Hirayama M. Useful characteristics and commercial applications of fructo-oligosaccharides. Biochemical Society Transactions 1991; 19 (3): 561–565
54. Praznik W, Spies T. Fructo-oligosaccharides from Urginea maritima. Carbohydrate Research 1993; 243 (1); 91–97
55. Mitsuoka T, Hidaka H, Eida T. Effect of fructo-oligosaccharides on intestinal microflora. Nahrung 1987; 31 (5–6): 427–436
56. Bouhnik Y, Flourié B, Riottot M et al. Effects of fructo-oligosaccharides ingestion on fecal bifidobacteria and selected metabolic indexes of colon carcinogenesis in healthy humans. Nutrition and Cancer 1996; 26 (1): 21–29
57. Willard MD, Simpson RB, Delles EK et al. Effects of dietary supplementation of fructo-oligosaccharides on small intestinal bacterial overgrowth in dogs. American Journal of Veterinary Research 1994; 55 (5): 654–659
58. Pierre F, Perrin P, Champ M et al. Short-chain fructo-oligosaccharides reduce the occurrence of colon tumors and develop gut-associated lymphoid tissue in Min mice. Cancer Research 1997; 57 (2): 225–228
59. Glatzel H, Rüberg-Schweer M. Regional influence on cutaneous blood flow effected by oral spice intake. Nutr. Dieta 1968; 10: 194–214
60. Saetta JP, March S, Gaunt ME, Quinton DN. Gastric emptying procedures in the self-poisoned patients: are we forcing gastric content beyond the pylorus? Journal of the Royal Society of Medicine 1991; 84 (5): 274–276
61. Vale JA. Primary decontamination: vomiting, gastric irrigation or only medicinal charcoal? Therapeutische Umschau 1992; 49 (2): 102–106
62. Underhill TJ, Greene MK, Dove AF. A comparison of the efficacy of gastric lavage, ipecacuanha and activated charcoal in the emergency management of paracetamol overdose. Archives of Emergency Medicine 1990; 7 (3): 148–154
63. Ilett KF, Gibb SM, Unsworth RW. Syrup of ipecacuanha as an emetic in adults. Medical Journal of Australia 1997; 2 (3): 91–93
64. Pons J, Bouhours G. Use of anthraquinones derived from rhubarb in dentistry. Information Dentaire 1971; 53: 3201
65. Roberts F. Modern herbalism for digestive disorders. Thomsons, Northamptonshire, 1981

BILIARY SYSTEM

SCOPE

Apart from their use to provide non-specific support for recuperation and repair, specific phytotherapeutic strategies include the following.

Treatment of:

- cholecystitis (biliary infection);
- minor or early cholelithiasis (biliary stones);
- conjugated hyperbilirubinaemia.

Management of:

- established cholelithiasis;
- chronic and moderate hepatobiliary diseases.

Because of the use of secondary plant products, particular **caution** is necessary in applying phytotherapy to:

- biliary carcinoma;
- blocked bile duct;
- acute and severe hepatobiliary diseases.

BACKGROUND

Bile acids/salts and mechanisms of biliary flow

Whereas cholesterol accounts for more than 90–95% of the sterols in bile, bile acids and their salts are the most important solutes; they are essential in the management of cholesterol levels and themselves help determine the extent of bile flow. Bile acids are synthesized from cholesterol in the liver. There are three groups. Primary bile acids, in humans mainly cholic and chenodeoxycholic acids and their salts, are produced directly. Secondary bile salts are created by the action of intestinal bacteria on primary bile salts with deoxycholate and lithocholate being formed from cholate and chenodeoxycholate, respectively. Tertiary bile salts are the result of modification of secondary bile salts by intestinal flora or hepatocytes; in humans these include the sulphate ester of lithocholate and ursodeoxycholate and the 7-beta-epimer of chenodeoxycholate.[1]

Bile flow rates and composition are subject to a wide variety of neural, endocrine and paracrine influences. One of the main stimulants of bile flow are bile acids themselves, either in their primary form or reabsorbed as secondary or tertiary forms in the enterohepatic circulation (see below). The cholagogic effects of bile acids have led to their prescription in hepatobiliary disorders. One derivative, ursodeoxycholic acid, has been shown in controlled clinical studies to be a useful agent in the management of patients with primary biliary cirrhosis, autoimmune chronic active hepatitis[2] and cystic fibrosis.[3]

Cholestasis

Infective conditions may lead to cholestasis or reduced bile flow. This has been attributed to the effects of lipopolysaccharide endotoxins.[4] Chronic alcoholics may have hypotonic gallbladder, with increased speed of bile secretion and low biliary levels of cholic acid, cholesterol and bilirubin. Patterns of bile stagnation can occur with increasing severity of alcoholism, especially when associated with cirrhosis.[5]

In one study serum cholestanol/cholesterol proportions were determined in 79 patients with inflammatory bowel (colonic and ileal) diseases, such as ulcerative colitis and Crohn's disease, and 23 with irritable bowel syndrome as controls. The findings suggested that the increased cholestanol proportion in colonic inflammatory bowel diseases is determined mainly by impaired biliary elimination of this sterol, while in ileal disease the dominating change in sterol balance is activated cholesterol synthesis. Increased serum cholestanol is a novel finding in colonic inflammatory bowel diseases, apparently indicating the presence of subclinical cholestasis in a marked number (20–50%) of inflammatory bowel disease patients.[6]

Therapeutic stimulation of bile flow could thus be justified in the management and treatment of any of the above circumstances (see below).

It appears that a substantial amount of urate is also eliminated by the biliary route in humans. Gout and other urate-associated conditions linked to decreased renal urate excretion may therefore benefit from measures that increase biliary urate excretion.[7]

Toxicity of bile acids

Because it is known that high concentrations of bile acids are cytotoxic, it has been speculated that their raised presence in serum and tissues in hepatobiliary diseases contributes to the pathological progression of these disorders. Bile acids are a causative factor in chronic gastritis.[8] Recent evidence suggests that oral administration of ursodeoxycholate, being a relatively non-toxic bile acid, can replace more hydrophobic hepatotoxic bile acids in the circulating pool and by doing so, ameliorate the harmful effects of the latter.[9] Although one further clinical study suggests that beneficial effects are not universal,[10] these data highlight the implications for health of the development or retention of relatively toxic bile metabolites.

Enterohepatic circulation

An important aspect of bile acid function and toxicity is the constant reabsorption from the intestine into the portal circulation and back to the liver and biliary system – the enterohepatic circulation. Both primary and secondary bile acids are involved in this recycling. In modern medicine a high degree of recycling is assumed but it is likely that humans living a more primitive lifestyle with much higher levels of fibre intake had lower reabsorption rates. The implications of enterohepatic circulation are best understood with reference to the kinetics of drugs like the morphine alkaloids and digoxin which are largely eliminated from the body through the bile. Increased retention of bile in the enterohepatic circulation is known to increase the half-life of these and other drugs in the body. It is likely, therefore, that the level of bile products (with the formation of tertiary bile acids) and other, potentially toxic metabolites may increase unless the enterohepatic circulation is at as low a level as possible. In practice, this is most likely to follow a relatively fast intestinal transit time, associated with a high-fibre diet.

Bile and cholesterol

Although they are generally cholagogic, the presence of bile acids in the enterohepatic cycle acts to decrease the biliary secretion of cholesterol, presumably through a process of negative feedback, and this is likely to control excessive cholesterol secretion in gallstone conditions. As with other hepatic conditions, replacement therapy with bile acids like chenodeoxycholic and ursodeoxycholic acids is promoted as a treatment, leading even to dissolution of existing gallstones.[11]

Of wider significance is the finding that reduction in the absorption of bile acids from the gut, associated with, for example, diarrhoea, leads to an increase in cholesterol synthesis and cholesterol esterification rate by the liver.[12,13]

Effects of bile acids in the intestinal tract

Both primary and secondary bile acids have secretagogue effects on the intestinal mucosa, changing net fluid transport across the villi from absorption to secretion.[14] There is also an atropine-inhibited (i.e. cholinergic) stimulation of intestinal contractions[15] and an increased mucosal vasodilation (blood flow increasing by around 50%) which is not inhibited by atropine.[16] Secondary bile acids in particular are thought to increase permeability at the zonulae occludentes which bind endothelial cells together at their luminal borders so that normal subepithelial hydrostatic pressure is raised sufficiently to reverse net sodium, chloride and water absorption to net secretion.[17]

Bile has sometimes been referred to as the body's own laxative or 'endolaxative'. Indeed, it is established that bile acids (especially secondary bile acids – see below) can be responsible for bowel looseness and their effects should be borne in mind in cases of unexplained chronic diarrhoea.[18,19]

Bile has a wider range of actions on the intestinal mucosa. Where there is clear reduction in bile levels, there is a reduction in thickness of the mucus blanket, reduced numbers of mucus-associated enterocytes (suggesting a reduced endothelial turnover rate) and lymphocytes and increased populations of bacterial organisms. The implication is that normal bile function is a vital part of the body's gut-related defences.[20] It has also been demonstrated that bacterial endotoxin absorption is increased in the absence of bile salts from the intestine.[21]

Bacterial action on bile acids – consequences and implications

The generally positive functions of primary bile acids become rather more mixed in their effects once bacterial deconjugation and dehydroxylation occur. Secondary bile acids are produced at a very early age – the process is clearly under way even in month-old infants[22] – and are an entirely normal range of metabolites. It is clear that most bacterial deconjugation occurs in the colon[23] but in various less ideal circumstances invasive bacterial populations can lead to secondary bile product formation in the small intestine.

Secondary bile acids have a decidedly irritating effect on the intestinal wall. Exposure of the intestinal wall to deconjugated bile acids stimulates local inflammatory mechanisms, accompanied by the release of prostaglandin E_2 and leukotriene C_4. Such effects are particularly pronounced if there is already latent or active inflammatory disease of the intestinal wall, particularly in small intestinal Crohn's disease.[24] The irritant effect of secondary bile products is especially apparent if their quantities are increased due to stasis in the small intestine. Among a number of ultrastructural alterations to the intestinal mucosa, they increase the numbers of lysosomal vascular structures, fused microvilli and dilated endoplasmic reticulum, which among other implications leads to a reduced absorption of solutes including glucose and other carbohydrates[25,26] and, significantly, fluid absorption:[27] diarrhoea is thus possible. Secondary bile metabolites substantially increase the absorption rates of urea and oxalates from the gut.[28]

There are more insidious potential effects too. Secondary bile acids and their metabolites increase colonic cell proliferation.[29] The carcinogenic effect is clearly linked to changes in the nature of bacterial populations in the gut rather than to the nature of the bile acids or indeed other starting materials in the gut.[30] However, there is also little doubt that decreased reabsorption of bile acids (for example, as seen with increasing old age) does increase the likelihood that carcinogenic and other pathogenic bile metabolites will be produced.[31]

Dietary factors are known to affect the balance between intestinal flora and bile metabolism. For example, consumption of sugars was shown in nine volunteers on a crossover basis to significantly prolong transit time through the colon and significantly raise the faecal levels of both primary and secondary bile metabolites.[32] On the other hand, the consumption of 16 g of wheat bran a day on a double-blind 6-month crossover basis by ulcerative colitis sufferers in remission was shown to decrease the faecal concentration of bile acids by almost half. No such effect was observed with psyllium seed.[33]

There are some potential benefits in bacterial action on bile acids. Anaerobic bacteria, for example, can produce volatile fatty acids which are known to non-specifically inhibit pathogenic bacterial populations.[34]

Bile acids in diseases

Disturbed and pathological states can change the dynamics of bile and other intestinal relationships. In malnutrition, for example, morphological changes in the intestinal wall lead to increased sensitivity to the effects of secondary bile acids, poor absorption of fats and other nutrients, all of which is compounded by changes in intestinal flora.[35]

The impact of inflammatory intestinal diseases like Crohn's is even more pronounced. The damage induced by the disease on the intestinal wall leads to reduced bile acid reabsorption[36] and compensatory increased cholesterol synthesis by the liver,[36] a reaction that probably explains the high level of biliary disease like gallstones in sufferers from Crohn's.[37,38] The link between inflammatory bowel disease and cholestasis has already been mentioned.

Similar negative impact on enterohepatic circulation follows small intestinal resection which has been shown to lead to increased synthesis of both bile acids and cholesterol.[39]

The association between biliary and intestinal functions is further highlighted in the condition primary sclerosing cholangitis, a disease characterized by inflammation and obliterative fibrosis of bile ducts. In 70% of cases it is associated with ulcerative colitis. In about two-thirds, there are circulating IgG antibodies to a peptide shared by epithelial cell walls in both bile ducts and colon. Another suggested cause is portal bacteraemia secondary to diseased bowel wall. The addition of bile acids to the gut has been proposed as a treatment.[40,41,42]

PHYTOTHERAPEUTICS

Plant constituents, cholesterol and bile function

In spite of its obvious significance, the dynamics of cholesterol has been little studied. In part, this is because observations are difficult. There is considerable interchange of cholesterol and its metabolites and analogues and it has proved impossible to track cholesterol through the body. A useful insight, however, has been made in studies of the metabolism of plant sterols. Plant sterols are structurally similar to cholesterol but, because of poor intestinal absorption, are ordinarily not present in the liver. However, there does appear to be some competition in the movement of plant sterols and cholesterol. For example, the proportions of plant sterols are significantly lower in cholesterol-rich gallstones than in bile but stones with low cholesterol content are proportionately richer in plant sterols.[43] One sterol studied, sitostanol, parallels the secretion from and distribution of cholesterol in the liver (e.g. both requiring bile salts for secretion in bile) so that it can be used as a physiologic analogue of unesterified cholesterol to trace the transport of sterols through the liver.[44] Such studies, for example, indicate that high-density lipoproteins (HDLs) are necessary along with bile acids for cholesterol elimination in bile.[45] The use of plant sterols (in this case campesterol and sitosterol) as markers of cholesterol absorption and biliary secretion was also seen in a study referred to above, showing subclinical cholestasis as a feature of bowel inflammatory disease.[37]

When serum concentrations and metabolism of cholesterol were studied in human vegetarians, cholesterol absorption was found to be normal and synthesis was slightly enhanced, though without increase in serum cholesterol precursors. The serum concentrations of total and low-density lipoprotein cholesterol were decreased but in addition to the obvious lower intake of cholesterol itself, it appeared that the higher intake of plant sterols interfered with cholesterol absorption and thus increased endogenous cholesterol synthesis. Thus, cholesterol saturation and bile acid composition of the bile were not changed. Biliary excretion of plant sterols was apparently relatively inefficient.[46]

Interactions between cholesterol transport and plant constituents extend to another major group. Saponins have been implicated in interference with the absorption of cholesterol, bile acids and fats, leading to reduced animal growth, but also have shown potential in the reduction of blood cholesterol levels. There is evidence of interference with the absorption of vitamins A and E.[47] Their cholesterol-lowering effect may also be linked to their binding of bile salts and increasing their faecal excretion, thus increasing bile salt synthesis by endogenous cholesterol.[48] Further studies to investigate the effects of saponins on bile, cholesterol and lipid metabolism are clearly warranted. One steroidal sapogenin that has been studied, diosgenin, is, like the sterols, also similar enough in structure to cholesterol to interfere with its esterification in the liver.[49] This may contribute to a marked increase observed in biliary cholesterol relative to phospholipids when it was fed for 7 days to rats.[50]

The role of dietary plant lipids in cholesterol elimination has also been studied. In rats a sunflower seed oil-enriched diet has been shown to reduce liver cholesterol levels and increase faecal excretion of cholesterol.[51]

There is the prospect of increased retention of bile acids in the body with the use of tannins as bowel astringents. Although this may have some beneficial effects (see above), the chances are that negative or even toxic metabolites may also accumulate and on balance this prospect adds to the usual caution against using large doses of tannins for a long time.

Choleretics and cholagogues

There is a traditional differentiation made between cholagogues and choleretics. The former are agents that stimulate the release of bile that has already been formed in the biliary system. Bile acids are the main endogenous cholagogues; fatty foods the most obvious exogenous factors.

Choleretics stimulate bile production by hepatocytes and most have effective cholagogue properties as well. Cholecystokinin, secretin and some of the other humoral agents are involved endogenously. Bitters and some of the botanical agents referred to below are likely to have choleretic activity.

There is very little interest in choleretic and cholagogue treatments in conventional medicine, at least in the English-speaking world. Among agents incidentally discovered, NSAIDs, especially aspirin (in one study at a level of 100 mg/kg), cause choleresis in animals.[52] Magnesium sulphate (Epsom salts), sometimes used for constipation, has at doses of 500 mg been shown to exert a direct effect on the motor activity of the gallbladder in dogs.[53]

Research on herbal choleretics and cholagogues has largely come from Germany and Eastern Europe. It is not comprehensive and most practice in this area is informed by traditional reputation. Given the difficulty in knowing what actually happens in the liver and the potential risks of counterproductive treatments (see below), this is not an ideal situation.

Among the work that has been done, it has been shown that the ethanolic extract of *Chelidonium majus* (greater celandine) in isolated liver culture significantly caused choloresis by increasing bile acid-independent flow.[54,55] A survey of the literature shows that *Cynara scolymus* (artichoke) possesses choleretic, diuretic and hypocholesterolaemic properties. The main active components of this plant are mono- and dicaffeylquinic acids, flavonoids and sesquiterpenes. The most suitable raw material is fresh leaves in the plant's first year of growth.[56] Phenolic acids in *Mentha longifolia* were found to possess significant in vivo choleretic and CNS stimulative effects.[57] The potential of *Curcuma comosa* rhizome as a choleretic and hypocholesterolaemic treatment has been supported in experimental studies.[58] This activity was later linked to a phloracetophenone glucoside.[59]

CHOLERETICS AND CHOLAGOGUES

Plant remedies traditionally used as choleretics and cholagogues

Berberis vulgaris (barberry), *Berberis aquifolium* (Oregon grape), Chelidonium (greater celandine), Chelone (balmony), Chionanthus (fringe-tree), Dioscorea (wild yam), *Euonymus atropurpureus* (wahoo), Taraxacum (dandelion), Veronicastrum (black root), Peumus (boldo).

Indications for choleretics and cholagogues

- Non-impacted gallstones
- Moderate cholecystitis (gallbladder infection)
- Conjugated hyperbilirubinaemia (jaundice due to decreased excretion of conjugated bilirubin through the bile duct)

Other traditional indications for choleretics and cholagogues

- 'Bilious' conditions associated with heaviness in the epigastrium, nausea, susceptibility to alcohol and fats, headaches
- 'Toxic' conditions associated with intestinal congestion, especially in skin and autoimmune diseases
- Constipation

Contraindications for choleretics and cholagogues

The effects of choleretic and cholagogue agents may be different in the diseased liver than the response produced in the normal liver. For example, experimental evidence suggests that the use of choleretic agents where hepatobiliary damage (e.g. cholangitis) is caused by obstructive jaundice might further depress hepatic functions.[60]

The use of choleretics and cholagogues is either contraindicated or at least inappropriate in the following.

- Obstructed bile ducts (due to impacted gallstones, cholangitis or cancer of bile duct or pancreas)
- Unconjugated hyperbilirubinaemia (jaundice following haemolytic diseases, hereditary disease like Gilbert's and Crigler–Najjar syndromes)
- Acute or severe hepatocellular disease (e.g. following viral hepatitis, cirrhosis, adverse reactions to drugs, e.g. anaesthetics, steroids, oestrogen, chlorpromazine)
- Septic cholecystitis (where there is a risk of peritonitis)
- Intestinal spasm or ileus
- Liver cancer

Traditional therapeutic insights into the use of choleretics and cholagogues

Stimulating bile flow has been seen as one of the main eliminative strategies in traditional medi-cine, reflecting the importance attached by even the most primitive cultures to the role of the liver (the name of the organ was often as evocative as it is in English).

However, bile stimulation was often accompanied by vigorous approaches to eliminating it from the gut as well; the almost universal reliance in folk medicine on emetics and purgatives as first-resort approaches to the treatment of acute disease almost certainly had the effect, intended or otherwise (and in the case of emetics it was often intended), of radically removing bile from the body. It is now easy in modern medicine to dismiss the use of such drastic procedures as useless or dangerous but, unlike the use of bleeding, which was often likely to be counterproductive, emesis and catharsis were almost prehuman measures and established themselves over millennia in the most demanding court of efficacy, the survival from acute disease.

Given what is now known of the retentive qualities of the enterohepatic cycle, the certainty that modern diets and lifestyle have significantly lengthened intestinal transit time compared to that of early humans, thus extending enterohepatic recycling further, it is likely that many modern practitioners might look with some envy at their forebears' ability to get rid of this pool of potentially or actually toxic metabolites. However, emesis and catharsis were seen as an option for the most robust constitutions and apart from the obvious inappropriateness, they are contraindicated in the more chronic and low-vitality conditions most often seen in the modern clinic.

Modern techniques to eliminate the bile pool generally involve dietary and other measures to decrease intestinal transit time combined with the use of choleretics and cholagogues. Some of the latter actually have laxative effects in any case, either because they contain the appropriate constituents or, more often, because their release of more bile is in itself laxative.

Application

Choleretics and cholagogues are best taken before meals, preferably about 30 minutes, but immediately before will suffice. They may, however, have contradictory effects if taken with or after food. As many rely at least in part on the effect of bitter constituents, they should be taken in fluid form.

Long-term therapy is probably not appropriate and clinical experience is that for maximum benefit, they are best applied for short duration, of up to 2 weeks at a time, sometimes much shorter.

Advanced phytotherapeutics

Choleretics and cholagogues may also be usefully applied in some cases (depending on other factors) of:

- constipation (not due to intestinal spasm nor responding to conventional measures);
- migraine;
- acne rosacea;
- inflammatory bowel disease;
- dysbiotic conditions of the gut;
- chronic skin diseases;
- autoimmune diseases (especially where associated with any of the above – see relevant sections).

References

1. Hay DW, Carey MC. Chemical species of lipids in bile. Hepatology 1990; 12 (3 pt 2): 6–14
2. Heathcote EJ, Cauch-Dudek K, Walker V et al. The Canadian multicenter double-blind randomized controlled trial of ursodeoxycholic acid in primary biliary cirrhosis. Hepatology 1994; 19 (5): 1149–1156
3. Van Demeeberg PC, Houwen RHJ, Sinaasappel M et al. Low-dose versus high-dose in cystic fibrosis-related cholestatic liver disease: results of a randomized study with 1-year follow-up. Scandinavian Journal of Gastroenterology 1997; 32 (4): 369–373
4. Trauner M, Nathanson MH, Rydberg SA et al. Endotoxin impairs biliary glutathione and HCO-3-excretion and blocks the choleretic effect of nitric oxide in rat liver. Hepatology 1997; 25 (5): 1184–1191
5. Mikhailovskaya AY, Loranskaya TI, Vasilevskaya LS. Liver bile-secreting function in chronic alcoholics and means of correction of its disorders. Voprosy Pitaniya 1995; (5): 34–36
6. Hakala K, Vuoristo M, Miettinen TA. Serum cholestanol, cholesterol precursors and plant sterols in different inflammatory bowel diseases. Digestion 1996; 57 (2): 83–89
7. Kountouras J, Magoula I, Tsapas G, Liatsis I. The effect of mannitol and secretin on the biliary transport of urate in humans. Hepatology 1996; 23 (2): 229–233
8. Kolarski V, Petrova-Shopova K, Vasileva E et al. Erosive gastritis and gastroduodenitis – clinical, diagnostic and therapeutic studies. Vutr Boles 1987; 26 (3): 56–59
9. Leveille-Webster C. Bile acids: what's new? Seminars in Veterinary Medicine and Surgery (Small Animal) 1997; 12 (1): 2–9
10. De Maria N, Colantoni A, Rosenbloom E, Van Thiel DH. Ursodeoxycholic acid does not improve the clinical course of primary sclerosing cholangitis over a 2-year period. Hepatogastroenterology 1996; 43 (12): 1472–1479
11. Hofmann AF. Bile acids as drugs: principles, mechanisms of action and formulations. Italian Journal of Gastroenterology 1995; 27 (2): 106–113
12. Akerlund JE, Reihner E, Angelin B et al. Hepatic metabolism of cholesterol in Crohn's disease. Effect of partial resection of ileum. Gastroenterology 1991; 100 (4): 1046–1053
13. Stahlberg D, Reihner E, Angelin B, Einarsson K. Interruption of the enterohepatic circulation of bile acids stimulates the esterification rate of cholesterol in human liver. Journal of Lipid Research 1991; 32 (9): 1409–1415
14. Gaginella TS, Haddad AC, Go VL, Phillips SF. Cytotoxicity of ricinoleic acid (castor oil) and other intestinal secretagogues on isolated intestinal epithelial cells. Journal of Pharmacology and Experimental Therapeutics 1977; 201 (1): 259–266
15. Karlstrom L. Evidence of involvement of the enteric nervous system in the effects of sodium deoxycholate on small-intestinal transepithelial fluid transport and motility. Scandinavian Journal of Gastroenterology 1986; 21 (3): 321–330
16. Karlstrom L. Mechanisms in bile salt-induced secretion in the small intestine. An experimental study in rats and cats. Acta Physiologica Scandinavica 1986; 549: 1–48
17. Wanitschke R. Intestinal filtration as a consequence of increased mucosal hydraulic permeability. A new concept for laxative action. Klinische Wochenschrift 1980; 58 (6): 267–278
18. Pickert A, Muller M. Chologenic diarrhea. Deutsche Medizinische Wochenschrift 1991; 116 (20): 796–797
19. Ford GA, Preece JD, Davies IH, Wilkinson SP. Use of the SeHCAT test in the investigation of diarrhoea. Postgraduate Medical Journal 1992; 68 (798): 272–276
20. Kalambaheti T, Cooper GN, Jackson GD. Role of bile in non-specific defence mechanisms of the gut. Gut 1994; 35 (8): 1047–1052
21. Cahill CJ, Pain JA, Bailey ME. Bile salts, endotoxin and renal function in obstructive jaundice. Surgery Gynecology Obstetrics 1987; 165 (6): 519–522
22. Jonsson G, Midtvedt AC, Norman A, Midtvedt T. Intestinal microbial bile acid transformation in healthy infants. Journal of Pediatric Gastroenterology and Nutrition 1995; 20 (4): 394–402
23. Bruwer M, Stern J, Stiehl A, Herfarth C. Changes in fecal bile acid excretion after proctocolectomy. Zeitschrift für Gastroenterologie 1996; 34 (2): 105–110
24. Casellas F, Guarner F, Antolin M et al. Abnormal leukotriene C4 released by unaffected jejunal mucosa in patients with inactive Crohn's disease. Gut 1994; 35 (4): 517–522
25. Wehman HJ, Lifshitz F, Teichberg S. Effects of enteric microbial overgrowth on small intestinal ultrastructure in the rat. American Journal of Gastroenterology 1978; 70 (3): 249–258
26. Lifshitz F, Wapnir RA, Wehman HJ et al. The effects of small intestinal colonization by fecal and colonic bacteria on intestinal function in rats. Journal of Nutrition 1978; 108 (12), 1913–1923
27. Fukushima T, Ishiguro N, Tsujinaka Y et al. Bile acid deconjugation in intestinal obstruction studied by breath test. Japan Journal of Surgery 1977; 7 (2): 73–81
28. Dobbins JW, Binder HJ. Effect of bile salts and fatty acids on the colonic absorption of oxalate. Gastroenterology 1976; 70 (6): 1096–1100
29. Parsonnet J. Bacterial infection as a cause of cancer. Environmental Health Perspectives 1995; 103 (supp 8): 263–268
30. Kanazawa K, Konishi F, Mitsuoka T et al. Factors influencing the development of sigmoid colon cancer. Bacteriologic and biochemical studies. Cancer 1996; 77 (8 supp): 1701–1706
31. Salemans JM, Nagengast FM, Tangerman A et al. Effect of ageing on postprandial conjugated and unconjugated serum bile acid levels in healthy subjects. European Journal of Clinical Investigation 1993; 23 (3): 192–198
32. Kruis W, Forstmaier G, Scheurlen C, Stellaard F. Effect of diets low and high in refined sugars on gut transit, bile acid metabolism, and bacterial fermentation. Gut 1991; 32 (4): 367–371
33. Ejderhamn J, Hedenborg G, Strandvik B. Long-term double-blind study on the influence of dietary fibres on faecal bile acid excretion in juvenile ulcerative colitis. Scandinavian Journal of Clinical and Laboratory Investigation 1992; 52 (7): 697–706
34. Tazume S, Ozawa A, Yamamoto T et al. Ecological study on the intestinal bacteria flora of patients with diarrhea. Clinical Infectious Diseases 1993; 16 (supp 2): 77–82
35. Behar M. The role of feeding and nutrition in the pathogeny and prevention of diarrheic processes. Bulletion of the Pan American Health Organization 1975; 9 (1): 1–9
36. Ejderhamn J, Rafter JJ, Strandvik B. Faecal bile acid excretion in children with inflammatory bowel disease. Gut 1991; 32 (11); 1346–1351
37. Hutchinson R, Tyrrell PN, Kumar D et al. Pathogenesis of gall stones in Crohn's disease: an alternative explanation. Gut 1994; 35 (1): 94–97
38. Murray FE, McNicholas M, Stack W, O'Donoghue DP. Impaired fatty-meal-stimulated gallbladder contractility in patients with Crohn's disease. Clinical Science (Colch) 1992; 6: 689–693
39. Akerlund JE, Bjorkhem I, Angelin B et al. Apparent selective bile acid malabsorption as a consequence of ileal exclusion: effects on bile acid, cholesterol, and lipoprotein metabolism. Gut 1994; 35 (8): 1116–1120
40. Stiehl A. Ursodeoxycholic acid in the treatment of primary sclerosing cholangitis. Annals of Medicine 1994; 26 (5): 345–349
41. Boberg KM, Lundin KE, Schrumpf E. Etiology and pathogenesis in primary sclerosing cholangitis. Scandinavian Journal of Gastroenterology 1994; 204: 47–58
42. Mandal A, Dasgupta A, Jeffers L et al. Autoantibodies in sclerosing cholangitis against a shared peptide in biliary and colon epithelium. Gastroenterology 1994; 106 (1): 185–192
43. Miettinen TE, Kesaniemi YA, Gylling H et al. Noncholesterol sterols in bile and stones of patients with cholesterol and pigment stones. Hepatology 1996; 23 (2): 274–280
44. Robins SJ, Fasulo JM, Pritzker CR, Patton GM. Hepatic transport and secretion of unesterified cholesterol in the rat is traced by the plant sterol, sitostanol. Journal of Lipid Research 1996; 37 (1): 15–21

45. Robins SJ, Fasulo JM. High density lipoproteins, but not other lipoproteins, provide a vehicle for sterol transport to bile. Journal of Clinical Investigation 1997; 99 (3): 380–384
46. Vuoristo M, Miettinen TA. Absorption, metabolism, and serum concentrations of cholesterol in vegetarians: effects of cholesterol feeding. American Journal of Clinical Nutrition 1994; 59 (6): 1325–1331
47. Jenkins KJ, Atwal AS. Effects of dietary saponins on fecal bile acids and neutral sterols, and availability of vitamins A and E in the chick. Journal of Nutritional Biochemistry 1994; 5 (3): 134–137
48. Oakenfull D, Sidhu GS. Could saponins be a useful treatment for hypercholesterolaemia? European Journal of Clinical Nutrition 1990; 44: 79–88
49. Juarez-Oropeza MA Diaz-Zagoya JC, Rabinowitz JL. In vivo and in vitro studies of hypocholesterolemic effects of diosgenin in rats. International Journal of Biochemistry 1987; 19: 679–683
50. Roman ID, Thewles A, Coleman R. Fractionation of livers following diosgenin treatment to elevate biliary cholesterol. Biochimica Biophysica Acta 1995; 1255 (1): 77–81
51. Fukushima M, Nakano M. Effects of sunflowers on lipid metabolism in rats. Bioscience Biotechnology and Biochemistry 1994; 58 (12): 2278–2280
52. Nussinovitch M, Zahavi I, Marcus H, Hackelman B, Dinari G. The choleretic effect of nonsteroidal anti-inflammatory drugs in total parenteral nutrition-associated cholestasis. Israel Journal of Medical Sciences 1996; 32 (12): 1262–1264
53. Sterczer A, Voros K, Karsai F. Effect of cholagogues on the volume of the gallbladder of dogs. Research in Veterinary Science 1996; 60 (1): 44–47
54. Vahlensieck U, Hahn R, Winterhoff H et al. The effect of Chelidonium majus herb extract on choleresis in the isolated perfused rat liver. Planta Medica 1995; 61 (3): 267–271
55. Táborská E, Bochoráková H, Dostál J, Paulová H. The greater celandine (Chelidonium majus L.) – review of present knowledge. Ceska A Slovenska Farmacie 1995; 44 (2): 71–75
56. Dranik LI, Dolganenko LG, Slapke J, Thoma H. Chemical composition and medical usage of Cynara scolymus L. Rastitel'nye Resursy 1996; 32 (4): 98–104
57. Mimica-Dukic N, Jakovljevic V, Mira P et al Pharmacological study of Mentha longifolia phenolic extracts. International Journal of Pharmacognosy 1996; 34 (5): 359–364
58. Piyachaturawat P, Gansar R, Suksamrarn A. Choleretic effect of Curcuma comosa rhizome extracts in rats. International Journal of Pharmacognosy 1996; 34 (3): 174–178
59. Suksamrarn A, Eiamong S, Piyachaturawat P, Byrne LT. A phloracetophenone glucoside with choleretic activity from Curcuma comosa. Phytochemistry (Oxford) 1997; 45 (1): 103–105
60. Fujii H, Yamamoto M, Mogaki M et al. Glucagon responses in rabbits with obstructive jaundice and a low energy status in the liver. Surgery Today (Tokyo) 1994; 24 (11): 982–986

THE LIVER

SCOPE

Apart from their use to provide non-specific support for recuperation and repair, specific phytotherapeutic strategies include the following.

Treatment of:

- postpartum symptoms of liver distress, e.g. after consumption of fatty foods and alcohol;
- moderate acute and chronic hepatitis.

Management of:

- chronic and acute hepatotoxin poisoning;
- acute and chronic hepatitis;
- cirrhosis.

Because of its use of secondary plant products, particular **caution** is necessary in applying phytotherapy to primary and secondary liver carcinoma.

ORIENTATION

There are few guides to the use of hepatics in conventional Western medicine. This is a concept more familiar in mainland Europe and further East but has become a more popular concept with the marketing of milk thistle seed.

Hepatics are remedies which are claimed to help reduce damage caused to the liver from hepatic stressors and disease. The liver is an extremely active organ in the metabolism of ingested materials and it is known to be particularly vulnerable to the effects of agents that are not readily metabolized or excreted. These are known to include many modern drugs but there are obvious prospects that other less understood agents, agrochemicals and other modern environmental pollutants are likely to damage the liver. Although severe hepatic damage is not common, constant exposure to new industrial agents, particularly if at relatively high levels and when combined with other well-known burdens on the liver, alcohol and high-fat diets, might lead to a modern syndrome of functional liver distress.

There are more natural stressors to liver function as well. It can be argued that animals have evolved in constant exposure to a multitude of environmental lipid-soluble *xenobiotics*, notably from ingested plants (see also Adverse effects of herbal drugs, p.96). As one defence, animals possess a number of cytochromes P-450 which can metabolize (and thus eliminate) these agents. One potential disadvantages of this system is that cytochrome P-450 may in unusual circumstances transform some of these xenobiotics into new chemically reactive metabolites and free radicals, which attack tissue constituents, and may lead to mutation, cancer or tissue necrosis, particularly of the liver whose content of cytochrome P-450 is particularly high.[1]

Because of the central role of the liver in immunological function and detoxification, there may also be a significant population of patients, perhaps presenting with other conditions (notably skin and bowel diseases, chronic allergic states, autoimmune disease and other chronic inflammatory disorders), where liver damage may have occurred. The increased incidence of viral hepatitis is, however, perhaps the major cause of long-term hepatic disorders.

The mechanisms of chronic liver damage may include immunological disturbances, due to modification of the antigenic properties of hepatocytes, with the possibility of such pathologies as chronic active hepatitis and primary biliary cirrhosis.

As hepatic damage usually starts with classic pathological processes of fatty infiltration, in theory a good hepatic should have appropriate antioxidant properties. As these need to be focused in liver tissue, they should also be readily absorbed, require little extra liver metabolism and preferably should be retained in the enterohepatic circulation.

PHYTOTHERAPEUTICS

Evidence of beneficial effects on the liver

Many plants have been experimentally shown to have hepatoprotective effects, generally in protecting against the effects in animals of hepatotoxins such as carbon tetrachloride (CCl_4), D-galactosamine, paracetemol and Amanita mushrooms. There may indeed be a general benefit in plant material given the widespread occurrence of some of the constituents researched.

The ubiquitous flavonoid quercetin is one of a number of antioxidants which have been shown to reduce the high level of chromosomal aberrations found in cases of viral hepatitis associated with environmental pollution.[2]

Several plant hormones and analogues have been shown to inhibit xanthine oxidase, a flavoprotein enzyme, which catalyses the oxidation of hypoxanthine to xanthine and then xanthine to uric acid and whose serum levels are increased in hepatitis, mild hepatic intoxication, tumours and DNA damage induced by cytotoxic agents; these constituents were considered potentially useful for the treatment of these diseases as well as gout.[3] In investigation of the stems of *Bougainvillea spectabilis*, used in folk medicine for hepatis, spinasterol and quercetin were isolated and characterized from the plant leaves. Quercetin showed a strong activity on xanthine oxidase inhibition (IC_{50} = 7.23 μm). A further nine naturally occurring flavonoids were then tested for the same effects and showed similar activity, in decreasing order: baicalein, wogonin, baicalin, capillarisin, d-catechin, d-epicatechin, hesperidin, liquiritin, puerarin.[4] Caffeic acid was found to be another active principle exhibiting strong inhibition of xanthine oxidase (IC_{50} = 39.21 μm). A further 12 naturally occurring phenolics (esculetin, scopoletin, scoparone, barbaloin, berberine chloride, sinomenine, osthole, paeonol, honokiol, magnolol, methyleugenol and 6-gingerol) were tested for their inhibitory effects on xanthine oxidase. The results showed that esculetin displayed the strongest activity.[5]

Oral administration of the flavonoids daidzin, daidzein and puerarin, from the Chinese herb *Pueraria lobata*, was effective in lowering blood alcohol levels and shortened sleep time induced by alcohol ingestion.[6,7]

A polyphenolic complex in the Eastern folk remedy *Maackia amurensis* displays hepatoprotective and choleretic action. The agent has antioxidative properties, inhibits the development of cytolysis and necrosis of hepatocytes, improves hepatic excretory function, increases bile secretion, bilirubin, cholesterol and bile acid excretion and also has a marked choleretic activity in vivo.[8] The preparation prevents the destruction of cytochrome P-450 caused by CCl_4, increases its stability and catalytic activity and stimulates conjugation reactions of endo- and xenobiotics.[9]

Evidence of the benefits of antioxidant activity in liver disease has been provided by a study on 199 patients with liver disease receiving antituberculosis treatment which showed that the inclusion into the treatment schedule of the antioxidant tocopherol and the infusion of the Chinese herb Astragalus exerted pronounced hepatoprotective effects.[10]

Boldo (*Peumus boldus*), a Chilean tree traditionally employed for the treatment of liver ailments, has recently been the subject of increasing attention. The recent demonstration that boldine is an effective antioxidant in both biological and non-biological systems reinforces the view that this is a potentially useful substance in many disease states featuring free radical-related oxidative injury.[11]

The milk thistle seed, *Silybum marianum*, widely used in Europe for its hepatic reputation, has been found to contain a flavolignan constituent silymarin with antifibrotic activity.[12] Glycyrrhizin, a major component of licorice, has been used intravenously for the treatment of chronic hepatitis B in Japan and improves liver function with occasional complete recovery from hepatitis.[13] In vitro studies suggest a hitherto unique mechanism involving intracellular transport across Golgi membranes.[14] In addition, weak binding activity to steroid receptors have been demonstrated.[15] Derivatives of glycyrrhizinic acid promote a decrease in the rate of lipid peroxide oxygenation and in the inhibition of liver enzyme activity (BHMT, ALT, AST) and also increase choleresis.[16] There is also evidence of a choleretic action,[17] also involving glycyrrhizin.

Piperine, an active alkaloidal constituent of the extract obtained from *Piper longum* and *P. nigrum*, was evaluated for its antihepatotoxic potential against CCl_4 and other agents and was found to have an appreciable benefit but at levels lower than silymarin.[18]

The water extract from the root of *Salvia miltiorhiza* showed a protective effect on cultured rat hepatocytes against CCl_4-induced necrosis. Lithospermate B, a tetramer of caffeic acid, was isolated and found to be an active constituent. Lithospermate B was also found to have a potent hepatoprotective activity not only in vitro but also in in vivo experimental liver injuries induced by CCl_4 or D-galactosamine-lipopolysaccharide.[19] Various other metabolites of caffeic acid formed in the liver are likely to account for many beneficial effects in that organ; these metabolites include cyclolignan derivatives as oxidation products, ferulic and isoferulic acid as methylation products and esculetin as a cyclization product.[20]

Acanthoic acid, a pimaradiene diterpene isolated from *Acanthopanax koreanum*, strongly inhibited the production of proinflammatory mediators interleukin-1 and tumour necrosis factor, as well as the release of superoxide anions and hydrogen peroxide from human monocytes/macrophages in vitro. An additional antifibrotic effect was demonstrated through in vitro and in vivo inhibition of collagen production by lung fibroblasts and lung tissue and granuloma formation and fibrosis in experimental silicosis, serum GOT and GPT in rats with cirrhosis and hepatic fibrosis and nodular formation.[21]

The Phyllanthus genus has been known to contain a number of biologically active constituents such as an angiotensin-converting enzyme inhibitor and HIV reverse transcriptase inhibitors.[22] *Phyllanthus amarus* has shown antihepatitis B virus activity. *P. ussuriensis*, a Korean native species, has been used to treat several infectious diseases, including hepatitis in folk medicine, and antihepatotoxic effects have been confirmed in vitro.[23] It inhibited hepatitis B virus polymerase activity, decreased episomal hepatitis B virus DNA content and suppressed virus release into culture medium. A number of mechanisms have been elucidated.[24]

Evidence of hepatoprotective effects also arises from studies on traditional remedies: *Artemisia spp*,[25,26] *Azadirachta indica* leaf extract,[27] *Picrorrhiza kurroa*,[28] *Osbeckia octandra*,[29] *Gynostemma pentaphyllum*,[30] Schisandra,[31] *Inula britannica* L. subsp. *japonica*,[32] *Salvia plebeia*.[33] Other plant hepatoprotectors have been reviewed.[34,35]

Even chlorophyllin, a food-grade derivative of the green plant pigment chlorophyll, has been demonstrated as being a potent inhibitor of hepatic aflatoxin B_1 (AFB_1)-DNA adduction and hepatocarcinogenesis.[36]

Another hitherto little explored hepatic activity may also be a feature of some herbal preparations: extracts of *Thuja occidentalis* and *Echinacea purpurea* stimulated Kupffer cell phagocytosis in vitro.[37]

Hepatic induction of antitumour effects

The central role of liver function in a range of defence mechanisms (for example, the transport of IgA and IgA immune complexes by the liver from serum to bile may provide a host defence against enteric pathogens[38]) raises the possibility that hepatics might have wider applications. Out of various spices and leafy vegetables screened for their influence on the carcinogen-detoxifying enzyme glutathione-S- transferase (GST) in Swiss mice, cumin seeds, poppy seeds, asafoetida, turmeric, kandathipili, neem flowers, manathakkali leaves, drumstick leaves, basil leaves and ponnakanni leaves increased GST activity by more than 78% in the stomach, liver and oesophagus – high enough to be considered as protective agents against carcinogenesis.[39] Several naturally occurring flavonoids and other polyphenols, prominently tannic acid, were also shown to exert varying degrees of concentration-dependent inhibition on uncharacterized rat liver GST.[40] Sesquiterpenes such as beta-caryophyllene, beta-caryophyllene oxide, alpha-humulene, alpha-humulene epoxide I and eugenol, all found in cloves, have demonstrated significant activity as inducers of GST in the mouse liver and small intestine,[41] as has myristicin, a major aromatic constituent of parsley.[42]

Capsaicin (0.5 μm) inhibited the formation by liver microsomal fractions of all metabolites of 4-(methylnitrosamino)-1-(3-pyridyl)-1-butanone (NNK), a potent carcinogen in tobacco and tobacco smoke. With other similar results, such findings suggest that it possesses antimutagenic and anticarcinogenic properties through the inhibition of xenobiotic metabolizing enzymes.[43]

HEPATICS

Plant remedies traditionally used as hepatics

Silybum marianum (milk thistle), Cynara (artichoke), Bupleurum (chai hu), Schisandra (wu wei zi).

Indications for hepatics

- Viral and other hepatitis and sequelae
- Adverse effects of alcohol and excess fat consumption
- Exposure to industrial pollutants
- In anticipation of or along with the prescription of powerful medications
- Cirrhosis and other chronic liver diseases

Other traditional indications for hepatics

Many dermatological, enteric and bowel, rheumatic, catarrhal and other chronic inflammatory diseases.

Contraindications for hepatics

Most widely used hepatics in European phytomedicine appear to have few contraindications. They are generally mild treatments and, as antioxidants, may have wider benefits. To some extent they may merely extend the known beneficial effect on the liver of plant foods. Nevertheless, some of the remedies mentioned above may have individual characteristics that need consideration. The use of hepatics may be inappropriate in liver carcinoma.

Traditional therapeutic insights into the use of hepatics

Diseases with early morning symptoms may be associated with liver disturbances on the assumption that the liver has been particularly active overnight during sleep. The occurrence of such signs might in itself be an indication for the use of hepatic remedies.

Traditional enquiry might also elicit how well a patient handled alcohol and dietary fats. Although difficulties here might rather suggest the use of cholagogues, hepatics would be particularly indicated if symptoms like headaches were associated with such consumption.

Hepatics are very often employed in the treatment of migraine, often seen traditionally as a liver condition.

Western practitioners are reminded of the ancient Greek humoral concept of 'black bile' (lit: *melancholia*) and the early view of clinical depression as a somatic rather than a psychological phenomenon. Using hepatics and other treatments for liver and digestive function as part of a fresh approach to the management of depression can be surprisingly productive in some cases.

Application

Hepatics are best applied before breakfast in the morning and before the last meal of the day, to take account of the extra liver activity during the night. However, they may also be taken before meals throughout the day.

Long-term therapy is quite appropriate for those like milk thistle and artichoke which have established their safety.

Advanced phytotherapeutics

Hepatics may also be usefully applied in some cases (depending on other factors) of:

- migraine;
- acne rosacea;
- autoimmune diseases (especially where associated with any of the above – see relevant sections).

There is also a strong case for their use in anticipation of, or association with, the prescription of powerful chemotherapeutic agents in, for example, the treatment of tuberculosis, cancer, psychoses and frequent recourse to general anaesthetics.

For evidence of adverse effects of herbal products on the liver, see p.97.

PHYTOTHERAPY FOR LIVER CONDITIONS

Acute viral hepatitis

The most important causes of acute hepatitis are the hepatitis A, B and C viruses. Other viruses, including Epstein–Barr virus and cytomegalovirus, may also cause acute hepatitis. All these viruses have a viral envelope and hence have some susceptibility to Hypericum (St John's wort) which is active against enveloped viruses.

Acute hepatitis can be treated using herbal medicine. In the case of hepatitis A, treatment can lead to rapid recovery and protect against posthepatitis syndrome. For hepatitis B and C, herbal treatment will mainly help to prevent the disease becoming chronic. The small amounts of alcohol involved from using extracts and tinctures will not be a problem to most patients. However, if there is a difficulty with alcohol then tablets, capsules and/or infusions or decoctions can be prescribed. As with other acute infections, oral herbal treatment should not be administered while there is vomiting.

It is hoped that individual strategies will be devised for each patient, taking some of the insights in this and other chapters into account, but essential aspects of treatment are as follows.

Example treatment

A typical treatment for acute hepatitis could be:

Echinacea angustifolia	1:2	35 ml
Hypericum perforatum (high in hypericin)	1:2	25 ml
Silybum marianum	1:1	20 ml
Phyllanthus amarus	1:2	20 ml
	Total	100 ml

Dose 5 ml with water four times a day.
Picrorrhiza tablets 500 mg, three per day can also be prescribed. (Gastrointestinal side effects such as cramping and diarrhoea should be watched for.)
Achillea and Zingiber tea (4 g of Achillea and 1 g of dried (not fresh) Zingiber per cup), three cups per day.

- Diaphoretics are indicated in all acute infections accompanied by fever. These include Tilia (lime flowers), Sambucus (elder) and Achillea (yarrow) and are best taken as an infusion. Diaphoretics are assisted by combination with a diffuse stimulant such as Zingiber (ginger).

- Antiviral agents, which for hepatitis include *Hypericum perforatum* (St John's wort), Phyllanthus and Thuja.

- Immune-enhancing herbs, especially Echinacea and Picrorrhiza.

- Hepatoprotective agents to minimize liver damage such as Silybum (St Mary's thistle), Bupleurum, *Taraxacum radix* (dandelion root), Cynara (globe artichoke) and Picrorrhiza.

- Posthepatitis syndrome should mainly be treated with the hepatoprotectives listed above.

Chronic viral hepatitis

Chronic viral hepatitis or chronic persistent hepatitis usually results from infection with hepatitis B or C. Especially with hepatitis C, some features of the disease may resemble autoimmune hepatitis. (Frank autoimmune liver disease is known as chronic active hepatitis.

A general treatment approach for autoimmune disease is outlined on p.140).

TREATMENT

Treatment of chronic viral hepatitis shares many similarities with the treatment of acute viral hepatitis. Essential features of treatment are:

- immune-enhancing agents such as Echinacea and Picrorrhiza, but also consider Astragalus for any chronic infection;
- hepatoprotective agents as described previously but also consider using Schisandra and prescribing Silybum in a more concentrated form such as Silymarin tablets;
- antiviral agents (see above). The use of Phyllanthus may be suitable for chronic viral hepatitis; see p. 191.

Cirrhosis of the liver

In cirrhosis, widespread death of liver cells, which can result from many causes but is most commonly due to alcohol abuse, is accompanied and followed by progressive fibrosis and distortion of liver architecture. Since alcohol is forbidden, herbal treatment should be in the form of tablets, capsules, infusions and/or decoctions. The main herbal treatment is based around hepatic trophorestoratives, especially concentrated tablets of *Silybum marianum*. Other important herbs in this category include Schisandra, *Taraxacum radix* (dandelion root), Cynara (globe artichoke), Bupleurum and Picrorrhiza. Berberine-containing herbs can also be indicated. Although cirrhosis is a progressive disease, the rate of progression varies and the outlook is related to many factors. In this context, herbal treatment can make a significant positive contribution.

Gallstones and biliary pain

Slow intestinal transit has been linked to gallstone formation in normal-weight women.[44]

Bile is often supersaturated before breakfast and this could explain the naturopathic practice of recommending lemon juice (a liver and gallbladder stimulant) before breakfast.

Most patients with gallstones have no symptoms and current medical thinking is that there is no distinct advantage in treating asymptomatic gallstones.[45] Oral dissolution therapy with bile salts is still used as a treatment but is reserved for patients with non-calcified cholesterol gallstones, a patent cystic duct and who do not require urgent surgery. These considerations also define the conditions for successful herbal treatment of gallstones. Patients who receive conventional oral therapy usually have a high rate of gallstone recurrence. This underlines the need in herbal therapy for long-term treatment concurrent with appropriate dietary and lifestyle changes.

The essential elements of treatment are as follows.

- Bitter herbs to improve digestive and gallbladder function, e.g. *Artemisia absinthium* (wormwood), Gentiana or Picrorrhiza.
- Choleretic herbs to improve bile flow, e.g. Chelidonium (greater celandine), Cynara (globe artichoke), *Taraxacum radix* (dandelion root) and Silybum (St Mary's thistle).
- Cholagogue herbs to improve gallbladder motility, e.g. Chelidonium (greater celandine), Cynara and *Mentha piperita* (peppermint). A terpene mixture similar to oil of peppermint has been shown to dissolve gallstones.[46]
- Spasmolytic herbs, e.g. *Viburnum opulus* (cramp bark), Matricaria (chamomile) and *Mentha piperita*, can help to relieve gallbladder pain.
- Long-term use of herbs containing steroidal saponins such as Dioscorea (wild yam) and smilax (sarsaparilla) is best avoided since these herbs can increase cholesterol levels in bile.[47]
- A short course of copious olive oil and lemon juice is often recommended to discharge gallstones. However, such a therapy should only be attempted if the gallstones are not calcified, the cystic duct is patent, the gallbladder is functional and herbal therapy to soften the stones has been given for at least 6 months.

Case history

A male patient aged 69 had been experiencing recurrent attacks of biliary pain for several months. A blood test showed the presence of high levels of bilirubin, perhaps due to temporary obstruction caused by the passage of a stone, and X-rays revealed gallbladder inflammation and gallstones. The patient was offered surgery but wanted to try herbal treatment first.

He was advised to follow a low-fat diet and the following formula was prescribed.

Silybum marianum	1:1	25 ml
Cynara scolymus	1:2	25 ml
Taraxacum officinale radix	1:2	20 ml
Picrorrhiza kurroa	1:2	10 ml
Mentha piperita	1:2	20 ml
	Total	100 ml

Dose 5 ml with water three times a day.
After a few months of treatment all symptoms had abated. The patient continued treatment for another 6 months, during which time he was free of symptoms. Since that time (several years) he has not had any herbal treatment but still remains free of gallbladder symptoms.

Poor liver function

The liver plays a vital role in detoxification and many other metabolic processes in the body. Phytotherapeutic and naturopathic thinking recognizes a condition where liver function is below optimum, although no medically observable liver disease or liver damage may be present. Because of the importance of the liver, a poorly functioning liver can have a wide-ranging impact on health.

Symptoms which may be due to poor liver function include sluggish digestion, fat intolerance, nausea, chronic constipation and chemical, food or drug intolerances. A poorly functioning liver may also contribute to a number of disease states such as psoriasis, autoimmune disease, irritable bowel syndrome, allergies and cancer. Patients will probably reveal a history of past liver infection, infestation or damage, alcohol or drug abuse or exposure to medical drugs or environmental pollutants such as pesticides. Drug side effects are more likely to occur in patients with poor liver function.

Depending on the symptoms, treatment is based on the following.

- Hepatoprotective and hepatic trophorestorative herbs, especially if there is a history of liver damage or exposure to toxins. Principal herbs include Silybum (St Mary's thistle), Cynara (globe artichoke) and Taraxacum (dandelion root). Schisandra is particularly useful since it also enhances the detoxifying capacity of the liver. These herbs will assist in cases of nausea and intolerances from any cause.
- Choleretic herbs to boost liver function are particularly indicated if digestive symptoms are predominant. They will also boost detoxification by the bile and therefore can be valuable in conditions such as psoriasis and cancer. Most of the hepatoprotective herbs listed above have a gentle choleretic activity but strongly choleretic herbs include Hydrastis (golden seal), *Berberis vulgaris* (barberry), Chelidonium (great celandine) and bitter herbs. These strongly choleretic herbs will cause nausea and irritability in a patient who has some history of liver damage. They should therefore be avoided at first in these circumstances and only introduced after prior treatment with hepatic trophorestoratives.
- Depurative herbs are also indicated in cases where hepatic detoxification may be inadequate. Those which act principally via the liver and digestion include Arctium (burdock), *Rumex crispus* (yellow dock) and Fumaria (fumitory).

Case history

A female patient aged 38 wished to take the contraceptive pill. She found that even a low-dose pill still caused symptoms of female hormone excess such as abdominal bloating, weight gain, nausea and depression. She had a past history of liver damage due to hydatid worm cysts during childhood.

Treatment consisted of:

Silybum marianum	1:1	30 ml
Taraxacum officinale radix	1:2	35 ml
Schisandra chinensis	1:2	35 ml
	Total	100 ml

Dose 5 ml with water twice a day.
The patient found she could take the pill without any adverse effects as long as she also took the herbal treatment.

References

1. Pessayre D. Cytochromes P450 and formation of reactive metabolites. Role in drug induced hepatotoxicity. Therapie (Paris) 1993; 48 (6): 537–548
2. Peresadin NA, Frolov VM, Pinskii LL. Correction with antioxidants of cytogenetic disturbances in viral hepatitis. Likars'ka Sprava 1995; 1–2: 76–79
3. Sheu S-Y, Chiang H-C. Inhibitory effects of plant growth regulators on xanthine oxidase. Anticancer Research 1996; 16 (1): 311–315
4. Chang W-S, Lee Y-J, Lu F-J, Chiang H-C. Inhibitory effects of flavonoids on xanthine oxidase. Anticancer Research 1993; 13 (6A): 2165–2170
5. Chang W-S, Chang Y-H, Lu F-I, Chaing H-C. Inhibitory effects of phenolics on xanthine oxidase. Anticancer Research 1994; 14 (2A): 501–506
6. Lin RC, Guthrie S, Xie CY et al. Isoflavonoid compounds extracted from Pueraria lobata suppress alcohol preference in a pharmacogenetic rat model of alcoholism. Alcoholism, Clinical and Experimental Research 1996; 20 (4): 659–663
7. Xie CI, Lin RC, Antony V et al. Daidzin, an antioxidant isoflavonoid, decreases blood alcohol levels and shortens sleep time induced by ethanol intoxication. Alcoholism, Clinical and Experimental Research 1994; 18 (6): 1443–1447

8. Vlasova TV, Vengerovskii AI, Saratikov AS. Maackia amurensis polphenols, effective hepatoprotective and cholagogue agents. Khimiko-Farmatsevticheskii Zhurnal 1994; 28 (3): 56–59
9. Bengerovskii AI, Sadykh IM, Saratikov AS. Effects of polyphenols from Maackia amurensis on antitoxic function of the liver. Eksperimental'naya i Klinicheskaya Farmakologiya 1993; 56 (5): 47–50
10. Skakun NL, Blikhar EI. Effect of antioxidants on lipid peroxidation and on liver function in patients with pulmonary tuberculosis. Farmakologiia I Toksikologiia 1986; 49 (5): 112–114
11. Speisky H, Cassels BK. Boldo and boldine: an emerging case of natural drug development. Pharmacology Research 1994; 29 (1): 1–12
12. Boigk G, Stroeter L, Waldschmidt J et al. Silymarin retards collagen accumulation in rat secondary biliary fibrosis. Journal of Hepatology 1995; 23 (supp 1): 142
13. Sato H, Goto W, Yamamura J et al. Therapeutic basis of glycyrrhizin on chronic hepatitis B. Antiviral Research 1996; 30 (2–3): 171–177
14. Takahara T, Watanabe A, Shiraki K. Effects of glycyrrhizin on hepatitis B surface antigen: a biochemical and morphological study. Journal of Hepatology 1994; 21 (4): 601–609
15. Tamaya T, Sato S, Okada H. Inhibition by plant herb extracts of steroid bindings in uterus, liver and serum of the rabbit. Acta Obstetrica et Gynecologica Scandinavica 1986; 65 (8): 839–842
16. Nasyrov KhM, Chepurina LS, Kireeva RM. Study of hepatoprotective and choleretic activity of glycyrrhizinic acid derivatives. Eksperimental'naya i Klinicheskaya Farmakologiya 1995; 58 (6): 60–63
17. Raggi MA, Bugamelli F, Nobile L et al. The choleretic effects of licorice: identification and determination of the pharmacologically active components of Glycyrrhiza glabra. Bollettino Chimico Farmaceutico 1995; 134 (11): 634–638
18. Koul IB, Kapil A. Evaluation of the liver protective potential of piperine, an active principle of black and long peppers. Planta Medica 1993; 59 (5): 413–417
19. Hase K, Kasimu R, Basnet P et al. Preventive effect of lithospermate B from Salvia miltiorhiza on experimental hepatitis induced by carbon tetrachloride or D-galactosamine- lipopolysaccharide. Planta Medica 1997; 63 (1): 22–26
20. Gumbinger HG, Vahlensieck U, Winterhoff H. Metabolism of caffeic acid in the isolated perfused rat liver. Planta Medica 1993; 59 (6): 491–493
21. Kang H-S, Kim Y-H, Lee C-S et al. Suppression of interleukin-1 and tumor necrosis factor-alpha production by acanthoic acid, (-)-pimara-9(11),15-dien-19-oic acid, and its antifibrotic effects in vivo. Cellular Immunology 1996; 170 (2): 212–221
22. Munshi A, Mehrotra R, Ramesh R, Panda SK. Evaluation of anti-hepadnavirus activity of Phyllanthus amarus and Phyllanthus maderaspatensis in duck hepatitis B virus carrier Pekin ducks. Journal of Medical Virology 1993; 41 (4): 275–281
23. Moon Y-S, Lim WS, Lee MK et al. Antihepatotoxic effect of callus cultures of the P. ussuriensis. Seoul University Journal of Pharmaceutical Sciences 1995; 20: 21–31
24. Lee C-D, Ott M, Thyagarajan SP et al. Phyllanthus amarus down-regulates hepatitis B virus mRNA transcription and replication. European Journal of Clinical Investigation 1996; 26 (12): 1069–1076
25. Janbaz KH, Gilani AH. Evaluation of the protective potential of Artemisia maritima extract on acetaminophen- and CC14-induced liver damage. Journal of Ethnopharmacology 1995; 47 (1): 43–47
26. Yin J, Wennberg RP, Miller M. Induction of hepatic bilirubin and drug metabolizing enzymes by individual herbs present in the traditional Chinese medicine, yin zhi huang. Developmental Pharmacology and Therapeutics 1993; 20 (3–4): 186–194
27. Chattopadhyay RR, Sarkar SK, Ganguly S et al. Hepatoprotective activity of Azadirachta indica leaves on paracetamol induced hepatic damage in rats. Indian Journal of Experimental Biology 1992; 8: 738–740
28. Dhawan BN. Picroliv – a new hepatoprotective agent from an Indian medicinal plant, Picrorrhiza kurroa. Medicinal Chemistry Research 1995; 5 (8): 595–605
29. Thabrew MI, Hughes RD, Gove CD et al. Protective effects of Osbeckia octandra against paracetamol-induced liver injury. Xenobiotica 1995; 9: 1009–1017
30. Li L, Jiao L, Lau BH. Protective effect of gypenosides against oxidative stress in phagocytes, vascular endothelial cells and liver microsomes. Cancer Biotherapy 1993; 8 (3): 263–272
31. Liu GT. Pharmacological actions and clinical use of fructus schizandrae. Chinese Medical Journal (Engl) 1989; 102 (10): 740–749
32. Iijima K, Kiyohara H, Tanaka M et al. Preventive effect of taraxasteryl acetate from Inula britannica subsp. japonica on experimental hepatitis in vivo. Planta Medica 1995; 61 (1): 50–53
33. Lin C-C, Lin J-K, Chang C-H. Evaluation of hepatoprotective effects of 'Chhit-Chan-Than' from Taiwan. International Journal of Pharmacognosy 1995; 33 (2): 139–143
34. Rumyantseva ZhN, Gudivok YS. Search for hepatoprotectors among preparations of plant origin. Rastitel'nye Resursy 1993; 29 (1): 88–97
35. Rakhmanin YA, Kushnerova NF, Gordeichuk TN et al. Metabolic responses of the liver exposed to carbon tetrachloride and their correction with plant antioxidants. Gigiena i Sanitariya 1997; (1): 30–32
36. Breinholt V, Schimerlik M, Dashwood R, Bailey G. Mechanisms of chlorophyllin anticarcinogenesis against aflatoxin B1: complex formation with the carcinogen. Chemical Research in Toxicology 1995; 4: 506–514
37. Vömel T. Effect of a plant immunostimulant on phagocytosis of erythrocytes by the reticulohistiocytary system of isolated perfused rat liver. Arzneimittel-Forschung 1985; 35 (9): 1437–1439
38. Kleinman RE, Harmatz PR, Walker WA. The liver: an integral part of the enteric mucosal immune system. Hepatology 1982; 2 (3): 379–384
39. Aruna K, Sivaramakrishnan VM. Plant products as protective agents against cancer. Indian Journal of Experimental Biology 1990; 11: 1008–1011
40. Zhang K, Das NP. Inhibitory effects of plant polyphenols on rat liver glutathione S-transferases. Biochemical Pharmacology 1994; 47 (11): 2063–2068
41. Zheng GQ, Kenney PM, Lam LK. Sesquiterpenes from clove (Eugenia caryophyllata) as potential anticarcinogenic agents. Journal of Natural Products 1992; 55 (7): 999–1003
42. Zheng GQ, Kenney PM, Zhang J, Lam LK. Inhibition of benzo[a]pyrene-induced tumorigenesis by myristicin, a volatile aroma constituent of parsley leaf oil. Carcinogenesis 1992; 13 (10): 1921–1923
43. Miller CH, Zhang Z, Hamilton SM, Teel RW. Effects of capsaicin on liver microsomal metabolism of the tobacco-specific nitrosamine NNK. Cancer Letters 1993; 75 (1): 45–52
44. Heaton, KW, Emmett PM, Symes LJ et al. An explanation for gallstones in normal-weight women: slow intestinal transit. Lancet 1993; 341 (8836): 8–10
45. Johnston, DE, Kaplan, MM. Pathogenesis and treatment of gallstones. New England Journal of Medicine 1993; 328 (6): 412–421
46. Bell, GD,Doran, J. Gall stone dissolution in man using an essential oil preparation. British Medical Journal 1979; 1 (6155): 241, 24
47. Thewles A, Parslow RA, Coleman R. Effect of diosgenin on biliary cholesterol transport in the rat. Biochem. J 1993; 291 (3): 793–798

CARDIOVASCULAR SYSTEM

Scope

Apart from their use to provide non-specific support for recuperation and repair, specific phytotherapeutic strategies include the following.

Treatment of:

- mild to moderate hypertension;
- angina;
- palpitations.

Management of:

- chronic, non-severe hypertension;
- atheromatous cardiovascular conditions;
- recuperation after cardiovascular attacks;
- venous insufficiency;
- congestive heart failure.

Because of its use of secondary plant products, particular **caution** is necessary in applying phytotherapy in cases of:

- warfarin, heparin and other anticoagulant prescription;
- digitalis glycoside prescription.

ORIENTATION

Old and new perspectives on the circulatory system

A phytotherapeutic perspective on the circulatory system has to take two parts. Most of what modern medicine understands of the system arises from preoccupation with disease states such as hypertension, hypercholesterolaemia, atherosclerosis, clotting disturbances and thrombosis and coronary diseases that were barely understood in an earlier era. Nevertheless, as this chapter will show, herbal remedies show considerable promise across many of these modern conditions and their use for this purpose has been considerably modified compared with their traditional indications. Three of the best-selling herbal products in Europe, Ginkgo, garlic and Crataegus (hawthorn), are traditional remedies highly adapted to new and productive ends.

Nevertheless, to understand more effectively the potential of medicinal plants in affecting circulatory functions an appreciation of the earlier traditional perspective will be helpful. It is immediately obvious that before modern instruments, human experience of the circulatory system and the effects of treatments upon it was very different. As shall be seen, the insights developed in these early times usefully inform modern prospects.

The circulatory apparatus of William Harvey provided a mechanistic framework for modern advances that was, however, of little application to everyday practice in his time. The common experience was that there was vital movement within the body, as measured by pulse, heartbeat and breathing, and that there was a red fluid whose presence was clearly essential. It was relatively easy to link this with the main manifestation of moving blood: the heat of the living body and the variations in that heat in health and disease. In short, blood pulsated and warmed and was generally linked with the common speculation that there must be circulation of energies, fluids and nutrients around the body. Circulation was marked by

- pulsation
- heat
- blood and reddened complexion and, when in good shape, by a general vital potency.

The heart was obviously associated with all this but as much as a resonator with the vital pulse as its director. It was the wider pulse itself (reflected in the driving rhythms of early tribal music) that was important in early experience of the circulatory system; it was clearly linked to wider vital events: activity, excitement, emotional stimulation and, in medicine, notably the fever.

Therapeutics in fever focused on dispersing agents to distribute excessive heat and circulation and (as 'diaphoretics') to diffuse the poisons clearly involved through the sweat glands. The detoxifying theme recurred in many traditional concepts of 'blood poisons' as a cause of inflammatory diseases, and the use of 'blood cleansers' or 'blood purifiers', often very vigorously, to treat them.

Also requiring eliminatives (mainly diuretics and laxatives) was oedema, one of the most common indications of poor circulation in the past. As briefly elaborated in Chapter 1, the traditional perspective closely linked circulatory function with elimination.

Traditional views also linked circulation with the assimilation and processing of nutrients. The vital pulse and heat were weakened in debility and exhaustion, conditions associated with coldness and pallor. The main treatments were in effect 'blood tonics', warming nutrients (often since found to be rich in mineral nutrients).

There will be profit in revisiting these perspectives in developing modern strategies for the treatment of circulatory problems using herbal remedies. This is even more justified when the phenomenon of circulation itself is reviewed.

Circulation as currents

Where there has been speculation about the nature of circulatory system in traditional medicine, it has tended to infer broad currents rather than the route map of William Harvey. The closest to the latter were the meridians of Chinese medicine, although even these were speculative phenomena not associated with anatomical conduits.[1] The phenomenological perspective of tradition turns out, however, to be closer to the reality than the conventional understanding of arteries, veins and capillaries might suggest.

As far as most tissue cells are concerned, blood flow is not through vessels at all. When plasma filters through the capillary walls to bathe the tissues, it does not diffuse freely. In most tissues, cells are embedded in a gelatinous matrix, formed of complexes of hyaluronic acid which is largely impermeable to aqueous fluids. Movement of plasma is thus confined through clefts and cleavages in the matrix. The interstitial matrix thus both maintains tissue integrity and restricts the free flow of the circulation – oedema is the main symptom of breakdown in this important construct.

The effect of the interstitial matrix on circulatory dynamics is profound. As far as tissues are concerned, circulation is not a Harveyian affair at all, it is more a diffusive process marked by local and wider oceanic currents. Factors that affect tissue circulation are thus different from those that preoccupy modern cardiovascular medicine. Atherosclerosis and thrombosis cause serious local circulatory harm, of course, but they impact on general circulation only when very severe. More important for circulatory health in the tissues are such factors as capillary wall integrity, the local responses to local environmental changes of powerful vasoactive agents like the kinins and histamine, venous or lymphatic stasis or congestion with subsequent oedema and toxicity.

Antipathogenic benefits of increased tissue perfusion?

A glance at any pathology text will confirm that the cellular processes of disease are remarkably consistent. Pathological deterioration starts with biochemical lesions, then a variety of stages supervene including intracellular lesions, cell hypertrophy and a range of possible degenerative changes, cellular swelling due to water influx into the cell, fatty change or accumulation, atrophy, necrosis, possibly leading to inflammation, or calcification. Most detectable disease states in the body are classified by one or more of these processes. Atherosclerosis, for example, involves fatty infiltration and then calcification of the tissues in the arterial walls.

Moreover, the very first initiating trauma is even more consistent. The most likely first step in tissue damage is a relative deficiency of oxygenated blood and fluids. Physical injury is the most likely initiating trauma followed by an accumulation of external or endogenous toxic substances. In both the first and last cases poor tissue perfusion is critical. There are a number of ways in which tissue circulation can be interrupted but there is a clear prima facie case for maintaining tissue perfusion as a core disease-preventing strategy.

One of the most fascinating prospects for the revival of traditional herbal and dietary approaches is in the number of ways in which plant constituents, like flavonoids, anthocyanins, sesquiterpenes and pungent principles, appear to act beneficially on local circulatory processes.

It is a consistent theme throughout history that the 'heating' remedies were literally life enhancing (see pp.4 and 10). The pungent remedies like cayenne, ginger and raw garlic had reputations that transcended the merely mundane. It is known that they do increase tissue perfusion and blood flow. Everyday subjective experiences of increased body heat after eating spicy food can be confirmed with thermometers. Reference to the ginger monograph (see p.394) reveals a number of studies demonstrating a thermogenic effect, involving such mechanisms as increased catecholamine production and cytokine activity. Supplementing rats' diet with garlic powder increased rectal temperatures, blood noradrenaline levels and mitochondrial activity in brown adipose tissues, an activity that was inhibited by beta-adrenergic blockers.[2]

The prospects for closer investigation are intriguing. It is most probable that the traditional remedies most often used for their tissue warming benefits will show really exciting properties in the treatment of, or prophylaxis against, a range of degenerative diseases that may include atherosclerosis and other cardiovascular diseases. The fact that most are common ingredients of the diet adds even more to this project.

A promise of what may be in store for cayenne, ginger, cinnamon, turmeric and the like is the remarkable story of garlic, now possibly the most intensively studied of all medicinal plants and foods.

Garlic

The chemistry of *Allium sativum* is complex and the multitude of garlic products available in the marketplace reflect this complexity.[3] These types of preparations can be divided into three main groups, to which is added fresh garlic.

1. Carefully dried **garlic powder** which preserves the compound alliin (S-allylcysteine sulphoxide) and the enzyme alliinase. On disintegration of tablets or capsules containing this powder in the digestive tract, alliin comes into contact with alliinase and is converted to allicin. (This mimics the chemical process that occurs when a fresh clove of garlic is crushed). Allicin is unstable and breaks down further into compounds such as diallyl sulphides, ajoene and the vinyl dithiins (the metabolic pathways for allicin in the human body are not fully understood).

2. **Aged garlic extracts** or 'odourless' garlic products which are produced by a fermentation process. These preparations contain modified sulphur compounds such as S-allylcysteine.

3. Steam-distilled preparations of garlic (garlic oil) which are rich in diallyl sulphides.

Most of the published clinical studies on garlic have used 'garlic powder' preparations, although trials on aged garlic extracts, fresh garlic and garlic oil are also in the literature.

Lipid-lowering effects

Many studies have demonstrated the lipid-lowering effects of garlic and the results of two metaanalyses supported the premise that garlic acted as a lipid-lowering agent. The first of these examined five selected clinical trials on various garlic preparations with a total of 410 patients.[4] The authors concluded that the best available evidence suggests that garlic, in an amount approximating one half to one clove per day, decreased total serum cholesterol levels by about 9%. About a year later a second metaanalysis was published by Silagy and Neil.[5] These scientists included 16 clinical trials with a total of 952 patients. Again, a variety of garlic preparations were included in the metaanalysis. They found that garlic lowered cholesterol levels by 12% and that dried garlic powder preparations also lowered serum levels of triglycerides. Since the metaanalysis of Silagy and Neil, two negative clinical trials on garlic powder have been published[6,7] and one negative trial on garlic oil.[8] On the other hand, there are many new positive studies as well. Only careful consideration given to dose and dosage form in a large clinical trial will resolve this issue.

Antiatherogenicity

Perhaps the real value of garlic in the prevention and treatment of cardiovascular disease lies elsewhere. For example, a double-blind, placebo-controlled study on 23 patients found that garlic powder tablets reduced the atherogenicity of low density lipoprotein.[9] In a controlled retrospective study on 202 healthy adults, divided equally between those taking garlic powder and controls, in which measures of the elastic properties of the aorta were used, the garlic reduced age-related increases in aortic stiffness.[10]

Antihypertensive

A metaanalysis of eight clinical trials (415 patients), all using the same garlic powder preparation, found that garlic caused a modest but significant reduction in both systolic and diastolic blood pressures.[11] However, only three of the trials were specifically conducted in hypertensive patients and many had other methodological shortcomings.

Antithrombotic

A platelet-inhibiting effect has been described for garlic. In a double-blind, placebo-controlled study on 60 volunteers with elevated cerebrovascular risk factors and increased spontaneous platelet aggregation, it was demonstrated that 800 mg of garlic powder per day over 4 weeks led to a significant reduction in platelet aggregation and circulating platelet aggregates.[12] This inhibition of platelet aggregation by garlic powder was confirmed by another research group.[13] However, the confounding issue of the various dosage forms of garlic was highlighted by a study of an oil extract of garlic, which found no significant effect on platelet aggregation.[14] In contrast, consumption of a fresh clove of garlic daily for a period of 16 weeks reduced serum thromboxane by about 80%.[15]

One of the compounds responsible for the antiplatelet effect of garlic powder could be ajoene.[16] This compound inhibits aggregation induced by all known platelet agonists in all species studied and prevents the amplification of platelet responses. Unlike aspirin, it acts by modifying the platelet membrane structure.

A review of published studies found that garlic consistently increased fibrinolytic activity after single or multiple doses. Garlic oil and garlic powder were both active, sometimes after only a single dose. The average increase in the reviewed studies was 58%.[17] A 1991 controlled study using raw garlic demonstrated a significant increase in clotting time and fibrinolytic activity after 2 months in normal volunteers.[18]

Adverse effects

A number of case reports have reflected these effects of garlic on bleeding parameters. A spontaneous spinal epidural haematoma associated with platelet dysfunction from excessive garlic ingestion was reported.[19] A patient taking garlic prior to cosmetic surgery experienced bleeding complications and had a clotting time of 12.5 minutes. After cessation of garlic, her clotting time dropped to 6 minutes and there were no complications during a second procedure.[20]

The value of garlic as a prevention and treatment for cardiovascular diseases will best be determined by controlled clinical trials using cardiovascular morbidity or mortality as endpoints. In the meantime, garlic can be prescribed on the basis that it does favourably influence haemorheological parameters (blood flow characteristics) and some cardiovascular risk factors but perhaps not levels of serum cholesterol. Attention should be paid to the type of garlic preparation used; the strongest published evidence to date is for garlic powder preparations, although other preparations will also be of value. Caution should be exercised when prescribing garlic to patients who are also taking other blood-thinning medications such as aspirin or warfarin and garlic intake should be discontinued 10 days before surgery.

Plant phenolics and the vasculature

When Szent-Gyorgy in the 1930s identified the flavonoid constituents of citrus fruits as a necessary co-factor with ascorbic acid in the prevention of scurvy, he opened an investigation which has actually increased in intensity in recent years. Interest in the flavonols such as rutin and its aglycone quercetin has been augmented by a growing fascination with other phenolic molecules, the oligomeric procyanidins and the polyphenolics linked to the tannins, all very common constituents in dietary fruit and vegetables as well as in herbal remedies.

Flavonoids, a group of phenolic constituents found widely in plants, including most fruits and vegetables, have been found to possess a number of anti-inflammatory effects, including, especially for rutin and others from the flavonol subgroup, effects on the microvasculature[21] (see also p.31).

Rutin, quercetin-3-rutoside, is a flavonoid glycoside with quercetin as an aglycone and rhamnose and glucose as sugar moieties. It is very widely distributed in the plant kingdom. It is official in many pharmacopoeias and is widely sold as a health supplement, sometimes in association with vitamin C. In experiments it has been shown to increase survival times of rats fed a thrombogenic diet and in other animals to reduce oedema, reduce cholesterol-induced atheroma and inhibit the carcinogenic action of benzo(a)pyrene.[22] Like ascorbic acid, it is an oxygen radical scavenger and has been shown to reduce the mutagenicity of dusts and asbestos[23] and other stressors.[24–27]

Commercial products with a similar structure, hydroxyethylrutosides or oxerutins (containing principally tri-0-(b-hydroxyethyl) rutoside, as well as a mixture of mono-, di-and tetra-0-(b-hydroxyethyl) rutosides), are marketed for the treatment of chronic venous insufficiency There are a number of reports demonstrating positive effects on capillary permeability,[28–30] on venous insufficiency[31,32] and venous hypertension.[33] Other researchers have reported an improvement in oxygen perfusion of tissues surrounding varicosed veins.[34]

The development of synthetic rutosides has followed the finding that natural rutin is poorly absorbed. However, rutin is now known to be rapidly metabolized by bacteria in the intestine, via quercetin, to 3,4-dihydroxyphenylacetic acid (3,4-DPA), a small phenolic compound with antioxidative properties. Early doubts about the efficacy of such flavonoid molecules (e.g.[35]) have therefore not been sustained.

Congestive heart failure

The original observations by William Withering of the benefits of foxglove in the treatment of dropsy by a country herbalist led to the synthesis of the digitalis glycosides, still the basis of the primary drug treatment for congestive heart failure. Given its seriousness and the potency of these plant extractives, it has generally been accepted that crude herbal drugs no longer have a place in the rational treatment of the condition.

Nevertheless, there is a consistent tradition for the use of herbs with cardiac glycosides such as *Convallaria majalis* (lily of the valley) around the world and pharmacological cases have been made for their use as more broad-spectrum gentler remedies (see p.47). Indeed, the use of crude *Digitalis folium* was favoured by some doctors in Britain over the synthetic isolate until relatively recently. There is also evidence that a wider range of plants may have supportive benefits in the condition. *Terminalia arjuna* (500 mg three times per day) demonstrated substantial benefits in the treatment of refractory congestive heart failure linked to dilated cardiomyopathy in a placebo-controlled double-blind crossover trial.[36]

The cardioglycoside effect may not even be entirely exogenous. Plasma digoxin-like factors (as defined by crossreactivity with digoxin antibody) and in vitro inhibition of ouabain binding have been detected after consumption of several herbal teas. The herb pleurisy root was found with particularly high direct values.[37] Such factors may constructively be used to improve the often uncertain record of synthetic digoxin prescription and eventually help develop gentler supportive strategies for the management of the condition.

Nevertheless, until clearer awareness of these dynamics is achieved it is difficult to recommend particular strategies.

PHYTOTHERAPY FOR CARDIOVASCULAR CONDITIONS

Essential hypertension

In about 90% of cases with hypertension there is no identifiable cause and the term 'essential hypertension' is used. In the remaining cases a cause can be identified and these are known as 'secondary hypertension'. The main cause is kidney disease; other causes include coarctation of the aorta, endocrine diseases and pregnancy. Generally, the treatment for secondary hypertension is the same as for essential hypertension but the cause should also be treated if possible. It is important to ensure that patients presenting with essential hypertension do not have a secondary cause. Many patients with hypertension have coexisting cardiovascular risk factors which should also be treated.

Although the milder stages of essential hypertension should probably not be considered as a disease, subjects with hypertension are more likely than those with normal blood pressure to have a number of cardiovascular diseases. In particular, hypertension is a risk factor for the development of coronary heart disease. As such, it is desirable to treat even mild hypertension.

Treatment should aim for gradual reduction in blood pressure. The kidneys will have become adapted to the previously high levels (indeed, an approach to understanding essential hypertension is that it may be a mechanism to ensure adequate kidney function when this is failing). Sudden reduction could lead to other problems. In this sense natural approaches, if effective, can be doubly suitable.

It is apparent to most practitioners that hypertension is an indication for a broad therapeutic strategy, including dietary and lifestyle advice. Some of the features of this advice are therefore outlined below. It is not advisable to attempt to treat severe (greater than 180/110), malignant or accelerated hypertension with only natural approaches; synthetic prescription drugs can be necessary to avoid serious harm in such cases.

Treatment

Diet and lifestyle

Although the physiological mechanisms responsible for the lowering of BP as a result of exercise have not been elucidated, strong epidemiological and experimental evidence supports a link between the two.[38] Aerobic exercise that uses large muscle groups for 20–60 minutes a day for a minimum of 3 days a week is advisable, although there may have to be a gradual build-up to these levels and all stages should be closely monitored.

Obesity and hypertension are strongly linked. There is a continuous linear relationship between excess body fat, blood pressure and the prevalence of hypertension.[39] A cause-and-effect relationship has also been demonstrated. Hence weight loss should always be attempted. The waist:hip ratio has been found to be a more accurate predictor of hypertension than either body weight or body mass index.[40]

The role of sodium (salt) restriction in treating hypertension has been controversial. However, double-blind studies by MacGregor and co-workers clearly show that even a modest reduction in salt intake leads to a fall in blood pressure; in older patients this is equivalent to results with diuretic therapy.[41] An editorial in the *British Medical Journal* was also supportive of the value of salt intake reduction.[42]

Randomized, controlled trials indicate a specific BP lowering effect of lactovegetarian diets.[39] A non-vegetarian diet rich in fruit and vegetables and low-fat dairy products also significantly reduced BP.[43] Although the effects of caffeine on BP are considered to be temporary, many practitioners suggest a reduction in caffeine intake to reduce aggravating factors.

Potassium supplementation or the use of a high-potassium, high-magnesium salt have been shown to reduce BP.[39,44] Increased calcium intake may also be of value[45] and 6 g per day of fish oil had a mild lowering effect.[46]

Relaxation techniques could be valuable,[45] although their acceptance has been hampered by poorly designed and ambiguous studies.[47]

Some self-prescribed non-prescription drugs may cause or exacerbate hypertension. These include ephedrine, pseudoephedrine and other decongestant and weight loss agents.[48]

Herbs

Most of the herbal treatments for hypertension probably act as peripheral vasodilators. They are all slow to exert their activity, except perhaps for Coleus. Important herbs for this condition include the following.

- Crataegus (hawthorn) – as well as reducing high blood pressure this herb has a trophic effect on the heart muscle. This is important because left ventricular heart failure is often caused by prolonged hypertension. The leaves are apparently more potent than the berries for reducing high blood pressure.

- *Allium sativum* (garlic) – as well as confirmed antihypertensive effects (see p.199) this plant also favourably influences other cardiovascular risk factors. Allicin-releasing preparations are most proven in blood pressure management.

- *Coleus forskohlii* – can have a pronounced lowering effect on high blood pressure. Only varieties containing forskolin should be used. Coleus also has pronounced antiplatelet activity, which may be desirable in some cases.

- Valeriana (valerian) – whether this herb acts as a peripheral or central vasodilator or if the activity is due to a general calming effect on the nervous system is not known. It is usually prescribed for stressed patients.

- *Olea europaea* (olive leaves) – has been proven to lower high blood pressure in clinical trials provided the dose is sufficiently high.

- *Viburnum opulus* (cramp bark) – this herb is thought to relax smooth muscle and has been used to augment antihypertensive prescriptions as a vasorelaxant.

- *Achillea millefolium* (yarrow) – is used by some herbalists to specifically lower an elevated diastolic blood pressure

- *Taraxacum officinale* (dandelion leaves) – has diuretic activity and high levels of potassium and can be useful especially for the treatment of elevated systolic pressure in the elderly.

Other herbs which are also commonly used to lower high blood pressure include Tilia species (lime flowers) and *Viscum album* (mistletoe). The Ayurvedic herb Rauwolfia is a powerful treatment for hypertension but is usually limited to prescription only.

Case history

A female patient aged 48 sought assistance for palpitations, anxiety, angina and mild hypertension. Her ECG did not reveal the presence of a cardiac arrhythmia and her palpitations were less severe in recent times. On examination her blood pressure was 170/95 despite her use of the prescribed drugs Trandate and Plendil.
After treatment over a few months, the following formula was settled upon.

Ginkgo biloba	standardized extract	20 ml
Panax notoginseng	1:2	20 ml
Crataegus folia	1:2	25 ml
Corydalis ambigua	1:2	20 ml
Hypericum perforatum	1:2	25 ml
Passiflora incarnata	1:2	20 ml
Salvia miltiorrhiza	1:2	20 ml
	Total	150 ml

Dose 7.5 ml with water three times a day.
Over the ensuing months her blood pressure was typically 135/85. She had no problems with palpitations and her anxiety and angina had improved.
The rationale for the formula was as follows:

- *Panax notoginseng*, Crataegus and Salvia for her heart and angina.
- The above herbs and Ginkgo, Corydalis and Passiflora for palpitations.
- Corydalis, Passiflora and Hypericum for anxiety.
- Crataegus and the above herbs for anxiety for her hypertension.

Angina

Angina pectoris is a manifestation of ischaemia of the heart muscle which is usually caused by diseased coronary arteries or other reduction in coronary blood flow. It is mostly a distressing rather than dangerous symptom but there is an increased risk of heart attack and a small proportion will have fatal or serious attacks soon after diagnosis. It is therefore not a condition to be treated casually. Conventional prescription drugs may be necessary, although these most often work well with herbal treatments. It is theoretically possible to argue that the frequent use of daily aspirin can be replaced by high phenol and polyphenolic consumption from fruit and vegetables (see Chapter 2) but without firm evidence it is unwise to interfere with a strategy that has good clinical evidence of efficacy. Reduction in smoking, hypertension, obesity, any high cholesterol or lipidaemia and a measured increase in exercise is strongly advisable if these measures can be introduced without serious perturbation.

Treatment

The key herb is Crataegus (hawthorn). Preparations from the leaves and flowers and/or berries may be used. As well as being proven in clinical trials to reduce myocardial oxygen demand (see the hawthorn monograph, p.439), Crataegus is antioxidant, cardioprotective and a coronary artery vasodilator. The clinical trials have shown that Crataegus is safe to combine with conventional drugs.

The Ayurvedic herb *Inula racemosa* (a close relative of elecampane – *Inula helenium*) has been shown to benefit angina in clinical trials. It is said by some authors to be a 'herbal beta-blocker'. The key Ayurvedic herb for heart conditions is *Terminalia arjuna* and this can also be of value in the treatment of angina.

Salvia miltiorrhiza (dan shen) is a Chinese herb which has been clinically studied for angina and other heart conditions. Its benefits include cardioprotective, vasodilator and antiplatelet activities.

Antiplatelet herbs such as *Coleus forskohlii, Allium sativum* (garlic), Zingiber (ginger) and *Curcuma longa* (turmeric) may have value even if the patient is taking aspirin, because of their differing mechanisms. (They do not appear to decrease prostacyclin production. They also have other properties which may be beneficial; e.g. Coleus is a vasodilator and Curcuma is antioxidant. However, care should be taken to ensure that bleeding time is not excessively prolonged.

Many scientists now concede the benefits of red wine in reducing heart disease. However, increased consumption of alcohol is undesirable for other reasons. Grape seed extract (100 mg/day) can therefore provide a suitable substitute for red wine intake.

Capsicum spp. (cayenne) has fibrinolytic activity and was traditionally used to improve myocardial blood supply.

Other vasodilating and relaxing herbs which are prescribed include Tilia species (lime flowers) and *Viburnum opulus* (cramp bark). For angina exacerbated by stress and anxiety, Valeriana and Corydalis or similar calming herbs can be prescribed.

Hyperlipidaemia

Hyperlipidaemia may involve hypercholesterolaemia (elevated serum cholesterol) or hypertriglyceridaemia (evaluated serum triglycerides). In adults less than 65 years of age, a cholesterol concentration greater than 6 mmol/l (240 mg/dl) or a triglyceride concentration greater than 2.8 mmol/l (250 mg/dl) clearly indicates hyperlipidaemia. However, in the presence of other independent risk factors for atherosclerosis, levels lower than these may require treatment (a 'desirable' cholesterol level is less than 5.2 mmol/l). Low high-density lipoprotein (HDL) cholesterol, below 0.9 mmol/l (35 mg/dl), is also a risk factor for atherosclerosis.

While there is no doubt that hyperlipidaemia, especially hypercholesterolaemia, is associated with increased incidence of premature ischaemic heart disease,[49] intervention with drug therapy, especially in some populations, is still controversial, as for example in healthy women[50] and the elderly (where high cholesterol levels may even be protective of health.[51]) However, the benefits of treating raised cholesterol in most patients with coronary heart disease after a myocardial infarction (secondary prevention) are clear.[52]

Treatment

Diet and lifestyle

Dietary treatment should be the first-line therapy for hyperlipidaemia, especially in those population groups where the benefit of more aggressive therapy has not been established. All common and most of the rarer types of hyperlipidaemia respond to diet therapy. Saturated fat intake should be reduced. Fibre, especially soluble fibre from fruit, vegetables, legumes, oats and rice, should be increased. Fish consumption, especially of oily fish, should be increased. There is probably benefit in the use of monounsaturated vegetable oils such as olive oil, and cholesterol intake should be reduced. Alcohol intake should be light and binge drinking avoided.[53]

Herbs

Key herbs to consider are Curcuma (turmeric), *Commiphora mukul* (guggul), *Allium sativum* (garlic) and Cynara (globe artichoke).

These herbs can be supported by saponin-containing herbs which are believed to sequester cholesterol in the digestive tract. Gymnema is rich in saponins and has been found to reduce cholesterol in clinical trials on diabetics (see Chapter 2); saponins from *Medicago sativa* (alfalfa) have also been shown to lower cholesterol.

Mucilages are a class of polysaccharide related to soluble fibre. Soluble fibre such as guar gum is thought to lower cholesterol by the following mechanism. Bacterial flora in the large bowel metabolize soluble fibre to produce short-chain fatty acids (SCFA). Some of these SCFA are carried by the portal venous system to the liver where they influence hepatic metabolism to decrease cholesterol biosynthesis. Patients can supplement their soluble fibre intake with mucilages such as Ulmus (slippery elm), Althaea (marshmallow root) and seeds or hulls from *Plantago species* (psyllium, ispaghula).

Green tea consumption has been shown to significantly reduce serum cholesterol and triglycerides and increase HDL.[54]

Palpitations

Palpitations (undue awareness of the beating of the heart) can be a significant source of anxiety to the sufferer. The awareness is most commonly brought about by a benign change in the rhythm or rate of the heart, amplified in the resonant chamber of a tense thoracic cavity. However, sinus tachycardia or less benign arrhythmias such as ventricular or atrial tachycardia, heart block or atrial fibrillation may be responsible. These factors should be excluded in diagnosis.

Treatment

Diet and lifestyle

A key element in palpitations is likely to be diaphragmatic spasm, unconscious tension of this large muscle and others in the wall of the chest. Palpitations (along with hyperventilation, some nervous dyspepsias and swallowing difficulties) are therefore an important indication for a coordinated programme of breathing exercises, best initiated under instruction. Patients should avoid excessive nicotine and caffeine intake. Intake of chocolate, cheese and synthetic food preservatives should be reduced. Vasodilator drugs and asthma or nasal treatments containing sympathomimetic (e.g. ephedrine) drugs should be reviewed. Excessive intake of the herbs Ephedra, Panax and Paulinia (guarana) and Cola should be avoided. Methods to reduce emotional stress should be advised.

Herbs

The combination of benign arrhythmias or ectopic beats with thoracic tension may be treated with *Leonurus cardiaca* (motherwort), Corydalis, Ginkgo, *Salvia mitiorrhiza* (dan shen) and particularly Crataegus.

Emotional and mental tensions may be reduced with the above combined with herbs such as Valeriana, Scutellaria (skullcap), Passiflora, *Piper methysticum* (kava) and Hypericum (St John's wort).

The dyspeptic and reflux conditions often associated with this syndrome should be treated with the appropriate upper digestive relaxants (see p.172).

Varicose veins

Weakness of the vein wall and poor venous tone can lead to venous valves becoming incompetent. Varicosed veins are the superficial sign of what may be a wider venous insufficiency. Although there are few prospects for cosmetically changing established varicosities, natural treatments stress the need to maintain good venous and connective tissue tone so as to reduce further trouble and improve venous return from the lower body.

Treatment

Diet and lifestyle

Fruit and vegetable intake should be high to maintain optimum levels of flavonols and other supportive elements. Regular walking and resting or sleeping with the legs elevated is often to be recommended. Elastic stockings should be useful, especially if applied first thing in the morning. Cold water applied to the legs from the knee to the foot can help to stimulate circulation and tone the area.

Herbs

Aesculus hippocastanum (horsechestnut)[55] and *Ruscus* (butcher's broom), taken internally and also applied topically in a cream, are key aspects of treatment. These herbs are proven to increase venous tone. Aesculus should not be applied to broken skin.

Crataegus and *Vitis vinifera* (grape seed extract) will also help maintain venous tone.

Melilotus (sweet clover) has antioedema activity and improves venous return.

Circulatory herbs, especially Achillea (yarrow) and Ginkgo, can be very helpful.

Other herbs beneficial on topical application include Symphytum (comfrey), Calendula and Hamamelis (witchhazel).

Stasis dermatitis and stasis ulceration

Stasis dermatitis (varicose eczema) develops in the legs as a result of chronic oedema and venous incompetence. It usually begins as a scaling associated with itching over the medial aspect of the ankle and can progress to become stained as a result of extravasation of blood.

Stasis ulceration (varicose ulcer) is a further complication of stasis dermatitis. The ulcers are shallow and can be quite large. They often result from damage such as knocking the leg and can take months or longer to heal. Bacterial infection is present.

Treatment

Treatment is essentially as for varicose veins but the following additions or modifications are important to prevent further damage and heal any ulcer.

Aesculus or Ruscus should not be applied topically. The best topical treatments consist of Calendula and Echinacea as a lotion and Calendula cream applied on the good skin around the edge of the ulcer.

Inclusion of Centella (gotu kola) for healing and Echinacea for its immune effects in the oral treatment can be beneficial.

References

1. Porkert M. The theoretical foundations of Chinese medicine. MIT Press, Massachusetts, 1978; pp 197–212
2. Oi Y, Okamoto M, Nitta M et al. Alliin and volatile sulfur-containing compounds in garlic enhance the thermogenesis by increasing norepinephrine secretion in rats. Journal Of Nutritional Biochemistry 1998; 9 (2): 60–66
3. Sendl A. Allium sativum and Allium ursinum: Part 1 Chemistry, analysis, history, botany. Phytomedicine 1995; 4: 323–339
4. Warshafsky S, Kamer RS, Sivak SL. Effect of garlic on total serum cholesterol. Annals of Internal Medicine 1993; 119: 599–605
5. Silagy C, Neil A. Garlic as a lipid lowering agent – a meta-analysis. Journal of the Royal College of Physicians of London 1994; 28 (1): 39–45
6. Simons LA, Balasubramaniam S, Von Konigsmark M et al. On the effect of garlic on plasma lipids and lipoproteins in mild hypercholesterolaemia. Atherosclerosis 1995; 113: 219–225
7. Isaacsohn JL, Moser M, Stein EA et al. Garlic powder and plasma lipids and lipoproteins. Archives of Internal Medicine 1998; 158: 1189–1194
8. Berthold HK, Sudhop T, Von Bergmann K. Effect of a garlic oil preparation on serum lipoproteins and cholesterol metabolism: a randomized controlled trial. JAMA 1998; 279 (23): 1900–1902
9. Orekhov AN, Pivovarova EM, Tertov VV. Garlic powder tablets reduce atherogenicity of low density lipoprotein. A placebo-controlled double-blind study. Nutr Metab Cardiovasc Dis 1996; 6: 21–31
10. Breithaupt-Grogler K, Ling M, Boudoulas H et al. Protective effect of chronic garlic intake on elastic properties of aorta in the elderly. Circulation 1997; 96 (8): 2649–2655
11. Silagy CA, Neil HAW. A meta-analysis of the effect of garlic on blood pressure. Journal of Hypertension 1994; 12 (4): 463–468
12. Kiesewetter H, Jung F, Jung EM et al. Effect of garlic on platelet aggregation in patients with increased risk of juvenile ischaemic attack. European Journal of Clinical Pharmacology 1993; 45: 333–336
13. Legnani C, Frascaro M, Guazzaloca G et al. Effects of a dried garlic preparation on fibrinolysis and platelet aggregation in healthy subjects. Arzneimittel- Forsching 1993; 43 (2): 119–122
14. Morris J, Burke V, Mori TA et al. Effects of garlic extract on platelet aggregation: a randomized placebo-controlled double-blind study. Clinical and Experimental Pharmacology and Physiology 1995; 22: 414–417
15. Ali M, Thomson M. Consumption of a garlic clove a day could be beneficial in preventing thrombosis. Prostaglandins, Leukotrienes and Essential Fatty Acids 1995; 53: 211–212
16. Rendu F. L'ajoene, un antiagrégant efficace et subtil. Acta Botanica Gallica 1996; 143 (2/3): 149–154
17. Reuter HD. Allium sativum and allium ursinum: Part 2 Pharmacology and medicinal application. Phytomedicine 1995; 2 (1): 73–91
18. Gadkari JV, Joshi VD. Effect of ingestion of raw garlic on serum cholesterol level, clotting time and fibrinolytic activity in normal subjects. Journal of Postgraduate Medicine 1991; 37 (3): 128
19. Rose KD, Croissant PD, Parliament CF et al. Spontaneous spinal epidural hematoma with associated platelet dysfunction from excessive garlic ingestion: A case report. Neurosurgery 1990; 26 (5): 880–882
20. Burnham BE. Garlic as a possible risk for postoperative bleeding. Plastic and Reconstructive Surgery 1995; 95 (1): 213
21. Lewis DA. Anti-inflammatory drugs from plant and marine sources. Birkhäuser Verlag, Basel 1989, pp 137–164
22. Leung AY. Rutin. In: Leung Ay (ed.) Encyclopedia of common natural ingredients used in food, drugs and cosmetics. John Wiley, New York, 1980
23. Korkina LG, Durnev AD, Suslova TB, Cheremisina ZP, Daugel-Dauge NO, Afanas-ev IB. Oxygen radical-mediated mutagenic effect of asbestos on human lymphocytes: suppression by oxygen radical scavengers. Mutation Research 1992; 265 (2): 245–253
24. Deschner EE, Ruperto J, Wong G, Newmark HL. Quercetin and rutin as inhibitors of azoxymethanol-induced colonic neoplasia. Carcinogenesis 1991; 12 (7): 1193–1196
25. Negre-Salvayre A, Reaud V, Hariton C, Salvayre R. Protective effect of alpha-tocopherol, ascorbic acid and rutin against peroxidative stress induced by oxidized lipoproteins on lymphoid cell lines. Biochemical Pharmacology 1991; 42 (2): 450–453
26. Steele VE, Kelloff GJ, Wilkinson BP, Arnold JT. Inhibition of transformation in cultured rat tracheal epithelial cells by potential chemopreventive agents. Cancer Research 1990; 50 (7): 2068–2074
27. Teofili L, Pierelli L, Iovino MS et al. The combination of quercetin and cytosine arabinoside synergistically inhibits leukemic cell growth. Leukemia Research 1992; 16 (5): 497–503
28. Blumberg S, Clough G, Michel C. Effects of hydroxyethylrutosides on the permeability of frog mesenteric capillaries. Presentation to the AGM of the British Microcirculation Society, Dept of Physiology, Charing Cross and Westminster Medical School, London, 1987
29. Burnand K. Effect of hydroxylethyl rutosides on transcutaneous PO2 measurements. Proceedings of the Surgical Research Society Leeds, 1987
30. Wismer R. The actions of tri-hydroxyethylrutoside on the permeability of the capillaries in man. Praxis 1963; 52: 1412

31. Fitzgerald D. A clinical trial of froxerutin in venous insufficiency of the lower limb. Practitioner 1967; 198: 406
32. Halborg-Sorenson A, Hansen H. Chronic venous insufficiency treated with hydroxyethylrutosides. Angiologica 1970; 7: 192
33. Belcaro G, Rulo A, Candiani C. Evaluation of the microcirculatory effects of Venoruton in patients with chronic venous hypertension by laserdoppler flowmetry, transcutaneous PO2 and PCO2 measurements, leg volumetry and ambulatory venous pressure measurements. Vasa 1989; 18 (2): 146–151
34. McEwan AJ, McArdle CS. Effort of hydroxyethylrutosides on blood oxygen levels and venous insuffiency symptoms in varicose veins. British Medical Journal 1971; 2: 138–141
35. Haeger K. The debatable value of flavonoids in venous insufficiency. Zbl Phlebol. 6, 23
36. Bharani A, Ganguly A, Bhargava KD. Salutary effect of Terminalia Arjuna in patients with severe refractory heart failure. International Journal of Cardiology 1995; 49 (3): 191–199
37. Longerich L, Johnson E, Gault MH. Digoxin-like factors in herbal teas. Clinical and Investigative Medicine 1993; 16 (3): 210–218
38. Yeater RA, Ullrich IH. Hypertension and exercise; where do we stand? Postgraduate Medicine 1992; 91 (5): 429–434
39. Beilin L. Epidemiology of hypertension. Medicine International 1993; 24: 351–355
40. Kochar MS. Hypertension in obese patients. Postgraduate Medicine 1993; 93 (4): 193–200
41. Cappuccio FP, Markandu ND, Carney C et al. Double-blind randomised trial of modest salt restriction in older people. Lancet 1997; 350: 850–854
42. Thelle DS. Salt and blood pressure revisited. British Medical Journal 1996; 321: 1240–1241
43. Appel LJ, Moore TJ, Obarzanek E et al. A clinical trial of the effects of dietary patterns on blood pressure. New England Journal of Medicine 1997; 336 (16): 1117–1124
44. Geleijnse JM, Witteman JCM, Bak AAA et al. Reduction in blood pressure with a low sodium, high potassium, high magnesium salt in older subjects with mild to moderate hypertension. British Medical Journal 1994; 309: 436–440
45. Blake GH, Beebe DK. Management of hypertension; useful nonpharmacologic measures. Postgraduate Medicine 1991; 90 (1): 151–158
46. Bonaa KH, Bjerve KS, Straume B et al. Effect of eicosapentaenoic and docosahexaenoic acids on blood pressure in hypertension. New England Journal of Medicine 1990; 322 (12): 795–801
47. Ramsay LE, Yeo WW, Chadwick IG et al. Non-pharmacological therapy of hypertension. British Medical Bulletin 1994; 50 (2): 494–508
48. Bradley JG. Nonprescription drugs and hypertension; which ones affect blood pressure? Postgraduate Medicine 1991; 89 (6): 195–202
49. Verschuren WMM, Jacobs DR, Bloemberg BPM et al. Serum total cholesterol and long-term coronary heart disease mortality in different cultures; Twenty-five-year follow-up of the seven countries study. JAMA 1995; 274 (2): 131–136
50. Walsh JM, Grady D. Treatment of hyperlipidemia in women. JAMA 1995; 274 (14): 1152–1158
51. Weverling-Rijnsburger AWE, Blauw GJ, Lagaay AM et al. Total cholesterol and risk of mortality in the oldest old. Lancet 1997; 350: 1119–1123
52. Oliver M, Poole-Wilson P, Shepherd J et al. Lower patients' cholesterol now. British Medical Journal 1995; 310: 1280–1281
53. Cullum A. The link between diet and CHD. Practitioner 1994; 238: 855–857
54. Imai K, Nakachi K. Cross sectional study of effects of drinking green tea on cardiovascular and liver diseases. British Medical Journal 1995; 310: 693–696
55. Bombardelli E, Morazzoni P. Aesculus hippocastanum L. Fitoterapia 1996; 67 (6): 483–510

RESPIRATORY SYSTEM

SCOPE

Apart from their use to provide non-specific support for recuperation and repair, specific phytotherapeutic strategies include the following.

Treatment of:

- inflammatory catarrhal conditions of the upper respiratory mucosa (e.g. common colds, rhinitis, sinusitis, otitis media);
- acute bronchial and tracheal infections;
- allergic rhinitis;
- nervous coughing patterns.

Management of:

- chronic obstructive pulmonary diseases (e.g. chronic bronchitis, bronchiectasis, emphysema, silicosis);
- asthma;
- chronic tracheitis;
- coughing due to persistent local irritation.

Because of its use of secondary plant products, particular **caution** is necessary in applying phytotherapy in cases of known allergic reactions to specific medicinal plant products.

RATIONALE AND ORIENTATION

To the Chinese the lungs were the internal organs most in contact with the exterior. So as well as ascribing to them the source of the body's rhythm and the site of the catalysis of vital energies, they were seen to be the organs in charge of defences. In earlier times the role of the respiratory system was obvious; the first cry was generally taken to be the first sign of life, the bronchial gasp on the deathbed the last, and everywhere like a never-ending nightmare was the hacking bloody cough of consumption or tuberculosis, the disease that once cast its baleful influence over the popular imagination like cancer and AIDS now do, the constant reminder of how fatal debility followed weakening of the lungs. It was obvious that the lungs, even more than the stomach, were prey to contagion, the expressive medieval precursor to viruses and bacteria. It was also obvious that the key to resistance lay not in attacking the alien invaders but in strengthening innate resources. Traditional strategies for treating respiratory disease were notably founded on supportive and tonifying remedies. Given that the modern virus remains as elusive as it ever was, an emphasis on supporting defences may seem appropriate again.

This is one area where the divide between traditional and modern approaches is particularly great. There are very few modern endorsements of early treatment strategies. Modern medical science, which at first embraced such agents in the earlier part of this century, now sees no role for their use. For example, modern editions of *Martindale's Extra Pharmacopoeia* claim that: 'There is little evidence to show that expectorants are effective'. Some modern drugs may have expectorant activity, such as bromhexine, but they are usually referred to as 'mucolytic'. The impact of traditional remedies on the respiratory system is relatively poorly researched. Reliable external measures of change in mucosal functions are elusive; many respiratory diseases are either self-limiting or are among some of the most persistent conditions in the clinic. Even in asthma, where peak flow rates provide a simple measure of benefit, the complexity of the condition and the usual presence of confounding and violent influences makes easy characterization of the condition and the measurement of all but the most powerful across-the-board remedies unreliable.

A sense that traditional approaches should be relegated to history is possibly reinforced in the medical psyche by the knowledge that one of the most dramatic advances of modern drugs was in controlling at last the old scourge of tuberculosis. However, this dismissal is not as conclusive as once thought. Tuberculosis is making a serious comeback on the world stage, attacking first the very impoverished and malnourished as it always did. As modern drugs struggle with this new manifestation, there may once again be value in looking at the lessons from the past, that treatment should be based on supportive remedies in a regime of convalescence. With the luxury of choice, with the option of taking modern drugs where these are necessary but also being able to select more supportive strategies at other times, there is real value in reviewing the treatments forged out of desperate but not always unsuccessful battles with disease in earlier times. These lessons are fortunately quite well learnt.

The dominant feature of respiratory conditions is how readily changes in their behaviour are appreciated subjectively. The often immediate effects of eating and drinking different foods and drinks, of temperature and humidity changes and of the various treatments used through history have been the main guide in determining therapeutic strategy. From such experience has come the view of the respiratory mucosa and musculature as being particularly sensitive to reflex responses, notably from the upper digestive tract, from the pharynx to the stomach. There is a persistent tradition in many cultures that respiratory problems are extensions of digestive dysfunctions. Embryology supports such links, with the bronchial tree starting as a diverticulum of the pharyngeal zone of the alimentary duct and sharing common vagal innervation, and recent associations between asthma and H_2 receptors in the stomach[1] add further support to such connections.

PHYTOTHERAPEUTICS

Part of the problem with expectorants probably arises from confusion over their definition. Another aspect of the dismissal of expectorants stems from the difficulties involved with measuring their efficacy.

The four definitions of expectorants given below highlight the difficulties. The dictionary meaning is only concerned with the actual oral production of phlegm or sputum. Since the majority of mucus produced from the lungs is swallowed, this definition is clearly unsatisfactory. Definitions from the pharmacologists Boyd and Lewis are more useful but probably the best definition comes from Brunton, a 19th century pharmacologist.

Definitions of expectorants

- Oxford Dictionary – 'Promoting the ejection of phlegm by coughing or spitting.'
- Boyd (1954) – 'An expectorant may be pharmacologically defined as a substance which increases the output of demulcent respiratory tract fluid.'
- Lewis (1960) – 'Expectorants increase the secretions of the respiratory tract and so reduce the viscosity of the mucus which can then act as a demulcent. By virtue of the presence of increased quantities of fluid mucus, expectorants produce a "productive cough" which is less exhausting and less painful to the patient.'
- Brunton (1885) – 'Remedies which facilitate the removal of secretions from the air passages. The secretion may be rendered more easy of removal by an alteration in its character or by increased activity of the expulsive mechanism.' Brunton's functional definition best explains the various ways in which medicinal plants can act as expectorants.

Why expectorants?

Many respiratory conditions are characterized by abnormal mucus (catarrh) which can narrow airways. This abnormal mucus may be thick and tenacious and hence very difficult to clear from the airways.

If expectorants can render this catarrh more fluid and/or assist in its expulsion, then a clinical benefit should be achieved.

Expectorants can help to relieve debilitating cough. The presence of an irritation in the airways (such as tenacious abnormal mucus) invokes the cough reflex. (The cough reflex is most sensitive in the trachea and larger airways. The sensitivity progressively decreases in the finer airways and in the very fine airways there is no reflex at all. So in alveolitis, there is little stimulation of the cough reflex, whereas for tracheitis the stimulus is strong.) By clearing abnormal mucus or by changing its character and making it more demulcent, expectorants can allay cough and are therefore antitussive.

From the incomplete scientific case and lack of a consensus orthodox view, it is clear that in the respiratory system the traditional therapeutic case dominates. In many instances however, the traditional case is strong and consistent across cultures and aeons. It includes mechanisms that are rational and which are usually immediately apparent. The following are categories of herbal remedies acting on the respiratory tract.

Topical agents

Throat applications

The surfaces at the back of the mouth and pharynx are the first point of contact for ingested or inhaled pathogens and irritants; the dense masses of lymphatic tissue in the region confirm their important role in defence. The use of gargles, lozenges and cough drops to mobilize local defences can be an effective way to encourage the body's response to a wide range of respiratory infections. In the case of sore throats, demulcent remedies, e.g. licorice and marshmallow,[2] and astringents such as Rubus (blackberry leaf) and Hamamelis (witchhazel) could at least reduce irritation and there are a range of remedies with more substantial reputations as topical antiinflammatories. These can be used as levers to improve resistance and recovery in rhinitis, sinusitis and otitis as well as treating more local inflammations. Rather than attempting local antisepsis, remedies such as tinctures of Calendula and myrrh, sage and thyme, balm of Gilead, propolis and Tolu balsam appear to mobilize activity in the surrounding lymphatic tissues, through the mildly provocative effect of their resins and essential oils.

Inhalations

The obvious topical applications for the respiratory mucosa, traditional approaches included smoking

(Datura for asthma, for example, a high-risk treatment not recommended today), inhaling steam from herbal infusions to relieve congestion and simple humidification. When the technology for extracting essential oils was developed medical inhalations were frequent applications. Most apparent activity is found with the oils from mints (especially menthol), Eucalyptus, camphor, the Melaleuca family (tea tree – *M. alternifolia*, cajaput – *M. leucadendron*, niaouli – *M. viridiflora*) and the pine family (turpentine – *Pinus palustris, P. sylvestris, P. excelsa*) and these were widely used for symptomatic relief of respiratory congestion, although in the case of menthol there are doubts as to the real benefits.[3] It is possible that some volatile principles could exert antiinflammatory effects (steam inhaled from chamomile flower infusions in some allergic rhinitis and pine oils in bronchitis, for example). Small doses of volatile oils may have a complex combination of activities, either reducing or stimulating ciliary activity[4] or mucosal secretions.[5]

Stimulating (reflex) expectorants

These are remedies that provoke increased mucociliary activity by reflex stimulation of the upper digestive wall. The classic examples were originally used as emetics. It was noted that this drastic action was accompanied by a noticeable expectoration. In fact, traditional practitioners in Britain used emesis as a technique to clear the lungs in chronic bronchitis until quite recent times. Application of these remedies in subemetic doses was thus a consistent feature in all major herbal traditions. Herbs like ipecacuanha, squills and Lobelia have been standards in Western medicine. There is some limited modern investigation of mechanisms involved. For example, ipecac-induced emesis is thought to be mediated through both peripheral and central 5-HT_3 receptors.[6] Other plants have been used as stimulating expectorants although not used as emetics; members of the Primula, Bellis, Saponaria and Polygala genuses are often included in this category in Western traditions. High saponin levels seem to be a common feature of this group.

Warming expectorants and mucolytics

Many of the spices were highly prized in the cold damp climates of northern Europe for their apparent ability to counteract associated chest problems. In particular, ginger had an almost mythical reputation; where this or imported cinnamon, aniseed, fennel and cloves were not available, Europeans resorted to garlic, mustard and horseradish for the same ends. Even cayenne or chilli peppers were used for this purpose, although generally taken to be too drying in most cases. The effect of the pungent spices probably includes increased blood flow to the respiratory mucosa, a reflex irritation of the upper digestive mucosa (as with the stimulating expectorants) and, especially in the sulphur-containing garlic and mustard family, a decrease in the thickness of mucus by altering the structure of its mucopolysaccharide constituents; the sensation usually is of a clearing of catarrh and the shifting of congestion up from the lungs.[7] A simple infusion of fresh ginger and cinnamon remains one of the most effective home treatments for the common cold.

Respiratory demulcents

These herbs contain mucilage and have a soothing and antiinflammatory action on the lower respiratory tract. Although the mechanism is not clear, an opposite effect to that of the stimulating expectorants has been postulated; i.e. the effect is a reflex one from the demulcent effect of the pharynx and upper digestive tract, again involving common embryonic origins and vagal innervation.

The major respiratory demulcent herbs are *Althaea officinalis* (marshmallow root or leaves) and other members of the Malvaceae (mallows), *Ulmus spp* (slippery elm), members of the Plantago genus, *Cetraria islandica* (Iceland moss) and *Chondrus crispus* (Irish moss). Tussilago (coltsfoot) and Symphytum (comfrey) were very widely popular before concerns about pyrrolizidine alkaloids constrained their sales.

Pronounced antitussive activity has been demonstrated experimentally with oral doses of 1000 mg/kg body weight of extract of *Althaea officinalis* (marshmallow), with comparable effects at 50 mg/kg of the isolated polysaccharides.[8] These animal studies might suggest enormous doses necessary for clinical effect but if, as implied, the effect is a mechanical one, then it is likely that only marginal increases in dose would be necessary to have similar impact in larger animals like humans.

Respiratory demulcents were popular for children's cough and generally for dry, irritable and ticklish coughing. They were seen as intrinsically contraindicated in wet, damp chest problems, although they can sometimes be quite well suited to these if there is an irritable element.

Respiratory spasmolytics

Respiratory spasmolytics relax the bronchioles of the lungs. Traditionally they included the Solanaceous plants (the nightshade family) with powerful atropine-related antiparasympathetic constituents: Datura, Atropa and Solanum were the prominent antiasthmatics of early history. As could now be explained pharmacologically, these remedies tended also to dry up the mucosa and had other less desirable effects so less powerful remedies were also popular. *Ephedra sinica* (ma huang) from Asia was popular when it reached Europe and works through a sympathomimetic action. Other gentle remedies include culinary herbs like hyssop and especially thyme,[7] horehound and the North American gumplant, *Grindelia comporum*.

Anticatarrhals

There are a range of popular herbal treatments for a range of respiratory mucosal conditions whose action still remains mysterious. Indications for their use range from catarrhal congestion to some types of mucosal hypersensitivity such as hayfever and allergic rhinitis.

Antitussives

Antitussives are remedies that allay coughing. Some may work through soothing irritability (respiratory demulcents); others are claimed to relieve coughs at source, by removing congestive mucus or other mobile provocations (expectorants).

However, the term 'antitussive' is often used specifically to refer to remedies that depress the cough reflex and in particular, in herbal terms, to those with appreciable levels of cyanogenic glycosides. The notable example in Western tradition is *Prunus serotina* (wild cherry). Another tradition was to use opiates and the gentle version of that strategy, Lactuca (wild lettuce), is still applied to the problem in some traditions. Such cough suppressants are not ideal treatments and could even be counterproductive if they reduce cleansing of the lungs. However, there are many cases where they provide helpful relief and they may be the only solution for coughing not due to mobilizable irritants (e.g. nervous cough on the one hand, tumours on the other).

Antiallergic herbs

The principal antiallergic herbs for respiratory tract allergies are Ephedra, Albizzia and *Scutellaria baicalensis* (Baical skullcap). Urtica (nettles) is another herb with antiallergic properties which can sometimes be useful, especially for allergic rhinitis.

Multipurpose remedies

As can be seen from the above, some herbs may fall into several categories. This is either because they contain several active components or a group of active components are acting in several different ways. For example, Verbascum (mullein) contains saponins which are expectorant, mucilage which is demulcent and iridoids which are anticatarrhal. Lobelia, although an emetic and stimulating expectorant, was used as primarily a relaxant remedy in 19th century North America; it thus has a broad-spectrum of effects on the respiratory system. Probably the broadest acting remedy in common use, however, is Glycyrrhiza (licorice) which combines a saponin stimulant effect, a soothing effect and appreciable antiinflammatory properties.

STIMULATING EXPECTORANTS

Plant remedies traditionally used as stimulating (reflex) expectorants

Cephaelis (ipecacuanha), *Lobelia inflata* (lobelia), Urginea (squills), *Primula veris* (cowslip), Bellis (daisy), Saponaria (soapwort), *Polygala senega* (snakeroot), Glycyrrhiza (licorice).

Indications for stimulating expectorants

- Cough linked to bronchial congestion
- Bronchitis, emphysema

Other traditional indications for stimulating expectorants

- In some cases as emetics in higher doses (×10 expectorant dose)

Contraindications for stimulating expectorants

Although there is no firm evidence of unsuitability, as gastric irritants they can transiently upset some individuals (immediately relieved by withdrawing or changing the remedy). In addition, the use of stimulating expectorants should be kept under review in cases of:

- dry and irritable conditions of the lungs;
- asthma;
- young children;
- dyspeptic conditions.

Application

Stimulating expectorants are best taken in hot infusions or as tinctures or fluid extracts, before food.

Long-term therapy with stimulating expectorants is appropriate in the management of chronic bronchial conditions as long as digestive functions are not affected.

Advanced phytotherapeutics

Stimulating expectorants may also be usefully applied in some cases (depending on other factors) of rheumatic and connective tissue diseases.

WARMING EXPECTORANTS (MUCOLYTICS)

Plant remedies traditionally used as warming expectorants

Pimpinella anisum (aniseed), *Cinnamomum zeylanicum* (cinnamon), Foeniculum (fennel), Zingiber (ginger), *Allium sativum* (garlic), *Angelica archangelica* (angelica).

Indications for warming expectorants

- Productive cough associated with cold
- Bronchitis, emphysema
- Profuse catarrhal conditions

Other traditional indications for warming expectorants

- As aromatic digestives (see p.171)
- Congestive chronic infections and inflammatory conditions

Contraindications for warming expectorants

The use of warming expectorants may be contraindicated or inappropriate in gastrooesophageal reflux.

Traditional therapeutic insights into the use of warming expectorants

There is a close association in traditional medicine between catarrhal congestion and the digestive/assimilative functions. The warming remedies were seen to act seamlessly across both respiratory and digestive functions treating disturbances in either or both together. Symptoms most often found with catarrhal conditions might include abdominal distension, loss of appetite and loose stools.

Applications

Warming expectorants are best taken immediately before meals. They are particularly effective taken in hot aqueous infusions.

Long-term therapy with warming expectorants is usually acceptable.

RESPIRATORY DEMULCENTS

Plant remedies traditionally used as respiratory demulcents

Althaea (marshmallow), Tussilago (coltsfoot), Plantago spp (ribwort and plantain), Verbascum (mullein, esp. leaf), Chondrus (Irish moss), Cetraria (Iceland moss), Glycyrrhiza (licorice).

Indications for respiratory demulcents

- Dry, non-productive, irritable cough
- Coughing in children
- Asthmatic wheezing and tightness

Other traditional indications for respiratory demulcents

- As mucilaginous digestive remedies (see p.169)
- The effects of dryness on the respiratory system

Contraindications for respiratory demulcents

The use of respiratory demulcents may be contraindicated or inappropriate in profuse catarrhal or congestive conditions of the mucosa.

Traditional therapeutic insights into the use of respiratory demulcents

As with other respiratory remedies, there is a close association between effects here and on the digestive tract. Respiratory demulcents are at their most appropriate if there are parallel indications in the gut: dry inflamed conditions like gastritis and oesophagitis associated with hyperacidity, dry constipation and its various associated problems.

Application

Respiratory demulcents are best taken before meals. They are particularly effective taken in cold aqueous infusions.

Long-term therapy with respiratory demulcents is usually well tolerated.

RESPIRATORY SPASMOLYTICS

Plant remedies traditionally used as respiratory spasmolytics

Ephedra (ma huang), *Datura stramonium* (jimson weed), *Atropa belladonna* (deadly nightshade), *Solanum dulcamara* (bittersweet), Hyssopus (hyssop), *Thymus vulgaris* (thyme), *Lobelia inflata* (lobelia), *Marrubium vulgare* (horehound), *Grindelia camporum* (gumplant), *Euphorbia hirta* (pill-bearing spurge), *Coleus forskohlii*, Glycyrrhiza (licorice), *Inula* (ele campane).

Indications for respiratory spasmolytics

- Tight, breathless, non-productive coughing
- Wheezing and other asthmatic symptoms

Other traditional indications for respiratory spasmolytics

- Many of the gentler remedies were used as relaxants.
- The Solanaceous plants have potent neuroactive properties.

Contraindications for respiratory spasmolytics

The use of respiratory spasmolytics may be contraindicated or inappropriate in the following:

- in the case of solanaceous plants: glaucoma, urinary retention, paralytic ileus, intestinal atony and obstruction
- in the case of ephedra: appetite disorders, glaucoma, prescription of MA01-inhibitors

Application

Respiratory spasmolytics may be taken at any time of the day as required for immediate effect.

Long-term therapy with respiratory spasmolytics is acceptable in the case of the gentler examples but not for the solanaeous plants or Ephedra, and in all cases, there should be attention to treatment of underlying causes rather than relying on symptomatic relief.

ANTICATARRHALS

Plant remedies traditionally used as anticatarrhals

Euphrasia spp (eyebright), *Plantago lanceolata* (ribwort), *Sambucus nigra* (elder), *Nepeta hederacea* (ground ivy), *Solidago virgaurea* (goldenrod), *Verbascum thapsis* (mullein flowers) and *Hydrastis canadensis* (goldenseal).

Indications for anticatarrhals

- Catarrhal conditions, especially in the upper respiratory tract
- Sinusitis, otitis media
- Allergic rhinitis and other hypersensitivity conditions

Contraindications for anticatarrhals

Anticatarrhals are generally regarded as gentle and safe.

Application

Anticatarrhals are best taken before meals.

Long-term therapy with anticatarrhals is usually well tolerated.

ANTITUSSIVES

Plant remedies traditionally used as antitussives

Prunus serotina (wild cherry bark), Lactuca (wild lettuce).

Indications for antitussives

- Non-productive, severe or persistent cough refractory to expectorants
- Nervous cough
- Cough due to external irritation or obstruction (e.g. tumour)

Contraindications for antitussives

Antitussives should be used only as needed and limited as soon as practical.

Application

Antitussives are best taken before meals.

Long-term therapy with antitussives is not advisable.

PHYTOTHERAPY FOR RESPIRATORY CONDITIONS

Allergic and non-allergic rhinitis

Rhinitis is an inflammation of the lining of the nose characterized by one or more of the following symptoms: nasal congestion, nasal discharge, sneezing and itching. Acute infectious rhinitis (and sinusitis) is usually due to the common cold and the appropriate treatment is described later in this chapter. Chronic infectious rhinitis is treated using the same approach as described under chronic sinusitis. Allergic rhinitis is triggered by inhaled allergens and may be perennial or seasonal (hayfever). Non-allergic or vasomotor rhinitis has no identified medical cause, although in naturopathic traditions it is understood as being caused or exacerbated by diet. Rhinitis may also be drug induced by overuse of nasal sprays containing decongestants.

In the herbal treatment of rhinitis, it is important to identify whether or not inhaled allergens are involved, since this determines the approach to treatment.

Treatment

The approach to the herbal treatment of rhinitis is to control symptoms and remove causes. Avoidance measures to reduce exposure to aeroallergens should be part of this treatment.

Dietary exclusions should be tried for both allergic and non-allergic rhinitis. Herbalists believe that diet can create a state of hypersensitivity and catarrh of the mucous membranes which predisposes to rhinitis. The dietary components which contribute to this process do not necessarily give a positive reaction on the RAST or skin prick test. They include dairy products, wheat, salt and refined carbohydrates. Excessive consumption of these should be avoided by sufferers of rhinitis and complete exclusion of one component, e.g. dairy, should be tried for at least 1 month.

Essential aspects of treatment are as follows.

- Immune-enhancing herbs such as Echinacea. This is especially the case for allergic rhinitis.

- Antiallergic herbs, e.g. Albizzia, only in the case of allergic rhinitis.

- Upper respiratory anticatarrhal herbs for both types of rhinitis, e.g. Euphrasia, Hydrastis and *Plantago lanceolata*.

- When treating seasonal allergic rhinitis, treatment must be commenced 6 weeks before the season starts and continued through the season. Any helpful dietary exclusions should also follow this time pattern.

- Stress can exacerbate rhinitis and should be treated if it is considered to be a factor with tonic herbs, nervine tonics, sedative herbs and adaptogens as appropriate (see p.231).

- Treatment of rhinitis at a deeper level may involve the use of depuratives, e.g. Galium (cleavers), lymphatics, e.g. Phytolacca (poke root) and choleretics and hepatics.

Case history

A 30-year-old female patient with chronic persistent rhinitis. Symptoms were worse in the morning with clear nasal discharge and irritated eyes. She was sensitive to house dust mite and had suffered tonsillitis, adenoids and otitis media as a child. She regularly took antihistamines. Treatment consisted of a dairy-free diet, protective measures against house dust mite and the following herbs.

Echinacea angustifolia	1:2	30 ml
Picrorrhiza kurroa	1:2	5 ml
Zingiber officinale	1:2	5 ml
Euphrasia officinalis	1:2	25 ml
Scutellaria baicalensis	1:2	20 ml
Albizzia lebbeck	1:2	15 ml
	Tot al	100 ml

Dose 8 ml with water twice a day.
Hydrastis 500 mg tablets, one tablet three times a day.
After 3 months of herbs, her antihistamine use was greatly reduced and symptoms were very much improved.

Common cold and influenza

Viral infections of the respiratory tract can be minor self-limiting, frequent and recurrent or terminally dangerous. Their unpredictable course makes reliable treatment recommendations notoriously difficult. However, the often instant benefits following some remedies and the experience of improving resistance to frequent winter viral infections in some individuals does provide support for some of the recommendations below.

Treatment

The basic treatment approaches for the common cold and influenza are similar. However, in the case of more severe forms of influenza, treatment is more vigorous (e.g. higher or more repeated doses). Essential aspects of treatment are as follows.

- Diaphoretics and heating remedies to manage and improve febrile responses. For the most direct agents, circulatory stimulants Zingiber (ginger, especially fresh grated) and cinnamon taken in hot water can dramatically improve mucosal symptoms and fend off the sensation of cold. For more gentle but sustained effects, especially in children, hot teas of Mentha piperita (peppermint), *Eupatorium perfoliatum* (boneset), *Nepeta cataria* (catmint), Achillea (yarrow), Tilia (lime flowers) and Sambucus (elderflower) are well-established diaphoretic approaches which in the context of a cold can exert surprisingly different effects than when consumed at other times. *Asclepias tuberosa* (pleurisy root) is indicated if there are pulmonary or bronchial complications. *Allium sativum* (garlic, taken raw) may also be useful as a general and warming defensive agent.

• Immune-enhancing herbs such as Echinacea, Andrographis and Picrorrhiza to support the body's fight against the virus. Note that Astragalus and tonics such as *Panax ginseng* are contraindicated in the acute stage of infection.

• Anticatarrhal herbs for upper respiratory catarrh, especially Euphrasia (eyebright), Sambucus (elder) and Hydrastis (golden seal). Traditionally, Hydrastis was said to be contraindicated in the acute stage of infection so its use may be best in the later stages of the secondary bacterial infection.

• Hypericum (St John's wort) as an antiviral treatment for influenza.

Acute and chronic sinusitis

With sinusitis, the drainage of the sinuses is blocked, usually by congestion and mucosal oedema. This results in stasis which allows a bacterial infection to take hold. Pain is caused by either negative pressure (due to absorption of gases by the vasculature) or positive pressure of mucosal congestion.

Factors involved in the aetiology of chronic sinusitis include pollution, occupational dust exposure, tobacco smoke, adenoids, allergy (especially in children), rhinitis, cold and damp weather, dental problems, trauma and flying. A deviated nasal septum or other structural causes may be present. Herbalists also believe that dietary factors can cause excessive mucus discharge which may cause and sustain the disease. Particularly implicated are dairy products, salt and wheat. Stasis and congestion may be aggravated if the patient has inadequate fluid intake.

Treatment

The treatment approaches for acute and chronic sinusitis are similar. For acute sinusitis the dose should be higher and given more frequently and treatment may need to be supplemented with diaphoretics, etc. as for acute rhinitis if fever is present.

Acute and chronic sinusitis

• Supporting the immune system in its fight against the bacteria with immune-enhancing herbs such as Echinacea, Andrographis and Picrorrhiza.

• Anticatarrhal (e.g. euphrasia) and decongestant (e.g. Ephedra) herbs to clear the stasis.

• Mucolytic herbs to clear the stasis such as *Allium sativum* (garlic) and Armoracia (horseradish).

• Particularly indicated is Hydrastis (golden seal) which has antimicrobial and anticatarrhal properties and is a mucous membrane trophorestorative. Regularly chewing a Hydrastis tablet can be very beneficial but they are exceedingly bitter.

• A steam inhalation containing antimicrobial and antiinflammatory essential oils, e.g. tea tree, pine, aniseed oils, or chamomile flowers, may be useful.

Chronic sinusitis only

• Chronic sinusitis may represent a vicarious elimination and this can be treated with depuratives, e.g. Galium (cleavers), and lymphatics, e.g. Phytolacca.

• Exposure to the environmental factors listed above should be reduced and a dairy-free, low-salt diet should be tried for at least 3 months.

• The sinuses are relatively inaccessible regions of the body and once a chronic infection has taken hold it can be difficult to eradicate. The following topical treatment can be beneficial.

Capsicum annuum	1.3	20 ml
Lobelia inflata	1:8	20 ml
Hydrastis canadensis	1:3	20 ml
Commiphora mol-mol	1:5	20 ml
Myrica cerifera	1:2	20 ml
	Total	100 ml

Work over the affected sinuses for 10 minutes once to twice a day. Keep away from the eyes. Use a glove or wash hands after using.
The Capsicum and Myrica act as decongestants, the myrrh is antiseptic and lobelia assists penetration. The properties of Hydrastis are given above. If Lobelia is unavailable, substitute with a saponin-containing herb such as Bupleurum or Aesculus (horsechestnut).

• Patients with chronic sinusitis should avoid antihistamines and steroid-based decongestant drugs as these will weaken immunity in the region further.

Case history

A male patient aged 36 presented with chronic sinusitis which followed from a bout of the common cold. There was a history of allergic rhinitis with chronic use of antihistamines and nasal steroids. Antibiotics had failed to resolve the condition which had been present for 4 years. The patient had a high dairy intake and had been a cigarette smoker.
Treatment consisted of the following.

Echinacea angustifolia	1:2	40 ml
Euphrasia officinalis	1:2	30 ml
Hydrastis canadensis	1:3	25 ml
Phytolacca decandra	1:5	5 ml
	Total	100 ml

Dose 5 ml with water three times daily
In addition, allicin-releasing garlic tablets (5000 mg fresh weight equivalent) three per day and Picrorrhiza 500 mg tablets, two per day, were prescribed. The patient was placed on a dairy-free and low-salt diet and advised not to use antihistamines and steroid decongestant drugs. The above sinus rub was also prescribed.
After a period of 6 months of treatment, symptoms were considerably improved.

Chronic tonsillitis and chronic sore throat

Chronic sore throat may be a symptom of other disorders, e.g. sinusitis. However, it may exist in its own right as a chronic bacterial infection in a patient with or without tonsils.

Treatment

The approaches to the herbal treatment of chronic tonsillitis and chronic sore throat are similar. The main aspects of treatment are as follows.

- Immune-enhancing herbs. Being a chronic condition, Astragalus may be used as well as Echinacea, Picrorrhiza and Andrographis.
- Lymphatic and depurative herbs.
- A local treatment such as a throat spray or lozenge using herbs such as:

  Glycyrrhiza (licorice) – soothing, antiinflammatory, topically antiviral
  Salvia (sage) – astringent and antiseptic
  Propolis – antiseptic, healing and anaesthetic
  Kava – anaesthetic
  Echinacea – immune enhancing, antiinflammatory
  Capsicum – stimulant, antiseptic
  Hydrastis (golden seal) – antiseptic, mucous membrane trophorestorative
  Althaea (marshmallow root) – demulcent
  Myrrh – antiseptic, induces local leucocytosis

- A dairy-free diet rich in fruit and vegetables should be observed.

Case history

A male patient aged 65 complained of a chronic sore throat which had been present for years. Other conditions were also being treated, but for the sore throat he was prescribed:

- *Echinacea angustifolia 1:2* 5 ml once a day with water
- A gargle consisting of:

Echinacea angustifolia	1:2	40 ml
Propolis	1:5	30 ml
Salvia officinalis	1:2	30 ml
	Total	100 ml

Dose 2 ml in 10 ml water as a gargle on the affected area of the throat twice a day. Swallow after use.
After 8 weeks the sore throat was considerably improved. With continuing treatment it has almost gone.

Otitis media

Inflammation of the middle ear, or otitis media, can be divided into acute, chronic or serous.

Viral upper respiratory tract infection is most commonly associated with the onset of acute otitis media, although the major infection present is bacterial. Symptoms can include pain, purulent discharge from the ear, hearing loss, vertigo, tinnitus and fever. Examination will demonstrate a red, dull and bulging or perforated ear drum.

Chronic otitis media with discharge from the ear can result from ineffectively treated acute or recurrent otitis media. The infection is clearly bacterial.

Serous otitis media or secretory otitis media (or 'glue ear') is an enigmatic disorder that usually occurs in children. Examination of the ear drum shows that it is retracted ('sucked in') and there is fluid in the middle ear cavity which can lead to conductive hearing loss. Allergy, nasal infection and chronic sinus infection may be involved and it is associated with increased frequency of respiratory infections. Medical treatment can involve the use of grommets to drain the middle ear cavity. The overuse of antibiotics is probably ill advised, although bacterial infection may play a role in some patients with this disorder.

Treatment

The treatments of acute and chronic otitis media are similar to the treatments of acute and chronic sinusitis respectively (with the exclusion of the topical treatment containing Capsicum).

Secretory otitis media (SOM) should be regarded as an allergic disorder, as well as possibly a vicarious elimination. A dairy-free, low-salt diet should be tried or otherwise a full elimination diet. However, the presence of microorganisms which contribute to the inflammation or the malfunction of the eustachian tube should also be considered. If adenoids are implicated, then the SOM should be treated similarly to tonsillitis. The following herbs should be emphasized during treatment.

- Antiallergic and decongestant herbs such as Albizzia, Ephedra and *Scutellaria baicalensis*.
- Upper respiratory anticatarrhal herbs such as Euphrasia, Solidago, Hydrastis, *Plantago lanceolata* and *Glechoma hederacea*.
- Depurative and lymphatic herbs such as Galium (cleavers) and Phytolacca.
- Immune-enhancing herbs, particularly Echinacea and Astragalus, to correct the presence of allergy and possibly infection.
- Chewing on a Hydrastis tablet (difficult for children because of its bitterness) will accentuate its mucous membrane trophorestorative and antibacterial effects on the upper respiratory tract.

Acute bronchitis

Acute bronchitis is an acute inflammation of the trachea and bronchi caused by bacteria. It commonly follows the common cold, influenza, measles or whooping cough. Patients with chronic bronchitis are particularly prone to develop episodes of acute bronchitis (where their sputum turns from grey or white to yellow or green). Other factors which can predispose to this kind of bacterial infection include cold, damp, dust and cigarette smoking.

Initially there is an irritating, unproductive cough which eventually progresses over a few days to copious, mucopurulent sputum. Infection usually starts in the trachea and progresses to the bronchi and with this spread there is a general febrile disturbance with temperatures of 38–39°C. Gradual recovery should occur over the next 4–8 days. However, it may progress to bronchiolitis or bronchopneumonia.

Treatment

Being an acute disorder, it is important to give frequent doses of herbs and, if possible, to follow the progression of the infection, adapting the treatment to the various stages.

- Antiseptic herbs such as *Inula helenium*, *Thymus vulgaris* and *Allium sativum* (garlic) should be prescribed throughout the course of the infection and preferably should be continued for 1 week into recovery to prevent relapse.
- During the dry, unprotective cough phase, demulcents such as Althaea glycetract should be prescribed.
- Diaphoretic herbs are indicated during the febrile phase, particularly *Asclepias tuberosa* (pleurisy root) which is almost a specific for acute lower respiratory tract infections. It is often combined with Zingiber to enhance its effectiveness. Other diaphoretics such as Tilia and Achillea can also be prescribed.
- Expectorant herbs, which include *Inula helenium*, *Thymus vulgaris*, Polygala and other saponin-containing herbs, Foeniculum (fennel), Pimpinella (aniseed) and Marrubium (white horehound) can be prescribed throughout the course of the disorder.
- Anticatarrhal herbs, especially Verbascum, *Plantago lanceolata* and Hydrastis, may be indicated when the sputum is particularly copious or if the productive cough lingers beyond the acute stage.
- Antitussive herbs should be used to help the cough, especially at night, and *Prunus serotina* (wild cherry) is particularly indicated if tracheitis predominates.

Whooping cough

Whooping cough or pertussis is a highly infectious disease caused by *Bordetella pertussis*. About 90% of cases occur in children under 5 years.

The first stage consists of respiratory infection lasting about 1 week during which conjunctivitis, rhinitis and an unproductive cough are present. Diagnosis is difficult at this stage, since it resembles other respiratory infections.

The coughing stage follows and is characterized by severe bouts of coughing. Each paroxysm consists of many short sharp coughs, gathering in speed and duration and ending in a deep inspiration when the characteristic whoop may be heard. The paroxysms can end with vomiting. This stage can last from one to several weeks. The sputum is particularly tenacious and difficult to expectorate.

Treatment

The treatment approach is similar to acute bronchitis but different aspects of the treatment are emphasized.

• Immune-enhancing herbs such as Echinacea and Andrographis and respiratory antiseptic herbs such as *Inula helenium*, *Thymus vulgaris* and *Allium sativum* (garlic) should be prescribed throughout to treat the infection and prevent complications.

• Drosera (sundew) is a specific for pertussis and has antispasmodic, demulcent and expectorant properties.

• In the coughing stage expectorant herbs such as *Inula helenium*, *Thymus vulgaris*, *Lobelia inflata*, Polygala, Glycyrrhiza (licorice) and other saponin-containing herbs, Foeniculum (fennel), Pimpinella (aniseed) and Marrubium (white horehound) should be emphasized to loosen the tenacious sputum.

• Also, antitussive and demulcent herbs are required to dampen and soothe the cough reflex. If vomiting is occurring, these should be extended by gastrointestinal spasmolytics such as *Viburnum opulus*.

• Respiratory spasmolytics which also have expectorant activity, such as Grindelia and *Inula helenium*, should also be emphasized in the coughing stage. A combination of Inula, Glycyrrhiza and Lobelia is worth trying for the most severe symptoms.

• Mucolytic herbs such as *Allium sativum* and Armoracia may be required to help loosen the tenacious sputum.

Chronic bronchitis and emphysema

Although chronic bronchitis and pulmonary emphysema are distinct disorders, they often coexist in the patient and it can be difficult to determine the relative importance of each condition in the individual case. The term 'chronic obstructive pulmonary disease' (COPD) often applies to a combination of the two. In emphysema, the fine architecture of the alveoli is damaged, leading to impairment of ventilatory capacity. There is probably little that can be done to reverse this destruction (although some natural therapists feel that bioavailable silica and herbs rich in this mineral, such as Equisetum, can help restore lung architecture).

In contrast, chronic bronchitis is a syndrome which can develop in response to long-term exposure to various types of irritants to the bronchial mucous membranes. These include cigarette smoke, dust and automobile or industrial air pollution, especially in conjunction with a damp climate. Acute infection is usually a precipitating or aggravating factor and chronic infection is usually present, with regular acute episodes. Hence, there are many factors in chronic bronchitis which are treatable and long-term herbal treatment can dramatically alter the course of chronic bronchitis.

In chronic bronchitis, ventilatory capacity is reasonably preserved but hypoxia, pulmonary hypertension and right ventricular failure occur early – 'the blue bloater'. In emphysema, the impairment of ventilatory capacity and exertional dyspnoea lead to the sufferer being labelled a 'pink puffer'. A mixed syndrome is most common and all patients should be treated along the following lines, regardless of their clinical label. The treatment outcome will, however, depend on how much the changes in their lungs can be reversed.

Treatment

In chronic bronchitis there is overactivity of the mucus-secreting glands and goblet cells. The vast excess of mucus coats the bronchial walls and clogs the bronchioles. Exacerbating this, many ciliated columnar cells are replaced by goblet cells in response to the chronic irritation. Therefore the excessive mucus is also less able to be cleared from the lungs. Hence, the use of expectorants is emphasized in the treatment of chronic bronchitis, despite the fact that an easily productive cough can be a feature of this disease. (In some patients sputum may be scanty and tenacious, which also requires treatment with expectorants.)

• Bronchial irritation must be avoided. Giving up smoking and a change in occupation or climate may be necessary. Mucus-producing foods such as dairy products and bananas should be reduced.

• The chronic infection should be treated and acute infections prevented by immune-enhancing herbs, especially Echinacea and Astragalus (discontinue Astragalus during acute febrile infections). Many chronic bronchitis patients are constitutionally cold, so the cold herbs Picrorrhiza and Andrographis should be avoided. Heating herbs such as cinnamon may be helpful and could be used in conjunction with these cold herbs.

• Expectorant herbs, such as *Inula helenium*, *Thymus vulgaris*, Polygala, and other saponin-containing herbs, Foeniculum (fennel), Pimpinella (aniseed) and

Marrubium (white horehound) can be prescribed throughout the course of the disorder. The diffusive stimulant properties of Zingiber will potentiate the activity of expectorants.

• Respiratory antiseptic herbs which also have expectorant or mucolytic properties are particularly indicated, such as *Inula helenium, Thymus vulgaris* and *Allium sativum*.

• Since the goblet cells are oversecreting, anticatarrhal herbs such as Verbascum, *Plantago lanceolata* and Hydrastis can help to reduce this oversecretion.

• If there is an unproductive cough at night, a separate formula containing demulcents such as Althaea glycetract and Glycyrrhiza and antitussives such as Glycyrrhiza and Bupleurum may be prescribed.

• Inhalation of peppermint and eucalyptus oils combined can help loosen mucus and dilate airways to make breathing easier.

• Bronchodilating herbs such as Coleus and Lobelia may be helpful. Ephedra should probably be avoided. Those with expectorant activity such as Grindelia can be chosen.

• Since chronic inflammation is present, antiinflammatory herbs such as Glycyrrhiza, Bupleurum and Rehmannia may be of value, as well as omega-3 fatty acids (as found in linseed oil).

• Support for the heart and general circulation with Crataegus and Ginkgo (see p.202) may be required.

Case history

A male patient, 66 years, has received herbal treatment for chronic bronchitis for 7 years. During this time there has been considerable improvement in the patient's condition and friends often now comment on how well he looks. The frequency of acute episodes has substantially reduced and his lung function parameters have improved. Although treatment varied over this time period, a representative herbal treatment is as follows.

• Immune formula (mainly)

Echinacea angustifolia/purpurea blend	1:2	45 ml
Arctium lappa	1:2	15 ml
Achillea millefolium	1:2	20 ml
Withania somnifera	1:2	20 ml
	Total`	100 ml

Dose 5 ml tds

• Lung formula

Glycyrrhiza glabra	1:1	15 ml
Inula helenium	1:2	20 ml
Zingiber officinale	1:2	10 ml
Foeniculum vulgare	1:2	15 ml
Thymus vulgaris	1:2	20 ml
Grindelia camporum	1:2	20 ml
	Total	100 ml

Dose 5 ml tds.

Bronchiectasis

The term 'bronchiectasis' describes an abnormal dilation of the bronchi which becomes a focus for chronic infection. In most cases it develops as a complication of a severe bacterial infection and then follows a chronic course. Clinical features include chronic cough, often with copious purulent sputum, and febrile episodes with malaise and night sweats which can last from a few days to weeks, and sometimes haemoptysis. The disorder can be debilitating. Although continual use of antibiotics is inadvisable, many patients are placed on this regime.

Treatment

Essential aspects of the treatment of bronchiectasis are as follows.

• Immune-enhancing herbs such as Echinacea, Andrographis and Astragalus.

• Respiratory antiseptic herbs such as *Inula helenium, Thymus vulgaris* and *Allium sativum*.

• Diaphoretics such as *Asclepias tuberosa* (pleurisy root) during the febrile episodes.

• Tonics such as Panax, Eleutherococcus or Withania if debility is present.

• Anticatarrhal herbs, such as Verbascum, *Plantago lanceolata* and Hydrastis.

• Expectorant herbs such as *Inula helenium, Thymus vulgaris,* Polygala and other saponin-containing herbs, Foeniculum (fennel), Pimpinella (aniseed) and Marrubium (white horehound).

• Note that Astragalus, Panax and Eleutherococcus should be discontinued during any febrile phases.

Case history

A male patient, 59 years, with bronchiectasis. He coughs up an egg cup of sputum every morning and experiences occasional febrile episodes and acute viral infections.

Herbal treatment consisted of the following.

- *Echinacea angustifolia* 500 mg tablets, two tablets 2–4 times daily. The Echinacea liquid disagreed with this patient hence the tablets. The higher dose was taken during febrile episodes and acute infections.

Aesculus hippocastanum	1:2	15 ml
Foeniculum vulgare	1:2	10 ml
Thymus vulgaris	1:2	30 ml
Ginkgo biloba standardized extract		20 ml
Inula helenium	1:2	25 ml
	Total	100 ml

Dose 8 ml twice a day.

The Ginkgo and Aesculus were mainly for circulatory problems but Aesculus also has expectorant properties due to its saponin content.

- Garlic, 1–2 fresh crushed cloves per day.
- A dairy-free diet was followed.

Treatment over 2 years has resulted in a substantial improvement of this patient's condition. Febrile episodes and acute infections are rare, and his sense of well-being is greatly improved.

References

1. Gonzalez H, Ahmed T. Suppression of gastric H2-receptor mediated function in patients with bronchial asthma and ragweed allergy. Chest 1986; 89(4): 491–496
2. Kurz H. Antitussiva und Expektoranzien. Wissenschaftliche Verlagsgesellschaft, Stuttgart, 1989
3. Eccles R, Morris S, Tolley NS. The effects of nasal anesthesia upon nasal sensation of airflow. Acta Otolaryngolica (Stockholm) 1988; 106: 152–155
4. Dorow P. Welchen Einfluss hat Cineol auf die mukoziliare Clearance? Therapiewoche 1989; 39: 2652–2654
5. Lorenz J, Ferlinz R. Expektoranzien: Pathophysiologie und Therapie der Mukostase. Arzneimitteltherapie 1985; 3: 22–27
6. Minton NA. Volunteer models for predicting antiemetic activity of 5-HT3-receptor antagonists. British Journal of Clinical Pharmacology 1994; 37(6): 525–530
7. Muller-Limmroth W, Frohlich HH. Effect of various phytotherapeutic expectorants on mucociliary transport. Fortschritte der Medizin 1980; 98(3): 95–101
8. Nosál'ova G, Strapková A, Kardosová A et al. Antitussive action of extracts and polysaccharides of marsh mallow (Althea officinalis L., var. robusta). Pharmazie 1992; 47(3): 224–226

URINARY SYSTEM

SCOPE

Apart from their use to provide non-specific support for recuperation and repair, specific phytotherapeutic strategies include the following.

Treatment of:

- urinary infections
- functional disturbances of micturition

Management of:

- interstitial cystitis;
- urinary stones;
- oedema with renal involvement;
- benign prostatic hypertrophy;
- moderate autoimmune kidney disease

Because of its use of secondary plant products, **extreme caution** is necessary in applying phytotherapy in cases of:

- renal failure;
- urinary obstruction;
- severe glomerulonephritis.

ORIENTATION

Herbal diuretics

Plants have been used as diuretic remedies thoughout history (Pliny the Elder mentions that many plants have diuretic properties in his *Naturalis Historia*[1]). However, the early indications for such use were often different – urinary stones, nephritis, cystitis, strangury, urinary retention and incontinence[2] – with severe oedema associated with dropsy, ascites and lymphatic disease quite often encountered and hypertension being quite unknown. The excruciating pain of urinary stones would of course be well known and would have driven many urgent treatments. Because of the severity of such conditions, diuretic remedies would have been more drastic than nowadays. Remedies would have been given in much higher doses, for shorter duration. The diuretic effects of purgatives were well understood (this reputation is supported by observations that anthraquinone derivatives induce experimental diuresis associated with the inhibition of ATPases in the kidney medulla[3]) and these may well have been used in desperate attempts to relieve the symptoms of ascites in advanced liver failure (a not uncommon condition given the frequency of hepatitis). Indeed, the drastic treatment, in at least one case, of dropsy forms the basis of one of medicine's best historical stories. When William Withering found that the active principle of one effective remedy for dropsy was the cardioactive foxglove he initiated a whole new medical tradition as well as confirming that dropsy was a symptom of heart failure rather than of the kidneys.

Inducing appreciable consistent diuresis does actually involve relatively drastic pharmacological activity and modern diuretic drugs are powerful agents. Examples of plants with direct diuretic effects producing consistent activity in controlled conditions in the literature are rare, and there are some studies that specifically show a negative effect in these circumstances.[4–7] Examples where a diuretic effect has been observed experimentally include a study showing significant increase in 24-hour urine volume, urine and serum sodium levels in nine mild hypertensives administered a whole-plant preparation of *Phyllanthus amarus*.[8] In another study, *Aerua lanata* flowers at doses of 10 g induced significant diuresis in 70% of subjects in uncontrolled clinical conditions.[9] A study on a product based on asparagus and parsley root has also shown limited diuretic effect in the management of congestive heart failure.[10] The benefits of the Indian remedy *Terminalia arjuna* bark extract at 500 mg every 8 hours, as adjuvant therapy to conventional medications, have been attested in a double-blind crossover trial on 12 patients with chronic congestive heart failure.[11]

There is some evidence of diuretic effects of various popular diuretics in experimental animals but only at very high doses (40 ml/kg)[12] and 1 g/kg,[13,14] at levels far outside any therapeutic range. Other plants with experimental diuretic effects in animals have been observed at various dosages include Taraxacum (dandelion),[15] members of the Equisetum family,[16] Orthosiphon leaf,[17] and Orthosiphon,[18] various Solidago species,[19,20] *Agrimonia eupatoria* (agrimony),[21] *Lactuca virosa* (wild lettuce)[22] and Parietaria (pellitory).[23] Diuretic activity (including renal vasodilation and urinary sodium excretion) has been observed in experimental studies on *Clerodendron trichotomum*,[24] and *Rehmannia radix*.[25] However, studies on *Alpinia speciosa*[26] and *Polygonum punctatum*[27] showed no diuretic properties in spite of other pronounced pharmacological activities and the main effect in rats of administering oral doses of *Opuntia ficusindica* infusions was a marked loss of potassium, with only modest diuresis and sodium loss at lower concentrations.[28]

The modest research evidence apart, the experience of even mild herbal prescriptions having sometimes dramatic diuretic effects is well known to practitioners and this is one of the most common reactions to treatment that patients report. One conclusion that can be drawn is that diuretic responses are variable, perhaps reflecting other indeterminate susceptibilities in the individual patient.

Aquaretics and diuretic depuratives

Two variations on the diuretic theme have emerged from earlier Western traditions. In German practice, the concept of 'aquaretic' has been used to describe diuretic agents that excrete water from the body, most probably associated with potassium, but not other electrolyte, excretion. They may exert their effect due to increased bloodflow to the kidney.[29] Most herbal diuretics in tradition are likely to be of this class. They are thus not easily comparable with modern diuretics that interfere with resorption at the distal tubule of the nephron, leading to wider electrolyte elimination, and thus may be less effective in treating hypertension and oedematous conditions.

In the case of hypertension the main benefit of herbal aquaretics may be in replacing the potassium lost through the use of modern diuretic prescriptions. High potassium levels relative to sodium has been shown to be a feature of herbal drugs with traditional diuretic activity.[30] Compared to a ratio in the average diet of 2:1, herbal remedies like Urtica (nettle tops), Equisetum (horsetail), Betula (birch), Sambucus (elder), Agrimonia (agrimony), *Phaseolus vulgaris* (bean pods), Matricaria (chamomile) and tilia (lime flowers) had ratios greater than 150:1 potassium to sodium, especially in decoction form. It is difficult with current information to link high potassium levels to any aquaretic or diuretic effect but given that diuresis is almost by definition accompanied by potassium loss, then to have an effective potassium supplement seems convenient.

In the case of oedema, phytotherapeutic strategies should emphasize activity on other body functions (see below) rather than any diuretic impact.

A second concept of 'diuretic depurative' is more compatible with the general meaning of diuretics in Western herbal tradition; it implies that the remedy removes metabolites and waste products as well as water, that is, as an aid to excretion.

There is one very gentle diuretic mechanism that may underlie the effect of many plants.

Osmotic diuresis

The principle of osmotic diuresis has been established since the end of the 19th century when Ustimowitsch, Falck and Richet stressed the influence of urinary solutes on urine flow, although over a century earlier Segalas and Wohler observed that an extra load of urea, or any other substance that is excreted by the kidney, causes a diuresis.[31]

The osmotic plant-based diuretic mannitol is used, by intravenous injection, in acute oliguric renal failure.[32] Mannitol is found in some plants, including the popular diuretic *Agropyron repens* (couch grass); however, its absorption from the gut wall is limited and it is unlikely to play a significant role in the effect of couch grass. Nevertheless, a number of similar sugar molecules may account for a gentle diuretic effect of many herbal remedies, as well as, more generally, fruits and vegetables. For example, the plant starch inulin is used in commercial preparations to measure glomerular filtration rate and in experiments of kidney microperfusion as a marker of tubular water reabsorption. A number of plant extracts of inulin have been shown to have a comparable effect.[33]

The kidneys and oedema

Although clearly active in the elimination of water from the body and the control of fluid levels within the tissues, the impact of the kidneys in oedema is not always obvious, compared with a failing heart, a cirrhotic liver or lymphatic or venous insufficiency in their relevant syndromes. Nevertheless, in all such cases prescription of conventional diuretic drugs is commonplace and it is widely assumed that the kidney is centrally involved in most cases.

This assumption has mixed support in the scientific literature. For example, renal complications of liver cirrhosis are certainly implicated in the development of ascites. These complications include inadequate renal prostaglandin production and the negative effect on the kidney of raised nitric oxide production. Such complications may actually reduce the effect of diuretics but they remain indicated in the treatment of ascites as long as they are effective.[34] In phytotherapy, however, the main effort now would be on using hepatics and other treatments for the liver (see p.190).

Although undoubtedly effective symptomatically, the value of diuretics used alone for congestive heart failure in the long term has been challenged, because of their possible excitation of the renin-angiotensin system. Concomitant prescription of ACE inhibitors has been proposed and positively evaluated, because they suppress this excitation.[35] As seen below, herbal diuretics are unlikely to raise the same concerns but may be only second-tier treatments compared to the cardioactive glycosides.

The localized oedema of lymphatic and venous insufficiency is treated in phytotherapy with particular remedies said to act on the vessel walls. These may have incidental diuretic effects (see p.31).

In phytotherapy, there are few traditional strategies that are likely to bear directly on the kidney cortex itself, with emphasis placed instead on activity lower down the urinary system. Nevertheless, little is known about the full impact of plant constituents on this organ and although there are very few cases where actual nephrotoxicity occurs, a general caution in using herbal treatments is advisable where the kidneys are already damaged.[36]

Beneficial effects of plant remedies on the kidney

Kidney disease such as glomerulonephritis and cystic disease presents awesome and possibly overwhelming odds for the phytotherapist. By definition the kidney in such cases, especially where the basement membrane is involved, is vulnerable to further damage with any new active metabolite and the practitioner needs to proceed with extreme caution. Nevertheless, there is experimental evidence, mainly from China and Japan, suggesting that some herbal remedies might have beneficial effects in such cases, including such conditions as nephrotic syndrome (Chinese herbs Astragalus and Angelica,[37] diabetic nephropathy (*Abemoschus manihot*[38]) and other kidney diseases.[39–43] *Andrographis paniculata* has shown experimental ability to reduce pyuria and haematuria as complications of urinary stone destruction[44] and magnesium lithospermate B, a component of Lycopus and Lithospermum species, has shown potential as a new therapeutic agent for inhibiting the progression of renal dysfunction.[45] The use of various Chinese bitter ('cooling and drying') herbs has been shown to improve biochemical markers associated with free radical damage in patients with chronic glomerulonephritis compared with matched controls.[46]

Other plant materials have shown apparent antinephrotoxic activity and may provide the basis for strategies following the adverse effects of heavy metals, antibiotics, analgesic and other prescription drugs, Amanita mushroom and aflatoxins and industrial agents. Protective effects of *Arctostaphlos uva-ursi*, *Orthosiphon stamineus* and *Polygonum aviculare* have been noted against the nephrotoxic effects of mercuric chloride,[47] and beneficial effects against the nephrotoxin aminoglycoside in elderly patients have also been noted in controlled studies for *Cordyceps sinensis*.[48] Aqueous rhubarb extract (at 150 mg/day) reduced proteinurea and glomerulosclerosis in rats exposed to experimental chronic renal fibrosis in controlled trials.[49]

DIURETICS (AQUARETICS AND DIURETIC DEPURATIVES)

Note: Most plants used primarily for their effects on the urinary system are collectively referred to as 'diuretics' in many texts. Nevertheless, this covers a broad range of traditional activities and probably very variable actual diuretic effects and the terms 'aquaretics' and 'diuretic depuratives' (see above) may be more accurate. However, the conventional terminology will be used here, as demarcation between the two categories is inadequate.

Plant remedies traditionally used as diuretics

Eupatorium purpureum (gravel root), *Agropyron repens* (couch grass), *Eryngium maritimum* (sea holly), *Zea mays* (corn silk), *Aphanes arvensis* (parsley piert), *Daucus carota* (wild carrot), *Parietaria diffusa* (pellitory), *Taraxacum officinale* (dandelion), *Apium graveolens* (celery).

Indications for diuretics

- Dysuria and oliguria linked to urinary infections or stones
- Heart failure (as an adjunct to cardioactive glycosides)
- Ascites (combined with hepatic remedies)
- Nocturnal enuresis and other functional disturbances of micturition
- Urinary stones

Other traditional indications for diuretics

- Haematuria
- Arthritis and skin disorders

Contraindications in the use of diuretics

The use of diuretic herbs may be inappropriate and possibly even contraindicated in the following:

- renal failure;
- diabetes.

Other traditional therapeutic insights into the use of diuretics

The traditional treatment of arthritic disease often involved using herbs that were otherwise considered diuretics. There is a more modern tradition that suggests these act to increase the elimination of metabolic acid wastes, like uric acid, factors popularly associated with arthritic disease. The precise explanation for the apparent efficacy of remedies like birch, celery seed and nettle leaf in arthritic diseases may be more complex.

This tradition is a reminder of the wider assumption that diuretics were among the eliminative strategies applied to a range of toxic conditions associated especially with inflammatory diseases and persistent or recurrent infections (see p.140). Any hint of fluid retention accompanying such conditions would be a traditional indication for diuretics.

Application

Diuretics, when prescribed overtly as such, are best taken in relatively high quantities at any time relative to eating. However, dramatic diuresis in some cases may follow quite small doses of many herbs, perhaps directed to other ends.

Phased treatments may be appropriate, for example, early morning and lunchtime dosages as part of a strategy for treating nocturnal enuresis.

Long-term therapy with many diuretics is quite acceptable.

Advanced phytotherapeutics

Diuretics may also be usefully applied in some cases (depending on other factors) of:

- osteoarthritis;
- dermatitis;
- other chronic inflammatory diseases accompanied by fluid retention;
- premenstrual syndrome.

URINARY ANTISEPTICS

Plant remedies traditionally used as urinary antiseptics

Arctostaphylos uva-ursi (bearberry), *Barosma betulina* (buchu), *Juniperus communis* (juniper), *Berberis vulgaris* (barberry), *Hydrastis canadensis* (golden seal), *Piper cubeba (cubeb)*.

Indications for urinary antiseptics

- Urinary infections or stones
- Prostatitis
- Interstitial cystitis

Contraindications in the use of urinary antiseptics

The use of urinary antiseptic herbs may be inappropriate and possibly even contraindicated in the following:

- kidney disease;
- renal failure;
- pregnancy.

Application

Urinary antiseptics may be taken before or with meals. It may be found that taking whole ground preparations in capsule form may be more effective than tinctures, but this is not a critical matter. Long-term therapy with many urinary antiseptics is not advisable.

PHYTOTHERAPY FOR URINARY CONDITIONS

Urinary stones

A theme that emerges from recent research is the complexity of mineral and electrolyte disturbance, involving other body systems, that can underlie urinary stone formation. For example, the pathogenesis of renal calculi may involve relative changes in concentrations of other urinary trace elements, notably copper and phosphorus,[50] that clearly reflect wider metabolic changes.

Oxalate stone formation may be associated with a high oxalate:calcium ratio in the urine and may be linked to low dietary calcium intake or defects in oxalate transport mechanisms in the gut or kidney. Gut factors may be particularly important, as evidenced by the hyperoxaluria, low urine volume, low urinary ionic strength, lower urinary citrate levels and increased incidence of oxalate stones seen with extensive disease in or resection of the small intestine.[51] In practice, phytotherapists are more productively directed to applying their array of digestive remedies for oxalate stones than focusing solely on the urinary tract.

There is also substantial evidence of interaction between urinary urates and oxalates so that higher urinary levels of the former, following disturbances of purine metabolism including gout, can lead to 'salting out' of calcium oxalate stones; drugs like allopurinol, that reduce urinary urates, also reduce oxalate stones.[52] This calls into question the use, in the case of incipient or actual oxalate calculi (for example, in cases of severe small intestinal disease as above), of some plants, like the seeds of *Apium graveolens* (celery) and *Petroselinum crispum* (parsley), *Eupatorium purpureum* (gravel root), *Betula spp* (birch) and *Urtica dioica* (nettle leaf), that are considered to increase urinary excretion of urates.

Other studies suggest that urate stones themselves may be linked to low blood urate levels following enhanced tubular secretion of urate within the kidney. In such cases agents increasing urate excretion would be clearly contraindicated and alkalinization of urine may be the most effective treatment.[53]

In pregnancy, hyperuricuria and hypercalciuria, changes in metabolic inhibitors of lithiasis formation, urinary stasis, relative dehydration and the presence of infection all increase the likelihood of stone formation.[54]

Haematuria in children may be a sign of relative hypercalcuria and hyperuricuria, although the long-term implications of this are not clear.[55]

Herbal remedies and urinary stones

In seven plants (*Verbena officinalis, Lithospermum officinale, Taraxacum officinale, Equisetum arvense, Arctostaphylos uva-ursi, Arctium lappa* and *Silene saxifraga*) studied for their effects on experimental risk factors for urinary stones (citraturia, calciuria, phosphaturia, pH and diuresis), moderate solvent action on uric stones was linked to the alkalinizing capacity of the herb infusions and to possible urinary antiseptic activity.[56]

Other Asiatic herbal products have been shown to reduce experimental renal stone formation.[57,58,59] In Ayurveda, *Crataeva nurvala* is highly acclaimed for its use in the management of urinary tract disorders, especially kidney stones. Research has demonstrated a range of activity on urinary structures, including improved performance in clinical studies of benign prostatic hyperplasia[60] and with urinary stones[61,62] and in reducing oxalate stone formation,[63] with the steroid lupeol being a possible active constituent.[64] A pharmacological study found that Crataeva influenced small intestinal Na, K-ATPase which in turn influenced the transport of minerals.[65] This is a reminder that oxalate problems may well originate from the digestive tract (see above).

Herbal teas in general have been recommended as alternatives to the usual black tea consumption because of the latter's association with increased risk of formation of calcium oxalate stones but this is unlikely to reflect a general benefit of plant extractives as such.[66]

Urinary infections

Lower urinary tract infections are one of the most amenable indications for phytotherapy, although there are some difficult exceptions. Several plant constituents have at least theoretical antiseptic effects when eliminated in the urinary tract (including simple fructose itself) and a number of plants have firm clinical reputations for long-term efficacy in uncomplicated urethritis and cystitis, especially when caused by Gram-negative bacteria like *Escherichia coli* (accounting for 80% of adult cases), *Staphyloccocus saprophyticus*, Klebsiella and Proteus.

It is also possible to treat higher tract infections, pyelonephritis with or without ureteritis and, in the case of men, bacterial prostatitis, although in such cases complications may make progress more difficult and in chronic pyelonephritis, involvement of the kidney parenchyma may lead to the dangers of kidney damage.

When urinary tract infections are complicated by pregnancy, diabetes, immunosuppression or other abnormalities, prudence will determine that these are addressed before simple urinary antiseptics are applied. Except in pregnancy and severe kidney disease, however, the treatments are rarely contraindicated. They may also show effectiveness in urinary tract conditions linked to fungal (e.g. Candida) and parasitic infections (e.g. following malaria, leishmaniasis, trichomoniasis and bilharziasis) and for those without obvious infective cause. In the latter case at least alkalinization of the urine is a helpful accompaniment, conventionally with half a teaspoon of sodium bicarbonate in water every 3–4 hours but also with increased consumption of fruit juice (and vegetable juice especially).

Urinary infection probably requires adhesion of the bacteria to the otherwise glassy surface of the urinary tract and those usually responsible have mechanisms to do this. Constituents of berries of the heather family, notably *Vaccinium macrocarpon* (cranberry), and *V. myrtillus* (blueberry, bilberry), appear at least in vitro to interfere with this adhesion mechanism.[67] An antibacteriuric effect of cranberry juice has been demonstrated in a double-blind controlled clinical study in elderly women.[68] Another plant constituent with clinical antiadhesive properties, at least in the gut and in synthetic form, is berberine (from the Berberis genus and golden seal used traditionally for cystitis).[69]

It is also possible that herbs may help in the condition known as interstitial cystitis. This difficult condition, marked by inflammatory infiltration in the bladder wall but no obvious infection, is generally thought to be an autoimmune disorder. However, an infective cause has not been ruled out,[70] and in spite of its name, it appears that there is no increased bladder permeability.[71] There do appear to be changes in neurotransmitter sensitivity (increasing resistance to atropine and histamine and a switch towards purinergic transmission in parasympathetic nerve terminals)[72] and impairment of bladder perfusion in patients has also been observed, especially when the bladder was full.[73] It is for these reasons that in herbal treatments urinary antiseptics are often combined with other agents with an apparent benefit on the bladder wall (e.g. Equisetum, *Crataeva nurvula* and Althaea).

Benign prostatic hyperplasia

Another popular application of herbal remedies is to the symptoms of benign prostatic hyperplasia. The early association of the symptoms of prostatic enlargement (urinary frequency, retention and diminished flow) with ageing in men led to the inevitable association of remedies that reduced these symptoms with rejuvenating male tonics and promoters of male potency. Given the eternal demand for such agents, it is not surprising that they feature in most traditions. In some it is difficult to distinguish the stimulant aphrodisiac from the prostatic remedy; whereas Cola (kola nuts) and *Pausinystalia yohimbe* (yohimbe), used in male virility ceremonies in west Africa, are obvious stimulants (the former a high caffeine source once briefly combined with the cocaine-containing Coca leaves in the stimulant tonic drink of that name), it is less easy to distinguish the modest euphoric effects of high doses of the central American plant *Turnera aphrodisiaca* (damiana) from its reputation in aiding at least some of the problems of older men. *Panax ginseng* (Asiatic ginseng) was used particularly for elderly men in traditional Asian cultures and is still favoured for prostatic enlargement symptoms – it has potential hormonal activity as a rationale. The most notable remedy from the southern USA is *Serenoa serrulata* (saw palmetto), initially used as a male tonic but with increasing evidence of benefits in benign prostatic hyperplasia. Saw palmetto is widely prescribed by urologists in Germany for early symptoms of benign prostatic hyperplasia, along with *Urtica dioica* (nettle root) and *Cucurbita pepo* (pumpkin seed).[74] It is possible that plant constituents could reduce the conversion of testosterone in the prostate in similar ways to the modern alpha-reductase inhibitors or could interact with relevant receptors or have other antiinflammatory effects in the organ. The evidence so far for these two remedies is reviewed in their monographs (see pp.490 and 523). The African remedy *Pygeum africanum* has been beneficial in clinical trials and is very popular in France. However, it has been classified as an endangered species. *Crataeva nurvala* (see above) improves bladder tone and decreases bladder emptying and is a useful symptomatic treatment for urinary obstruction including that linked to prostatic enlargement.

References

1. Melillo L. Diuretic plants in the paintings of Pompeii. American Journal of Nephrology 1994; 14(4–6): 423–425
2. Aliotta G, Capasso G, Pollio A et al. Joseph Jacob Plenck (1735–1807). American Journal of Nephrology 1994; 14(4–6): 377–382
3. Zhou XM, Chen QH. Biochemical study of Chinese rhubarb. XXII. Inhibitory effect of anthraquinone derivatives on Na+-K+-ATPase of the rabbit renal medulla and their diuretic action. Yao Hsueh Hsueh Pao 1988; 23(1): 17–20
4. Doan DD, Nguyen NH, Doan HK et al. Studies on the individual and combined diuretic effects of four Vietnamese traditional herbal remedies (Zea mays, Imperata cylindrica, Plantago major and Orthosiphon stamineus). Journal of Ethnopharmacology 1992; 36(3): 225–231
5. Goonaratna C, Thabrew I, Wijewardena K. Does Aerua lanata have diuretic properties? Indian Journal of Physiological Pharmacology 1993; 37(2): 135–137
6. Black HR, Ming S, Poll DS et al. A comparison of the treatment of hypertension with Chinese herbal and Western medication. Journal of Clinical Hypertension 1986; 2(4): 371–378
7. Laranja SM, Bergamaschi CM, Schor N. Evaluation of three plants with potential diuretic effect. Revista da Associacao Medica Brasileira 1992; 38(1): 13–16
8. Srividya N, Periwal S. Diuretic, hypotensive and hypoglycaemic effect of Phyllanthus amarus. Indian Journal of Experimental Biology 1995; 33(11): 861–864
9. Udupihille M, Jiffry MT. Diuretic effect of Aerua lanata with water, normal saline and coriander as controls. Indian Journal of Physiological Pharmacology 1986; 30(1): 91–97
10. Von Beitz G, Hippe SK, Schremmer D. Asparagus-P, das pflanzliche Diuretikum in der Herz-Kreislauf-Therapie. Naturheilpraxis 1996; 2: 247–252
11. Bharani A, Ganguly A, Bhargava KD. Salutary effect of Terminalia Arjuna in patients with severe refractory heart failure. International Journal of Cardiology 1995; 49(3): 191–199
12. De Ribeiro RA, De Barros F, De Melo MM et al. Acute diuretic effects in conscious rats produced by some medicinal plants used in the state of Sao Paulo, Brasil. Journal of Ethnopharmacology 1988; 24(1): 19–29
13. Cáceres A, Girón LM, Martínez AM. Diuretic activity of plants used for the treatment of urinary ailments in Guatemala. Journal of Ethnopharmacology 1987; 19(3): 233–245
14. Cáceres A, Saravia A, Rizzo S et al. Pharmacologic properties of Moringa oleifera. 2: Screening for antispasmodic, antiinflammatory and diuretic activity. Journal of Ethnopharmacology 1992; 36(3): 233–237

15. Racz-Kotilla E, Racz G, Solomon A. The action of Taraxacum officinale extracts on the body weight and diuresis of laboratory animals. Planta Medica 1974; 26: 212–217
16. Pérez Gutiérrez RM, Laguna GY, Walkowski A. Diuretic activity of Mexican equisetum. Journal of Ethnopharmacology 1985; 14(2–3): 269–272
17. Englert J, Harnischfeger G. Diuretic action of aqueous Orthosiphon extract in rats. Planta Medica 1992; 58(3): 237–238
18. Casadebaig-Lafon J, Jacob M, Cassanas G et al. Adsorbed plant extracts, use of extracts of dried seeds of Orthosiphon stamineus benth. Pharmaceutica Acta Helvetiae 1989; 64(8): 220–224
19. Leuschner J. Anti-inflammatory, spasmolytic and diuretic effects of a commercially available Solidago gigantea herb extract. Arzneimittel-Forschung 1995; 45(2): 165–168
20. Chodera A, Dabrowska K, Sloderbach A et al. Effect of flavonoid fractions of Solidago virgaurea L on diuresis and levels of electrolytes. Acta Poloniae Pharmaceutica 1991; 48(5–6): 35–37
21. Giachetti D, Taddei E, Taddei I. Diuretic and uricosuric activity of Agrimonia eupatoria L. Bollettino Societa Italiana Biologia Sperimentale 1986; 62(6): 705–711
22. Gu WZ, Deng LJ. Studies on the chemical constituents of the essential oil in the seed of Lactuca setiva L. and its diuretic action. Chung Yao Tung Pao 1987; 11: 33–5, 63
23. Giachetti D, Taddei E, Taddei I. Diuretic and uricosuric activity of Parietaria judaica L. Bollettino Societa Italiana Biologia Sperimentale 1986; 62(2): 197–202
24. Lu GW, Miura K, Yukimura T, Yamamoto K. Effects of extract from Clerodendron trichotomum on blood pressure and renal function in rats and dogs. Journal of Ethnopharmacology 1994; 42(2): 77–82
25. Lee HS, Kim ST, Cho DK. Effects of rehmanniae radix water extract on renal function and renin secretion rate in unanesthetized rabbits. American Journal of Chinese Medicine 1993; 21(2): 179–186
26. Mendonca VL, Oliveira CL, Craveiro AA et al. Pharmacological and toxicological evaluation of Alpinia speciosa. Memorias do Instituto Oswaldo Cruz 1991; 86(supp 2): 93–97
27. Simões CM, Ribeiro-do-Vale RM, Poli A et al. The pharmacologic action of extracts of Polygonum punctatum Elliot (= P. acre HBK). Journal de Pharmacie de Belgique 1989; 44(4): 275–284
28. Perfumi M, Tacconi R. Effect of Opuntia ficus-indica flower infusion on urinary and electrolyte excretion in rats. Fitoterapia 1996; 67(5): 459–464
29. Robbins JE, Tyler VE. Herbs of Choice, Haworth Press, New York, 1999, P 89
30. Szentmihályi, K, Kéry A, Then M et al. Potassium-sodium ratio for the characterisation of medicinal plant extracts with diuretic activity. Phytotherapy Research 1998; 12: 163–166
31. Richet GC. Osmotic diuresis before Homer W. Smith: a winding path to renal physiology. Kidney International 1994; 45(4): 1241–1252
32. Archer DP, Freymond D, Ravussin P. Use of mannitol in neuroanesthesia and neurointensive care. Annales françaises d' Anesthésie et de Réanimation 1995; 14(1): 77–82
33. Dias-Tagliacozzo GM, Dietrich SMC, Mello-Aires M. Measurement of glomerular filtration rate using inulin prepared from Vernonia herbacea, a Brazilian native species. Brazilian Journal of Medical and Biological Research 1996; 29(10): 1393–1396
34. Roberts LR, Kamath PS. Ascites and hepatorenal syndrome: pathophysiology and management. Mayo Clinic Proceedings 1996; 71(9): 874–881
35. Taylor SH. Refocus on diuretics in the treatment of heart failure. European Heart Journal 1995; 16(supp): 7–15
36. Markell MS. Herbal therapies and the patient with kidney disease. Quarterly Review of Natural Medicine 1997; Fall: 189–200
37. Li L, Wang H, Zhu S. Hepatic albumin's mRNA in nephrotic syndrome rats treated with Chinese herbs. Chung Hua I Hsueh Tsa Chih 1995; 75(5): 276–279
38. Yu JY, Xiong NN, Guo HF. Clinical observation on diabetic nephropathy treated with alcohol of Abelmoschus manihot. Chung Kuo Chung Hsi I Chieh Ho Tsa Chih 1995; 15(5): 263–265
39. Li P, Fujio S. Effects of chai ling tang on proteinuria in rat models. Journal of Traditional Chinese Medicine 1995; 15(1): 48–52
40. Zheng JF, Chen SY. Observations on therapeutic effects of huangdan decoction and Tripterygium Wilfordii compound tablet on membranous glomerulonephritis in rats. Journal of Tongji Medical University 1995; 15(1): 31–34
41. Shida K, Imamura K, Katayama T et al. Clinical efficacy of sairei-to in various urinary tract diseases centering on fibrosis. Hinyokika Kiyo 1994; 40(11): 1049–1057
42. Kawachi H, Takashima N, Orikasa M et al. Effect of traditional Chinese medicine (sairei-to) on monoclonal antibody-induced proteinuria in rats. Pathology International 1994; 44(5): 339–344
43. Ren G, Chang F, Lu S et al. Pharmacological studies of Polygonum capitatum Buch Ham. ex D. Don. Chung Kuo Chung Yao Tsa Chih 1995; 20(2): 107–109, 128
44. Muangman V, Viseshsindh V, Ratana-Olarn K, Buadilok S. The usage of Andrographis paniculata following Extracorporeal Shock Wave Lithotripsy (ESWL). Journal of the Medical Association of Thailand 1995; 78(6): 310–313
45. Yokozawa T, Zhou JJ, Hattori M et al. Effects of a Dan Shen component, magnesium lithospermate B, in nephrectomized rats. Nippon Jinzo Gakkai Shi 1995; 37(2): 105–111
46. Yu EK. Anti-free radical damage of chronic glomerulonephritis with febrifugal and diuretic medicinal herbs. Chung Kuo Chung Hsi I Chieh Ho Tsa Chih 1993; 13(8): 464–6, 452
47. Shantanova LN, Mondodoev AG, Lonshakova KS, Nikolaev SM. Pharmacotherapeutic effectivity of plant nephrophyte polyextractions in cases of mercuric chloride necronephrosis. Rastitel'nye Resursy 1996; 32(1–2): 110–117
48. Bao ZD, Wu ZG, Zheng F. Amelioration of aminoglycoside nephrotoxicity by Cordyceps sinensis in old patients. Chung Kuo Chung Hsi I Chieh Ho Tsa Chih 1994; 14(5): 271–273, 259
49. Zhang G, El Nahas AM. The effect of rhubarb extract on experimental renal fibrosis. Nephrology Dialysis Transplantation 1996; 11(1): 186–190
50. Rodgers AL, Barbour LJ, Pougnet BM et al. Re-evaluation of the 'week-end effect' data: possible role of urinary copper and phosphorus in the pathogenesis of renal calculi. Journal of Trace Elements in Medicine and Biology 1995; 9(3): 150–155
51. Sutton RA, Walker VR. Enteric and mild hyperoxaluria. Mineral and Electrolyte Metabolism 1994; 20(6): 352–360
52. Grover PK, Ryall RL. Urate and calcium oxalate stones: from repute to rhetoric to reality. Mineral and Electrolyte Metabolism 1994; 20(6): 361–370
53. Hisatome I, Tanaka Y, Kotake H et al. Renal hypouricemia due to enhanced tubular secretion of urate associated with urolithiasis: successful treatment of urolithiasis by alkalization of urine K+, Na(+)-citrate. Nephron 1993; 65(4): 578–582
54. Swanson SK, Heilman RL, Eversman WG. Urinary tract stones in pregnancy. Surgical Clinics of North America 1995; 75(1): 123–142
55. Stapleton FB. Hematuria associated with hypercalciuria and hyperuricosuria: a practical approach. Pediatric Nephrology 1994; 8(6): 756–761
56. Grases F, Melero G, Costa-Bauza A, Prieto R, March JG. Urolithiasis and phytotherapy. International Urology and Nephrology 1994; 26(5): 507–511
57. Yamaguchi S, Jihong L, Utsunomiya M et al. The effect of takusha and kagosou on calcium oxalate renal stones in rats. Hinyokika Kiyo 1995; 41(6): 427–431
58. Hirayama H, Wang Z, Nishi K et al. Effect of Desmodium styracifolium-triterpenoid on calcium oxalate renal stones. British Journal of Urology 1993; 71(2): 143–147
59. Kawamura K, Moriyama M, Nakajima C et al. The inhibitory effects of Takusha on the formation, growth and aggregation of calcium oxalate crystals in vitro. Hinyokika Kiyo 1993; 39(8): 695–700
60. Deshpande PJ, Sahu M, Kumar P. Crataeva nurvala Hook and Forst (Varuna) – the Ayurvedic drug of choice in urinary disorders. Indian Journal of Medical Research 1982; 76(supp): 46–53

61. Prabhakar YS, Kumar DS. The Varuna tree, Crataeva nurvala, a promising plant in the treatment of urinary stones. A review. Fitoterapia 1990; 61(2): 99–111
62. Varalakshmi P, Shamila Y, Latha E. Effect of Crataeva nurvala in experimental urolithiasis. Journal of Ethnopharmacology 1990; 28(3): 313–321
63. Anand R, Patnaik GK, Kulshreshtha DK et al. Antiurolithiatic activity of Crataeva nurvala ethanolic extract on rats. Fitoterapia 1993; 64(4): 345–350
64. Anand R, Patnaik GK, Kulshreshtha DK et al. Antiurolithiatic and diuretic activity of lupeol, the active constituent isolated from Crataeva nurvala (Buch. Ham). Proceedings of the 24th Indian Pharmacological Society Conference, Ahmedabad, Gujarat, India, 1991; A10
65. Varalakshmi P, Latha E, Shamila Y et al. Effect of Crataeva nurvala on the biochemistry of the small intestinal tract of normal and stone-forming rats. Journal of Ethnopharmacology 1991; 31(1): 67–73
66. McKay DW, Seviour JP, Comerford A et al. Herbal tea: an alternative to regular tea for those who form calcium oxalate stones. Journal of the American Dietetic Association 1995; 95(3): 360–361
67. Ofek I, Goldhar J, Zafiri D et al. Anti-Escherischia adhesin activity of cranberry and blueberry juice. New England Journal of Medicine 1991; 324: 1559
68. Avorn J, Monane M, Gurwitz JH et al. Reduction of bacteriuria and pyuria after ingestion of cranberry juice. JAMA 1994; 271: 751–754
69. Rabbani GH, Butler T, Knight J et al. Randomised controlled trial of berberine sulfate therapy for diarrhea due to enterotoxigenic Escherichia coli and Vibrio cholerae. Journal of Infectious Diseases 1987; 155: 979–984
70. Warren JW. Interstitial cystitis as an infectious disease. Urology Clinics of North America 1994; 21(1): 31–39
71. Ruggieri MR, Chelsky MJ, Rosen SI et al. Current findings and future research avenues in the study of interstitial cystitis. Urology Clinics of North America 1994; 21(1): 163–176
72. Paella S, Artibani W, Ostardo E et al. Evidence for purinergic neurotransmission in human urinary bladder affected by interstitial cystitis. Journal of Urology 1993; 150(6): 2007–2012
73. Irwin P, Galloway NT. Impaired bladder perfusion in interstitial cystitis: a study of blood supply using laser Doppler flowmetry. Journal of Urology 1993; 149(4): 890–892
74. Bombardelli E, Morazzoni P. Cucurbita pepo L. Fitoterapia 1997; 68(4): 291–302

NERVOUS SYSTEM

SCOPE

Apart from their use to provide non-specific support for recuperation and repair, specific phytotherapeutic strategies include the following.

Treatment in some circumstances of:

- stress symptoms;
- psychosomatic conditions;
- anxiety states, panic attacks;
- neuralgia;
- nervous exhaustion;
- insomnia;
- visceral spasm.

Management of:

- herpes infections;
- moderate visceral pain;
- mild to moderate depressive conditions;
- nervous debility;
- dose reduction for prescription hypnotics and sedatives.

As with any pharmacological agent, particular **caution** is necessary in applying phytotherapy in cases of:

- severe psychosis;
- prescription of powerful antipsychotics, antiepileptics, anaesthetics;
- addictive personality

ORIENTATION

Receptor activity

Although herbal remedies are not exactly comparable to conventional drugs in terms of directness of action, it is most likely that the primary effect of plant constituents on the nervous system is similarly on the synaptic junctions between nerve and nerve and nerve and muscle or other tissue. The receptor sites involved, whether on the presynaptic or postsynaptic membranes, are the communication junctions in the nervous system where its modulation is generally effected. The transmitter chemicals involved are among the most powerful molecules in the body and play a major part in the functions of other body systems; as seen in the relevant chapters of this book, plant constituents have been widely shown to engage with receptors in the hormonal, immunological and other control systems in the body. These systems form a whole whose study, psychoneuroimmunology, has attracted the attention of the more imaginative medical researchers since the 1960s. The ability of plant constituents to engage cell receptors is also a particular feature of activity within the digestive system (see p.163), which in clinical reality is probably the most accessible interface to the chemical control of the nervous system for herbal remedies.

There are ample opportunities for herbal constituents to interact with synaptic function in the nervous system. Various herbal extracts have been shown in vitro to act on adrenergic, muscarinic, 5-HT_1A and 5-HT_2 receptors, dopamine (D_1 and D_2), the benzodiazepine and the gamma-amino-n-butyric acid (GABA) binding sites.[1,2] Particular examples of such activity follow; apart from familiar Western plants, much of the literature cited reflects the fact that most published research in this area emanates from China and Japan. While these experimental examples might not always reflect real clinical effects, they are given here to reflect the wide spectrum of possible activities of herbal remedies.

Calcium channel activity

Modifications of the movement of calcium ions through channels in the cell wall is a common factor in many receptor mechanisms. As well as the calcium channel-blocking effect of opioid alkaloids like protopine and tetrandene ([3] and see the Analgesic section below), this has also been observed in vascular tissues for ginseng saponins.[4,5] A coumarin, scoparone, from Capillaris also inhibits calcium influx.[6] From the Chinese remedy *Dictamnus dasycarpus*, calcium channel block was found with fraxinellone and dictamine, two constituents with vasorelaxant effect.[7]

Adrenergic effects

The adrenergic effects of alkaloids of Ephedra, ephedrine and pseudoephedrine have been understood for many years. Beta-2-adrenergic receptor stimulation has also been mooted to explain the effect of *Angelica sinensis* in reducing experimental pulmonary hypertension;[8] Rehmannia and *Plastrum testudinis* have also shown such activity in vitro.[9] The nociceptive effect of processed aconite was demonstrated as involving adrenergic rather than opioid receptors[10] and hypaconitine appears to be the most active of the alkaloids.[11] The bronchorelaxant (antiasthmatic) effect of coumarins in the fruit of *Cnidium monnieri* is mediated by a beta-2-receptor and blocked by propranolol.[12] Alismol, a sesquiterpenoid from *Alisma orientale*, demonstrated in vitro inhibition of noradrenaline release at adrenergic postsynaptic membranes.[13]

Acetylcholine receptors

Acetylcholine is a common synaptic transmitter in the body. Acetylcholine-sensitive or 'cholinergic' receptors are divided into many types, depending on their other sensitivities. 'Nicotinic' receptors are also sensitive to the alkaloid from *Nicotinana tabacum* (tobacco). 'Muscarinic' receptors are also sensitive to muscarine from the fly agaric mushroom. The atropine-like alkaloids in plants of the Solanaceae (such as deadly nightshade, henbane and jimson weed) block muscarinic receptors in the parasympathetic nervous system. The effect of dried orange peel on digestive activity was blocked by atropine, suggesting activity on the muscarinic receptors.[14] The traditional analgesic effect of *Atractylodes lancea* in cases of muscle pain has led to the isolation of an alcohol, beta-eudesmol, which has been shown to block muscle nicotinic receptors in vitro;[15] this may be linked to an observed presynaptic depression of the regenerative release of acetylcholine in neuromuscular junctions.[16] An action on the presynaptic membrane calcium channels to facilitate acetylcholine release at motor neuron terminals, apparently for the first time, is demonstrated for a lectin fraction of *Pinellia ternata*.[17] Pinellia was also shown to stimulate vagal and thus gastric activity in vivo, an activity antagonized by apomorphine.[18]

GABA and benzodiazepine receptors

The benzodiazepine valium was named in recognition of recent research that had established valerian as manifesting some tranquillizing properties. Although there are no chemical similarities between valerian constituents and benzodiazepines, some pharmacological similarities have emerged, with evidence that like the benzodiazepines, valerian acts in part through an effect on the receptors on inhibitory neurons sensitive to gamma-amino butyric acid (GABA) (see also p.163). GABA-A and benzodiazepine receptor binding has been shown as a feature of a number of herbal remedies.[19,20] For example, *Salvia miltiorrhiza* (dan shen), much researched in Beijing as a postulated treatment for ischaemic damage after strokes,[21] and in the repair of other nerve tissue damage,[22,23] has effects which apparently include stimulating GABA release[24,25] and blocking calcium input.[26] GABA secretion is depressed by a lactone fraction from *Coriaria spp*.[27] Dipsacus saponin C has experimental antinociceptive effects; GABA-A, N-methyl-D-aspartic acid (NMDA) and non-NMDA receptors, but not opioid and GABA-B receptors, appeared to be involved in this activity.[28]

Dopaminergic receptors

Tetrahydrocolumbamine from *Polygala tenuifolia* inhibits dopamine receptors, in part competitively,[29] as does tetrahydropalmatine from Corydalis (and see below). In the monograph on chaste tree on p.328, other evidence for dopaminergic receptor activity is outlined.

Analgesic activity

Analgesics present a major challenge to the modern herbalist. Painkillers are by definition relatively powerful agents. Natural analgesics are likely to have been identified early in human history for their immediate benefits in pain relief and/or for their psychoactive properties. Obvious examples are the opium poppy (morphine alkaloids), the nightshade family (atropine alkaloids), willow, poplar and birch barks among other sources of salicylates and phenols, as well as the many psychoactive plants (coca, cannabis, psylocybin, mescaline, etc.). Most are now only legally prescribable by doctors, if at all, and it would appear that there is little scope for relatively gentle remedies to compete with the improved targeting of synthetic analgesics.

There are, however, a number of traditional remedies with general and specific analgesic reputations that have been less well exploited in modern times and which are relatively well tolerated in clinical use. Although not as powerful as some of the modern synthetic analgesics, they do show sufficient activity to be taken seriously and are particularly likely to be helpful in pain linked to inflammation and to visceral and vascular spasm. The research papers cited in the following examples demonstrate that even in the demanding area of analgesia there is ample evidence to support useful clinical intervention by the medical herbalist. Nevertheless, none of the following remedies are safe for widespread use by the public; their use is to be confined to the most experienced practitioner who can take account of all factors, including the increased likelihood of adverse effects.

Eschscholtzia californica (Californian poppy)

A traditional medicinal plant of the Indians, now used mainly by the rural population of western USA for its mild analgesic and sedative properties (and as the state flower of California). In studies on a prescription drug in Germany, Phytonoxon N containing *E. californica* and *Corydalis cava* (see below) at 4:1 relative concentration, investigators have identified interactions with opioid receptors,[30] as well as other neurotransmitter activity.[31] Aqueous-alcoholic extracts from *E. californica* also were shown to inhibit the enzymatic degradation of catecholamines as well as the synthesis of adrenaline, dopamine beta-hydroxylase and monoamine oxidase (MAO-B).[32]

One separate study of the effects of the aqueous extract of the plant shows that at 25 mg/kg it had an anxiolytic action when administered intraperitoneally in mice, as measured by changes in behavioural parameters; at higher levels the effect became more sedative.[33]

A key alkaloidal constituent, chelerythrine, is a well-known protein kinase C inhibitor with antitumour activity.[34] Activation of protein kinase C in spinal cord dorsal horn neurons contributes to persistent pain following noxious thermal[35] and chemical stimulation; chelerythrine produced significant reductions of nociceptive responses in one study.[36] Another Canadian study suggests that chelerythrine can attenuate the development of morphine dependence.[37] It demonstrates a range of effects on protein phosphorylation in different tissues[38] and also demonstrates a range of potent antiinflammatory activities.[39–42]

Chelerythrine and and another alkaloidal constituent, sanguinarine, exhibited affinity for rat liver vasopressin V1 receptors and are competitive inhibitors of [3H]-vasopressin binding. These alkaloids represent two of the first non-peptidic structures providing original chemical leads for the design of synthetic vasopressin compounds.[43]

Corydalis cava et spp (yan hu suo)

This remedy has been widely used in China and the East for pain, especially of dysmenorrhoea and the abdomen. In the studies on Phytonoxon N referred to above for *E. californica*, *Corydalis cava* was generally the stronger of the two ingredients.

Whole Corydalis extract demonstrated antispasmodic activity in acetylcholine-induced contractions at around half that seen for papaverine.[44] Alkaloidal constituents have shown a range of activities. Isocoryne, like other phthalide isoquinoline alkaloids, produced an inhibitory effect on GABA-activated currents.[45] Cavidine, protopine, corlumine, yenhusomine and dehydrocavidine have exhibited spasmolytic activity.[46] Dehydrocorydaline appears to block noradrenaline release and an experimental antiulceration action is posited.[47] Intravenous tetrahydropalmatine induces hypotension and bradycardia in rats and acts, apparently through 5-HT_2 and/or D_2 receptor antagonism in the hypothalamus,[48] at levels comparable to one-tenth the dose of haloperidol.[49] It also has powerful antiinflammatory effects.[50,51,52] Tetrahydroberberine inhibited the rabbit platelet aggregation triggered by arachidonic acid and an inhibition of venous thrombosis in vivo.[53] Various tetrahydroprotoberberine alkaloids have been shown to be selective alpha- 1-adrenoceptor antagonists in vascular smooth muscle.[54] Protopine isolated from Corydalis inhibited norepinephrine-induced tonic contraction in rat thoracic aorta in a concentration-dependent manner, probably by suppressing the calcium influx through both voltage- and receptor-operated calcium channels.[55]

Traditional vinegar-processed preparations of the fresh Corydalis tuber have been shown to have stronger analgesic effects in vivo than those of the dried preparation.[56] There appeared to be higher concentrations of total alkaloids in the fresh specimen.[57]

Evodia rutaecarpa (wu zhu yu)

This remedy was traditionally used for pain, especially arising from abdominal and digestive causes with headaches and abdominal pain, including dysmenorrhoea. Evodia extract at various concentrations showed biphasic effects on the secretion of interleukin-1-beta, interleukin-6, tumour necrosis factor alpha, and granulocyte-macrophage colony stimulating factor by mononuclear cells in vitro. The effect was more stimulating at lower doses.[58]

At least some of the effectiveness of Evodia has been linked to the fraction containing Evodiamine and rutaecarpine.[59] A cholinergic mechanism has been implicated in this activity;[60,61] on the other hand, in the case of Evodia's vasodilatory activity, an alpha-adrenoceptor blocking and 5-HT antagonizing action are suggested,[62] as well as for the powerful cardiotonic and uterotonic evodiamine[63,64] and for the vasorelaxant and hypotensive dehydroevodiamine.[65,66,67] This has itself demonstrated multiple receptor activities.[68] Direct action on muscarinic receptors has been linked to its antidiarrhoeal action.[69]

However, other antiinflammatory fractions have also been identified;[70] antihistamine and antinociceptive effects were reported for methanolic extracts of various Evodia species, though this was not directly correlated with alkaloidal content as such.[71]

Among a number of plants tested Evodia showed a strong inhibitory effect on acetylcholinesterase in vitro[72] and an antiscopolamine effect in vivo. This antiamnesic effect was more potent than that of tacrine which is the only drug for Alzheimer's disease approved by the FDA.[73] The active component was identified as dehydroevodiamine hydrochloride.

Stephania tetrandra (han fang ji)

This Chinese medicinal herb has been used traditionally as a remedy for neuralgia and arthritis, especially febrile rheumatic disease, but its use in modern times is complicated by the apparently frequent substitution by Aristolochia. Tetrandrine, a key constituent alkaloid, has more recently been used to treat hypertension.

The vasodilatory action of tetrandrine[74] is associated with in vitro observations of direct calcium channel block in vascular smooth muscle cells,[75] lymphocytes,[76] cardiac cells ,[77,78] rat glioma cells[79] and bovine chromaffin cells.[80] In vivo investigations demonstrate that tetrandrine inhibits KCl-induced intracellular Ca flow; it also inhibits norepinephrine-induced vasocontraction in the presence of extracellular calcium.[81] Findings suggest that tetrandrine is a structurally unique natural product calcium entry blocker.[82] Hypotensive activity for tetrandrine has also been supported in experimental studies.[83,84]

Tetrandrine has been used in China as a treatment for silicosis, and antisilicosis benefits have figured largely in Chinese research e.g.[85] Its mechanism is unclear but it has been found to scavenge superoxide (O_2-) radicals produced from xanthine/xanthine oxidase, and has inhibited lipid peroxidation.[86–90]

Bisbenzylisoquinoline alkaloids are known to affect immune as well as inflammatory responses and have been used for the treatment of inflammatory symptoms in China. In a study aimed at elucidating the inhibitory effects of two alkaloids, fangchinoline and isotetrandrine inhibited inflammatory mediators including cytokines and IL-1-beta.[91]

Another constituent, tetrahydropalmatine, has analgesic, sedative and tranquillizing effects, involving dopamine receptor antagonist and depleting activity.[92]

Herbal sedatives and hypnotics

In conventional pharmacological terms, sedatives reduce nervous activity and hypnotics promote sleep. There is obviously overlap in practice between the two categories, and both imply a degree of depression of nervous activity and consequent dangers (as seen most obviously in the barbiturates). There is a third category of calming agent that was postulated as an ideal anxiolytic strategy: the tranquillizer. This was originally defined as a treatment whose effect was confined to the reticular activating system that determined the level of arousal in the central nervous system, and did not otherwise sedate. Although the benzodiazepines were hailed as tranquillizers on their discovery, this ideal has been clearly compromised and these remedies are now seen to have appreciable sedative and hynoptic effects as well.

Many traditional herbal remedies have various degrees of sedative and tranquillizing activity and some have had this effect supported in experimental and clinical studies. However, it is probably misleading to apply the strict pharmacological definitions to them; their effects are much broader in clinical experience, with strong sedation rare. For the purposes of this text, therefore, the terms 'herbal sedatives and hypnotics' will be used to describe remedies that are actually relaxing, with little evidence of depressive activity. This herbal dimension is even more obvious in the next category.

Relaxants and antispasmodics

Most medical preoccupation has been with the nervous system as an entity in itself, with the goal of better analgesics, sedatives, tranquillizers and antipsychotics. Traditional interest in such areas was of course also strong and many plants were favoured for their powerful psychoactive properties. However, probably the most widespread use of neuroactive plants, or nervines, nowadays is for their effects on innervated structures rather than on nervous tissue alone.

The antispasmodic (or spasmolytic) is a modern descriptor of the effect of an agent on visceral muscle in vitro, often the isolated guinea pig ileum. The technique is widely used as a model to indicate muscarinic or related receptor activity as above, but is a property with little therapeutic application. By contrast, herbal antispasmodics, spasmolytics or relaxants are remedies used to reduce the symptoms of tension in the body. Pre-Cartesian insights into the human condition had no separation between body and mind and this particular holistic view is a constant feature of Asian medicine still. Apart from the obvious psychoactives, remedies were not seen to be acting on the nervous system as such; rather there were many remedies that treated various manifestations of turbulence in the body linked to what nowadays would be described as 'stress-related' conditions.

Even though using other terms, early texts described such conditions as classic hypertension ('*Liver qi* rising'), nervous headaches, palpitations, breathless attacks and hyperventilation ('constriction of the chest'), nervous dyspepsia, dysphagia, irritable bowel and urinary frequency.

The remedies selected for these conditions were seen as somatic in emphasis. The markers for application and effectiveness were physical symptoms. Nowadays modern herbalists refer to many of them as antispasmodics or spasmolytics or, more recently, 'visceral relaxants'. They are offered to the modern stressed patient as a welcome antidote to the culture of tranquillizers and sedatives, treatments working from the 'neck down' to reduce the physical effects of tension without befuddling the brain or impugning their sanity. Western remedies like those listed later have all developed reputations as useful management measures in helping patients handle and even overcome psychosomatic disorders, perhaps combined with appropriate breathing exercises and adrenaline-reducing aerobic activity. Some Chinese remedies like *Uncaria rhycholphylla* were targeted at such conditions and hold out the promise of modern applications.

PHYTOTHERAPEUTICS

Nervine tonics and nervous trophorestoratives

Herbal medicine has had to adapt significantly from its traditional roots. There is evidence that in many earlier cultures there were different perspectives on anxiety and tension syndromes. Whether there was genuinely less opportunity for the modern diagnosis in highly structured communities living on the edge of survival or whether such symptoms were not recognized as such is arguable. There is, however, less emphasis on treatments to relieve stress conditions in most traditional texts.

There were also no powerful synthetic agents that relieved pain and distress. It is thus an entirely modern notion that herbs could provide gentle back-up for sufferers with nervous or mental problems.

In the West, where such adjustments have been made over many decades, the group of remedies that has emerged to meet modern needs is sometimes referred to as 'nervines'. In recognition of the common observation that many conditions of tension are linked with fatigue, debility and depression, there is also a category of remedies that were seen to restore energies and build up strength. These have sometimes been referred to as 'trophorestoratives'. It was a general principle that some tonifying element be included in most nervine prescriptions, so as to aim for lasting value rather than just short-term alleviation.

ANALGESICS

Plant remedies traditionally used as analgesics

Corydalis spp (yan hu suo), *Eschscholtzia californica* (Californian poppy), *Evodia rutaecarpa* (wu zhu yu), *Gelsemium sempervirens* (yellow jasmine), *Paederia scandens* (ji shi teng), *Schefflera arboricola* (qi ye lian), *Stephania tetrandra* (han fang ji). Topically: *Bryonia alba* (white bryony).

Indications for herbal analgesics

- Pain associated with inflammation (e.g. arthritis, chondritis, tendinitis, myalgia)
- Pain associated with visceral spasm (e.g. gallbladder, urinary and intestinal colic)
- Pain associated with vascular spasm (e.g. migraine, spasmodic dysmenorrhoea)
- Neuralgic pain (in limited cases)

Other traditional indications for analgesics

- Primitive anaesthesia

Contraindications for herbal analgesics

As powerful agents, herbal analgesics should be restricted in their application to experienced and well-trained practitioners only. There is a theoretically increased risk of neurotoxicity and other adverse effects (although little known incidence) and there is always the possibility that individual examples could be withdrawn from use by regulatory authorities; this is most likely after cases of irresponsible use. The following cases should be approached with particular caution.

- Concurrent prescription of powerful analgesics
- Pain in children
- Neurological disease
- Depression and psychosis
- Liver and kidney disease
- History of allergic or anaphylactic reactions

Application

Herbal analgesics may be taken as required or before food. There is likely to be a longer delay compared with synthetic analgesics and the temptation to dose excessively must be resisted.

Long-term therapy with analgesics is not advisable.

Advanced phytotherapeutics

Herbal analgesics may also be usefully applied in some cases (depending on other factors) of inflammatory disease.

HERBAL SEDATIVES AND HYPNOTICS

Plant remedies traditionally used as sedatives and hypnotics

Corydalis spp (yan hu suo), *Humulus lupulus* (hops), *Lactuca virosa* (wild lettuce), *Passiflora incarnata* (passionflower), *Piper methysticum* (kava), *Piscidia erythrina* (Jamaican dogwood), *Scutellaria laterifolia* (skullcap)[93, 94]

Indications for herbal sedatives and hypnotics

- Moderate tension and anxiety syndromes (short-term or intermittent use)
- Insomnia (difficulty in getting off to sleep first thing at night)
- Weaning off conventional sedative prescriptions

Other traditional indications for sedative and hypnotics

- Restlessness disturbing convalescence

Contraindications for herbal sedatives and hypnotics

As generally milder than prescribed sedatives, herbal equivalents should not be seen as immediate substitutes in the more serious indications. It would be unwise and even dangerous to drop the use of strong sedative medication without careful planning, preferably with the cooperation of the prescribing physician.

- Depression
- Insomnia marked by increasing restlessness during the early hours of the morning

Traditional therapeutic insights into the use of sedatives and hypnotics

In what were usually harsher and more robust times, the need for sedatives was often urgent, and opium extracts were the most favoured. The main tradition of use of moderate herbal sedatives were as short-term components of convalescent management, particularly to help with sleep. There was apparently little use of sedatives for wider lifestyle management.

Application

Herbal sedatives and hypnotics may be taken as required, at bedtime or before food.

Prescription of herbal sedatives should be limited. In the first place they are part of an essentially negative strategy that aims to substitute stupor for resolution of underlying problems. Although most unlikely to lead to addiction, compared with modern sedatives, the body may habituate to herbal sedatives and hypnotics with diminishing benefits.

Advanced phytotherapeutics

Herbal sedatives and hypnotics may also be usefully applied in some cases (depending on other factors) of inflammatory disease.

ANTISPASMODICS AND RELAXANTS

Plant remedies traditionally used as antispasmodics and relaxants

Dioscoria spp (wild yam), *Leonurus cardiaca* (motherwort), *Lobelia inflata* (lobelia), *Matricaria recutita* (chamomile), *Passiflora incarnata* (passionflower), *Piper methysticum* (kava), *Scutellaria lateriflora* (scullcap), *Tilia spp* (lime flowers), *Valeriana officinalis* (valerian), *Viburnum opulus* (cramp bark). (See also Aromatics and Volatile Antispasmodics, pp 171–172).

Indications for antispasmodics and relaxants

- Anxiety, irritability and restlessness, including in children
- Sleeplessness due to anxiety and irritability
- Nervous dyspepsia
- Irritable bowel and intestinal colic
- Tension headaches and migraines
- Spasmodic dysmenorrhoea

Contraindications for antispasmodics and relaxants

As a group these remedies are generally safe and well tolerated.

Traditional therapeutic insights into the use of antispasmodics and relaxants

Early use of antispasmodics also appears to have been dominated by their emergency indications, notably urinary and biliary colic. The use of milder relaxant treatments was mainly as tisanes for children and in the largely unrecorded but vast realm of family care. As expected, systematic classifications of medicine throughout history are generally silent on this area of popular healthcare.

Relaxants were obviously indicated for functional overactivities, indications like dyspeptic and colicky conditions were probably the most common (and carminatives like the spices the most frequent tisanes). Headaches, teething and restlessness in children and menstrual pains were likely to make up most of the remaining indications. These were usually treated within the home by local remedies with recipes handed down through the family.

It remains true to this day that often the most effective relaxant therapy is a cup of hot herbal infusion.

Some remedies are more sedative than others in this class (see above). These might be added to a relaxant prescription to increase its impact. However, sedation may be depleting: the more a remedy is chosen for its sedative effects, the shorter the treatment should be and the more tonifying remedies should be added (see following section). The latter should also be a major element in prescriptions for the increasing proportion of tension conditions linked with fatigue, debility, depression and exhaustion.

Application

Antispasmodics and relaxants (and also those aromatics and volatile antispasmodics used for this purpose) may be best taken as hot infusions, though the ordinary teabag may not be sufficiently strong compared with the traditional brew and in acute cases, traditional doses were very high indeed. However, the following herbs probably work better in aqueous ethanolic extracts: *Dioscoria spp*, *Lobelia inflata*, *Passiflora incarnata*, *Piper methysticum*, *Valeriana officinalis*, *Viburnum opulus*.

Long-term therapy is generally well tolerated and may be appropriate, although the use of more sedative remedies should be reduced.

NERVINE TONICS (NERVOUS TROPHORESTORATIVES)

Plant remedies traditionally used as trophorestoratives

Avena officinalis (oatstraw), *Hypericum perforatum* (St John's wort), *Scutellaria lateriflora* (skullcap), *Turnera aphrodisiaca* (damiana), *Verbena officinalis* (vervain), *Withania somniferum* (Indian ginseng).

Indications for trophorestoratives

(see also Tonics, p.155).

- Nervous exhaustion
- Neuralgia, herpes infections
- Depressive states
- Insomnia (waking up in the small hours after getting off to sleep easily)

Other traditional indications for trophorestoratives

- Convalescence
- Neurasthenia

Contraindications for trophorestoratives

True trophorestoratives are almost nutritional in their effects, with few risks of adverse effects except in those patients with extremely debilitated constitutions (see also the discussion on tonics).

Traditional therapeutic insights into the use of trophorestoratives

Neurasthenia encompassed a wider range of disorders than nervous exhaustion. In days before psychoanalysis and neurology, it included symptoms where the nervous tissues were seen to be affected such as neuralgia and neuritis, depression, anxiety states and neurosis. The trophorestoratives were thus often combined with other tonics and convalescent foods such as molasses, yeast and malt extract (now known as rich sources of the B vitamins), oatmeal and other cereals.

Application

Trophorestoratives may be taken as required or before food.

Long-term therapy with trophorestoratives is generally the norm.

References

1. Liao JF, Jan YM, Huang SY et al. Evaluation with receptor binding assay on the water extracts of ten CNS-active Chinese herbal drugs. Proceedings of the National Science Council of the Republic of China B 1995; 3: 151–158
2. Ishihara S, Yamada K, Hayashi T et al. Effects of kamikihito, a traditional Chinese medicine, on neurotransmitter receptor binding in the aged rat brain determined by in vitro autoradiography: changes in dopamine D1 and serotonin 5-HT2A receptor binding. Biological and Pharmaceutical Bulletin 1994; 17(8): 1132–1134
3. Ko FN, Wu TS, Lu ST et al. Ca(2+)-channel blockade in rat thoracic aorta by protopine isolated from Corydalis tubers. Japan Journal of Pharmacology 1992; 58(1): 1–9
4. Low AM, Berdik M, Sormaz L et al. Plant alkaloids, tetrandrine and hernandezine, inhibit calcium-depletion stimulated calcium entry in human and bovine endothelial cells. Life Science 1996; 58, 25: 2327–2335

5. Kwan CY. Vascular effects of selected antihypertensive drugs derived from traditional medicinal herbs. Clinical and Experimental Pharmacology and Physiology 1995; 22(suppl 1): S297–299
6. Yamahara J, Kobayashi G, Matsuda H et al. Vascular dilatory action of the Chinese crude drug. II. Effects of scoparone on calcium mobilization. Chemical and Pharmaceutical Bulletin (Tokyo) 1989; 37(2): 485–489
7. Yu SM, Ko FN, Su MJ et al. Vasorelaxing effect in rat thoracic aorta caused by fraxinellone and dictamine isolated from the Chinese herb Dictamnus dasycarpus Turcz: comparison with cromakalim and Ca2+ channel blockers. Naunyn Schmiedebergs Archives of Pharmacology 1992; 345(3): 349–355
8. Sun RY, Yan YZ, Zhang H, Li CC. Role of beta-receptor in the radix Angelicae sinensis attenuated hypoxic pulmonary hypertension in rats. Chinese Medical Journal (Engl) 1989; 102(1): 1–6
9. Yi NY, Feng GP, Yu YM et al. The action of radix Rehmanniae and Plastrum testudinis on beta-adrenergic receptor-cAMP system. Chinese Medical Journal (Engl) 1987; 100(11): 893–898
10. Isono T, Oyama T, Asami A et al. The analgesic mechanism of processed Aconiti tuber: the involvement of descending inhibitory system. American Journal of Chinese Medicine 1994; 22(1): 83–94
11. Kimura M, Muroi M, Kimura I et al. Hypaconitine, the dominant constituent responsible for the neuromuscular blocking action of the Japanese-sino medicine 'bushi' (aconite root). Japan Journal of Pharmacology 1988; 48(2): 290–293
12. Chen Z, Duan X. Mechanism of the antiasthmatic effect of total coumarins in the fruit of Cnidium monnieri (L.) Cuss. Chung Kuo Chung Yao Tsa Chih 1990; 15(5): 304–305, 320
13. Matsuda H, Yamahara J, Kobayashi G et al. Effect of alismol on adrenergic mechanism in isolated rabbit ear artery. Japan Journal of Pharmacology 1988; 46(4): 331–335
14. Huang ZH, Yang DZ, Wei YQ. Effect of atropine on the enhancing action of Fructus Aurantii Immaturus on the myoelectric activity of small intestine in dogs. Chung Kuo Chung Hsi I Chieh Ho Tsa Chih 1996; 16(5): 292–294
15. Kimura M, Nojima H, Muroi M, Kimura I. Mechanism of the blocking action of beta-eudesmol on the nicotinic acetylcholine receptor channel in mouse skeletal muscles. Neuropharmacology 1991; 30(8): 835–841
16. Chiou LC, Chang CC. Antagonism by beta-eudesmol of neostigmine-induced neuromuscular failure in mouse diaphragms. European Journal of Pharmacology 1992; 216(2): 199–206
17. Shi YL, Xu YF, Zhang H. Effect of Pinellia ternata lectin on membrane currents of mouse motor nerve terminals. Science in China B 1994; 37(4): 448–453
18. Niijima A, Okui Y, Kubo M et al. Effect of Pinellia ternata tuber on the efferent activity of the gastric vagus nerve in the rat. Brain Research Bulletin 1993; 32(2): 103–106
19. Yamada K, Hayashi T, Hasegawa T et al. Effects of Kamikihito, a traditional Chinese medicine, on neurotransmitter receptor binding in the aged rat brain determined by in vitro autoradiography (2): changes in GABAA and benzodiazepine receptor binding. Japan Journal of Pharmacology 1994; 66(1): 53–58
20. Sugiyama K, Kano T, Muteki T. Intravenous anesthetics, acting on the gamma-amino butyric acid (GABA) A receptor, potentiate the herbal medicine 'saiko-keishi-to'-induced chloride current. Masui 1997; 46(9): 1197–1203
21. Kuang P, Wu W, Zhu K. Evidence for amelioration of cellular damage in ischemic rat brain by radix salviae miltiorrhizae treatment – immunocytochemistry and histopathology studies. Journal of Traditional Chinese Medicine 1993; 13(1): 38–41
22. Zhu MD, Cai FY. The effect of Inj. Salviae Miltiorrhizae Co. on the retrograde axoplasmic transport in the optic nerve of rabbits with chronic IOP elevation. Chung Hua Yen Ko Tsa Chih 1991; 27(3): 174–178
23. Hu Y, Ge Y, Zhang Y et al. Treatment of 100 cases of nerve deafness with injectio radix salviae miltiorrhizae. Journal of Traditional Chinese Medicine 1992; 12(4): 256–258
24. Chang HM, Chui KY, Tan FW et al. Structure-activity relationship of miltirone, an active central benzodiazepine receptor ligand isolated from Salvia miltiorrhiza Bunge (Danshen). Journal of Medical Chemistry, 1991; 34(5): 1675–1692
25. Kuang P, Xiang J. Effect of radix salviae miltiorrhizae on EAA and IAA during cerebral ischemia in gerbils: a microdialysis study. Journal of Traditional Chinese Medicine 1994; 14(1): 45–50
26. Tao Y, Kuang P, Zuo P. Inhibitory effect of 764–3 on Ca2+ uptake in rat brain synaptosomes. Journal of Traditional Chinese Medicine 1996; 16(4): 288–292
27. Zhu X, Zhu C, Wu Y. Coriaria lactone on gamma-aminobutyric acid secretion and glutamic acid decarboxylase and its receptor binding in rat. Chung Hua I Hsueh Tsa Chih 1995; 75(6): 363–365, 384
28. Suh HW, Song DK, Son KH et al. Antinociceptive mechanisms of dipsacus saponin C administered intracerebroventricularly in the mouse. General Pharmacology 1996; 27(7): 1167–1172
29. Shen XL, Witt MR, Dekermendjian K, Nielsen M. Isolation and identification of tetrahydrocolumbamine as a dopamine receptor ligand from Polygala tenuifolia Willd. Yao Hsueh Hsueh Pao 1994; 29(12): 887–890
30. Reimeier C, Schneider I, Schneider W, Schäfer HL, Elstner EF. Effects of ethanolic extracts from Eschscholtzia californica and Corydalis cava on dimerization and oxidation of enkephalins. Arzneimittelforschung 1995; 45(2): 132–136
31. Schäfer HL, Schäfer H, Schneider W, Elstner EF. Sedative action of extract combinations of Eschscholtzia californica and Corydalis cava. Arzneimittelforschung 1995; 45(2): 124–126
32. Kleber E, Schneider W, Schäfer HL, Elstner EF. Modulation of key reactions of the catecholamine metabolism by extracts from Eschscholtzia californica and Corydalis cava. Arzneimittelforschung 1995; 45(2): 127–131
33. Rolland A, Fleurentin J, Lanhers MC et al. Behavioural effects of the American traditional plant Eschscholtzia californica: sedative and anxiolytic properties. Planta Medica 1991; 57(3): 212–216
34. Herbert JM, Augereau JM, Gleye J, Maffrand JP. Chelerythrine is a potent and specific inhibitor of protein kinase C. Biochemical and Biophysical Research Communications 1990; 172(3): 993–999
35. Meller ST, Dykstra C, Gebhart GF. Acute thermal hyperalgesia in the rat is produced by activation of N-methyl-D-aspartate receptors and protein kinase C and production of nitric oxide. Neuroscience 1996; 71(2): 327–335
36. Yashpal K, Pitcher GM, Parent A, Quirion R, Coderre TJ. Noxious thermal and chemical stimulation induce increases in 3H-phorbol 12,13-dibutyrate binding in spinal cord dorsal horn as well as persistent pain and hyperalgesia, which is reduced by inhibition of protein kinase C. Journal of Neuroscience 1995; 15(5 Pt 1): 3263–3272
37. Fundytus ME, Coderre TJ. Chronic inhibition of intracellular Ca2+ release or protein kinase C activation significantly reduces the development of morphine dependence. European Journal of Pharmacology 1996; 300(3): 173–181
38. Lombardini JB. Paradoxical stimulatory effect of the kinase inhibitor chelerythrine on the phosphorylation of approximately 20 K M(r) protein present in the mitochondrial fraction of rat retina. Brain Research 1995; 673(2): 194–198
39. Herbert JM, Savi P, Laplace MC, Dumas A, Dol F. Chelerythrine, a selective protein kinase C inhibitor, counteracts pyrogen-induced expression of tissue factor without effect on thrombomodulin down-regulation in endothelial cells. Thrombosis Research 1993; 71(6): 487–493
40. Lane T, Novales-Li P. Chelerythrine inhibits the secretory response of human blood platelets without specifically inhibiting protein kinase C. Tokai Journal of Experimental and Clinical Medicine 1996; 21(2): 61–67
41. Shah BH, Shamim G, Khan S, Saeed SA. Protein kinase C inhibitor, chelerythrine, potentiates the adrenaline-mediatated aggregation of human platelets through calcium influx. Biochemistry and Molecular Biology International 1996; 38(6): 1135–1141

42. Pavlakovic G, Eyer CL, Isom GE. Neuroprotective effects of PKC inhibition against chemical hypoxia. Brain Research 1995; 676(1): 205–211
43. Granger I, Serradeil-le Gal C, Augereau JM, Gleye J. Benzophenanthridine alkaloids isolated from Eschscholtzia californica cell suspension cultures interact with vasopressin (V1) receptors. Planta Medica 1992; 58(1): 35–38
44. Boegge SC, Kesper S, Verspohl EJ, Nahrstedt A. Reduction of ACh-induced contraction of rat isolated ileum by coptisine, (+)-caffeoylmalic acid, Chelidonium majus, and Corydalis lutea extracts. Planta Medica 1996; 62(2): 173–174
45. Chernevaskaja NI, Krishtal OA, Valeyev AY. Inhibitions of the GABA-induced currents of rat neurons by the alkaloid isocoryne from the plant Corydalis pseudoadunca. Toxicon 1990; 28(6): 727–730
46. Bhakuni DS, Chaturvedi R. The alkaloids of Corydalis meifolia. Journal of Natural Products 1983; 46(4): 466–470
47. Kurahashi K, Fujiwara M. Adrenergic neuron blocking action of dehydrocorydaline isolated from Corydalis bulbosa. Canadian Journal of Physiology and Pharmacology. 1976; 54(3): 287–293
48. Lin MT, Chueh FY, Hsieh MT, Chen CF. Antihypertensive effects of DL-tetrahydropalmatine: an active principle isolated from Corydalis. Clinical and Experimental Pharmacology and Physiology 1996; 23(8): 738–742
49. Chueh FY, Hsieh MT, Chen CF, Lin MT. DL-tetrahydropalmatine-produced hypotension and bradycardia in rats through the inhibition of central nervous dopaminergic mechanisms. Pharmacology 1995; 51(4): 237–244
50. Matsuda H, Tokuoka K, Wu J, Shiomoto H, Kubo M. Anti-inflammatory activities of dehydrocorydaline isolated from Corydalis Tuber. Natural Medicines 1997; 51(4): 293–297
51. Matsuda H, Tokuoka K, Wu J, Shiomoto H, Kubo M. Inhibitory effects of dehydrocorydaline isolated from corydalis tuber against type I-IV allergic models. Biological and Pharmaceutical Bulletin 1997; 20(4): 431–434
52. Pang Z, Wang B, Huang H. Study on pharmacokinetics of tetrahydropalmatine in corydalis yanhusuo. Xi'an Yike Daxue Xuebao 1995; 16(3): 284–286
53. Xuan B, Wang W, Li DX. Inhibitory effect of tetrahydroberberine on platelet aggregation and thrombosis. Chung Kuo Yao Li Hsueh Pao 1994; 15(2): 133–135
54. Ko F-N, Chang Y-L, Chen C-M, Teng C-M. (Racemic)-govadine and (Racemic)-THP, two tetrahydroprotoberberine alkaloids, as selective alpha-1-adrenoceptor antagonists in vascular smooth muscle cells. Journal of Pharmacy and Pharmacology 1996; 48(6): 629–634
55. Ko FN, Wu TS, Lu ST, Wu YC, Huang TF, Teng CM. Ca(2+)-channel blockade in rat thoracic aorta by protopine isolated from Corydalis tubers. Japan Journal of Pharmacology 1992; 58(1): 1–9
56. Liu L, Li G, Zhu F, Wang L, Wang Y, Comparison of analgesic effect between locally vinegar-processed preparation of fresh rhizoma Corydalis and traditionally vinegar-processed rhizoma Corydalis. Chung Kuo Chung Yao Tsa Chih 1990; 15(11): 666–667, 702
57. Wang Y, Zhu F, Zhang J et al. Chemical evaluation of vinegar-processing method for fresh rhizoma Corydalis. Chung Kuo Chung Yao Tsa Chih 1990; 15(9): 526–528
58. Chang CP, Chang JY, Wang FY, Tseng J, Chang JG. The effect of Evodia rutaecarpa extract on cytokine secretion by human mononuclear cells in vitro. American Journal of Chinese Medicine 1995; 23(2): 173–180
59. Yamahara J, Yamada T, Kitani T, Naitoh Y, Fujimura H. Antianoxic action and active constituents of evodiae fructus. Chemical and Pharmaceitical Bulletin (Tokyo) 1989; 37(7): 1820–1822
60. Yamahara J, Yamada T, Kitani T, Naitoh Y, Fujimura H. Antianoxic action of evodiamine, an alkaloid in Evodia rutaecarpa fruit. Journal of Ethnopharmacology 1989; 27(1–2): 185–192
61. Yu LL, Liao JF, Chen CF. Effect of the crude extract of Evodiae Fructus on the intestinal transit in mice. Planta Medica 1994; 60(4): 308–312
62. Chiou WF, Liao JF, Chen CF. Comparative study of the vasodilatory effects of three quinazoline alkaloids isolated from Evodia rutaecarpa. Journal of Natural Products 1996; 59(4): 374–378
63. Shoji N, Umeyama A, Takemoto T, Kajiwara A, Ohizumi Y. Isolation of evodiamine, a powerful cardiotonic principle, from Evodia rutaecarpa Bentham (Rutaceae). Journal of Pharmaceutic Sciences 1986; 75(6): 612–613
64. King CL, Kong YC, Wong NS, Yeung HW, Fong HH, Sankawa U. Uterotonic effect of Evodia rutaecarpa alkaloids. Journal of Natural Products 1980; 43(5): 577–582
65. Chiou WF, Liao JF, Shum AY, Chen CF. Mechanisms of vasorelaxant effect of dehydroevodiamine: a bioactive isoquinazolinocarboline alkaloid of plant origin. Journal of Cardiovascular Pharmacology 1996; 27(6): 845–853
66. Chiou WF, Chou CJ, Shum AY, Chen CF. The vasorelaxant effect of evodiamine in rat isolated mesenteric arteries: mode of action. European Journal of Pharmacology 1992; 215(2–3): 277–283
67. Yang MC, Wu SL, Kuo JS, Chen CF. The hypotensive and negative chronotropic effects of dehydroevodiamine. European Journal of Pharmacology 1990; 182(3): 537–542
68. Chiou WF, Liao JF, Shum AY, Chen CF. Mechanisms of vasorelaxant effect of dehydroevodiamine: a bioactive isoquinazolinocarboline alkaloid of plant origin. Journal of Cardiovascular Pharmacology 1996; 27(6): 845–853
69. Yu LL, Liao JF, Chen CF. Effect of the crude extract of Evodiae Fructus on the intestinal transit in mice. Planta Medica 1994; 60(4): 308–312
70. Matsuda H, Wu JX, Tanaka T, Iinuma M, Kubo M. Antinociceptive activities of 70% methanol extract of evodiae fructus (fruit of Evodia rutaecarpa var. bodinieri) and its alkaloidal components. Biological and Pharmaceutical Bulletin 1997; 20(3): 243–248
71. Kubo M, Chen Y, Hirose N, Asano T, Matsuda H. Studies on Evodiae Fructus I. Qualitative evaluation of various Evodiae Fructus by pharmacognostical and pharmacological methods. Natural Medicines 1995; 49(4): 451–454
72. Kim HJ, Jang YP, Kim YC. A constituent from Evodiae fructus having inhibitory effect on acetylcholinesterase. Seoul University Journal of Pharmaceutical Sciences 1995; 20: 1–11
73. Park CH, Kim SH, Choi W et al. Novel anticholinesterase and antiamnesic activities of dehydroevodiamine, a constituent of Evodia rutaecarpa. Planta Medica 1996; 62(5): 405–409
74. Kamiya T, Sugimoto Y, Yamada Y. Vasodilator effects of bisbenzylisoquinoline alkaloids from Stephania cepharantha. Planta Medica 1993; 59(5): 475–476
75. Wu SN, Hwang TL, Jan CR, Tseng CJ. Ionic mechanisms of tetrandrine in cultured rat aortic smooth muscle cells. European Journal of Pharmacology 1997; 327(2–3): 233–238
76. Leung YM, Berdik M, Kwan CY, Loh TT. Effects of tetrandrine and closely related bisbenzylisoquinoline derivatives on cytosolic Ca2+ in human leukaemic HL-60 cells: a structure-activity relationship study. Clinical and Experimental Pharmacology and Physiology 1996; 23(8): 653–659
77. Liu QY, Karpinski E, Pang PK. Tetrandrine inhibits both T and L calcium channel currents in ventricular cells. Journal of Cardiovascular Pharmacology 1992; 20(4): 513–519
78. Perez G, Cassels B, Reisin IL. Inhibition of Maxi K channels from coronary smooth muscle by tetrandrine, a hypotensive alkaloid. Biophysical Journal 1997; 72(2): 263
79. Imoto K, Takemura H, Kwan CY, Sakano S, Kaneko M, Ohshika H. Inhibitory effects of tetrandrine and hernandezine on Ca-2+ mobilization in rat glioma C6 cells. Research Communications in Molecular Pathology and Pharmacology 1997; 95(2): 129–146
80. Weinsberg F, Bickmeyer U, Wiegand H. Effects of tetrandrine on calcium channel currents of bovine chromaffin cells. Neuropharmacology 1994; 33(7): 885–890
81. Liu QY, Li B, Gang JM, Karpinski E, Pang PK. Tetrandrine, a Ca++ antagonist: effects and mechanisms of action in vascular smooth muscle cells. Journal of Pharmacology and Experimental Therapeutics 1995; 273(1): 32–39

82. King VF, Garcia ML, Himmel D et al. Interaction of tetrandrine with slowly inactivating calcium channels. Characterization of calcium channel modulation by an alkaloid of Chinese medicinal herb origin. Journal of Biological Chemistry 1988; Feb 15 263(5): 2238–44
83. Kawashima K, Hayakawa T, Oohata H et al. Antihypertensive effect of synthetic tetrandrine derivatives in SHR rats. General Pharmacology 1991; 22(1): 165–168
84. Kawashima K, Hayakawa T, Miwa Y et al. Structure and hypotensive activity relationships of tetrandrine derivatives in stroke-prone spontaneously hypertensive rats. General Pharmacology 1990; 21(3): 343–347
85. Liu B-C, He Y-X, Miao Q, Wang H-H, You B-R. The effects of tetrandrine (TT) and polyvinylpyridine-N-oxide (PVNO) on gene expression of type I and type III collagens during experimental silicosis. Biomedical and Environmental Sciences 1994; 7(3): 199–204
86. Shi X, Mao Y, Saffiotti U et al. Antioxidant activity of tetrandrine and its inhibition of quartz-induced lipid peroxidation. Journal of Toxicology and Environmental Health 1995; 46(2): 233–248
87. Cao Z-F. Scavenging effect of tetrandrine on active oxygen radicals. Planta Medica 1996; 62(5): 413–414
88. Cao Z-F, Zhu X-Q. Antioxidant action of tetrandrine: an alkaloid from the roots of Radix stephania tetrandra, S. Moore. Journal of the Science of Food and Agriculture 1997; 73(1): 106–110
89. Kang H-S, Kim Y-H, Lee C-S, Lee J-J, Choi I, Pyun K-H. Anti-inflammatory effects of Stephania tetrandra S. Moore on interleukin-6 production and experimental inflammatory disease models. Mediators of Inflammation 1996; 5(4): 280–291
90. Seow WK, Ferrante A, Goh DB, Chalmers AH, Li SY, Thong YH. In vitro immunosuppressive properties of the plant alkaloid tetrandrine. International Archives of Allergy and Applied Immunology 1988; 85(4): 410–415
91. Onai N, Tsunokawa Y, Suda M et al. Inhibitory effects of bisbenzylisoquinoline alkaloids on induction of proinflammatory cytokines, interleukin-1 and tumor necrosis factor-alpha. Planta Medica 1995; 61(6): 497–501
92. Zhu XZ. Development of natural products as drugs acting on central nervous system. Memorias do Instituto Oswaldo Cruz 1991; 86(Suppl 2): 173–175
93. Della Loggia R, Tubaro A, Redaelli C. Evaluation of the activity on the mouse CNS of several plant extracts and a combination of them Rivista di Neurologia 1981; 51(5): 297–310
94. Della Loggia R, Zilli C, Del Negro P, Redaelli C, Tubaro A. Isoflavones as spasmolytic principles of Piscidia erythrina. Progress in Clinical Biology Research 1988; 280: 365–368

FEMALE REPRODUCTIVE SYSTEM

SCOPE

Apart from their use to provide non-specific support for recuperation and repair, specific phytotherapeutic strategies include the following.

Treatment of:

- irregular menstruation and dysmenorrhoea (painful periods);
- some cases of menorrhagia (heavy menstrual bleeding);
- premenstrual syndromes;
- menopausal syndrome;
- impaired lactation;
- postnatal syndromes;
- some cases of infertility;
- functional ovarian cysts;
- some cases of vaginitis, cervicitis, vulvitis.

Management of:

- fibroids and endometrial polyps;
- endometriosis and pelvic inflammatory diseases;
- polycystic ovary.

Because of its use of secondary plant products and for ethical and legal reasons, particular **caution** is necessary in applying phytotherapy in cases of:

- delayed menstruation
- pregnancy and lactation;
- venereal disease;
- ovarian cancers;
- hormone antagonist treatment for cancer (e.g. tamoxifen).

ORIENTATION

Introduction

The female reproductive system provides perhaps the most substantial challenge to modern medical procedures and at the same time potentially the richest prospects for an inspired phytotherapy. Modern medicine finds disorders of the system difficult to treat conservatively. The reproductive structures themselves are the most dramatic examples of structure following function and, indeed, where function is notably rhythmic. Beyond this is the historical and social reality; women have often been the herbal practitioners in society, they have necessarily had to focus a great deal on matters of their own reproductive health, fertility and, as midwives, childbirth and childrearing. They have mastered the skills of intuitive diagnosis and treatment of functions that are notably difficult to isolate and measure and nowadays often do feel particularly aggrieved about the medicalization of their reproductive functions.

The medical challenge

It has proven difficult to devise modern treatments for disorders of the female reproductive system that are genuinely appropriate to the task. It has always been hard to get a true measure of the job in the first place. Many problems start with dysfunctions in menstrual cycles or with hormonal disruptions, for which treatment outcome measures are not agreed and where subjective distress is not matched by technological monitoring. Even pathologies are more variable than consistent. Endometriosis is almost unclassifiable and, with fibroids, largely inexplicable; there are more categories of ovarian cysts and tumours than can easily be grasped; pelvic inflammatory conditions are almost defined by their unchartability.

Treatments therefore tend to bluntness. The primary recourse is to hormones, hormone analogues or hormone antagonists. These often have a crude effect on reproductive tissues that can be beneficial. However, they cannot interact comfortably with the astonishing choreography of multiple hormonal interactions that shape normal reproductive functions. They work by blocking this complexity, changing the force of negative feedback from subtle rhythm generation to the dictator of an artificial regime. As with almost everything else in this area, clear indicators of the wider impact of such treatments are hard to obtain but many women do not feel happy with them. Other conventional treatments are even more intrusive. Surgery is probably used for gynaecological and obstetric problems more extensively than for any other area of medicine. Although the days of routine hysterectomies, ovariectomies and mastectomies may be passing, it is still the case that surgery is undertaken too quickly for many sufferers, simply for want of any alternatives. Other measures – antibiotics for pelvic inflammatory disease, short-wave diathermy, dilation and curettage and laser oblation – appear often to be used without a clear treatment strategy and without an evidence base of efficacy.

One only needs to review the social history of obstetrics in the modern world, the move by women in many countries to reclaim home births, the move to less medicalized labour wards in hospitals, the increasing restoration of the midwife as arbiter of labour management, the exceptionally high professional liability insurance premiums required of obstetricians, to see that medicine has not always served women's needs well. There appears to be a case for a different approach to their healthcare, one ideally that involves them better.

Structures and functions

Neither reproductive functions nor structures are fixed through life. In the case of the female, there is additional variability due to the need to ensure ideal conditions for pregnancy. In most mammals ovulation, and the associated transformation of the reproductive system, only occurs in certain situations and at certain times of the year (early hunter nomad women also probably ovulated only when food and circumstances were acceptable). Nevertheless, there is in the human female the mechanism for constant menstrual cycles which switches on in adolescence and, circumstances permitting (adequate food is still important), is maintained to the sixth decade of life. The menstrual cycle is a transformative cycle, generated by the interplay of secretory sites, the hypothalamus, the anterior pituitary and the ovaries, and of the hormones they produce. It leads to real changes in reproductive structures so that the relevant anatomy actually changes through the month. The hormone secretions appear to be the outcome of a rhythmic pulse.[1] The anatomical changes in the ovarian hormone secretors, the development and ripening of the follicle to ovulation and the formation of the new secretory apparatus, the corpus luteum, out of the remnants of the follicle are rate-limiting elements in the equation and, with the functional pulsation, can be seen to provide the structural mechanism for the 'ovarian clock'. If pregnancy occurs the corpus luteum is enabled to increase its activity, so priming the whole body towards the major shifts in both structure and function required to support a developing embryo and eventually give birth.

The main characteristic of the female reproductive system therefore is its mobility and changeability. Many disorders of it are thus functional disorders and most start that way. Dysfunctions are medical challenges in their own right. There is by definition no physical damage or pathological change to observe as functional measures (such as biochemical markers like metabolite and hormone levels) are notoriously unreliable in complex systems. There is more subjective impression than objective monitoring. Treatments that aim to correct such dysfunctions can do so in two ways: suspend normal activity, in this case often with hormonally active agents – the contraceptive pill or hormone replacement therapy, for example, or hormonal antagonists; or engage it at that level. In this case treatments should be interactive, should support rather than interfere with normal checks and balances and should in part be directable by the subjective pilot, the woman herself. Even when treating actual pathologies a strategy which also supported the return to underlying functional rhythms could be commended.

The herbal strategy: prompts to self-organization

As there is a particular paucity of hard scientific data for the herbal treatment of female reproductive problems, practitioners have to be guided by case evidence. In treating menstrual disorders, this can be striking. Typically a woman suffering dysmenorrhoea, irregular menstruation, premenstrual syndrome or menorrhagia will be given a mixture of traditional women's remedies. For 1 or 2 months there are likely to be unfamiliar changes in the menstrual cycle, occasionally even a worsening of the original problem. Then from the third or fourth cycle there is often a real sense that a normal rhythm is emerging. It is as if the original software program has been rebooted: the disturbance is diminished or even disappears. Most importantly, it is often possible to stop the medication soon after this point without relapse.

Such cases, and there are many in practice, are very illuminating. Whatever mechanisms are involved, and these can only be speculative, there appears to be a strong self-corrective tendency to the menstrual cycle. It is of course very robust and consistent among women all over the world and in all sorts of circumstances. A tendency to self-organization would be consistent with the behaviour of other complex dynamic systems in biology (see p.16). It is also highly reassuring. It suggests that to return to normal, menstrual function requires only the lightest nudge, even a placebo nudge (see p.88). (It is also striking, however, how often women through the ages spontaneously chose plants with high levels of steroidal molecules for this work.)

The herbal nudge to self-correction is a feature of other gynaecological treatment strategies. Menopausal disturbances are another example. A typical scenario might involve a woman in her late 40s with increasing menstrual difficulties, premenstrual syndrome, congestive dysmenorrhoea and/or emotional turbulence. She thinks they may be signs of impending menopause but of course cannot be sure. A herbal treatment that might include *Vitex agnus castus* (chaste berry), Hypericum (St John's wort) or *Chamaelirium luteum* (helonias root) could be given, with one of two possible endpoints. Either periods stop and a smooth menopause, with hopefully few symptoms, could be under way in a few months or normal menstrual cycles could be resumed over the same time frame. The treatment seems to prompt the body to revert to its program, whatever that might be. Again, there is the assumption of self-organization, extended in this context to the view that menopause is programmed to be a smooth transition, that menopausal syndrome is an aberration (this could be argued if even one woman had a quiet and positive menopause; in fact a good proportion of women do).

Similar assumptions underpin the traditional herbal treatment of infertility, of difficulties after childbirth and with lactation and even of more overtly pathological states, functional ovarian cysts, some cases of endometriosis and the management of fibroids and pelvic inflammatory disease. Even when faced with more serious pathologies where conventional medical treatment is already under way, such as breast and cervical cancers, polycystic ovaries, the aftermath of hysterectomies, provided that there is some prospect of returning normal ovarian-pituitary dialogue and rhythms, then herbal prompts to this end are plausible and attractive strategies towards improved health.

Emmenagogues and abortifacients

Women in earlier times lived very different lives with radically different aspirations compared with their descendants in modern societies. Childbirth and childrearing were generally more central to their lives. Infertility was one of the worst social problems a woman could suffer, often seriously threatening her position in the community. In all cultures considerable effort was put into treatments to improve fertility. These might well have worked to the principles set out above. Nevertheless, childbirth needed to be paced. For those who were normally fertile the priority became birth control. The absence at the due time of a period was not always welcome and there would be a regular demand in most communities for remedies that could prompt menstruation when delayed: emmenagogues. These would clearly need to be uterine stimulants and might need to be taken in heroic dosages. In modern times they might be classified as abortifacients.

Many herbs passed down as 'women's remedies' were probably for this purpose, although the term 'emmenagogue' has come in popular books to refer to menstrual regulators in general and is no longer a reliable pointer to such an effect. In reviewing the modern application of traditional women's remedies, it will be useful to keep this category of remedies in mind, however. Although generally taken in small doses in modern times, they may be contraindicated in pregnancy or where pregnancy is being sought and may be more stimulating than the menstrual modulators described earlier. In the Anglo-American tradition, they could include Caulophyllum (blue cohosh), *Cimicifuga racemosa* (black cohosh), *Mitchella repens* (squaw vine), *Ruta graveolens* (rue), *Thuja occidentalis* (arbor-vitae), *Mentha pulegium* (pennyroyal), *Gossypium herbaceum* (cotton root), *Artemisia spp* (the wormwoods) as well as the stimulating laxatives and cathartic remedies. Uterostimulant action has also been shown for Chinese herbs *Carthamus tinctorius*, *Angelica sinensis* and *Leonurus sibiricus* with H_1 and alpha-adrenergic receptors as postulated mediators.[2] Some traditional effects on reproductive structures and functions have been linked with herbal activities on various prostaglandin receptors and functions that may also constitute stimulation of this type.[3]

The use of emmenagogues as abortifacients cannot be recommended in this text. Ethicolegal issues aside, getting the dose and timing right to terminate an early pregnancy was undoubtedly either a skilled or a messy affair and the possibility of embryo-damaging mistakes is theoretically high.

PHYTOTHERAPY IN GYNAECOLOGICAL AND OBSTETRIC CONDITIONS

Premenstrual syndrome

Premenstrual syndrome (PMS) is a variety of psychological, behavioural and physical symptoms which occur in the luteal phase of the menstrual cycle. Most women experience some change in their bodies premenstrually but in about 8% this can be severe.

The symptoms experienced vary from woman to woman and Abrahams has created five distinct subgroups (see Table).[4] This classification is relevant since a pilot clinical trial conducted in England found that the herb *Vitex agnus castus* (chaste berry) gave good results for PMS-A, PMS-D and PMS-H. A second larger clinical trial with Vitex found no statistical significance over placebo, although there was a tendency to improvement for breast tenderness and symptoms of fluid retention (see the monograph on Vitex, p.328).[5] Given that Vitex appears to reduce high levels of prolactin in the blood,[6] it may be that PMS associated with this condition may be the most appropriate indication.

PMS-A	PMS-C	PMS-D	PMS-H	PMS-P
Nervous tension	Increased appetite	Depression	Fluid retention	Aches and pains
Irritability	Headaches	Forgetfulness	Weight gain	Reduced pain threshold
Mood changes	Fatigue	Crying	Swelling of extremities	
Anxiety	Dizziness	Confusion	Breast tenderness	
	Heart pounding	Insomnia	Abdominal bloating	

Treatment

The aims of herbal treatment in PMS are as follows.

• Correct any hormonal imbalance. Vitex is often prescribed throughout the cycle on a long-term basis. Usual dose is 2 ml of a 1:2 extract taken with water on rising.

• Correct EFA status. Evening primrose oil at doses of 3000–4000 mg per day. According to Abraham it is particularly indicated in PMS-C which is associated with a prostaglandin deficiency.

• Treat the main physical symptoms as they occur, e.g. treat fluid retention with diuretics such as Taraxacum leaves (dandelion), aches and pains with herbal analgesics such as Salix (willow bark) or Gelsemium and sweats with Salvia (sage). Ginkgo throughout the cycle was found to be useful for breast symptoms. Sometimes symptomatic treatment will not be necessary if the other aims are addressed.

• Treat the emotional disturbances. This can often be the most important part of the therapy. Treatment is usually throughout the cycle. Tonics such as Hypericum (St John's wort) can help with depressive symptoms and sedatives such as Valeriana (valerian) for anxiety or insomnia.

• Compensate for the adverse effects of stress on the body using adaptogenic herbs such as Eleutherococcus (Siberian ginseng) and Withania. Sources of stress should be examined and dealt with if possible and diet should be balanced and mainly consist of unprocessed foods.

• Treat the liver if signs of sluggishness are apparent, e.g. difficulty digesting fats, tendency to constipation, history of liver disease, tendency to nausea, preference for light or no breakfasts, etc. The liver is the site of the breakdown of female hormones and a sluggish liver may contribute to hormonal imbalance. Herbs to use include Taraxacum root and Silybum (St Mary's thistle).

Dysmenorrhoea

Dysmenorrhoea means painful menstruation and two types are recognized:

1. spasmodic dysmenorrhoea in which the pain is directly related to the onset of menstruation and is uterine in origin;
2. secondary or congestive dysmenorrhoea which occurs before or late in menstruation and may arise in the uterus or in some other organ.

Treatment

• Since Vitex (chaste berry) enhances progesterone production, it can aggravate spasmodic dysmenorrhoea and should not be used. However, if a woman with spasmodic dysmenorrhoea also suffers from PMS with congestive symptoms, e.g. breast tenderness, Vitex will help both disorders when used in the long term.

• Herbs which support oestrogen function in the body (they may not be intrinsically oestrogenic themselves) are indicated and include *Chamaelirium luteum* (helonias root) and Dioscorea (wild yam). These herbs will help long term.

• Lamium (white dead nettle) is a specific which may decrease the condition when given long term.

• Short-term treatment consists of uterine spasmolytics and herbs which decrease prostaglandin production. The former include *Angelica sinensis* (dong quai), Dioscorea, Rubus (raspberry leaves) and *Viburnum species* (cramp bark or black haw). Achillea (yarrow) is spasmolytic and will check excessive bleeding if taken long term. The latter include Zingiber (ginger), Curcuma (turmeric) and Salix (willow bark). These prostaglandin-decreasing herbs are not powerful analgesics, so it is best to start their use about a week before menstruation. Cimicifuga (black cohosh) is an antiinflammatory and hormonal herb which is also indicated and Corydalis is a useful analgesic.

Abnormal uterine bleeding

Excessive or abnormal bleeding from the uterus is a symptom, not a disease. The pattern of bleeding can vary, as can the cause. Metrorrhagia, where the bleeding is irregular in amount, acyclical in nature and often prolonged in duration, is usually due to a pathological condition of the uterus. A number of conditions, largely dysfunctional in nature, can respond to herbal treatment and are described below. Where abnormal bleeding is due to an organic cause, treatment should be directed at that cause. Such problems may be beyond the scope of herbal treatment.

Menorrhagia

This is excessively profuse or prolonged bleeding occurring with a normal cycle. The iron status of women with menorrhagia should always be checked. Fibroids (see below) are the most likely cause but underlying causes must be investigated.

Treatment may include Vitex (chaste berry), *Chamaelirium luteum* (helonias root), antihaemorrhagic herbs, e.g. Achillea (yarrow), *Panax notoginseng* (Tienchi ginseng) and Equisetum (horsetail) and uterine antihaemorrhagics such as Capsella (shepherd's purse) and Trillium (beth root).

Functional secondary amenorrhoea

This is the absence of menses for 6 months or for longer than three of the patient's normal menstrual cycles. First exclude pregnancy, lactation, drugs, premature menopause, poor diet or excessive exercise as causes. Other organic causes should also be excluded.

Herbal treatment of amenorrhoea is aimed at:

- correcting hypothalamic malfunction and the resultant hormonal imbalance using Vitex (chaste berry), *Chamaelirium luteum* (helonias root) and Caulophyllum (blue cohosh);
- treating the effects of depression with nervine tonics such as Hypericum (St John's wort);
- treating the effects of stress with adaptogens, nervine tonics and sedative herbs;
- treating debility with tonic herbs such as Withania and *Panax ginseng*. *Angelica sinensis* (dong quai) is specifically indicated where amenorrhoea follows menorrhagia or is associated with anaemia.

Difficulty with conception

This has a number of causes, many of which are not treatable by herbs. It should firstly be established if the problem truly exists with the women. If this is the case, the cause or causes should be isolated, if this is possible. Endometriosis is a common cause which will be treated as a separate subject.

Some categories of difficult conception are listed below with the corresponding herbal approach to treatment.

- Excessive anovulatory cycles. Treat with *Chamaelirium luteum* (helonias root), Vitex (chaste berry) and nervine tonics. Caulophyllum (blue cohosh), Cimicifuga (black cohosh) and *Angelica sinensis* may also be tried.

- Defective luteal function, possibly associated with latent or frank hyperprolactinaemia. Treat mainly with Vitex and Caulophyllum.

- Cervical mucus may be too viscous. Promote oestrogen with Chamaelirium and Dioscorea. Cervical mucus may be 'hostile' for reasons other than hormonal. If this is suspected, recommend an alkaline diet (low protein, high fruit and vegetables). Lifestyle factors should be addressed (see below) and alkalinizing herbs such as Apium (celery seed) prescribed together with oestrogen-promoting herbs which will help to stabilize vaginal flora.

- Immunological rejection of sperm. Sperm carries foreign proteins and a woman will often mount an immunological reaction against the sperm of her partner. With a consistent partner, this reaction usually abates but sometimes it does not. Treat with immune-regulating herbs such as Echinacea. Also attend to any factors which may be causing immune system dysregulation.

- After investigation of difficulty with conception, no known factor can be identified in 20–30% of cases. Emotions can affect hypothalamic-pituitary hormone secretion and release. Stress and other emotional stimuli are known to increase prolactin release, which may affect reproductive function. Emotional factors may be involved in producing oviductal spasm which is sometimes observed in diagnostic tests. Obesity or being underweight and overall health may determine whether conception occurs or not. Lifestyle factors such as excessive or too little exercise, diet, tea, coffee, alcohol, smoking and drugs should be investigated. Treatment should be based on the above considerations and could include Vitex, Caulophyllum (blue cohosh) and *Chamaelirium luteum* (helonias root) for the hormonal side, *Viburnum opulus* for oviductal spasm and tonics, adaptogens, nervine tonics and sedatives as appropriate.

Pelvic inflammatory disease (PID)

This is infection of the uterus, fallopian tubes and adjacent pelvic structures which is not associated with surgery or pregnancy. It is also known as chronic salpingitis. The most common organisms involved are *Chlamydia trachomatis* and *Neisseria gonorrhoeae*.

Treatment

- Immune-enhancing herbs such as Echinacea and Picrorrhiza.
- *Chamaelirium luteum* (helonias root) and Dioscorea to support the female organs.
- Hydrastis (golden seal) is a mucous membrane tonic useful for chronic infections of the oviducts.
- Corydalis may assist to relieve the pain.

The above approach to treatment is compatible with and will actually assist conventional antibiotic treatment.

Uterine myoma (fibroids)

Uterine fibroids are benign, slow-growing smooth muscle tumours. They are probably the most common neoplasm in women. Medically they are treated by luteinizing hormone releasing hormone (LHRH) analogues or by surgery. The most common problem they cause is menorrhagia. Endometrial ablation is a new medical technique which can relieve this aspect to the problem.

Treatment

Herbal approaches are aimed at controlling the tumour growth (shrinking the tumour is unlikely, but may occur) and alleviating symptoms caused by the fibroids. Vitex (chaste berry) is a major part of treatment and can be given in high doses, e.g. 5 ml twice a day, if the fibroids are severe. Liver herbs may help the breakdown of excessive oestrogen. Antihaemorrhagic and uterine antihaemorrhagic herbs are indicated for the menorrhagia. Herbs which have been traditionally used to control benign growths include Echinacea, Thuja (arbor-vitae) and Chelidonium (greater celandine). *Ginkgo biloba* standardized extract can relieve pain associated with fibroids. Oestrogen-promoting herbs such as *Chamaelirium luteum* (helonias root) and Dioscorea (wild yam) should be avoided. To modify the effects of oestrogen, the intake of phytooestrogens and oestrogenic lignans should be increased.

Case history

A patient aged 43 presented with uterine fibroids characterized by menorrhagia and pain, especially with menstruation. She did not want surgery and asked for herbs to control her symptoms.
Treatment was as follows (based on 1 week).

Capsella bursa-pastoris	1:2	20 ml
Achillea millefolium	1:2	25 ml
Thuja occidentalis	1:5	20 ml
Echinacea angustifolia	1:2	20 ml
Panax notoginseng	1:2	15 ml
	Total	100 ml

Dose 5 ml with water three times a day.
She was also prescribed Vitex 1:2, 2.5 ml with water twice a day, with the first dose on rising in the morning.
Ginkgo biloba 50:1 standardized extract, 40 mg per tablet, two tablets per day, was also prescribed.
After 10 weeks of treatment there was considerable improvement in the menorrhagia and pain. Herbal treatment was maintained for continued symptom control.

Endometriosis

Endometriosis is the presence of functioning endometrial tissue in an abnormal location. This may occur between the muscle fibres of the myometrium (uterine endometriosis) or in various locations in the pelvic cavity. The ectopic endometrium forms a cyst which can often rupture, resulting in inflammation and formation of multiple adhesions.

Treatment

The most important herb for the treat of endometriosis is *Vitex agnus castus* (chaste berry). Higher doses may be necessary, similar to those recommended for uterine fibroids.

Because of the prostaglandin abnormalities, evening primrose oil can also be indicated. Recent clinical trials tend to support its value in endometriosis. Other herbs indicated for the symptoms include:

- *Viburnum opulus* (cramp bark), Corydalis, Caulophyllum (blue cohosh), *Angelica sinensis* (dong quai), *Rubus idaeus* (raspberry leaf) and Zingiber (ginger) for dysmenorrhoea and chronic pelvic pain;
- Pulsatilla for ovarian and ovulation pain;
- *Centella asiatica* (gotu kola) and *Saliva miltiorrhiza* (dan shen) to reduce formation of adhesions;
- antihaemorrhagic and uterine antihaemorrhagic herbs for the menorrhagia;
- sedative, nervine tonic and adaptogenic herbs for the exacerbating effects of stress;
- antiinflammatory herbs such as Zingiber (ginger) Glycyrrhiza (licorice) and Rehmannia.

Herbs which may influence the underlying pathology include:

- Vitex, because of its regulating effect on ovarian function;
- liver herbs, especially Schisandra and Silybum (St Mary's thistle), to accelerate the breakdown of oestrogen;
- immune-enhancing herbs to help prevent and resolve endometrial cysts, e.g. Echinacea, Picrorrhiza and Phytolacca (poke root);
- herbs to control benign growths, e.g. Thuja (arbor-vitae) and Echinacea.

To modify the effects of oestrogen, the intake of phytooestrogens and oestrogenic lignans should be increased.

In general the oestrogen-promoting herbs such as *Chamaelirium luteum* (helonias root) and Dioscorea (wild yam) should be avoided.

Benign breast disorders

Many terms have been used in the past to describe benign breast disorders. These include such descriptions as benign mammary dysplasia, cystic mastopathy, chronic cystic mastitis and cystic epithelial hyperplasia. Often they were grouped under the term 'fibrocystic breast disease' but this nomenclature is now considered to be inappropriate and benign breast disease can be more appropriately categorized as the following:

- fibroadenoma;
- cystic disease of the breast.

A new concept has been proposed to describe benign breast disorders. They are seen as aberrations of normal breast development and involution. This is based on the fact that most benign breast disorders are not neoplastic growths but rather arise on the basis of normal changes occurring in the breast throughout the various stages of reproductive life. They are no more benign neoplasms than is endometriosis.

Fibroadenoma

Treatment

Vitex is the main treatment, because of its regulating effect on ovarian function. Herbs for growths such as Thuja (arbor-vitae) and Echinacea are also indicated. Oestrogen-promoting herbs such as *Chamaelirium luteum* (helonias root) and Paeonia may be beneficial because a fibroadenoma is an aberration of normal lobule development. Given the increased risk of breast cancer, once the fibroadenoma is resolved the intake of phytooestrogens and oestrogenic lignans should be increased. The stress aspect should also be addressed by prescribing nervine tonics, sedatives or tonics as the case history dictates.

Case history

Jenny was 31 and had a breast lump which was diagnosed as a fibroadenoma. Her GP recommended 3 months' observation but the surgeon wanted the lump removed. Being concerned at the prospect of surgery, she decided to try herbal treatment during the observation period.
Treatment was as follows (based on 1 week).

Echinacea angustifolia	1:2	30 ml
Scutellaria lateriflora	1:2	30 ml
Paeonia lactiflora	1:2	25 ml
Thuja occidentalis	1:5	15 ml
	Total	100 ml

Dose 5 ml with water three times a day.
Vitex 1:2, 2 ml with water on rising, was also prescribed.

Treatment was continued for 3 months. When she returned to the surgeon, he could find no trace of the fibroadenoma.

Breast cysts

Treatment

The herbal treatment of breast cysts is similar to the approach used for fibroadenoma, except that oestrogen-promoting herbs are best avoided. Vitex is the most important herb and the alleviation of the negative physiological effects of stress should also be emphasized. Abstinence from stimulants, as described above, should also be observed. To modify the effects of oestrogen, intake of phytooestrogens and oestrogenic lignans should be increased. This could also reduce the risk of breast cancer.

Menopause

The climacteric or menopause is a period of waning ovarian function which marks the end of the reproductive lifespan. As such, it is a normal event in the life of a woman and should not be regarded as a disease. The aim of herbal treatment is to assist the adjustment to this important change and provide symptomatic alleviation of the effects of oestrogen withdrawal. It is not intended that herbal treatment for the menopausal change should be prescribed indefinitely, although it may be required for several years until the body has adapted to the new hormonal levels.

Not all women have menopausal symptoms but about 70% experience hot flushes and 40% suffer from depression. Other symptoms such as sweating, fatigue, irregular menstruation and insomnia occur in 20–40% of perimenopausal women. Fewer than one-third of women experiencing menopause have symptoms sufficiently distressing to seek aid.

Treatment

The main aims of herbal assistance with the menopausal change are as follows.

- To assist the body to adapt to the new hormonal levels by reducing the effects of oestrogen withdrawal. This is achieved by prescribing saponin-containing herbs such as *Chamaelirium luteum* (helonias root), Dioscorea (wild yam) and Cimicifuga (black cohosh). *Alchemilla vulgaris* (ladies mantle) is also indicated in this context. Panax (ginseng) is a tonic saponin-containing herb with some evidence for oestrogenic activity; however, it may aggravate irritability and insomnia and should be used cautiously.

- To provide support for the nervous system using tonic and nervine tonic herbs. Hypericum (St John's wort) is almost a specific for menopausal depression. Avena (oats) is also popular.

- To abate the intensity of the hot flushes or sweating. The important herb here is Salvia (sage) although cardiovascular herbs such as Crataegus (hawthorn) and *Leonurus* (motherwort) also can be useful.

- Vitex has a role to play for the perimenopausal woman with PMS-like symptoms (which may or may not be premenstrual due to menstrual irregularity). Some herbalists are of the opinion that Vitex also helps allay other menopausal symptoms such as flushes. Its influence on pituitary function might be the key here.

- Phytooestrogen intake should be increased through soya products and herbal teas, but it should not be excessive as this may interfere with the main herbal treatment.

Despite its popularity, there is little traditional or clinical evidence to support the claim that *Angelica sinensis* (dong quai) has a specific role in menopause. However, its tonic effect will be of some value. Although popular, evening primrose oil appears to have no place in a therapeutic regime for the menopause.

The above approach will generally reduce the severity of menopausal symptoms in a majority of cases. Many women will find that although hot flushes still occur, their intensity and frequency are so reduced as not to be a problem. A small percentage of women cannot be helped by the above approach, presumably because their levels of oestrogen are too low or have dropped too rapidly. After menopause, oestrogen is manufactured in fat and muscle tissue from adrenal hormones. Such unresponsive cases may respond to adrenal support using herbs such as Panax, Rehmannia and Glycyrrhiza (licorice).

Case history

A woman, 47 years old, presented with hot flushes, sweating, depression and interrupted sleep caused by the hot flushes. She was irritable, low in energy and under stress at work. The hot flushes started 18 months ago.

The following formula was prescribed (based on 1 week):

Hypericum perforatum	1:2	20 ml
Chamaelirium luteum	1:2	20 ml
Dioscorea villosa	1:2	20 ml
Crataegus oxyacantha (fruit)	1:2	15 ml
Withania somnifera	1:2	25 ml
	Total	100 ml

Dose 5 ml with water three times a day.

After 1 month of treatment there was little change but by the end of the second month there were considerable reductions in the frequency and severity of the hot flushes. She was less irritable and depressed. After 1 year of treatment the herbs were stopped and no return of menopausal symptoms occurred.

Therapy during pregnancy

After taking into account the professional reluctance to prescribe herbs in pregnancy, there are nevertheless a number of herbs invaluable for the treatment of some common problems of pregnancy.

Morning sickness

In the first trimester, Zingiber (ginger) can provide effective relief in mild to moderate cases of morning sickness. About 10 drops (approx 0.3 ml) of a 1:2 extract with water can rapidly relieve nausea. This can be repeated up to nine times more in a day if required. More severe cases may require liver herbs such as Silybum (St Mary's thistle) and Taraxacum (dandelion root). *Mentha piperita* (peppermint), Filipendula (meadowsweet) and Ballota (black horehound) are also useful herbs. For morning sickness and nausea which extends into the second trimester, Rubus (raspberry leaf) is usually an effective treatment.

Threatened miscarriage

Vitex (chaste berry) is indicated for threatened miscarriage if progesterone levels are relatively low. Otherwise key herbs are *Chamaelirium luteum* (helonias root) and Dioscorea (wild yam). Other herbs which are usually indicated are *Viburnum opulus* or *prunifolium* for cramping or bearing down sensations and Capsella (shepherd's purse) for bleeding.

Varicose veins

Varicose veins are more likely to develop during pregnancy, probably because of the weakening effect on connective tissue of higher levels of female hormones. The main basis of treatment is therefore to maintain connective tissue and safe herbs which do this include Vaccinium (bilberry) and Crataegus (hawthorn). A cream containing Aesculus and Hamamelis (witch-hazel) can be applied to problem areas.

Preparation for childbirth

To help the mother prepare for birth, *Rubus idaeus* (raspberry leaf) and Mitchella (squaw vine) can be taken continuously after the first trimester. It is not known how these herbs act but Rubus probably builds up the strength of the myometrium (uterine muscle), which leads to an easy birth. The value of Rubus in pregnancy has been proven in many cases and there is no evidence for any deleterious effect. During labour, Rubus should be taken with increased frequency, up to six 5 ml doses in a day. *Viburnum opulus* (cramp bark) may also be prescribed if there is a problem with dilation of the cervix.

Therapy following pregnancy

Herbs and breastfeeding

Herbs which promote milk include: Galega (goats rue), Foeniculum (fennel), Trigonella (fenugreek), Vitex (chaste berry), Verbena (vervain), Urtica (nettles) and *Euphorbia pilulifera*.

Herbs which decrease milk include Salvia (sage), *Mentha piperita* (peppermint) and Lycopus (gypsywort or bugleweed).

Some herbal components may be passed in the milk. A breastfed baby can sometimes be effectively treated by medicating the mother, especially if there is infant colic.

Postnatal depression

Postnatal depression is caused by a combination of female hormonal effects with the adrenal depletion which can follow pregnancy and childbirth. Treatment is based around Vitex, tonics and nervine tonics.

A typical treatment is as follows (based on 1 week).

Panax ginseng	1:2	10 ml
Hypericum perforatum	1:2	25 ml
Glycyrrhiza glabra (high in glycyrrhizin)	1:1	15 ml
Withania somnifera	1:2	30 ml
Verbena officinalis	1:2	20 ml
	Total	100 ml

Dose 5 ml with water three times a day.

Also Vitex 1:2, 2 ml with water once a day on rising.

References

1. Filicori M, Tabarelli C, Casadio P et al. Interaction between menstrual cyclicity and gonadotrophin pulsatility. Horm Research 1998; 49: 3–4, 169–172
2. Shi M, Chang L, He G. Stimulating action of Carthamus tinctorius L., Angelica sinensis (Oliv.) Diels and Leonurus sibiricus L. on the uterus. Chung Kuo Chung Yao Tsa Chih 1995; 20(3): 173–175, 192
3. Li W, Zhou CH, Lu QL. Effects of Chinese materia medica in activating blood and stimulating menstrual flow on the endocrine function of ovary-uterus and its mechanisms. Chung Kuo Chung Hsi I Chieh Ho Tsa Chih 1992; 12(3): 165–168, 134
4. Abraham GE. Nutritional factors in the etiology of the premenstrual tension syndromes. Journal of Reproductive Medicine 1983; 28(7): 446–464
5. Mills S, Turner S A double-blind clinical trial on a herbal remedy for premenstrual syndrome: a case study. Complementary Therapy Medicine 1993; 1(2): 73–77
6. Böhnert KJ. The use of Vitex agnus castus for hyperprolactinaemia. Quarterly Review of Natural Medicine 1997; Spring: 19–21

JOINT DISEASES

SCOPE

Apart from their use to provide non-specific support for recuperation and repair, specific phytotherapeutic strategies include the following.

Treatment of:

- early and transient joint inflammation;
- gout.

Management of:

- long-standing joint disease with joint damage.

Because of its use of secondary plant products, particular **caution** is necessary in applying phytotherapy in cases of:

- very aggressive joint inflammations.

ORIENTATION

Background

Degeneration of one or more joints in the body affects almost all persons from the fifth decade of life and there are equally universal clinical signs by the age of 70. There is evidence of the problem occurring in the bone record from the distant past as well and it is a condition found in almost all vertebrates, even dinosaurs, whales, fish and birds. It is probable that the joint structures reach the limit of their regenerative capacity earlier than other body tissues. They certainly operate at the limit of engineering tolerance and circulatory renewal at the best of times. A number of environmental conditions, life circumstances, traumatic events, infections and other diseases and genetic factors might reduce the regenerative capacity even further.

In fact, surprisingly little is known of the aetiology of osteoarthritis. Wear and tear is a factor in prolonged overuse of a certain joint but use is generally better than inactivity (long-distance runners have no worse incidence of the disease but even moderate forced inactivity can accelerate the condition). The immediate event is a disturbance in the behaviour of the chondrocyte, normally a very quiescent and isolated cell responsible for maintaining the cartilage of the joint, leading to its mitosis, then an interactive stimulation of neighbouring osteoblasts to produce the bony overgrowth. Whatever provokes the chondroblasts, it is fair, in the absence of hard evidence, to look at the widest systemic evidence for disturbance around the body and the interpretations of such events by earlier observers.

In looking at the wider picture to understand localized osteoarthritis, one is taking a similar path to that for the more overtly inflammatory arthritic conditions, the diffuse connective tissue diseases: rheumatoid arthritis, Sjögren's and Behçet's syndromes, polymyalgia rheumatica, the lupus erythematoses, polymyositis and the like, as well as the spondylitic diseases, ankylosing spondylitis, Reiter's syndrome and psoriatic arthropathy. These all share a substantial immunological component and their treatment is best taken along with other diseases of this type (see p.144). Nevertheless, even these diseases, inasmuch as the joints are involved, can be approached with some of the following points in mind.

As with skin diseases (see p.252), the verdict of the ancients on joint diseases was unanimous. Arthritis represented a toxic accumulation at the site. There was probably an appreciation that joints were uniquely vulnerable structures, fairly obvious 'bottlenecks' in the circulatory flow; the notion of a 'toxic logjam' at such sites seems commonplace, evidenced in part by the topical treatments usually applied.

Counterirritation

There was, of course, an immediate imperative in joint pain. It quickly affected mobility and threatened survival. It was also easily focused upon. If the problem represented a local toxic accumulation then local measures to improve circulation were the obvious treatment. Applying heat to the joint would most often reduce pain. Applying stronger heating measures could often have a longer term benefit. Thus throughout the world drastic heating measures were applied to affected joints. At the least, hot poultices or baths with mustard, pepper or cayenne would be used as rubefacients (a milder effect can be had with proprietary liniments and embrocations). For more dramatic effects stronger remedies were used, those that in Galenic terms (see p.5) would be classified as 'hot in the fourth degree', that 'corrode and cause blisters if outwardly applied'.

Blistering in arthritis was a common technique. A very strong mustard or cayenne application might do it and flaying with stinging nettles was favoured in ancient Europe (even birds and some animals will expose themselves to ant bites in certain circumstances) but more corrosive substances like croton oil and formic acid (found in ant bites and stinging nettle) became favoured as they were isolated. Blistering was used, for example, among the new industrial working classes of 19th-century Britain who still favoured their rural herbal traditions and would visit the recently urbanized herbalist because in this way, and without effective social security or system of disability payments, they would be able to get back to work more quickly (they often did not pay until such results were achieved either!). The application could produce a large blister in minutes; lancing this could yield an impressive quantity of fluid. The fact that pain could be instantly reduced and mobility often at least temporarily improved led to the obvious supposition that the blister fluids carried toxins away and that the associated and obvious heating brought in more healing circulation to do the rest. In modern central Europe blistering applications have sometimes been replaced with precision-depth epidermal puncture devices followed by irritant applications; fluids pass through the puncture holes without blisters having to form. Similar simple devices are also used in traditional Chinese medicine.

Counterirritation is often in modern accounts explained as resulting from some form of stimulation of nerve receptors leading to reflex analgesia. This does not do justice to the technique or to its therapeutic context; indeed, both rubefacients and blistering agents, expertly applied, are intrinsically comforting sensations. A better speculation might be that counterirritation is a proinflammatory technique; the increased vasoactivity and stimulation of other inflammatory mediators can be seen as constituting a therapeutic inflammation, doing painlessly what the body itself does with pain, swelling and disability. It is a principle, espoused by Samuel Thomson in 19th-century North America (see p.12), that fever and its local counterpart, inflammation, are not the disease themselves but the body's defence against disease. Like Thomson's cayenne and Galen's heating remedies generally, the topical counterirritations, whether simply warming liniments and embrocations or blistering heating packs, were recognition that the best therapy was to improve upon nature's defences and even extend them.

In modern practice blistering is rarely acceptable. However, good results can often be had with heating poultices, footbaths or handbaths, using an agent like powdered mustard. For a poultice, a slurry made with the yellow powder sold to make English mustard can be smeared on a gauze and held over the affected joint under a hot wet flannel pad. Occasional glimpses of the area under the dressing should warn if blistering is impending but the most common reaction is a mild erythema only. Fifteen to 20 minutes should be enough application. For a hand or footbath a dessertspoonful of mustard powder is put into a bowl of hot water just large enough to immerse the affected limb; this in turn is best placed in a larger bowl of hot water better to maintain the temperature for up to 20 minutes. It is still possible to obtain cayenne plasters from specialist suppliers, rubber material impregnated with cayenne, and it may be possible to make one's own substitute. Russian ointment includes cayenne for a particularly robust liniment. Otherwise strong muscle rubs or the Asian product 'Tiger Balm' will provide moderate relief for arthritic joints. Most accessibly, many embrocations and liniments are available in pharmacies and elsewhere, mostly based on mentholated ointments with various rubefacient constituents, like eucalyptus and wintergreen oils, added, although these are likely to have only mild benefits.

The above approaches are most indicated for the low level of inflammatory activity associated with osteoarthritis. They may also be indicated in more volatile inflammations of rheumatic disease but are sometimes not. Gout is another joint condition that is usually contraindicated. If the joint is too inflamed and hot already, these techniques may be aggravatory. Sensitivity to liniments or heat may be a good guide not to proceed further.

Internal treatments

As indicated earlier, a consistent theme in traditional medicine was to remove toxic accumulations from affected joints. Equally consistent was the view that this was particularly a burden on the kidneys. Many traditional treatments for arthritis were also diuretic remedies, perceived as helping the body remove toxic waste through the urine. In European medicine herbs such as Apium (celery), Betula (birch), Taraxacum (dandelion) and Filipendula (meadowsweet) were widely used diuretics in the treatment of arthritic disease.

The juxtaposition of kidney function and joint disease was elaborated in the European naturopathic and North American Eclectic traditions in their focus on acid/alkali balance (the kidneys of course are dedicated largely to maintaining electrolyte equilibrium in the body fluids). The concept has permeated folk culture: acids are bad for joints, alkalis good.

It is widely understood that the body has to eliminate acid metabolites and that joint problems are a classic outcome of failure to do this. Under such circumstances it makes sense to reduce acidic foods from the diet; not (and this is one detail causing much confusion) foods that taste acidic like citrus and other fruits but foods that leave an acidic residue after digestion, due to a preponderance of sulphates and phosphates. Proteins are the major example of the latter. One guide is to test the acidity of ash after combustion

PRAL of certain food groups and combined foods[1]

Food group	*PRAL (mEq/100 g)*
Fats and oils	0
Fish	7.9
Fruits and fruit juices	–3.1
Grain products	
Bread	3.5
Flour	7.0
Noodles	6.7
Meat and meat products	9.5
Milk and dairy products	
Milk and non-cheese products	1.0
Cheeses with lower protein content[a]	8.0
Cheeses with higher protein content[b]	23.6
Vegetables	–2.8

a Less than 15 g protein per 100 g
b More than 15 g protein per 100 g

of the food, given that digestion is enzymatically an analogous process; in this test lemons leave an alkaline ash, cheese, meat and eggs an acidic ash.

However, estimates based on the acid or alkaline nature of the mineral ash of the food do not take into account the incomplete intestinal absorption of various nutrients. A study published in Germany provides a simple new model based on the potential renal acid loads (PRAL) of various foods.[1] Provided that growth, mineral losses through the skin and transient metabolic variations do not apply (which is the case for healthy, non-pregnant adults under normal living conditions), the model will be valid.

The PRAL of various foods is calculated from their sodium, potassium, calcium, magnesium, phosphorus, chloride and sulphur content, taking into account the known percentage absorption rates for protein (in the case of sulphur) and minerals. It is expressed as milliequivalents (mEq) per 100 g. The PRAL content averages for various food groups are shown in the box. A positive value means that the food is acidic and a negative value indicates alkalinity.

The most acidic food was parmesan cheese (PRAL 34.2) and the most alkaline food was raisins (PRAL –21.0). Plant-based beverages such as wine, tea and coffee are generally alkaline if taken without milk. However, some beers and cola drinks were acidic. Mineral water could be quite alkaline (PRAL –1.8) depending on its origin. The most alkaline fruit was the banana (PRAL –5.5), closely followed by apricots (PRAL –4.8). The most alkaline vegetable was spinach (PRAL –14.0), mainly due to its very high calcium content. The least alkaline vegetables were cucumber and asparagus. Processed meats were the most acidic form of meat or fish consumption and lentils and peas were also mildly acidic. Nuts were variable: hazelnuts were alkaline and peanuts and walnuts were acidic. Egg yolks were highly acidic (PRAL 23.4) and chocolate and cake were moderately so.

The herbal diuretics mentioned above can be understood as usefully complementing a high-alkali diet based on vegetables and fruits in reducing the rate of joint deterioration in many sufferers from osteoarthritis.

The diuretic herbs may be augmented by inflammatory modulators traditionally used in arthritic disease. Salix (willow) and Populus (poplar) have appreciable levels of antiinflammatory salicylates. Others are less obvious in their rationale and rely on traditional reputation to support their use; Harpagophytum (devil's claw), Guaiacum (lignum-vitae), *Cimicifuga racemosa* (black cohosh), *Curcuma longa* (turmeric), *Boswellia serrata*[1,2] and Juniperus (juniper) may feature. The efficacy of some of the above together has been established in a double-blind controlled clinical trial[3] and evidence for similar combinations exists elsewhere.[4] Zingiber (ginger) and Zanthoxylum (prickly ash) might be added in cases where cold and poor circulation are identified as factors.

A number of other alterative remedies are used non-specifically for arthritis. Notable in European tradition is Urtica (nettle), for which there is now some evidence of efficacy available.[5]

Gout

Arthritic disease caused by accumulation of urate crystals at joints provides a particular indication for herbal remedies. There are a number which are claimed to increase elimination of urates from the kidneys, notably Apium (celery), Urtica (nettle) and Betula (birch). There is no doubt that prescriptions based on such herbs appear to ease the symptoms and even help to prevent recurrence. They thus provide a simple and probably safe treatment (with the possible exception of Apium in the very long term), especially when combined with a low purine diet (reduced red meat, offal, oily fish, red wines and port) so that urate metabolites are as reduced as far as possible.

References

1. Various authors. Report of Boswellia symposium. Phytomedicine 1996; 3(1): 67–90
2. Etzel, R. Special extract of Boswellia serrata (H15) in the treatment of rheumatoid arthritis. Phytomedicine 1996; 3(1): 91–94
3. Mills, SY, Jacoby RK, Chacksfield M, Willoughby M. Effect of a proprietary herbal medicine on the relief of chronic arthritic pain: a double blind study. British Journal of Rheumatology 1996; 35: 874–878
4. Von Kruedener S, Schneider W, Elstner EF. A combination of Populus tremula, Solidago virgaurea and Fraxinus excelsior as an anti-inflammatory and antirheumatic drug. Arzneimittel-Forschung 1995; 45(2): 169–171
5. Chrubasik, S, Enderlein, W, Bauer R, Grabner W. Evidence for antirheumatic effectiveness of Herba Urticae dioicae in acute arthritis: a pilot study. Phytomedicine 1997; 4(2): 105–108

SKIN DISEASES

Scope

Apart from their use to provide non-specific support for recuperation and repair, specific phytotherapeutic strategies include the following.

Treatment of:

- eczema;
- some cases of psoriasis and immunological skin diseases;
- contact and other allergic skin disease;
- superficial fungal infections;
- acne and furunculosis.

Management of:

- chronic psoriatic disease;
- rosacea.

Because of its use of secondary plant products, **caution** is necessary in applying phytotherapy topically over some:

- broken skin;
- mucosal surfaces.

Note: contact sensitivity reactions are possible to almost any ingredient in the vehicles (e.g. creams and ointments) for topical applications to skin disease.

ORIENTATION

Internal and external applications

Herbal medicine provides two unique approaches to the treatment of skin inflammations. There are particular physical and pharmacological properties in plant constituents that possess topical benefits directly on external applications. Secondly, there are developed medicinal strategies for treating skin problems as manifestations of internal disease, such that most herbal prescriptions are taken orally. For both reasons and in spite of a lack of new clinical research data, phytotherapy can be recommended as a dermatological strategy. Nevertheless, skin diseases are among the most complex and inconsistent categories in medicine. There are many (e.g. malignant tumours, bullous diseases, alopecia areata, pigmentary disorders) that are probably beyond conservative treatment, others (e.g. pityriasis rosea, lichen planus) that usually do not need treatment at all and some that are wholly unpredictable. It is unrealistic to claim consistent performance for phytotherapy either. What is offered below is a number of pragmatic options, productively to be considered along with conventional prescription, as well as other complementary approaches, dietary and psychotherapeutic treatments.

The nature of the beast

There are few clear guides to understanding skin diseases. The origin of a proportion can be traced to simple sources, bacterial, viral or fungal infections for example (although a good practitioner would still puzzle out the reason why) or toxic exposures, but the great majority are largely mysterious. Even attempts to distinguish external (exogenous) and endogenous disease are not very helpful. It may look a simple matter that someone has a contact dermatitis to this, that or the other or that eliminating milk products apparently resolves eczema but the internal reasons for such sensitivity are left unaddressed. For most skin disease, it is almost impossible to pick out substantative causative factors. Although dermatology is an impressive discipline in terms of differential diagnosis (distinguishing plantar psoriasis from tinea pedis or sarcoidosis from granuloma anulare), there is remarkably little to say about the causes of most skin diseases and the speciality is remarkably bereft of curative strategies. Topical and systemic corticosteroids largely replaced coal-tar products in the 1950s but these remain the pillars of dermatological treatment, although palliative only.

It is clear that much skin disease is very complex. Notable are those linked to immunological disorders. Psoriasis is specifically an immunological skin disease but there are many others with greater or lesser association with internal autoimmune disorders: discoid lupus erythematosus, scleroderma, dermatomyositis. Already in some such cases links have been made between the skin symptoms and events deep in the body (see also p.145). These conditions are also the most inconsistent and refractory; remission may be possible in some individuals but relapses are at least as common and neither change is likely to show much pattern. Clinical experience is that each individual case history is unlike any other and that the landmarks of deterioration, used by practitioners as clues to the construction of a therapeutic strategy, show few common themes.

Although the various skin inflammations diagnosed as eczema are more likely to be considered as local defects, a dermatitis only, it is also certain that these can reflect a wide variety of environmental, dietary and psychological/emotional influences. Again it is hard to avoid the conclusion that the skin manifests deeper disorders, that treatment seems more appropriate directed from the inside out.

Traditional observers of skin disease were almost unanimous in seeing it as a wider disturbance within. Given the paucity of treatment options in conventional dermatology, it may be time to reconsider some of the older strategies.

A suitable case for cleansing

An almost universal view of skin diseases in the past was that they were signals of inner toxicities, accumulations of irritants that the normal eliminatory functions had failed to remove. The variety of possible problems reflected a great variety of toxicities and most developed traditions had a wide range of diagnoses and treatments. The metaphors used were those found elsewhere in these humoral systems. In the meteorological analogies used, toxicity was often equated with 'damp', which in turn reflected disorders of the digestive system and liver. The fluctuation in some skin problems was seen to reflect the influence of 'wind', the consequence of disturbances in metabolic balance, in the balance of heating and cooling. Those that currently would be classified as allergic eczemas might be considered 'dry' in earlier times, with reference to the gut and respiratory system. Skin disease could also be predominantly 'hot' or 'cold'. In other words, treatments might extend across the whole range of traditional materia medica, depending on details of the indication, mostly though applying remedies that were also seen to be eliminative.

Folk traditions were generally less sophisticated but the concept of skin disease as a toxicity symptom was consistent. In European traditions, for example, skin problems were treated with 'blood cleansers' and 'blood purifiers' and the terms 'depurative' and 'dyscratic' are also derived from this perspective. In China some remedies are seen as simply good at eliminating poison and were often used as folk treatments for skin diseases. The more acute and severe the skin inflammations, the more robust the remedy used.

Unfortunately there is a gaping lack of modern clinical research for the traditional internal strategies for skin disease. The one notable exception is, however, encouraging.

Two double-blind controlled clinical trials published by a London team of dermatologists and immunologists in 1992 showed significant efficacy of a herb formulation taken internally. In one study 40 adult patients with chronic, refractory, widespread atopic dermatitis in crossover between active treatment and placebo herbs showed that substantial benefits followed the use of the Chinese herbs.[1] In a second, 47 children with a chronic extensive morbilliform variant of non-exudative atopic eczema were given Chinese herbs and placebo herbs in random order, each for 8 weeks, with an intervening 4-week washout period. In 37 who completed the study, the difference in benefits was clear.[2] Follow-up studies in both cases were also positive. One year after the trial, all subjects on treatment in the first study showed significant benefit; although none were able to discontinue permanently, most had reduced dosage. By contrast, mean scores for untreated individuals showed deterioration.[3] A 1-year follow-up on the children's trial showed that over 50% of subjects showed significant lasting benefit and 20% were able to stop treatment with complete remission.[4]

Inevitable safety issues have been raised, not least by the authors of the papers themselves (who recommend routine monitoring of liver function tests and tight exclusion criteria for treatment). For example, two cases of acute hepatic illness have been associated with the use of Chinese herbs for eczema[5] and one case of severe cardiomyopathy was reported after a 2-week course of such treatment.[6] Nevertheless, actual reports in the clinical trials were not alarming. In the follow-up of the children trial after a year of continuous treatment, two subjects taking treatment had raised asymptomatic AST levels but there were no abnormalities in either full blood counts or biochemical parameters in any adult patient on continued treatment after a year.

The implications of such work on wider medical thinking have been slow to emerge. However, it has led to considerable effort in developing licensed medicines for eczema and other skin diseases. If this is successful and a new range of effective prescription drugs is launched it could revolutionize medical practice. It also demonstrates that it is possible to design appropriate studies applying traditional diagnoses as inclusion criteria and it is fervently to be hoped that more studies will be forthcoming.

Topical treatments

Reference to Chapter 2 will lead the reader to many plant constituents with appreciable direct action on body tissues. There is a wide range of herbal applications to skin lesions, where the skin barrier is damaged. The section on topical applications (p.133) should also be consulted. In summary, the following characteristics of herbal remedies are relevant.

Demulcents

Helpful in reducing pruritus (itching) and inflammatory pain due to skin disease. In some cases longer term healing can result.

Astringents

Sometimes dramatically helpful where the skin is broken and discharging. As well as providing temporary relief, a strong astringent application can reduce discharge, reduce sepsis and promote healing.

Antiinflammatories

The most obvious recourse for topical treatments of most skin diseases.

Antiseptics

For at least containing fungal conditions (like tinea and candida) and bacterial infections (erysipelas, furunculosis).

PHYTOTHERAPY

A strategic approach

A good practitioner will have no set treatments for skin diseases. It is of course helpful to have a good diagnosis, so that treatment can be better directed. However, even then one reverts quickly to first principles. How are the fundamental body functions? In particular, is there evidence of difficulties in digestive, hepatobiliary and bowel or other eliminatory functions? If there is an immunological component, as in autoimmune or allergic conditions, then events at the gut wall are even more likely to be factors; they should be tracked down assiduously, with techniques such as rigorous experimental dietary eliminations to elucidate particular difficulties. The priority of treatment is to work at such 'primary lesions'. It may then be helpful to apply a humoral classification; is there evidence of patterns that might once have been classified as damp, dryness, cold, heat and/or wind (see p.147)? Remedies that dry, moisten, cool, heat or balance respectively could then feature in the prescription.

The treatment of acne and furunculosis may particularly suggest bowel treatments; rosacea and allergic drug eruptions, heptobiliary and bowel remedies. Particularly in such cases one would understandably revert to traditional alterative remedies (see below), especially if their role overlapped with what had been determined as primary problems.

Healing crises?

Skin disease is particularly prone to exacerbations during treatment. It can take very little to provoke this adverse result and 'healing crises' are common in homoeopathic and dietary treatments of skin disease (e.g. in fasting). Some proponents of the latter disciplines claim these are a good thing, a sign that 'toxins are coming out'. An immersion in pathophysiological mechanisms of skin inflammation would discourage this view and it is not even internally consistent as a notion. Skin inflammation is by definition an extraordinary event, involving a range of traumata in the dermal tissues that have little intrinsic value. If in traditional terms skin diseases suggest inadequacies in the ordinary eliminatory and processing functions then having even more toxins coming out of the skin, even briefly, does not recommend itself.

There is only one exception to the inadequacy of the healing crisis as a technique in treating skin disease. In cases of low-grade chronic skin trouble, where lack of activity is a characteristic of the condition, promoting subacute or acute crises has been a traditional manoeuvre to render the condition a little more vulnerable to treatment. In most other cases, clinical experience suggests exacerbations beyond a few initial days rarely lead to benefits in the long term; indeed, the opposite is normally true.

A good herbal practitioner will therefore aim for the minimum exacerbation, promoting the defective functions so as to diffuse the pathology. Given the readiness with which exacerbation does occur, a treatment strategy that led to progressive relief without a healing crisis would be something of a triumph.

ALTERATIVES

Plant remedies traditionally used as alteratives

Arctium lappa (burdock root), *Berberis aquifolium* (Oregon grape root), *Fumaria officinalis* (fumitory), *Galium aparine* (cleavers), *Iris versicolor* (blue flag), *Juglans regia* (walnut), *Rumex crispus* (yellow dock root), *Scrophularia nodosa* (figwort), *Trifolium pratense* (red clover flowers), *Urtica dioica* (nettle), *Viola tricolor* (heartsease).

Indications for alteratives

- Skin disease traditionally associated with toxaemia or septicaemia (e.g. furunculosis, some cases of acne)
- Many cases of eczema;
- Some cases of urticaria;
- Most other skin diseases (as components of wider acting prescriptions).

Other traditional indications for alteratives

- Joint diseases
- Connective tissue diseases
- Any wider detoxification regime (e.g. spring fasts)

Contraindications for alteratives

Alteratives can in many cases be provocative to skin disease. Care needs to be taken to reduce the prospects for major exacerbations (see 'Healing crises?' above).

Traditional therapeutic insights into the use of alteratives

Alteratives were seen primarily to detoxify, to help eliminatory and processing functions reduce the metabolic waste products accumulating. It was seen to be better to stimulate elimination than processing or at least to conduct therapy in that order. Increased processing without elimination would be exacerbatory. Similarly, any remedy that led to increased constipation or other elimination would often be accompanied by exacerbation. Arctium (burdock) is notable for its potential for exacerbation; it should be used carefully, well combined with, or preceded by, more eliminatory remedies.

Application

Long-term therapy with alteratives is often appropriate and is usually safe.

References

1. Sheehan MP, Rustin MHA, Atherton DJ et al. Efficacy of traditional Chinese herbal therapy in adult atopic dermatitis. Lancet 1992; 340(ii): 13–17
2. Sheehan MP, Atherton DJ. A controlled trial of traditional Chinese medicinal plants in widespread non-exudative atopic eczema. British Journal of Dermatology. 1992; 126(2): 179–184
3. Sheehan MP, Stevens H, Ostlere LS et al. Follow-up of adult patients with atopic eczema treated with Chinese herbal therapy for 1 year. Clinical and Experimental Dermatology 1995; 20(2): 136–140
4. Sheehan MP, Atherton DJ. One-year follow up of children treated with Chinese medicinal herbs for atopic eczema. British Journal of Dermatology. 1994; 130(4): 488–493
5. Kane JA, Kane SP, Jain S. Hepatitis induced by traditional Chinese herbs; possible toxic components. Gut 1995; 36(1): 146–147
6. Ferguson JE, Chalmers RJ, Rowlands DJ. Reversible dilated cardiomyopathy following treatment of atopic eczema with Chinese herbal medicine. British Journal of Dermatology 136(4): 592–593

Part 3

Materia Medica

Introduction

GENERAL CONSIDERATIONS

In this book the monographs on individual herbs are designed to be user friendly and hence are divided into two sections:

- a summary monograph which provides at a glance a definition, background material and clinically relevant information;
- a technical data section which extensively reviews the botany, pharmacology, clinical trial data, safety data and regulatory status in selected countries.

If the reader requires only information about the clinical applications of a particular herb and the general sources from which this information is derived, he or she need only refer to the summary monograph. On the other hand, if more detailed technical information is required, this is available in the technical data section. The review of the technical material has been conducted as widely and as comprehensively as possible at the time of writing. However, due to limits on space, for certain herbs such as ginkgo, St John's wort and ginseng, it was not possible to review all the published studies known to the authors. In these instances, a selection was made of what were considered to be the most important publications.

SPECIFIC HEADINGS

The monographs are headed and ordered according to the English common name of each herb. This is followed by the currently accepted botanical name of the plant from which the herb is derived.

SYNONYMS

Other English common names, alternative botanical names and common names in several other languages are listed.

WHAT IS IT?

This section includes historical and background information about the herb, the plant parts commonly used and other relevant details.

EFFECTS

This section describes in simple language how the herb acts.

TRADITIONAL VIEW

The traditional view reviews the traditional uses of the herb. As recounted elsewhere in this book, traditional use data are more than just anecdotal information and can often provide valuable insights into the therapeutic potential of a particular plant. This section is referenced so that the sources of this traditional use information are apparent.

SUMMARY ACTIONS

The actions are important because they encompass the traditional pharmacology of herbal medicine and link the therapeutic requirements of the patient to the choice of herbs (see Ch. 7). Only those actions which are considered to be well supported are listed.

CAN BE USED FOR

This section is divided into two parts. The part headed 'indications supported by clinical trials' summarizes those indications for which it is felt that there is good justification from clinical trial data.

The part headed 'Traditional therapeutic uses' is not just a repetition of the 'Traditional view' section. Rather, these traditional uses have been selected as being those most relevant and supported by contemporary practice.

This section effectively covers the clinical uses which can be recommended in practice.

MAY ALSO BE USED FOR

Again, this section is often divided into two parts. The part headed 'extrapolations from pharmacological studies' lists clinical indications which might be reasonably expected to follow from sound pharmacological data. Unfortunately, these extrapolations are often made in herbal writings but not stated to be such. This can leave the reader confused as to which recommended indications come from sound clinical or traditional data and which are merely speculative.

The second part headed 'Other applications' lists applications of interest which may not strictly involve medical conditions, e.g. cosmetic applications, or potential medical applications which derive from the extrapolation of limited clinical, folk or traditional information.

The information in this section should be read in the spirit that it is speculative but may provide a useful solution to a particular therapeutic problem.

PREPARATIONS

The various preparations of the herb which can be used in therapy are described.

DOSAGE

The dosages of specific preparations are given. In general, this information is based on those dosage regimes used in clinical trials with successful outcomes, reliable traditional sources such as the various pharmacopoeias and compendiums and expert committees such as Commission E and the scientific committee of ESCOP (European Scientific Cooperative on Phytotherapy).

DURATION OF USE

This section provides information about the duration of safe use of the herb.

SUMMARY ASSESSMENT OF SAFETY

This section summarizes the safety data detailed in the 'Technical data' section.

TECHNICAL DATA

BOTANY

A brief description of the plant is provided.

KEY CONSTITUENTS

The main phytochemical content of the plant is summarized and levels of particular constituents are provided where available. Chemical diagrams of some key constituents are included.

PHARMACODYNAMICS

This section reviews pharmacodynamic studies of various extracts of the herb (using different solvents) and of isolated key constituents. This information is grouped under relevant headings. In general, in vitro studies are provided first, followed by animal studies. It should be kept in mind that, because of their chemical complexity and uncertain pharmacokinetics, in vitro studies of herbal extracts do not necessarily provide clinically relevant information. In particular, some in vitro studies (and also animal studies) use excessive concentrations or doses, which are difficult to relate to normal therapeutic regimes. The reader is cautioned to refer to the original publication, taking these and other relevant factors into account, before drawing conclusions about use in humans.

The pharmacodynamic section also includes studies on healthy volunteers which were seeking to establish information about the human pharmacodynamics of the herb in question.

PHARMACOKINETICS

The known pharmacokinetics of key constituents is reviewed, giving emphasis to human studies.

CLINICAL TRIALS

Emphasis is given to randomized, controlled, double-blind clinical trials. However, open (not blinded) and uncontrolled (no control group) trials are also briefly summarized. Where a number of clinical trials have been subjected to metaanalysis, this publication is primarily reviewed rather than those individual trials included in the metaanalysis.

TOXICOLOGY AND OTHER SAFETY DATA

Studies investigating the acute, subacute and chronic toxicity of the herb or its key constituent are reviewed where available. Data on teratogenic effects are generally unavailable for herbs but these have been included where known.

Information pertaining to contraindications, special warnings and precautions, interactions with conventional drugs, use in pregnancy and lactation, effects on ability to drive and use machines, side effects and overdose is also provided. The general approach taken here is rational and cautious but not excessively so. Many reputed contraindications and concerns for herbs have little basis in fact. Similarly, adverse reactions are often attributed to herbs when other possibilities have not been conclusively ruled out. There is no doubt that a certain hostility towards herbal medicine which permeates some scientific publications has led to safety concerns about particular herbs on the flimsiest of evidence.

On the issue of safety during pregnancy and lactation, there is often little information available. However, the authors have adopted the view that a lack of information should not automatically preclude the use of a herb during pregnancy, especially if there is a traditional precedent for use during pregnancy or lactation.

CURRENT REGULATORY STATUS IN SELECTED COUNTRIES

Inclusion in relevant pharmacopoeias is noted and the view of the German Commission E monograph (where available) is summarized.

Commission E monographs are defined as positive, negative or null, which broadly classifies the herb as 'approved' (positive) or 'unapproved' (negative or null). In the view of the Commission E, a positive monograph indicates that the herb is reasonably safe and effective when used according to the dosage, contraindications and other warnings and provisions specified in the monographs. Negative assessment was made by the Commission for herbs if no plausible evidence of efficacy (including in traditional medicine in Germany) was available or when safety concerns outweighed the potential benefits. If there is neither a risk nor sufficiently documented efficacy, the monograph is termed null by Commission E and the herb is considered 'unapproved'. The negative and null monographs contain an application section which outlines historical and/or current use in Germany which has not been documented in scientific literature. This section does not imply approval by Commission E. The majority of the Commission E monographs pertain to single herbs but some also apply to fixed combinations and component characteristics. Fixed combinations refer to formulas containing multiple herbal ingredients. Component characteristics refer to herbs added to combinations for which the efficacy of the formula may depend on the safety and efficacy of a particular ingredient.

Information is also provided about the regulatory status of the herb in the UK, USA and Australia.

Under UK law, the legislative requirements relating to the prescribing, supply and administration of medicines are set out in the Medicines Act 1968 and in secondary legislation made under this Act, such as the Prescriptions Only Medicines Order 1997 and the Medicines (Pharmacy and General Sale – Exemption) Order 1980. Medicines are divided into three categories: those available on general sale (the General Sale List (GSL)), pharmacy medicines and prescription-only medicines. Other legislation which governs the use of herbs, such as Statutory Instrument SI 2130 and the Medicines (Retail Sale or Supply of Herbal Remedies) Order 1977, is mentioned where relevant.

In the USA, the federal Food and Drug Administration (FDA) regulated dietary supplements (including herbal medicines) as foods within the 1958 Food Additive Amendments to the Federal Food, Drug, and Cosmetic Act (FD&C Act). 'Generally Recognized As Safe' (GRAS) for human consumption was a rating provided by this legislation. GRAS status for a herbal product implies general recognition of its safety based on long-term and/or widespread traditional use without significant side effects. The GRAS status listed in the monographs includes herbs and components listed in Sect. 582.10 (Spices and other natural seasonings and flavorings) and 582.20 (Essential oils, oleoresins (solvent-free), and natural extractives (including distillates)) of Title 21, Code of Federal Regulations. Substances included in Sec. 172.510 (Natural flavoring substances and natural substances used in conjunction with flavors) are not included.

More recently, with passage of the Dietary Supplements Health and Education Act of 1994 (DSHEA), Congress amended the FD&C Act to include several provisions which apply only to dietary supplements and dietary ingredients of dietary supplements. As a result of these provisions, dietary ingredients used in dietary supplements are no longer subject to the premarket safety evaluations required of other new food ingredients or for new uses of old food ingredients. They must, however, meet the requirements of other safety provisions.

In Australia, herbal medicines are subject to federal legislation, defined by the Therapeutic Goods Act and Regulations, and State and Territories legislation reflected in the Standard for the Uniform Scheduling of Drugs and Poisons (SUSDP). Part 4 of Schedule 4 of the Therapeutic Goods Regulations lists herbs which are considered to be more toxic in nature. These herbs cannot be included in over-the-counter products without prior evaluation by an expert committee.

References

In order to save space, references for the monographs are provided in an abbreviated form.

Andrographis
(*Andrographis paniculata* (Burm. f.) Nees)

SYNONYMS

Chiretta, king of bitters (Engl), kalmegh (Bengali, Hindi), kirata (Sanskrit), chuan xin lian (Chin), senshinren (Jap).

WHAT IS IT?

Andrographis, commonly known as kalmegh (meaning 'king of bitters'), is grown in hedgerows and gardens in India where it is highly valued by the local people as a medicine. It has often been used as a substitute for the bitter herb *Swertia chirata* and, as such, also has the common name of chirayta. At one point, Andrographis was advertised in England as a substitute for quinine (possibly due to its bitterness). However, this was discontinued due to lack of significant antimalarial activity. The whole herb including the root has been used for medicinal purposes in India but use of the leaf or aerial parts is more common. As well as Ayurveda, Andrographis is prominent in the materia medica of other traditional medical systems, including those of China and Thailand.

EFFECTS

Stimulates the immune system, especially phagocytic activity; stimulates bile production and flow; protects the liver from toxins; counters the damaging effects of free radicals.

TRADITIONAL VIEW

In Ayurvedic medicine, Andrographis is used for its bitter tonic, stomachic, antipyretic and laxative properties. It is said to increase appetite, strengthen digestion and diminish flatulence, hyperacidity and biliousness.[1] The herb is utilized for the treatment of many conditions, including diabetes, debility and hepatitis.[2] The roots and leaves have a reputation for being depurative and anthelmintic.[3] In traditional Chinese medicine, Andrographis is bitter and 'cold' and is used to clear *Heat* from the *Blood* (especially in the lungs, throat and urinary tract) and to detoxify *Fire Poison* (manifesting as skin sores and carbuncles). In addition to gastrointestinal complaints, it is prescribed for throat infections, cough with thick sputum and snake bites.[4,5] Since Andrographis is regarded as a 'cold' herb, it is ideally suited to treating acute infections, which are 'hot' conditions.

SUMMARY ACTIONS

Bitter tonic, choleretic, immunostimulant, hepatoprotective, antipyretic, antiinflammatory, antiplatelet, abortifacient, antioxidant.

CAN BE USED FOR

INDICATIONS SUPPORTED BY CLINICAL TRIALS

Bacterial and viral respiratory infections including the common cold and pharyngotonsillitis, enteric infections; for prevention of urinary tract infections following shock wave lithotripsy; prophylaxis of common cold.

TRADITIONAL THERAPEUTIC USES

Loss of appetite, atonic dyspepsia, flatulence, diarrhoea, dysentery, gastroenteritis, bowel complaints of children; liver infections; diabetes; general debility and for convalescence after fevers; respiratory and skin infections.

MAY ALSO BE USED FOR

EXTRAPOLATIONS FROM PHARMACOLOGICAL STUDIES

To boost immune function in bacterial and viral infections; protection against hepatotoxicity; to enhance the detoxifying capacity of the liver; to alleviate inflammation.

PREPARATIONS

Dried or fresh herb as a decoction, infusion and liquid extract for internal use. The leaf juice is also used in Ayurveda.

DOSAGE

Being very bitter, some people may find Andrographis difficult to take in liquid preparations. Whichever way it is taken, the daily preventative dose for an adult is about 2–3 g or its equivalent (4–6 ml per day of 1:2 liquid extract). During infection, the effective dose is nearer to 6 g per day (up to 12 ml per day of 1:2 liquid extract). Standardization for andrographolides is preferable.

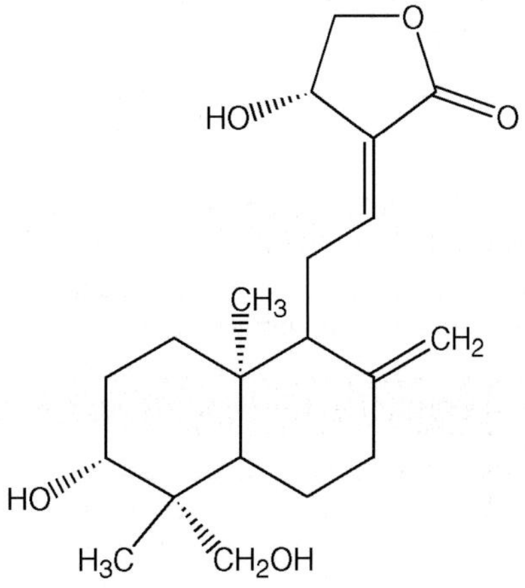

Since Andrographis is energetically 'cold', it is preferably taken in combination with 'warm' herbs when used during winter as a preventative treatment, especially if the user has a 'cold' constitution. Warming herbs include ginger, Astragalus and tulsi (*Ocimum sanctum*).

DURATION OF USE

May be taken long term.

SUMMARY ASSESSMENT OF SAFETY

No significant adverse effects from ingestion of Andrographis are expected, although high doses may cause gastric discomfort. Andrographis is contraindicated during pregnancy.

TECHNICAL DATA

BOTANY

Andrographis paniculata is an annual shrub belonging to the Acanthaceae family. It grows to a height of 1 metre with branches that are sharply quadrangular, often narrowly winged towards the apical region. The leaves are lanceolate (5–8 cm long) and the flowers are small, solitary in panicles, with a corolla ranging from white to rose pink in colour and hairy externally. The fruit is approximately 2 cm long, linear-oblong in shape and acute at both ends. The seeds are numerous, yellowish-brown and glabrous.[6] Andrographis grows wild as an undershrub in tropical moist deciduous forests[6] and is also cultivated as a rainy season crop.[2]

KEY CONSTITUENTS

- Diterpenoid lactones, collectively referred to as andrographolides and consisting of aglycones (such as andrographolide) and glucosides (such as neoandrographolide and andrographiside):[7,8]
- Diterpene dimers,[7] flavonoids.[9]

Many of the diterpenoid lactones are bitter (such as andrographolide) but neoandrographolide is not bitter.[8]

HO, O, O, CH3, CH2, HO, H3C, CH2OH

Andrographolide

PHARMACODYNAMICS

Antiinfective and immunostimulating activity

Although Andrographis is widely used in infections and infestations, the weight of evidence is that its value here is mainly as an immune-enhancing treatment. Early reports in China attributed an antibacterial activity to the plant which has not recently been confirmed. The andrographolides are certainly devoid of antibacterial activity.[5]

No direct antibacterial activity could be demonstrated for an aqueous extract of Andrographis against Salmonella, Shigella, *E. coli*, group A streptococci and *S. aureus* in vitro. Animal studies using orally administered Andrographis (0.12–0.24 g/kg) for 6 months failed to demonstrate bactericidal activity.[10] Serum taken from 10 healthy volunteers after a single oral dose of Andrographis (ranging from 1 g to 6 g) showed no bactericidal activity against a number of organisms.[10] However, alcoholic extract of Andrographis did show significant activity against an *E. coli* enterotoxin-induced secretory response (which causes diarrhoea) in in vivo models.[11]

Liquid extract of Andrographis root demonstrated strong in vitro anthelmintic activity against human *Ascaris lumbricoides*.[12] Subcutaneous administration of a decoction of Andrographis leaves to infected dogs reduced nematode larvae in the blood by 85%.[13]

Dehydroandrographolide succinic acid monoester (DASM), a drug derived from andrographolide, has been found to inhibit HIV in vitro. This effect was observed on several HIV strains and DASM was nontoxic to other cells in the active concentration range. However, the diterpenoid lactones of Andrographis (dehydroandrographolide and andrographolide) were devoid of anti-HIV activity.[14] Moreover, in vitro studies with aqueous extracts of Andrographis showed little or no inhibition of HIV-1. Modes of inhibition studied comprised inhibition of HIV-1 protease,[15] inhibition of interaction between HIV-1 gp 120 and immobilized CD4 receptor, inhibition of HIV-1 reverse transcriptase and inhibition of glycohydrolase enzymes.[16]

An immunostimulant action, especially on phagocytosis, has been demonstrated by a decoction of Andrographis in vitro and in vivo after injection of the soluble derivatives.[5] Isolated andrographolide and Andrographis liquid extract stimulated both antigen-specific and non-specific immune responses in mice. The liquid extract produced stronger immunostimulation.[17] Prolonged survival in animals after snakebite was observed after pretreatment with extracts of Andrographis.[18]

Hepatoprotective and choleretic activity

Andrographolide showed protective activity against chemically induced toxicity on rat hepatocytes in vitro. The hepatoprotective effect was greater than silymarin.[19]

Intraperitoneal administration of andrographolide, andrographiside and neoandrographolide (100 mg/kg) to mice protected against hepatic damage caused by carbon tetrachloride and tert-butyl hydroperoxide. Andrographiside and neoandrographolide had the greatest effect on reducing lipid peroxidation and were comparable to silymarin.[20] Similar studies indicate that andrographolide is the major active antihepatotoxic principle in Andrographis.[21] Intraperitoneal administration of three diterpene constituents of Andrographis showed protective effects on hepatotoxicity induced in mice by various chemical agents. The protective effect of andrographiside and neoandrographolide was as strong as silymarin and could be due to the sugar groups acting as strong antioxidants.[22] Andrographolide exhibited hepatoprotective activity after oral or intraperitoneal administration to rats with chemically induced acute hepatitis. Treatment with the herb led to complete normalization of five biochemical parameters and improved the histopathological changes in the liver.[23]

Oral administration of Andrographis extract and andrographolide to rats demonstrated a protective action against carbon tetrachloride-induced hepatic toxicity. The leaf extract showed stronger activity than andrographolide.[24] Pre- and posttreatment with oral doses of Andrographis (0.5 g/kg/day) normalized alcohol-induced increases in serum transaminase activity in rats. The researchers concluded that Andrographis has a protective as well as a curative effect on alcohol-induced toxic liver damage.[25] Significant hepatoprotective activity was demonstrated for an alcohol extract of Andrographis and two of its diterpenes, andrographolide and neoandrographolide, against the hepatotoxicity caused by *Plasmodium berghei* infection in animals. This hepatotoxicity is thought to be mediated through free radical damage. The protective effect of Andrographis is thought to be due, in part, to reactivation of superoxide dismutase which in turn counteracts peroxidative damage. Andrographis may also cause induction of hepatic drug-metabolizing systems which detoxify hepatotoxins.[26] The following study supports this latter point. Administration of Andrographis (0.5 g/kg per day) or andrographolide (5.0 mg/kg per day) to rats for 7–30 consecutive days caused a significant induction of the liver microsomal drug-metabolizing enzymes aniline hydroxylase, N-demethylase and O-demethylase. However, a single dose caused inhibition of aniline hydroxylase activity only and had no effect on N- and O-demethylase.[27]

Andrographolide produced a dose-dependent choleretic effect (increased bile flow, bile salt and bile acids) in rats and guinea pigs after oral administration[28] and after intraperitoneal injection in rats.[29] The effect was stronger than silymarin.[28] Aqueous extract of Andrographis orally administered to rats at 3.75 ml/kg increased bile flow and liver weight. The maximal increase in flow and weight was reached after 2 days and levels remained constant after longer treatment periods. Pretreatment at the same dose for 5 days shortened experimentally induced sleeping time in mice. These activities provide further evidence that Andrographis may cause induction of hepatic drug-metabolizing enzymes.[30]

Cardiovascular activity

A study of an aqueous extract administered by intravenous administration suggested that Andrographis may limit the expansion of the ischaemic focus, may exert a marked protective effect on reversible ischaemic myocardium and could demonstrate a weak fibrinolytic action.[31] Andrographis was found to alleviate myocardial ischaemia-reperfusion injury.[32] The mechanism was probably via a decrease in the harmful effect of oxygen free radicals.[33] A study on rabbits found that Andrographis alleviated atherosclerotic arterial stenosis induced by both deendothelialization and a high cholesterol diet. In addition, it lowered the restenosis rate after experimental angioplasty.[34]

An aqueous extract of Andrographis given by intraperitoneal infusion to rats exhibited a dose-dependent hypotensive effect on systolic blood pressure in spontaneously hypertensive rats and normotensive controls.[35] A crude water extract of Andrographis and two semipurified n-butanol and aqueous fractions significantly reduced mean arterial blood pressure in anaesthetized rats without decreasing heart rate. The hypotensive substance in the crude water extract appeared to be concentrated in the butanol fraction.[36] The dosages stated in this work suggest Andrographis was administered by injection.

Antifertility activity

Oral administration of Andrographis leaf powder (20 mg/day for 60 days) to male rats produced an antifertility effect, possibly due to an antispermatogenic and/or antiandrogenic mechanism.[37] A later study using levels of 10 mg and 20 mg per day for 24 and 48 days resulted in biochemical changes in the testes and male accessory organs.[38] These results were not duplicated in a similar study using a standardized dried ethanol extract of Andrographis at 20, 200 and 1000 mg/kg per day for 60 days. The authors concluded that the variation in results may be due to differences in plant material used in the two studies, i.e. dried leaf powder and a dried ethanol extract. Andrographis did not produce subchronic testicular toxicity.[39]

A controlled experiment in female mice fed with 2 g/kg per day found Andrographis prevented pregnancy in 100% of those treated.[40]

Antiinflammatory, antipyretic and analgesic activities

Several in vivo studies have shown antipyretic and antiinflammatory effects for andrographolides (by oral administration or injection). The antiinflammatory activity of andrographolides may be due to promotion of ACTH and consequent enhancement of adrenocortical function.[5] Andrographolide administered orally (30, 100 and 300 mg/kg) significantly reduced inflammation in a number of animal models, including adjuvant-induced arthritis.[41] The addition of andrographolide to an endothelial cell culture together with tumour necrosis factor (TNF) effected a concentration-dependent reduction of the TNF-induced enhancement of endothelial monocyte adhesion, which is part of the inflammatory process.[42]

Oral doses of andrographolide at 300 mg/kg demonstrated analgesic activity; at 100 and 300 mg/kg significant antipyretic effects were also observed after 3 hours. In addition, this dose had significant antiulcerogenic activity against aspirin-induced ulceration in rats.[43]

Other activity

Aqueous extract of Andrographis (10 mg/kg) was found to prevent glucose-induced hyperglycaemia in rabbits but it failed to prevent glucose absorption from the gut.[44] Oral administration of Andrographis extract and andrographolide produced a dose- and time-dependent activation of brush-border membrane-bound hydrolases (lactase, maltase, sucrase) in rats. This suggests that Andrographis accelerates intestinal digestion and absorption of carbohydrate (as opposed to simple glucose).[45]

Methanol extract of Andrographis showed potent cell differentiation-inducing activity on mouse leukaemia cells in vitro. (This implies anticarcinogenic activity.) Some of the isolated diterpenes also demonstrated activity.[7]

PHARMACOKINETICS

Oral doses of radiolabelled andrographolide given to mice were rapidly absorbed and distributed to organs, especially gallbladder, kidney, ovary and lung. Andrographolides levels appeared to be low in spleen, heart and brain. Approximately 90% was excreted in the urine and faeces after 24 hours and 94% after 48 hours. At 48 hours, radiolabelled andrographolide only accounted for approximately 11% of urine and liver fractions, the remainder consisting of metabolites.[46]

CLINICAL TRIALS

Respiratory infections

Chinese clinical studies of bacterial and viral respiratory infections demonstrated good effects after oral administration of Andrographis or andrographolides, implying an immunostimulant action.[5] Investigations from the Sichuan Traditional Medicine Research Institution showed Andrographis had a beneficial effect in the treatment of infectious diseases associated with cold symptoms. The major finding in this study was a lowered body temperature after treatment with Andrographis: of 84 cases of common cold, 70 achieved normal body temperature within 48 hours.[47]

A randomized double-blind study on 152 patients with pharyngotonsillitis found 6 g per day of Andrographis for a week to be as effective as paracetamol in providing relief of fever and sore throat. For both groups the differences between baseline symptoms and final evaluation were significant ($p<0.0001$). Lower doses of Andrographis were not as effective.[48]

Tablets containing a total of 1200 mg Andrographis extract (standardized to 4% andrographolides) or placebo were given to 61 patients suffering symptoms of common cold in a double-blind, placebo-controlled clinical trial. After 4 days of treatment, measured symptoms were significantly reduced in the Andrographis-treated group compared to placebo: strength of disease (p=0.0001), tiredness (p=0.0001), sweating/shivering (p=0.001), sore throat (p=0.0001) and muscular ache (p=0.0001). For clinical signs (rhinitis, sinus pains and headaches, lymphatic swellings), there was no significant difference between the treated and placebo groups at day 4. However, if the groups are compared over time (i.e. day 0 versus day 4) there was a significant decrease in the intensity of these signs only for the Andrographis-treated group (p<0.05). (The overall reduction in the symptom score over time was also significant (p<0.01).) The authors concluded that Andrographis treatment can significantly shorten the course and duration of the common cold.[49]

In an earlier controlled trial, improvement of hospital inpatients suffering from common cold and sinusitis was significantly better in the Andrographis group compared to placebo (p<0.001).[50] In a randomized, double-blind, placebo-controlled clinical trial, 107 healthy children received either Andrographis extract tablets (200 mg per day of extract, standardized to 11.2 mg andrographolide) or placebo for 3 months during the winter season. This dose corresponds to about 1 g of the original herb. Analysis after the first month indicated no significant change for Andrographis treatment. However, by the third month there was a significant decrease in the incidence of colds compared to placebo (30% versus 62%; p<0.01). The relative risk of catching a cold was 2.1 times lower for the Andrographis group.[51]

In a randomized, double-blind, placebo-controlled pilot study conducted by the Swedish Herbal Institute, 50 outpatients with symptoms of common cold were treated with placebo or tablets containing Andrographis extract (1020 mg per day, about 6 g of herb). The patients were instructed to make their first clinic visit not later than 3 days after the occurrence of cold symptoms. After 5 days of therapy, subjective evaluation demonstrated a significantly reduced number of sick leave days (p<0.03), improved symptoms (p<0.025) and hastened recovery (p<0.05) for the Andrographis group. Side effects were very few and mild.[52]

Enteric infections

Many Chinese studies using oral administration of Andrographis or andrographolides in acute bacillary dysentery and enteritis have shown a marked benefit.[5] Patients with acute diarrhoea were treated with powdered leaves and stems of Andrographis. The Andrographis was effective in reducing the number of Shigella but was less effective for cholera compared to tetracycline. Oral administration of 1 g every 12 hours for 2 days was more effective than giving a dose of 500 mg every 6 hours for 2 days.[53]

Other conditions

An open study in Thailand compared parameters of urinary tract infection in patients undergoing shock wave dissolution of kidney stones (lithotripsy). The study found that 1 g of Andrographis was as effective as the antibiotics cotrimoxazole and norfloxacin in the reduction of pyuria and haematuria.[54]

Sixty-three patients with cardiac and cerebral vascular diseases were observed at 3 hours and/or 1 week after taking Andrographis extracts. Results showed that platelet aggregation induced by ADP was significantly inhibited (p<0.001). The aggregation rate was also lower at 1 week. In other volunteers taking Andrographis, serotonin release from platelets was decreased (p<0.01) but plasma serotonin levels remained unchanged. A rise in platelet cyclic AMP levels might be the mechanism behind the antiplatelet activity of Andrographis.[55]

A majority of the 20 patients with infective hepatitis showed marked improvement in symptoms after approximately 24 days' treatment with Andrographis decoction (equivalent to 40 g of herb per day). Significant decreases in various liver function tests were also observed. Overall, 80% of cases were cured and 20% were relieved.[56]

TOXICOLOGY

No toxic effect was observed after administration of a decoction of Andrographis leaves to rabbits.[13] The LD_{50} values of the andrographolides and their derivatives indicate Andrographis has a low toxicity: 13.4 g/kg for oral administration of the total andrographolides, greater than 40 g/kg for oral andrographolide.[5]

CONTRAINDICATIONS

Pregnancy.

SPECIAL WARNINGS AND PRECAUTIONS

None known.

INTERACTIONS

No adverse interactions known.

USE IN PREGNANCY AND LACTATION

The antifertility effect in female mice (albeit at high doses) suggests that Andrographis should not be used during human pregnancy.

EFFECTS ON ABILITY TO DRIVE AND USE MACHINES

No adverse effects.

SIDE EFFECTS

High doses may cause gastric discomfort, anorexia and emesis but generally there are few side effects and it is not toxic. Two cases of urticaria were reported in the pilot trial of 50 patients treated with 1020 mg of Andrographis extract.[52]

OVERDOSE

No effects known.

CURRENT REGULATORY STATUS IN SELECTED COUNTRIES

Andrographis is official in the Pharmacopoeia of the People's Republic of China (English Edition 1997). Andrographis was official in the second edition of the *Indian Pharmacopoeia* (1966) but was not included in the third edition (1985).

Andrographis is not covered by a Commission E monograph and is not on the UK General Sale List.

Andrographis does not have GRAS status. However, it is freely available as a 'dietary supplement' in the USA under DSHEA legislation (1994 Dietary Supplement Health and Education Act).

Andrographis is not included in Part 4 of Schedule 4 of the Therapeutic Goods Act Regulations of Australia.

References

1. A Panel of Vaidyas. Clinical application of Ayurvedic remedies, Indian medical science series no. 3, 4th edn. Sri Satguru Publications, Delhi 1998, p 100.
2. Kapoor LD. CRC handbook of Ayurvedic medicinal plants. CRC Press, Boca Raton, 1990, p 39.
3. Chopra RN, Chopra IC, Handa KL et al. Chopra's indigenous drugs of India, 2nd edn reprint. Academic Publishers, Calcutta, 1982, p 278.
4. Bensky D, Gamble A. Chinese herbal medicine materia medica. Eastland Press, Seattle, 1986, p 136.
5. Chang H, But P. Pharmacology and applications of Chinese material medica, vol 2. World Scientific, Singapore, 1987, pp 918–928.
6. Thakur RS, Puri HS, Husain A. Major medicinal plants of India. Central Institute of Medicinal and Aromatic Plants, Lucknow, 1989, p 61.
7. Matsuda T, Kuroyanagi M, Sugiyama S et al. Chem Pharm Bull 1994; 42 (6): 1216–1225.
8. Tang W, Eisenbrand G. Chinese drugs of plant origin. Springer Verlag, Berlin, 1992, pp 97–103.
9. Zhu PY, Liu GQ. Chin Trad Herb Drugs 1984; 15: 373–376.
10. Leelarasamee A, Trakulsomboon S, Sittisomwong N. J Med Assoc Thai 1990; 73 (6): 299–304.
11. Gupta S, Chaudhry MA, Yadava JNS. Int J Crude Drug Res 1990; 28 (4): 273–283.
12. Raj RK. Ind J Physiol Pharmacol 1975; 19 (1): 47–49.
13. Dutta A, Sukul NC. J Helminthol 1982; 56 (2): 81–84.
14. Chang RS, Ding L, Chen GQ et al. Proc Soc Exp Biol Med 1991; 197 (1): 59–66.
15. Xu H, Wan M, Loh B et al. Phytother Res 1996; 10: 207–210.
16. Collins RA, Ng TB, Fong WP et al. Life Sci 1997; 60 (23): 345–351.
17. Puri A, Saxena R, Saxena RP et al. J Nat Prod 1993; 56 (7): 995–999.
18. Martz W. Toxicon 1992; 30 (10): 1131–1142.
19. Visen PK, Shukla B, Patnaik GK et al. J Ethnopharmacol 1993; 40 (2): 131–136.
20. Kapil A, Koul IB. Hepatoprotective agents from Indian traditional plants. In: Pushpangadan P et al (eds) Glimpses of Indian ethnopharmacology. (Proceedings of the First National Conference on Ethnopharmacology. Tropical Botanic Garden and Research Institute, Kerala, India: 1995, pp 283–297
21. Handa SS, Sharma A. Indian J Med Res 1990; 92: 276–283.
22. Kapil A, Koul IB, Banerjee SK et al. Biochem Pharmacol 1993; 46 (1): 182–185.
23. Handa SS, Sharma A. Indian J Med Res 1990; 92: 284–292.
24. Choudhury BR, Poddar MK. Methods Find Exp Clin Pharmacol 1984; 6 (9): 481–485.
25. Choudhury BR, Poddar MK. Methods Find Exp Clin Pharmacol 1983; 5 (10): 727–730.
26. Chander R, Srivastava V, Tandon JS. Int J Pharmacog 1995; 33 (2): 135–138.
27. Choudhury BR, Haque SJ, Poddar MK. Planta Med 1987; 53 (2): 135–140.
28. Shukla B, Visen PKS, Patnaik GK et al. Planta Med 1992; 58 (2): 146–149.
29. Tripathi GS, Tripathi YB. Phytother Res 1991; 5: 176–178.
30. Chaudhuri SK. Indian J Exp Biol 1978; 16: 830–832.
31. Zhao HY, Fang WY. J Tongji Med Univ 1990; 10 (4): 212–217.
32. Guo ZL, Zhao HY, Zheng XH. J Tongji Med Univ 1994; 14 (1): 49–51.
33. Guo ZL, Zhao HY, Zheng XH. J Tongji Med Univ 1995; 15 (4): 205–208.
34. Wang DW, Zhao HY. Chin Med J 1994; 107 (6): 464–470.
35. Zhang CY, Tan BK. Clin Exp Pharmacol Physiol 1996; 23 (8): 675–678.
36. Zhang CY, Tan BK. J Ethnopharmacol 1997; 56 (2): 97–101.
37. Akbarsha MA, Manivannan B, Hamid KS et al. Indian J Exp Biol 1990; 28 (5): 421–426.
38. Akbarsha MA, Manivannan B. Indian J Compar Animal Physiol 1993; 11 (2): 103–108.
39. Burgos RA, Caballero EE, Sanchez NS. J Ethnopharmacol 1997; 58 (3): 219–224.
40. Zoha MS, Hussain AH, Choudhury SA. Bangladesh Med Res Counc Bull 1989; 15 (1): 34–37.
41. Madav S, Tandan SK, Lal J. Fitoterapia 1996; 67 (5); 452–458.
42. Habtemariam S. Phytother Res 1998; 12: 37–40.
43. Madav S, Tripathi HC, Tandan SK. Ind J Pharm Sci 1995; 57 (3): 121–125.
44. Borhanuddin M, Shamsuzzoha M, Hussain AH. Bangladesh Med Res Counc Bull 1994; 20 (1): 24–26.
45. Choudhury BR, Poddar MK. Methods Find Exp Clin Pharmacol 1985; 7 (12): 617–621.

46. Zheng ZY, Wan YD, He GX. Chin Trad Herb Drugs 1982; 13: 417–420.
47. Pharmacology Department, Sichan, 1975, cited in Melchior J, Palm S, Wikman G. Phytomed 1996/7; 3 (4): 315–318.
48. Thamlikitkul V, Dechatiwongse T, Theerapong S et al. J Med Assoc Thai 1991; 74 (10): 437–442.
49. Hancke J, Burgos R, Caceres D. Phytother Res 1995; 9: 559–562.
50. Hancke J, Ibarra M. Article under publication, cited in Melchior J, Palm S, Wikman G. Phytomed 1996/7; 3(4): 315–318.
51. Caceres DD, Hancke JL, Burgos RZ et al. Phytomed 1997; 4 (2): 101–104.
52. Melchior J, Palm S, Wikman G. Phytomed 1996/7; 3 (4): 315–318.
53. Chaicharntipyuth C, Thanangkul P. The Eighth Conference, December 15, Faculty of Pharmacy, Chulalongkorn University, Bangkok, 1989.
54. Muangman V, Viseshsindh V, Ratana-Olarn K et al. J Med Assoc Thai 1995; 78 (6): 310–313.
55. Zhang YZ, Tang JZ, Zhang YJ. Chung-Kuo Chung Hsi I Chieh Ho Tsa Chin 1994; 14 (1): 28–30.
56. Chaturvedi GN, Tomar GS, Tiwari SK et al. Ancient Sci Life 1982; 2: 208–215.

Arnica flowers (*Arnica montana* L.)

SYNONYMS

Leopard's or wolf's bane, mountain tobacco (Engl), Arnicae flos (Lat), Arnikablüten, Berwohlverleih (Ger), fleurs d'arnica (Fr), polmonaria di montagna (Ital), guldblomme (Dan).

WHAT IS IT?

Arnica has been traditionally used externally for the treatment of sprains and bruises and taken internally mainly in the form of homoeopathic preparations. The macerated oil of Arnica flowers, known as 'Arnica oil', is also often used topically. The bright yellow aromatic flowers of Arnica are native to the mountain pastures in central Europe. *Arnica montana* is a protected species in Germany; its declining occurrence in Europe may be related to soil quality. For this reason another closely related species (*A. chamissonis* ssp *foliosa*) is also used. Products adulterated with Mexican Arnica (*Heterotheca inuloides*), a common substitute, should be avoided.

EFFECTS

In external use for bruising, sprains, swellings, muscle pain, symptoms of varicose veins and haemorrhoids, Arnica stimulates the peripheral blood supply and has antiinflammatory and oedema-reducing activity.

TRADITIONAL VIEW

Traditionally Arnica has been a popular remedy, used externally for sprains, bruises, painful swellings, injuries and wounds. Topical application was avoided in cases of tender or broken skin. It was often used diluted and the surface deliberately not covered with bandages. Arnica was used internally as a stimulant and diuretic but to a much less extent due to its allergenic and irritant effects.[1–3]

SUMMARY ACTIONS

Antiinflammatory, antiecchymotic (against bruises), analgesic, antiseptic.

CAN BE USED FOR

INDICATIONS SUPPORTED BY CLINICAL TRIALS

Topically for chronic venous insufficiency and muscle ache.

TRADITIONAL THERAPEUTIC USES

Externally for bruises, sprains, swellings, unbroken chilblains, haematomas, inflammations, dislocations, oedema associated with fractures; haemorrhoids; rheumatic, muscle and joint complaints; inflamed insect bites; surface phlebitis and symptoms of varicose veins.[2,3]

MAY ALSO BE USED FOR

EXTRAPOLATIONS FROM PHARMACOLOGICAL STUDIES

Topically for antimicrobial activity.

OTHER APPLICATIONS

Externally for alopecia neurotica[4] and in hair preparations to prevent dandruff and to stimulate the circulation in the scalp.[5]

PREPARATIONS

To prepare a poultice: 2–3 g of Arnica is covered with approximately 150 ml of hot water and after 10 minutes strained. Bandages, gauze or cotton are soaked in the infusion and then placed on the affected area of the body.

'Arnica oil' is obtained by macerating one part Arnica flowers in five parts vegetable oil. Arnica tincture (1:5, 45%) is also used topically as a lotion or incorporated into creams or ointments.

DOSAGE

- Lotion: dilute a 1:5 tincture by five times with water and apply 2–3 times per day.
- Ointment should contain 10–25% tincture or about 15% 'Arnica oil'; apply 2–3 times per day.

DURATION OF USE

Not for prolonged application.

SUMMARY ASSESSMENT OF SAFETY

Arnica is toxic if taken internally (except diluted homoeopathic preparations). Contact dermatitis can occur. Arnica preparations should not be applied to open wounds or near the eyes or mouth.

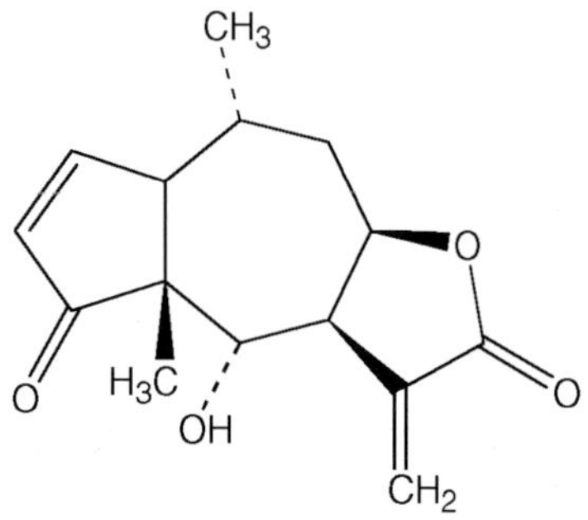

Helenalin

TECHNICAL DATA

BOTANY

Arnica, a member of the Compositae or Asteraceae (daisy) family, is a perennial herb with a horizontally growing rhizome. It grows to 30–60 cm, the lower leaves are up to 17 cm long, elliptical in shape, five-veined and form a rosette at the base of the stem. The flower heads number 1–3 and are up to 8 cm wide. They consist of peripheral, lingulate flowers, which are yellow-orange, and central tubular flowers.[6,7]

KEY CONSTITUENTS

- Sesquiterpene lactones of the pseudoguaianolide type (0.2–1.5%), including helenalin and 11-alpha, 13-dihydrohelenalin and their esters.[8]
- Flavonoids (0.4–0.6%),[8] essential oil-containing alkanes.[9]
- Phenolic acids, coumarins, carotinoids;[9] non-toxic pyrrolizidine alkaloids.[10]

PHARMACODYNAMICS

Antiinflammatory activity

Results from in vitro studies suggest that the mechanism of the antiinflammatory activity possibly occurs at several sites:[11]

- uncoupling of oxidative phosphorylation in polymorphonuclear neutrophils;
- elevation of cAMP in neutrophils and liver cells;
- inhibition of lysosomal enzymatic activity in neutrophils and liver cells.

Polymorphonuclear neutrophil chemotaxis was inhibited at low concentrations, whereas cyclooxygenase activity was inhibited at a higher concentration by a series of sesquiterpene lactones, including helenalin and dihydrohelenalin.[11]

Many sesquiterpene lactones, including those from Arnica, have demonstrated antiinflammatory activity after intraperitoneal injection (2.5 mg/kg/day) in animal models such as carrageenan-induced paw oedema and chronic adjuvant arthritis. The alpha-methylene-gamma-lactone structure was required for inhibitory activity in both models and the 6-hydroxy group of helenalin was required for potency in the former model. Inhibition of writhing reflex (an indication of analgesic activity) was also observed.[12]

Antimicrobial activity

Components of the essential oil of Arnica have demonstrated potent activity against Gram-positive and Gram-negative bacteria and against *Candida spp*, in vitro.[13] Helenalin and helenalin acetate were also active in vitro against Gram-positive bacteria and *Proteus vulgaris*.[14]

The polyacetylenes from the root have shown broad-range antimicrobial activity against pathogenic fungi (*Trichophyton spp*, *Microsporum gypseum*, *Epidermophyton spp*) and bacteria (*Staph. aureus*, *Pseudomonas aeruginosa*, *E. coli*) in vitro.[15]

Antitumour activity

In a screening of 21 flavonoids and five sesquiterpene lactones from *Arnica spp*, helenalin demonstrated the strongest cytotoxic activity of the sesquiterpene lactones. The flavonoids showed moderate to low cytotoxicity compared with the reference compound.[16] The effect of flavones and flavonols from *Arnica spp* on the cytotoxicity of helenalin was investigated in the human lung carcinoma cell line. At non-toxic concentrations, all flavonoids (except kaempferol) significantly reduced helenalin-induced cytotoxicity.[17] Sesquiterpene lactones of Arnica inhibited Walker 26 carcinosarcoma and Ehrlich ascites tumour growth in vivo.[18]

Other activity

The stabilization of lysosomal membrane in liver cells by sesquiterpene lactones was dependent on the alpha-methylene-gamma-lactone structure.[11] Helenalin and 11-alpha,13-dihydrohelenalin in vitro have inhibited human platelet function via thiol-dependent pathways. The reduction in platelet sulphydryl groups is probably associated with reduced phospholipase A_2 activity.[19]

Arnica extracts applied to animal smooth muscle in vitro inhibited experimentally induced spasm.[20]

Phagocytosis of *Staphylococcus epidermidis* by horse and pig leucocytes was stimulated by Arnica extract in vitro. Injection of Arnica extract enhanced phagocytosis in mice and protected against *Listeria monocytogenes* infection.[21]

Helenalin, dihydrohelenalin and epoxyhelenalin (20 mg/kg/day in mice) produced a lowering of serum cholesterol (30%) and serum triglycerides (25%). Thiol-bearing enzymes of lipid synthesis were inhibited by these compounds in vitro, suggesting they alkylate thiol nucleophiles by a Michael-type addition.[22]

PHARMACOKINETICS

No data available.

CLINICAL TRIALS

A placebo-controlled, double-blind, randomized clinical study of 89 patients with pronounced symptoms of chronic venous insufficiency tested the efficacy of an Arnica gel (containing 20% Arnica tincture). After 3 weeks, the symptom of feeling heaviness in the legs (which is strongly associated with peripheral oedema) together with objective measurements of oedema and venous tone were assessed. The 'heavy leg' feeling improved significantly more in the Arnica group compared to placebo; in addition, venous tone and oedema were improved for the Arnica group. The efficacy of Arnica in the treatment of symptoms associated with varicose veins is believed to be due to a protective effect against oedema.[23]

Twelve male volunteers externally applied preparations for muscle ache. Arnica gel was more effective than placebo gel.[24]

TOXICOLOGY

The oral median lethal dose of helenalin varies from 85 mg/kg in hamsters to 150 mg/kg in sheep. It is a toxic sesquiterpene lactone for mammals.[10]

CONTRAINDICATIONS

Not to be taken internally. Apply only to unbroken skin, withdraw on first sign of dermatitis. Avoid use on those with Arnica or other Compositae allergy (including chamomile, yarrow, Calendula).

SPECIAL WARNINGS AND PRECAUTIONS

Not for internal use. Not for prolonged application.

INTERACTIONS

Not known.

USE IN PREGNANCY AND LACTATION

For topical use only: no adverse effects expected if used within the recommended guidelines.

EFFECTS ON ABILITY TO DRIVE AND USE MACHINES

None known.

SIDE EFFECTS

Topical application of Arnica, mostly the tincture, has been known to cause allergic or irritant contact dermatitis since 1844. The sesquiterpene lactones are the proven sensitizing components. There have also been reports of crossreactivity to other Compositae plants.[25] Arnica ointments and plasters are considered to pose a much lower risk than other types of applications.[26] Prolonged treatment of damaged skin can cause oedematous dermatitis with the formation of pustules. Extended use may cause eczema. In treatment involving higher concentrations, primary toxic skin reactions with the formation of vesicles or even necrosis may occur.[27]

OVERDOSE

The symptoms of overdose after oral ingestion include dizziness, diarrhoea, trembling, increased heart rate, cardiac rhythm disturbances and collapse. Arnica poisoning has been observed to cause death due to circulatory paralysis with secondary respiratory arrest.[28] If taken internally, report to physician or hospital immediately.

Discontinue external application if dermatitis occurs.

CURRENT REGULATORY STATUS IN SELECTED COUNTRIES

A draft monograph of Arnica is being prepared and may appear subsequent to the 1997 edition of the *European Pharmacopoeia*.

Arnica for external use is covered by a positive Commission E monograph and has the following applications: injuries and accidents, for example, for haematomas, dislocations, sprains, bruising, oedema associated with fractures, in rheumatic muscle and joint complaints, inflammation of the mucous membranes of the mouth and throat, furuncles, inflamed insect bites and surface phlebitis.

Arnica is not on the UK General Sale List.

Arnica does not have GRAS status. However, it is freely available as a 'dietary supplement' in the USA under DSHEA legislation (1994 Dietary Supplement Health and Education Act).

Arnica for internal use is included in Part 4 of Schedule 4 of the Therapeutic Goods Act Regulations of Australia. External use of Arnica is unrestricted.

References

1. Grieve M. A modern herbal, vol 1. Dover Publications, New York, 1971, p 55.
2. Felter HW, Lloyd JU. King's American dispensatory, 18th edn, 3rd revision, vol 1, 1905. Reprinted by Eclectic Medical Publications, Portland, 1983, pp 279–281.
3. Felter HW. The eclectic materia medica, pharmacology and therapeutics, 1922. Reprinted by Eclectic Medical Publications, Portland, 1983, pp 206–207.
4. British Herbal Medicine Association's Scientific Committee. British herbal pharmacopoeia, BHMA, West York, 1983, p 31.
5. Sanderson L. How to make your own herbal cosmetics. Keats Publishing, New Canaan, 1977, p 51.
6. Chiej R. The Macdonald encyclopedia of medicinal plants. Macdonald, London, 1984, entry no. 40.
7. Launert EL. The Hamlyn guide to edible and medicinal plants of Britain and Northern Europe. Hamlyn, London, 1981, p 210.
8. Wagner H, Bladt S. Plant drug analysis: a thin layer chromatography atlas, 2nd edn. Springer-Verlag, Berlin, 1996, p 197.
9. Bisset NG (ed). Herbal drugs and phytopharmaceuticals. Medpharm Scientific Publishers, Stuttgart, 1994, pp 84–85.
10. De Smet PAGM, Keller K, Hansel R (eds). Adverse effects of herbal drugs, vol 1. Springer-Verlag, Berlin, 1992, pp 194, 238.
11. Hall IH, Starnes CO, Lee KH et al. J Pharm Sci 1980; 69 (5): 537–543.
12. Hall IH, Lee KH, Starnes CO et al. J Pharm Sci 1979; 68 (5): 537–542.
13. Kellner W, Kober W. Arzneim-Forsch 1955; 5: 224.
14. Willuhn G, Rottger PM, Quack W. Pharm Ztg 1982; 127: 2183–2185.
15. Reisch J et al. Arzneim-Forsch 1967; 17: 816.
16. Woerdenbag HJ, Merfort I, Passreiter CM et al. Planta Med 1994; 60 (5): 434–437.
17. Woerdenbag HJ, Merfort I, Schmidt TJ et al. Phytomed 1995; 2 (2): 127–132.
18. Hall IH, Lee KH, Starnes CO et al. J Pharm Sci 1978; 67 (9): 1235–1239.
19. Schroder H, Losche W, Strobach H et al. Thromb Res 1990; 57 (6): 839–845.
20. Brunelin-Geray J, Debelmas AM. Plant Med Phytother 1969; 3: 15–19.
21. Buschmann H. Fortschr Veterinaermed 1974; 20: 98–103.
22. Hall IH, Lee KH, Starnes CO et al. J Pharm Sci 1980; 69 (6): 694–697.
23. Quartz P, Landgrebe W, Wohling D et al. Paper presented at the 6th Phytotherapy Congress, Berlin, Oct 5–7, 1995.
24. Moog-Schulze JB. Tijdschr Integr Geneeskunde 1993; 9: 105–112.
25. Hormann HP, Korting HC. Phytomed 1994; 1: 161–171.
26. Hormann HP, Korting HC. Phytomed 1995; 4: 315–317.
27. German Federal Minister of Justice. German Commission E for human medicine monograph, Bundes-Anzeiger (German Federal Gazette) no. 228, dated 05.12.1984.
28. Hänsel R, Hass H. Therapie mit Phytopharmaka. Springer-Verlag, Berlin: 1983, p 272.

Astragalus
(*Astragalus membranaceus* (Fisch.) Bge.)

SYNONYMS

Membranous milk-vetch root (Engl, Astragali Radix (Lat), huang qi (Chin), ogi (Jap), hwanggi (Kor), astragel (Dan).

WHAT IS IT?

The root of *Astragalus membranaceus* has been used for many hundreds of years in traditional Chinese medicine. The *Pharmacopoeia* of the People's Republic of China defines *A. membranaceus* and *A. membranaceus* var. *mongholicus* (synonym: *A. mongholicus*) as the medicine Radix Astragali. Another species of the Astragalus genus which grows in the mountainous districts of Iran and Iraq yields tragacanth gum from its thorny stems. Although many species are used as forage for livestock and wild animals, some species (including the locoweeds) are known to cause intoxication in livestock which can be passed to humans through milk and meat. *Astragalus membranaceus* is not one of these selenium-accumulating species.

EFFECTS

Restores and strengthens the body's immune response; increases vitality.

TRADITIONAL VIEW

In traditional Chinese medicine Astragalus is classified as a herb that tonifies the *Qi* (energy) and *Blood* (nutrition), hence it is used for postpartum fever and recovery from severe loss of blood. It tonifies the *Spleen* (hence is used for fatigue linked to decreased appetite), raises the *Yang Qi* of the *Spleen* and *Stomach* (hence used for organ prolapse and uterine bleeding) and promotes urination, tissue healing and the discharge of pus. Its properties are sweet and slightly warm.[1] Traditionally, Astragalus would be taken as the powdered, dried root or as a decoction.

SUMMARY ACTIONS

Immunostimulant, tonic, adaptogenic, cardiotonic, diuretic, hypotensive, antioxidant.

CAN BE USED FOR

INDICATIONS SUPPORTED BY CLINICAL TRIALS

Impaired immunity especially if associated with leucopoenia; adjunct in treatment of cancer; viral infections including common cold, cervical erosion associated with herpes simplex virus infection.

TRADITIONAL THERAPEUTIC USES

Postpartum fever and recovery from severe loss of blood; fatigue; decreased appetite; organ prolapse, uterine bleeding; to raise vitality;[1] palpitation with shortness of breath; spontaneous sweating; prostration; chronic diarrhoea.[2]

MAY ALSO BE USED FOR

EXTRAPOLATIONS FROM PHARMACOLOGICAL STUDIES

General prevention of infection; autoimmune diseases; conditions resulting in immune suppression, e.g. patients receiving chemotherapy; viral infections (e.g. infection with Japanese encephalitis, coxsackie B2 and B3, parainfluenza virus type I, viral myocarditis); general debility; hypertension; protection against oxidative damage.

OTHER APPLICATIONS

Skin care, cosmetics and hair tonics for its healing, nourishing and vasodilating properties.[3]

PREPARATIONS

Dried root for decoction, liquid extract and tablets; powdered root.

DOSAGE

- 10–30 g per day of the dried root by decoction. Larger doses are used in traditional Chinese medicine as required, for example to treat paralysis.[1]
- 4–8 ml per day of the 1:2 liquid extract.

DURATION OF USE

May be taken long term for most applications but is contraindicated during acute infections.

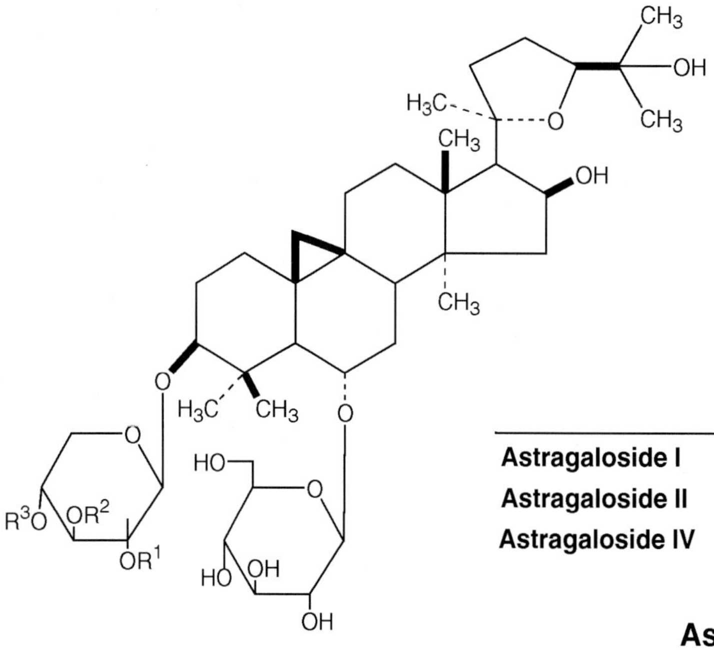

	R^1	R^2	R^3
Astragaloside I	$COCH_3$	$COCH_3$	H
Astragaloside II	$COCH_3$	H	H
Astragaloside IV	H	H	H

Astragalosides

SUMMARY ASSESSMENT OF SAFETY

No adverse effects are expected if used as recommended. Can aggravate acute infections.

TECHNICAL DATA

BOTANY

Astragalus is a member of the Leguminosae (pea) family, the Papilionoideae subfamily and grouped in the same tribe as the licorice genus.[4] *Astragalus mongholicus* is a perennial herb growing 60–150 cm high. The leaves are pinnate with 25–37 leaflets and elliptic. The racemes are axillary, the calyx is 5 mm long and tubular. The root is flexible, long and covered with a tough, wrinkled, yellowish-brown epidermis. The woody interior is of a yellowish-white colour.[5]

KEY CONSTITUENTS

- Triterpenoid saponins (astragalosides), flavonoids, polysaccharides.[6]
- Phytosterols, essential oil, amino acids (gamma-aminobutyric acid, canavanine).[7]

PHARMACODYNAMICS

Immune function

Astragalus markedly enhanced the cytotoxicity of natural killer cells,[8] potentiated interleukin-2-generated LAK (lymphokine-activated killer) cell cytotoxicity manifested by tumour cell lysis[9] and reversed tumour-associated macrophage suppression in urological tumours,[10] all in vitro. Using an in vitro local graft-versus-host reaction as a test assay for T-cell function, Astragalus extract restored the reaction in nine of 10 cancer patients.[11] Saponins from Astragalus stimulated the natural killer cell activity of human peripheral blood lymphocytes and restored steroid-inhibited natural killer cell activity, both in vitro.[12] Astragalus saponins reduced nicotinic acetylcholine receptor antibodies in blood cell cultures from myasthenia gravis patients.[13]

Oral doses of Astragalus in mice enhanced several aspects of immunity, including increased thymus weight, potentiation of phagocytic function, superoxide anion production by peritoneal macrophages and proliferation of splenocytes.[14] Protective effects on immune suppression in mice were observed after coadministration of Astragalus with a carcinogen.

Macrophage numbers and white cell function were raised to the same as or greater than normal levels.[15] Coadministration of Astragalus with an antitumour agent resulted in similar protection against the immunosuppression induced by the antitumour agent.[16] Oral administration of Astragalus (5 g/kg per day for 7 days) increased phagocytic activity[17] and significantly increased the lymphocyte transformation rate in a suppressed cellular immunity model.[18] Astragalus promoted interleukin-2 production in splenic lymphocytes of blood-deficient mice.[19] A protective effect of Astragalus extract after oral administration against Japanese encephalitis virus infection in mice was demonstrated. The authors proposed that the protective effect of Astragalus is based on a non-specific mechanism during the early stage of infection, before shifting to antibody production, and that macrophages play an important role by inducing the production of active oxygen.[20]

High oral doses of Astragalus decoction given to healthy subjects (15.6 g/day for 20 days) significantly increased serum IgM, IgE and cAMP.[21] Two months of oral treatment in subjects susceptible to the common cold greatly increased levels of IgA and IgG in nasal secretions and administration for 2 weeks or 2 months enhanced the induction of interferon by peripheral white blood cells.[22]

The polysaccharides of Astragalus show considerable immune-enhancing activity in vitro but whether this has relevance to oral use of Astragalus is questionable. Astragalus polysaccharides potentiated the immune-mediated antitumour activity of interleukin-2[23] and the activity of monocytes.[24] Astragalus polysaccharides improved the responses of lymphocytes from normal subjects and cancer patients[25] and enhanced natural killer cell activity of normal subjects and SLE patients.[26] The polysaccharide fraction F3 potentiated the lymphokine-activated killer cell-inducing activity of interleukin-2 in cancer and AIDS patients.[27]

Antiviral activity

The antiviral activity of Astragalus is most likely to be due to increased immunity and possibly enhanced interferon production.[2] In support of this, Astragalus demonstrated slight inhibitory activity against adenovirus type 7 in vitro. Natural and recombinant interferon enhanced the inhibitory activity of Astragalus.[28] It also promoted the production of interferon by mouse lung against parainfluenza virus type I and Newcastle disease virus in vitro.[29] Astragalus exhibited potent hepatitis B surface antigen-inactivating activity in vitro,[30] inhibited the activity of murine retroviral reverse transcriptase and human DNA polymerases[31] and had a protective effect on cultured beating heart cells infected with coxsackie B2 virus.[32]

Oral or intranasal administration of Astragalus decoction protected mice from infection with parainfluenza virus type I.[14,22,33] Results from a series of in vivo experiments indicated that the effect of Astragalus resembled that of both bronchitis vaccine and the interferon mediator tilorone.[22]

Astragalus increased the survival rate and improved some abnormal electrophysiological parameters in acute coxsackie B3 viral myocarditis in vivo.[34] In vitro and in vivo studies indicate Astragalus may act by decreasing the secondary damage caused by calcium ion influx, thereby improving the abnormal myocardial electric activity, as well as inhibiting the replication of coxsackie B3 virus RNA in the myocardium.[35,36]

In contrast with other work, an inhibitory effect on virus RNA replication in vivo was not correlated with the induction of beta-interferon[37] but was greater than a calcium channel blocker (verapamil) and a steroidal antiinflammatory drug (dexamethasone) in vitro.[38] Routine therapy combined with oral administration of Astragalus to viral myocarditis patients significantly enhanced immune parameters when compared to patients receiving routine therapy alone.[39]

Adaptogenic and tonic activity

Addition of Astragalus enhanced growth, metabolism and longevity in cell cultures.[2] It lowered oxygen consumption in mitochondria, enhanced tolerance to stress and prolonged the life of human embryonic kidney cells in culture.[40]

Administration of Astragalus over 2 weeks to mice markedly increased plasma cAMP.[41]

Astragalus decoction improved learning performance in animal maze tests[42] and improved memory in two models (50 g/kg per day, 7 days, intragastric).[43] Administration over 15 days inhibited field search behaviour, decreased spontaneous activity and increased sleep time.[42] Decoction of Astragalus improved endurance in mice and increased weight gain compared to controls.[1] A mixture of ginseng and Astragalus demonstrated antifatigue activity in mice. This activity was partly due to an improvement of energy metabolism.[44] Oral administration of Astragalus increased the turnover of proteins in serum and liver in animals treated daily for 10 days.[45] Astragalus lowered collagen content in the aorta and lung of old rats to near levels found in young animals.[46] Oral administration of Astragalus increased plasma cAMP in healthy subjects.[47]

Cardiovascular activity

Astragalus saponins demonstrated a positive inotropic action on the isolated heart and decreased the resting potential of cultured myocardial cells, suggesting the inotropic effect may be exerted through modulation of Na^+–K^+–ATPase.[48]

Oral administration of aqueous extract of Astragalus countered the rise in blood pressure and plasma renin activity in a hypertensive model.[49] Intragastric administration of Astragalus produced a hypotensive effect in another experimental model.[50] Gamma-aminobutyric acid was isolated as the hypotensive constituent.[51]

Cardiac output increased in 20 patients with angina pectoris after 2 weeks of treatment with Astragalus.[52] Astragalus strengthened left ventricular function and had an anti-OFR (oxygen free radical) effect in acute myocardial infarction patients compared to controls. The decrease in the preejection period: left ventricular ejection time ratio was closely correlated with the increased superoxide dismutase activity of red blood cells and the decreased lipid peroxidation of plasma. This anti-OFR activity of Astragalus may be one of the mechanisms behind its cardiotonic activity.[53]

Haemorrheological activity

Astragalus extract demonstrated a protective effect on erythrocyte deformability in vitro for blood taken from normal subjects and patients with systemic lupus erythematosus.[54] Astragalus significantly enriched the blood as measured by improvement in haemorrheological indexes,[55] and, in a 'blood stagnation' experimental model, decreased whole-blood specific viscosity and increased plasma specific viscosity.[56]

Hepatoprotective activity

Astragalus saponins were protective against chemically induced liver injury in vitro and in vivo.[57] Astragalus exhibited hepatoprotective activity and increased the activity of hepatic lysozymes, tissue dehydrogenase and liver glycogen.[58–60]

Antioxidant activity

Astragalus flavonoids demonstrated a protective effect on mammalian cell damage caused by the hydroxyl radical, inhibited lipid peroxides and increased superoxide dismutase activity in vitro.[61] Three Astragalus saponins demonstrated superoxide anion scavenging activity in vitro.[62]

Other activity

Astragalus inhibited aldose reductase,[63] promoted the replication of hepatic DNA,[64] inhibited mitochondrial oxygen consumption caused by lipid peroxidation[65] and stimulated the motility of human sperm[66] in vitro. Methanolic extract of Astragalus strongly inhibited the growth of the human intestinal bacterium *Clostridium perfringens* in vitro.[67]

Oral administration of Astragalus normalized the imbalance in intestinal flora in an experimental model of senility.[68]

Oral administration of a concentrated solution of Astragalus strengthened small intestine movement and muscle tonus, especially in the jejunum.[69] This activity supports its traditional use in organ prolapse.

Oral administration of Astragalus increased urine output and sodium excretion[70] and demonstrated a protective effect against experimental nephritis by markedly reducing proteinuria and nephrosis.[71]

Coincubation with *Astragalus membranaceus* and *Ligustrum lucidum* abolished the suppressed macrophage function in murine renal cell carcinoma cultures. Intraperitoneal injection of a preparation containing 500 μg of each herb to tumour-bearing mice resulted in increased survival rate compared to controls. The antitumour activity may have been exerted via augmentation of phagocyte and LAK cell activities.[72]

PHARMACOKINETICS

No data available.

CLINICAL TRIALS

Immune function

Patients with small cell lung cancer underwent long-term treatment with chemotherapy, radiotherapy, immunotherapy and herbal medicine consisting of *Panax ginseng* leaf and Astragalus root in an open trial. The combined treatment raised the survival rates considerably, with some patients gaining 3–17 years in survival.[73]

In an open randomized clinical trial, 115 patients with leucopaenia received a high dose of a concentrated Astragalus preparation (equivalent to 30 g of Astragalus per day) or a low dose (equivalent to 10 g per day) over a period of 8 weeks. There was a significant rise of average WBC counts in both groups after treatment ($p<0.001$). The average WBC count for the high-dose group was significantly higher than for the low-dose group ($p<0.05$). On the basis of these findings, the author suggested that Astragalus is an effective treatment for leucopaenia and increasing the dosage could enhance its effectiveness.[74] In an open study, 1000 subjects received Astragalus either orally, as a nasal spray or in a compound formula. A prophylactic effect for the common cold was observed, as evidenced by decreased incidence and shortened duration of infection.[22]

In a comparative clinical study, shen-qi (ginseng-Astragalus) injection used with chemotherapy reduced toxic chemotherapy effects, increased body weight and increased cellular immune function compared to chemotherapy alone in 176 patients with malignant tumours of the digestive tract.[75]

Antiviral activity

Administration of Astragalus in an open trial to a large number of patients with chronic viral hepatitis resulted in a success rate of 70%. In most cases, elevated serum GPT levels returned to normal after 1–2 months.[76]

In a double-blind clinical trial, 235 patients with typical chronic cervicitis (associated with viral infection) received one of the following substances applied locally by gauze: two groups using recombinant interferon-alpha-1 (at 5 µg or 10 µg), both interferon (5 µg) and Astragalus extract (0.5 ml of a 1:1 extract) or Astragalus alone (0.5 ml of a 1:1 extract). These treatments were applied twice per week for 3 weeks. The Astragalus plus interferon group showed a similar improvement to the higher dose interferon group, with approximately 60% of patients demonstrating complete cure or marked improvement. Only 8% of patients treated with Astragalus alone had marked improvement and no patients were completely cured. These results suggest that Astragalus acted synergistically with interferon therapy.[77] An earlier double-blind trial showed a similar result for 164 patients with cervical erosion associated with herpes simplex virus infection.[78]

Natural killer activity increased significantly in patients with coxsackie B viral myocarditis treated with intramuscular injections of Astragalus for 3–4 months. General condition and symptoms improved and alpha- and gamma-interferon levels increased in comparison with pretreatment levels. Patients treated with conventional therapy demonstrated no improvement.[79]

Other conditions

Astragalus and *Angelica sinensis* root together with a high-protein diet improved protein imbalance and serum protein in nephrotic patients in an uncontrolled study.[80]

In a comparative trial, 92 patients suffering from ischaemic heart disease were treated with Astragalus, *Salvia miltiorrhiza* or the antianginal drug nifedipine. Results were superior for the Astragalus-treated group, as demonstrated by marked relief from angina pectoris and improvement in several objective clinical parameters. The treatment of ischaemic heart disease by Astragalus was significantly more effective compared to the control group ($p< 0.05$).[81]

In a double-blind, placebo-controlled clinical trial of 507 elderly people, oral administration of Astragalus in combination with *Polygonum multiflorum* and *Salvia miltiorrhiza* demonstrated significant anti-ageing effects. Improvements were noted in vigour, strength, vision, cellular immunity and serum lipofuscin levels. The total effective rate was 76.6% compared to 34.5% for placebo ($p<0.001$).[82]

TOXICOLOGY

Aqueous extract of Astragalus at a level of 1.25 mg/ml modestly increased the incidence (16%) of aberrant cells in vitro.[83] No adverse effects were observed within 48 hours after oral administration of Astragalus at 75 and 100 g/kg. The LD_{50} of Astragalus in mice by the intraperitoneal route was determined to be 39.8 g/kg.[2]

CONTRAINDICATIONS

Not advisable in acute infections.

SPECIAL WARNINGS AND PRECAUTIONS

None.

INTERACTIONS

None known.

USE IN PREGNANCY AND LACTATION

No adverse effects expected.

EFFECTS ON ABILITY TO DRIVE AND USE MACHINES

No adverse effects.

SIDE EFFECTS

None known.

OVERDOSE

Not known.

CURRENT REGULATORY STATUS IN SELECTED COUNTRIES

Astragalus is official in the *Pharmacopoeia* of the Republic of China (English edition, 1997) and the *Japanese Pharmacopoeia* (English edition, 1996).

Astragalus is not covered by a Commission E monograph and is not on the UK General Sale List.

Astragalus does not have GRAS status. However, it is freely available as a 'dietary supplement' in the USA under DSHEA legislation (1994 Dietary Supplement Health and Education Act).

Astragalus is not included in Part 4 of Schedule 4 of the Therapeutic Goods Act Regulations of Australia.

References

1. Bensky D, Gamble A. Chinese herbal medicine materia medica. Eastland Press, Seattle, 1986, pp 457–459.
2. Chang H, But P. Pharmacology and applications of Chinese materia medica, vol 2. World Scientific, Singapore, 1987, pp 1041–1046.
3. Leung AY, Foster S. Encyclopedia of common natural ingredients used in food, drugs and cosmetics, 2nd edn. John Wiley, New York, 1996, p 52.
4. Mabberley DJ. The plant book, 2nd edn. Cambridge University Press, Cambridge, 1997, pp 64, 396–398.
5. World Health Organization. Medicinal plants in China. World Health Organization, Regional Office for the Western Pacific, Manilla, 1989, p 47.
6. Tang W, Eisenbrand G. Chinese drugs of plant origin. Springer Verlag, Berlin, 1992, pp 191–197.
7. Katsura E, Katoh Y, Yamagishi T. Hokkaidoritsu Eisei Kenkyushoho 1983; 33: 136–137.
8. Jing JP, Lin WF. Chin J Microbiol Immunol 1983; 3: 293–296.
9. Wang Y, Qian XJ, Hadley HR et al. Mol Biother 1992; 4 (3): 143–146.
10. Rittenhouse JR, Lui PD, Lau BHS et al. J Urol (Paris) 1991; 146 (2): 486–490.
11. Sun Y, Hersh EM, Talpaz M et al. Cancer 1983; 52 (1): 70–73.
12. You L, Zhou Y, Zhang Y et al. Zhongguo Mianyixue Zazhi 1990; 6 (1): 60–63.
13. Tu LH, Huang DR, Zhang RQ et al. Chin Med J (Engl) 1994; 107 (4): 300–303.
14. Sugiura H, Nishida H, Inaba R et al. Nippon Eiseigaku Zasshi 1993; 47 (6): 1021–1031.
15. Jin R, Mitsuishi T, Akuzawa Y et al. Kitakanto Med J 1994; 44 (2): 125–133.
16. Jin R, Wan LL, Mitsuishi T. Chung Kuo Chung Hsi I Chieh Ho Tsa Chih 1995; 15 (2): 101–103.
17. Isotopes Laboratory, Beijing Institute of Tuberculosis. Xinyiyaexue Zazhi 1974; 8: 12.
18. Wang JY, Zhong JX, Zhou ZH et al. Chin J Integr Trad West Med 1987; 7 (9): 543.
19. Chen YC. Chung Kuo Chung Yao Tsa Chih 1994; 19(2): 739–741.
20. Kajimura K, Takagi Y, Ueba N et al. Biol Pharm Bull 1996; 19 (9): 1166–1169.
21. Institute of Basic Medical Sciences, Chinese Academy of Medical Sciences. Chung Hua I Hsueh Tsa Chih 1979; 59: 31–34.
22. Institute of Epidemic Prevention, Chinese Academy of Medical Sciences: Med Commun 1978; 4: 4.
23. Chu D, Sun Y, Lin J et al. Chung Hsi I Chieh Ho Tsa Chih 1990; 10 (1): 34–36.
24. Chu DT, Sun Y, Lin JR. Chung Hsi I Chieh Ho Tsa Chih: 1989; 9 (6): 351–354.
25. Wang DC. Chung Hua Chung Liu Tsa Chih 1989; 11 (3): 180–183.
26. Zhao XZ. Chung Kuo Chung Hsi I Chieh Ho Tsa Chih 1992; 12: 669–671, 645
27. Chu DT, Lin JR, Wong W. Chung Hua Chung Liu Tsa Chih 1994; 16 (3): 167–171.
28. Peng J, Wu SH, Zhang LL et al. Zhongguo Yixue Kexueyuan Xuebao 1984; 6 (2): 116–119.
29. Institute of Epidemic Prevention, Chinese Academy of Medical Sciences. Studies on Epidemic Prevention 1976; 3: 204.
30. Zheng MS et al. Chin Trad Herbal Drugs 1987; 18 (10): 459–461.
31. Ono K, Nakane H, Meng ZK et al. Chem Pharm Bull (Tokyo) 1989; 37 (7): 1810–1812.
32. Yuan WL, Chen HZ, Yang YZ et al. Chin Med J (Engl) 1990; 103 (3): 177–182.
33. Institute of Epidemic Prevention, Chinese Academy of Medical Sciences. Studies on Epidemic Prevention 1976; 2: 124.
34. Rui T, Yang YZ, Zhou TS. Chung Kuo Chung Hsi I Chieh Ho Tsa Chih 1994; 14 (5): 262, 292–294.
35. Peng TQ, Yang YZ, Kandolf R. Chung Kuo Chung Hsi I Chieh Ho Tsa Chih 1994; 14 (11): 664–666.
36. Guo Q, Peng TQ, Yang YZ. Chung Kuo Chung Hsi I Chieh Ho Tsa Chih 1995; 15 (8): 483–485.
37. Peng T, Yang Y, Riesemann H et al. Chin Med Sci J 1995; 10 (3): 146–150.
38. Guo Q, Peng T, Yang Y et al. Virologia Sinica 1996; 11 (1): 40–44.
39. Huang ZQ, Qin NP, Ye W. Chung Kuo Chung Hsi I Chieh Ho Tsa Chih 1995; 15 (6): 328–330.
40. Xiong ZY. Zhejiang J Trad Chin Med 1983; 18 (5): 235–238.
41. Isotopes Section of the Pharmacology Department, Basic Sciences Research Unit, Capital Hospital of the Chinese Academy of Medical Sciences et al. Med Res Commun 1977; 10: 27.
42. Pan SY, Hou JY, Jiang MY et al. Chung Yao Tung Pao 1986; 11 (9): 559–561.
43. Hong GX, Qin WC, Huang LS. Chung Kuo Chung Yao Tsa Chih 1994; 19 (11): 687–688, 704.
44. Nagai K, Hanazuka M, Hizume S et al. Jap Pharmacol Therapeut 1992; 20 (9): 47–53.
45. Liu J et al. Chin Trad Herbal Drugs 1981; 12 (6): 264–265.
46. Xu P, Jin G, Shen X. Chung-Kuo Chung Yao Tsa Chih 1991; 16 (1): 49–50.
47. Institute of Basic Medical Sciences, Chinese Academy of Medical Sciences. Zhonghua Yixue Zazhi 1979; 1: 23.
48. Wang Q. Chung Kuo Chung Yao Tsa Chih 1992; 17 (9): 557–559.
49. Song DJ, Gu DG, Mao SY et al. Chin Trad Herbal Drugs 1989; 20 (8): 361–364.
50. Chengdu Institute for Drug Control. Chengdu Medical and Health Information 1971; 1: 90.
51. Hikino H, Funayama S, Endo K. Planta Med 1976; 30 (4): 297–302.
52. Lei ZY, Qin H, Liao JZ. Chung Kuo Chung Hsi I Chieh Ho Tsa Chih 1994; 14 (4): 199–202.
53. Chen LX, Liao JZ, Guo WQ. Chung Kuo Chung Hsi I Chieh Ho Tsa Chih 1995; 15 (3): 141–143.
54. Dai JH, Liang ZJ, Qin WZ et al. Guizhou Med J 1987; 11 (1): 23–24.
55. Xue JX, Jiang Y, Yan YQ. Chung Kuo Chung Yao Tsa Chih 1993; 18 (10): 621–630, 640.
56. Xue JX, Yan YQ, Jiang Y. Chung Kuo Chung Yao Tsa Chih 1994; 19 (2): 108–110, 128.
57. Zhang YD, Shen JP, Zhu SH et al. Yao Hsueh Hsueh Pao 1992; 27(6): 401–406.
58. Han DW, Xu RL, Yeung SCS. Abst Chin Med 1988; 2 (1): 114–115.
59. Zhang ZL, Wen QZ, Liu CX et al. J Ethnopharmacol 1990; 30 (2): 145–150.

60. Yan XW et al. 1962 Symposium of the Chinese Pharmaceutical Association 1962, p 332.
61. Wang D, Shen W, Tian Y et al. Chung Kuo Chung Yao Tsa Chih 1995; 20 (4): 240–242, 254.
62. Liu XJ, Jiang M, Yu Z et al. Tianran Chanwu Yanjiu Yu Kaifa 1991; 3 (4): 1–6.
63. Zhang JQ, Zhou YP. China J Chin Materia Medica 1989; 14 (9): 557–559.
64. Mu DW. Yixueyanjiu Tongxun 1985; 10: 289–290.
65. Hong CY, Lo YC, Tan FC et al. Am J Chin Med 1994; 22 (1): 63–70.
66. Hong CY, Ku J, Wu P. Am J Chin Med 1992; 20 (3–4): 289–294.
67. Ahn YJ, Kwon JH, Chae SH et al. Micro Ecol Health Dis 1994; 7 (5): 257–261.
68. Yan M, Song H, Xie N et al. Chung Kuo Chung Yao Tsa Chih 1995; 20 (10): 624–626.
69. Yang DZ. Chung Kuo Chung Hsi I Chieh Ho Tsa Chih 1993; 13 (10): 582, 616–617.
70. Deng ZF et al. Chin Med J 1961; 1: 7.
71. Jia JS et al. 2nd National Symposium on Pathophysiology of the Chinese Society of Physiology, 1963, p 63.
72. Lau BHS, Ruckle HC, Botolazzo T et al. Cancer Biother 1994; 9 (2): 153–161.
73. Cha RJ, Zeng DW, Chang QS et al. Chung Hua Nei Ko Tsa Chih 1994; 33 (7): 462–466.
74. Weng XS. Chung Kuo Chung Hsi I Chieh Ho Tsa Chih 1995; 15 (8): 462–464.
75. Li NQ. Chung Kuo Chung Hsi I Chieh Ho Tsa Chih 1992; 12 (10): 579, 588–592.
76. Zhou QJ. Chinese medicinal herb in the treatment of viral hepatitis. In: Chang HM, Yeung HW, Tso WW et al (eds) Advances in Chinese medicinal materials research. World Scientific, Singapore, 1985, p 216.
77. Qian ZW, Mao SJ, Cai XC et al. Chin Med J 1990; 103 (8): 647–651.
78. Qian ZW, Mao SJ, Cai XC et al. Chin J Integr Trad West Med 1987; 7 (5): 268–269, 287.
79. Yang YZ, Jin PY, Guo Q et al. Chin Med J 1990; 103 (4): 304–307.
80. Li L, Yu H, Pan J. Chung Hua Nei Ko Tsa Chih 1995; 34 (10): 670–672.
81. Li SQ, Yuan RX, Gao H. Chung Kuo Chung Hsi I Chieh Ho Tsa Chih 1995; 15 (2): 77–80.
82. Du X, Zhang ZL. Chung Hsi I Chieh Ho Tsa Chih 1986; 6 (5): 258–259, 271–274.
83. Tadaki S, Yamada S, Miyazawa N et al. Jap J Toxicol Environ Health 1995; 41 (6): 463–469.

Bearberry (*Arctostaphylos uva ursi* (L) Spreng.)

SYNONYMS

Arctostaphylos officinalis Wimm., *Arbutus uva ursi* L. (botanical synonyms), mountain cranberry, green manzanita, uva ursi (Engl), Uvae ursi folium (Lat), Bärentraube (Ger), busserole, raisin d'ours (Fr), uva d'orso, uva ursina (Ital), melbær (Dan).

WHAT IS IT?

The Arctostaphylos genus contains 50 species which are indigenous to western North America, *A. uva ursi* has circumpolar distribution and is found in central and northern Europe as well as in North America.[1,2] Bearberry leaves have been used as a urinary antiseptic in the UK since the 13th century.[1] It is also a traditional herb of the Native Americans who used the leaves for ceremonial smoking. However, their main use was in the form of a tea to treat venereal disease and inflammation of the genitourinary tract.[3] The berries of *Arctostaphylos species* have provided food not only for wildlife such as birds and bears but also for humans. *Arctostaphylos species* suppress the growth of neighbouring plants due to the hydroquinone formed from the arbutin in their leaves, bark and roots.[3]

EFFECTS

Antibacterial, astringent and antiinflammatory effects in the genitourinary tract.

TRADITIONAL VIEW

Bearberry was traditionally used for its astringent property and was considered of great value in diseases of the bladder and kidneys, strengthening and imparting tone to the urinary passages and alleviating inflammation of the urinary tract.[4] Uses by Eclectic physicians included chronic irritation of the bladder, enuresis, excessive mucous and bloody discharges in the urine, chronic diarrhoea, dysentery, menorrhagia, leucorrhoea, diabetes, chronic gonorrhoea and strangury.[5]

SUMMARY ACTIONS

Urinary antiseptic, astringent, antiinflammatory.

CAN BE USED FOR

INDICATIONS SUPPORTED BY CLINICAL TRIALS

Cystitis, recurrent cystitis (in conjunction with other herbs).

TRADITIONAL THERAPEUTIC USES

Urinary infections such as cystitis, urethritis, prostatitis, pyelitis; lithuria; diarrhoea and intestinal irritations; any condition requiring an astringent action including chronic diarrhoea. The specific indication listed in the *British Herbal Pharmacopoeia* 1983 is acute catarrhal cystitis with dysuria and highly acid urine[6] but in light of recent pharmacological data, the requirement for acidic urine may not be correct.

MAY ALSO BE USED FOR

EXTRAPOLATIONS FROM PHARMACOLOGICAL STUDIES

Internally and externally as adjuvant treatment of inflammatory conditions such as contact dermatitis, inflammatory oedema and arthritis.

OTHER APPLICATIONS

Whitening agent for the skin and may assist in the control of hyperpigmentary disorders.[7]

PREPARATIONS

Dried leaves as a cold infusion or liquid extract for internal or external use. Cold water extraction of powdered leaves results in better levels of arbutin and lower levels of tannins compared to hot water extraction.[8]

DOSAGE

- Up to 12 g dried leaf per day, equivalent to 400–840 mg arbutin prepared as an infusion or cold macerate.
- Bearberry tablets (0.7 g, standardized to contain 70 mg arbutin): two tablets, 2–3 times per day.
- 4–8 ml of 1:2 liquid extract per day, 10–17 ml of 1:5 tincture per day.

Studies have shown that the antimicrobial effect of bearberry occurs when the urine has an alkaline pH.

However, the majority of urinary tract infections produce an acid urine. Alkalinization of the urine may therefore be beneficial in conjunction with herbal therapy using bearberry. This can be achieved, at least in the short term, by concurrent administration of bicarbonate or proprietary urinary alkalinizing products. An alkaline-forming diet, high in fruit and vegetables, could also be taken during treatment. Consumption of plenty of water during treatment is also advised.

DURATION OF USE

Due to its high tannin content, bearberry is not suitable for prolonged internal use.

SUMMARY ASSESSMENT OF SAFETY

There is a very low risk associated with the short-term administration of bearberry but its use should be avoided during pregnancy and lactation.

TECHNICAL DATA

BOTANY

Arctostaphylos uva ursi is a small, evergreen, prostrate, mat-forming shrub belonging to the Ericaceae (heath) family. The leathery leaves are alternate, obovate from a wedge-shaped base, 1–2 cm long, dark green on the upper surface and pale green underneath. The small pink flowers with a bell-shaped corolla are arranged in drooping clusters. The fruit is shiny, small, round and scarlet-red.[4,9]

KEY CONSTITUENTS

- Hydroquinone glycosides (4–15%),[10] including arbutin and methylarbutin.[11]
- Polyphenols (predominantly gallotannins); phenolic acids, flavonoids, triterpenes.[11]

Interestingly, arbutin is found at high concentrations in some plants capable of surviving extreme and sustained dehydration.[12]

The *German Pharmacopoeia* (DAB 10) sets a lower limit of 6% for arbutin content. Bearberry samples containing less than 6% arbutin should be regarded as adulterated and probably contain other species of Arctostaphylos.

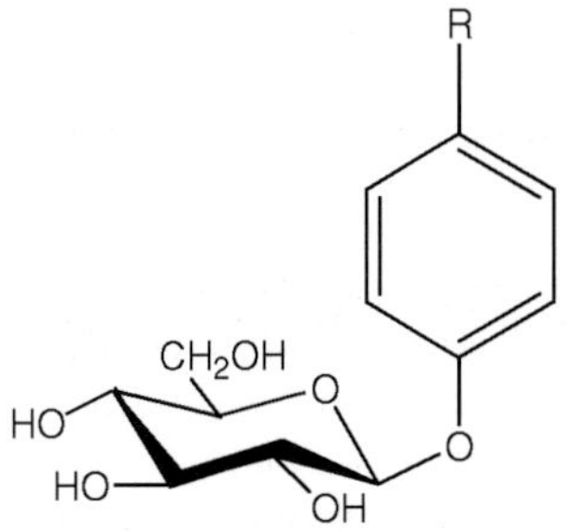

R

CH$_2$OH

HO

HO

O

O

OH

	R
Arbutin	OH
Methylarbutin	OCH_3

Hydroquinone derivatives

PHARMACODYNAMICS

Antimicrobial activity

There is some debate as to whether the antimicrobial effect of bearberry is due to hydroquinone esters such as arbutin or free hydroquinone.[11] The antimicrobial activity of arbutin and aqueous extract of bearberry were tested in vitro against bacterial strains implicated in urinary tract infections. The antibacterial activity of arbutin was directly correlated with the beta-glucosidase activity of the bacteria. (This enzyme converts arbutin into free hydroquinone.) The highest enzyme activity was found in Streptococcus, Klebsiella and Enterobacter, the lowest in *E. coli*.[13] Arbutin (128 mg/l) inhibited three of eight clinical isolates of *Pseudomonas aeruginosa* tested in vitro.[14] Arbutin and hydroquinone inhibited the growth of *Ureaplasma urealyticum* and *Mycoplasma hominis* in vitro.[15] These bacteria are associated with non-gonococcal urethritis.

Piceoside, a glucoside isolated from bearberry, did not demonstrate antibacterial activity in vitro, but its aglycone p-hydroxyacetophenone showed activity against *Proteus vulgaris, Enterobacter aerogenes* and *Bacillus subtilis*.[16] Bearberry extracts have shown antimicrobial activity in vitro against *Escherichia coli, Proteus vulgaris, Enterobacter aerogenes, Streptococcus faecalis, Staphylococcus aureus, Salmonella typhi* and *Candida albicans*.[17] The summer and autumn leaves are more potent than the winter leaves.[18]

The antibacterial activity of various agents was tested in vitro using 74 different strains of bacteria isolated from the urinary tract including *E. coli, Proteus mirabilis, Pseudomonas aeruginosa, Staphylococcus aureus* and species of Enterobacter, Citrobacter and Klebsiella. Urine was collected from healthy volunteers 3 hours after oral administration of 0.1 g or 1.0 g of arbutin;

several synthetic antibiotics were also tested. Of all test substances, only gentamicin, nalidixic acid and urine collected after intake of 1.0 g of arbutin and adjusted to pH 8 were active against all strains used.[19]

A study of the dry leaf extract of bearberry on the course of acute bacterial pyelonephritis (caused by *E. coli*) in white rats showed that, at a dose of 25 mg/kg, bearberry extract had a marked antibacterial and nephroprotective effect.[20]

Samples of normal urine and urine collected from healthy subjects who had consumed bearberry tea were compared for resistance to bacterial contamination. Urine from bearberry tea drinkers was more bacteriostatic than normal urine samples. However, the addition of arbutin to normal urine did not result in the same bacteriostatic activity. A series of solutions were then tested for inhibition of growth of strains of *Staph. aureus* and *E. coli* in vitro. The samples included hydroquinone, methylhydroquinone and arbutin solutions, normal urine and urine from bearberry tea drinkers, all at normal pH and pH elevated to 8.0 by the addition of potassium hydroxide. Only hydroquinone or methylhydroquinone solutions inhibited bacterial growth at normal pH. However, incubation of bacteria with bearberry tea drinkers' urine at pH 8 also resulted in inhibition of bacterial growth. The inhibitory effect could also be achieved at pH 8 by urine from subjects given pure arbutin.[21] The authors concluded that antibacterial activity will only occur when the excretion products of arbutin (hydroquinone paired with glucuronate and sulphate) appear in sufficiently high concentrations in an alkaline urine. It was suggested that, at an alkaline pH, these excretion products of arbutin release small amounts of free hydroquinone in the presence of bacteria, thereby rendering antibacterial activity to the urine. The maximum antibacterial effect from the hydroquinone glucuronides and sulphate formed from arbutin is obtained about 3–4 hours after taking the herb.[22] Free hydroquinone is only excreted in trace amounts, which is desirable given the toxic potential of this agent.

Urine produced by a healthy individual on a meat and fish diet is in the pH range 4.5–6.0; a vegetarian diet will make urine more alkaline. A urine of pH > 7 during a urinary tract infection indicates infection by a microorganism capable of urea splitting, with release of ammonia.[23] Urea-splitting organisms include *Proteus spp*, *Klebsiella spp*, some *Citrobacter spp*, some *Haemophilus spp*, *Bilophila wadsworthia*, the yeast *Cryptococcus neoformans* and several other bacteria and fungi.[24] On the basis of the above research, infection with these organisms should be susceptible to treatment with bearberry. Alkalinization of the urine with buffering agents such as Ural (containing sodium bicarbonate, sodium citrate, citric acid and tartaric acid) in conjunction with bearberry intake may prove to be clinically effective for the treatment of cystitis caused by non-urea splitting bacteria.

Antiinflammatory and antiallergic activities

Arbutin inhibited phospholipase A_2 after partial rehydration of lyophilized liposomes in vitro but did not inhibit the enzyme in the presence of excess water.[12] Coadministration of arbutin (oral) and indomethacin (subcutaneous) showed an inhibitory effect on swelling in a delayed-type hypersensitivity model which was stronger than that of indomethacin alone.[25] In the same model, arbutin plus prednisolone or dexamethasone showed stronger effects than either of the antiinflammatory drugs alone.[26] Arbutin may therefore have a synergistic antiinflammatory activity on type IV allergic reaction-induced inflammation. In the same model, oral administration of bearberry methanolic extract (100 mg/kg) demonstrated an inhibitory effect on swelling. When administered simultaneously with subcutaneous prednisolone, the inhibitory effect was more potent than that of prednisolone alone.[27]

Although ointments containing 1% and 2% aqueous extract of bearberry did not inhibit the ear swelling caused by experimentally induced contact dermatitis or carrageenan-induced paw oedema in rats and mice, they did increase the antiinflammatory effect of a steroid ointment (dexamethasone). The coadministration of bearberry did not increase the side effects of dexamethasone.[28] Topical doses of bearberry might also increase the antiinflammatory effects of other steroid-like compounds such as plant-derived saponins.

Effect on melanin synthesis

Arbutin at a concentration of 5×10^{-5} M decreased melanin content to approximately 39% when compared to untreated melanoma cells in vitro, without affecting cell growth. Tyrosinase activity also dropped significantly in the arbutin-treated cells. (This enzyme is involved in melanin synthesis). Arbutin was not hydrolysed to hydroquinone, suggesting that the observed inhibitory effect was for arbutin itself, not hydroquinone.[29] Further studies have revealed that the depigmenting mechanism of arbutin in humans involves inhibition of melanosomal tyrosinase activity, rather than the suppression of expression and synthesis of tyrosinase.[30]

A 50% methanolic extract of bearberry inhibited melanin synthesis in vitro. Both the bearberry extract and arbutin had an inhibitory effect on tyrosinase activity and inhibited the production of melanin by both tyrosinase and autoxidation.[7] Bearberry extract could have a bleaching effect on freckles and may assist in the control of hyperpigmentary disorders.

Other activity

Oral doses of arbutin (50 mg/kg) suppressed experimentally induced cough reflex. The effect of arbutin was stronger than that of the non-narcotic antitussive dropropizine and comparable to that of codeine.[31]

Oral administration of a bearberry infusion (3 g/l) to healthy rats fed a standard diet containing calcium (8 g/kg) and magnesium (2 g/kg) did not induce significant diuresis, nor affect calcium or citrate concentration levels.[32]

Aqueous and methanolic extracts of bearberry have demonstrated molluscicidal activity against the freshwater snail *Biomphalaria glabrata* (the intermediate host of schistosomiasis). The methanol extract was active at a concentration of 50 ppm.[33]

A methanol extract of bearberry showed algicidal activity when tested in ponds. It is believed the tannins precipitated the algal proteins.[34]

PHARMACOKINETICS

Arbutin is easily hydrolysed by dilute acids (e.g. after oral ingestion), yielding D-glucose and hydroquinone, but gallotannin prevents enzymes such as beta-glucosidase from splitting arbutin.[35] Beta-glucosidase is not present in mammalian cells but is present in some microorganisms which occur in the gastrointestinal tract or possibly in the infected urinary tract.[36]

Urinary excretion of phenolic metabolites after oral administration of either bearberry leaf tea or arbutin occurs within 1–2 hours and reaches a maximum 4 hours after administration. In healthy subjects given bearberry tea, 70–75% of the administered dose was excreted within 24 hours. Arbutin is altered after passage through the body; it only occurs in trace amounts in urine when high doses are given and free hydroquinone is only excreted in trace amounts, if at all. It is suggested that arbutin is hydrolysed to free hydroquinone in the stomach or intestine, is conjugated by phase II liver enzymes and appears in the urine paired with glucuronate or sulphate.[21]

In a crossover study with six healthy volunteers, enteric-coated bearberry tablets demonstrated the same bioavailability within a 24-hour period as an equivalent bearberry extract. The release of arbutin metabolites was retarded by at least 3 hours with the tablets. In a pilot study conducted prior to this main study, no free hydroquinone was found in the urine of volunteers, although the above hydroquinone derivatives were found.[37] This study was designed to compare the bioavailability of enterically coated tablets containing bearberry extract with uncoated tablets.

Some other studies investigating the elimination of arbutin in rats have arrived at different conclusions, which casts doubt on their validity. In these studies, orally administered arbutin was excreted unchanged in urine[38] and oral administration of bearberry tea resulted in elimination of six unidentified phenolic compounds, but no hydroquinone. No degradation products were observed after perfusion of isolated rat liver with arbutin, thus leading to the conclusion that it was hydrolysed in the kidneys.[39] The results of these studies are not supported by the above human studies. Moreover, in the case of the orally administered arbutin, the authors may have actually measured arbutin metabolites and mistakenly assigned them as arbutin. Arbutin is probably hydrolysed in the digestive tract of humans, not the liver or kidneys.

CLINICAL TRIALS

Urinary disorders

In a double-blind, placebo-controlled, randomized clinical trial, 57 women who had experienced at least three episodes of cystitis during the preceding year received either herbal medicine or placebo. The herbal medicine consisted of bearberry extract (standardized for arbutin and methylarbutin content) and extract of dandelion root and leaf (dose of individual herbs not specified). Treatment for 1 month significantly reduced the recurrence of cystitis during the 1-year follow-up period, with no incidence of cystitis in the herbal group and a 23% occurrence in the placebo group ($p<0.05$). No side effects were reported.[40]

TOXICOLOGY

Hydroquinone is a recognized toxic compound. However, arbutin and bearberry extracts are considerably less toxic than hydroquinone, as evidenced by the studies cited below.

The oral LD_{50} of hydroquinone in 2% aqueous solution has been reported as between 320 and 550 mg/kg in various laboratory animals.[41] Hydroquinone is non-mutagenic in the Ames test but induces chromosome aberrations or karyotypic effects in eukaryotic cells.[42] In contrast, arbutin did not induce mutations in concentrations up to 10^{-2} M in a gene mutation assay. An increase in mutation frequency was observed with concentrations of 10^{-3} M and higher when arbutin was preincubated with beta-glycosidase. Hydroquinone, used as a positive control, also exhibited clear effects. In vivo, hydroquinone administered by intraperitoneal injection induced elevated micronucleus incidences. However, there was no induction of micronuclei in bone marrow when arbutin was administered orally (0.5–2.0 g/kg). This research suggests that arbutin itself is not mutagenic but any generated hydroquinone could exert its mutagenic potential.[36]

CONTRAINDICATIONS

According to the *British Herbal Compendium*, bearberry is contraindicated in kidney disorders[11] but there are few data to support this and the contraindication probably arose out of a theoretical caution.

According to the Commission E, bearberry is contraindicated in pregnancy and lactation and for children under 12 years of age.[43]

SPECIAL WARNINGS AND PRECAUTIONS

Bearberry is not suitable for prolonged use.

INTERACTIONS

Bearberry should not be given together with treatments that will lead to the production of an acidic urine since this will reduce the antibacterial effect. Bearberry will work best when urine has an alkaline pH.

The high tannin levels will cause interference of the absorption of various nutrients.

USE IN PREGNANCY AND LACTATION

Should not be used in pregnancy or lactation.[43,44] The transfer of arbutin or hydroquinone to breast milk is not advisable.[43]

EFFECTS ON ABILITY TO DRIVE AND USE MACHINES

No adverse effects.

SIDE EFFECTS

Hydroquinone depigmenting creams may cause exogenous ochronosis (hyperpigmentation)[45] and/or allergic contact dermatitis.[46] However, these side effects have not been reported for cosmetic creams containing bearberry.

Due to the high tannin content, internal use of bearberry may cause cramping, nausea, vomiting and constipation.

OVERDOSE

No effects documented.

CURRENT REGULATORY STATUS IN SELECTED COUNTRIES

Bearberry is official in the *European Pharmacopoeia* (1997).

Bearberry is covered by a positive Commission E monograph and has the following application: inflammatory disorders of the lower urinary tract.

Bearberry is on the UK General Sale List and in France the herb is accepted for the internal treatment of benign urinary infections and to promote the renal elimination of water.

Bearberry does not have GRAS status. However, it is freely available as a 'dietary supplement' in the USA under DSHEA legislation (1994 Dietary Supplement Health and Education Act). Bearberry has been present in the following over-the-counter (OTC) drug products: weight control drug products and orally administered menstrual drug products. The FDA, however, advises: 'that based on evidence currently available, there is inadequate data to establish general recognition of the safety and effectiveness of these ingredients for the specified uses'.

Bearberry is not included in Part 4 of Schedule 4 of the Therapeutic Goods Act Regulations of Australia.

References

1. Mabberley DJ. The plant book, 2nd edn. Cambridge University Press, Cambridge, 1997, p 53.
2. Evans WC. Trease and Evans' pharmacognosy, 14th edn. WB Saunders, London, 1996, p 223.
3. Brinker FJ. Eclectic dispensatory of botanical therapeutics, vol 2, section 1: native healing gifts. Eclectic Medical Publications, Sandy, 1995; pp 19–23.
4. Grieve M. A modern herbal, vol 1. Dover Publications, New York, 1971, pp 89–90.
5. Felter HW, Lloyd JU. King's American dispensatory, 18th edn, 3rd revision, vol 2, 1905. Reprinted by Eclectic Medical Publications, Portland, 1983; pp 2038–2040.
6. British Herbal Medicine Association's Scientific Committee. British herbal pharmacopoeia. BHMA, West York, 1983; pp 29–30.

7. Matsuda H, Nakamura S, Shiomoto H et al. Yakugaku Zasshi 1992; 112 (4): 276–282.
8. Frohne D. Pharm Ztg 1980; 125: 2582–2583.
9. Launert EL. The Hamlyn guide to edible and medicinal plants of Britain and Northern Europe. Hamlyn, London 1981; p 128.
10. Wagner H, Bladt S. Plant drug analysis – a thin layer chromatography atlas, 2nd edn. Springer-Verlag, Berlin, 1996; p 248.
11. British Herbal Medicine Association. British herbal compendium, vol 1. BHMA, Bournemouth, 1992, p 211–213.
12. Oliver AE, Crowe LM, De Araujo PS et al. Biochim Biophys Acta 1996; 1302 (1): 69–78.
13. Jahodar L, Jilek P, Patkova M et al. Cesk Farm 1985; 34 (5): 174–178.
14. Ng TB, Ling JM, Wang ZT et al. Gen Pharmacol 1996; 27 (7): 1237–1240.
15. Robertson JA, Howard LA. J Clin Microbiol 1987; 25 (1): 160–161.
16. Jahodar L, Kolb I. Pharmazie 1990; 45(6): 446.
17. Holopainen M, Jabodar L, Seppanen-Laakso T et al. Acta Pharm Fenn 1988; 97 (4): 197–202.
18. Skvortsov SS, Khan-Fimina VA. Fitontsidy Mater Soveshch 1969; 6: 207–209.
19. Kedzia B, Wrocinski T, Mrugasiewicz K et al. Med Dosw Mikrobiol 1975; 27: 305–314.
20. Nikolaev SM, Shantanova LN, Mondodoev AG et al. Rastitel'Nye Resursy 1996; 32 (3): 118–123.
21. Frohne D. Planta Med 1970; 18: 1–25.
22. German Federal Minister of Justice. German Commission E for human medicine monograph, Bundes-Anzeiger (German Federal Gazette) no. 228, dated 05.12.84 and no. 109, dated 15.06.1994.
23. Bouchier IAD, Morris JS (eds). Clinical skills – a system of clinical examination, 2nd edn. WB Saunders, London, 1982, p 243.
24. Baron EJ, Peterson LR, Finegold SM. Bailey and Scott's diagnostic microbiology, 9th edn. Mosby Year Book, St Louis, 1994, p 106.
25. Matsuda H, Tanaka T, Kubo M. Yakugaku Zasshi 1991; 111 (4–5): 253–258.
26. Matsuda H, Nakata H, Tanaka T et al. Yakugaku Zasshi 1990; 110 (1): 68–76.
27. Kubo M, Ito M, Nakata H et al. Yakugaku Zasshi 1990; 110 (1): 59–67.
28. Matsuda H, Nakamura S, Tanaka T et al. Yakugaku Zasshi 1992; 112 (9): 673–677.
29. Akiu S, Suzuki Y, Asahara T et al. Nippon Hifuka Gakkai Zasshi 1991; 101 (6): 609–613.
30. Maeda K, Fukuda M. J Pharmacol Exp Ther 1996; 276 (2): 765–769.
31. Strapkova A, Jahodar L, Nosalova G. Pharmazie 1991; 46 (8): 611–612.
32. Grases F, Melero G, Costa-Bauza R et al. Int Urol Nephrol 1994; 26 (5): 507–511.
33. Schaufelberger D, Hostettmann K. Planta Med 1983; 48 (2): 105–107.
34. Ayoub SMH, Yankov LK, Hussein-Ayoub SM. Fitoterapia 1985; 56 (4): 227–229.
35. Budavari S, O'Neil MJ, Smith A et al (eds). The Merck index: an encyclopedia of chemicals, drugs and botanicals, 12th edn. Merck, Whitehouse Station, NJ, 1996, p 131.
36. Mueller L, Kasper P. Mutat Res 1996; 360 (3): 291–292.
37. Paper DH, Koehler J, Franz G. Pharm Pharmacol Lett 1993; 3: 63–66.
38. Jahodar L, Leifertova I, Lisa M. Pharmazie 1983; 38(11): 780–781.
39. Leifertova I, Lisa M, Jahodar L et al. Rozvoj Farm Ramci Ved-Tech Revoluce, Sb Prednasck Sjezdu Cesk Farm Spol, 1979; 7th p41–43. Meeting date 1977; Publisher: University of Karlova, Prague.
40. Larsson B, Jonasson A, Fianu S. Curr Ther Res Clin Exp 1993; 53 (4): 441–443.
41. Woodard G, Hagan CE, Radomski JL. Fed Proc 1949; 8: 348.
42. Devillers J, Boule P, Vasseur P et al. Ecotoxicol Environ Saf 1990; 19 (3): 327–354.
43. German Federal Minister of Justice. German Commission E for human medicine monograph, Bundes-Anzeiger (German Federal Gazette) no. 109, dated 15.06.94; no. 19, dated 28.01.1994.
44. Scientific Committee of ESCOP. ESCOP monographs: Uvae ursi folium. European Scientific Cooperative on Phytotherapy, Exeter, 1997.
45. Howard KL, Ferner BB. Cutis 1990; 45 (3): 180–182.
46. Engasser PG, Maibach HI. J Am Acad Dermatol 1981; 5 (2): 143–147.

Berberis bark and Hydrastis root (*Berberis vulgaris* L., *Hydrastis canadensis* L.)

SYNONYMS

Berberis vulgaris: barberry (Engl), Berberidis cortex (Lat), Berberitze, Sauerdorn (Ger), epinevinette, vinettier (Fr), berberi (Ital), almindelig Berberis (Dan).

Hydrastis canadensis: golden seal (Engl), Hydrastidis rhizoma (Lat), Goldsiegel, Kanadische Gelbwurzel (Ger), guldsegl (Dan).

WHAT IS IT?

There are more than 500 species of the Berberis genus and *B. vulgaris*, the common or European barberry, is indigenous to Europe and naturalized in Britain. Many parts of the plant have been utilized: the fine wood for turning, root and stems providing dyestuff for fabrics, leather and wood (also formerly a hair dye); the fruit has been used in jams.[1] The root and stem bark are used medicinally.

Hydrastis canadensis was known to the Cherokee nation long before the settlement of America by Europeans. They employed its underground portion for dyeing and as an internal remedy and acquainted the early settlers with most of its properties.[2] The plant is indigenous to central and eastern North America but its population is now much reduced through over-exploitation.[3,4] Because of the high price commanded by the root and rhizome, it is susceptible to adulteration. Hydrastis was a very prominent herb in the Eclectic tradition.

The activities of Berberis and Hydrastis are thought to be mainly due to their isoquinoline alkaloids, in particular berberine and hydrastine (the latter occurs only in Hydrastis). Other plants also contain berberine but will not be examined in this monograph. It is preferable to use cultivated sources of Hydrastis because of its endangered status.

EFFECTS

Berberis vulgaris: controls gastrointestinal infections; improves the flow of bile.

Hydrastis canadensis: in addition to the above, restores the integrity of mucous membranes of the respiratory and digestive tract.

TRADITIONAL VIEW

Berberis vulgaris has had a long history of use in Western herbalism. A decoction was taken in the spring months as a blood purifier and used externally as a mouth and eyewash. The Eclectics regarded Berberis primarily as a tonic but it was also used for conditions affecting the liver and gallbladder, diarrhoea, dysentery and parasitical infections including malaria.[5,6]

Hydrastis canadensis was specifically indicated for catarrhal states of the mucous membranes, when unaccompanied by acute inflammation (except in the case of acute purulent otitis media, where it was considered to work better than in the chronic condition) and also if there was muscular debility. As a bitter stomachic, it was used to sharpen appetite and aid digestion and was considered valuable for disordered states of the digestive apparatus, especially when functional in character. It was considered a valuable local agent in affections of the nose and throat. Hydrastis was also used in cutaneous diseases, especially when dependent upon gastric difficulties; concurrent internal and external use was said to hasten the cure.[7] In addition, Hydrastis was recommended for submucosal myoma, haemorrhagic endometriosis and heavy menstrual bleeding.[8]

SUMMARY ACTIONS

Berberis vulgaris: antimicrobial, cholagogue, choleretic, antiemetic, mild laxative, bitter.

Hydrastis canadensis: stomachic, reputed oxytocic, antihaemorrhagic, anticatarrhal, trophorestorative for mucous membranes, antimicrobial, bitter, antiinflammatory, depurative, vulnerary, choleretic.

CAN BE USED FOR

INDICATIONS SUPPORTED BY CLINICAL TRIALS

From clinical trials on berberine: acute infectious diarrhoea; trachoma (as eyedrops); giardiasis; hypertyraminaemia; adjunct in the treatment of non-insulin dependent diabetes mellitus; cutaneous leishmaniasis (topically).

TRADITIONAL THERAPEUTIC USES

Berberis vulgaris: jaundice (when there is no obstruction of the bile ducts); biliousness, cholecystitis, gallstones; functional derangement of the liver; digestive stimulant, diarrhoea; in larger doses for constipation.[5,6,9]

Hydrastis canadensis: catarrhal states of the mucous membranes when unaccompanied by acute inflammation (except in acute purulent otitis media); disordered states of the gastrointestinal tract (particularly gastritis, peptic ulcer, diarrhoea) including conditions with hepatic symptoms; as a tonic during convalescence; haemorrhagic conditions of the uterus and pelvis (but it was considered too slow for active postpartum haemorrhage); internally and externally for skin disorders, especially with gastrointestinal involvement; discharges from the genitourinary tract (e.g. leucorrhoea, gonorrhoea); disorders of the ear, nose, mouth, throat; externally for superficial disorders of the eye (but has no value in intraocular affection).[7]

MAY ALSO BE USED FOR

EXTRAPOLATIONS FROM PHARMACOLOGICAL STUDIES

Berberine-containing herbs may also be used for: bacterial and fungal infections; protozoal infections (cutaneous and visceral leishmaniasis, amoebic dysentery, malaria, giardiasis, trichomoniasis); tapeworm infestation; possibly as an adjunct in treatment of congestive heart failure, arrhythmia; possibly in prevention of cancer; thrombocytopaenia.

Hydrastis: the above indications plus anorexia and conditions requiring increased flow of gastric juices; conditions of visceral and/or smooth muscle spasm.

OTHER APPLICATIONS

Hydrastis was used as a component of eyewashes and both Hydrastis and Berberis are used in bitter tonic preparations. Berberine salts are used in ophthalmic products, usually in eyedrops and eyewashes.[10] Despite the traditional contraindication for Hydrastis in acute respiratory infections, it is often used in this way, particularly in modern practice in the USA. Despite popular use, Hydrastis has no value in masking drug-screening tests.

PREPARATIONS

Dried or fresh stem bark or root bark (Berberis) or rhizome and rootlets (Hydrastis) for decoction, liquid extract and tincture for internal or external use.

DOSAGE

- *Berberis vulgaris*: 1.5–3 g per day of the dried root or stem bark or 3–6 ml per day of the 1:2 liquid extract, 7–14 ml per day of the 1:5 tincture.
- *Hydrastis canadensis*: 0.7–2 g per day of the dried rhizome/root or 2–4 ml per day of the 1:3 tincture, 3.5–7 ml per day of the 1:5 tincture.

Higher doses of both herbs are necessary in acute conditions.

DURATION OF USE

Both may be taken long term within the recommended dosage.

SUMMARY ASSESSMENT OF SAFETY

No adverse effects from ingestion of either Berberis or Hydrastis are expected when used within the recommended dosage. Berberine-containing plants are not recommended for use during pregnancy.

TECHNICAL DATA

BOTANY

Berberis vulgaris, a member of the Berberidaceae family, is a deciduous shrub 0.75–1.75 m tall with thick, creeping roots and a very branched, greyish stem. The leaves are arranged in clusters on short axillary shoots, obovate to oblong-obovate, up to 4 cm long with spiny-toothed margins and short petioles. Its yellow flowers are six-sepalled and six-petalled, falling in loose clusters. The edible berries are red, oblong and about 1 cm in size.[11,12]

Hydrastis canadensis, a member of the Ranunculaceae (buttercup) family, is a small perennial. The stems are purplish and hairy above ground but below the soil the root hairs and rhizome are yellow. The yellow rhizome is characteristically marked with depressions caused by the falling away of the annual stems (hence golden seal, as in the impression in wax once used to seal letters). The rhizome is about 5 cm in length, producing a profusion of yellow roots at its sides, 30 cm or more in length. The stems bear two or three large, slightly hairy five-part leaves. The small solitary, greenish white or rose-coloured flower develops into a berry-like fruiting head, bright red in colour when fully ripe, resembling a raspberry and containing 10–30 black seeds.[13]

The Ranunculaceae and Berberidaceae are part of the same order (Ranunculales).

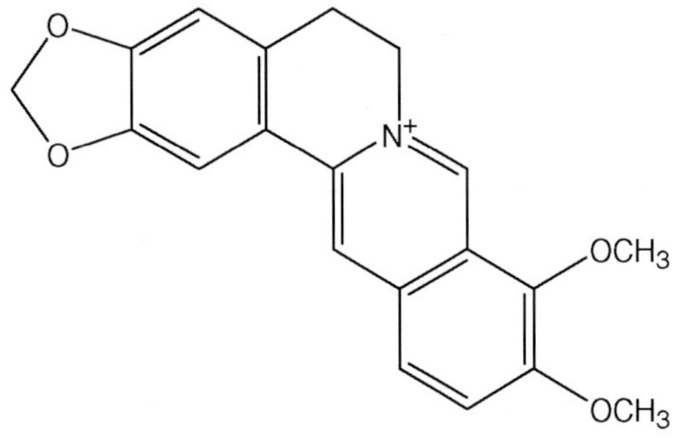

Berberine

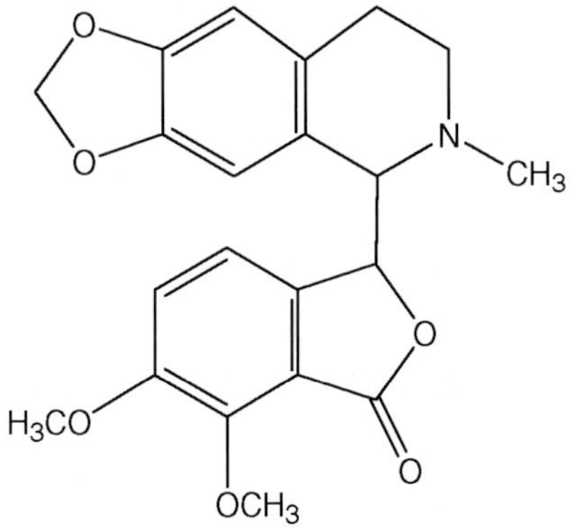

Hydrastine

KEY CONSTITUENTS

Berberis vulgaris (root bark)

- Alkaloids (up to not greater than 13%), including those of the isoquinoline group: protoberberines (berberine (up to 6%), jatrorrhizine, palmatine) and bisbenzylisoquinolines (total <5%, including oxyacanthine).[14]

Hydrastis canadensis

- Alkaloids (2.5–6%), including those of the isoquinoline group, the protoberberines: (berberine (2–4.5%), canadine (0.5–1%), hydrastine (3.2–4%).[14]

PHARMACODYNAMICS OF KEY CONSTITUENTS

The activities of Berberis and Hydrastis are thought to be due to the presence of their isoquinoline alkaloids. A review of the pharmacological activities of these alkaloids indicated that berberine has the following activities:[15]

- antimicrobial, antifungal, antiparasitic;
- antidiarrhoeal, intestinal antisecretory, inhibits enterotoxins, cholera toxin antagonist;
- antiarrhythmic, positive inotropic (cardiotonic);
- cytotoxic, antimitotic, antitumoral, increases the action of antitumorals, inhibits the action of carcinogens;
- cholagogue, choleretic, increases bilirubin excretion;
- mydriatic (dilates the pupil), increases lacrimal secretion;
- anticariogenic;
- inhibits acetylcholinesterase;
- hypoglycaemic.

Hydrastine has the following activities:[16]

- choleretic;
- sedative;
- antibacterial;
- vasoconstrictive.

Antimicrobial and antiparasitic activity

Berberine sulphate blocked the adhesion of a uropathogenic strain of *E. coli*, in vitro. The reduction in adherence is related to the loss of the synthesis and expression of fimbriae (hairlike appendages) on the surface of the berberine-treated bacteria. Inhibition of microbial adherence results in termination of infection and may explain the antiinfectious activity of berberine in *E. coli* urinary tract infections, since the direct antimicrobial activity of berberine against *E. coli* is relatively low (see Table 1).[17]

Berberine sulphate demonstrated antimycotic activity against several fungal species. Concentrations of 10–25 mg/ml inhibited the growth of Alternaria, *Aspergillus flavus, Asp. fumigatus, Candida albicans*, Curvularia, Drechslera, Fusarium, Mucor, Penicillium, *Rhizopus oryzae* and Scopulariopsis. The growth of Syncephalastrum was inhibited by a concentration of 50 mg/ml.[18]

Berberine and protoberberine derivatives exhibited a potency comparable to that of quinine in vitro against two clones of human malaria, *Plasmodium berghei* and *P. falciparum*. None of the compounds, however, were active against *P. berghei*-parasitized mice.[19] Berberine sulphate inhibited the growth of *Entamoeba histolytica, Giardia lamblia* and *Trichomonas vaginalis* in vitro and induced morphological changes in the parasites.[20] Berberine chloride (1 μg/ml) significantly inhibited the growth of *Leishmania donovani* promastigotes by approximately 50%, in vitro. A concentration of 5 µg/ml resulted in complete inhibition of growth. *L. donovani* causes visceral leishmaniasis.[21]

Berberine demonstrated significant activity (greater than 50% suppression of lesion size) against *Leishmania braziliensis panamensis* in golden hamsters.[22] In both the 8-day and long-term models of *Leishmania donovani* infection in hamsters, berberine markedly diminished the parasitic load, rapidly improved the haematological picture and was less toxic than pentamidine. Berberine was found to interact in vitro with nuclear DNA from *L. donovani* promastigotes.[23] Berberine sulphate administered into the lesion (1% four times per week) was

Table 1 In vitro sensitivity of microorganisms to berberine sulphate[28–30]

Test organism	Causative agent for the following conditions in humans	Inhibitory concentration µg/ml
Bacteria		
Bacillus cereus	Food poisoning	50.0*
B. pumilus	As for *B. subtilis*	25.0
B. subtilis	Food poisoning and various infections including septicaemia	25.0
Clostridium tetani	Tetanus	50
Corynebacterium diphtheriae	Diphtheria	6.2
Escherichia coli	Toxic strains can cause enteritis, peritonitis, infections of the urinary tract	>100.0
Klebsiella spp	Infections of the respiratory tract	>100.0
K. pneumoniae	Responsible for severe pneumonitis	25.0
Pseudomonas pyocyanea	Various suppurative (pus-forming) infections.	>100.0
Proteus spp	Infant diarrhoea, urinary tract infection, suppurative lesions	>100.0
Salmonella paratyphi	Enteric fever	>100.0
S. schottmuelleri	Enteric fever	>100.0
S. typhimurium	Gastroenteritis, food poisoning in Western countries	>100.0
S. typhi	Typhoid fever	>100.0
Shigella boydii	Bacillary dysentery	12.5
Staphylococcus aureus	Abscesses, endocarditis, pneumonia, osteomyelitis, septicaemia	6.2–50.0
S. albus	Occasionally endocarditis and infection of central nervous system	50.0
Streptococcus pyogenes	Variety of suppurative diseases including acute pharyngitis, impetigo and non-suppurative diseases including rheumatic fever	12.5
Vibrio cholerae	Cholera	25–50.0
Mycobacterium tuberculosis	Tuberculosis	200**
Fungi		
Candida albicans	Thrush and candidiasis and infection involving various parts of the body	12.5
C. tropicalis	As for *C. albicans*	3.1+
Saccharomyces cerevisiae	Associated with endocarditis and occasionally pulmonary infection	100[a]
Microsporum gypseum	Tinea	50[b]
Sporotrichum schenkli	Sporotrichosis (a granulomatous disease of the skin, occasionally of internal organs and bones)	6.2+
Trichophyton mentagrophytes	Attacks skin, hair and nails including dermatophytosis (a skin eruption)	100[b]
Cryptococcus neoformans	Cryptococcosis (an infection involving lungs, bones or skin but often the CNS (meningitis)	150[b]
Other		
Entamoeba histolytica	Protozoa responsible for amoebiasis	200

** Liquid medium unless otherwise stated. Inoculation size varied between 107 and 5 × 107 cells/ml, pH adjusted to 8.0 unless stated otherwise. Maximum concentration of berberine sulphate used was 100 µg/ml.*

*** Solid medium, plate diffusion assay. Minimum concentration that gave a zone of inhibition of diameter 7 mm at pH 7.0.*

+pH 7.0

[a]pH 7.0; test tube. Minimum concentration of berberine sulphate

[b] Solid medium, Sabouraud's glucose agar, tube test; pH 5.8

found to be highly effective against cutaneous leishmaniasis in dogs. Cutaneous leishmaniasis (oriental sore) is caused by the protozoan *Leishmania tropica* infection.[24]

Berberine hydrochloride demonstrated a high degree of activity against *E. histolytica* in vitro with a minimum amoebicidal concentration of 10 μg/ml. Oral administration of berberine (100 mg/kg) to rats with experimental amoebiasis (protozoal infection) reduced the infection by 83%. Berberine also reduced the level of infection to 20% in infected hamsters.[25] Studies have shown that certain antimicrobial agents can block the adherence of microorganisms to host cells at doses much lower than those needed to kill cells or inhibit cell growth. At concentrations below the minimum inhibitory concentration, berberine caused an increase in release of lipoteichoic acid (LTA) from streptococci. LTA is the major ligand responsible for the adherence of the bacteria to host cells, including host cell receptors (fibronectin). Release of LTA from the streptococcal cells means a loss of LTA and a corresponding reduction in the capacity of the bacteria to adhere to the host. Berberine also interfered with bacterial adherence by directly preventing the complexing of LTA with fibronectin or by dissolving the complexes once they were formed.[26]

The effect of hydrastine on the protoscolices (larvae) of the tapeworm *Echinococcus granulosus* was measured in vitro and in vivo. Hydrastine at 0.3% concentration produced 70% mortality of the larvae in both experiments.[27]

Antidiarrhoeal activity

Oral doses of berberine (>25 mg/kg) and Geranium extract showed significant inhibition of diarrhoea in mice and both substances inhibited spontaneous peristalsis in rat intestine. Comparison to atropine and papaverine indicated that the antidiarrhoeal activity of berberine differs from that of Geranium extract.[31]

The effect of berberine on *E. coli*-induced intestinal fluid accumulation was observed in rats. Oral administration of berberine (0.1 mg) together with the *E. coli* enterotoxin resulted in significant ($p<0.01$) reduction in fluid accumulation. Treatment with berberine prior to or after administration of the enterotoxin was ineffective.[32]

Intragastric administration of berberine sulphate reduced the purging effects of castor oil or *Cassia angustifolia* leaf in mice. It did not affect the gastrointestinal transport of Chinese ink in normal mice.[33]

The goal of drug therapy of diarrhoeal diseases is to decrease stool water. This can be done in two ways: increase the absorption of water and electrolytes or decrease the stimulated secretion. Berberine probably does the latter.[34] Berberine does not significantly alter normal ileal water and electrolyte transport as measured in vivo[35] and in vitro.[36] However, it inhibited secretion caused by *V. cholerae* and *E. coli* heat-labile enterotoxins, even when administered after the enterotoxin had bound to intestinal mucosa. The antisecretory effect is therefore not dependent upon the type of enterotoxin.[37] Two studies have been contradictory as to whether berberine alters cholera toxin-induced stimulation of the adenylate cyclase-cAMP system.[36,37] Hence the precise mechanism of action of berberine is not known but its site of action appears to be distal to second messenger production and may be at a level common to all stimuli of colonic chloride secretion.[38]

Cardiovascular activity

An in vitro study indicated that berberine inhibits voltage-dependent and ATP-sensitive potassium channels. The hypoglycaemic and antiarrhythmic activity of berberine might be due to its potassium channel-blocking effects.[39] Intravenous administration of berberine (1 mg/kg) decreased the amplitude of delayed after-depolarizations and blocked arrhythmias in rabbit ventricular muscles. The mechanism of antiarrhythmic activity of berberine may therefore be due to suppression of delayed after-depolarizations caused by a decrease in sodium influx.[40]

Administration of berberine sulphate increased the number of thrombocytes, decreased the activity of factor XIII and promoted blood coagulation in intact and gamma-irradiated rats and mice.[41]

Berberine inhibited platelet aggregation and platelet adhesiveness in rats with reversible middle cerebral artery occlusion. Thromboxane B_2 levels after treatment with berberine were lower than levels in untreated ischaemic controls. The decline of platelet aggregation and decrease of thromboxane B_2 may be one of the important factors behind the antiischaemic activity of berberine.[42]

Berberine markedly inhibited clot retraction in vitro, which may be due to direct inhibition of calcium ion influx.[43]

Cytotoxic activity

Berberine demonstrated cytotoxic activity in a particular yeast strain in vitro, blocking mutation in the DNA strand-break repair pathway,[44] and caused growth inhibition in vitro in human hepatoma cells, increasing glucocorticoid receptor levels compared to control cells.[45]

Berberine activated macrophages to be highly cytostatic against tumour cells[46] and caused morphological changes to human leukaemia cells, in vitro.[47] The DNA fragmentation of the cells was characteristic of apoptosis, the programmed death function of the cell.[47]

Protoberberines have been identified as poisons of topoisomerases I and II (enzymes involved in DNA replication and transcription) which supports their in vitro antitumour activity.[48]

Antiinflammatory activity

Ethanol extract of Berberis, three alkaloidal fractions and isolated alkaloids (berberine and oxyacanthine) were applied by intraperitoneal route in acute inflammation models. The ethanol extract demonstrated the highest antiinflammatory activity. The ethanol extract also demonstrated antiinflammatory activity in chronic inflammation (adjuvant arthritis). The two fractions containing only protoberberines and berberine suppressed a delayed-type hypersensitivity reaction. The other fraction (containing protoberberines and bisbenzylisoquinoline alkaloids) and berberine reduced the antibody response against sheep red blood cells (SRBC) in vivo.[49]

Berberine inhibited cellular proliferation of human peripheral lymphocytes in vitro. Some effects of berberine, especially its antiinflammatory activity, may arise in part from the inhibition of DNA synthesis in activated lymphocytes.[50]

Antispasmodic activity

Berberine reduced the tonic contraction induced by carbachol in isolated longitudinal muscle of gastric fundus. It mainly acts by inhibiting extracellular calcium entry induced by both carbachol and potassium chloride.[51] Comparative examinations were made on the relationship between isoquinoline alkaloids and the antispasmodic action on isolated mouse intestine and uterus. Berberine, palmatine, jatrorrhizine, dihydroberberine and dihydropalmatine caused marked contraction of uterus. Only tetrahydroberberine, tetrahydropalmatine and tetrahydrojatrorrhizine showed strong papaverine-like spasmolytic activity on intestines.[52]

Other activity

Acute doses (2.5 mg) of berberine hydrochloride to rats by oral administration significantly increased ($p<0.05$) the secretion of bilirubin in experimental hyperbilirubinaemia without affecting the functional capacity of the liver. Chronic administration of 5 mg/day for 8 days abolished the effect, resulting in normal biliary bilirubin excretion.[53]

An in vitro study conducted on the sebaceous glands of the hamster ear found that lipogenesis was suppressed 63% by 10^{-4} M berberine ($p<0.01$). Lipogenesis was also suppressed by wogonin, a flavonoid in *Scutellaria baicalensis*. Herbal medicines containing berberine and/or wogonin may therefore be useful in the treatment of acne vulgaris, especially topically. Berberine also increased the incorporation of radiolabelled carbon into the lipid free fatty acid fraction. It is likely then that berberine inhibits lipogenesis at the level of synthesis of triglyceride from free fatty acid.[54]

Berberine significantly improved scopolamine-induced amnesia in rats. The antiamnesic effect of berberine may be related to the increase in activity in the peripheral and central cholinergic neuronal systems.[55]

Berbamine by intraperitoneal administration demonstrated suppressive effects on the delayed hypersensitivity and mixed lymphocyte reactions and significantly prolonged allograft survival compared with untreated transplanted mice. Berbamine may therefore have potential as an agent in clinical transplantation.[56] In an earlier study on berberine, it significantly inhibited the proliferative response of spleen cells to mitogens and reduced the amount of haemolytic plaque-forming cells. The ratio of CD4+ cells to CD8+ cells of spleen T-lymphocytes was decreased, which may be one of the mechanisms of action.[57]

Intragastric administration of berberine sulphate significantly inhibited the increased vascular permeability induced by intraperitoneal acetic acid in mice. Subcutaneous administration markedly inhibited the increased vascular permeability in rats and inhibited mouse ear swelling.[33]

PHARMACODYNAMICS OF THE HERBS

Antimicrobial activity

A more efficient inhibition of growth was observed for a 1:4 tincture of Berberis compared to 0.2% berberine chloride solution against a variety of microorganisms in vitro. This effect of the Berberis tincture was the result of a higher concentration of berberine (0.31%) and the presence of other chemical components, including alkaloids.[58]

Effects on smooth muscle

Berberine causes a slow diminution of tone, amplitude, rate and response to acetylcholine in rat uterus. Hydrastine increased the rate of uterine contraction, with slowly decreasing tone and amplitude. Berberine and hydrastine together produced a rapid decrease in tone and amplitude, similar to that produced by Hydrastis extract.[59] The author suggested that, although commonly regarded as a uterine stimulant, Hydrastis was in fact a uterine sedative. Hydrastis extract and total crude alkaloids of Hydrastis demonstrated antispasmodic action on isolated mouse intestine and uterus.[60]

In contrast, an alcohol extract of Hydrastis produced a vasoconstrictive effect but inhibited contraction of rabbit aorta induced by adrenaline, serotonin and histamine in vitro. However, berberine and hydrastine did not show this vasoconstrictive effect. Berberine demonstrated some inhibiting activity on aortic contraction induced by adrenaline but hydrastine was inactive.[61] The observed vasoconstrictive effect of Hydrastis extract may be due to the presence of hydrastinine, a decomposition product of hydrastine.

The four major alkaloids of Hydrastis (berberine, hydrastine, canadine and canadaline) were tested on rabbit aorta strips for adrenolytic activity (inhibition of adrenaline-induced contraction). The total extract had a lower adrenolytic potency than the alkaloid mixture and the authors suggested that berberine, canadine and canadaline act synergistically and the presence of other compounds (in particular hydrastine) probably counteracts their activity.[62]

The major alkaloids of Hydrastis (berberine, hydrastine, canadine and canadaline) evoked contractile activity on isolated guinea pig ileum through an indirect cholinergic mechanism, acting on acetylcholine release from nerve endings. They demonstrated differing contractile potencies depending on chemical structure.[63]

In confirmation of earlier research, an ethanolic extract of Hydrastis exhibited reversible relaxant activity on spontaneous contractions in non-pregnant rat uterus and also on contractions induced by serotonin, oxytocin and acetylcholine.[64] The extract also relaxed carbachol precontracted guinea pig trachea. An ethanolic extract of Hydrastis induced strong relaxation in rabbit bladder detrusor muscle but the four major individual alkaloids were inactive.[65]

Other activity

Berberis tincture increased contractions in isolated rabbit intestine and demonstrated cholagogue activity in guinea pigs and cholekinetic activity in rats.[66]

Extract of *Berberis aristata* root inhibited the PAF-induced aggregation of rabbit platelets in a dose-dependent manner in vitro. It also inhibited the radiolabelled PAF binding to rabbit platelets in a competitive manner.[67]

Conflicting results have been recorded for Berberis in pyresis. An early study demonstrated an antipyretic effect in rabbits with fever for Berberis decoction.[68] However, in a later study water, chloroform and hexane extracts showed no activity.[69]

A study of the action of bitters was conducted in 1956 on the stomach of a man named Tom, who had an occluded oesophagus and a gastric fistula.[2] Bitters were administered by mouth and swallowed into the blind oesophagus; the resulting salivary volume and gastric secretion were compared with direct administration into the stomach. In the 96 experiments conducted it was found that there was considerable variation in the effect of the bitters. Hydrastis was the most active herb and gentian was virtually inactive at the levels tested.[70]

PHARMACOKINETICS

Oral administration of 50 mg/100 g to rabbits resulted in a maximum level of berberine in the blood after 8 hours. Berberine was still found in the blood after 72 hours. Levels were highest in the heart, pancreas and liver and it was excreted through the stools and the urine.[71]

A study investigated the concentration of berberine in rat plasma after oral administration of aqueous extracts of *Coptis spp*. Coadministration with aqueous extract of Glycyrrhiza did not influence the bioavailability of berberine from the Coptis extract.[72]

CLINICAL TRIALS (MAINLY USING BERBERINE)

Diarrhoea and cholera

An early uncontrolled clinical study suggested that berberine therapy may be useful for cholera and severe diarrhoea.[73] A parallel open clinical trial comparing berberine and antidiarrhoeal drugs was conducted on 100 children suffering from gastroenteritis of less than 5 days' duration. Fifty children up to 6 months old received 25 mg of berberine four times a day; older children received 50 mg initially and 25 mg every 6 hours; another 50 children received one of several antidiarrhoeal drugs. The state of hydration and number of stools passed were used to assess the treatment. Berberine demonstrated effective antidiarrhoeal action and compared well with the standard antidiarrhoeal drugs. Patients on berberine improved faster.[74]

In a randomized, placebo-controlled, double-blind clinical trial, the effects of berberine, tetracycline and tetracycline plus berberine were studied on 400 patients presenting with acute watery diarrhoea. Of this number, 185 patients had cholera and 215 non-cholera diarrhoea. At the dosage used (100 mg four times daily) berberine did not show significant anti-secretory activity in either group. A reduction in diarrhoeal stool volume and cyclic AMP concentrations in stools was observed, although not significant.[75]

In a later trial, a larger dosage of berberine of 200 mg four times daily plus tetracycline was compared to tetracycline alone in a randomized, double-blind clinical design conducted on 74 patients infected with *V. cholerae*. No statistically significant differences were observed between the two groups.[76]

One hundred and sixty-five adult men with diarrhoea caused by *Escherichia coli* or *Vibrio cholerae* were treated in a randomized, controlled clinical trial. In patients with *E. coli* diarrhoea, mean stool volume decreased significantly ($p<0.05$) in the first 8 hours after treatment with 40 mg of berberine when compared to controls. Over the 24-hour period a 48% reduction was observed. Only limited effects against diarrhoea caused by *V. cholerae* were observed, however, and no significant difference was found between patients treated with 1200 mg berberine plus tetracycline and those treated with tetracycline alone.[77] The clinical efficacy and safety of potential antisecretory and antimicrobial drugs in the treatment of diarrhoea caused by *Vibrio cholerae* and enterotoxigenic *E. coli* were investigated in randomized, placebo-controlled clinical trials. Berberine, among other antidiarrhoeal agents, reduced stool volumes in diarrhoeal patients without significant side effects. Berberine was more effective in enterotoxigenic *E. coli* diarrhoea than in cholera.[78]

The conclusion which can be drawn from these clinical studies is that berberine has value for some forms of acute infectious diarrhoea, particularly *E. coli* infection, but has no value in the treatment of *V. cholerae* infection (cholera).

Other gastrointestinal effects

Small intestine transit time in 20 healthy human subjects was significantly delayed after oral administration of 1.2 g of berberine ($p<0.01$). Therefore the antidiarrhoeal property of berberine might be additionally mediated by its ability to delay small intestinal transit.[79]

A clinical trial compared the effect of an antiulcer drug (ranitidine) and four antibacterial drugs, one of which was berberine (300 mg twice daily), on patients with *H. pylori*-associated duodenal ulcer disease. Although the antibacterial drugs were more effective in *H. pylori* clearance and improvement of gastritis, ranitidine proved more effective in ulcer healing. (Acid secretion may therefore be of more importance in ulcer formation than *H. pylori*.)[80]

Trachoma

Fifty-one patients with clinically active trachoma lesions (stages I and II) were treated for 8 weeks with eyedrops of either 0.2% berberine chloride or the anti-trachoma drug, sulfacetamide. Sulfacetamide eye-drops gave the best clinical results but the infective agent (*Chlamydia trachomatis*) remained present in the conjunctiva and relapses of symptoms occurred. Berberine-treated patients showed only very mild ocular symptoms and were negative for infective agent. Also, no relapses occurred among these patients.[81]

A double-blind, placebo-controlled clinical trial was conducted on 96 children with trachoma stage IIa or IIb over a period of 3 months. Berberine eyedrops (0.2%) were compared with berberine plus neomycin, sulfacetamide and a placebo. In patients treated with berberine alone, 84% were clinically cured ($p<0.001$) but only 50% were microbiologically cured. The response rate was higher in those treated with berberine and neomycin and lower in the sulfacetamide group. Berberine treatment was better tolerated than sulfacetamide.[82]

Giardiasis

Berberine was administered at a dose of 5 mg/kg/day for 6 days to 25 giardiasis patients between the ages of 1 to 10 years; 68% became negative for the presence of Giardia cysts. In a similar group receiving placebo, only 25% experienced a parasitological cure. Flagyl (metronidazole) at a dosage of 10 mg/kg/day for 6 days was 100% effective in another nine patients.[83]

A clinical trial conducted on children (5 months to 14 years) with giardiasis compared the effect of berberine with established antigiardial drugs. A group of 42 patients received 10 mg/kg/day of berberine orally for 10 days; 90% of patients had negative stool specimens upon completion of treatment, although a small number of cases relapsed 1 month later. This result compared favourably with the other three antigiardial drugs investigated.[84]

Liver cirrhosis

Patients with cirrhosis of the liver have high plasma concentrations of tyramine which can cause cardiovascular and neurologic complications. An uncontrolled clinical trial investigated the effect of oral berberine on hypertyraminaemia in cirrhotic patients over several months. Oral administration of berberine (600–800 mg/day) corrected hypertyraminaemia and prevented the elevation of plasma tyramine levels following chemical tyramine stimulation. This effect was probably due to inhibition of bacterial tyrosine decarboxylase in the intestine.[85]

Diabetes mellitus

An uncontrolled clinical trial investigated the effect of berberine on 60 patients with type II diabetes mellitus. The patients varied in severity of this disorder. Oral doses (0.3–0.5 g three times a day) were prescribed for 1–3 months, together with a therapeutic diet prescribed for 1 month. Major symptoms of diabetes disappeared, patients' strength improved, blood pressure became normal and blood lipids decreased. Fasting glycaemic levels in 60% of patients were controlled. Further testing in animal models indicated that treatment with berberine led to healthier pancreatic tissue compared to controls. It is suggested that the mechanism of action of berberine may be associated with promoting regeneration and functional recovery of β-cells.[86]

Other effects

Ten patients with cutaneous leishmaniasis received a 1% berberine salt solution intralesionally at weekly intervals for a period of 2 months. A blood sample was taken from the patients before and after treatment. The lesions showed evidence of healing after the second injection. Two patients dropped out of this uncontrolled trial and of the remaining eight, healing was complete by 4–8 weeks.[87]

Berberine bisulphate given on its own and in a combined treatment at a dose of 15 mg/day for 15 days increased platelet count in patients with primary and secondary thrombocytopaenia.[88] Two hundred and fifteen patients with chloroquine-resistant malaria were randomized into three groups: 82 patients received pyrimethamine and berberine chloride (1.5 g per day), 64 patients received pyrimethamine and tetracycline and 69 patients received pyrimethamine and cotrimoxazole. The clearance rate of asexual parasitaemia after treatment was 74% in the berberine group, 67% in the tetracycline group and 48% in the cotrimoxazole group. Berberine was more effective in clearing the parasite than the other antimicrobial agents when used in conjunction with pyrimethamine.[89]

Twelve patients with refractory congestive heart failure were studied before and during berberine intravenous infusion at rates of 0.02 and 0.2 mg/kg per minute for 30 minutes. The lower infusion dose produced no significant circulatory changes, apart from a reduction in heart rate. The higher dose produced significant changes indicative of cardiotonic activity.[90]

Popular literature has suggested that Hydrastis can be used to mask banned drug use, but this is not the case. The performance of a particular assay (CEDIA) for screening amphetamines, barbiturates, benzodiazepines, cocaine, opiates, phencyclidine and tetrahydrocannabinol in urine was evaluated. Only minimal or selective interferences were observed with the following adulterants, which were added to potentially invalidate the screening results: Hydrastis tea, lemon juice, Visine and low concentrations of bleach and Drano.[91]

TOXICOLOGY

The oral LD_{50} in mice of berberine is 329 mg/kg.[60] Oral doses of up to 100 mg/kg of berberine sulphate have been well tolerated in animal studies without lasting effects. However, prolonged administration caused organ damage and death after 8–10 days.[92,93]

The oral LD_{50} of *Hydrastis canadensis* extract in mice is 1620 mg/kg.[60]

The LD_{50} of berberine sulphate in mice by intraperitoneal route is 24.3 mg/kg. In high doses, berberine causes haemorrhagic nephritis and eventually death by respiratory failure.[94]

CONTRAINDICATIONS

Berberine-containing plants are not recommended for use during pregnancy[95,96] or for jaundiced neonates.[96]

Berberine was traditionally contraindicated for use in diarrhoea[6] but the above pharmacological and clinical studies on berberine indicate the efficacy and safety of therapeutic doses.

Hydrastis is said to be contraindicated in hypertensive conditions.[6]

SPECIAL WARNINGS AND PRECAUTIONS

None required.

INTERACTIONS

A Chinese study investigating the effect of berberine on the protein binding of bilirubin in vitro found that berberine exerted a 10-fold effect in comparison with phenylbutazone, a potent displacer of bilirubin. Chronic intraperitoneal administration of berberine (10–20 mg/g/day × 7) to rats resulted in a significant decrease in mean bilirubin serum protein binding.[96]

Hence, berberine may reinforce the effects of other drugs which displace the protein binding of bilirubin. This might also explain the contraindication for pregnancy, rather than any reputed uterine-contracting effects.

USE IN PREGNANCY AND LACTATION

Berberine-containing plants are not recommended for use during pregnancy.

EFFECTS ON ABILITY TO DRIVE AND USE MACHINES

No negative influence is expected for either herb.

SIDE EFFECTS

The use of berberine for diarrhoea in children has resulted in cases of poor tolerance due to emesis. However, the berberine was often given in combination with other compounds which may contribute to this adverse reaction.[95]

At doses higher than 0.5 g, berberine may cause dizziness, nose bleeds, dyspnoea, skin and eye irritation, gastrointestinal irritation, nausea, diarrhoea, nephritis and urinary tract disorders.[94]

OVERDOSE

Death from berberine poisoning has occurred.[94]

CURRENT REGULATORY STATUS IN SELECTED COUNTRIES

Berberis bark is covered by a negative Commission E monograph. In the opinion of the Commission E there is no evidence for the efficacy of the herb and there are risks associated with plant parts containing berberine. Side effects are possible if more than 0.5 g of berberine is ingested.

Berberis is on the UK General Sale List.

Berberis does not have GRAS status. However, it is freely available as a 'dietary supplement' in the USA under DSHEA legislation (1994 Dietary Supplement Health and Education Act).

Berberis is not included in Part 4 of Schedule 4 of the Therapeutic Goods Act Regulations of Australia.

Development of a monograph on Hydrastis is pending and may appear in the *United States Pharmacopoeia – National Formulary* subsequent to June 1999.

Hydrastis canadensis is not covered by a Commission E monograph but it is on the UK General Sale List.

Hydrastis does not have GRAS status. However, it is freely available as a 'dietary supplement' in the USA under DSHEA legislation (1994 Dietary Supplement Health and Education Act). Hydrastis has been present in the following over-the-counter (OTC) drug products: digestive aid products, weight control products, orally administered menstrual products, antiseptic products and counterirritant products. Hydrastis has also been present as an ingredient in products offered over the counter (OTC) for use as an aphrodisiac. However, the FDA advises: 'that based on evidence currently available, there is inadequate data to establish general recognition of the safety and effectiveness of these ingredients for the specified uses'.

Hydrastis is not included in Part 4 of Schedule 4 of the Therapeutic Goods Act Regulations of Australia.

References

1. Mabberley DJ. The plant book, 2nd edn. Cambridge University Press, Cambridge, 1997, p 84.
2. Osol A, Farrar GE et al. The dispensatory of the United States of America, 24th edn. JB Lippincott, Philadelphia, 1947, pp 543–545.
3. Mabberley DJ. The plant book, 2nd edn. Cambridge University Press, Cambridge, 1997, p 352.
4. Concannon JA, DeMeo TE. Endangered Species Bulletin 1997; 22 (6): 10–12.
5. Felter HW, Lloyd JU. King's American dispensatory, 18th edn, 3rd revision, vol 1, 1905. Reprinted by Eclectic Medical Publications, Portland, 1983, pp 345–346.
6. British Herbal Medicine Association's Scientific Committee. British herbal pharmacopoeia. BHMA, West York, 1983, pp 39–40.
7. Felter HW, Lloyd JU. King's American dispensatory, 18th edn, vol 2. Eclectic Medical Publications, Portland, 1983, pp 1020–1030.
8. Spaich W. Moderne Phytotherapie. Karl F. Haug Verlag, Heidelberg, 1977, pp 232–234.
9. Grieve M. A modern herbal, vol 1. Dover Publications, New York, 1971, pp 82–84.
10. Leung AY, Forster S. Encyclopedia of common natural ingredients used in food, drugs and cosmetics, 2nd edn. John Wiley, New York, 1996, pp 67, 282.
11. Chiej R. The Macdonald encyclopedia of medicinal plants. Macdonald, London, 1984, entry no. 54.
12. Launert EL. The Hamlyn guide to edible and medicinal plants of Britain and Northern Europe. Hamlyn, London, 1981, p 24.
13. Veringa L, Zaricor BR. Goldenseal/etc. A pharmacognosy of wild herbs. Ruka Publications, Santa Cruz, 1978, pp 20–22.
14. Wagner H, Bladt S. Plant drug analysis: a thin layer chromatography atlas, 2nd edn. Springer-Verlag, Berlin, 1996, p 10.
15. Simeon S, Rios JL, Villar A. Plantes méd phytothér 1989; 23 (3): 202–250.
16. British Herbal Medicine Association. British herbal compendium, vol 1. BHMA, Bournemouth, 1992, pp 119–120.

17. Sun D, Abraham SN, Beachey EH. Antimicrob Agents Chemother 1988; 32 (8): 1274–1277.
18. Mahajan VM, Sharma A, Rattan A. Sabouraudia 1982; 20 (1): 79–81.
19. Vennerstrom JL, Klayman DL. J Med Chem 1988; 31 (6): 1084–1087.
20. Kaneda Y, Torii M, Tanaka T et al. Ann Trop Med Parasitol 1991; 85 (4): 417–425.
21. Ghosh AK, Rakshit MM, Ghosh DK. Ind J Med Res 1983; 78: 407–416.
22. Vennerstrom JL, Lovelace JK, Waits VB et al. Antimicrob Agents Chemother 1990; 34 (5): 918–921.
23. Ghosh AK, Bhattacharyya FK, Ghosh DK. Exp Parasitol 1985; 60 (3): 404–413.
24. Ahuja A, Purohit SK, Yadav JS et al. Ind J Public Health 1993; 37 (1): 29–31.
25. Dutta NK, Iyer SN. J Ind Med Assoc 1968; 50 (8): 349–352.
26. Sun D, Courtney HS, Beachey EH. Antimicrob Agents Chemother 32 (9): 1370–1374.
27. Chen QM, Ye YC, Chai FL et al. Chung Kuo Chi Sheng Chung Hsueh Yu Chi Sheng Chung Ping Tsa Chih 1991; 9 (2): 137–139.
28. Amin AH, Subbaiah TV, Abbasi KM. Can J Microbiol 1969; 15: 1067–1076.
29. Palasuntheram C, Sangara Iyer K, De Silva LB et al. Ind J Med Res 1982; 76 (suppl): 71–76.
30. Pizzorno JE, Murray MT. A textbook of natural medicine, vol 1. John Bastyr College Publications, Seattle, 1987, V: Hydras-2.
31. Takase H, Yamamoto K, Ito K et al. Nippon Yakurigaku Zasshi 1993; 102 (2): 101–112.
32. Khin-Maung U, Nwe-Nwe-Wai J. Diarrhoeal Dis Res 1992; 10 (4): 201–204.
33. Zhang MF, Shen YQ. Chung Kuo Yao Li Hsueh Pao 1989; 10 (2): 174–176.
34. Donowitz M, Wicks J, Sharp GW. Rev Infect Dis 1986; 8 (suppl 2): S188–S201.
35. Swabb EA, Tai YH, Jordan L. Am J Physiol 1981; 241 (3): G248–G252.
36. Tai YH, Feser JF, Marnane WG et al. Am J Physiol 1981; 241 (3): G253–G258.
37. Sack RB, Froehlich JL. Infect Immun 1982; 35 (2): 471–475.
38. Taylor CT, Baird AW. Br J Pharmacol 1995, 116(6): 2667–2672.
39. Hua Z, Wang XL. Yao Hsueh Hsueh Pao 1994; 29 (8): 576–580.
40. Wang YX, Yao XJ, Tan YH. J Cardiovasc Pharmacol 1994; 23 (5): 716–722.
41. Ziablitskii VM, Romanovskaia VN, Umurzakova RZ et al. Eksp Klin Farmakol 1996; 59 (1): 37–39.
42. Wu JF, Liu TP. Yao Hsueh Hsueh Pao 1995; 30 (2): 98–102.
43. Chu ZL, Huang CG, Lai FS. Chin Pharmacol Bull 1994; 10 (2): 114–116.
44. Pasqual MS, Lauer CP, Moyna P et al. Mutat Res 1993; 286 (2): 243–252.
45. Chi CW, Chang YF, Chao TW et al. Life Sci 1994; 54 (26): 2099–2107.
46. Kumazawa Y, Itagaki A, Fukumoto M et al. Int J Immunopharmacol 1984; 6 (6): 587–592.
47. Kuo CL, Chou CC, Yung BY. Cancer Lett 1995; 93 (2): 193–200.
48. Sanders MM, Liu AA, Li TK et al. Biochem Pharmacol 1998; 56 (9): 1157–1166.
49. Ivanovska N, Philipov S. Int J Immunopharmacol 1996; 18 (10): 553–561.
50. Ckless K, Schlottfeldt JL, Pasqual M et al. J Pharm Pharmacol 1995; 47 (12A): 1029–1031.
51. Lin WC, Change HL. Res Commun Mol Pathol Pharmacol 1995; 90 (3): 333–346.
52. Imaseki I, Kitabatake Y, Taguchi H. Yakugaku Zasshi 1961; 81: 1281–1284.
53. Chan MY. Comp Med East West 1977; 5 (2): 161–168.
54. Seki T, Morohashi M. Skin Pharmacol 1993; 6 (1): 56–60.
55. Peng WH, Hsieh MT, Wu CR. Jpn J Pharmacol 1997; 74(3): 261–266.
56. Luo CN, Lin X, Li WK et al. J Ethnopharmacol 1998; 59 (3): 211–215.
57. Luo CN, Lin X, Li WK et al. Phytother Res 1997; 11: 585–587.
58. Pepeljnjak S, Petricic J. Pharmazie 1992; 47 (4): 307–308.
59. Gibbs OS. Fed Proc 1947; 6: 322.
60. Haginiwa J, Harada M. Yakugaku Zasshi 1962; 82: 726–731.
61. Palmery M, Leone MG, Pimpinella G et al. Pharmacol Res 1993; 27 (suppl 1): 73–74.
62. Palmery M, Cometa MF, Leone MG. Phytother Res 1996; 10 (suppl 1): S47–S49.
63. Cometa MF, Galeffi C, Palmery M. Phytother Res 1996; 10 (suppl 1): S56–S58.
64. Cometa MF, Abdel-Haq H, Palmery M. Phytother Res 1998; 12 (suppl 1): S83–S85.
65. Bolle P, Cometa MF, Palmery M et al. Phytother Res 1998; 12 (suppl 1): S86–S88.
66. Rentz E. Arch Exp Pathol Pharmakol 1948; 205: 332–338.
67. Tripathi YB, Shukla SD. Phytother Res 1996; 10 (7): 628–630.
68. Nikoronow M. Acta Polon Pharm 1939; 3: 23–56
69. Khattak SG, Gilani SN, Ikram M. J Ethnopharmacol 1985; 14 (1): 45–51.
70. Wolf S, Mack M. Drug Stand 1956; 24 (3): 98–101.
71. Bhide MB, Chavan SR, Dutta NK. Ind J Med Res 1969; 57 (11): 2128–2131.
72. Ozaki Y, Suzuki H, Satake M. Yakugaku Zasshi 1993; 113 (1): 63–69.
73. Lahiri SC, Dutta NK. J Ind Med Assoc 1967; 48 (1): 1–11.
74. Sharda DC. J Ind Med Assoc 1970; 54: 22–24.
75. Khin-Maung U, Myo-Khin, Nyunt-Nyunt-Wai et al. Br Med J (Clin Res Ed) 1985; 291 (6509): 1601–1605.
76. Khin-Maung-U, Myo-Khin, Nyunt-Nyunt-Wai et al. J Diarrhoeal Dis Res 1987; 5 (3): 184–187.
77. Rabbani GH, Butler T, Knight J et al. J Infect Dis 1987; 155 (5): 979–984.
78. Rabbani GH. Dan Med Bull 1996; 43 (2): 173–185.
79. Yuan J, Shen XZ, Zhu XS. Chung Kuo Chung Hsi I Chieh Ho Tsa Chih 1994; 14 (12): 718–720.
80. Hu FL. Chung Hua I Hsueh Tsa Chih 1993; 73 (4): 217–219, 253.
81. Babbar OP, Chhatwal VK, Ray IB et al. Ind J Med Res 1982; 76 (suppl): 83–88.
82. Mohan M, Pant CR, Angra SK et al. Ind J Ophthalmol 1982; 30 (2): 69–75.
83. Choudhry VP, Sabir M, Bhide VN. Ind Pediatr 1972; 9 (3): 143–146.
84. Gupte S. Am J Dis Child 1975; 129 (7): 866.
85. Watanabe A, Obata T, Nagashima H. Acta Med Okayama 1982; 36 (4): 277–281.
86. Ni YX, Liu AQ, Gao YF et al. Chin J Integr Med 1988; 8 (12): 711–713.
87. Purohit SK, Kochar DK, Lal BB et al. Ind J Public Health 1982; 26 (1): 34–37.
88. Chekalina SI, Umurzakova RZ, Saliev KK et al. Gematol Transfuziol 1994; 39 (5): 33–35.
89. Sheng WD, Jiddawi MS, Hong XQ et al. East Afr Med J 1997; 74 (5): 283–284.
90. Marin-Neto JA, Maciel BC, Secches AL et al. Clin Cardiol 1988; 11 (4): 253–260.
91. Wu AHB, Forte E, Casella G et al. J Forensic Sci 1995; 40 (4): 614–618.
92. Kulkarni SK, Dandiya PC, Varandani NL. Jpn J Pharmacol 1972; 22 (1): 11–16.
93. Turova AD, Leskov AI, Bichevina VI. Lekarstv Sredstva iz Rast 1962; pp 303–307.
94. German Federal Minister of Justice. German Commission E for human medicine monograph, Bundes-Anzeiger (German Federal Gazette) no. 43, dated 02.03.1989
95. De Smet PAGM, Keller K, Hansel R et al (eds). Adverse effects of herbal drugs, vol 1. Springer-Verlag, Berlin, 1992, p 101.
96. Chan E. Biol Neonate 1993; 63 (4): 201–208.

Bilberry fruit (*Vaccinium myrtillus* L.)

SYNONYMS

Whortleberry (Engl), Myrtilli fructus (Lat), Heidelbeeren, Blaubeeren (Ger), petit myrte, baies de myrtille (Fr), baceri mirtillo (Ital), blåbær (Dan).

WHAT IS IT?

Bilberry fruit is well known as a food, in particular, as a jam. The Vaccinium genus contains hundreds of species, many with edible berry-like fruits (including the American cranberry, *V. macrocarpon*). The name bilberry is derived from a Danish word meaning dark berry. Bilberry has been used in Europe to colour wine and to dye wool. During World War II, bilberry jam was consumed by RAF pilots to improve their night vision. Both the leaves and the ripe blue-black fruits are used medicinally but this monograph only covers the use of the fruit.

EFFECTS

Assists vision; decreases vascular permeability; protects against oxidative stress; astringent and antiinflammatory to mucosa of the gastrointestinal tract.

TRADITIONAL VIEW

Bilberry fruit was used to treat diarrhoea, dysentery, gastrointestinal inflammation, haemorrhoids and vaginal discharges and to 'dry up' breast milk. The fruit has also been used to treat scurvy and for urinary complaints.[1]

SUMMARY OF ACTIONS

Vasoprotective, antioedema, antioxidant, antiinflammatory, astringent.

CAN BE USED FOR

INDICATIONS SUPPORTED BY CLINICAL TRIALS

Peripheral vascular disorders of various origins, including Raynaud's syndrome; venous insufficiency, especially of the lower limbs; venous disorders during pregnancy, including haemorrhoids; symptoms caused by decreased capillary resistance; conditions involving increased capillary fragility, such as nosebleed; diabetic and hypertensive retinopathies; postoperative complications of minor surgery (such as ear, nose, throat); vision disorders due to impaired photosensitivity or altered microcirculation of the retina, including myopia, retinitis, hemeralopia, simple glaucoma; improvement in night vision (uncontrolled trials); dysmenorrhoea.

TRADITIONAL THERAPEUTIC USES

Digestive disorders (diarrhoea, dyspepsia, gastrointestinal infections and inflammations); haemorrhoids.

MAY ALSO BE USED FOR

EXTRAPOLATIONS FROM PHARMACOLOGICAL STUDIES

For capillary repair and to protect damaged capillaries; to treat and protect against ischaemic injury; antioxidant including inhibition of lipid peroxidation; wound healing (internal and topical); stabilization of connective tissue; gastric disorders requiring repair of gastric mucosal barrier (ulceration, gastritis, oesophagitis); as an antiplatelet agent.

OTHER APPLICATIONS

Topical treatment for inflammation of the mucous membranes of the mouth and throat;[2] inclusion in cosmetics (toners and skin products).[3]

PREPARATIONS

Dried or fresh fruit as a decoction, liquid extract and tablets for internal use. Decoction or extract for topical use. Available as a concentrated extract standardized for anthocyanin content and prepared from the fresh fruit.

Stability testing of solid and liquid forms of purified bilberry extract under drastic conditions (such as mild and strong acid solution at elevated temperatures) did not produce important changes in the relative anthocyanin composition. Mild conditions did not produce significant degradation of the anthocyanins.[4]

DOSAGE

- 3–6 ml of 1:1 liquid extract per day.
- Tablets providing 50–120 mg of anthocyanins per day (equivalent to about 20–50 g of fresh fruit) have been typically used in clinical trials.

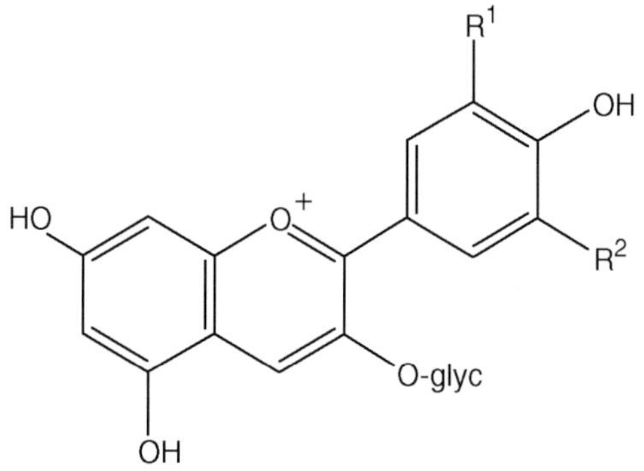

	R^1	R^2
Delphinidin 3-O-glycoside	OH	OH
Cyanidin 3-O-glycoside	OH	H
Petunidin 3-O-glycoside	OH	OCH_3
Peonidin 3-O-glycoside	OCH_3	H
Malvidin 3-O-glycoside	OCH_3	OCH_3

glyc = arabinoside, glucoside or galactoside

Anthocyanins

DURATION OF USE

May be taken long term for most applications.

SUMMARY ASSESSMENT OF SAFETY

No significant adverse effects from ingestion of bilberry are expected, although ingestion of the whole fresh fruit (as opposed to extracts) may irritate the intestinal lining in sensitive individuals.

TECHNICAL DATA

BOTANY

Vaccinium myrtillus, a member of the Ericaceae (heath) family, is a small shrub approximately 30–40 cm high with erect, branched flowering stems. The alternate, light green leaves are flat, oval and pointed with a toothed margin; flowers contain 4–5 white or pink petals. The fruit is a deep violet, fleshy berry enclosing crescent-shaped seeds.[5]

KEY CONSTITUENTS

- Anthocyanins (0.5%), also known as anthocyanosides, including C-3 glucosides of delphinidin, malvidin, pelargonidin, cyanidin and petunidin,[6] some of which are blue pigments responsible for the colour of the ripe fruits.
- Catechin, epicatechin, condensed tannins,[7] oligomeric procyanidins (procyanidin B1–B4).[8]
- Flavonoids, phenolic acids, pectins.[7,8]

PHARMACODYNAMICS

Vascular protective and antioedema activity

Anthocyanins improved functional disturbances of the fine blood vessels, especially capillaries,[9] were more effective in protecting damaged capillaries than flavonoids[10] and stimulated capillary repair.[11] Bilberry extract in vivo reduced microvascular impairments due to ischaemia-reperfusion injury, resulting in preservation of endothelium, attenuation of leucocyte adhesion and improvement of capillary perfusion.[12]

Oral administration of bilberry extract (equivalent to 180 mg/kg anthocyanins per day) for 12 days maintained normal permeability of the blood–brain barrier and limited the increase in vascular permeability in the skin and aorta wall after induced hypertension. Interaction with collagen within blood vessel walls is believed to be partly responsible for this vasoprotective activity.[13]

Oral administration of bilberry extract (equivalent to 72–144 mg/kg anthocyanins) demonstrated significant vasoprotective and antioedema effects in vivo. Activity was stronger and longer lasting than that of rutin and was not due to a specific antagonism of inflammatory mediators such as histamine or bradykinin. The antioedema activity was also observed after topical application (but resulted in persistent coloration due to the anthocyanins).[14]

Intravenous administration of bilberry extract (equivalent to 1.8–3.6 mg/kg anthocyanins) induced arteriolar vasomotion in cheek pouch and skeletal muscle of hamsters. By enhancing arteriolar rhythmic diameter changes, bilberry may play a role in the redistribution of microvascular blood flow and interstitial fluid formation.[15]

Effects on vision

Anthocyanins have demonstrated an affinity for the pigmented epithelium of the retina in vitro.[16] Bilberry hastens the regeneration of rhodopsin (visual purple) in vitro and in vivo after injection.[17] Rhodopsin is a light-sensitive pigment found in the rods of the retina.

It must be quickly regenerated in order to maintain visual sensitivity.

Bilberry anthocyanins significantly accelerated adaptation to the dark and improved visual acuity in dim light in healthy subjects compared to placebo.[18] In a placebo-controlled trial, individuals taking anthocyanins demonstrated significantly better night vision than those taking placebo.[19] In a double-blind, placebo-controlled study on 40 healthy subjects, a single dose of bilberry extract (equivalent to 86 mg anthocyanins) induced a more efficient pupillary photomotor response which was evident 2 hours after treatment.[20] Bilberry extract improved night vision in uncontrolled trials conducted with air-traffic controllers, pilots and automobile drivers.[21]

Antioxidant activity

Anthocyanins demonstrated in vitro antioxidant activity in a number of models, including scavenging of superoxide anions and inhibition of lipid peroxidation.[22] Bilberry extract also demonstrated antioxidant activity in vitro by inhibiting the potassium ion loss induced by free radicals in human erythrocytes and by inhibiting cellular reactions induced by oxidant compounds.[23,24]

A concentration-dependent inhibition of oxysterol formation (cholesterol oxides) was observed in vitro for bilberry extract after photo-induced oxidation of human low density lipoproteins (LDL). This antioxidant activity was confirmed by the partial restoration of the normal electrophoretic mobility of LDL. Oxysterols are the main contributors to the atherogenicity and cytotoxicity of oxidized LDL.[25] Aqueous extract of bilberry also demonstrated potent protective activity on human LDL particles during in vitro copper-mediated oxidation.[26]

Wound-healing activity

Bilberry extract was reported to accelerate the process of spontaneous healing of experimental wounds after topical application.[27] Topical bilberry extract significantly improved the healing of experimental skin wounds after healing had been delayed by a steroidal antiinflammatory agent. The wound-healing activity was more potent than that of the selected triterpenoids of *Centella asiatica*.[28]

Antiplatelet activity

Bilberry extract demonstrated strong antiplatelet activity in vitro and, at dosages equivalent to up to 144 mg/kg anthocyanins, prolonged bleeding time without affecting blood coagulation in vivo.[29] Inhibition of platelet aggregation was demonstrated from the blood of healthy subjects after oral administration of an extract equivalent to 173 mg anthocyanins per day for 30–60 days. The mechanism of action may depend on an increase in the concentration of cAMP and/or a decrease in the concentration of platelet thromboxane.[30]

Other activity

Anthocyanins have demonstrated collagen-stabilizing activity in vitro.[31] Two anthocyanins from bilberry protected collagen against non-enzymatic proteolytic activity in vitro and therefore may protect collagen from degradation during inflammatory processes.[32] Anthocyanins stimulated mucopolysaccharide biosynthesis in experimentally induced granuloma in vivo.[33]

Bilberry extract induced active phagocytosis and intense cell regeneration from human umbilical cord and demonstrated growth-promoting activity for fibroblasts and smooth muscle cells in vitro.[34,35]

Anthocyanins (cyanidin, delphinidin and malvidin 3-O-glucosides) and their aglycones inhibited phosphodiesterases from several tissues in vitro and were more active than isobutylmethylxanthine. The highest activity was observed on retinal phosphodiesterase.[36–38] Inhibition of phosphodiesterase leads to increased cyclic AMP and cyclic GMP in tissue.

Components of the hexane/chloroform fraction of bilberry extract exhibited potential anticarcinogenic activity by inducing the phase II detoxification enzyme quinone reductase in vitro. The crude extract, anthocyanin and oligomeric procyanidin fractions were not highly active.[39]

Cyanidin chloride (an anthocyanin from bilberry) demonstrated promising antiulcer activity in vivo. Gastric mucus production was increased without affecting gastric secretion.[40,41] Bilberry extract (equivalent to 9–72 mg/kg anthocyanins) demonstrated significant dose-dependent antiulcer activity, in some cases exhibiting stronger activity than carbenoxolone or cimetidine.[28]

PHARMACOKINETICS

Pharmacokinetic studies after oral administration of bilberry extract indicate that although the anthocyanins have low bioavailability, plasma peak levels are within the therapeutic range. Absorption from the gastrointestinal tract was about 5% and there was no hepatic first-pass effect. Plasma concentrations of anthocyanins reached peak levels after 15 minutes and then rapidly declined within 2 hours. Elimination occurred mainly through the bile.[42]

CLINICAL TRIALS

Peripheral vascular disorders and venous disorders

Uncontrolled trials dating back to 1964 demonstrated the efficacy of bilberry in the treatment of peripheral vascular disorders.[18] In later trials, bilberry extract (equivalent to 86–173 mg anthocyanins per day) improved oedema and subjective symptoms of lower limb varicose syndrome,[43] reduced protein exudate of varicose ulcers[33] and decreased the total drainage time after reactive hyperaemia in chronic venous insufficiency.[44] Bilberry extract (57–115 mg anthocyanins per day for 2–3 months) provided relief for venous disorders including haemorrhoids during pregnancy.[45,46] A review of uncontrolled trials from 1979 to 1985 on a total of 568 patients with venous insufficiency of the lower limbs concluded that bilberry extract caused rapid disappearance of symptoms and improvements in venous microcirculation and lymph drainage.[47] Mobilization of finger joints was improved in patients with Raynaud's syndrome.[48]

Bilberry extract (equivalent to 173 mg anthocyanins per day) or placebo was administered for 30 days in a single-blind, placebo-controlled clinical trial on 60 patients with venous insufficiency. Significant reduction in the severity of symptoms (oedema, sensation of pain, paraesthesia, cramping pain) was observed for the treated group after 4 weeks' treatment ($p<0.01$).[49]

In a double-blind, placebo-controlled trial, 47 patients with peripheral vascular disorders of various origins were treated with bilberry extract (equivalent to 173 mg anthocyanins per day) or placebo for 30 days. The treated group experienced a reduction in subjective symptoms including paraesthesia, pain, heaviness and oedema.[48]

Microcirculation disorders including retinopathy

In uncontrolled trials, bilberry extract (equivalent to 57–288 mg anthocyanins per day) improved symptoms caused by decreased capillary resistance (petechiae, bruising and faecal occult blood),[34] reduced the microcirculatory changes induced by cortisone therapy in patients with asthma and chronic bronchitis[50] and improved diabetic retinopathy with a marked reduction or even disappearance of retinic haemorrhages.[51] Postoperative complications from surgery of the nose were reduced in patients who received bilberry extract (equivalent to 115 mg anthocyanins per day) administered for 7 days before and 10 days after surgery.[52]

In a placebo-controlled trial, bilberry extract (equivalent to 115 mg anthocyanins per day for 12 months) improved early-phase diabetic retinopathy as indicated by a reduction of hard exudate at the posterior pole.[53]

In a double-blind, placebo-controlled clinical trial, 14 patients with diabetic and/or hypertensive retinopathy received bilberry extract (equivalent to 115 mg anthocyanins per day) or placebo for 1 month. Significant improvements in the ophthalmoscopic and angiographic patterns were observed in 77–90% of treated patients.[54]

Visual disorders

In uncontrolled trials conducted as early as 1964, bilberry extract (including isolated anthocyanins), alone or in combination with beta-carotene and retinol, improved vision in healthy subjects and in patients with visual disorders such as myopia.[21,55] Enlargement of visual range was observed for patients with pigmentary retinitis[56] and retinal sensitivity was improved in patients with hemeralopia (defective vision in bright light).[57]

Visual perception improved in 76% of myopic patients receiving bilberry extract (equivalent to 54 mg anthocyanins per day) and retinol for 15 days.[58] Similar results were obtained for patients with simple glaucoma.[59]

Bilberry extract (equivalent to 115 mg anthocyanins per day) for 90 days improved darkness adaptation in all myopic patients and improved day vision in those suffering from light to medium myopia.[60]

Other conditions

In uncontrolled trials, bilberry extract was administered postoperatively in conjunction with antiinflammatory and analgesic drugs to patients who had undergone haemorrhoidectomy. Bilberry reduced postoperative symptoms (itching and oedema).[61,62]

In a placebo-controlled trial, bilberry extract (equivalent to 115 mg anthocyanins per day for 180 days) was effective in reducing nosebleed caused by abnormal capillary fragility of the mucous membranes.[63]

In a double-blind, placebo-controlled trial, 30 women with chronic primary dysmenorrhoea were treated with bilberry extract (equivalent to 115 mg anthocyanins per day) for 3 days before and during menstruation. Bilberry significantly reduced symptoms of dysmenorrhoea such as pelvic and lumbosacral pain, mammary tension, headache, nausea and heaviness of lower limbs ($p<0.01$).[64]

TOXICOLOGY

In early studies using the anthocyanins of bilberry, no teratogenic effects from daily doses of 600 mg per day in rats, mice and rabbits were observed.[65]

Bilberry extract (standardized to contain 36% anthocyanins) had low acute toxicity by the oral route in experimental models. The LD_{50} was greater than the equivalent of 720 mg/kg anthocyanins in rats and mice. Long-term oral administration of doses containing up to the equivalent of 180 mg/kg anthocyanins per day for 6 months did not produce toxic effects. No evidence of mutagenic or teratogenic effects was observed.[66]

Weak activity was observed for bilberry extract in the Ames mutagenicity test, probably due to the presence of quercetin.[67]

CONTRAINDICATIONS

None known.

SPECIAL WARNINGS AND PRECAUTIONS

Very high doses should be used cautiously in patients with haemorrhagic disorders and in those taking warfarin or antiplatelet drugs.

INTERACTIONS

Possible interaction with warfarin and antiplatelet drugs, but only for very high doses.

USE IN PREGNANCY AND LACTATION

No adverse effects expected.

EFFECTS ON ABILITY TO DRIVE AND USE MACHINES

No adverse effects.

SIDE EFFECTS

A surveillance study was conducted on over 2000 patients with venous disorders and retinal microcirculation disorders who consumed on average the equivalent of 115 mg anthocyanins per day for 1–2 months. About 4% of patients reported mild side effects affecting the gastrointestinal, cutaneous or nervous systems.[66]

OVERDOSE

No effects known.

CURRENT REGULATORY STATUS IN SELECTED COUNTRIES

Bilberry was added to the *French Pharmacopoeia* in 1992 and is on the UK General Sale List. Bilberry fruit is covered by a positive Commission E monograph and has the following applications:

- non-specific, acute diarrhoea;
- topical treatment of mild inflammation of the mucous membranes of the mouth and throat.

Bilberry does not have GRAS status. However, it is freely available as a 'dietary supplement' in the USA under DSHEA legislation (1994 Dietary-Supplement Health and Education Act).

Bilberry is not included in Part 4 of Schedule 4 of the Therapeutic Goods Act Regulations of Australia.

References

1. Grieve M. A modern herbal, vols 1 and 2. Dover Publications, New York, 1971, pp 99–100.
2. German Federal Minister of Justice. German Commission E for human medicine monograph, Bundes-Anzeiger (German Federal Gazette) no. 76, dated 23.04.1987, no. 50, dated 13.03.1990.
3. Smeh NJ. Creating your own cosmetics – naturally. Alliance Publishing Garrisonville, 1995, pp 81, 142.
4. Martinelli EM, Scilingo A, Pifferi G. Anal Chim Acta 1992; 259 (1): 109–113.
5. Chiej R. The Macdonald encyclopedia of medicinal plants. Macdonald, London, 1984, entry no. 321.
6. Wagner H, Bladt S. Plant drug analysis: a thin layer chromatography atlas, 2nd edn. Springer-Verlag, Berlin, 1996, p 282.
7. Bisset NG (ed). Herbal drugs and phytopharmaceuticals. Medpharm Scientific Publishers, Stuttgart, 1994, pp 351–352.
8. Brenneisen R, Steinegger E. Pharm Acta Helv 1981; 56 (7): 180–185.
9. Terrasse J, Moinade S. Presse Med 1964; 72: 397–400.
10. Demure G. PhD thesis in medicine: Etude expérimentale et clinique d'un nouveau facteur vitaminique P: les Anthocyanosides. Clermont, France, 1964.
11. Bombardelli E. Therapia Angiol 1976; 5: 177.
12. Bertuglia S, Malandrino S, Colantuoni A. Pharmacol Res 1995; 31 (3–4): 183–187.
13. Detre Z, Jellinek H, Miskulin M et al. Clin Physiol Biochem 1986; 4: 143–149.
14. Lietti A, Cristoni A, Picci M. Arzneim-Forsch 1976; 26 (1): 829–835.
15. Colantuoni A, Bertuglia S, Magistretti MJ et al. Arzneim-Forsch 1991; 41 (9): 905–909.
16. Wegmann R, Maeda P, Tronche P et al. Ann Histochim 1969; 14: 237–256.

17. Cluzel C, Bastide P, Wegman R et al. Biochem Pharmacol 1970; 19: 2295–2302.
18. Jayle GE, Aubert L. Therapie 1964; 19: 171–185.
19. Jayle GE, Aubury M, Gavini G et al. Ann Ocul 1965; 198: 556–562.
20. Vannini L, Samuelly R, Coffano M et al. Boll Ocul 1986; 65 (suppl 6): 569–577
21. Morazzoni P, Bombardelli E. Fitoterapia 1996; 67 (1): 3–29.
22. Meunier MT, Duroux E, Bastide P. Plant Med Phytother 1989; 23 (4): 267–274.
23. Maridonneau I, Braquet P, Garay RP. In: Farkas L, Gabor M, Kallay F et al (eds) Flavonoids and bioflavonoids. Elsevier, Amsterdam, 1982, pp 427–436.
24. Mavelli I, Rossi L, Autuori F et al. Oxy radicals and their scavenger systems. In: Cohen G, Greenwald RA (eds) Proceedings of the 3rd International Conference on Superoxide and Superoxide Dismutase, New York, October, 1982. Elsevier, New York, 1983, pp 326–329.
25. Francesca Rasetti M, Caruso D, Galli G et al. Phytomed 1996/1997; 3 (4): 335–338.
26. Laplaud PM, Lelubre A, Chapman MJ. Fundam Clin Pharmacol 1997; 11 (1): 35–40.
27. Curri SB, Liteti A, Bombardelli E. Giorn Minerva Derm 1976; 111: 509–515
28. Cristoni A, Magistretti MJ. Il Farmaco Ed Pr 1987; 42 (2): 29–43.
29. Morazzoni P, Magistretti MJ. Fitoterapia 1990; 61 (1): 13–21.
30. Pulliero G, Montin S, Bettini V et al. Fitoterapia 1989; 60 (1): 69–75.
31. Ronziere MC, Herbage D, Garrone R et al. Biochem Pharmacol 1981; 30: 1771–1776.
32. Monboisse JC, Braquet P, Randoux A et al. Biochem Pharmacol 1983; 32: 53–58.
33. Mian E, Curri SB, Leitti A et al. Minerva Med 1977; 68 (52): 3565–3581.
34. Piovella C, Curri BS, Piovella M et al. Therapia Angiol 1979; 35: 119.
35. Piovella F, Ricetti MM, Almasio P et al. Minerva Angiol 1981; 6: 135–140.
36. Ferretti C, Magistretti MJ, Robotti A et al. Pharmacol Res Commun 1988; 20 (suppl 2): 150.
37. Ferretti C, Blengio M, Malandrino S et al. XIth International Symposium on Medicinal Chemistry, Jerusalem, Israel, 1990.
38. Pifferi G, Malandrino S, Morazzoni P et al. XVIth International Conference of the Groupe Polyphenols, Lisbon, 1992. Polyphenols Actualities 1992; 8: 60.
39. Bomser J, Madhavi DL, Singletary K et al. Planta Med 1996; 62 (3): 212–216.
40. Magistretti MJ, Conti M, Cristoni A. Arzneim-Forsch 1988; 38 (5): 686–690.
41. Cristoni A, Malandrino S, Magistretti MJ. Arzneim-Forsch 1989; 39 (5): 590–592.
42. Morazzoni P, Livio S, Scilingo A et al. Arzneim-Forsch 1991; 41 (1): 128–131.
43. Ghiringhelli C, Gregoratti F, Marastoni F. Minerva Cardioang 1977; 26: 255–276.
44. Corsi C, Pollastri M, Tesi C et al. Fitoterapia 1985; 56 (suppl 1): 23.
45. Grismondi GL. Minerva Gin 1981; 33 (2–3): 221–230.
46. Teglio L, Tronconi R, Mazzanti C et al. Quad Clin Ostet Ginecol 1987; 42 (3): 221–231.
47. Berta V, Zucchi C. Fitoterapia 1988; 59 (suppl 1): 27.
48. Allegra C, Pollari G, Criscuolo A. Minerva Angiol 1982; 7: 39–44.
49. Gatta L. Fitoterapia 1988; 59 (suppl 1): 19.
50. Carmignani G. Lotta Contro Tuberce Malatt Polm Sociali 1983; 53: 732–735
51. Orsucci PL, Rossi M, Sabbatini G et al. Clin Ocul 1983; 4: 377–381
52. Mattioli L, Dallari S, Galetti R. Fitoterapia 1988; 59 (suppl 1): 41.
53. Repossi P, Malagola R, De Cadihac C. Ann Ottalmol Clin Ocul 1987; 113 (4): 357–361.
54. Perossini M, Guidi G, Chiellini S et al. Ann Ottalmol Clin Ocul 1987; 113 (12): 1173–1190.
55. Gandolfo E. Boll Ocul 1990; 69 (1): 57–72.
56. Fiorini G, Biancacci A, Graziano FM. Ann Ottalmol Clin Ocul 1965; 91 (6): 371–386.
57. Zavarise G. Ann Ottalmol Clin Ocul 1968; 94 (2): 209–214.
58. Virno M, Recori Giraldi J, Auriemma L. Boll Ocul 1986; 65 (4): 789–796.
59. Caselli L. Arch Med Interna 1985; 37: 29–35.
60. Contestabile MT, Appolloni R, Suppressa F et al. Boll Ocul 1991; 70 (6): 1157–1169.
61. Pezzangora V, Barina R, De Stefani R et al. Gaz Med Ital 1984; 143 (6): 405–409.
62. Oliva E, Nicastro A, Sorcini A et al. Aggior Med Chir 1990; 8: 1
63. Massenzo D, Gentile A, Mosciaro O. Riv Ital Otl Aud Fon 1992; 12 (1): 65–68.
64. Colombo D, Vescovini R. Giorn Ital Ost Gin 1985; 7 (12): 1033–1038.
65. Pourrat H, Bastide P, Dorier P et al. Chim Ther 1967; 2: 33–38.
66. Eandi M. 'Post marketing investigation on Tegens® preparation with respect to side effects', 1987; cited in Morazzoni P, Bombardelli E. Fitoterapia 1996; 67 (1): 3–29.
67. Schimmer O, Kruger A, Paulini H et al. Pharmazie 1994; 49 (6): 448–451.

Black cohosh (*Cimicifuga racemosa* (L.) Nutt.)

SYNONYMS

Actaea racemosa L. (botanical synonym), bugbane, black snakeroot (Engl), Cimicifugae rhizoma (Lat), schwarzes Wanzenkraut, Cimicifugawurzelstock (Ger), cimicaire, actée à grappes (Fr), sølvlys (Dan).

WHAT IS IT?

The common names of *Cimicifuga racemosa* rhizome, black snakeroot and rattle snakeroot, refer to its use in its native country, North America, to treat snakebite including that of rattlesnake. The generic name Cimicifuga comes from the Latin 'to chase insects away' and reflects on a reputed use of the European species. In recent years the root of black cohosh has become a popular treatment for menopausal symptoms, with its registration in proprietary medicines in Germany.

EFFECTS

Oestrogen-like effect, binds to oestrogen receptors; suppresses luteinizing hormone (LH).

TRADITIONAL VIEW

Black cohosh, a favourite of the Eclectic physicians, was used for myalgia, neuralgia (not of spinal origin), chorea, female reproductive tract disorders (amenorrhoea, dysmenorrhoea, ovarian pain, menorrhagia) and rheumatic conditions (arthralgia, muscular rheumatism). Other conditions treated included whooping cough, tinnitus and mastitis.[1,2] Black cohosh is also used to treat premenstrual syndrome and secondary amenorrhoea in Germany.[3,4]

SUMMARY ACTIONS

Antirheumatic, antispasmodic, oestrogenic, uterine tonic.

CAN BE USED FOR

INDICATIONS SUPPORTED BY CLINICAL TRIALS

Treatment of climacteric symptoms and symptoms arising from ovarian insufficiency.

TRADITIONAL THERAPEUTIC USES

Used particularly for arthritis and rheumatism, neuralgia, sciatica; menstruation disorders (amenorrhoea, dysmenorrhoea, menorrhagia, ovarian pain); respiratory tract disorders, whooping cough, asthma; tinnitus.

MAY ALSO BE USED FOR

EXTRAPOLATIONS FROM PHARMACOLOGICAL STUDIES

Adjunct in the treatment of conditions requiring reduction in LH levels (e.g. infertility, miscarriage, cyst formation, ovarian tumorigenesis, polycystic ovary syndrome).

PREPARATIONS

Dried or fresh rhizome for decoction, liquid extract for internal use.

DOSAGE

Two dosage approaches are evident. The first is based on traditional doses:

- 0.5–1 g of dried root/rhizome 3–4 times per day;[5]
- 1.5–3 ml of 1:2 liquid extract per day; 3.5–7 ml of 1:5 tincture per day;
- 6–12 ml of 1:10 tincture per day.[5]

The second is based on recent experiences with German products:

- ethanol extract equivalent to 40 mg of dried rhizome and root per day;[3]
- 40–200 mg of dried rhizome and root per day;[6]
- 0.4–2 ml of 1:10 tincture in 60% ethanol per day.[6]

DURATION OF USE

May be taken long term within the recommended dosage, although the Commission E recommends not more than 6 months.

SUMMARY ASSESSMENT OF SAFETY

No adverse effects from ingestion of black cohosh are expected when used at the recommended dosage. It is not recommended during pregnancy except for assisting birth.

TECHNICAL DATA

BOTANY

Black cohosh is a member of the Ranunculaceae (buttercup) family and grows to an average height of 150 cm.[7] It produces feathery racemes of white blossoms which droop gracefully and a dry fruit containing numerous seeds. The leaves have three-pointed, trilobate leaflets. The fleshy, dark brown/black rhizome is a creeping underground stem, from which follow dark brown roots.[7,8]

KEY CONSTITUENTS

- Triterpene glycosides (saponins) of the cycloartane type, including actein and cimicifugoside.[9]
- Isoflavones (formononetin), caffeic and isoferulic acids.[10]
- 15–20% resins (cimicifugin),[10] fatty acids.[6]

Recent research disputes the presence of formononetin (and kaempferol) in black cohosh extracts, although other flavonoids were present.[11]

PHARMACODYNAMICS

Hormonal activity

Prolonged injections of black cohosh extract in rats and mice increased the weight of the uterus and established menstrual cycles in juvenile and climacteric animals.[12] Black cohosh extract demonstrated a selective reduction of serum LH in ovariectomized rats. FSH (follicle-stimulating hormone) and prolactin levels were unchanged. Intraperitoneal administration of black cohosh extract (24 mg dried extract/day) resulted in significant inhibition of LH secretion after the third day. Fractionated extraction of black cohosh and subsequent testing with three fractions indicated that the LH-suppressive substances reside in the dichloromethane extract. The intact glycosidal components of this extract were more active with regard to LH suppression than the aglycone form. Oral administration of the non-hydrolysed extract demonstrated a significant inhibition of LH, although much lower than that achieved by injection.[13] (This does not necessarily mean the aglycone is inactive as the glycoside may provide enhanced bioavailability with cleavage, yielding an active aglycone.)[14]

Serum levels of LH in ovariectomized rats were reduced after intraperitoneal administration of a trichloromethane fraction of a black cohosh methanolic extract. The trichloromethane fraction also demonstrated an ability to bind to oestrogen receptors in vitro. This fraction was further separated into three subfractions, two of which suppressed LH secretion in vivo and displaced oestrogen in vitro. This indicates that at least two groups of compounds may be responsible for the endocrine activity of black cohosh. One active compound identified was the isoflavone formononetin. Despite activity in the oestrogen receptor assay, formononetin failed to reduce the serum levels of LH in ovariectomized rats.[15] These results suggest that formononetin may act as an oestradiol antagonist (binding to the receptor but not producing an effect) rather than an agonist (binding to and activating the receptor) and hence not affect LH secretion.[16]

Water and chloroform fractions prepared from a black cohosh methanol extract were tested in ovariectomized rats by intraperitoneal injection over several days (chronic administration). The chloroform fraction demonstrated a strong LH-suppressing effect after 3 days; the water fraction was inactive. Further fractionation of the chloroform extract led to the conclusion that the LH-suppressive effect of black cohosh extract is caused by at least three different synergistically acting compounds.[17]

Two commercial black cohosh extracts were tested for their ability to compete with oestradiol for the antigen binding sites on an antibody (IgG) directed against oestradiol (radioimmunoassay). Both extracts ran parallel with the displacement curve obtained with oestradiol, which supports the presence of oestrogenic compounds in black cohosh.[18] However, no oestrogenic activity was found after oral or subcutaneous administration of black cohosh extract (6, 60, 600 mg/kg) to groups of immature mice and ovariectomized rats respectively.[19]

One hundred and ten women experiencing menopausal symptoms who had received no hormone replacement therapy for at least 6 months, received either a standardized black cohosh extract (four tablets* per day) or placebo. After 8 weeks of treatment, LH levels were significantly reduced ($p<0.05$) in the black cohosh group but FSH levels were unchanged.[17*]

Other activity

Unlike oestradiol, black cohosh extract did not stimulate growth of mammary tumour cells in vitro. In fact a dosage of 2.5 μg/ml led to a strong inhibition of proliferation.[20] The simultaneous incubation of tumour cells with tamoxifen (anticarcinogenic agent, oestrogen antagonist) and black cohosh displayed a much stronger inhibition of growth than of either substance

*Refer to the Clinical trials subsection below for an explanation of dosage.

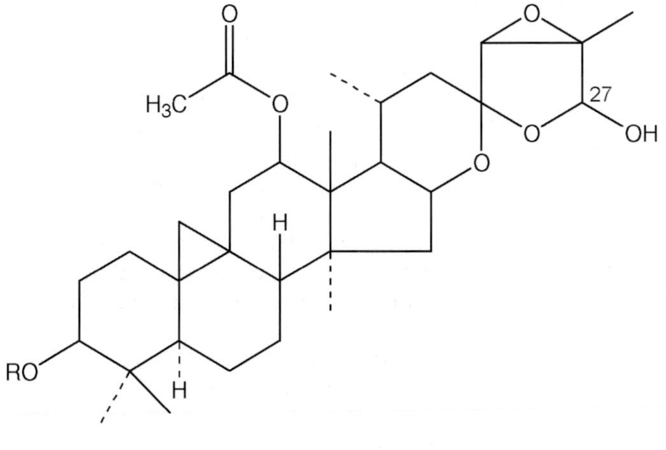

	R
Actein	β-D-xylosyl
Acetylacteol	H

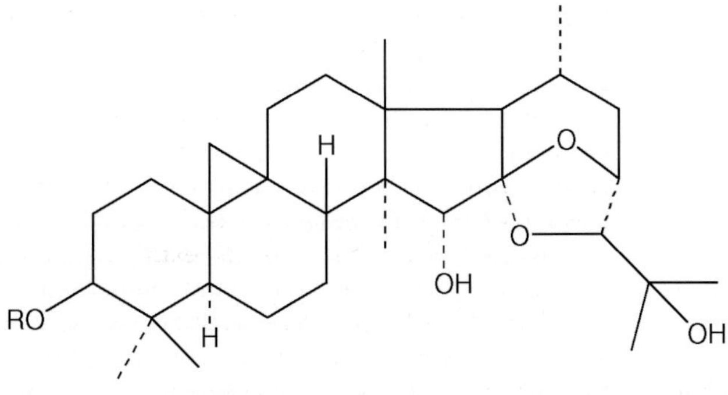

	R
Cimicifugoside	β-D-xylosyl
Cimigenol	H

alone.[21] (Oestrogen is contraindicated in patients with oestrogen receptor-positive breast carcinoma, since it promotes the growth of the tumour cells.)

Pretreatment with cimicifugoside inhibited blastogenesis in mouse splenic lymphocytes and brought about a decrease in the number of plaque-forming colonies using sheep erythrocytes (SRBC). The anti-SRBC response in the plaque-forming assay was suppressed in mice after pretreatment by intraperitoneal administration and delayed hypersensitivity was suppressed after intravenous administration. The immunosuppressive activity of cimicifugoside is directed toward B-cell function with larger doses being required for suppression of T-cell function.[22]

Black cohosh extract and several fractions obtained from it demonstrated hypotensive activity after intravenous administration at 1 mg/kg to rabbits. The hypotensive activity was observed in particular with the resinous part and may be due to actein. A hypotensive effect was not observed in human subjects (by intravenous administration), although a peripheral vasodilatory effect was evident, even in subjects with peripheral arterial disease.[23] Oral administration of black cohosh extract (2 g/kg) inhibited 5-hydroxytryptophan-induced diarrhoea in mice.[24]

PHARMACOKINETICS

No data available.

CLINICAL TRIALS

The clinical studies outlined below were conducted using a German proprietary medicine with lower doses than those used traditionally. These studies date back to the 1950s and definitive information about the level of dried herb equivalent within the tablets is not always available. The tablets are quoted as consisting of 2 mg of a dried ethanol/water extract of black cohosh and containing 1 mg of a marker triterpene glycoside (27-deoxyactein). The liquid product was a tincture, also containing 1 mg per dose (approximately 20 drops) of a marker triterpene glycoside (27-deoxyactein). Current regulatory information indicates that these tablets now contain 24.8–42.7 mg dried herb equivalent, containing 0.8–1.2 mg triterpene glycosides.

Menopause

Standardized black cohosh extract was used with success in the 1950s and 1960s for the treatment of menopausal symptoms, menstrual disturbances in young women (secondary but not primary amenorrhoea) and symptoms arising from ovarian dysfunction or insufficiency. The Kupperman Index is an indicator of climacteric symptoms, originally defined in 1953. Medical opinion of the 1970s led to a correction of the index, reducing it to only two essential symptoms (hot flushes and genital atrophy) and disregarding psychosomatic symptoms (insomnia, nervousness, depression) as not specific to menopause. A new score, the Menopause Rating Scale (MRS) has been proposed, which adopts most of the symptoms of the Kupperman Index and adds the symptoms: alteration of libido, urological complaints and vaginal dryness. It also provides an individual profile of each patient.[25,26] In the clinical trials listed below, the symptoms measured by the Kupperman Index are indicated where known or described as 'full' or 'modified' according to the above.

Observation of 110 case studies in the late 1950s indicated black cohosh extract was useful as a supplementary medication in the treatment of menopausal symptoms. Positive results were obtained with standardized black cohosh extract (30 drops of tincture or 1–2 tablets, each three times per day) in 33 of 61 patients with climacteric symptoms due to menopause and in eight of 10 patients with induced menopause as a result of surgery. Only minor improvements were observed in the younger women who had undergone surgery. Black cohosh did not have a positive effect on the remaining 21 patients with menstrual irregularities (amenorrhoea, oligomenorrhoea) and dysmenorrhoea.[27]

In an uncontrolled trial, 62 menopausal women were treated with a low dose of standardized black cohosh extract (60 drops of tincture per day, decreasing to 30 over time). The patients initially also received hormone treatment, which was discontinued over the course of treatment where possible (except for those with complete hormone deficiency). The following patients were considerably better after treatment: eight of eight premenopausal women with hypomenorrhoea or oligomenorrhoea, 15 of 18 women in their first to second year of menopause, 21 of 21 women in their third year of menopause, seven of seven women with postoperative climacteric symptoms with intact ovaries and eight of eight women with postoperative climacteric symptoms after removal of ovary/ovaries. Women with symptoms of depression, short-term memory loss and tinnitus responded well to treatment.[28]

In an uncontrolled study conducted by 131 general practitioners, patients with climacteric symptoms were treated with standardized black cohosh extract (80 drops per day of tincture, over 6–8 weeks). About 40% of the 629 women who completed the study were also taking oestrogen therapy and/or psychotropic drugs. After 4 weeks, significant improvement of climacteric symptoms was observed in 80% of patients and symptoms had largely disappeared after 6–8 weeks of treatment. Nervousness, sleeplessness and depression showed similar improvement. About 7% of patients complained of continuing stomach problems.[29]

In two uncontrolled studies (36 and 50 patients respectively),[30,31] gynaecologists treated climacteric symptoms in patients, some with contraindications to or opposition to hormone replacement therapy. Patients received standardized black cohosh extract (80 drops per day of 1:5 tincture for 12 weeks). After 4 weeks, significant improvement ($p<0.001$) was observed in the first study, as indicated by a reduction in the Kupperman Index.[30] In the second study, significant improvement was seen in the full Kupperman Index ($p<0.001$). Improvement was also recorded for psychiatric symptoms, with decreased fatigue and depression ($p<0.001$) and increased energy ($p<0.001$).[31]

Fifty women with pronounced menopausal symptoms were treated with the view to replacing their 6 monthly hormone injection treatment with standardized black cohosh extract (four tablets per day) in an uncontrolled trial. A significant decrease in the menopause index ($p<0.001$) followed from 12 weeks of black cohosh treatment and 56% of patients required no additional hormone injections.[32]

Forty-one patients with menopausal symptoms were administered placebo and then standardized black cohosh extract (three tablets per day initially for 1 week and then a reduced dose) in a single-blind study. A noticeable decrease of symptoms was observed for 31 women while taking black cohosh compared to only four while on placebo. Three patients reported stomach complaints.[33]

Sixty patients under 40 years of age who had undergone hysterectomy and who had at least one intact ovary but complained of climacteric symptoms were randomized into four groups. They received either oestriol, conjugated oestrogens, oestrogen-gestagen sequential therapy or standardized black cohosh extract (four tablets per day) for 24 weeks in an open trial. In all groups the modified Kupperman Index was significantly lower ($p<0.01$), but a decrease in LH and FSH could not be confirmed statistically. There were no significant differences between the various groups.[34]

In an open controlled study, 60 patients received either standardized black cohosh extract (80 drops per day of tincture), oestrogen (0.625 mg/day) or diazepam (2 mg/day) over 12 weeks. Signs of oestrogen stimulation of the vaginal mucosa, improvement in vaginal cytological indices (such as eosinophilic index) and in skin and hair problems were observed for the black cohosh and oestrogen groups. A decrease was observed in all three treatment groups for the SDS Index, which evaluates depression, and the modified Kupperman Index. Black cohosh was considered at least as effective as conjugated oestrogen and both treatments were better than diazepam for vegetative and psychological alterations.[35]

In a randomized, double-blind, placebo-controlled comparative clinical trial, 80 women with climacteric symptoms received standardized black cohosh extract (four tablets per day), conjugated oestrogens (0.625 mg/day) or placebo for 12 weeks. At the end of treatment, patients receiving black cohosh had improved compared to both the oestrogen and placebo groups. Neurovegetative symptoms (measured using the full Kupperman Index) and psychological complaints (Hamilton Anxiety Scale) for these patients were significantly improved ($p<0.001$). The black cohosh treatment group also showed significant improvement ($p<0.01$) in the proliferation status of vaginal epithelium. Oestrogen treatment yielded no effect compared to placebo, although the applied dose was considered too low.[36]

Arthritis

In a randomized, double-blind, placebo-controlled trial 82 male and female patients with osteoarthritis and rheumatoid arthritis received a licensed over-the-counter herbal medicine (two tablets per day) or placebo for a period of 2 months. The formula contained black cohosh, willow bark, guaiacum resin, sarsaparilla and poplar bark. Although there was no significant difference between the two groups for most symptoms, a significant decrease ($p<0.05$) in pain scores occurred for those taking the herbal formula. Many patients reported a decline in health related to cold, damp, windy weather experienced near the end of the trial which may have altered the findings. A relative improvement in mood scores was also noted for those taking the herbal tablets.[37] The authors of this study advised that the results may not be relevant to the activity of black cohosh, as the formulation predominantly comprised herbs containing salicylate derivatives.

TOXICOLOGY

A constituent isolated from the chloroform fraction of black cohosh extract, likely to be actein, did not provoke acute toxicity when administered by intragastric and hypodermic routes in rabbits. A minimum lethal dose of greater than 1 g/kg was observed in rats by intragastric administration.[23] Testing of standardized black cohosh extract for genotoxic-mutagenic activity and chronic toxicity was negative.[38]

During the years 1953 to 1957, approximately 3200 pregnancies were followed to investigate prenatal influences on foetal development and survival. A listing of congenital malformations and survival in relation to the first trimester use of specific drugs and vaccines revealed no striking discrepancy between the treated group and control groups. This study included black cohosh which was used in three pregnancies, one of which included a malformation. The degree of severity was not defined.[39]

CONTRAINDICATIONS

Pregnancy and lactation (see below). Avoid herbs with oestrogenic activity in women with oestrogen-dependent tumours (e.g. breast cancer).

SPECIAL WARNINGS AND PRECAUTIONS

None required.

INTERACTIONS

The antiproliferative effect of black cohosh extract in combination with tamoxifen was assessed in vitro on 17-beta-oestradiol-stimulated MCF-7 human breast cancer cells.[40] Dilutions of black cohosh extract in the range 10^{-3} to 10^{-5} augmented the antiproliferative action of 10^{-5} tamoxifen. Whether this interaction also applies in vivo has not been established.

USE IN PREGNANCY AND LACTATION

Contraindicated, except for assisting birth.

EFFECTS ON ABILITY TO DRIVE AND USE MACHINES

No negative influence is expected.

SIDE EFFECTS

High doses cause a frontal headache, with a dull, full or bursting feeling. This headache is the most characteristic effect observed when giving even therapeutic doses.[41] Stomach complaints of low frequency have been observed in clinical trials.[29,33]

Other reputed adverse reactions have been reported. A 45-year-old woman who had been taking herbal preparations containing black cohosh, chaste tree and evening primrose oil for 4 months had three seizures within a 3-month period. The herbal preparations were stopped and the patient was treated with anticonvulsants.[42] A baby was born with basal ganglia and parasagittal hypoxic injury. The pregnancy had been normal. During the homebirth a herbal mixture containing black cohosh and blue cohosh was given to the mother. The labour was normal, but 30 minutes after birth the baby had to be rushed to hospital after suffering seizures and acute tubular necrosis. A combination of maternal vasodilation and hypotension with increased uterine activity could have resulted in a reduction of placental blood flow.[43] It is not clear that the herbal mixture caused this outcome. Black cohosh was regarded by the Eclectics as an excellent partus praeparator if given for several weeks before birth.[44]

OVERDOSE

Overdose of black cohosh is potentially dangerous; it is likely to produce vertigo and visual and nervous disturbance.[45] Overdose has produced nausea and vomiting[8] (perhaps because it is closely allied with the poisonous plants *Actaea spicata* (baneberry) and white cohosh (*A. alba*)).[46]

CURRENT REGULATORY STATUS IN SELECTED COUNTRIES

Black cohosh is covered by a positive Commission E monograph with the following applications: neurovegetative complaints of premenstrual, dysmenorrhoeic or climacteric origin. Black cohosh is on the UK General Sale List, with a maximum single dose of 200 mg.

Black cohosh does not have GRAS status. However, it is freely available as a 'dietary supplement' in the USA under DSHEA legislation (1994 Dietary Supplement Health and Education Act). Black cohosh has been present in OTC menstrual drug products. The FDA advises: 'that based on evidence currently available, there is inadequate data to establish general recognition of the safety and effectiveness of these ingredients for the specified uses'.

Black cohosh is not included in Part 4 of Schedule 4 of the Therapeutic Goods Act Regulations of Australia.

References

1. British Herbal Medicine Association. British herbal pharmacopoeia. BHMA, Cowling, 1983, p 66.
2. Felter HW, Lloyd JU. King's American dispensatory, 18th edn, 3rd revision, vol 1, 1905. Reprinted by Eclectic Medical Publications, Portland, 1983, pp 529–533.
3. German Federal Minister of Justice. German Commission E for human medicine monograph, Bundes-Anzeiger (German Federal Gazette) no. 43, dated 02.03.1989
4. Harnischfeger G, Stolze H. Erfahrungsheilkunde 1981; 30 (6): 439–444.
5. Pharmaceutical Society of Great Britain. British pharmaceutical codex 1934. The Pharmaceutical Press, London, 1934, p 324.
6. British Herbal Medicine Association. British herbal compendium, vol 1. BHMA, Bournemouth, 1992, p 34.
7. Chiej R. The Macdonald encyclopedia of medicinal plants. Macdonald, London, 1984, entry no. 87.
8. Grieve MA. A modern herbal, vol 1. Dover Publications, New York, 1971, p 211.
9. Hostettmann K, Marston, A. Chemistry and Pharmacology of natural products: saponins. Cambridge University Press, Cambridge, 1995, p 280.
10. Wagner H, Bladt S. Plant drug analysis: a thin layer chromatography atlas, 2nd edn. Springer-Verlag, Berlin, 1996, p 336.
11. Struck D, Tegtmeier M, Harnischfeger G. Planta Med 1997; 63: 289.
12. Gizycki H. Z Exptl Med 1944; 113: 635–644.
13. Jarry H, Harnischfeger G. Planta Med 1985; 51 (1): 46–49.
14. Jarry H, Gorkow Ch, Wuttke W. Treatment of menopausal symptoms with extracts of Cimicifuga racemosa: in vivo and in vitro evidence for estrogenic activity. In: Loew D, Rietbrock N (eds) Phytopharmaka in Forschung und klinischer Anwendung. Steinkopff (Verlag), Darmstadt, 1995, p 104.
15. Jarry H, Harnischfeger G, Düker EM. Planta Med 1985; 51 (4): 316–319.
16. Jarry H, Gorkow Ch, Wuttke W. Treatment of menopausal symptoms with extracts of Cimicifuga racemosa: in vivo and in vitro evidence for estrogenic activity. In: Loew D, Rietbrock N (eds) Phytopharmaka in Forschung und klinischer Anwendung. Steinkopff (Verlag), Darmstadt, 1995, p 108.
17. Duker EM, Kopanski L, Jarry H et al. Planta Med 1991; 57 (5): 420–424.
18. Jarry H, Gorkow Ch, Wuttke W. Treatment of menopausal symptoms with extracts of Cimicifuga racemosa: in vivo and in vitro evidence for estrogenic activity. In: Loew D, Rietbrock N (eds) Phytopharmaka in Forschung und klinischer Anwendung. Steinkopff (Verlag), Darmstadt, 1995, pp 109–110.
19. Einer-Jensen N, Zhao J, Andersen KP et al. Maturitas 1996; 25 (2): 149–153.
20. Nesselhut T, Schellhase C, Dietrich R et al. Arch Gynecol Obstet 1993; 254 (1–4): 817–818.
21. Nesselhut T. Expert forum on Remifemin®: report and results from endocrinology expert forum in Luneburg, May 1993. Available from Schaper & Brummer GmbH & Co., Salzgitter (Ringelheim).
22. Hemmi H, Ishida N. J Pharmacobiodyn 1980; 3 (12): 643–648.
23. Genazzani E, Sorrentino L. Nature 1962; 194: 544–545.
24. Yoo JS, Jung JS, Lee TH et al. Korean J Pharmacogn 1995; 26 (4): 355–359.
25. Hauser GA. Schweiz Med Wochenschr 1997; 127 (4): 122–127.
26. Hauser GA. Fortschr Med 1996; 114 (5): 49–52.
27. Heizer H. Med Klin 1960; 55: 232–233.
28. Kesselkraul O. Med Monatsschr 1957; 11 (2): 87–88.
29. Stolze H. Gyne 1982; 3 (1): 14–16.
30. Daiber W. Arztl Praxis 1983; 35 (65): 1946–1947.

31. Vorberg G. Z Allg Med 1984; 60 (13): 626–629.
32. Petho A. Arztl Praxis 1987; 47: 1551–1553.
33. Foldes J. Arztl Forsch 1959; 13: 623–624.
34. Lehmann-Willenbrock E, Riedel HH. Zentralbl Gynakol 1988; 110 (10): 611–618.
35. Warnecke G. Med Welt 1985; 36 (22): 871–874.
36. Stoll W. Therapeutikon 1987; 1: 23–31.
37. Mills SY, Jacoby RK, Chacksfield M et al. Br J Rheumatol 1996; 35 (9): 874–878.
38. Liske E, Duker E. Ars Medici 1993; 83 (7): 426–430.
39. Mellin GW. Am J Obst Gynec 1964; 90 (7, pt 2): 1169–1180.
40. German Patent DE 196 52 183 CI. Verwendung eines Extraktes aus Cimicifuga racemosa. Schaper & Brümmer Gmbh & Co KG, 38259 Salzgitter, DE.
41. Felter HW. The eclectic materia medica, pharmacology and therapeutics, 1922. Reprinted by Eclectic Medical Publications, Portland, 1983, p 466.
42. Shuster J. Hosp Pharm 1996; 31(12): 1553–1554.
43. Gunn TR. NZ Med J 1996; 109 (1032): 410–411.
44. Felter HW. The eclectic materia medica, pharmacology and therapeutics, 1922. Reprinted by Eclectic Medical Publications, Portland, 1983, p 469.
45. Mills SY. The A-Z of modern herbalism. Thorsons, London, 1989, p 39.
46. Grieve M. A modern herbal, vol 1. Dover Publications, New York, 1971, p 81.

Buchu
(*Agathosma betulina* (Bergius) Pill.)

SYNONYMS

Barosma betulina (Bergius) Bartl. et Wendl. (botanical synonym), bucco (Engl), Barosmae folium (Lat), Bukkostrauch, Buccoblätter (Ger), buchu (Fr), diosma (Ital), bukko (Dan).

WHAT IS IT?

Buchu is a South African herb that is extensively used in diuretic preparations and may also be used in laxative, stomachic and carminative formulas. The Hottentots use buchu leaves to perfume their bodies. (The Agathosma genus is native to South Africa, especially the southwest Cape region.) The oil is used as a component of artificial fruit flavours, especially blackcurrant, and it may be found in trace amounts in a wide variety of food products and beverages.

The leaves are the part most commonly used for therapeutic purposes and should be harvested whilst the plant is flowering and fruiting. They possess a strongly aromatic taste and a curious peppermint-like odour.

EFFECTS

Disinfects the urinary tract and acts as a mild diuretic.

TRADITIONAL VIEW

Buchu was used to treat gravel, inflammation and catarrh of the bladder.[1] According to the Eclectics, buchu is an aromatic stimulant and tonic that promotes the appetite, relieves nausea and flatulence and acts as a diuretic and diaphoretic. Its principal use was in the treatment of chronic diseases of the genitourinary tract including chronic inflammation of the mucous membranes of the bladder, irritable conditions of the urethra, in urinary discharges (particularly mucus or mucopurulent discharges), abnormally acidic urine with a constant desire to urinate with little relief from micturition, and incontinence associated with a diseased prostate.[2]

SUMMARY ACTIONS

Urinary antiseptic, mild diuretic.

CAN BE USED FOR

TRADITIONAL THERAPEUTIC USES

Urinary tract infection, dysuria, cystitis, urethritis and prostatitis.

MAY ALSO BE USED FOR

OTHER APPLICATIONS

Buchu may be included as an aroma or taste enhancer in herbal tea mixtures.[3]

PREPARATIONS

Dried leaf as a decoction, liquid extract, tincture or tablets for internal use. As with all essential oil-containing herbs, use of the fresh plant or carefully dried herb is advised. Keep covered if infusing the herb to retain the essential oil.

DOSAGE

- 3–6 g of the dried leaf per day or as infusion.
- 2–4 ml of 1:2 liquid extract per day, 5–10 ml of 1:5 tincture per day.

DURATION OF USE

May be taken long term for most applications.

SUMMARY ASSESSMENT OF SAFETY

May occasionally cause gastrointestinal irritation if taken on an empty stomach. Other species of Agathosma contain high levels of pulegone and are contraindicated in pregnancy.

TECHNICAL DATA

BOTANY

Agathosma betulina, a member of the Rutaceae (citrus) family, is a low shrub that can grow to a height of 2 m. The leaves are rhomboid-obovate in shape, 12–20 mm long and 4–25 mm broad, with a blunt and recurved apex. Numerous small oil glands are scattered throughout the lamina and large oil glands are situated at the base of each marginal indentation and at the apex. The flowers have five whitish petals and the brown fruits contain five carpels.[4] The leaves become brittle and coriaceous when dried and when moistened become mucilaginous.[4] They have a spicy odour and a pungent and spicy taste.[5]

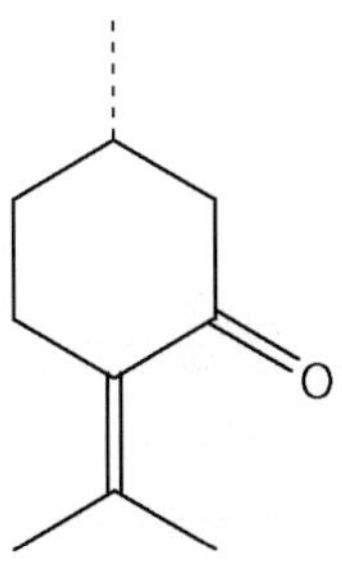

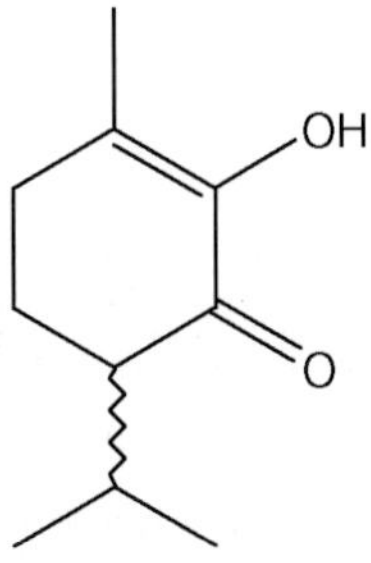

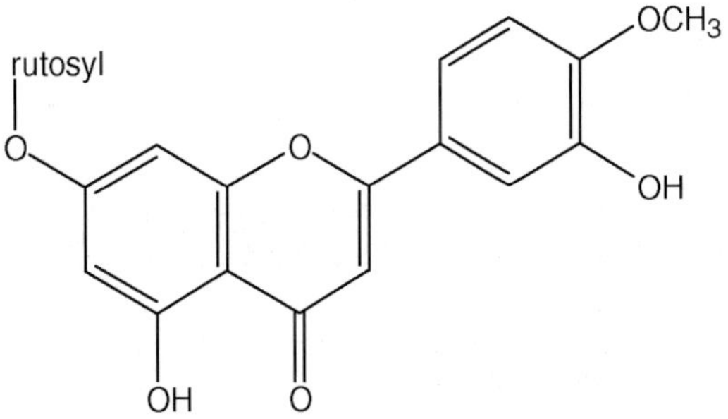

KEY CONSTITUENTS

- Essential oil (2%), consisting mainly of the monoterpene diosphenol. Other components include: limonene, (–)-isomenthone, (+)-menthone, (–)-pulegone, terpinen-4-ol and the sulphur-containing p-menthan-3-on-8-thiol which is responsible for the blackcurrant flavour.[5]
- Flavonoids, especially diosmin and rutin.[6]

Note: Other species such as *Agathosma crenulata* are not suitable for medicinal use due to their lower diosphenol content and higher pulegone content in the essential oil.[7]

PHARMACODYNAMICS

An in vitro study demonstrated some activity for the alcoholic extract of buchu against microflora typical of urinary tract infections.[8] However, only the essential oil showed considerable activity against all the test organisms.

PHARMACOKINETICS

No data available.

CLINICAL TRIALS

No clinical studies on the urinary antiseptic and diuretic effects traditionally attributed to buchu are available.

TOXICOLOGY

There are no reports of cases of poisoning and no toxicology data are available.

CONTRAINDICATIONS

None known.

SPECIAL WARNINGS AND PRECAUTIONS

None known.

INTERACTIONS

None known.

USE IN PREGNANCY AND LACTATION

Some writers suggest that buchu is contraindicated in pregnancy.[6] However, this would only be the case for buchu substitutions (such as *Agathosma crenulata*) which contain much higher levels of pulegone in their essential oil.[7,9]

EFFECTS ON ABILITY TO DRIVE AND USE MACHINES

None known.

SIDE EFFECTS

Occasional gastrointestinal intolerance and irritation if taken on an empty stomach.[6]

OVERDOSE

No effects known.

CURRENT REGULATORY STATUS IN SELECTED COUNTRIES

Buchu is covered by a null Commission E monograph. It is on the UK General Sale List.

Buchu does not have GRAS status. However, it is freely available as a 'dietary supplement' in the USA under DSHEA legislation (1994 Dietary Supplement Health and Education Act). Buchu has been present as an ingredient in OTC weight control drug products and orally administered menstrual drug products. The FDA, however, advises that: 'based on evidence currently available, there is inadequate data to establish general recognition of the safety and effectiveness of these ingredients for the specified uses'.

Buchu is not included in Part 4 of Schedule 4 of the Therapeutic Goods Act Regulations of Australia.

References

1. Grieve M. A modern herbal, vol 1. Dover Publications, New York, 1971, pp 133–134.
2. Felter HW, Lloyd JU. King's American dispensatory, 18th edn, 3rd revision, vol 1, 1905. Reprinted by Eclectic Medical Publications, Portland, 1983, pp 891–892.
3. German Federal Minister of Justice. German Commission E for human medicine monograph, Bundes-Anzeiger (German Federal Gazette), no. 22a, dated 01.02.1990.
4. Evans WC. Trease and Evans' Pharmacognosy, 14th edn. WB Saunders, London, 1996, p 272.
5. Bisset NG (ed). Herbal drugs and phytopharmaceuticals Medpharm Scientific Publishers, Stuttgart, 1994, pp 102–103.
6. British Herbal Medicine Association. British herbal compendium, vol 1. BHMA, Bournemouth, 1992, pp 43–45.
7. Kaiser R, Lamparsky D, Schudel P. J Agric Food Chem 1975; 23 (5): 943–950.
8. Didry N, Pinkas M. Plantes méd phytothér 1982; 16 (4): 249–252.
9. Tisserand R, Balacs T. Essential oil safety: a guide for health care professionals. Churchill Livingstone, Edinburgh, 1995, p 124.

Bupleurum
(*Bupleurum falcatum* L.)

SYNONYMS

Hare's ear root (Engl), Bupleuri radix (Lat), chai hu (Chin), saiko (Jap), siho (Kor), segl-hareøre (Dan).

WHAT IS IT?

Several species of Bupleurum have been officially used in traditional Chinese medicine, mainly *B. falcatum* L., *B. chinense* DC and *B. scorzonerifolium* Willd. Although other species may be used, the toxic plant *B. longiradiatum* should not be used medicinally. Recent pharmacological research on Bupleurum root has highlighted its antiinflammatory activity, which appears to be mediated through the enhanced release and potentiation of hormones from the adrenal cortex. There are gaps in the research evidence but it is possible that Bupleurum acts to mobilize the body's own equivalent of steroidal antiinflammatory mechanisms.

EFFECTS

Supports the body's antiinflammatory responses; modulates immune function; protects the liver, stomach and kidneys from toxic damage; decreases gastric ulcer development.

TRADITIONAL VIEW

In traditional Chinese medicine Bupleurum is classified as a herb that resolves *Lesser Yang Heat* patterns, relaxes constrained *Liver Qi*, disharmony between the *Liver* and the *Spleen* and raises the *Yang Qi* in *Spleen* or *Stomach Deficiency*. Hence Bupleurum is used to treat alternating chills and fever, liver enlargement, prolapse of the uterus and rectum and irregular menstruation.[1] Traditional texts list its properties as bitter and cool and it acts as a diaphoretic (i.e. in fever management) and to regulate and restore gastrointestinal and liver function.

SUMMARY ACTIONS

Antiinflammatory, hepatoprotective, antitussive, diaphoretic.

CAN BE USED FOR

INDICATIONS SUPPORTED BY CLINICAL TRIALS

Influenza, common cold, feverish conditions (uncontrolled studies).

TRADITIONAL THERAPEUTIC USES

Alternating chills and fever; liver enlargement; prolapse of the uterus and rectum; epigastric pain, nausea, indigestion; irregular menstruation. Often combined with Astragalus for debility and prolapse.

MAY ALSO BE USED FOR

EXTRAPOLATIONS FROM PHARMACOLOGICAL STUDIES

Chronic inflammatory disorders, especially autoimmune disease involving the liver or kidneys; acute or chronic liver diseases, chemical liver damage, poor liver function; gastric ulceration; reactive hypoglycaemia.

PREPARATIONS

Dried root for decoction, liquid extract and tablets; powdered root.

DOSAGE

- 3–12 g per day of the dried root by decoction.
- 4–8 ml per day of the 1:2 liquid extract.

DURATION OF USE

May be used in the long term if taken within the recommended dosage.

SUMMARY ASSESSMENT OF SAFETY

Minor side effects may occur in sensitive individuals.

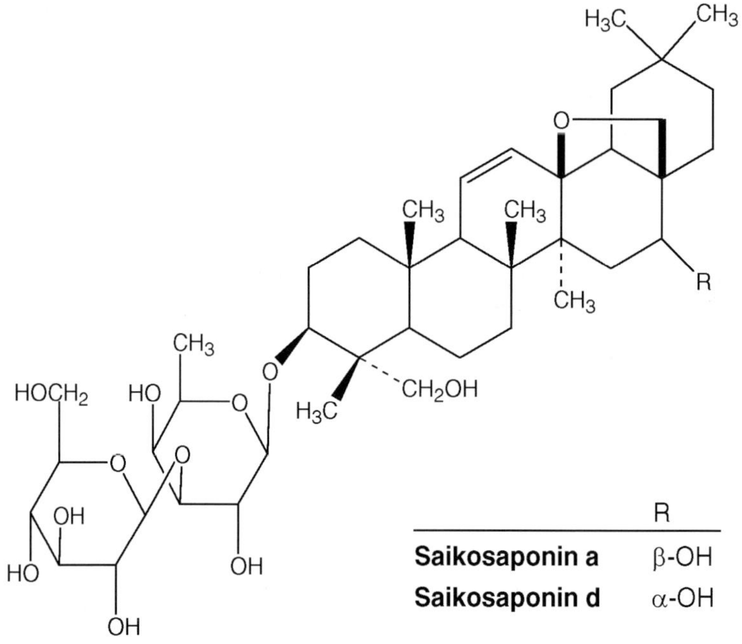

	R
Saikosaponin a	β-OH
Saikosaponin d	α-OH

TECHNICAL DATA

BOTANY

The Bupleurum genus is a member of the Umbelliferae (carrot) family and consists of shrubs and herbs with entire leaves, often parallel veined, hence the name hare's ear.[2] *Bupleurum chinensis* grows 45–85 cm high and may or may not be branched. Leaves are alternate, broad-linear to broad-lanceolate (3–9 cm long, 0.6–1.3 cm wide) with a marginal vein. Umbels are compound, axillary and terminal and contain yellow flowers. Fruit is ovoid, the brown root is conical, 6–15 cm long and 0.3–0.8 cm in diameter.[3]

KEY CONSTITUENTS

Bupleurum falcatum

- Triterpenoid saponins (saikosaponin a, b_1, b_2, b_3, b_4, c, d, e, and f) and sapogenins.[4]
- Phytosterols,[4] pectin-like polysaccharides (bupleurans).[5]

Since the highest levels of saikosaponins are found in *Bupleurum falcatum* (2.8%) and *B. chinensis* (1.7%), these species are preferred.[6,7] Saikosaponins a and d are considered to be the most biologically active.

PHARMACODYNAMICS

Many pharmacological studies have been conducted on isolated saikosaponins. Although these studies are relevant to the medicinal use of Bupleurum, some important qualifications should be considered. In much of the research saikosaponins are tested in vitro or administered by injection. Since a major active form of saikosaponins in the bloodstream is probably the sapogenins (i.e. saponin aglycones), the relevance of in vitro research to the oral use of Bupleurum is uncertain. Similarly, the relevance of injected saikosaponins to the oral use of Bupleurum is not entirely clear, although it appears that oral doses do have some similar though milder activity.[8–10]

Antiinflammatory activity

The antiinflammatory activity of the saikosaponins appears to be related, at least in part, to their ability to both induce secretion of endogenous corticosterone and potentiate its antiinflammatory activity. Saikosaponins and some of their gastric and intestinal metabolites have demonstrated this activity following oral doses in mice.[10] Saikosaponin d caused an increase in serum corticosterone in rats when administered orally.[9] Combined oral administration of Bupleurum extract and corticosterone acetate increased antiinflammatory activity compared to corticosterone alone, as indicated by the increase in activity of liver tyrosine aminotransferase (LTA).[4] This effect was also demonstrated clinically[4] and confirmed in a later study on rats which found that individual injection of saikosaponins a, d or f (ssa, ssd, ssf) or cortisone acetate did not induce LTA activity in adrenalectomized rats.[11] However, coadministration of the same dose of cortisone acetate with either ssa, ssd or ssf significantly induced LTA activity, suggesting that these saikosaponins potentiate the action of cortisone.[11]

Saikosaponins a, b_1, b_2, b_3, b_4, d and saikogenins F and G were all found to increase plasma corticosterone levels in rats 30 minutes after IP injection.[9] Ssa and ssd had the strongest effect and the activity of the saikosaponins was considerably greater than the saikogenins. Saikosaponin c (ssc) was inactive.[9]

Injection of ssa and ssd, but not ssc, raised plasma corticosterone and ACTH levels in rats pretreated with dexamethasone.[12] Dexamethasone is a potent and long-lasting inhibitor of ACTH secretion by a feedback mechanism to the hypothalamus and pituitary. This suggests that the site of action of saikosaponins is the hypothalamic-pituitary system. The use of an antihistamine showed that the saponin-induced corticosterone secretion was not due to histamine release.[12] Another study found that injection of saikogenin A (sgA) increased plasma ACTH levels, possibly through its effect of increasing cyclic AMP levels in the pituitary, but not the hypothalamus.[13] Injections of ssd significantly increased adrenal weight and decreased thymus weight in both dexamethasone-treated and normal rats.[14] However, this effect was abolished in rats with no pituitary, suggesting a mechanism of action involving the pituitary or hypothalamus.[14] The authors suggested that saikosaponins may be used to reduce the dose of glucocorticoid drugs and to prevent glucocorticoid-induced adrenal suppression.

The antiinflammatory action of saikosaponins has been demonstrated in several experimental models. Oral doses of a mixture of saikosaponins were shown to have significant antiinflammatory activity using the granuloma pouch,[4,15] dextran-induced oedema[15] and cotton pellet methods.[8] (In one study plasma corticosteroid levels decreased and adrenal weight remained unchanged, contrary to previous findings.)[8] However, some negative results have also been recorded for oral doses of saikosaponins in tests for antiinflammatory activity.[4]

Saikosaponins administered by injection demonstrated potent antiinflammatory activities in several models.[6,8] Saikosaponins a and d antagonized the inflammatory effects of implanted cotton pellets and were as active as prednisolone.[6] Combined injection of doses of ssd and dexamethasone produced an antiinflammatory effect on cotton-induced granuloma in rats.[16] However, individual administration of the same doses of ssd and dexamethasone were inactive.[16] The antiinflammatory activity of the saikosaponins may not be limited to their interaction with endogenous corticosteroids. An in vitro study found that some saikosaponins inhibit the production of prostaglandins.[17]

The ability of saikosaponins to raise blood glucose levels was demonstrated in several pharmacological studies following both oral and injected doses.[6,9,12] This is probably a direct consequence of their ability to increase levels of endogenous glucocorticoids. Since saikosaponins also increase liver glycogen stores,[6] Bupleurum may prove to be useful in the treatment of reactive hypoglycaemia.

Immune-modulating activity

Saikosaponins and saikogenins given by injection stimulate immune function. If significant activity were established for oral doses, this would indicate a useful and unusual combination of antiinflammatory and immune-enhancing activities for Bupleurum.

Injections of ssa, ssd and saikogenin D caused a marked increase in the number and activation of macrophages in the peritoneum of mice.[18] Since saikogenin D is a metabolite of ssd, it is probable that ssd also possesses oral activity in this regard. The same compounds were found to enhance the non-specific resistance of mice infected with *Pseudomonas aeruginosa* but not *Listeria monocytogenes*.[19] Peritoneal macrophages from mice treated with ssd showed intense spreading and significantly increased phagocytic activity.[20]

Pretreatment of mice with ssd injections increased the antibody response after immunization with sheep red blood cells (SRBC).[21] Saikosaponin d also enhanced spleen cell proliferative responses to T-cell mitogens both before and after immunization with SRBC, but decreased the response to B-cell mitogens.[21] Macrophages from ssd-treated mice showed increased spreading activity and lysosomal enzyme activity. Interleukin-1 production was also increased in a dose-dependent manner.[21] Similar results were also found in another study by the same research group, who also observed increased intracellular killing of yeasts by macrophages obtained from ssd-treated mice.[22]

Hot water extracts of Bupleurum demonstrated mitogenic activity on lymphocytes in vitro. The mitogenic substances were likely to be large molecular weight polyphenolic compounds and polysaccharides.[23] Further testing determined that the mitogenic substance was a polyphenolic compound and that the structure was modified during the extraction to increase the stable free radical components.[24]

Hepatoprotective activity

Although Bupleurum is traditionally used as a liver treatment, the hepatoprotective activity of saikosaponins after oral doses has not been clearly demonstrated.[4] However, injected doses of saikosaponins a and d demonstrated marked hepatoprotective activity in several animal models.[25–27] Decoctions of Bupleurum administered subcutaneously were also hepatoprotective.[28] Saponins isolated from *B. scorzonerifolium* demonstrated hepatoprotective activity on D-galactosamine-induced cytotoxicity in cultured rat hepatocytes.[29]

The hepatoprotective mechanism of the saikosaponins is not known. However, they have been shown to increase hepatic protein synthesis in vivo and in vitro.[30,31] Increased protein synthesis may enhance the ability of the hepatocyte to withstand a toxic insult.

Nephroprotective activity

Injection of ssd significantly decreased urinary protein excretion in rats with chemically induced proteinuria (and symptoms similar to nephrotic syndrome).[32] Urinary protein was reduced by up to 48% in animals treated with ssd and the degree of abnormality in glomerular epithelial cells was lower. It was suggested that ssd protects the basement membrane of the glomerulus.[32]

Injection of various saikosaponins demonstrated antinephritic activity following administration of an antiglomerular basement membrane serum to rats.[33] Urinary protein excretion and elevation of serum cholesterol were prevented and histopathological changes such as hypercellularity and adhesion were significantly inhibited.[33] Additional experimentation revealed that the antinephritic mechanisms of saikosaponins were partly due to antiplatelet and corticosterone-releasing activities and an inhibition of the decrease in free radical scavengers such as glutathione peroxidase.[33]

Other activity

Both bupleurans and saikosaponins exhibit decreased gastric ulcer development in a number of models.[5,6,34] The saikosaponins may act by inhibiting gastric secretion.[35] Saikosaponins have also been found to decrease the corrosive and protein-denaturing effects of tannic acid and to improve the integrity of the gastric mucosa of rats.[36] However, as might be expected of saponins, high doses of saikosaponins cause gastric irritation.[6]

Many saponins are known to lower cholesterol and this activity has also been demonstrated for the saikosaponins.[6,30] It has been suggested that saikosaponins and saikogenins lower cholesterol by increasing cholesterol excretion in bile.[6]

Oral administration of Bupleurum decoction and saikosaponins demonstrated antipyretic activity.[6] Injection of saikosaponins demonstrated a potent antitussive effect on guinea pigs.[37]

Saikosaponin d inactivated enveloped viruses such as measles and herpes viruses but had no effect on a naked virus (polio).[38] Despite this, a toxic effect on host cells was noted, leading to the conclusion that ssd is not a useful antiviral agent.[38] Saikosaponins a and d demonstrated cytotoxic activity on human hepatoma cell lines in vitro.[39,40] Saikosaponin b_2 inhibited the proliferation of B16 melanoma cells in vitro. The apoptosis induced by saikosaponin b_2 may be due to downregulation of protein kinase C activity.[41]

PHARMACOKINETICS

The pharmacokinetics of oral doses of saponins are complex and not completely understood. While low levels of triterpenoid saponins may be absorbed into the bloodstream unchanged, it is also likely on current evidence that significant quantities of triterpenoid saponin metabolites are absorbed in most cases. These metabolites are usually formed by the action of gastric and intestinal secretions and/or bowel flora. The pharmacological implications of these observations are not fully understood.

Oral administration of saikosaponins at a dosage which was 10 times that of intramuscular injection demonstrated a similar antiinflammatory activity in the granuloma pouch method.[8] This indicates that the saponins and/or their metabolites probably exhibit poor absorption profiles (about 10% absorption). Saikosaponins a, c and d are transformed into 27 metabolites in the gastrointestinal tract of mice.[10,42] Therefore 30 compounds are potentially available for absorption into the bloodstream. However, ssa and its monoglycoside (prosaikogenin F) and aglycone (saikogenin F) were detectable in the plasma of rats when ssa was administered orally.[31] The plasma concentration of ssa peaked after 30 minutes at 74 μg/l and ssa was undetectable after 1.5 hours.[31] In contrast, the ssa metabolites were both found to peak after 8 hours at about 2 μg/l and were undetectable after 12 hours.[31] This implies that after oral doses of ssa there is a short but intense plasma concentration (and therefore activity) of ssa itself, followed by more prolonged and less intense activities of its metabolites. These findings need to be confirmed in human studies. Total faecal excretion of injected doses of saikosaponins after 2 and 7 days accounted for about 50% and 85% respectively of the administered dose.[6] This suggests that saikosaponin metabolites undergo enterohepatic recycling.

CLINICAL TRIALS

Despite the considerable number of pharmacological studies on the saikosaponins, controlled clinical studies on either Bupleurum or saikosaponins are lacking.

In an uncontrolled clinical study of 143 patients treated with *B. chinensis*, fever subsided within 24 hours in 98.1% of influenza cases and 87.9% of common cold cases. In another study of 40 patients with pathological fever, Bupleurum produced an antipyretic effect in 97.5% and achieved a reduction of 1–2°C in body temperature in 77.5%.[6] Intravenous injection of *B. chinensis* (10–20 ml, 1–2 times a day for adults, 5–10 ml per day for children) was found to give satisfactory therapeutic effects in 100 cases of infectious hepatitis in an uncontrolled study.[6] In chronic hepatitis with hepatomegaly, an injection of Bupleurum and *Salvia miltiorrhiza* was used, with vitamins B and C taken orally. Each course lasted 10 days with 4–5 days' interval between courses. After treatment, patients usually showed marked improvement in mental state, appetite and subjective symptoms. Amelioration or disappearance of pain over the liver area was achieved in 4–5 days in most patients.[6]

TOXICOLOGY

Like most saponins, crude saikosaponins show medium toxicity after IP administration (LD_{50} 112 mg/kg in mice, 58.3 mg/kg in guinea pigs) but low toxicity by the oral route (LD_{50} 4.7 g/kg in mice).[15,37] Aqueous extract of Bupleurum root did not show any toxic effect in rats and mice at oral doses of 6 g/kg.[43] Repeated oral administration at 1.5 and 3.0 g/kg/day over 21 days caused slight decreases in red blood cell count and liver weight.[43]

Bupleurum extract decreased the mutagenicity of the mutagens benzo(alpha)pyrene and aflatoxin B in the Ames test against two *Salmonella typhimurium* strains.[44]

CONTRAINDICATIONS

Bupleurum is contraindicated in *Deficient Yin* cough (i.e. cough in debility) or *Liver Fire* ascending to the head (i.e. some cases of headache and hypertension). Bupleurum can occasionally cause nausea or vomiting; if this happens, use the smallest dose possible.[1]

SPECIAL WARNINGS AND PRECAUTIONS

Bupleurum has a sedative effect in some patients.

INTERACTIONS

None known.

USE IN PREGNANCY AND LACTATION

No adverse effects expected.

EFFECTS ON ABILITY TO DRIVE AND USE MACHINES

Not known.

SIDE EFFECTS

Bupleurum has a sedative effect in some patients and may also increase bowel movements and flatulence, especially in larger doses.[6] Bupleurum can occasionally cause nausea and reflux in sensitive patients – this is a property common to most saponin-rich herbs.

A traditional Chinese formula known as Minor Bupleurum Combination has been found to induce pneumonitis in some patients.[45–47] Whether this effect is due to Bupleurum or to other herbs in the formula is not clear. Minor Bupleurum Combination also appears to cause liver damage in rare cases.[48] A further 15 cases of interstitial pneumonitis due to ingestion of this herbal preparation have since been reported.[49]

OVERDOSE

Not known.

CURRENT REGULATORY STATUS IN SELECTED COUNTRIES

Bupleurum is official in the *Pharmacopoeia of the People's Republic of China* (English edition, 1997) and the *Japanese Pharmacopoeia* (English edition, 1986).

Bupleurum is not covered by a Commission E monograph and is not on the UK General Sale List.

Bupleurum does not have GRAS status. However, it is freely available as a 'dietary supplement' in the USA under DSHEA legislation (1994 Dietary Supplement Health and Education Act).

Bupleurum is not included in Part 4 of Schedule 4 of the Therapeutic Goods Act Regulations of Australia.

References

1. Bensky D, Gamble A. Chinese herbal medicine materia medica. Eastland Press, Seattle, 1986, pp 68–69.
2. Mabberley DJ. The plant book, 2nd edn. Cambridge University Press, Cambridge, 1997, p 107.
3. World Health Organization. Medicinal plants in China. World Health Organization, Regional Office for the Western Pacific, Manilla, 1989, p 61.
4. Tang W, Eisenbrand G. Chinese drugs of plant origin. Springer Verlag, Berlin, 1992, pp 223–232.
5. Yamada H, Sun XB, Matsumoto T et al. Planta Med 1991; 57 (6): 555–559.
6. Chang H, But P. Pharmacology and applications of Chinese materia medica, vol 2. World Scientific, Singapore, 1987, pp 967–974.
7. Dong YY, Luo SQ. Chung Kuo Chung Yao Tsa Chih 1989; 14 (11): 678–681, 703–704.
8. Yamamoto M, Kumagai A, Yamamura Y. Arzneim-Forsch 1975; 25 (7): 1021–1023.
9. Yokoyama H, Hiai S, Oura H. Chem Pharm Bull (Tokyo) 1981; 29 (2): 500–504.
10. Nose M, Amagaya S, Ogihara Y. Chem Pharm Bull (Tokyo) 1989; 37 (10): 2736–2740.
11. Hashimoto M, Inada K, Ohminami H et al. Planta Med 1985; 51 (5): 401–403.
12. Hiai S, Yokoyama H, Nagasawa T et al. Chem Pharm Bull (Tokyo) 1981; 29 (2): 495–499.
13. Cheng JT, Tsai CL. Biochem Pharmacol 1986; 35 (15): 2483–2487.
14. Hiai S, Yokoyama H. Chem Pharm Bull (Tokyo) 1986; 34 (3): 1195–1202.
15. Shibata M. Yakugaku Zasshi 1970; 90 (3): 398–404.
16. Abe H, Sakaguchi M, Arichi S. Nippon Yakurigaku Zasshi 1982; 80 (2): 155–161.
17. Ohuchi K, Watanabe M, Ozeki T et al. Planta Med 1985; 51 (3): 208–212.
18. Kumazawa Y, Takimoto H, Nishimura C et al. Int J Immunopharmacol 1989; 11 (1): 21–28.
19. Kumazawa Y, Kawakita T, Takimoto H et al. Int J Immunopharmacol 1990; 12 (5): 531–537.
20. Ushio Y, Abe H. Int J Immunopharmacol 1991; 13 (5): 493–499.
21. Ushio Y, Oda Y, Abe H. Int J Immunopharmacol 1991; 13 (5): 501–508.
22. Ushio Y, Abe H. Jpn J Pharmacol 1991; 56 (2): 167–175.
23. Oka H, Ohno N, Iwanaga S et al. Biol Pharm Bull 1995; 18 (5): 757–765.
24. Ohtsu S, Izumi S, Iwanaga S et al. Biol Pharm Bull 1997; 20 (1): 97–100.
25. Abe H, Sakaguchi M, Yamada M et al. Planta Med 1980; 40 (4): 366–372.
26. Abe H, Sagaguchi M, Odashima S et al. Naunyn Schmiedebergs Arch Pharmacol 1982; 320 (3): 266–271.
27. Abe H, Orita M, Konishi H et al. J Pharm Pharmacol 1985; 37 (8): 555–559.
28. Lin CC, Chiu HF, Yen MH et al. Am J Chin Med 1990; 18 (3–4): 105–112.
29. Matsuda H, Murakami T, Ninomiya K et al. Bioorg Med Chem Lett 1997; 7 (17): 2193–2198.
30. Yamamoto M, Kumagai A, Yamamura Y. Arzneim-Forsch 1975; 25 (8): 1240–1243.
31. Fujiwara K, Ogihara Y. Life Sci 1986; 39 (4): 297–301.
32. Abe H, Orita M, Konishi H et al. Eur J Pharmacol 1986; 120 (2): 171–178.
33. Hattori T, Ito M, Suzuki Y. Nippon Yakurigaku Zasshi 1991; 97 (1): 13–21.
34. Sun XB, Matsumoto T, Yamada H. J Pharm Pharmacol 1991; 43 (10): 699–704.
35. Shibata M, Yoshida R, Motoashi S et al. Yakugaku Zasshi 1973; 93 (12): 1660–1667.
36. Hung CR, Wu TS, Chang TY. Chin J Physiol 1993; 36 (4): 211–217.
37. Takagi K, Shibata M. Yakugaku Zasshi 1969; 89 (5): 712–720.
38. Ushio Y, Abe H. Planta Med 1992; 58 (2): 171–173.
39. Motoo Y, Sawabu N. Cancer Lett 1994; 86 (1): 91–95.
40. Okita K, Li Q, Murakamio T et al. Eur J Cancer Prev 1993; 2 (2): 169–175.
41. Zong Z, Fujikawa-Yamamoto K, Tanino M et al. Biochem Biophys Res Commun 1996; 219 (2): 480–485.
42. Shimizu K, Amagaya S, Ogihara Y. J Pharmacobiodyn 1985; 8 (9): 718–725.
43. Tanaka S, Takahashi A, Onoda K et al. Yakugaku Zasshi 1986; 106 (8): 671–686.
44. Kim JM, Ji HW, Jung YM. Korean J Vet Public Health 1994; 18 (3): 261–268.
45. Tsukiyama K, Tasaka Y, Nakajima M et al. Nippon Kyobu Shikkan Gakkai Zasshi 1989; 27 (12): 1556–1561.
46. Takada N, Arai S, Kusuhara N et al. Nippon Kyobu Shikkan Gakkai Zasshi 1993; 31 (9): 1163–1169.
47. Daibo A, Yoshida Y, Kitazawa S et al. Nippon Kyobu Shikkan Gakkai Zasshi 1992; 30 (8): 1583–1588.
48. Itoh S, Marutani K, Nishimina T et al. Dig Dis Sci 1995; 40 (8): 1845–1848
49. Mizushima Y, Oosake R, Kobayashi M. Phytother Res 1997; 11: 295–298.

Chamomile, German
(*Matricaria recutita* (L.) Rauchert)

SYNONYMS

Matricaria chamomilla L., *Chamomilla recutita* (L.) Rauschert (botanical synonyms), German chamomile, wild chamomile, matricaria (Engl), Matricariae flos (Lat), Kamillenblüten, Feldkamille (Ger), fleur de camomile, matricaire (Fr), camomilla (Ital), kamille (Dan).

WHAT IS IT?

A number of plants have 'chamomile' as part of their common name, including the corn chamomile (*Anthemis arvensis*), and although sweet or Roman chamomile (*Chamaemelum nobile* = *Anthemis nobilis*) is also used medicinally, German chamomile is the medicinal chamomile considered here. *Matricaria recutita* has been known and used since ancient times. The flower heads were used widely in pharmaceutical and medicinal preparations, beverages and cosmetics and the essential oil for perfumes. In the Mediterranean it is common to order chamomile tea in restaurants or bars, even in a concentrated 'expresso' form. Eclectic physicians preferred the use of German to Roman chamomile which is also known to cause allergic reactions such as contact dermatitis and anaphylactic reaction. Roman chamomile can be an adulterant in German chamomile dried herb.

EFFECTS

Antiinflammatory; inhibits spasm in the digestive tract; inhibits the occurrence of ulceration; promotes wound healing; stimulates skin metabolism.

TRADITIONAL VIEW

Chamomile has been considered to have two specific fields of action: the nervous system (as a calming treatment) and the gastrointestinal tract (decreasing irritation and as a carminative and spasmolytic). It is believed to affect both sensory and motor nerves and was used to treat nervous manifestations of dentition and conditions with a morbid susceptibility to pain. Other important applications were nervous conditions affecting the gastrointestinal tract and amenorrhoea and large doses of chamomile infusion could produce free diaphoresis, which was even said to relieve dysmenorrhoea and prevent clotting.[1] Chamomile was also considered to be anticatarrhal and used to treat catarrhal affections of the ears, nose and eyes.[1,2] It was used commonly in external applications: haemorrhoids, mastitis, mammary abscess, leucorrhoea and leg ulcers. The traditional use with children clearly indicates chamomile was considered a very gentle and safe herb.[2,3] The Eclectic physicians prescribed chamomile for medicinal use during pregnancy.[1]

SUMMARY ACTIONS

Antiinflammatory, antispasmodic, mild sedative, antiulcer, antimicrobial, vulnerary, diaphoretic.

CAN BE USED FOR

INDICATIONS SUPPORTED BY CLINICAL TRIALS

- Topical application: eczema; for wound healing.
- Internally: in combination with pectin for the treatment of acute, non-complicated diarrhoea; in combination with other herbs for the treatment of infantile colic.

TRADITIONAL THERAPEUTIC USES

Flatulent and nervous dyspepsia, travel sickness, nervous diarrhoea; nasal catarrh; dysmenorrhoea, amenorrhoea; restlessness and anxiety; use during dentition.

MAY ALSO BE USED FOR

EXTRAPOLATIONS FROM PHARMACOLOGICAL STUDIES

Acute or chronic inflammation; spasm or ulceration of the gastrointestinal tract; restlessness, anxiety, mild sleep disorders.

OTHER APPLICATIONS

Cosmetics (sensitive skin, antiinflammatory and antiacne products), bath preparations and hair care products.[4]

PREPARATIONS

Infusion of dried herb or liquid extract for internal use; infusion of dried herb, liquid extract or essential oil for external use or as an ingredient in ointments, creams, bath additives, mouthwashes and sprays. As with all essential oil-containing herbs, use of the fresh plant or carefully dried herb is advised. Keep covered if infusing the herb to retain the essential oil.

Topical studies have generally used chamomile extracts from high bisabolol chemotypes. Given the pharmacological properties of (–)-alpha-bisabolol and matricine (chamazulene), it is important to use these varieties.

DOSAGE

- 2–4 g three times per day of dried flower heads or in infusion.
- 3–6 ml per day of 1:2 liquid extract, 7–14 ml per day of 1:5 tincture; 50% ethanol is the preferred extraction solvent.
- Infusions or semisolid preparations containing 3–10% w/w of the flowers or equivalent for external use as wash or gargle.

DURATION OF USE

No restriction on long-term use.

SUMMARY ASSESSMENT OF SAFETY

Except in extremely rare cases of contact allergy in susceptible patients, chamomile is a safe herb.

TECHNICAL DATA

BOTANY

Matricaria recutita, a member of the Compositae (daisy) family, is an annual which can grow as tall as 1 m in the right soil (usually up to 60 cm). The alternate leaves are bipinnatisect, delicately lobed and thread-like, ending in a point. The flower consists of 12–16 white ligules (ray florets, 10–15 mm long) surrounding the central mound of tiny yellow flowers (disc florets, five-lobed) which are embedded in a hollow, conical receptacle. The flower head is 1.2–2.4 cm in diameter. The light-coloured fruits are very small achenes, without outside oil glands.[5,6]

KEY CONSTITUENTS

- Essential oil (0.5–1.5%), containing (–)-alpha-bisabolol (also known as levomenol), chamazulene, bisabolol oxides A, B, C; cis- and trans-en-yn-dicycloethers.[7] The chamazulene is formed from matricine during steam distillation.[8]
- Flavonoids (0.5–3%), particularly apigenin 7-glucoside, flavonoid aglycones,[7] coumarins (herniarin and umbelliferone), phenolic acids, mucilage,[9] GABA.[10]

The content of these active constituents varies considerably between different chemical races or varieties of chamomile.[11] The *European Pharmacopoeia* recommends that chamomile contain not less than 4 ml/kg of blue essential oil.[12]

PHARMACODYNAMICS

Antiinflammatory activity

Chamazulene inhibited the formation of leukotriene B_4 in intact neutrophils in a dose-dependent manner and blocked the chemical peroxidation of arachidonic acid. Matricine did not show these effects, even at higher concentrations. Matricine had no effect on the cyclooxygenase and 12-lipoxygenase activities in human platelets.[13] In vitro studies have recently determined that at least part of the antiinflammatory activity of chamomile extracts is due to constituents which inhibit the formation of 5-lipoxygenase and cyclooxygenase and have antioxidant activity. Bisabolol and apigenin appear to be responsible for this activity.[14] Oral intake of matricine has demonstrated antiinflammatory activity in the carrageenan test on rat paw.[15] Matricine was nearly as effective as (–)-alpha-bisabolol up to 3 hours after oral administration. Chamazulene was significantly less active than both matricine and (–)-alpha-bisabolol.[16] Matricine, together with most of the components in chamomile oil, especially bisabolol, has demonstrated antiinflammatory activity when tested topically on skin.[17]

(–)-Alpha-bisabolol demonstrated antiinflammatory activity in a number of experimental inflammatory models: rat paw oedema, adjuvant arthritis of the rat, ultraviolet erythema of the guinea pig and yeast fever in rats.[18] cis-En-yn-dicycloether inhibited the development of dextran-induced oedema in rats.[19] Several polysaccharides of chamomile have demonstrated antiinflammatory activity when applied topically.[20]

The antiinflammatory activity of an aqueous alcoholic extract of fresh chamomile, an aqueous alcoholic extract of dried chamomile, the essential oil and isolated components of the essential oil, by topical administration, were investigated using croton oil-induced dermatitis in mouse ear. The extract prepared from dried flowers showed a mild but significant antiinflammatory activity (24%) but the extract based on fresh chamomile was more active (32%) and

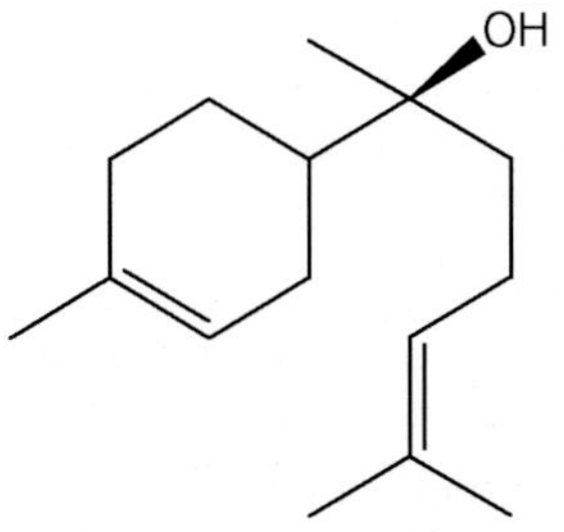

(–)-α-Bisabolol

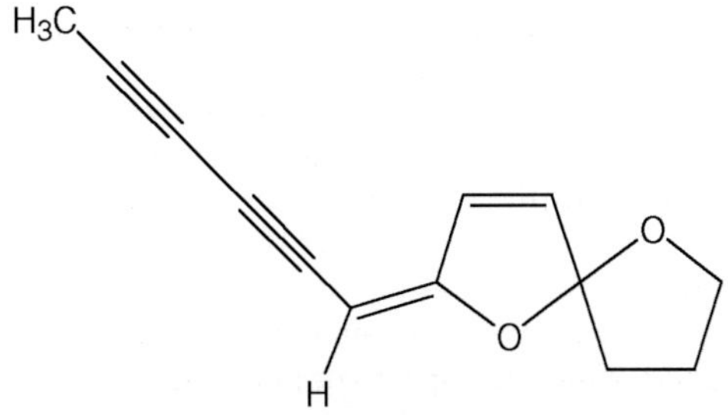

cis-En-yn-dicycloether

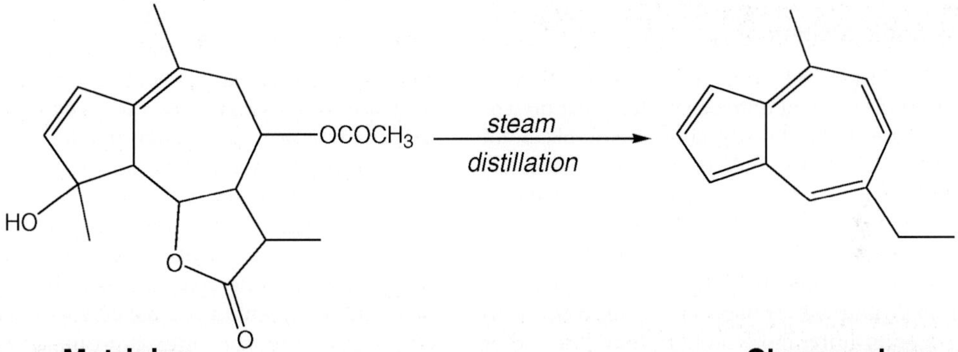

Matricine

steam distillation

Chamazulene

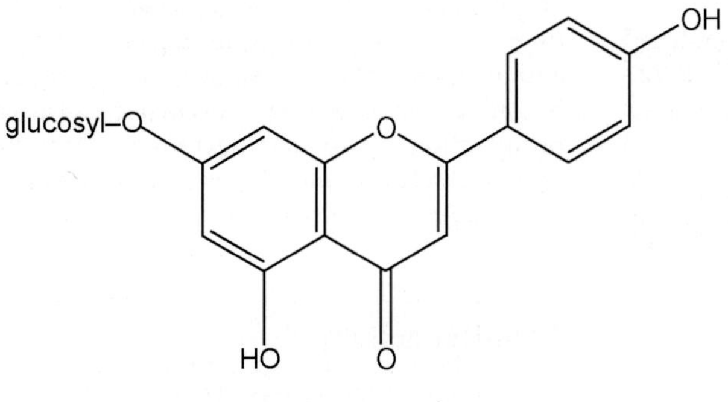

Apigenin-7-glucoside

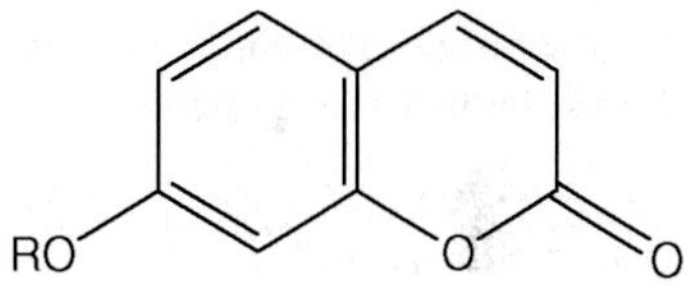

	R
Herniarin	CH_3
Umbelliferone	H

equalled the activity of the reference drug, benzydamine. The essential oil solution did not show significant inhibition of oedema. The antiinflammatory activity of apigenin was 10 times higher than that of matricine, which was 10 times higher than chamazulene. The differences in antiinflammatory activity of the various preparations may be attributed to the varying concentrations of matricine.[21]

Aqueous alcoholic extract of dried chamomile demonstrated significant reduction of oedema (23.4%) compared to controls, after topical administration to mice in the croton oil ear test. The non-steroidal antiinflammatory agent benzydamine produced a similar reduction at a dose corresponding to twice its usual clinical dose. Hydrocortisone was the most active (56.4%).[22] An antiinflammatory effect was demonstrated by topical administration of standardized chamomile extract, the flavone fraction and isolated flavones (apigenin, luteolin and quercetin) in experimental dermatitis (croton oil in mouse ear). The lipophilic flavone fraction demonstrated stronger activity than the total chamomile extract. The action of apigenin was superior to that of the reference drugs indomethacin and phenylbutazone.[23]

The antiinflammatory efficacy of topical compounds was measured directly and objectively on the skin of healthy volunteers using the tesa-film stripping technique. Three pharmaceutical formulations were investigated: a chamomile cream, its cream base and a hydrocortisone ointment. Chamomile cream exhibited 70% of the activity of the hydrocortisone ointment.[24] Experimentally induced toxic contact dermatitis was topically treated with chamomile ointment and compared to ointment base and 1% hydrocortisone acetate. The chamomile ointment demonstrated a superior soothing effect in comparison to the cortisone cream on human skin.[25]

Antispasmodic activity

Chamomile extract and some constituents demonstrated a dose-dependent antispasmodic effect on isolated guinea pig ileum. (–)-Alpha-bisabolol, bisabolol oxides A and B and chamomile oil showed a papaverine-like antispasmodic activity, the essential oil showing the lowest effect. The cis-en-yn-dicycloether also showed activity, although not dose dependent. The flavones apigenin, luteolin, patuletin and quercetin demonstrated marked antispasmodic effects, with apigenin significantly more potent than the other flavones but less active than papaverine. The coumarins only demonstrated a weak effect.[26]

Antispasmodic activity has also been observed following oral administration of apigenin.[27] cis-En-yn-dicycloether demonstrated a more pronounced antispasmodic effect than papaverine on isolated guinea pig and rabbit intestine.[19] Chamomile extract (25 ml/l)[28] and chamomile oil (0.2 ml diluted in 400 ml methanol)[29] inhibited acetylcholine- and histamine-induced contractions in guinea pig ileum in vitro.

Sedative and CNS activity

Several fractions from aqueous extract of chamomile, including isolated apigenin, have demonstrated significant affinity for the central benzodiazepine receptor in vitro. Apigenin also demonstrated clear antianxiety activity and slight sedative activity without muscle relaxant effects after intraperitoneal administration in mice.[30] Fractions isolated from the methanol extract of chamomile were able to selectively bind to both central and peripheral benzodiazepine receptors in vitro. The displacing activity on radiolabelled muscimol binding observed for several of the fractions was found to be due to the presence of GABA in micromolar concentrations. The identity of other active compounds was not established. Some of the fractions not containing GABA produced a statistically significant reduction of locomotor activity in rats after intracerebroventricular injection.[10]

A dried preparation of chamomile infusion demonstrated a depressive effect on the CNS after intraperitoneal administration in mice. A dose-dependent decrease of basal locomotor activity was observed (90–360 mg/kg) without involving motor coordination and muscle relaxation. A significant sleeping-time potentiating effect was only observed at the two highest doses (160 and 320 mg/kg).[31] Inhalation of chamomile oil vapour decreased stress-induced increases of plasma ACTH level in ovariectomized rats compared to placebo. The plasma ACTH level decreased further when diazepam was administered along with inhaling chamomile oil vapour and the decrease was blocked by flumazenil. This suggests that chamomile oil may have an effect on GABA-ergic systems in rat brain and perhaps an activity similar to benzodiazepine agonists.[32]

The effect of olfactory stimulation on fluency, vividness of imagery and associated mood was studied with 22 subjects after exposure to either chamomile oil or placebo. Patients were asked to visualize positive and negative images after exposure to one oil, then the other. Chamomile oil did not affect the vividness of imagery ratings but significantly prolonged the time taken for subjects to visualize both positive and negative phrases, suggesting a sedative effect. Negative mood ratings following negative phrase presentation were less extreme after chamomile ($p=0.042$). Overall mood was higher (mean = +1) after chamomile in comparison with placebo (mean = 0) ($p=0.001$).[33]

Antiulcer activity

Chamomile extract demonstrated antipeptic activity in vitro.[34] (–)-Alpha-bisabolol inhibited the occurrence of ulceration induced by indomethacin, stress or ethanol in rats. A decrease in healing time of ulcers was also observed. A standardized chamomile extract also demonstrated ulcer-protective activity.[35] Oral administration of (–)-alpha-bisabolol demonstrated a significant protective effect ($p<0.05$) against gastric toxicity produced by acetylsalicylic acid in rats.[36]

Antimicrobial activity

Antimicrobial activity has been demonstrated for (–)-alpha-bisabolol in vitro[37] and chamomile oil (<0.05% v/v) against *Staphylococcus aureus, Bacillus subtilis* and *Candida albicans*[38] and herniarin in the presence of near UV light. Chamomile extracts demonstrated similar activity against *E. coli*.[39] The growth of *Staphylococcus aureus*, *Streptococcus mutans*, group B Streptococcus and *Streptococcus salivarius* was completely inhibited by chamomile extract at 10 mg/ml. The extract showed strong antibacterial activity against *Bacillus megatherium* and *Leptospira icterohaemorrhagiae*. The effective dose of each component (alpha-bisabolol, bisabolol oxides, dicycloethers, chamazulene) was much lower when the component was in combination with the others, as in the natural extract, indicating a synergistic effect.[40]

Other activity

Chamazulene and (–)-alpha-bisabolol, within the concentration range 10^{-9}–10^{-5} M, demonstrated very little influence on histamine release in isolated rat mast cells. At concentrations higher than 10^{-5} M they stimulated histamine release. En-yn-dicycloether had a moderately stimulating effect in concentrations lower than 10^{-4} M and a strong inhibiting effect on histamine release at higher concentrations.[41]

Chamazulene inhibited membrane lipid peroxidation in vitro in a concentration- and time-dependent manner. It also demonstrated hydroxyl radical scavenging activity.[42]

Diets containing chamomile flower (1.5% and 7%), several chamomile oils (0.2–0.35%) or guaiazulene (0.2%) stimulated liver regeneration in rats.[43]

The wound-healing activity of chamomile is closely linked to its antiinflammatory activity. Chamomile extract and its isolated constituents demonstrated wound-healing activity in several experimental models, including thermally damaged rat tail. (–)-Alpha-bisabolol promotes granulation and tissue regeneration.[37] Application of chamomile extract altered the metabolism of guinea pig skin cells, indicating possible stimulation of cellular regeneration and inhibition of inflammation.[44]

PHARMACOKINETICS

Chamazulene is formed from matricine in the gut of rats by the action of gastric acid following oral administration.[16]

Topical application of radioisotope-labelled (–)-alpha-bisabolol to the skin of nude mice resulted in half the radioactivity being found on the skin, with the remainder present in tissue and organs. Of the level measured in the tissues and organs, 90% was intact (–)-alpha-bisabolol. Further measurements indicated that (–)-alpha-bisabolol penetrated quickly into the skin. Five hours after the topical application it was displaced from outermost to innermost areas. A fast cutaneous absorption and a long therapeutic effect can be expected from (–)-alpha-bisabolol.[45] In contrast, a similar earlier study found that most of the bisabolol had been metabolized to a polar metabolite. Bisabolol was mainly excreted in the urine in the form of polar metabolites and to a slight extent as CO_2 in the exhaled air.[46]

Skin penetration studies of the chamomile flavones apigenin, luteolin and apigenin 7-O-beta-glucoside were carried out with nine healthy female volunteers. Application chambers were fixed on the upper arms. The decline of flavonoid concentration from the skin was measured over 7 hours. Apigenin showed the greatest flux (i.e. the greatest amount of flavonoid per time and area), followed by luteolin. Penetration of apigenin 7-O-beta-glucoside was negligible. A steady state was attained after 3 hours, indicating that the flavonoids penetrated through further skin layers. It was concluded that the flavonoids are not only adsorbed at the skin surface, but penetrate into deeper skin layers.[47,48]

CLINICAL TRIALS

Eczema, dermatitis and ulceration

Topical application of chamomile preparations have shown benefit in the treatment of eczema[49] and varicose eczema.[50] In a survey conducted in the early 1980s, 95% of 2477 general practitioners described good tolerance and therapeutic efficacy obtained from a chamomile cream (containing 2% standardized chamomile extract) in the treatment of eczema.[49] The treatment decreased inflammation[50] and allowed for a reduction in the level of topical corticosteroids used.[49]

Chamomile cream was compared to steroidal and non-steroidal dermal preparations in the maintenance therapy of eczema in an open bilateral comparative trial of 161 patients suffering from inflammatory dermatoses on hands, forearms and lower legs. During maintenance therapy over 3–4 weeks, the chamomile cream showed similar efficacy to 0.25% hydrocortisone. It demonstrated superior activity to the non-steroidal antiinflammatory agent (5% bufexamac) and a glucocorticoid preparation (0.75% fluocortin butyl ester).[51]

Chamomile extract demonstrated a statistically significant effect on wound healing in a double-blind, placebo-controlled clinical trial on 14 patients. The significant decrease of the weeping in the wound area and the drying tendency after dermabrasion of tattoos ($p<0.05$) indicated the therapeutic efficacy of chamomile.[52] In a randomized controlled trial, chamomile cream was preferred over almond cream by patients for the treatment of erythema and moist desquamation acquired after receiving radiotherapy.[53]

In an open uncontrolled clinical trial, patients with varicose ulcers were treated with a chamomile ointment alone and another group was treated with the ointment and a chamomile wash. Therapeutic response was good at 83% and 78%, respectively.[54]

Oral inflammation

In an uncontrolled trial with 36 patients, a chamomile mouthwash provided a cooling and astringent effect for the treatment of chronic oral inflammations, except in the case of glossodynia.[55] In an uncontrolled trial, a chamomile preparation was used therapeutically and prophylactically as an oral rinse in the treatment of oral mucositis caused by head and neck irradiation and systemic chemotherapy. Resolution of mucositis was accelerated by the chamomile rinse and prophylactic use was favourable.[56] In a double-blind, placebo-controlled clinical trial of 164 patients, chamomile mouthwash did not decrease the incidence of stomatitis induced from 5-fluoruracil-based chemotherapy.[57]

Other activity

Oral administration of chamomile tea during cardiac catheterization induced a deep sleep in 10 of 12 patients tested, despite the pain and anxiety experienced from the procedure. The chamomile tea had essentially no cardiac effects.[58]

In a prospective, double-blind, randomized, multicentre, parallel group study, 79 children with acute, non-complicated diarrhoea received either a preparation containing apple pectin and chamomile extract or placebo for 3 days, in addition to the usual rehydration and realimentation diet. At the end of treatment, the diarrhoea had ended significantly ($p<0.05$) more frequently in the pectin/chamomile group (85%) compared to the placebo group (58%). The pectin/chamomile combination significantly reduced the duration of diarrhoea by at least 5.2 hours ($p<0.05$). In contrast to placebo, a trend of continuous improvement was observed by parents for the pectin/chamomile group. The parents expressed their satisfaction more frequently (82%) with pectin/chamomile than with placebo (60%).[59]

The effect of a herbal instant tea preparation containing chamomile, vervain, licorice, fennel and lemon balm on infantile colic was assessed in a prospective double-blind study on babies about 3 weeks old. Tea or placebo up to 150 ml per dose was given to each infant with every episode of colic, but not more than three times a day. After the 7 days of the trial, the colic improvement scores were significantly better in the herbal tea group: 1.7 versus 0.7 for the placebo group ($p<0.05$). In addition, more babies in the treatment group had their colic eliminated: 57% compared to 26% for placebo ($p<0.01$).[60]

TOXICOLOGY

No toxicity was observed in mice administered a dried preparation of chamomile infusion by intraperitoneal injection up to 1440 mg/kg.[31] The acute oral LD_{50} value of chamomile oil in rats and the acute dermal LD_{50} value in rabbits exceeded 5 g/kg.[61]

Long-term oral administration of chamomile extracts produced no observable toxicity and produced no teratogenicity in rats. Cutaneous application of chamomile to rabbits or inhalation of chamomile extracts by guinea pigs daily for 3 weeks produced no observable toxicity.[62]

CONTRAINDICATIONS

Despite reports of skin reactions and dermatitis from topical use of chamomile, the likelihood of chamomile preparations causing a contact allergy is low. However, persons with known sensitivity to other members of the Compositae family (such as ragweed, daisies, chrysanthemums) should avoid topical application of chamomile or chamomile products.

SPECIAL WARNINGS AND PRECAUTIONS

See Contraindications section.

INTERACTIONS

None known.

USE IN PREGNANCY AND LACTATION

No adverse effects expected.

EFFECTS ON ABILITY TO DRIVE AND USE MACHINES

No negative influence is expected.

SIDE EFFECTS

Dermatitis and skin reactions

Chamomile was described as a trigger for eczema as early as 1921. However, varying reports of chamomile causing iatrogenic contact eczema have been noted. In a 1936 study on 539 patients, 3.1% displayed a sensitivity to chamomile on epidermal testing. No occurrences were reported in 260 patients over a period from 1957 to 1963. From 1964 to 1967 1.3% of 237 patients demonstrated an adverse reaction to external applications containing chamomile. Other authors concluded that chamomile was not a causative factor in their studies of 265 and 240 cases of iatrogenic contact eczema. However, a 1967 report indicated that 7.1% of 338 patients demonstrated iatrogenic contact eczema from chamomile preparations. It is unknown whether the chamomile preparation was the single identifiable harmful substance.[63]

A further clinical investigation was undertaken to clarify the possible adverse reaction to chamomile preparations. Among 200 patients, 21 (10.5%) reacted positively on epicutaneous tests to chamomile preparations, though only three patients reacted to chamomile extract. Only one patient clinically exhibited a contact eczema to a chamomile ointment used previously. Of the other 18 patients, 13 had a provable hypersensitivity to the preservatives and five patients probably to ointment bases and/or other constituents of the preparations. The authors felt that genuine chamomile allergy was not as prevalent as first thought.[63] A high (–)-alpha-bisabolol-containing chamomile extract demonstrated negative results in a contact allergy study in 540 patients with eczema. These results confirmed that the extract does not contain allergizing components which may be found in other chamomile products.[64]

A woman developed slight nausea and oedema and erythema in the periorbital regions after ingestion of a strong cup of chamomile tea. The skin changes continued to worsen over several days. The woman had used a hand cream containing chamomile and periodically drank chamomile tea over many years. Several months later the woman responded positively to a patch test with a solution containing a chamomile extract. This case was considered rare, as it was the first positive reaction observed amongst the testing of 830 dermatitis patients.[65]

To investigate Compositae dermatitis, sesquiterpene lactones and ether extracts of five European Compositae plants (Arnica, feverfew, German chamomile, yarrow and tansy) were added to routine patch testing of patients over 1 year; 4.5% of the 686 patients demonstrated Compositae sensitivity. Testing with the individual ingredients of the extract in these Compositae-allergic patients resulted in 75% positive reaction to chamomile.[66]

An earlier study found that application of Compositae ether extracts to the skin of 25 Compositae-sensitive patients revealed that two were allergic to chamomile. Crossreactions were seen to chamomile in a further 11 patients. The sesquiterpene lactones of Compositae plants are believed to be responsible for the sensitization, with the presence of an alpha-methylene group exocyclic to the gamma-lactone as the requisite for allergy,[67] which matricine does not contain. A total of 1032 patients randomly chosen from six patch test clinics were patch tested with a series of five ointments and the components of the ointment bases. Two patients demonstrated a positive reaction to a chamomile cream which was verified by additional tests with the herb itself.[68]

The above data suggest that the likelihood of chamomile preparations causing a contact allergy is low, but persons with known sensitivity to other members of the Compositae family should avoid contact with chamomile or chamomile products.

Conjunctivitis

Seven hayfever patients suffering from conjunctivitis demonstrated positive skin prick tests to chamomile tea extract, chamomile and mugwort pollen extracts. Conjunctival irritation was observed in all the patients with the chamomile tea extract. However, no symptoms were observed after oral ingestion of the infusion. IgE activity was detected and shown to be due to the chamomile pollen. Further testing in 100 hayfever controls revealed a positive immediate skin response to chamomile pollen for eight and five for chamomile tea. Only two demonstrated a positive conjunctival response. In conclusion, eye washing with chamomile tea can induce allergic conjunctivitis and the pollen contained in these infusions are the allergens responsible for the reactions.[69] Pollens and their proteins are unlikely to be present or active in aqueous alcohol extracts of chamomile.

Anaphylactic reaction

An 8-year-old atopic boy developed a severe anaphylactic reaction after the ingestion of chamomile tea infusion. The patient suffered from hayfever and bronchial asthma caused by a variety of pollens including mugwort. Further study suggested that a type I IgE-mediated mechanism based on a crossreaction with mugwort pollen was responsible for the patient's anaphylactic symptoms.[70] Given the widespread consumption of chamomile tea and the few reported cases of anaphylaxis, this type of reaction must be extremely rare. Moreover, the use of ethanolic extracts denatures the proteins in chamomile and renders this type of reaction unlikely.

OVERDOSE

Not known.

CURRENT REGULATORY STATUS IN SELECTED COUNTRIES

Chamomile is official in the *European Pharmacopoeia* (1997). Chamomile became official in the *United States Pharmacopeia-National Formulary* (USP23–NF18, 1995–June 1999).

Chamomile is covered by a positive Commission E monograph and has the following applications:

- externally: inflammation of the skin and mucous membranes and bacterial skin conditions, including those of the mouth and gums;
- inhalations: inflammation and irritation of the respiratory tract;
- baths and washes: complaints in the anal and genital regions;
- internally; gastrointestinal spasms and inflammatory conditions of the gastrointestinal tract.

Chamomile is on the UK General Sale List.

Chamomile and chamomile oil have GRAS status. Chamomile is also freely available as a 'dietary supplement' in the USA under DSHEA legislation (1994 Dietary Supplement Health and Education Act). Chamomile has been present in over-the-counter (OTC) digestive aid drug products. The FDA, however, advises: 'that based on evidence currently available, there is inadequate data to establish general recognition of the safety and effectiveness of these ingredients for the specified uses'.

Chamomile is not included in Part 4 of Schedule 4 of the Therapeutic Goods Act Regulations of Australia.

References

1. Felter HW, Lloyd JU. King's American dispensatory, 18th edn, 3rd revision, vol 2, 1905. Reprinted by Eclectic Medical Publications, Portland, 1983, pp 1246–1247.
2. British Herbal Medicine Association's Scientific Committee. British herbal pharmacopoeia. BHMA, West York, 1983, pp 139–140.
3. Grieve M. A modern herbal, vol 1. Dover Publications, New York, 1971, pp 187–188.
4. Smeh NJ. Creating your own cosmetics – naturally. Alliance Publishing, Garrisonville, 1995, pp 81, 82, 137.
5. Chiej R. The Macdonald encyclopedia of medicinal plants. Macdonald, London, 1984, entry no. 191.
6. Launert EL. The Hamlyn guide to edible and medicinal plants of Britain and Northern Europe. Hamlyn, London, 1981, pp 192–194.
7. Wagner H, Bladt S. Plant drug analysis: a thin layer chromatography atlas, 2nd edn. Springer-Verlag, Berlin, 1996, pp 159, 199.
8. Schmidt PC, Weibler K, Soyke B. Dtsch Apoth Ztg 1991; 131: 175–181.
9. British Herbal Medicine Association. British herbal compendium, vol 1. BHMA, Bournemouth, 1992, pp 154–157.
10. Avallone R, Zanoli P, Corsi L et al. Phytother Res 1996; 10 (suppl 1): S177–S179.
11. Carle R, Isaac O. Dtsch Apoth Ztg 1985; 125 (43 supp 1): 2–8.
12. European Pharmacopoeia, 3rd edn. European Department for the Quality of Medicines within the Council of Europe, Strasbourg, 1996, pp 1146–1147.
13. Safayhi H, Sabieraj J, Sailer E-R et al. Planta Med 1994; 60: 410–413.
14. Ammon HPT, Sabieraj J, Kaul R. Dtsch Apoth Ztg 1996; 136 (22): 17–30.
15. Shipochliev T, Dimitrov A, Aleksandrova E. Vet Med Nauki 1981; 18: 87–94.
16. Jakovlev V, Isaac O, Flaskamp E. Planta Med 1983; 49: 67–73.
17. Della Loggia, R. 24th International Symposium on Essential Oils, Berlin, July 1993.
18. Jakovlev V, Isaac K, Thiemer K et al. Planta Med 1979; 35: 125–140.
19. Breinlich J, Scharnagel K. Arzneim Forsch 1968; 18: 429–431.
20. Fuller E, Sosa S, Tubaro A et al. Planta Med 1993; 59(Suppl): A666–A667.
21. Della Loggia R, Carle R, Sosa S et al. Planta Med 1990; 56: 657–658.
22. Tubaro A, Zilli C, Redaelli C et al. Planta Med 1984; 50: 359.
23. Della Loggia R. Dtsch Apoth Ztg 1985; 125 (43 suppl 1): 9–11.
24. Albring M, Albrecht H, Alcorn G et al. Meth Find Exp Clin Pharmacol 1983; 5 (8): 575–577.
25. Nissen HP, Biltz H, Kreysel HW. Z Hautkr 1988; 63 (3): 184–190.
26. Achterrath-Tuckermann U, Kunde R, Flaskamp E et al. Planta Med 1980; 39: 38–50.
27. Redaelli C Formentini L, Santaniello E. Poster, International Research Congress on Natural Products as Medical Agents, Strasbourg, 1980. Cited in Carle R, Isaac O. Z Phytother 1987; 8: 67–77.
28. Forster HB, Niklas H, Lutz S. Planta Med 1980; 40 (4): 309–319.
29. Lis-Balchin M, Hart S, Deans SG et al. J Herbs Spices Med Plants 1996; 4 (2): 69–86.
30. Viola H, Wasowski C, Levi de Stein M et al. Planta Med 1995; 61: 213–215.
31. Della Loggia R, Traversa U, Scarcia V et al. Pharmacol Res Commun 1982; 14 (2): 153–162.
32. Yamada K, Miura T, Mimaki Y et al. Biol Pharm Bull 1996; 19 (9): 1244–1246.
33. Roberts A, Williams JM. Br J Med Psychol 1992; 65 (2): 197–199.
34. Thiemer K, Stadler R, Isaac O. Arzneim Forsch 1972; 22 (6): 1086–1087.
35. Szelenyi I, Isaac O, Thiemer K. Planta Med 1979; 35: 218–227.
36. Torrado S, Torrado S, Agis A et al. Pharmazie 1995; 50 (2): 141–143.
37. Carle R, Isaac O. Z Phytother 1987; 8: 67–77.
38. Aggag ME, Yousef RT. Planta Med 1972; 22: 140–144.
39. Ceska O, Chaudhary SK, Warrington PJ et al. Fitoterapia 1992; 58 (5): 387–394.
40. Cinco M, Banfi E, Tubaro A et al. Int J Crude Drug Res 1983; 21 (4): 145–151.
41. Miller T, Wittstock U, Lindequist U et al. Planta Med 1996; 62 (1): 60–61.
42. Rekka EA, Kouroundakis AP, Kourounakis PN. Res Commun Mol Pathol Pharmacol 1996; 92 (3): 361–364.
43. Gershbein LL. Food Cosmet Toxicol 1977; 15: 173–181.

44. Thiemer K, Stadler R, Isaac O. Arzneim Forsch 1973; 23 (6): 756–759.
45. Hahn B, Hölzl J. Arzneim-Forsch 1987; 37 (6): 716–720.
46. Hölzl J, Hahn B. Dtsch Apoth Ztg 1985; 125: 32–38.
47. Merfort I, Heilmann J, Hagedorn-Leweke U et al. Pharmazie 1994; 49 (7): 509–511.
48. Heilmann J, Merfort I, Hagedorn U et al. Planta Med 1993; 59 (suppl): A638
49. Patzelt-Wenczler R. Dtsch Apoth Ztg 1985; 125 (43 suppl 1): 12–13.
50. Homberg Pharma Germany, Division of Degussa: Kamillosan Scientific Information, Frankfurt.
51. Aertgeerts P, Albring M, Klaschka F et al. Z Hautkr 1985; 60 (3): 270–277.
52. Glowania HJ, Raulin Chr, Swoboda M. Z Hautkr 1987; 62 (17): 1262–1271.
53. Maiche AG, Grohn P, Maki-Hokkonen H. Acta Oncol 1991; 30: 395–396.
54. Aertgeerts J. Arztl Kosmetol 1984; 14 (6): 502–504.
55. Nasemann T. Z Allgemeinmed 1975; 51: (25): 1105–1106.
56. Carl W, Emrich LS. J Prosthet Dent 1991; 66: 361–369.
57. Fidler P, Loprinzi CL, O'Fallon JR et al. Cancer 1996; 77 (3): 522–525.
58. Gould L, Reddy RCV, Gomprecht RF. J Clin Pharmacol 1973; 13: 475–479.
59. De La Motte S, Bose-O'Reilly S, Heinisch M et al. Arzneim-Forsch 1997; 47 (11): 1247–1249.
60. Weizman Z, Alkrinawi S, Goldfarb D et al. J Pediatrics 1993; 122 (4): 650–652.
61. Opdyke DLJ. Food Cosmet Toxicol 1974; 12: 851–852.
62. Homberg Pharma Germany, Division of Degussa: Kamillosan Scientific Information, Frankfurt (Main).
63. Von Beetz D, Cramer H, Melhorn HC. Derm Mschr 1971; 157: 505–510.
64. Jablonska S, Rudzki E. Z Hautkr 1996; 71 (7): 542–546.
65. Rudzki E, Rebandel P. Contact Derm 1998; 38: 164–184.
66. Paulsen E, Andersen KE, Hausen BM. Contact Derm 1993; 29 (1): 6–10.
67. Hausen BM. Dermatologica 1979; 159: 1–11.
68. Bruynzeel DP, Van Ketel WG, Young E et al. Contact Derm 1992; 27: 278–279.
69. Subiza J, Subiza JL, Alonso M et al. Ann Allergy 1990; 65: 127–132.
70. Subiza J, Subiza JL, Hinojosa M et al. J Allergy Clin Immunol 1989; 84: 353–358.

Chaste tree
(*Vitex agnus-castus* L.)

SYNONYMS

Monk's pepper (Engl), Agni casti fructus (Lat), Keuschlammfrüchte (Ger), agneau chaste, gatillier (Fr), kyskhedstræ (Dan).

WHAT IS IT?

The ripe berries of chaste tree have long been regarded as a symbol of chastity, as they were used in the Middle Ages to suppress sexual excitability. The dried fruits have a peppery taste and were used in monasteries instead of pepper, supposedly to suppress libido. The remedy was considered primarily a herb for women's complaints, especially from the mid-1900s throughout Europe. Modern scientific interest developed in Germany in the 1930s.

EFFECTS

Enhances corpus luteal development (thereby correcting a relative progesterone deficiency) via a dopaminergic activity on the anterior pituitary (which inhibits prolactin); normalizes the menstrual cycle, encourages ovulation. Indicated for any kind of premenstrual aggravation. The inhibition of prolactin contrasts with the traditional use to promote breast milk.

TRADITIONAL VIEW

A tincture of the fresh berries was used traditionally by the Eclectics as a galactagogue and emmenagogue and was also said to 'repress the sexual passions'. Suggested uses from the Eclectics include impotence, sexual melancholia, sexual irritability with nervousness, melancholia or mild dementia.[1] The main traditional use of chaste tree occurred in Europe where it was widely used by women for a variety of gynaecological problems. Details of traditional use by women are very scanty (as is often the case with such remedies). However, it appears to have had a wide variety of applications and was an archetypal 'women's herb' in some Mediterranean traditions. The most persistent traditional indication is insufficient lactation.[2,3]

SUMMARY ACTIONS

Prolactin inhibitor, dopamine agonist, galactagogue, indirectly progesterogenic.

CAN BE USED FOR

INDICATIONS SUPPORTED BY CLINICAL TRIALS

Menstruation disorders including secondary amenorrhoea, metrorrhagia (from functional causes), oligomenorrhoea (lengthened cycle), polymenorrhoea (shortened cycle), especially when marked by progesterone deficiency (cystic hyperplasia of the endometrium) and latent hyperprolactinaemia; premenstrual tension (except type C, which is characterized by symptoms such as headache, craving for sweets, palpitations and dizziness), especially premenstrual mastalgia and fluid retention; other premenstrual aggravations (e.g. mouth ulcers, orofacial herpes, epilepsy); insufficient lactation; infertility due to decreased progesterone levels or hyperprolactinaemia; acne.

TRADITIONAL THERAPEUTIC USES

Promotion of lactation; menstrual irregularities; to decrease libido.

MAY ALSO BE USED FOR

EXTRAPOLATIONS FROM PHARMACOLOGICAL STUDIES

Relative progesterone deficiency; conditions where unopposed oestrogen plays a role: fibroids, endometriosis, follicular ovarian cysts; additional conditions caused by hyperprolactinaemia (e.g. some cases of erectile impotence in men, hypogonadism, galactorrhoea or irregular menstruation).

OTHER APPLICATIONS

Despite the progesterone-favouring effect of chaste tree, it is also used in the treatment of menopausal symptoms and for HRT withdrawal. Chaste tree is not restricted to women; it has been used to treat male disorders, particularly male acne. Other suggested uses include those conditions in which raised prolactin secretion is implicated: breast cysts, fibrocystic breast disease, benign prostatic hyperplasia.[4]

PREPARATIONS

Dried or fresh ripe berries for decoction or liquid extract for internal use.

DOSAGE

Low doses are used in Germany: 30–40 mg per day of herb in an appropriate preparation/water-alcohol solution. However, practitioners in the English-speaking countries tend to use the following approach: daily dose of 1–5 ml of a 1:5 tincture, 1– 4 ml of a 1:2 extract or chaste tree tablets (500 mg, 1–2 tablets). In severe cases, higher doses may be used in the short term but prolonged use of very high doses should be avoided.

It is common practice, and also recommended by German manufacturers, that chaste tree is taken as a single dose each morning before breakfast throughout the cycle. It is considered that hormonal regulation is more receptive to this regime.

DURATION OF USE

May be used long term if prescribed within the recommended therapeutic range. Chaste tree should be discontinued if the length of the menstrual cycle is excessively changed.

SUMMARY ASSESSMENT OF SAFETY

Only mild adverse effects from ingestion of chaste tree are expected when consumed within the recommended dosage range.

TECHNICAL DATA

BOTANY

Vitex agnus-castus, a member of the Verbenaceae (verbena) family, was indigenous to southern Europe but is now widely cultivated.[5] The shrub grows to 3–5 m and produces large dark green leaves radiating from a long, hairy stalk. The shoots terminate in a slender spike and are composed of whorls of violet flowers. The black spherical berries are about 5 mm in size and contain four seeds.[6]

KEY CONSTITUENTS

- Essential oil (0.7%, containing monoterpenes and sesquiterpenes);[7] flavonoids: methoxylated flavones including casticin.[8]
- Iridoid glycosides, including aucubin (0.3%), agnoside (0.6%).[9]

PHARMACODYNAMICS

It is important to bear in mind that the menstrual cycle is unique to the human female and that animal models as cited below may have limited applicability.

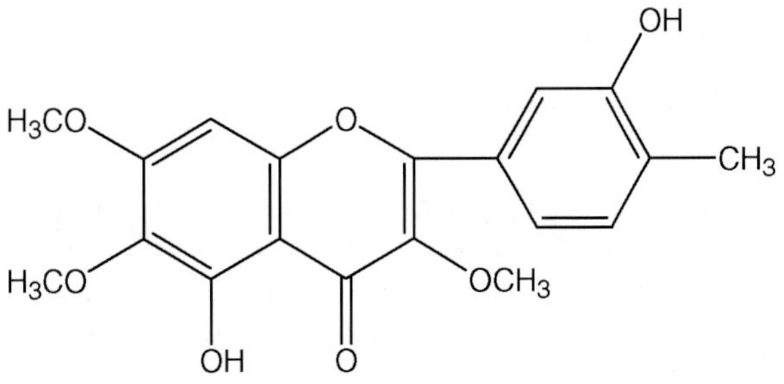

H3CO H3CO OH O OH CH3 OCH3

Casticin

Hormonal activity

Prolactin secretion from the anterior pituitary is inhibited by dopamine and stimulated by thyroxin-releasing hormone (TRH) released from the hypothalamus. Chaste tree and a synthetic dopamine agonist (lisuride) significantly inhibited basal and TRH-stimulated prolactin secretion in isolated rat pituitary cells. This inhibition could be blocked by adding a dopamine receptor blocker, which confirmed the dopaminergic effect of chaste tree.[10] In addition, a dopamine agonist (haloperidol) was able to counteract the prolactin-lowering effect of chaste tree, proving a dopaminergic mode of action.[11] Using the corpus striatum membrane dopamine receptor binding assay, it was determined that chaste tree extract contains an active principle which binds to the dopamine D_2 receptor. The action of chaste tree on pituitary hormone secretion in vitro was selective, since both basal or LHRH-stimulated gonadotrophin (FSH, LH) release remained unaffected.[12]

Chaste tree extract (containing 3.3 mg water-soluble substances per ml) yielded several fractions which contained prolactin-inhibiting substances, as tested in vitro with pituitary cells, indicating that more than one compound is responsible for the dopaminergic activity. Based on several tests, it was concluded that the dopaminergic substances in chaste tree extracts may have catechol structure and therefore undergo autooxidation easily after isolation. It is possible that chaste tree protects its dopaminergic substances by an endogenous production of antioxidants (which are eventually lost with increasing purification).[13]

An early experimental study found that at low doses, female guinea pigs given chaste tree orally for 90 days demonstrated a decrease of oestrogen effects and a promotion of progesterone effects which was presumably mediated through the pituitary gland: that is, FSH secretion was decreased and LH and prolactin secretion were increased. Corpus luteal development and glandular proliferation in breast tissue were enhanced and follicular development and uterine weight were slightly increased. At the high dose (about 20 times the low dosage) an inhibition of all gonadotrophic hormones and growth hormone resulted. Pituitary, adrenal and uterine weights were significantly decreased and breast tissue showed signs of atrophy.[14] This suggests that in the guinea pig, high doses of chaste tree probably inhibit all aspects of anterior pituitary function. Intravenous injection of chaste tree extract (containing 3.3 mg water-soluble substances per ml) markedly reduced stress-induced prolactin release in rats.[13] Administration of chaste tree extract (at the high dose of 0.3–2.3 g extract per kg body weight) to suckling rats led to a clear increase in young animals without milk. This was comparable to rats given bromocriptine, a drug which suppresses prolactin secretion. The authors believed a reduction in prolactin levels leads to the significant reduction in milk production. There were no indications of toxicity, including no change in body weight of the adults.[15]

In an open, placebo-controlled trial, 20 male subjects received special extract of chaste tree (120, 240 or 480 mg per day) or placebo for 14 days. There was a significant increase in a 24-hour prolactin secretion at the lowest dosage, in contrast to the higher dosages, which caused a small drop. On the last day of the trial, prolactin release over a 1-hour period after TRH stimulation was measured compared to placebo; a significant increase of prolactin at the lowest dosage and a significant drop at the highest dosage were recorded. This suggests the activity of chaste tree is dependent on dosage and the initial level of the prolactin concentration. Chaste tree did not alter the serum concentrations of the gonadotrophins (LH, FSH) or testosterone.[16,17]

Pretreatment before mating with powdered chaste tree (1–2 g/kg) had no antifertility effect (as measured by a reduction in the number of foetuses) in male and female rats and guinea pigs. In addition, chaste tree aqueous extract inhibited the spontaneous activity of the isolated rat uterus.[18] The flavonoid-rich fraction from the seeds of *Vitex negundo*, which contained largely methoxylated flavones similar to *Vitex agnus-castus*, showed antiandrogenic effects in vivo by intraperitoneal route.[19]

Antimicrobial activity

Ethanolic and etheric extracts of chaste tree demonstrated in vitro antimicrobial activity against the following strains, using the dilution method: *Staphylococcus aureus, Streptococcus faecalis* (6.5–20% extracts), *Salmonella spp, Escherichia coli* (10–20%), *Candida albicans, C. tropicalis, C. pseudotropicalis* and *C. krusei* (10–40%). High toxicity against the mycelial growth of *Trichophyton mentagrophytes, Epidermophyton floccosum, Microsporum canis, M. gypseum* (1.5–12%) and *Penicillium virdicatum* (9–23%) was also found.[20] Essential oil from chaste tree ripe fruit showed greater antimicrobial activity against *E. coli* and *Candida albicans* than against *Staph. aureus* or *Bacillus anthracoides*.[21]

PHARMACOKINETICS

No data available.

CLINICAL TRIALS

Hyperprolactinaemia is one of the most frequent causes for cyclical disorders, from corpus luteal insufficiency (shortened luteal phase, extended PMS and/or reduced progesterone secretion) to secondary amenorrhoea, and premenstrual mastalgia. Latent hyperprolactinaemia is present throughout the cycle but due to the removal of the inhibitory effect of progesterone at the end of the luteal phase, high quantities of prolactin are released under minor stress conditions as well as during deep sleep phases at night. Hyperprolactinaemia and corpus luteum insufficiency may both be implicated in PMS but there is insufficient evidence to link them invariably with the condition.

Menstruation disorders

Uncontrolled clinical studies on chaste tree date back to 1954. Improvement was noted in patients suffering from a variety of menstruation disorders, including secondary amenorrhoea, and was particularly marked for patients suffering from cystic hyperplasia of the endometrium (a disorder due to a relative progesterone deficiency). In a number of these patients ovulatory cycles were reestablished. Chaste tree was particularly indicated in patients with deficient corpus luteum function.[22] This work was supported in another study which demonstrated improvement in 63% of patients.[23] An improvement was observed in 66% patients with heavy or frequent bleeding.[24] For 33 cases of polymenorrhoea (shortened cycle), treatment with chaste tree lengthened the average cycle from 20 to 26 days. With 35 cases of oligomenorrhoea (infrequent menstruation) the average cycle was shortened from 39 to 31 days and for 58 cases of menorrhagia, average duration of bleeding decreased from 8 to 5 days. Treatment with chaste tree was long term, over many months.[25]

In a large, uncontrolled trial 1592 women with conditions defined as corpus luteum insufficiency were treated with chaste tree. Thirty-three percent were observed to be free of complaints and 51% were in satisfactory condition according to the physician's assessment. In the patients' assessment, 61% were assessed as good, 29% as satisfactory.[26] Thirteen patients with hyperprolactinaemia and cyclic disorders were treated for 3 months with a low-dose chaste tree preparation (60 drops per day, equivalent to 33.4 mg of herb). The menstrual cycle returned to normal in all patients. Prolactin levels were significantly reduced and in some patients prolactin levels even returned to the normal range.[27]

Observation of 551 patients by 153 gynaecologists over several menstrual cycles found the efficacy of chaste tree treatment to be good in 68.8% of cases. Three hundred and sixty-nine patients had symptoms of corpus luteal insufficiency or cyclic disorders; 210 had PMS. A majority of patients (81.1%) were relieved of complaints or stated that their condition had improved.[28] Thirty-seven women with luteal phase defects due to latent hyperprolactinaemia completed a double-blind, placebo-controlled trial testing the efficacy of a chaste tree preparation (20 mg per day). With this disorder, blood levels of prolactin may only be slightly raised but there is an excessive prolactin response following IV injection of TRH. The menstrual cycle is also abnormal; the luteal phase is much shorter although the total length of the cycle can be normal. Blood for hormonal analysis was taken at days 5–8 and day 20 of the menstrual cycle, before and after 3 months of therapy. Latent hyperprolactinaemia was analysed by monitoring prolactin release after IV injection of TRH. With chaste tree treatment, prolactin release following TRH was significantly reduced. Shortened luteal phases were normalized and luteal phase progesterone deficiencies were corrected. There were no changes in any other hormones except that luteal phase 17-beta-oestradiol (i.e. oestrogen) levels were higher in the chaste tree group. Two women receiving chaste tree became pregnant and PMS symptoms were significantly reduced in the chaste tree group.[29]

Premenstrual syndrome (PMS)

Pharmacological and clinical studies suggest that chaste tree corrects a relative progesterone deficiency created by latent hyperprolactinaemia. Many patients with premenstrual symptoms show latent hyperprolactinaemia associated with corpus luteum insufficiency. This may be the only aetiological factor in PMS which responds to chaste tree treatment. Therefore the reputation of chaste tree in the treatment of PMS may solely be based on its dopaminergic activity. This could explain the negative finding in the PMS clinical trial cited below but the high placebo effect in PMS makes such trials difficult to design and conduct.

Uncontrolled trials in the early 1960s indicate that chaste tree has had an effect on a variety of unusual premenstrual aggravations, including posttraumatic epilepsy,[30] mouth ulcers[31] and orofacial herpes simplex.[32] In a pilot controlled clinical trial, significant benefit was observed for all types of PMS except type PMS-C (characterized by symptoms such as headache, craving for sweets, palpitations and dizziness).[33]

In a double-blind, placebo-controlled trial, patients with PMS received chaste tree (1.8 g per day) or a soya-based placebo for 3 months. There was little difference found between chaste tree and placebo for the majority of symptoms associated with PMS. However, there was a tendency to improvement in the fluid retention group of symptoms, especially mastalgia, although not reaching statistical significance.[34] Given that PMS may have different aetiologies and demonstrates a high placebo effect in clinical trials, it may be impossible to prove a beneficial treatment except for symptoms such as fluid retention which define specific aetiologies or subgroups. Moreover, the soya-based placebo may have had pharmacological activity.

In a multicentre, randomized, double-blind, comparative trial, 175 women with PMS received either chaste tree or vitamin B_6 (pyridoxine) over three cycles. Patients received chaste tree (3.5–4.2 mg of a 9.5–11.5:1 extract) each day or one capsule of placebo twice daily on days 1–15 and one capsule of pyridoxine (100 mg) twice daily on days 16–35 of the menstrual cycle. Some patients did not complete the trial or were excluded from analysis. The premenstrual tension syndrome scale decreased for both treatments but chaste tree treatment was superior to pyridoxine overall. Characteristic symptoms (breast tenderness, oedemas, abdominal tension, headaches, constipation, depressed mood) were more significantly reduced by chaste tree than by pyridoxine. The efficacy of treatment was rated as excellent by about 25% of physicians for chaste tree but by only 12% for pyridoxine. Thirty-six percent of women treated with chaste tree felt free from complaints, compared to 21% of pyridoxine-treated patients. Nine patients recorded adverse events, four from the pyridoxine group and five receiving chaste tree. Of these adverse events, gastrointestinal disturbances were approximately equally distributed between the two study groups. Two chaste tree-treated subjects experienced skin reactions and one reported transient headache.[35] However, the significance of results of this study are difficult to assess in terms of the possible benefit of chaste tree for PMS because a placebo control group was not included in the experimental design.

Infertility

In two uncontrolled studies, the influence of chaste tree on corpus luteal function was investigated. When the data from these trials are combined, the effect of chaste tree was studied on 45 infertile women aged between 23 and 39. These women were considered to be capable of reproduction and had normal prolactinaemia (less than 20 ng/ml), but showed pathologically low serum progesterone levels of between 7.0 and 12.0 ng/ml at day 20 of the menstrual cycle. After 3 months, chaste tree treatment was considered to be successful in 39 of 45 cases. Seven women became pregnant, 25 women had normal serum progesterone levels at day 20 and another seven tended towards normal levels. These results generally coincided with a lengthening of the luteal (hyperthermic) phase and a positive change in the LHRH test dynamic.[36,37] The findings indicate an enhancement of corpus luteal function, which may have been inhibited as part of a latent hyperprolactinaemia syndrome.

Influence on lactation

A favourable effect was observed on milk production in 80% of 125 subjects treated with chaste tree in a case observation study.[38] In an open, controlled trial of 817 patients, a significant effect was observed from chaste tree treatment, with average milk production about three times that of controls after 20 days of treatment.[39]

Mastalgia

In the period 1968–1976, 1480 women with mastodynia (painful breasts) were treated with a homoeopathic formula containing chaste tree mother tincture for 3–6 months. An analysis of 444 women found 58% achieved a complete symptom-free state and 25% experienced a clear improvement.[40] In an uncontrolled trial, 52 patients with mastopathia received chaste tree extract (60 drops per day, equivalent to 33.4 mg of herb) over a period of at least three cycles. No pain was experienced by 46% of patients and in 29% the pain was decreased to a minimum.[41] These results from uncontrolled trials should be interpreted with caution, because a high placebo effect is likely.

In a double-blind clinical trial, 160 patients with premenstrual mastalgia received a homoeopathic formula also containing chaste tree, gestagen therapy (lynestrenol) or placebo. Significant difference was observed between the groups as treatment with phytotherapy gave good relief of symptoms in 74.5% of patients compared to 82.1% for lynestrenol and 36.8% for placebo. Treatment with phytotherapy was considered superior because of the lower incidence of side effects.[42] In an earlier trial with 20 patients using the same design but including crossover, a statistically significant reduction of symptoms was observed with chaste tree treatment. Short-lived nausea was reported.[43]

Acne

In a controlled trial of 161 patients with acne, both male and female, a minimum of 3 months' treatment with chaste tree resulted in an improvement for 70% of patients, a result which was significantly better than placebo.[44] The mechanism for the beneficial effect of chaste tree on acne is not known but may be due to a mild antiandrogenic effect.

TOXICOLOGY

No information available.

CONTRAINDICATIONS

Chaste tree is preferably not to be taken in conjunction with progesterone drugs, the contraceptive pill or HRT. Chaste tree may aggravate pure spasmodic dysmenorrhoea not associated with PMS. This may be due to the priming effect of progesterone on the endometrial prostaglandin release during the initial stages of menstruation. However, chaste tree is usually beneficial for spasmodic dysmenorrhoea associated with PMS and for congestive dysmenorrhoea.[45]

SPECIAL WARNINGS AND PRECAUTIONS

None required.

INTERACTIONS

None known definitely, but chaste tree may interact antagonistically with dopamine receptor antagonists.[46]

USE IN PREGNANCY AND LACTATION

Use cautiously in pregnancy and only in the early stages for insufficient corpus luteal function. Although the dopaminergic activity might suggest that chaste tree is best avoided during lactation, clinical trials have demonstrated its positive activity, albeit at low doses.

EFFECTS ON ABILITY TO DRIVE AND USE MACHINES

None known.

SIDE EFFECTS

After three endocrinologically normal cycles while undergoing unstimulated in vitro fertilization treatment, a woman took chaste tree at the beginning of a fourth unstimulated IVF treatment cycle. In this fourth cycle, her serum gonadotrophin and ovarian hormone measurements were disordered. One embryo resulted from the three eggs collected but a pregnancy did not ensue. She had symptoms suggestive of mild ovarian hyperstimulation syndrome in the luteal phase. Two subsequent cycles were endocrinologically normal. However, the authors' conclusion that chaste tree may not be suitable to promote normal ovarian function is probably premature.[47]

Rare occurrences of itching and urticaria have been reported.[46] In a large uncontrolled trial of 1592 women treated with chaste tree for conditions defined as corpus luteum insufficiency, 1% of patients terminated treatment because of side effects.[26] Observation of 551 patients treated with chaste tree by 153 gynaecologists indicated 5% of patients experienced side effects, predominantly nausea.[28] In a randomized, comparative trial for the treatment of PMS in 175 women, just over 13% of those treated with chaste tree and 6% of those treated with vitamin B_6 had mild side effects (gastrointestinal and lower abdominal complaints, skin eruptions, short-term headaches). These side effects were not considered serious.[35]

A 45-year-old woman who had been taking herbal preparations containing black cohosh, chaste tree and evening primrose oil for 4 months had three seizures within a 3-month period. The herbal preparations were stopped and the patient was treated with anticonvulsants.[48]

OVERDOSE

None known.

CURRENT REGULATORY STATUS IN SELECTED COUNTRIES

Chaste tree is covered by a positive Commission E monograph and can be used for the treatment of menstrual problems, premenstrual syndrome and mastodynia.

Chaste tree is not on the UK General Sale List.

Chaste tree does not have GRAS status. However, it is freely available as a 'dietary supplement' in the USA under DSHEA legislation (1994 Dietary Supplement Health and Education Act).

Chaste tree is not included in Part 4 of Schedule 4 of the Therapeutic Goods Act Regulations of Australia.

References

1. Felter HW, Lloyd JU. King's American dispensatory, 18th edn, 3rd revision, vol 2, 1905. Reprinted by Eclectic Medical Publications, Portland, 1983, p 2056.
2. Mills SY. Out of the earth: the essential book of herbal medicine. Viking Arkana (Penguin), London, 1991, pp 522–524.
3. Mills SY. Woman medicine: vitex agnus-castus, the herb. Amberwood, Christchurch, UK, 1992, pp 10–15.
4. Christie S, Walker AF. Eur J Herbal Med 1997; 3 (3): 29–45.
5. Mabberley DJ. The plant book, 2nd edn. Cambridge University Press, Cambridge, 1997, p 749.
6. Thomson WAR (ed). Healing plants. Macmillan, London, 1980, p 111.
7. Zwaving JH, Bos R. Planta Med 1996; 62: 83–84.
8. Wollenweber E, Mann K. Planta Med 1983; 48: 126–127.
9. Gorler K, Oehlke D, Soicke H. Planta Med 1985; 50: 530–531.
10. Sliutz G, Speiser P, Schultz AM et al. Horm Metab Res 1993; 25 (5): 253–255.
11. Winterhoff H. Abstracts of papers of the American Chemical Society 1996; 212 (1–2): AGFD 105.
12. Jarry H, Leonhardt S, Gorkow C et al. Exp Clin Endocrinol 1994; 102 (6): 448–454.
13. Wuttke W, Gorkow Ch, Jarry H. Dopaminergic compounds in vitex agnus castus. In: Loew D, Rietbrock N (eds) Phytopharmaka in Forschung und klinischer Anwendung. Steinkopff (Verlag), Darmstadt, 1995, pp 83–90.
14. Haller J. Z Geburtsh Gynakol 1961; 156 (3): 274–302.
15. Winterhoff H, Gorkow C, Behr B. Z Phytother 1991; 12 (6): 175–179.
16. Loew D, Gorkow C, Schrodter A et al. Z Phytother 1996; 17 (4): 237–240, 243.
17. Merz PG, Schrodter A, Rietbrock S et al. Prolaktinsekretion und Verträglichkeit unter der Behandlung mit einem Agnus-castus-Spezialextrakt (B1095E1). Erste Ergebnisse zum Einfluβ auf die Prolaktinsekretion. In: Loew D, Rietbrock N (eds) Phytopharmaka in Forschung und klinischer Anwendung. Steinkopff (Verlag), Darmstadt, 1995, pp 93–97.
18. Lal R, Sankaranarayanan A, Mathur VS et al. Bull Postgrad Inst Med Educ Res Chandigarh 1985; 19 (2): 44–47.
19. Bhargava SK. J Ethnopharmacol 1989; 27 (3): 327–339.
20. Pepeljnjak S, Antolic A, Kustrak D. Acta Pharm 1996; 46 (3): 201–206.
21. Mishurova SS, Malinovskaya TA, Akhmedov IB et al. Rastitel 'nye-Rastursy 1986; 22 (4): 526–530.
22. Probst V, Roth OA. Dtsch Med Wschr 1954; 79 (35): 1271–1274.
23. Roth OA. Med Klin 1956; 51: 1263–1265.
24. Kayser HW, Istanbulluoglu S. Hippokrates 1954; 25: 717–719.
25. Bleier W. Zbl Gynakol 1959; 81: 701–709.
26. Propping D, Bohnert KJ, Peeters M et al. Therapeutikon 1991; 5: 581–585.
27. Roeder D. Z Phytother 1994; 15 (3): 157–163.
28. Peters-Welte C, Albrecht M. TW Gynakol 1994; 7 (1): 49–52.
29. Milewicz A, Gejdel E, Sworen H et al. Arzneim-Forsch 1993; 43 (7): 752–756.

30. Ecker G. Landarzt 1964; 40: 872–874.
31. Hillebrand H. Landarzt 1964; 40 (36): 1577–1578.
32. Albus GA. Z Hautkr Geschlkrkh 1964; 36 (7): 220–223.
33. Promotional brochure. Gerard House, UK, 1988.
34. Turner S, Mills S. Compl Ther Med 1993; 1: 73–77.
35. Lauritzen CH, Reuter HD, Repges R et al. Phytomed 1997; 4 (3): 183–189.
36. Propping D, Katzorke T. Z Allge Med 1987; 63 (31): 932–933.
37. Propping D, Katzorke T, Belkien L. Therapiewoche 1988; 38 (41): 2992–3001.
38. Noack M. Dtsch Med Wschr 1943; 9: 204–206.
39. Mohr W. Hippokrates 1957; 28: 586–591.
40. Gregl A. Med Welt 1979; 30: 264–268.
41. Kress D, Thanner E. Med Klin 1981; 76 (20): 566–567.
42. Kubista E, Muller G, Spona J. Rev Fr Gynecol Obstet 1987; 82 (4): 221–227.
43. Kubista E, Muller G, Spona J. Zentralbl Gynakol 1983; 105 (18): 1153–1162.
44. Giss G, Rothenburg W. Z Haut Geschlechtskr 1968; 43 (15): 645–647.
45. Bone KB. Vitex agnus castus: scientific studies and clinical applications. MediHerb professional newsletter, no. 42, 43 October and November 1994. MediHerb Pty Ltd, PO Box 713, Warwick, Qld 4370, Australia.
46. German Federal Minister of Justice. German Commission E for human medicine monograph, Bundes-Anzeiger (German Federal Gazette), no. 226, dated 02.12.1992.
47. Cahill DJ, Fox R, Wardle PG et al. Hum Reprod 1994; 9 (8): 1469–1470.
48. Shuster J. Hosp Pharm 1996; 31: 1553–1554.

Chelidonium
(Chelidonium majus L.)

SYNONYMS

Greater celandine (Engl), Chelidonii herba (Lat), Schöllkraut, Goldwurz (Ger), chélidoine (Fr), cinerognolle (Ital), svaleurt (Dan), baiqucai (Chin).

WHAT IS IT?

Chelidonium has a long history of use as a therapeutic plant. It was mentioned by Pliny, to whom we owe the tradition of calling the plant Chelidonium, which is derived from the Greek *chelidon* (a swallow). This is because it comes into flower when the swallows arrive and fades when the swallows depart. Pliny reported that its acrid juice was used to remove films from the cornea of the eye and in the 14th century a drink made with Chelidonium was supposed to be good for the blood. Alchemists believed it was good for jaundice because of its intense yellow colour. Although the root contains the characteristic alkaloids and is used to a limited extent medicinally, the aerial parts are more widely used and are the focus of this monograph.

EFFECTS

Assists liver and gall function, protects against hepatic injury; spasmolytic to the gastrointestinal tract; stimulates bile flow; topical antimicrobial effect against fungal infections and warts; decreases benign tumours (topically and possibly internally).

TRADITIONAL VIEW

Chelidonium was used to treat conditions of the liver such as jaundice, hepatic congestion and biliary dyspepsia. It was also used for bilious and migraine headaches and haemorrhoids.[1] Chelidonium was often used in the form of poultices or ointments for the treatment of cutaneous conditions and traumatic inflammation.[1] The fresh milky juice was used topically in the treatment of warts, ringworms and corns.[1,2]

SUMMARY ACTIONS

Choleretic, cholagogue, spasmolytic, mild laxative, antiinflammatory, antiviral and vulnerary (topically).

CAN BE USED FOR

INDICATIONS SUPPORTED BY CLINICAL TRIALS

Disorders of the liver and gall bladder; cramp-like pain of the gastrointestinal tract and gall ducts, including irritable bowel syndrome; as an enema for colonic polyposis; as a topical application for warts (all uncontrolled studies).

TRADITIONAL THERAPEUTIC USES

Gallbladder disease, gallstones; liver disease, jaundice; to aid detoxification via the liver and bowel; hepatic and splenic congestion; migraine, bilious headaches and supraorbital neuralgia; skin conditions including warts, fungal growths and ringworm (especially the fresh juice); as a poultice or ointment for scrofula, cutaneous diseases and piles.[1]

In China Chelidonium is also used for gastritis, gastric ulcer, enteritis, jaundice, abdominal pain as well as bronchitis and whooping cough.[3,4]

MAY ALSO BE USED FOR

EXTRAPOLATIONS FROM PHARMACOLOGICAL STUDIES

The antiplatelet action suggests a beneficial action in migraine; inhibition of keratinocyte proliferation in psoriasis (topical use).

PREPARATIONS

Dried herb as a decoction, liquid extract and tablets for internal use. Decoction, extract or fresh juice for external use.

DOSAGE

1–2 ml of 1:2 liquid extract per day, 2–4 ml of 1:5 tincture per day. Short-term use of higher doses up to the equivalent of 3 g per day may be necessary (as per the Berlin clinical trial).

The dose used in China is 3–9 g per day or even higher. However, these doses are generally administered by decoction and this method may not efficiently extract the Chelidonium alkaloids.

DURATION OF USE

High doses should be restricted to short-term use and long-term use of normal doses is not preferred.

SUMMARY ASSESSMENT OF SAFETY

No significant adverse effects have been noted but excessive intake of the decoction may cause nausea and other gastrointestinal symptoms.

TECHNICAL DATA

BOTANY

Chelidonium majus, a member of the Papaveraceae (poppy) family, is a perennial herb approximately 50–90 cm in height with a branched woody taproot. The fragile stems are branched, with scattered hairs and contain an orange latex. The leaves are pinnatisect, with up to seven oblong or ovate leaflets with a bluish green underside. The flowers contain four bright yellow petals and are grouped in small clusters. The fruit capsule is one-celled, up to 5 cm long and contains black seeds with a white appendage.[5]

KEY CONSTITUENTS

- Isoquinoline alkaloids (0.35–1.3%),[6] including the major alkaloids chelidonine (>0.07%), chelerythrine, sanguinarine, berberine, coptisine and *dl*-stylopine; other alkaloids: sparteine (which is usually found in the Leguminosae (pea) family).[6,7]
- Flavonoids, phenolic acids.[7]

The isoquinoline group of alkaloids contains many structural types including benzophenanthridines (chelidonine, chelerythrine, sanguinarine) and protoberberines (berberine, coptisine).

PHARMACODYNAMICS

Hepatoprotective and choleretic activity

Oral administration of an alcohol extract of dried Chelidonium reduced carbon tetrachloride-induced liver injury in rats.[8] Significant reductions in elevated plasma levels of liver enzymes and bilirubin occurred in the treated group. A follow-up study was undertaken to clarify the underlying aspects of tissue recovery. There was an absence of fibrotic changes in the Chelidonium-treated rats which was thought to be related to a reduced degree of cellular necrosis and to a reduction in fibroblast-stimulating factors.[9]

Extracts of dried Chelidonium were tested for choleretic activity using the isolated perfused rat liver. The total extract of the herb significantly induced choleresis (bile flow). However, it did this without increasing the total output of bile acids (i.e. there was an increased flow of more dilute bile). In contrast, the phenolic and alkaloidal fractions of the total extract, tested individually and in combination, did not significantly increase bile flow, although small increases were observed. The authors concluded that the increased bile flow is due to an additive effect from all compounds in the total extract of Chelidonium and not one or two specific active constituents or fractions.[10]

Antimicrobial activity

An alkaloid fraction isolated from the dried roots of Chelidonium contained chelerythrine and sanguinarine. Chelerythrine and this fraction were found to be ineffective against Gram-negative bacteria in vitro. However, significant antimicrobial effect was observed against Gram-positive bacteria, such as *Staphylococcus aureus*, two strains of Streptococcus and also against the fungus *Candida albicans*.[11] Extracts of Chelidonium were found to have antiviral effects in vitro against adenovirus types 12 and 5 and herpes simplex virus type 1 (HSV-1). The most promising antiviral alkaloid was found in greater concentrations in the fresh and aerial plant samples. The alkaloid, which belongs to the benzophenanthridine group, was not identified.[12] Alkaloids from Chelidonium and sanguinarine solution inhibited the growth of *Trichomonas vaginalis* in vitro. Sanguinarine solution also caused the protozoa to undergo deformation followed by disintegration within 2 hours.[13]

An in vitro study demonstrated that alkaloids extracted from Chelidonium, chelerythrine and a mixture of chelerythrine and sanguinarine, had an antifungal effect on some Trichophyton strains, *Microsporum canis*, *Epidermophyton floccosum* and *Aspergillus fumigatus*.[14] Another in vitro study investigated the effect of Chelidonium extracts on several *Candida species* and other dermatophytes. Liquid extracts of Chelidonium prepared from dried plant material collected in late July and early September (Europe) were compared. Both extracts showed greater than average antifungal activity against organisms involved in skin infections. The July extract was effective against *Candida albicans* but the September extract showed no activity.[15]

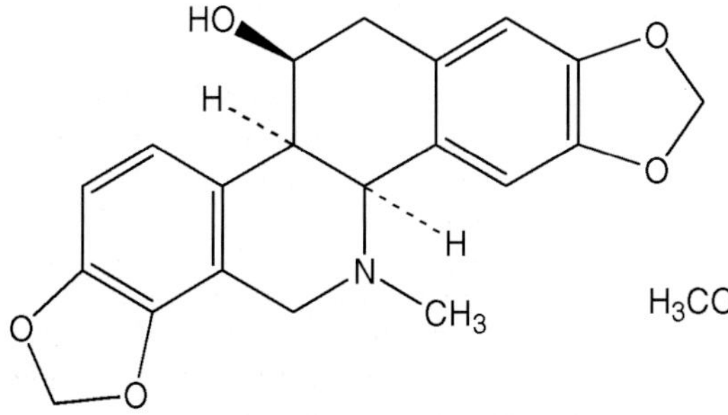

HO H H N CH3 O O O O

Chelidonine

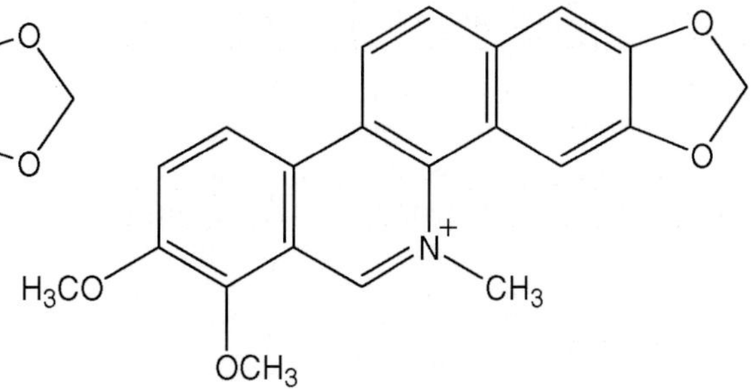

H_3CO OCH_3 N^+ CH_3 O O

Chelerythrine

O O O O N^+ CH_3

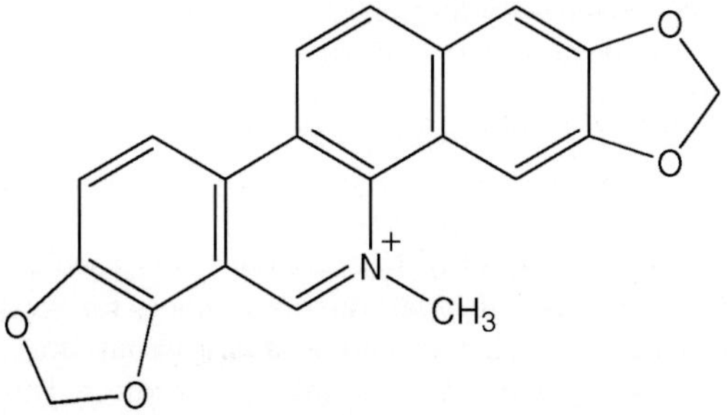

Sanguinarine

Antitumour activity

The activities of water and alcoholic extracts of Chelidonium, the partially purified methanol extract and chelidonine and protopine were screened on transplanted tumours in mice. The water-soluble, purified methanol extract of dried Chelidonium demonstrated high tumour inhibition with relatively mild cytotoxic side effects. Intraperitoneal administration of 700 mg/kg for 7 days resulted in 55% inhibition of sarcoma 180 and Ehrlich carcinoma. The aqueous extract showed insignificant activity and chelidonine and protopine (both of which are insoluble in water) showed insignificant tumour inhibition and were associated with considerable cytotoxic side effects. The crude methanol extract also showed more pronounced toxic side effects.[16]

An alcohol extract of rhizomes and roots of Chelidonium exhibited cytotoxicity against a carcinoma of the nasopharynx in vitro. One of the cytotoxic principles was found to be the alkaloid coptisine.[17] Chelidonium exerted an antimutagenic effect in vitro against several mutagens in the Ames test.[18] Chelidonine caused changes in the mitotic index of transplanted ascitic cells, showing marked antimitotic activity.[3] The numbers of stomach tumours in mice treated with Chelidonium extract after initial exposure to a carcinogen were significantly lower than untreated but exposed animals.[19]

Antiinflammatory activity

The alkaloids sanguinarine and chelerythrine are potent inhibitors of 5-lipoxygenase in polymorphonuclear leucocytes and 12-lipoxygenase in mouse epidermis. Extract of Chelidonium also inhibits 5-lipoxygenase. The inhibitory effects against lipoxygenase enzymes appear to be due to a specific enzyme interaction rather than non-specific redox mechanisms.[20] The Chelidonium alkaloids chelerythrine and sanguinarine have demonstrated antiinflammatory activity in the carrageenan rat paw oedema test.[11]

Other effects

Chelidonium extract and isolated components (coptisine and caffeolmalic acid) weakly antagonized experimentally induced contraction of isolated rat ileal smooth muscle.[21]

Radioreceptor assays have provided evidence that the alkaloids sanguinarine, chelerythrine, stylopine, allcryptopine and particularly protopine interact with the chloride channel of the $GABA_A$ receptor.[22] Biochemical studies in mice have shown that allocryptopine and protopine increase the brain concentration of the neurotransmitter GABA and the activity of its synthesizing enzyme GAD.[23]

Chelerythrine chloride exerts an in vitro antiplatelet effect that is believed to be due to the inhibition of thromboxane formation and phosphoinositide breakdown.[24]

The extract of Chelidonium inhibits human keratinocyte proliferation, with the alkaloid sanguinarine being the most potent constituent. The mechanism of action appears to be inhibition of the inflammatory mediators leukotriene B_4 and 12(S)-HETE, both of which have a known role in stimulating epidermal keratinocyte proliferation. Although tertiary benzophenanthridine alkaloids have demonstrated cytotoxic activity in low concentrations, sanguinarine and chelerythrine did not cause more damage to cell membranes than the antipsoriatic drug anthralin, as observed by the release of lactate dehydrogenase activity (an indicator of plasma membrane damage).[25]

The antinociceptive action of aminophenazone in mice was potentiated by the Chelidonium alkaloids allocryptopine, chelidonine and sanguinarine.[26]

PHARMACOKINETICS

No data available.

CLINICAL TRIALS

Spasmolytic and cholagogue effects

In an uncontrolled trial, a Chelidonium extract exerted good to very good results in two-thirds of patients treated for cholangitis, cholelithiasis and cholecystitis without stones. Forty patients received 3 ml per day (for 43–50 days) of a fresh plant tincture standardized to 20 mg alkaloids per 100 ml.[27] A clinical trial investigated the effect of a suspension of *Silybum marianum*, Chelidonium and Curcuma on 28 patients. In comparison to a control liquid, the herbal mixture demonstrated a greater increase in bile flow and pancreatic secretion.[28]

In 60 Berlin practices, 608 patients were treated and observed in an uncontrolled study over a 3-month period with a high-dose standardized preparation of dried Chelidonium, which acted as a plant-based spasmolytic. The main symptoms were cramp-like pains in the gastrointestinal tract (43%) or gall ducts (48.2%). Each Chelidonium tablet contained 2.85 mg of total alkaloids including 0.79 mg of chelidonine. The dose was initially five tablets/day and this was reduced to three tablets/day in patients who responded to treatment. The average duration of treatment necessary was 22 days and the longest treatment time was 2.5 months. A good or very good therapeutic effect on symptoms with a quick response was observed in 87.4% of cases. In most cases, symptom relief occurred within 30 minutes of taking the herbal medication (62.3%). In 46.1% of patients, the average duration of efficacy of each tablet dose was better than 3 hours. This study indicates the value of Chelidonium for the treatment of cramp-like abdominal pains associated with irritable bowel syndrome and other causes.[29]

Warts, polyps

In a small, uncontrolled trial an infusion of dried Chelidonium was administered as an enema for colonic polyposis. Administration of 10 or more enemas resulted in complete disappearance of colonic polyps in several cases.[30] In a later study, the fresh plant was made into a paste and administered 2 or 3 hours after an evacuant enema. In most cases, two or three courses (consisting of 10–20 enemas each) were deemed to be necessary. This regime was inefficient for treating malignant regenerated or degenerated polyps. Over a 2-year period treating 149 patients with various forms of polyposis, 87% showed improvement with 27% making a complete recovery.[31]

An alcohol extract of Chelidonium was used as a topical application to treat nursing mothers for warts, papillomas, condylomas and nodules in an uncontrolled trial. The extract was applied to the affected area approximately 200 times per day for 2–3 weeks or until improvement was observed. Complete resolution of the warts occurred after 15–20 days in 135 individuals.[32]

Bronchitis and whooping cough

Chelidonium was given as a syrup or extract (equivalent to 15 g of herb per day) to patients with chronic bronchitis in an uncontrolled study. The effective rate was around 80%. It was more effective in the simple type than the asthmatic type.[3] Chelidonium syrup or a decoction of the fresh herb was used to treat whooping cough in an uncontrolled study. Dosage: infants under 6 months 5–8 ml; 6–12 months 8–10 ml; 1–3 years 10–15 ml; 3–6 years 5–20 ml; and above 6 years 20–30 ml. Treatment was for a course of 8–10 days. Of 500 cases so treated, 355 were cured and 116 improved.[3]

Anticancer activity

Intravenous injection of Ukrain, a high-dose, water-soluble derivative of Chelidonium alkaloids, to nine men with proven lung cancer resulted in restoration of cellular immunity, characterized by an increase in the proportion of total T-cells and a significant decrease in the percentage of T-suppressor cells. Objective tumour regression was seen in four of the nine treated patients.[33] There are many other studies on Ukrain but results for this preparation are not relevant to the oral use of Chelidonium extracts. It is believed to modulate the immune system.

Chelidonium was one of three herbs used to examine the efficacy of traditional Chinese herbs on squamous cell carcinoma of the oesophagus. A 30 ml dose (equivalent to 30 g of crude herb) of a decoction of Chelidonium was given orally to 30 patients twice daily for 2 weeks prior to surgery. Histological examination of the excised tissue demonstrated a greater degree of stromal lymphoid cell infiltration and cancer tissue degeneration in the patients given Chelidonium than in patients given the herb plus endoxan or in the control patients. The antitumour action of Chelidonium was thought to be due to an activation of an immunological rejection mechanism.[34]

TOXICOLOGY

No harmful or toxic effects from therapeutic doses have been established. The LD_{50} of the decoction in mice by intraperitoneal injection is 9.5 g/kg[3] and the LD_{50} of the alkaloids in mice is 300 mg/kg (subcutaneous).[4]

In an antitumour experiment, intraperitoneal administration of a methanol extract of Chelidonium (350 mg/kg per day for 7 days) to mice resulted in a 20% mortality rate.[16]

CONTRAINDICATIONS

None known.

SPECIAL WARNINGS AND PRECAUTIONS

Given the nature of the alkaloid content of this herb, long-term use (except topical) is not preferred.

INTERACTIONS

None known.

USE IN PREGNANCY AND LACTATION

No adverse effects expected.

EFFECTS ON ABILITY TO DRIVE AND USE MACHINES

No adverse effects known.

SIDE EFFECTS

A case of haemolytic anaemia was reported after oral ingestion of Chelidonium extract. The patient was treated with corticosteroids, blood transfusions and haemodialysis and recovered after about 12 days.[35] In a case study published in 1997, hepatotoxicity after ingestion of a Chelidonium preparation (200 mg of dry extract with 4.0–4.4 mg total alkaloids per capsule) was described in a 28-year-old patient.[36]

When Chelidonium is used in traditional Chinese medicine, various degrees of dry mouth, dizziness, gastric discomfort, diarrhoea, abdominal distension, nausea and mild leucopaenia have been reported in a minority of patients. Symptoms generally disappeared within 3–5 days without discontinuation of the treatment.[3]

OVERDOSE

No effects known.

CURRENT REGULATORY STATUS IN SELECTED COUNTRIES

Chelidonium is covered by a positive Commission E monograph and can be used for cramp-like disorders of the biliary and gastrointestinal tracts.

Chelidonium is not on the UK General Sale List. Under the terms of the British Medicines Act 1968 and the Statutory Instrument SI 2130 (Retail Sale or Supply of Herbal Remedies) Order 1977 (Schedule Part III), the sale of Chelidonium is restricted to herbal practitioners. It may be prescribed at a maximum dosage of 2 g three times per day.

Chelidonium does not have GRAS status. However, it is freely available as a 'dietary supplement' in the USA under DSHEA legislation (1994 Dietary Supplement Health and Education Act).

Chelidonium is not included in Part 4 of Schedule 4 of the Therapeutic Goods Act Regulations of Australia.

References

1. Felter HW, Lloyd JU. King's American dispensatory, 18th edn, 3rd revision, vol 1, 1905. Reprinted by Eclectic Medical Publications, Portland, 1983, pp 491–493.
2. Grieve M. A modern herbal, vol 1. Dover Publications, New York, 1971, pp 178–179.
3. Chang HM, But PP. Pharmacology and applications of Chinese materia medica, vol 1. World Scientific, Singapore, 1987, pp 390–394.
4. Huang KC. The pharmacology of Chinese herbs. CRC Press, Boca Raton, 1993, pp 144–145.
5. Launert EL. The Hamlyn guide to edible and medicinal plants of Britain and Northern Europe. Hamlyn, London, 1981, p 26.
6. Wagner H, Bladt S. Plant drug analysis: a thin layer chromatography atlas, 2nd edn. Springer-Verlag, Berlin, 1996, p 10.
7. Colombo ML, Bosisio E. Pharmacol Res 1996; 33 (2): 127–134.

8. Mitra S, Gole M, Samajdar K et al. Int J Pharmacog 1992; 30 (2): 125–128
9. Mitra S, Sur RK, Roy A et al. Phytother Res 1996; 10 (4): 354–356.
10. Vahlensieck U, Hahn R, Winterhoff H et al. Planta Med 1995; 61 (3): 267–271.
11. Lenfeld J, Kroutil M, Marsalek E et al. Planta Med 1981; 43 (2): 161–165.
12. Kery A, Horvath J, Nasz I et al. Acta Pharm Hung 1987; 57 (1–2): 19–25.
13. Bodalski T, Pelozarska H, Ujec M. Arch Immunol Terapii Doswiadcjalny 1958; 6 (4): 705–711.
14. Hejtmánková N, Walterova D, Preininger V. Fitoterapia 1984; 55 (5): 291–294.
15. Vukusic I, Pepeljnjak S, Kustrak D et al. Planta Med 1991; 57 (suppl 2): A46.
16. Sokoloff B, Saelhof CC, Yoshichi MD et al. Growth 1964; 28: 225–231.
17. Kim HK, Farnsworth NR, Blomster RN et al. J Pharm Sci 1969; 58 (3): 372–374.
18. Shi GZ. Chung-Hua Yu Fang I Hsueh Tsa Chih 1992; 26 (3): 165–167.
19. Kim DJ, Ahn B, Han BS et al. Cancer Lett 1997; 112 (2): 203–208.
20. Vavreckova C, Gawlik I, Müller K. Planta Med 1996; 62 (5): 397–401.
21. Boegge SC, Kesper S, Verspohl EJ et al. Planta Med 1996; 62 (2): 173–174.
22. Häberlein H, Tschiersch KP, Boonen G et al. Planta Med 1996; 62 (3): 227–231.
23. Jagiello-Wójtowicz EWA, Feldo M, Kleinrok Z. Polish J Pharmacol Pharm 1992; 44 (suppl): 144.
24. Ko FN, Chen IS, Wu SJ et al. Biochim Biophys Acta 1990; 1052: 360–365.
25. Vavreckova C, Gawlik I, Müller K. Planta Med 1996; 62 (6): 491–494.
26. Jagiello-Wójtowicz EWA, Feldo M, Chodkowska A et al. Polish J Pharmacol Pharm 1992; 44 (suppl): 143.
27. Neumann-Mangoldt P. Med Welt 1977; 28 (4): 181–185.
28. Baumann JC, Heintze K, Muth HW. Arzneim-Forsch 1971; 21 (1): 98–101.
29. Kniebel R, Urlacher W. Zeit Allg Med 1993; 69 (25): 680–684.
30. Aminev AM, Stoliarenko AI. Vop Onkol 1960; 6 (8): 81–82.
31. Aminev AM. Am J Proctol 1963; 14 (1): 25–27.
32. Demchenko PF. Vrachebn Delo 1957; 12: 1335–1338.
33. Staniszewski A, Slesak B, Kolodzief J et al. Drugs Exp Clin Res 1992; 18 (suppl): 63–67.
34. Xian MS, Hayashi K, Lu JP et al. Acta Med Okayama 1989; 43 (6): 345–351.
35. Pinto Garcia V, Vicente PR, Barez A et al. Sangre (Barc) 1990; 35 (5): 401–403.
36. Greving I, Niedereichholz U, Meister V et al. Poster No. PO19, Europäischer Pharmakovigilanz Kongress, Berlin, February 1997.

Citrus seed extract (Citrus spp)

SYNONYMS

Grapefruit seed extract (Engl), citrus frφ (Dan).

WHAT IS IT?

Citrus seed extract is obtained from the seeds of *Citrus species*, especially the grapefruit (*Citrus paradisi*). Citrus seed extract is prepared in a hydrophilic organic solvent (particularly glycerol or propylene glycol) which is miscible with water and provides stability.[1]

EFFECTS

Antiseptic: effective against a wide variety of bacteria and fungi; preservative.

TRADITIONAL VIEW

Citrus seed extract has not been used traditionally.

SUMMARY ACTIONS

Antibacterial, antifungal, preservative.

CAN BE USED FOR

INDICATIONS SUPPORTED BY CLINICAL TRIALS

To reduce pathological organisms in the gastrointestinal tract, especially Candida, Geotrichum and haemolytic *Escherichia coli*.

MAY ALSO BE USED FOR

EXTRAPOLATIONS FROM PHARMACOLOGICAL STUDIES

As part of the treatment for conditions in which abnormal bowel flora may play a role, including irritable bowel syndrome and autoimmune diseases such as ulcerative colitis, Crohn's disease and ankylosing spondylitis; mouthwash to treat oral bacteria and to reduce plaque and tooth decay.

OTHER APPLICATIONS

Natural preservative for pharmaceuticals, food, cosmetics, paint; natural water decontaminant (but caution is advised as it will not inactivate viruses); antiseptic agent for eye lenses, cooking equipment;[2–4] antifungal and antialgae agent in the treatment of domestic water and pools, spas and ponds[1] and for use in paper making and industrial water treatment.[5]

PREPARATIONS

Citrus seed extract is available as a glycerol extract and can be added to creams, mouthwashes and drinking water as an antimicrobial agent. It can also be added to herbal formulas or water and taken orally for the treatment of gastrointestinal infections. The liquid form is absorbed on to microfine silica to form a powder which is used in tablets and capsules.

DOSAGE

3–10 ml per week of a 1:2 extract in a glycerol base.

DURATION OF USE

No problems known with long-term use.

SUMMARY ASSESSMENT OF SAFETY

No adverse effects are expected from ingestion of citrus seed extract within the recommended dosage.

TECHNICAL DATA

BOTANY

There are 12 different species of citrus belonging to the Rutaceae (Rue), family orange subfamily Aurantioideae. The flowers are usually in cymes with 4–5 sepals, 4–5 petals, eight or 10 stamens and a superior ovary. The fruit of Aurantioideae is a hesperidium: the fleshy parts are divided into segments.[6]

KEY CONSTITUENTS

Flavonoids (including naringin); plant acids including ascorbic acid, benzoic acid,[7] citric acid.

PHARMACODYNAMICS

Citrus seed extract is effective against a wide variety of potentially pathogenic bacteria and fungi.[8] The use of citrus seed extract as a natural preservative is based on its strong antimicrobial activity. The active constituents have not been satisfactorily identified and the antimicrobial activity of citrus seed extracts may reflect a synergy between several natural compounds.

Antibacterial activity

Ascorbic acid and citric acid are constituents of citrus seed extract. Their antimicrobial activity therefore provides information which supports such activity in citrus seed extract. Ascorbic acid at concentrations as low as 15.6 and 156 mg/ml demonstrated bactericidal effect on *Pseudomonas aeruginosa* cells in vitro and rendered them susceptible to the action of several antibiotics by altering the cell surface to render it increasingly permeable to antibiotic substances.[10]

The incubation of *E. coli* with 50 mg/ml ascorbic acid for 18 hours resulted in the loss of flagella, altered the cell wall, decreased adherence to epithelial cells and increased susceptibility to phagocytosis and bactericidal action.[11] In an in vitro investigation, the rate of inactivation of *Listeria monocytogenes* was found to be dependent on the pH and concentration of citric acid. At pH less than 4, citric acid enhanced the rate of inactivation of the bacteria.[12]

Citric acid with potassium sorbate demonstrated synergistic antibacterial or bacteriostatic activity towards a number of bacteria including lactic acid bacteria, *Lactobacillus plantarum, Yersinia enterocolitica* and Salmonella.[13] Citric acid and ascorbic acid applied individually or in mixtures demonstrated antimicrobial activity towards a variety of microorganisms in potato homogenate, including Enterobacteriaceae, *Pseudomonas spp, Lactobacillus spp*, moulds, yeasts, clostridium sulphite reducers, psychrotropic microorganisms and aerobic and anaerobic viable spores.[14]

An in vitro study of the effectiveness of citrus seed extract against 194 bacterial and 93 fungal strains observed that at 0.5% concentration, the growth of all microorganisms except for Klebsiella and Pseudomonas was inhibited. This included Gram-positive bacteria (*Streptococcus spp, Staph. aureus, Enterococcus spp.*), Gram-negative bacteria (*Enterobacter spp, E. coli*) and yeasts and moulds (*Candida, Geotrichum, Aspergillus* and *Penicillium spp*). Only increased concentrations of extract (1–2%) inhibited *Klebsiella* and *Proteus spp*. No effects were observed against *Pseudomonas spp*.[15]

A minimum inhibitory concentration (MIC) of citrus seed extract in vitro in the range of 10–500 ppm (parts per million) was observed for the following bacterial strains: *Escherichia coli, Salmonella typhi, Salmonella anatum, Salmonella cholerae-suis, Staphylococcus aureus, Staphylococcus pyogenes, Streptococcus faecalis, Corynebacterium spp, Proteus vulgaris, Bacillus subtilis, Mycobacterium spp, Pasteurella multocida*.[8] Concentrations in the range 1000–2000 ppm produced a bactericidal effect on *Pseudomonas aeruginosa* and *P. fluorescens*.[16] This contrasts with the above study which found that the extract did not inhibit the growth of Pseudomonas, which could be due to differing potencies of differing extracts.

Alcohol and chloroform extracts of *Citrus reticulata* (mandarin) seed were found to have mild activity at concentrations of 50, 500 and 1000 g/ml against several bacteria: *Staph. aureus, Salmonella typhi, P. aeruginosa* and *Strep. lactis*.[17]

Citrus seed extract was added to two batches of contaminated tank water to a concentration of 0.5%. The water was tested after 1 hour and in three microbiological tests the bacterial levels were substantially reduced. The three tests included:

1. total count (all strains of bacteria able to grow in the medium);
2. *Pseudomonas spp*;
3. coliform bacteria (species of Escherichia and Aerobacter, which demonstrate evidence of faecal contamination).[8]

A grapefruit seed extract demonstrated antimicrobial activity at concentrations down to 100 ppm against several species of bacteria and fungi which were applied to utensils (stainless steel cups, glass rods and cotton swabs). At 10 000 ppm all of the tested microorganisms were killed within 1–2 hours. A similar efficacy was observed for utensils contaminated with microorganisms in the presence of blood.[3]

A sample of a herbal cream was analysed for preservative efficacy following the guidelines of the *British Pharmacopoeia* (Appendix XVIC, 1993). The cream consisted of an oil in water emulsion, Calendula extract, tea tree oil (1%) and citrus seed extract (0.5%) and was tested against *Staph. aureus, P. aeruginosa, Candida albicans* and *Aspergillus niger*. The cream passed the BP requirements for the effective preservation of a topical product.[18]

Antifungal activity

Ascorbic acid enhanced the lethal effect of the antibiotic amphotericin B on two species of fungi: *Candida albicans* and *Cryptococcus neoformans*.[19] The MIC of citrus seed extract in vitro ranged from 500 to 2000 ppm for the following fungal strains: *Aspergillus flavus, Aspergillus niger, Aspergillus oryzae, Penicillium citrinum, Penicillium spp, Fusarium oxysporum, Fusarium spp, Pullularia pullulans, Trichophyton interdigital, Candida albicans*,[8] *Saccharomyces cerevisiae, Zygosaccharomyces rouxii and Hansenula anomala* var. *anomala*.[16]

The antimicrobial activity of a grapefruit seed extract against six fungi was stronger than that of five food preservatives.[9] Grapefruit seed extract exhibited significant activity against *Penicillium spp* in vitro.[20] Alcohol and chloroform extracts of *Citrus reticulata* (mandarin) seed were found to have mild activity against several fungi: *Fusarium solani, Alternaria solani,* and *Aspergillus niger*.[17]

PHARMACOKINETICS

Citrus seed extract is anticipated to exert a local effect on the skin or, after ingestion, in the gastrointestinal tract. No pharmacokinetic studies on citrus seed extract have been published.

CLINICAL TRIALS

Microbiological investigation of duodenal aspirates and faecal microflora of a group of patients with atopic eczema revealed significantly increased counts of haemolytic coliforms and staphylococci, *Candida spp, Geotrichum spp* and pathogenic *Clostridium spp*. These were generally associated with reduced counts of lactic acid-producing bacteria. Intermittent diarrhoea, constipation, flatulence, bloating and abdominal discomfort were also noted in a majority of cases. Initially patients received two drops of citrus seed extract twice a day which was, however, not sufficient to cause changes in faecal microflora. At the higher dose of 150 mg of powdered extract (equivalent to four drops of liquid) three times per day, significant activity was observed. The citrus seed extract was most effective in reducing the counts of Candida, Geotrichum and haemolytic *E. coli* in faecal microflora. The growth of *Staphylococcus aureus*, Lactobacillus and aerobic spore formers was slightly inhibited and there was no effect on Bifidobacteria and Klebsiella. No side effects were recorded and all patients noted a definite improvement in constipation, flatulence and abdominal discomfort after 4 weeks of treatment at the higher dose. The authors concluded that even higher doses may be more effective.[15]

TOXICOLOGY

An LD_{50} value of greater than 2.0 g/kg was obtained for acute and chronic oral administration in male and female mice. Normal growth of animals was observed during chronic administration and no abnormalities in main organs were observed from autopsy after the acute trials.[16]

CONTRAINDICATIONS

None known.

SPECIAL WARNINGS AND PRECAUTIONS

None required.

INTERACTIONS

None known.

USE IN PREGNANCY AND LACTATION

No data available.

EFFECTS ON ABILITY TO DRIVE AND USE MACHINES

No adverse effects expected.

SIDE EFFECTS

None known.

OVERDOSE

No toxic effects reported. Excessive doses of glycerol may cause dehydration.

CURRENT REGULATORY STATUS IN SELECTED COUNTRIES

Citrus seed extract is not covered by a Commission E monograph and is not on the UK General Sale List.

Citrus seed extract does not have GRAS Status. However, it is freely available as a 'dietary supplement' in the USA under DSHEA legislation (1994 Dietary Supplement Health and Education Act).

Citrus seed extract is not included in Part 4 of Schedule 4 of the Therapeutic Goods Act Regulations of Australia.

References

1. British Patent 9225625, December 1992 (lodged in Australia: Application No. 52242/93, December 1993), Legionella effective biocide for aqueous based systems, WR Grace and Co.
2. International Patent 9400160, January 1994, Ophthalmic compositions and methods for preserving and using same, Allergen Inc.

3. United States Patent 5425944, June 1995, Antimicrobial grapefruit extract, J Harich.
4. Japanese Patent 02247106, October 1990, Natural germicide preparation for spraying on cooking utensils – by extracting germicidal components from citrus fruit seed, Iwatani Industries KK.
5. United States Patent 4468372, Aug 1984, Hygienic air purifying device, J Harich.
6. Evans WC. Trease and Evans' pharmacognosy. 14th edn. WB Saunders, London, 1996, p 42.
7. Certificate of analysis no. 952863, conducted by Conmac Laboratory Services, 20th October 1995, held at MediHerb Pty Ltd.
8. Bone K. Modern Phytotherapist 1995; 2 (1): 10–12.
9. Nishina A, Kihara H, Uchibori T et al. J Antibact Antifung Agents 1991; 19: 401–404.
10. Rawal BD. Chemotherapy (Basel) 1978; 24: 166–171.
11. Papavassiliou J, Lianou P, Katsorchis T et al. Delt Hell Mikrobiol Hetair 1986; 31 (5–6): 165–169.
12. Buchanan RL, Golden MH. J Food Protection 1994; 57 (7): 567–570.
13. Restaino L, Komatsu KK, Syracuse J. J Food Sci 1981; 47: 134–139.
14. Giannuzzi L, Zaritzky NE. J Food Protection 1993; 56 (9): 801–807.
15. Ionescu G, Kiehl R, Wichmann-Kunz F et al. J Orthomolec Med 1990; 5 (3): 155–157.
16. Japanese Patent 06040834-A, May 1995, Antimicrobial spray – comprises extract of grapefruit seeds, Calfa Chem KK.
17. Ali R, Hasnain A, Khan KA. Karachi Univ J Sci 1990; 18 (1–2): 131–136.
18. Test results commissioned by MediHerb Pty Ltd, conducted by independent analysts: Biotest Laboratories Pty Ltd, Preservative Efficacy – QB Calendula Cream RD B.51202, February 1996.
19. Brajtburg J, Elberg S, Kobayashi GS et al. J Antimicrob Chemother 1989; 24: 333–337.
20. Park SW, Jeon JH, Kim HS et al. J Korean Soc Horticult Sci 1995; 36 (2): 179–184.

Devil's claw
(*Harpagophytum procumbens* DC ex Meissner)

SYNONYMS

Grapple plant (Engl), Harpagophyti radix (Lat), Teufelskralle, Trampelklette, Sudafrikanische (Ger), tubercule de griffe du diable (Fr), venustorn (Dan), duiwelsklou (Afrik).

WHAT IS IT?

Harpagophytum procumbens, a native to the savannah of the Kalahari of South Africa, Namibia and Botswana, has been wildcrafted and imported into Europe since 1953. The fruit is a capsule protected by numerous curved spines which, after splitting of the fruit, take on a claw-like appearance, hence the names harpagophytum (from the Greek *harpagos*, a grappling hook) and devil's claw. The secondary root tuber is the part used medicinally. It is also known as wood spider, grapple plant, burdock and Windhoeks' root. Recognition of the medicinal value of the plant by Europeans is traced to German soldiers, and later to GA Menhert during the Hottentot rebellion in 1904. Menhert observed the recovery of a Hottentot (who had been given up as lost by doctors) when treated by a local witch doctor. He then followed the witch doctor and discovered what plant was used and then spread the use of the root under the name 'harpagophytum tea'. Devil's claw root is mostly sold in small pieces or as a coarse powder.

EFFECTS

Reduces inflammation and pain; acts as a bitter tonic.

TRADITIONAL VIEW

Not much is known about the use of the herb in early traditional medicine. Devil's claw has been used in recent times in South Africa amongst Europeans, Euro-Africans, Bushmen, Hottentots and the Bantu for its purgative action, as a bitter tonic for digestive disturbances and for febrile illnesses, allergic reactions and migraine. Externally it has been used in the form of an ointment for ulcers, wounds, cutaneous lesions and boils. Amongst the Bushmen, Hottentots and Bantu, women ingest the pulverized root and apply ointment to the abdomen during labour to alleviate pain.[1,2]

SUMMARY ACTIONS

Antiinflammatory, analgesic, antirheumatic, bitter.

CAN BE USED FOR

INDICATIONS SUPPORTED BY CLINICAL TRIALS

Rheumatic and arthritic conditions.

TRADITIONAL THERAPEUTIC USES

Digestive disturbances, febrile illnesses, allergic reactions and to relieve pain. Externally for wounds, ulcers, boils and the relief of pain.

MAY ALSO BE USED FOR

EXTRAPOLATIONS FROM PHARMACOLOGICAL STUDIES

Cardiac arrhythmias.

PREPARATIONS

Decoction of dried root, tablets or liquid extract for internal use; dried root or liquid extract for external use as an ingredient in ointments and creams.

DOSAGE

In tablet form, devil's claw has been used in doses up to 6 g per day without side effects.[3] In view of this and other recent clinical trials, the doses given in the BHP 1983 are inadequate for antirheumatic and analgesic activity.[4] For these applications the equivalent of 3–6 g per day of the dried herb should be prescribed.[5,6] This corresponds to 6–12 ml per day of a 1:2 extract or 15–30 ml per day of 1:5 tincture. Tablets containing a 5:1 powdered extract should be taken at the rate of 600 mg to 1200 mg of extract per day. For gastrointestinal complaints, much lower doses can be used.

Recent studies have indicated that the analgesic and antiinflammatory effects of devil's claw are decreased by the acidity of the stomach. While these findings do not necessarily discount the use of galenical preparations (such as teas and liquid extracts), they do suggest that enteric-coated extracts of devil's claw may be more beneficial clinically. At the very least, devil's claw preparations should be administered between meals when gastric activity is at its lowest.

DURATION OF USE

No restriction on long-term use.

SUMMARY ASSESSMENT OF SAFETY

No adverse effects are expected if used as recommended but given its bitter properties, it should be prescribed with caution in patients with peptic ulcers.

TECHNICAL DATA

BOTANY

Harpagophytum procumbens, a member of the family Pedaliaceae, order Scrophulariales, is a weedy, perennial plant with creeping stems spreading from a tuberous rootstock. The greyish-green leaves are placed either alternately or directly opposite each other. Red-violet, yellow-violet or violet flowers are found at the juncture between leaf and stem. The characteristic fruits have long branching arms with anchor-like hooks (which assist their dissemination by animals). The primary root descends up to 2 m with secondary roots spreading out for up to 1.5 m on all sides, which allows it to conserve water.[2,7]

KEY CONSTITUENTS

- Iridoid glycosides (0.5–3.0%), primarily harpagoside (which has a bitter taste), isoharpagoside, harpagide (which has a slightly sweet taste), procumbide.[8]
- Sugars (over 50%), triterpenes, phytosterols, phenolic acids and glycosides, flavonoids.[6,9,10] The sugars lead to an unusually high water-soluble fraction of 50–70%.[6,10]

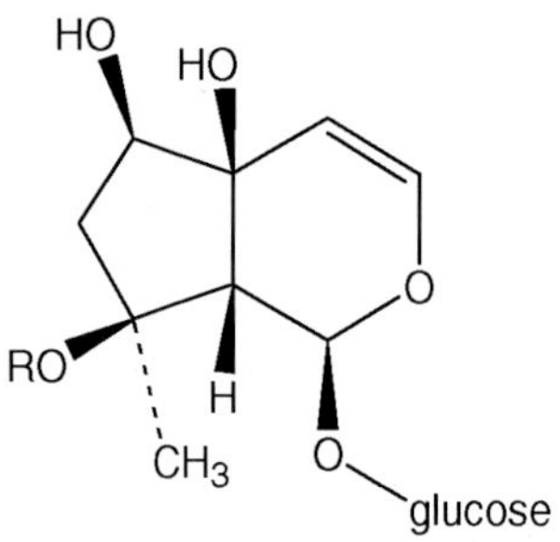

	R
Harpagoside	*trans*-cinnamoyl
Harpagide	H

The *European Pharmacopoeia* recommends that devil's claw contain not less than 1.2% of harpagoside, calculated with reference to the dried herb.[11] *H. zeyheri* is physically similar to *H. procumbens* and has become an inferior substitution species, despite its low level of active constituents.

PHARMACODYNAMICS

Antiinflammatory and antirheumatic activity

Many of the studies undertaken to examine the antiinflammatory effects of devil's claw have demonstrated limited activity in the standard inflammatory models. The antiinflammatory effect varies with the route of administration and nature of the condition (acute or subacute).

Antiinflammatory effects have been more convincingly demonstrated in the subacute animal models rather than the acute.[5] In subacute animal models utilizing formaldehyde-, Freund's adjuvant- and granuloma-induced experimental arthritis, aqueous and methanolic extracts of devil's claw appear to be efficient in reducing inflammation. In one study using the croton oil-induced granuloma pouch test in rats, the reduction in inflammation produced by a 12-day oral administration of aqueous and methanolic extracts of devil's claw at a dose of 200 mg/kg per day was similar to that of phenylbutazone.[12] In the formaldehyde-induced arthritis test, an effect comparable to 40 mg/kg per day of phenylbutazone was demonstrated with an aqueous extract of devil's claw at a dose of 20 mg/kg per day after 10 days of intraperitoneal administration.[13] Another study using different but similar models found that devil's claw did not produce significant effects on primary or secondary inflammatory reactions in rats.[14]

Little or no activity of oral doses of aqueous extracts of devil's claw or harpagoside has been demonstrated in acute models such as carrageenan-induced oedema.[5,12,13,15] However, intraperitoneal pretreatment with an aqueous extract of devil's claw produced significant, dose-dependent antiinflammatory effects in the carrageenan-induced acute oedema test.[16] The highest dose tested was more effective than pretreatment with 10 mg/kg of indomethacin.[16] Harpagoside did not appear to be involved in this antiinflammatory effect, since it did not protect against carrageenan inflammatory effects at levels corresponding to 400 mg of dried root. When devil's claw root was treated with acid at similar levels to the stomach, it lost all activity on intraperitoneal injection.[16] A later study confirmed the loss of antiinflammatory activity following passage through the stomach.[17]

Most non-steroidal antiinflammatory drugs (NSAIDs) act by inhibiting prostaglandin biosynthesis. Both in vitro and in vivo studies have demonstrated that devil's claw has minimal effects on production of these compounds. An in vitro study found that devil's claw at concentration up to 1×10^5 µg/ml does not alter the activity of cyclooxygenase, one of the major enzymes required for the production of prostaglandins.[15] A second study examined the effect of devil's claw at a dosage of 2 g per day of powder for 21 days on prostaglandin production during blood clotting in healthy humans. There were no significant differences in prostaglandin production between the before-and-after measurements.[18] These studies indicate that devil's claw is unlikely to act by a similar mechanism to NSAIDs and further suggest that devil's claw will not have the same irritant effects on the stomach which these drugs have.

Analgesic activity

Injection of devil's claw extract and harpagoside exhibited dose-dependent peripheral analgesic effects comparable to aspirin.[16] This activity was abolished by acid pretreatment of the herbal extract. In earlier work, intraperitoneal administration of harpagoside (20 mg/kg) produced an analgesic effect comparable to phenylbutazone (50 mg/kg).[13] However, harpagoside hydrolysed by emulsion (which would produce harpagogenin) was inactive.[13] No consistent analgesic effects were found in mice after oral doses of devil's claw extracts.[12]

PHARMACOKINETICS

The pharmacokinetics of devil's claw and the iridoid glycosides have not been established. Indeed, there is some controversy on the action of the stomach or acid hydrolysis on the extract and its active ingredients, as suggested by the above studies. Some authors suggest that the substances obtained after acid hydrolysis, especially harpagogenin, are the active compounds producing the antiinflammatory and antiarthritic properties, whereas other studies suggest that the extract, and harpagoside in particular, may be partially inactivated by the acid milieu of the stomach.[7,17] In other words, the basic issue is whether harpagoside and other iridoid glycosides (and perhaps other compounds in the root) are more active after oral doses than their respective hydrolysis products such as harpagogenin. Recent studies would suggest that this is the case.[16,17]

CLINICAL TRIALS

Antirheumatic activity

Several studies have demonstrated the efficacy of devil's claw in the relief of rheumatic and arthritic conditions. A few uncontrolled studies had positive outcomes for therapy with devil's claw.[7] For example, in a large open study on 630 patients with various rheumatic illnesses, 42–85% of patients showed significant improvement after 6 months of treatment with 3–9 g of the aqueous extract of devil's claw per day. The efficacy varied with the site of the arthritis; 80% of patients with arthritis in the large joints or spinal column experienced a significant improvement in symptoms whilst the remaining 20% experienced no therapeutic effect even at maximum dosage.[19] However, one open study on 13 patients with rheumatoid arthritis and psoriatic arthropathy found no benefit from devil's claw treatment.[20]

Two double-blind, placebo-controlled studies have also demonstrated the effectiveness of devil's claw as an antirheumatic agent. In the first study, 50 volunteers suffering from arthrosis were given a course of two capsules containing 400 mg of a hydroethanolic extract of devil's claw (with an iridoid glycoside content of 1.5%) three times daily for 3 weeks.[21] Individual patients were given from one to three courses of treatment. The extract produced a statistically significant decrease in the severity of pain when compared to placebo. Improvements were more frequent in moderate cases than in more severe cases of arthritis. The second study assessed the efficacy and tolerance of two capsules containing 335 mg of powdered devil's claw extract, with an iridoid glycoside content of 3.0%, three times daily for 2 months in 89 volunteers with articular pain. The results indicated a significant drop in the intensity of pain and increase in spinal mobility in the treated group. Side effects or changes in the biological parameters including blood tests were not observed during the period of the study.[22]

In a recent study, 118 patients with chronic back pain seeking treatment for acute attacks of pain were included in a 4-week randomized study on the safety and efficacy of an extract of devil's claw. Patients were given two tablets three times daily, with the treatment group consuming a dose equivalent to 6 g of crude devil's claw daily. The supplementary analgesic drug

Ultram (tramadol) was allowed during the study. The placebo and treatment groups were well matched in physical characteristics, severity, duration, nature and accompaniments of their pain as well as for laboratory indices of organ system function. The results revealed that nine of 51 patients who received devil's claw treatment were pain-free at the end of the treatment, compared to one of 54 patients who received placebo ($p=0.008$). The devil's claw group experienced a greater percentage reduction in the back pain index than the placebo group but this finding had only borderline statistical significance. The reduction in pain, however, was confined almost exclusively to the subgroup of patients whose pain did not radiate to one or both legs. The study demonstrated an absence of identifiable clinical, haematological or biochemical side effects in the treatment group.[3]

TOXICOLOGY

The aqueous and ethanolic extracts of devil's claw, and the isolated iridoids harpagoside and harpagide, have shown very low toxicity during acute and subacute toxicity studies. In one study, the acute oral LD_{50} of devil's claw was greater than 13.5 g/kg. In a study of subacute toxicity, no significant haematological or gross pathological findings were evident after 21 days of oral treatment with 7.5 g/kg of devil's claw. No hepatotoxic effects were observed with respect to liver weight, levels of microsomal protein and six liver enzymes after 7 days of oral treatment with 2.0 g/kg.[5]

CONTRAINDICATIONS

The Commission E advises the following contraindications: gastric and duodenal ulcers; with gallstones, to be used only after consultation with a doctor.

SPECIAL WARNINGS AND PRECAUTIONS

None required.

INTERACTIONS

None known.

USE IN PREGNANCY AND LACTATION

No adverse effects expected.

EFFECTS ON ABILITY TO DRIVE AND USE MACHINES

No negative influence is expected.

SIDE EFFECTS

Due to the lack of inhibitory effects of devil's claw on cyclooxygenase, the adverse effects often associated with NSAIDs are unlikely, even during long-term therapy.[5] Mild gastrointestinal disturbances may occur in sensitive individuals, especially at higher dosage levels.[19]

OVERDOSE

Not known.

CURRENT REGULATORY STATUS IN SELECTED COUNTRIES

Devil's claw is official in the *European Pharmacopoeia* (1997) and the *British Pharmacopoeia* (1998).

Devil's claw is covered by a positive Commission E monograph and has the following applications:

- lack of appetite, dyspeptic complaints;
- in supportive therapy for degenerative disorders of the musculoskeletal system.

It is on the UK General Sale List.

Devil's claw does not have GRAS status. However, it is freely available as a 'dietary supplement' in the USA under DSHEA legislation (1994 Dietary Supplement Health and Education Act).

Devil's claw is not included in Part 4 of Schedule 4 of the Therapeutic Goods Act Regulations of Australia.

References

1. Ragusa S, Circosta C, Galati EM et al. J Ethnopharmacol 1984; 11 (3): 245–257.
2. Van Wyk B-E, Van Oudtshoorn B, Gericke N. Medicinal plants of South Africa. Briza Publications, Arcadia, 1997; pp 144–145.
3. Chrubasik S, Zimpfer CH, Schutt U et al. Phytomed 1996; 3 (1): 1–10.
4. British Herbal Medicine Association's Scientific Committee. British herbal pharmacopoeia. BHMA, Cowling, 1983; p 111.
5. Scientific Committee of ESCOP. ESCOP monographs: harpagophyti radix. European Scientific Cooperative on Phytotherapy, Exeter, 1996.
6. British Herbal Medicine Association. British herbal compendium, vol 1. BHMA, Bournemouth, 1992; pp 78–80.
7. Wenzel P, Wegener T. Dtsch Apoth Ztg 1995; 135 (13): 1131–1144.
8. Wagner H, Bladt S. Plant drug analysis: a thin layer chromatography atlas, 2nd edn. Springer-Verlag, Berlin, 1996; p 76.
9. Burger JFW, Brandt EV, Ferreira D. Phytochem 1987; 26 (5): 1453–1457.
10. Ziller KH, Franz G. Planta Med 1979; 37: 340–348.
11. European pharmacopoeia, 3rd edn. European Department for the Quality of Medicines within the Council of Europe, Strasbourg, 1996; pp 716–717.

12. Erdos A, Fontaine R, Friehe H et al. Planta Med 1978; 34 (1): 97–108.
13. Eichler O, Koch C. Arzneim-Forsch 1970; 20: 107–109.
14. McLeod DW, Revell P, Robinson BV. Br J Pharmacol 1979; 66 (1): 140P–141P.
15. Whitehouse LW, Znamirowska M, Paul CJ. Can Med Assoc J 1983; 129 (3): 249–251.
16. Lanhers MC, Fleurentin J, Mortier F et al. Planta Med 1992; 58 (2): 117–123.
17. Soulimani R, Younos C, Mortier F et al. Can J Physiol Pharmacol 1994; 72 (12): 1532–1536.
18. Moussard C, Alber D, Toubin MM et al. Prostagland Leukotri Essential Fatty Acids 1992; 46 (4): 283–286.
19. Belaiche P. Phytotherapy 1982; 1: 22–28.
20. Grahame R, Robinson BV. Ann Rheum Dis 1981; 40 (6): 632.
21. Guyader M. Dissertation. Université Pierre et Marie Curie, Paris, 1984. Cited in Scientific Committee of ESCOP. ESCOP monographs: harpagophyti radix. European Scientific Cooperative on Phytotherapy, Exeter, 1996.
22. Lecomte A, Costa JP. Cited in: Scientific Committee of ESCOP. ESCOP monographs: harpagophyti radix. European Scientific Cooperative on Phytotherapy, Exeter, 1996.

Dong quai
(*Angelica sinensis* (Oliv.) Diels)

SYNONYMS

A. polymorpha var. *sinensis* (botanical synonym), dong quai (Engl), Radix Angelica sinensis (Lat), dang gui (Chin), toki (Jap), tanggwi (Kor), kinesisk kvan (Dan).

WHAT IS IT?

The root of dong quai is an extremely popular herb and has been used by the Chinese for thousands of years as a tonic and a spice. Its reputation in the West as a Chinese herb is second only to ginseng. Women have especially used dong quai to protect their health. *Angelica acutiloba*, which is indigenous to Japan, became a substitute in that country for genuine dong quai. The popular use of dong quai in the West as a herb to treat menopausal symptoms such as hot flushes appears to be ill advised. Nonetheless, it may have value in menopause as a tonic.

EFFECTS

Regulates menstruation, alleviates dysmenorrhoea; treats blood deficiency; relieves constipation by lubricating the bowel; treats and prevents cardiovascular disorders; protects the liver.

TRADITIONAL VIEW

Dong quai is sweet, acrid, bitter and warm. It strengthens the heart, lung and liver meridians and lubricates the bowel. Dong quai tonifies the *Blood*, regulates menstruation, invigorates and harmonizes the *Blood* and is used to treat congealed blood conditions, blood deficiency and *Deficient Blood* patterns. It is an important herb in the treatment of gynaecological problems.[1]

SUMMARY ACTIONS

Antiinflammatory, antianaemic, antiplatelet, female tonic, mild laxative, antiarrhythmic.

CAN BE USED FOR

INDICATIONS SUPPORTED BY CLINICAL TRIALS

To relieve dysmenorrhoea and treat infertility (uncontrolled trials); chronic hepatitis and cirrhosis (uncontrolled trial). No benefits were found in the treatment of menopausal symptoms.

TRADITIONAL THERAPEUTIC USES

Irregular menstruation, amenorrhoea, dysmenorrhoea; constipation; congealed blood (abdominal pain, traumatic injuries, swellings, contusions, bruising); blood deficiency (tinnitus, blurred vision, palpitations); as a tonic, especially for women.

MAY ALSO BE USED FOR

EXTRAPOLATIONS FROM PHARMACOLOGICAL STUDIES

For the prevention of atherosclerosis; as an antiplatelet agent.

PREPARATIONS

Dried root as a decoction; liquid extract or tablets for internal use.

DOSAGE

- 3–15 g per day of the dried root by decoction.
- 4–8 ml per day of a 1:2 liquid extract.

DURATION OF USE

May be taken long term.

SUMMARY ASSESSMENT OF SAFETY

No adverse effects from ingestion of dong quai are expected, providing the contraindications are observed.

TECHNICAL DATA

BOTANY

Dong quai, a member of the Umbelliferae (carrot) family, is a fragrant, perennial herb native to China, Korea and Japan which grows to a height of 0.5–1 m. The inferior leaves are tripinnate, superior leaves are pinnate, on long, sheathed petioles. The umbels number 10–14, with irregular rays, each umbel containing 12–36 white flowers. The root's exterior is grey-dark brown in colour and its surface is covered in wrinkles. The root consists of a head, body and tail.[2] Different properties are ascribed to these parts – the head is most tonic and the tail moves the blood most strongly. Such preparations are very expensive and the entire root is usually prescribed.

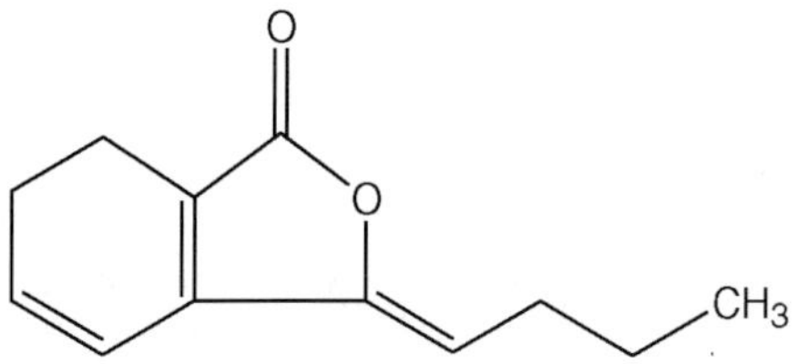

Ligustilide

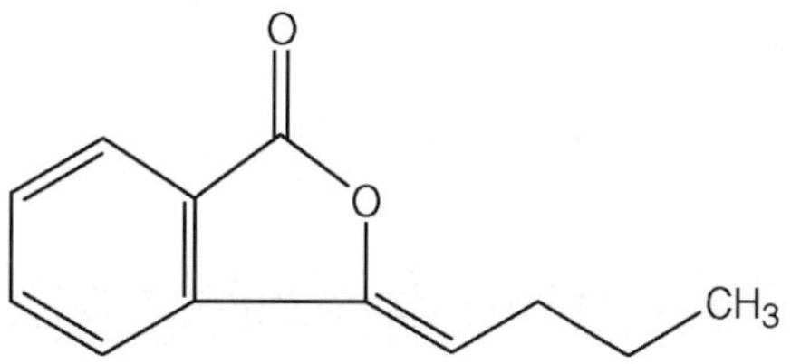

n-Butylidenephthalide

KEY CONSTITUENTS

- Essential oil (0.4–0.7%), mainly consisting of ligustilide and n-butylidene phthalide.[2]
- Phytosterols, ferulic acid, coumarins (angelol, angelicone).[2]

n-Butylidene phthalide is a component of the essential oil with a characteristic fragrance.[3]

PHARMACODYNAMICS

Effects on sexual function

The essential oil relaxed the isolated uterus but other components increased uterine contraction.[4] Some experiments on the whole root have shown a stimulant effect in vivo, while others have shown that it can relax or coordinate (make more rhythmic) uterine contractions, depending on uterine tone. The root is devoid of oestrogenic action[4,5] and its different parts have a similar spasmolytic effect on isolated rabbit uterus.

One study showed increased sexual activity in female animals and a reduction in signs of vitamin E deficiency in male mice.[6] Butylidene phthalide demonstrated antispasmodic activity by inhibiting rat uterine contractions. Its effect is non-specific, similar to papaverine but with a different mechanism of action.[7] Intraperitoneal injection of dong quai protected mice ovaries from the effects of gamma radiation.[8]

Cardiovascular activity

Dong quai has a quinidine-like action on the heart. It can prolong the refractory period and correct experimental atrial fibrillation induced by atropine, pituitrin, strophanthin, acetylcholine or electrical stimulation.[4] Ferulic acid is antiplatelet, as is the aqueous extract.[4] Both the aqueous extract of dong quai and ferulic acid inhibited platelet aggregation and serotonin release.[9]

Dong quai can prevent experimental coronary atherosclerosis in rabbits and rats.[4] It lowered blood pressure, dilated the coronary vessels, increased coronary flow, reduced blood cholesterol and reduced respiratory rate. Mixed in feed at 5%, it has reduced atherosclerosis formation in animals.[10] Dong quai exerted a stimulating effect on haematopoiesis in bone marrow.[10]

Immune function

Some studies have shown a pronounced inhibition of antibody production, while others have shown a sometimes weak stimulation of phagocytosis and lymphocyte proliferation.[4] Dong quai can somewhat counter the immunosuppressive effects of hydrocortisone in vivo but is not as effective as Astragalus.[11] Combined with Astragalus, it improved thrombocytopaenic purpura in rabbits.

Other activity

Ligustilide demonstrated an antiproliferative effect on smooth muscle cells in vitro[12] and a muscle relaxation effect in rats, which was believed to be of central origin.[13] Ligustilide (0.14 ml/kg IP) given to guinea pigs inhibited the asthmatic reaction induced by acetylcholine and histamine.[9]

In tests on vascular permeability in mice, oral dong quai showed an antiinflammatory effect[4] (this may partly explain its effects in dysmenorrhoea).

Feeding rats 5% dong quai for 4 weeks increased metabolism and oxygen utilization in the liver. Glutamic acid and cysteine oxidation were also enhanced.[4]

Sodium ferulate pretreatment by intragastric administration demonstrated hepatoprotective activity in mice.[14] A water extraction of dong quai protected the liver from carbon tetrachloride toxic hepatitis and prevented loss of liver glycogen.[6]

Dong quai protected against experimentally induced injury in rat lungs by decreasing alveolitis and the release of inflammatory factors.[15]

PHARMACOKINETICS

No data available.

CLINICAL TRIALS

Female reproductive tract conditions

Ligustilide at 450 mg per day was used to treat 112 cases of dysmenorrhoea in an uncontrolled trial. The effective rate was 77% compared to 38% for aqueous extract of dong quai.[16] In combination with Corydalis, *Paeonia lactiflora* and Ligusticum, dong quai showed a 93% improvement rate for the treatment of dysmenorrhoea in an uncontrolled trial. The decoction was given daily, starting 5 days before and until cessation of menstruation. (After treatment for about four cycles, 72% were 'cured'.)[17]

Infertility due to tubal occlusion was treated for up to 9 months with uterine irrigation of dong quai extract in an uncontrolled trial; 79% of patients regained tubal patency and 53% became pregnant.[18]

In a randomized, double-blind, placebo-controlled clinical trial, 71 postmenopausal women (FSH levels of > 30 mIU/ml with hot flushes) received either dong quai (4.5 g dried root per day) or placebo for 24 weeks. Dong quai did not produce oestrogen-like responses in endometrial thickness or in vaginal maturation. The incidence of symptoms dropped in both groups but there was no significant difference between dong quai and placebo.[19]

Other conditions

Dong quai has been successfully used to treat Buerger's disease and constrictive aortitis[1] and is often combined with dan shen in the treatment of angina, peripheral vascular disorders and stroke.

Dong quai improved abnormal protein metabolism, improved abnormal thymol turbidity test and increased plasma protein level in 60% of patients with chronic hepatitis or hepatic cirrhosis after 1–3 weeks of treatment in an uncontrolled trial.[20]

TOXICOLOGY

At concentrations higher than 2500 µg/ml, aqueous extracts of dong quai root exerted a general cytotoxicity to melanocytes in culture. Prior treatment of the dong quai extract to reduce its coumarin content resulted in reduced cytotoxicity.[21]

The oral LD_{50} of a concentrated dong quai extract in rats was measured at 100 g/kg body weight. According to information supplied by the author, this concentrated extract was 8 to 16:1.[2]

CONTRAINDICATIONS

Contraindications according to traditional Chinese medicine are as follows: diarrhoea caused by weak digestion, haemorrhagic disease, bleeding tendency or very heavy periods, first trimester of pregnancy, tendency to spontaneous abortion and acute viral infections such as colds and influenza.[2]

SPECIAL WARNINGS AND PRECAUTIONS

None required.

INTERACTIONS

The effects of dong quai on the pharmacodynamics and pharmacokinetics of warfarin were studied in rabbits. Single subcutaneous doses of warfarin (2 mg/kg) were administered with or without 3 days' treatment with oral dong quai extract (2 g/kg, twice daily). The dong quai treatment did not affect prothrombin time on its own but significantly lowered the value 3 days after coadministration with warfarin. No significant variation in the pharmacokinetic parameters of warfarin were observed after dong quai treatment for both single-dose administration or steady-state concentrations of warfarin.[22] Caution is therefore advised for patients receiving chronic treatment with warfarin.

USE IN PREGNANCY AND LACTATION

Contraindicated in the first trimester of pregnancy, especially in higher doses.

EFFECTS ON ABILITY TO DRIVE AND USE MACHINES

No adverse effects expected.

SIDE EFFECTS

None known.

OVERDOSE

No effects known.

CURRENT REGULATORY STATUS IN SELECTED COUNTRIES

Dong quai is official in the *Pharmacopoeia of the People's Republic of China* (English edition, 1997). It is not covered by a Commission E monograph and is not on the UK General Sale List.

Dong quai does not have GRAS status. However, it is freely available as a 'dietary supplement' in the USA under DSHEA legislation (1994 Dietary Supplement Health and Education Act). Dong quai has been used as an ingredient in products offered over the counter for use as an aphrodisiac. The FDA, however, advises that: 'based on evidence currently available, any OTC drug product containing ingredients for use as an aphrodisiac cannot be generally recognized as safe and effective'.

Dong quai is not included in Part 4 of Schedule 4 of the Therapeutic Goods Act Regulations of Australia.

References

1. Bensky D, Gamble A. Chinese herbal medicine materia medica. Eastland Press, Seattle, 1986, pp 474–476.
2. Zhu DP. Am J Chin Med 1987; 15 (3–4): 117–125.
3. Lin M, Zhu GD, Sun QM et al. Yao Hsueh Hsueh Pao 1979; 14 (9): 529–534.
4. Chang HM, But PP. Pharmacology and applications of Chinese materia medica, vol 1. World Scientific, Singapore, 1987, pp 489–505.
5. Lan TH, Chang YT, Sun CL et al. Acta Physiol Sin 1957; 21 (3): 205.
6. Zhu DPQ. Am J Chin Med 1987; 15 (3–4): 117–125.
7. Ko WC. Jpn J Pharmacol 1980; 30 (1): 85–91.
8. Zhang D, Shan S, Zhang L. Acta Acad Med Hubei 1996; 17 (3): 216–218.
9. Yin ZZ, Zhang LY, Xu LN. Yao Hsueh Hsueh Pao 1980; 15 (6): 321–326.
10. Huang KC. The pharmacology of Chinese herbs. CRC Press, Boca Raton, 1993, pp 247–248.
11. Luo B, Li SC, Cui WY et al. J Beijing Med Univ 1987; 19 (6): 419–422.
12. Kobayashi S, Mimura Y, Notoya K et al. Jpn J Pharmacol 1992; 60 (4): 397–401.
13. Ozaki Y, Sekita S, Harada M. Yakugaku Zasshi 1989; 109 (6): 402–406.
14. Wang H, Peng RX. Chung Kuo Yao Li Hsueh Pao 1994; 15 (1): 81–83.
15. Xu Q, Liu W, Lin Y. Acta Acad Med Hubei 1997; 18 (1): 20–23.
16. Gao YM, Zhang H, Duan ZX. J Lanzhou Med Coll 1988; 1: 36–38.
17. Liu MA, Qi CH, Yang JC. Beijing J Trad Chin Med 1988; 5: 30–31.
18. Fu YF, Xia Y, Shi YP et al. Jiangsu J Trad Chin Med 1988; 9 (1): 15–16.
19. Hirata JD, Swiersz LM, Zell B et al. Fertil Steril 1997; 68 (6): 981–986.
20. Zhou QJ. Chinese medicinal herbs in the treatment of viral hepatitis. In: Chang HM (ed) Advances in Chinese medicinal materials research. World Scientific, Singapore, 1985, p 217.
21. Raman A, Lin ZX, Sviderskaya E et al. J Ethnopharmacol 1996; 54 (2–3): 165–170.
22. Lo AC, Chan K, Yeung JH et al. Eur J Drug Metab Pharmacokinet 1995; 20 (1): 55–60.

Echinacea
(Echinacea spp)

SYNONYMS

Echinacea herba/radix (Lat), Sonnenhut, Igelkopf (Ger), racine d'échinaeace (Fr), Echinacea (Ital), solhat (Dan).

WHAT IS IT?

Three species of Echinacea, commonly known as purple coneflower, are used medicinally: *Echinacea angustifolia* DC. (narrow-leaved purple coneflower), *E. purpurea* (L.) Moench. (common or broad-leaved purple coneflower) and *E. pallida* (Nutt.) Nutt. (pale purple coneflower). *Echinacea purpurea* has become the most cultivated and widely used of the various species because the whole plant (root, leaf, flower, seed) can be used and also because it is more easily cultivated. The root and rhizome of *E. angustifolia* and *E. pallida* are used medicinally, although *E. pallida* is sometimes considered to be less active. In the past *E. pallida* preparations have been incorrectly labelled as *E. angustifolia*, particularly in Europe. *Parthenium integrifolium*, the Missouri snakeroot, is a documented adulterant of commercial Echinacea.

EFFECTS

Immunostimulant, mainly acting on non-specific immunity, hence may modulate immune function in allergy and autoimmunity; enhances resistance to infections, particularly of the upper respiratory tract; assists in recovery from chemotherapy; antiinflammatory, particularly by topical application.

TRADITIONAL VIEW

Information about the use of Echinacea first came from Native American tribes. Their use of Echinacea was adopted by the Eclectics, a group of practitioners who were prominent around the late 19th and early 20th centuries in the United States. By 1921 Echinacea (specifically the root of *E. angustifolia*) was by far the most popular treatment prescribed by Eclectic physicians. The Eclectics used Echinacea for about 50 years. However, given that their use was based on tribal knowledge and that they accumulated extensive clinical experience, their traditional use data is of a high quality. The best sources of these data are *King's American Dispensatory*[1] and Ellingwood.[2] The extensive range of conditions in these texts for which Echinacea was prescribed included snakebite, syphilis, typhus, septic wounds, diphtheria, scarlet fever, dysentery and even cancer. It is clear from these writers that the limitations on Echinacea use suggested by some modern authors are not supported. The conditions treated were mainly infections and envenomations of various kinds (which probably attest to Echinacea's influence on the immune system). However, the inclusion of tuberculosis and disorders related to autoimmunity such as diabetes, exophthalmic goitre, psoriasis and renal haemorrhage contrasts with contraindications proposed by some modern writers.

The Eclectics were also not averse to using Echinacea long term. For example, according to Ellingwood, Echinacea was recommended for the following chronic conditions: cancer, chronic mastitis, chronic ulceration, tubercular abscesses, chronic glandular indurations and syphilis. With regard to syphilis, Ellingwood writes. 'The longest time of all cases yet reported, needed to perfect the cure, was nine months.' He cites a dramatic case history of vaccination reaction where Echinacea was taken every 2 hours for up to 6 weeks.

SUMMARY ACTIONS

Immunomodulator, antiinflammatory, vulnerary, lymphatic. Any significant clinical antibacterial and antiviral activity probably follows indirectly from immune enhancement.

CAN BE USED FOR

INDICATIONS SUPPORTED BY CLINICAL TRIALS

Treatment of upper respiratory tract infections; beneficial for the prophylaxis of upper respiratory tract infections and infections in general, especially in patients with weakened immunity including those undergoing chemotherapy; recurrent candidiasis; sinusitis; topically for skin complaints.

TRADITIONAL THERAPEUTIC USES

Bacterial, viral and protozoal infections including infections of the digestive, respiratory and urinary tracts; mild septicaemia; states of weakened, suppressed or imbalanced immunity, including allergies and autoimmune disease; inflammatory and purulent conditions, including acne, abscess, furunculosis; envenomation. Topically for treating poorly healing wounds, inflamed skin conditions and bacterial infections.

MAY ALSO BE USED FOR

EXTRAPOLATIONS FROM PHARMACOLOGICAL STUDIES

To increase phagocytosis; antiviral activity, probably indirect. Topically: to improve wound healing, increase resistance to infection, increase connective tissue regeneration and for the prevention and/or treatment of photodamage by UV radiation.

OTHER APPLICATIONS

In modern usage, Echinacea is sometimes prescribed as adjunct therapy during cancer treatment.[3] Echinacea is also used in lip balms and toothpaste[4] and skin and hair care products, including facial toners, creams and lotions, especially for damaged skin.[5]

PREPARATIONS

Echinacea purpurea preparations include liquid extracts of fresh or dried whole plant or aerial parts; fresh or dried preparations of root and rhizome; stabilized juice of the flowering tops, mixtures of any of the above preparations and tablets and capsules based on any of the above plant parts or corresponding extracts.

For *E. angustifolia* or *E. pallida*, similar preparations are used, although the roots of these species are generally preferred.

DOSAGE

It should be noted that doses of Echinacea employed in some countries (especially Europe) are sometimes relatively low, which reflects more on a homoeopathic style of use for this herb.

Preventative doses or doses for chronic conditions:

- 1–3 g per day of *E. angustifolia* dried root, similar doses for *E. pallida* root.
- 1.5–4.5 g per day of *E. purpurea* dried root.
- 2.5–6 g per day of *E. purpurea* dried aerial parts.
- 3–5.5 ml per day of 1:1 fresh plant tincture of *E. purpurea* (which includes root and flowering tops) or of dried whole plant (1:1), which includes root and flowering tops.

According to the Commission E, the dose for *E. purpurea* fresh herb pressed juice is 8–9 ml per day.

- 2–6 ml per day of 1:2 liquid extract of *E. angustifolia* root.
- 3–9 ml per day of 1:2 liquid extract of *E. purpurea* dried root.
- 5–15 ml per day of 1:5 tincture of *E. angustifolia* root.
- 7.5–22.5 ml per day of 1:5 tincture of *E. purpurea* dried root.

For acute conditions, these dosages may be substantially increased in the short term; for example, *E. angustifolia* root can be taken up to 10–15 g per day (or its equivalent in liquid or tablet preparations).

DURATION OF USE

There is no evidence to suggest that long-term usage will have an adverse effect on immune function. Echinacea is probably a benign agent acting mainly on phagocytic activity (non-specific immunity).

SUMMARY ASSESSMENT OF SAFETY

Echinacea preparations may be safely prescribed for oral and topical use if the recommended dosage is not exceeded. Despite many reputed contraindications in the literature, the herb is unlikely to cause adverse effects in a wide range of applications including asthma, allergies and autoimmunity. However, care should be exercised when prescribing any preparation which includes the flowers to patients with known allergy to members of the Compositae (daisy) family.

TECHNICAL DATA

BOTANY

Echinacea is a member of the Compositae (daisy) family and grows to a maximum height of 50–180 cm, depending on the species. The distinctive flower head consists of white, rose or purple drooping ray florets and a conical disc made up of numerous tubular florets. *E. angustifolia* is most easily identified by its low habit and the coarse hair and relatively straight ray florets; *E. purpurea* by the large, egg-shaped, serrated leaves and the bright purple ray florets; *E. pallida* by the white pollen and the longer length of the paler ray florets.[6,7]

KEY CONSTITUENTS

Roots

- Alkylamides, mostly isobutylamides (which cause a characteristic tingling in the mouth).[8–11] Largely absent from *E. pallida*.[9]

- Caffeic acid esters: echinacoside (not present in *E. purpurea*), chicoric acid (significant quantities in *E. purpurea* only),[12] cynarin (in *E. angustifolia* only).[13]
- Essential oil;[14] polyacetylenes (including a distinctive series in *E. pallida*);[8,15] polysaccharides,[16] non-toxic pyrrolizidine alkaloids.[17]

Aerial parts

- Alkylamides as above.[18]
- Caffeic acid esters: including echinacoside (not present in *E. purpurea*), chicoric acid (abundant in *E. purpurea*), verbascoside (*E. angustifolia, E. pallida*), caftaric acid (*E. purpurea, E. pallida*), chlorogenic and isochlorogenic acids (*E. angustifolia, E. pallida*).[18]
- Flavonoids,[18] essential oil;[14] polysaccharides (notably in *E. purpurea*).[19]

PHARMACODYNAMICS

Immune-modulating activity

Echinacea extracts increased the phagocytotic index of human granulocytes in vitro.[20]

The juice of *E. purpurea* tops increased the in vitro phagocytosis of *Candida albicans* by granulocytes and monocytes. There was no effect on intracellular killing of bacteria or yeasts and the preparation did not induce the transformation of lymphocytes.[21] Expressed juice of *E. purpurea* (aerial parts) increased the number of granular leucocytes, segmented neutrophilic granulocytes and macrophages in vitro.[22] A similar preparation demonstrated a stimulating effect on the production of lymphokines by lymphocytes in vitro.[23] Peripheral blood adherent macrophages produced elevated cytokine levels (TNF-alpha, IL-1, IL-6, IL-10) when activated with fresh and dried plant juice of *E. purpurea* in vitro.[24]

E. purpurea extract enhanced cellular immune function of peripheral blood mononuclear cells from both normal individuals and patients with depressed cellular immunity (chronic fatigue syndrome, AIDS) in vitro. Natural killer cell activity and antibody-dependent cellular cytotoxicity were enhanced at concentrations as low as 1 μg/ml.[25]

Ethanolic extracts of all three species demonstrated an increase in phagocytic activity in vitro and after oral administration in the carbon clearance test. Of the three tested extracts, *E. purpurea* was the most active both in vitro and in vivo.[26,27] Lipophilic (fat-soluble) and hydrophilic (water-soluble) fractions of these ethanol extracts also demonstrated activity, although it was weaker than the complete ethanolic extracts. The lipophilic fractions from *E. angustifolia* and *E. pallida* were considerably more active than their hydrophilic fractions, both in vitro and in vivo. In contrast, the hydrophilic fraction of the ethanol extract of *E. purpurea* significantly stimulated phagocytosis in vitro and showed activity in vivo after oral doses, although not as great as the whole extract. Components of the lipophilic fraction included polyacetylenes, essential oil and alkylamides; the hydrophilic fraction contained caffeic acid derivatives. Polysaccharides were not present.[28] Immunostimulatory principles of Echinacea are therefore present in both the lipophilic and the hydrophilic fractions of a pure ethanolic extract.

Chicoric acid or an enriched alkylamide fraction from *E. angustifolia* and *E. purpurea* roots increased phagocytic activity in vivo after oral doses. Extracts of the aerial parts of the three species demonstrated lower activity than that of the roots.[27] In contrast, echinacoside from *E. angustifolia* and *E. pallida* (which is often used as a quality marker for these species) has not demonstrated immune-enhancing activity.[26] Intraperitoneal, intravenous or oral administration of a water-based extract of *E. angustifolia* in mice revealed no effect on unspecified cellular immunity.[29]

In both in vitro and in vivo tests, a plant combination (containing *E. angustifolia, Eupatorium perfoliatum, Baptisia tinctoria* and *Arnica montana*) demonstrated step-by-step stimulation of phagocytosis more

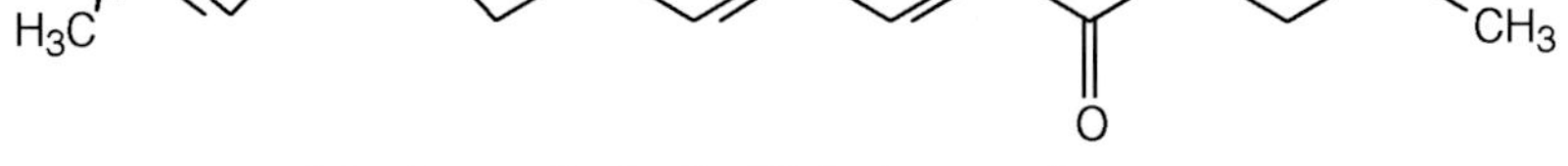

H_3C … N–H … CH_3 … CH_3 … O

Dodeca-2, 4, 8, 10-tetraenoic acid isobutylamides (mixture)

efficiently than did the single extract of *E. angustifolia*.[30] Phagocytosis of erythrocytes by Kupffer cells in vitro was significantly improved by a herbal mixture containing Thuja, Baptisia and *Echinacea purpurea*. Single extracts also demonstrated activity, with *E. purpurea* extract mainly influencing phagocytosis-dependent metabolism.[31]

No significant alteration in the production of cytokines was observed from culture supernatants of stimulated whole blood cells derived from 23 tumour patients undergoing a 4-week oral treatment with a preparation containing extracts of *Echinacea angustifolia, Eupatorium perfoliatum* and *Thuja occidentalis*, in comparison to a control group of tumour patients. No detectable effect on tumour patients' lymphocyte activity was observed.[32]

Twenty-four healthy men received 4.5 ml per day of standardized alcoholic extract of *E. purpurea* root (equivalent to 1 mg each of chicoric acid and alkylamides per day) or placebo for 5 days. A maximum stimulation of granulocyte phagocytosis was observed on the fifth day at 120% of the starting value. The rate of immune stimulation was much higher than that observed with administration by intramuscular injection.[33]

Immune-enhancing activity has been demonstrated for Echinacea polysaccharides in vitro.[34–37] These results, however, may not be translatable to effects in a living organism after oral administration due to gastrointestinal breakdown, poor absorption and poor tissue mobility. Polysaccharides are probably not present in pharmacologically significant quantities and are not absorbed in levels sufficient to achieve the concentrations used in the in vitro studies. Moreover, the quantity of polysaccharides present in preparations containing 50% ethanol or more will be negligible. In addition, some of the polysaccharides used in these studies were isolated from tissue culture and are different to those found naturally in Echinacea preparations.

Excessive extrapolations of the above pharmacological research, especially the in vitro studies on Echinacea polysaccharides, have led to unsupported statements concerning the immunological activity of Echinacea.[38] These include that Echinacea is mitogenic to T-lymphocytes, that ethanolic extracts of Echinacea are ineffective, that Echinacea will accelerate pathology in HIV/AIDS and that Echinacea will aggravate asthma.

In fact, the only immune activity for oral doses of Echinacea which is well supported by experimental findings is the non-specific enhancement of phagocytic activity.

Antiviral activity

Chicoric acid demonstrated antiviral activity against vesicular stomatitis viruses in vitro.[39] Expressed juice of *E. purpurea* (aerial parts) demonstrated an interferon-like antiviral activity against several viruses including influenza and herpes in vitro. Virus resistance did not develop in the presence of hyaluronidase, hence the virucidal activity was indirect. The activity was interferon-like without the induction of interferon.[40,41] Marked inhibition of herpes, influenza and poliovirus was demonstrated by an aqueous extract of *E. purpurea* in vitro.[42]

Purified root extracts from the three *Echinacea species* demonstrated antiviral activity towards herpes simplex virus and influenza virus in vitro. An indirect antiviral effect was also observed via stimulation of alpha- and beta-interferon production.[43]

Antiinflammatory and wound-healing activity

Alkylamides from Echinacea demonstrated inhibitory activity against cyclooxygenase and 5-lipoxygenase in vitro. The structure of the alkylamide determined the degree of activity.[30,44] An antiinflammatory effect was observed after the topical application of a crude polysaccharide fraction from *E. angustifolia* roots in the croton oil mouse ear test.[45]

Application of patches containing expressed juice of *E. purpurea* (aerial parts) to experimental wounds reduced oedema and subcutaneous hemorrhage. The preparation also significantly decreased the rate of necrosis of skin flaps by increasing peripheral circulation.[46] An ointment made from the expressed juice of *E. purpurea* (aerial parts) signifi-cantly improved wound healing in an experimental model.[47]

Topical application of an extract of *E. angustifolia* root inhibited oedema in the croton oil mouse ear test both at the maximum (6 hours) and in the decreasing phase (18 hours). Echinacea was more potent than the topical NSAID benzydamine.[48]

Antihyaluronidase activity

Early research found that expressed juice of *E. purpurea* (aerial parts) inhibited hyaluronidase in vitro[49] and may exert an indirect antihyaluronidase activity.[37] Caffeic acid esters obtained from *E. angustifolia* root demonstrated antihyaluronidase activity in vitro.[50] The possible antihyaluronidase activity may help increase the resistance of tissue to the spread of certain infections and, in conjunction with the increased presence of fibroblasts, facilitate connective tissue regeneration. This effect would most likely be observed for topical application of Echinacea preparations.

Antimicrobial activity

In early research echinacoside demonstrated weak antimicrobial activity against *Staphylococcus aureus* in vitro.[51] Polyacetylenes from *E. angustifolia* and *E. purpurea* root also demonstrated bacteriostatic and fungistatic activity against *E. coli* and *Pseudomonas aeruginosa*.[15] Pure acidic arabinogalactan isolated from *E. purpurea* plant cultures caused 90% destruction of Leishmania parasites by intracellular lysis.[28] *E. angustifolia* extract showed weak inhibitory activity in vitro against *Trichomonas vaginalis*[52] and *E. purpurea* extract inhibited the growth of *Epidermophyton interdigitale* in vitro.[53]

Other effects

Lipophilic fractions of *E. pallida* roots and of the essential oil of *E. angustifolia* root inhibited tumour cells in vitro.[54]

Caffeic acid esters protected collagen from free radical damage in vitro. The protection occurred via a scavenging effect on reactive oxygen species. The authors concluded that topical Echinacea preparations may be useful in the prevention or treatment of photodamage of the skin by ultraviolet radiation.[55]

PHARMACOKINETICS

No data available.

CLINICAL TRIALS

The many clinical trials on the expressed juice of Echinacea administered by injection have not been included in this monograph, since this mode of dosage application is not common in the English-speaking world.

A review of controlled clinical trials investigating the immunomodulatory efficacy of oral doses of Echinacea preparations for infections found the methodological quality of most studies was low.[56] The reviewers concluded that improvement in clinical studies on Echinacea could be achieved through clear definition of diagnostic criteria, detailed description of patient characteristics and baseline data, predefinition of one main outcome measure when judging respiratory tract infections, large sample sizes and use of chemically defined Echinacea preparations.[56] Studies that achieved a score of more than 50% on the reviewers' rating included references [57–60, 63, 66] and [67] which are reviewed below. (Studies of poor quality or some using preparations containing herbs and homoeopathic remedies are omitted from review in this monograph.)

Upper respiratory tract infections, common cold and influenza-like syndromes

In a randomized, double-blind placebo-controlled trial, 180 patients with upper respiratory tract infections received the equivalent of 1800 mg per day or 900 mg per day of *E. purpurea* root as a tincture or placebo. Patients receiving the high dose experienced significant relief of symptoms. Patients receiving the lower dose were not significantly different from the control.[57] (The therapeutic dosage for a 1:5 tincture of *E. purpurea* would therefore begin at 9 ml per day during an infection.)

Patients with upper respiratory tract infections (160) received either the equivalent of 900 mg per day of *E. pallida* root as a tincture or placebo in a randomized, double-blind, placebo-controlled trial.[58] The duration of illness was significantly shorter in the test group (9–10 days) compared to controls (13 days) and symptoms were significantly improved. Efficacy was similar to the higher *Echinacea purpurea* root dose used in the previous trial but it should not be concluded that *E. pallida* is more active since some aspects of this latter trial were unsatisfactory, such as the different frequency of bacterial and viral infections in the treatment and control groups.[56]

In a randomized, double-blind, placebo-controlled trial, 100 patients with upper respiratory tract infections received either placebo or 15–30 ml per day of a preparation containing 1:10 tinctures of *E. angustifolia*, *Eupatorium perfoliatum*, *Baptisia tinctoria* and homoeopathic *Arnica montana*. Three of the seven measured symptoms were significantly better in the test group.[59] In an earlier trial on 100 patients using a similar preparation and dosage, significant improvement was observed in the test group for a majority of symptoms.[60] In a similar trial design, 139 patients with upper respiratory tract infections received three tablets containing extracts of *E. angustifolia* and *E. pallida* root, *Thuja occidentalis* and *Baptisia tinctoria* three times a day or placebo. The majority of symptoms were significantly better in the test group.[61]

Prophylaxis of infection was studied in a randomized, double-blind, placebo-controlled trial during which 108 patients received either 4 ml twice a day of expressed juice of *E. purpurea* (aerial parts) or placebo over 8 weeks. There was a reduction in the intensity and incidence of infections, although it was not statistically significant. Patients with weakened immune systems (CD4/CD8 <1.5) received the most benefit.[62]

In a randomized, double-blind, placebo-controlled trial, 609 university students regularly received either placebo or 12 ml per day of a preparation containing 1:10 tinctures of *E. angustifolia, Eupatorium perfoliatum, Baptisia tinctoria* and homoeopathic *Arnica montana*. A modest reduction in the frequency of infections (15%) was observed in the treatment group.[63]

Since the review of Echinacea clinical trials, additional studies have been published. A randomized, double-blind, placebo-controlled trial examined the effect of the stabilized expressed juice of *E. purpurea* tops in 120 patients with initial symptoms of a common cold.[64] The dose of this preparation was 20 drops every 2 hours for the first day and then three times daily for up to 10 days. Patients taking Echinacea showed a more rapid recovery ($p<0.0001$) than those taking placebo (4 days for Echinacea versus 8 days for placebo). No specific adverse effects were reported for either group.

The safety and efficacy of two root extracts of Echinacea (*E. purpurea* or *E. angustifolia*) for preventing upper respiratory tract infections were assessed in a three-armed, randomized, double-blind, placebo-controlled trial on 302 healthy volunteers over 12 weeks.[65] Although there was a numerical tendency towards a lower infection rate in both Echinacea groups, statistical significance was not achieved. Participants in the treatment groups believed they had more benefit from Echinacea than those in the placebo group ($p=0.04$). Adverse effects reports were 18 for *E. angustifolia*, 10 for *E. purpurea* and 11 for placebo. One problem with this trial was the relatively low doses of Echinacea used (about 200 mg of dried root per day).

Antineoplastic therapy

In a randomized controlled trial, 25 of 50 female patients undergoing irradiation following breast cancer received the equivalent of 1.25 ml per day of a preparation containing extracts of *E. angustifolia* and *E. pallida* root, *Thuja occidentalis* and *Baptisia tinctoria*. Peripheral blood count and the incidence of infections did not significantly differ from the control group.[66] Again, this trial used a low test dose.

In a controlled, randomized study, 33 female patients with advanced breast cancer received a similar dose of preparation containing extracts of *E. angustifolia* and *E. pallida* root, *Thuja occidentalis* and *Baptisia tinctoria* in conjunction with chemoradiation therapy.[67] In comparison with 34 patients receiving only chemoradiation, recuperation of the haematopoietic system was promoted and there was a tendency to reduced infections, but only in cases of minor damage to the bone marrow.

Other diseases

In an uncontrolled study, 60 patients received the equivalent of 4.5 ml per day of expressed juice of *E. purpurea* (aerial parts) over 10 weeks in conjunction with an antifungal cream for the treatment of recurrent candidiasis. A 17% recurrence rate was observed in the treatment group compared to 60% for those receiving only antifungal cream.[68] A significant normalization of cell-mediated immunity was also observed for the Echinacea group.

Sixty patients suffering from acute sinusitis received either three tablets per day containing extracts of *E. angustifolia* and *E. pallida* root, *Thuja occidentalis* and tincture of *Baptisia tinctoria* together with doxycycline (a tetracycline antibiotic) or doxycycline alone in an open comparative study. X-ray and global assessment was much better for the group receiving the herbs.[69]

In a postmarketing surveillance study 4500 patients were examined by 500 doctors from all over Germany investigating the effect of an ointment containing Echinacea juice on a variety of skin complaints. In 86% of cases a favourable result was obtained.[70]

TOXICOLOGY

The expressed juice of *E. purpurea* was orally administered over 4 weeks to rats in doses many times the human therapeutic dose. Laboratory tests and necropsy findings showed no evidence of toxic effects. In vitro and in vivo tests showed no mutagenicity or carcinogenicity for the *E. purpurea* juice.[71] The acute toxicity of an *E. purpurea* root extract has been determined at a level of >3000 mg/kg in mice.[72]

CONTRAINDICATIONS

Extracts or expressed juice of the aerial parts may contain pollen proteins. Hence caution should be exercised in those with a tendency to allergic reactions, especially against Compositae.

The German Commission E monograph states that in principle, Echinacea should not be used in 'progressive conditions' such as tuberculosis, leukaemia, collagen disorders, multiple sclerosis, AIDS, HIV infection and other autoimmune disease. However, the key words here are 'in principle'. There are no clinical studies which document an adverse effect resulting from Echinacea use in any of these conditions.

The suggestion that Echinacea is contraindicated in autoimmune disease assumes that any enhancement of any aspect of immune function is detrimental. However, immune function is extraordinarily complex and a substance which acts largely on phagocytic activity may be safe or even beneficial in autoimmunity. Many theories have been proposed as to the causative factors in autoimmune disease. However, there is growing evidence that an inappropriate response to infectious microorganisms, through phenomena such as molecular mimicry, may be at work.[73,74] If this is the case, Echinacea may be beneficial in these disorders because it may decrease the chronic presence of microorganisms. There is now a large body of clinical observations, including those of the authors, that long-term Echinacea is at least not harmful in autoimmunity and is probably beneficial. Similarly, there is one published case study of long-term Echinacea use in chronic lymphocytic leukaemia which did not reveal adverse effects.[75]

Recently, an article in the *Australian Medical Observer* has cautioned that Echinacea is a danger to asthmatics.[76] This caution is apparently based on the concern that Echinacea increases the cytokine known as tumour necrosis factor-alpha (TNF-alpha) which increases the inflammatory process in asthma. However, the information for TNF-alpha comes from in vitro tests on Echinacea juice or polysaccharides. For a number of reasons discussed already, such studies are likely to have little relevance to normal oral use of Echinacea. This has been recently confirmed in a clinical study which found that oral therapy with Echinacea had no detectable effect on cytokine production by lymphocytes. Specifically, levels of TNF-alpha release were not changed by Echinacea.[32]

Although the Commission E recommends limitations on Echinacea use (including a contraindication in pregnancy) several writers and other authoritative sources do not support these restrictions. For example, the *British Herbal Pharmacopoeia* 1983[77] and the *British Herbal Compendium*[78] offer no contraindications for Echinacea. In fact, the indications in the Compendium for prophylaxis of colds and influenza and chronic viral and bacterial infections suggest long-term usage. Weiss suggests that Echinacea can do no harm and has no side effects.[79]

SPECIAL WARNINGS AND PRECAUTIONS

Caution is advised for transplant patients taking immunosuppressive drugs. Short-term therapy only is suggested.

There is no evidence to suggest that long-term use of Echinacea is detrimental to immune function. There is one published clinical study which has led some writers to suggest that Echinacea depletes the immune system when used continuously for periods longer than several days, a phenomenon known as tachyphylaxis. This is the study by Jurcic and co-workers (cited previously) which tested the effect of an *E. purpurea* tincture on the phagocytic activity of human granulocytes following intravenous or oral administration.[33] Confusion has arisen over this study because it was not appreciated that the test dose was only administered for 5 days. While Echinacea was given, phagocytic activity remained higher than controls. Only when the Echinacea was stopped did phagocytic activity decline to normal (pretest) values, demonstrating a typical wash-out effect. The study in fact demonstrated that there is a residual stimulating effect which lasted for about 2 days after Echinacea was stopped.

INTERACTIONS

None known.

USE IN PREGNANCY AND LACTATION

No data available.

EFFECTS ON ABILITY TO DRIVE AND USE MACHINES

None known.

SIDE EFFECTS

Side effects are generally not expected for oral or topical administration. As indicated below contact dermatitis may occur rarely in susceptible patients. Unsubstantiated reports of three deaths attributed to Echinacea products over a 6-year period occurred in the German media in 1996. However, no action was taken by the authorities as no causal link between the deaths and the taking of Echinacea could be established.[80]

A risk-benefit assessment of the stabilized juice of *Echinacea purpurea* tops for long-term oral immunostimulation found that adverse events on oral administration for up to 12 weeks are infrequent and consist mainly of unpleasant taste, especially for Echinacea lozenges, and some digestive symptoms. *E. purpurea* juice was well tolerated on long-term oral administration.[81]

A total of 1032 patients, randomly chosen from six patch test clinics, were patch tested with a series of five ointments and the components of the ointment bases. Two patients demonstrated a positive reaction to Echinacea. However, it is not certain that the reaction was to the plant material itself.[82] Anaphylaxis was attributed to a woman with allergy after taking, among other dietary supplements, a commercial extract of *E. purpurea* and *E. angustifolia*.[83] However, it was suggested that the pharyngeal irritation experienced by the patient may have been due to the alkylamide content of the preparation (the patient took twice the recommended amount).[84]

OVERDOSE

Not known.

CURRENT REGULATORY STATUS IN SELECTED COUNTRIES

A draft monograph of Echinacea is being prepared and may appear in the *European Pharmacopoeia* subsequent to the 1997 edition and in the *United States Pharmacopeia-National Formulary* subsequent to June 1999.

Echinacea angustifolia/pallida herb, *E. angustifolia* root and *E. purpurea* root are covered by null and negative Commission E monographs. *E. pallida* root and *E. purpurea* herb are covered by positive monographs. These herbs are listed with the following uses:

- to support the immune system with infections of the respiratory and lower urinary systems (*E. purpurea* herb);
- in supportive treatment of influenza-like infections (*E. pallida* root);
- externally for poorly healing wounds and chronic ulcerations (*E. purpurea* herb).

E. purpurea root is listed in the unapproved component characteristics section. The negative status of *Echinacea angustifolia/pallida* herb, *E. angustifolia* root and *E. purpurea* root is due to poor benefit:risk ratio and concerns about the risk from parenteral application (injection). The null status is due to a lack of substantiation of its activity for the listed conditions, leading to its therapeutic use not being recommended. Echinacea is on the UK General Sale List.

Echinacea does not have GRAS status. However, it is freely available as a 'dietary supplement' in the USA under DSHEA legislation (1994 Dietary Supplement Health and Education Act).

Echinacea is not included in Part 4 of Schedule 4 of the Therapeutic Goods Act Regulations of Australia.

References

1. Felter HW, Lloyd JU. King's American dispensatory, 18th edn, vol 1. Eclectic Medical Publications, Portland, 1983; pp 671–677.
2. Ellingwood F. American materia medica, therapeutics and pharmacognosy, vol 2. Eclectic Medical Publications, Portland 1993; pp 358–376.
3. Grieve M. A modern herbal, vol 1. Dover Publications, New York, 1971; pp 265.
4. Leung AY, Foster S. Encyclopedia of common natural ingredients used in food, drugs and cosmetics, 2nd edn. John Wiley, New York 1996; pp 216–219.
5. Smeh NJ. Creating your own cosmetics – naturally. Alliance Publishing, Garrisonville, 1995; pp 76, 82, 135–140, 142, 157.
6. Bauer R, Wagner H. Echinacea. Handbuch für Ärzte, Apotheker und andere Naturwissenschaftler, Wissenschaftliche Verlagsgesellschaft, Stuttgart, 1990; pp 30–32.
7. Lust JB. The herb book. Bantam Books, New York, 1974; p 177.
8. Bauer R, Khan IA, Wagner H. Planta Med 1988; 54: 426–430.
9. Bauer R, Remiger P. Planta Med 1989; 55: 367–371.
10. Bauer R, Remiger P, Wagner H et al. Phytochem 1989; 28: 505–508.
11. Bohlmann F, Grenz M. Chem Ber 1966; 99: 3197–3200.
12. Bauer R, Wagner H. Echinacea. Handbuch für Ärzte, Apotheker und andere Naturwissenchaftler, Wissenschaftliche Verlagsgesellschaft, Stuttgart, 1990; pp 94–95.
13. Bauer R, Alstat E. Planta Med 1990; 56: 533–534.
14. Bauer R, Wagner H. Echinacea species as potential immunostimulatory drugs. In: Farnsworth NR et al (eds) Economic and medicinal plant research, vol 5. Academic Press, London, 1991; pp 266–267.
15. Schulte KE, Ruecker G, Perlick J. Arzneim-Forsch 1967; 17: 825–829.
16. Giger E, Keller F, Baumann TW. Poster, 37th Annual Congress of the Society of Medicinal Plant Research, Braunschweig, September 5–10, 1989.
17. Röder E, Wiedenfeld H, Hille T et al. Dtsch Apoth Ztg 1984; 124: 2316–2318.
18. Bauer R, Remiger P, Wagner H. Dtsch Apoth Ztg 1988; 128: 174–180.
19. Bauer R, Wagner H. Echinacea species as potential immunostimulatory drugs. In: Farnsworth NR et al (eds) Economic and medicinal plant research, vol 5. Academic Press, London, 1991; pp 280–282.
20. Brandt L. Scand J Haematol 1967; 2 (suppl 2): 1–126.
21. Wildfeuer A, Mayerhofer D. Arzneim-Forsch 1994; 44 (3): 361–366.
22. Krause M. Dissertation, Berlin 1984. Cited in Bauer R, Wagner H. Echinacea species as potential immunostimulatory drugs. In: Farnsworth NR et al (eds) Economic and medicinal plant research, vol 5. Academic Press, London, 1991; pp 291–292.
23. Coeugniet EG, Elek E. Onkol 1987; 10 (suppl): 27–33.
24. Burger RA, Torres AR, Warren RP. Int J Immunopharmacol 1997; 19 (7): 371–379.
25. See DM, Broumand N, Sahl L et al. Immunopharmacol 1997; 35 (3): 229–235.
26. Bauer R, Jurcic K, Puhlmann J et al. Arzneim-Forsch 1988; 38 (2): 276–281.
27. Bauer R, Remiger P, Jurcic K et al. Z Phytother 1989; 10: 43–48.
28. Bauer R, Wagner H. Echinacea species as potential immunostimulatory drugs. In: Farnsworth NR et al (eds) Economic and medicinal plant research, vol 5. Academic Press, London, 1991; pp 292–296, 304, 306.
29. Schumacher A, Friedberg KD. Arzneim-Forsch 1991; 41 (2): 141–147.
30. Wagner H, Jurcic K. Arzneim-Forsch 1991; 41: 1072–1076.
31. Vomel T. Arzneim-Forsch 1985; 35: 1437–1439.
32. Elsasser-Beile U, Willenbacher W, Bartsch HH et al. J Clin Lab Anal 1996; 10 (6): 441–445.
33. Jurcic K, Melchart D, Holzmann M et al. Z Phytother 1989; 10: 67–70.
34. Wagner H, Proksch A, Riess-Maurer I et al. Arzneim-Forsch 1985; 35: 1069–1075.
35. Stimpel M, Proksch A, Wagner H et al. Infect Immunol 1984; 46: 845–849.

36. Luettig B, Steinmüller G, Gifford GE et al. J Nat Cancer Inst 1989; 81: 669–675.
37. Bauer R, Wagner H. Echinacea species as potential immunostimulatory drugs. In: Farnsworth NR et al (eds) Economic and medicinal plant research, vol 5. Academic Press, London, 1991; pp 286–288, 301.
38. Bone K. Alternat Med Rev 1997; 2 (2): 87–93.
39. Cheminat A, Zawatzky R, Becker H et al. Phytochem 1988; 27: 2787–2794.
40. Orinda D, Diederich J, Wacker A. Arzneim-Forsch 1973; 23: 1119–1120.
41. Wacker A, Hilbig W. Planta Med 1978; 33: 89–102.
42. May G, Willuhn G. Arzneim-Forsch 1978; 28: 1–7.
43. Beuscher N, Bodinet C, Willigmann I et al. Z Phytother 1995; 16 (3): 157, 165–166.
44. Wagner H, Breu W, Willer F et al. Planta Med 1989; 55: 566–567.
45. Tubaro A, Tragni E, Del Negro P et al. J Pharm Pharmacol 1987; 39 (7): 567–569.
46. Meissner FK. Arzneim-Forsch 1987; 37 (1): 17–18.
47. Kinkel HJ, Plate M, Tullner HU. Med Klin 1984; 79: 580.
48. Tragni E, Tubaro A, Melis C et al. Food Chem Toxicol 1985; 23 (2): 317–319.
49. Büsing KH. Arzneim-Forsch 1952; 2: 464–467.
50. Facino RM, Carini M, Aldini G et al. Farmaco 1993; 48 (10): 1447–1461.
51. Stoll A, Renz J, Brack A. Helv Chim Acta 1950; 33: 1877–1893.
52. Samochowiec E, Urbanska L, Manka W et al. Wiad Parazytol 1979; 25: 77–81.
53. Jung H-D, Schröder H. Arch Dermat Syphilis 1954; 197: 130–144.
54. Voaden DJ, Jacobson M. J Med Chem 1972; 15: 619–623.
55. Facino RM, Carini M, Aldini G et al. Planta Med 1995; 61 (6): 510–514.
56. Melchart D, Linde K, Worku F et al. Phytomed 1994; 1: 245–254.
57. Bräunig B, Dorn M, Knick E. Z Phytother 1992; 13: 7–13.
58. Bräunig B, Knick E. Naturheilpraxis 1993; 1: 72–75.
59. Dorn M. Natur Ganzheitsmed 1989; 2: 314–319.
60. Vorberg G, Schneider B. Ärztl Forsch 1989; 36: 3–8.
61. Reitz HD. Notabene Medici 1990; 20: 362–366.
62. Schöneberger D. Forum Immunol 1992; 2: 18–22.
63. Schmidt U. Natur Ganzheitsmed 1990; 3: 277–281.
64. Hoheisel O, Sandberg M, Bertram S et al. Eur J Clin Res 1997; 9: 261–268.
65. Melchart D, Walther E, Linde K et al. Arch Fam Med 1998; 7: 541–545.
66. Bendel R, Renner K, Stolze K. Strahlenther Onkol 1988; 164: 278–283.
67. Bendel R, Bendel V, Renner K et al. Onkol 1989; 12 (3) (suppl): 32–38.
68. Coeugniet EG, Kühnast R. Therapiewoche 1986; 36: 3352–3358.
69. Zimmer M. Therapiewoche 1985; 35: 4024–4028.
70. Corrigan D. Indian medicine for the immune system. Amberwood Publishing, Surrey, 1994; p 36.
71. Mengs U, Clare CB, Poiley JA. Arzneim-Forsch 1991; 41: 1076–1081.
72. German Federal Minister of Justice. German Commission E for human medicine monograph, Bundes-Anzeiger (German Federal Gazette), no. 162, dated 29.08.1992.
73. Bone KM. Treating autoimmune disease part 1. Modern Phytotherapist 1995; 1 (1): 1–8.
74. Bone KM. Treating autoimmune disease part 2. Modern Phytotherapist 1995; 1 (2): 15–27.
75. McLeod D. Case history of chronic lymphocytic leukaemia. Modern Phytotherapist 1996; 2 (3): 34–35.
76. Sharp R. Echinacea a danger to asthmatics. Medical Observer, 8 August, 1997: 1.
77. British Herbal Medicine Association. British herbal pharmacopoeia. BHMA, Cowling. 1983; pp 80–81.
78. British Herbal Medicine Association. British herbal compendium, vol 1. BHMA, Bournemouth, 1992; pp 81–83.
79. Weiss RF. Herbal medicine. Beaconsfield Publishers, Beaconsfield: 1988; pp 229–230.
80. Bauer R, Wagner H. Z Phytother 1996; 17: 251–252.
81. Parnham MJ. Phytomed 1996; 3 (1): 95–102.
82. Bruynzeel DP, Van Ketel WG, Young E et al. Contact Derm 1992; 27: 278–279.
83. Mullins RJ. MJA 1998; 168: 170–171.
84. Myers SP, Wohlmuth H. MJA 1998; 168: 583.

Evening primrose oil (*Oenothera biennis L.*)

SYNONYMS

Echte Nachtkerze (Ger), herbe aux ânes, onagre bisannuelle (Fr), stella di sera (Ital), kaempe natlys (Dan).

WHAT IS IT?

Evening primrose oil (EPO) is the fixed (fatty) oil obtained from the seed of the common evening primrose, *Oenothera biennis*. Flowers of this genus often open and release scent in the evenings and are pollinated by moths.[1] The seeds were recommended as a coffee substitute in wartime and have an aromatic flavour reminiscent of poppy seed oil.[2] Other parts of the plant have been used medicinally: leaves and bark for dyspepsia, liver and female complaints. The root can be eaten as a vegetable.[3] Evening primrose oil was developed as a source of gamma-linolenic acid (GLA) in response to an increased understanding of the role of eicosanoids in human disease processes.

EFFECTS

Antiinflammatory; corrects omega-6 essential fatty acid deficiency; improves vasodilator eicosanoid synthesis; corrects nerve blood flow and nerve conduction velocity deficits in diabetes.

TRADITIONAL VIEW

Evening primrose oil was not used traditionally.

SUMMARY ACTIONS

Antiinflammatory, antiallergic, corrects omega-6 essential fatty acid deficiency, hypotensive.

CAN BE USED FOR

INDICATIONS SUPPORTED BY CLINICAL TRIALS

Indications supported by trials using evening primrose oil: diabetic neuropathy; mastalgia. EPO may also be beneficial in the treatment of premenstrual syndrome, atopic dermatitis, rheumatoid arthritis, schizophrenia, Raynaud's phenomenon and ulcerative colitis although the results of clinical trials are not conclusive.

Indications suggested by trials using evening primrose oil and fish oil are hypertension, postviral fatigue syndrome, osteoporosis and Alzheimer's disease although more studies are necessary to fully confirm efficacy.

MAY ALSO BE USED FOR

EXTRAPOLATIONS FROM PHARMACOLOGICAL STUDIES

Impaired omega-6 essential fatty acid metabolism (especially diabetes); inflammatory disorders (including rheumatoid arthritis, ulcerative colitis, SLE); alcoholism.

OTHER APPLICATIONS

Used in cosmetic products such as hand lotions, soaps and shampoos.[4] Veterinary applications include skin disorders such as papulocrustous dermatitis, crusting dermatoses and non-seasonal atopic dermatitis.

PREPARATIONS

Oils like EPO (containing the polyunsaturated *cis* fatty acid, GLA) are difficult to preserve as they can easily be oxidized and become rancid, so EPO is best administered with a preservative such as vitamin E, protected from oxygen in soft gelatin capsules.

DOSAGE

Low to medium dosage should be used for conditions such as atopic dermatitis and mastalgia: 250–500 mg GLA per day (approximately 2.6 to 5.2 g per day of EPO).

Medium to high doses should be used for conditions such as diabetes, alcoholism, inflammatory disorders (including arthritis, ulcerative colitis) or cardiovascular disorders (hyperlipidaemia, hypertension): 0.4–2 g GLA per day (approximately 4.2–21 g per day of EPO). A suitable dose to begin treatment for rheumatoid arthritis is 500–600 mg GLA per day (approximately 5.2–6.3 g per day of EPO).

DURATION OF USE

Evening primrose oil should be used cautiously in the long term for patients with rheumatoid arthritis. Otherwise long-term use appears to be safe.

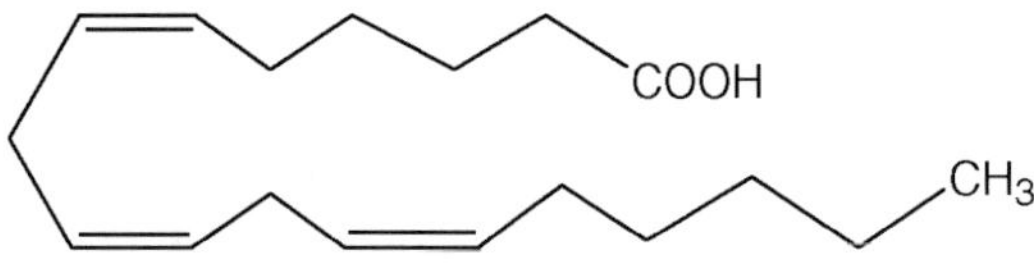

gamma - Linolenic acid

SUMMARY ASSESSMENT OF SAFETY

Evening primrose oil is very well tolerated, with very few side effects reported in clinical trials when administered at therapeutic doses over the short and medium term. Long-term use may potentiate the risk of arachidonate build-up in the treatment of rheumatoid arthritis. There is concern in some quarters regarding the administration of EPO where there is a history of epilepsy but this is not well supported by fact.

TECHNICAL DATA

BOTANY

Evening primrose is a member of the Onagraceae (willow herb) family, which grows to a height of about 1 m. It is an annual or biennial plant with lanceolate leaves and large, showy yellow flowers which are arranged in a terminal leafy spike. The flowers consist of four petals; the fruit is cylindrical and opens lengthwise by four valves.[5,6]

KEY CONSTITUENTS

- Fixed oil (15–20%), containing essential fatty acids: linoleic acid (65%), gamma-linolenic acid (8–10%).[7,8]
- Triacylglycerols in the oil, mainly comprising trilinolein (linoleic acid in all three esterified positions on the glycerol molecule) and dilinoleoyl-mono-gamma-linolenin (two linoleic acids, one GLA). The latter, known as DLMG, accounts for over half of the total amount of GLA.[9]

PHARMACODYNAMICS

Essential fatty acids (EFAs) are nutrients which play a role in the structure of cell membranes, helping to ensure their fluidity and flexibility, and modulate the behaviour of membrane-bound proteins. They are also precursors of the eicosanoids (prostaglandins, leukotrienes and thromboxanes) which function in platelet aggregation and inflammatory processes.

Omega-6 series	Omega-3 series
Linoleic acid (LA)	Alpha-linolenic acid (ALA)
↓	↓
Gamma-linolenic acid (GLA)	
↓	↓
Dihomogamma-linolenic acid (DGLA)	
↓	↓
Arachidonic acid (AA)	Eicosapentaenoic acid (EPA)
↓	↓
↓	↓
↓	Docosahexaenoic acid (DHA)

Since they contain two or more double bonds, EFAs are classified as polyunsaturated fatty acids. There are two types of EFA: the omega-6 series which is derived from linoleic acid (LA) and the omega-3 series which is derived from alpha-linolenic acid (ALA). These are named for the position of the double bond nearest to the methyl ($-CH_3$) group at the end of the molecule. Omega-3 fatty acids are found in fish oils and certain seeds (e.g. linseed).

Within the body LA and ALA are metabolized by a series of alternating desaturations and elongations, as shown below.

Arachidonic acid forms prostaglandin products of the 2-series (e.g. PGE_2) and leukotrienes with subscript 4 (LTB_4). DGLA and EPA can be converted to metabolites closely related to these eicosanoids: DGLA producing prostaglandins of the 1-series and leukotrienes of the 3-series; EPA producing prostaglandins of the 3-series and leukotrienes of the 5-series. The presence of these particular omega-3 and omega-6 fatty acids can result in decreased production of some arachidonate metabolites and increased levels of the other less inflammatory eicosanoids.

Although GLA has been found in higher concentrations from other sources, including borage oil, blackcurrant oil and fungal lipids, there is currently less evidence to support their clinical efficacy compared to EPO.[10]

Diabetes

Reduced nerve perfusion, indicated by a nerve conduction velocity deficit and reduced nerve blood flow is an important factor in the aetiology of diabetic neuropathy, a common complication of diabetes. Metabolic changes include a high polyol pathway flux (mediated by aldose reductase), increased advanced glycosylation, elevated oxidative stress and impaired omega-6 essential fatty acid metabolism. GLA improves vasodilator eicosanoid synthesis, correcting nerve blood flow and nerve conduction velocity deficits.

Combined treatment of EPO with aldose reductase inhibitors or antioxidants (such as ascorbate) markedly enhanced neuroactivity.[11] Depletion of polyunsaturated fatty acids derived from the omega-6 pathway may also lead to abnormalities of myelin turnover and membrane-bound proteins (e.g. enzymes, receptors) and other axonal structural abnormalities.[12]

Treatment with EPO can prevent or reverse motor nerve conduction velocity deficit (an indicator of peripheral neuropathy) in diabetic animals. This was achieved without changing the sorbitol, fructose or myoinositol levels in peripheral nerves and without having any effect on the control of blood sugar.[13,14] Evening primrose oil outperformed blackcurrant oil, borage oil and fungal oils in ameliorating nerve conduction velocity deficits in diabetic rats.[15] Treatment with EPO improved nerve blood flow measurements in rats with experimentally induced diabetes. Reduced production of nitric oxide may be responsible for the development of endoneurial ischaemia in diabetes and EPO may correct this deficiency in vivo.[16] Aspirin enhanced the neuroactivity of EPO in experimental diabetes, thus indicating that prostanoids are unlikely to mediate this neuroactivity.[17] Daily treatment with EPO caused oscillation of nerve conduction velocity in diabetic rats needing 10 days to stabilize. The latency suggests that neuroactivity of EPO may be mediated by its metabolic products synthesized in the body and not by ready-made constituents of the oil.[18]

Short-term biochemical changes have been noted from GLA treatment in insulin-dependent diabetic (IDDM) patients. At the 2 g/day dosage of GLA over 6 weeks, a decrease in serum triglycerides, cholesterol and plasma beta-thromboglobulin was observed. No changes were observed on platelet aggregation or thromboxane B_2 and PGE_1 released from platelets.[19]

Antiinflammatory activity

GLA and DGLA inhibit inflammation and excessive immune reactivity in a variety of models: adjuvant arthritis, experimental allergic encephalomyelitis, autoimmune disease (systemic lupus erythematosus), salmonella-associated arthritis and subacute, acute and chronic inflammation induced by Freund's adjuvant or urate crystal.[20–22] The GLA-enriched diet significantly suppressed the cellular phase of inflammation but had little effect on the fluid phase.[21] EPO raised gastric mucosal prostaglandin synthesis in humans but not in rats.[23,24] EPO, however, protected rats but not humans against aspirin-induced damage.[23,25] Four different doses of GLA in the form of either borage oil or EPO were fed to rats over 6 weeks and compared with corn oil. DGLA and GLA levels demonstrated a dose-dependent increase in liver, red blood cell and aorta phospholipids. The AA:DGLA ratio in tissues decreased with increasing intake of GLA. There was no significant difference in GLA or DGLA levels within groups given borage oil or EPO. The dose of GLA did not influence PGE_2 production in stimulated aortic rings or thromboxane levels in serum, although an increase in PGE_1 occurred in the stimulated aorta.[26]

In a study investigating the metabolism of GLA, 29 volunteers either adhered to a fat-controlled diet and received GLA supplementation or maintained a typical Western diet. Supplementation with GLA at 3–6 g/day resulted in increased GLA and DGLA in serum lipids. AA increased in all subjects. Neutrophil phospholipids were higher in DGLA but not GLA or AA. Neutrophils obtained from those supplemented with GLA synthesized less LTB_4 and platelet-activating factor. The increase in DGLA relative to AA within inflammatory cells such as neutrophils may decrease the production of AA metabolites and explain how GLA exerts its antiinflammatory activity.[27]

Bone metabolism

GLA and EPA were administered orally to different groups of rats in several ratios. Intestinal calcium absorption, calcium balance and bone calcium all increased significantly in the 3:1 (GLA:EPA) ratio group, compared to controls.[28] Several different ratios of GLA and EPA were administered to young rats, as a mixture of EPO and fish oil. Bone calcium content increased significantly in the group receiving the high GLA:EPA diet compared to controls receiving LA and ALA.[29]

Reproductive function

In a placebo-controlled trial during the reproductive period, male and female blue foxes were fed either a standard diet or one supplemented with EPO, zinc sulphate and vitamin E. A tendency for an increased litter size in the treatment group was found, mainly as an effect of male treatment.[30] Control male minks were mated with control and test female minks and test males were mated with control and test females. For those males supplemented with EPO, there was a tendency for a reduced rate of stillborns and loss of life during the first 21 days of life. EPO did not affect reproductive performance in females but there was a tendency for lower weight losses during lactation.[31]

Cytotoxic effects

The cytotoxicity of GLA and other fatty acids containing two, four, five and six double bonds were examined on human breast cancer cells in vitro. GLA and arachidonate, with three and four double bonds respectively, were the most cytotoxic fatty acids, compared to acids with six double bonds which were the least effective. The effectiveness of a given fatty acid in killing cancer cells correlated with the extent of lipid peroxidation of the added fatty acid in the cells.[32] GLA, AA and EPA were highly effective in killing human breast, lung and prostate tumour cells in vitro, while leaving normal cells viable.[33] GLA, AA and EPA enhanced free radical generation in tumour cells but not in normal cells in vitro.[34]

The growth of human breast carcinoma xenografts was studied in mice treated with dietary supplements of EPO and fish oil and compared to controls. Animals in the treatment group developed tumours which were significantly smaller than controls.[35]

Hypotensive effects

Vegetable oils including sunflower oil, linseed oil and EPO enhanced the hypotensive effect of antihypertensive drugs (dihydralazine, clonidine and captopril) in rats under experimental conditions.[36] Hypertension induced in rats was reversed by the addition of DGLA (5.0%) to the diet.[37] LA bioconversion to AA was decreased in the liver microsomes of spontaneously hypertensive rats compared to controls, due to a decrease in the desaturase enzymes.[38] The effect of salt loading on blood pressure (BP) development and its modification by dietary omega-3 and omega-6 fatty acids was studied in the borderline hypertensive rat. EPO abolished the pressor response, reducing BP below control levels.[39] GLA supplementation reduced cardiovascular responses to chronic stress in normal and borderline hypertensive rats.[40,41]

Other effects

In comparison to a corn oil placebo, EPO produced significant inhibition of gastric mucosal damage induced by pylorus ligation, NSAIDs or hypothermic restraint and had a marked cytoprotective effect against all necrotizing agents used.[42]

Analysis of fatty acid composition of the plasma of children with atopic bronchial asthma showed significantly higher levels of LA and lower levels of AA in comparison to healthy controls. No differences were observed in GLA and DGLA. There is therefore no justification for GLA supplementation on the basis of a 6-desaturation defect (and subsequently low levels of eicosanoid precursors from DGLA).[43]

Treatment of pregnant rats with ethanol and EPO led to a significant reduction in the embryopathic activity of ethanol.[44] EPO slowed the progression of renal failure in rats[45] and reduced the severity of experimental autoimmune glomerulonephritis in rats.[46]

PHARMACOKINETICS AND METABOLISM

Essential fatty acids are hydrolysed by lipases in the gastric and intestinal lumen. Long-chain polyunsaturated fatty acids (PUFAs) are taken up by tissues less rapidly than short-chain PUFAs. The liver is one of the most active organs in producing long-chain PUFAs (by a series of desaturation and elongation reactions). In this way less active organs such as the brain are provided with long-chain PUFAs secreted in very low density lipoprotein (VLDL). Insulin and thyroxin are necessary for the desaturation process but glucagon, adrenaline, ACTH and glucocorticoids inhibit desaturation.[47]

The pharmacokinetics of GLA in six healthy volunteers after the administration of EPO was recorded. EPO capsules were administered to each subject in the morning and the evening over several days. The values for accumulated concentration (24 hours) and C_{max} (maximum concentration) for GLA were significantly increased over baseline values. Other fatty acids such as DGLA and AA did not show a significant increase in their concentration. After the evening administration, T_{max} (time to reach maximum concentration) was shorter than after the morning dose. An influence of the administration of GLA on serum concentrations of DGLA and AA (and hence on the biosynthesis of prostaglandin PGE_1 and PGE_2) could not be clearly established in these healthy volunteers.[48]

VETERINARY STUDIES

Eleven cats with papulocrustous dermatitis randomly received either EPO or sunflower oil for 12 weeks. Cats in both groups improved during the period of treatment and the concentration of LA in erythrocyte phospholipid increased in the cats fed EPO. Six weeks after the treatment was withdrawn, the cats fed EPO had deteriorated less than those fed sunflower oil.[49] Fourteen cats with crusting dermatoses were treated with various combinations of EPO and fish oil. The cutaneous symptoms improved in those treated with either EPO alone or in combination with fish oil. The subsequent administration of a combination of the two oils resulted in a resolution of the dermatosis.[50]

A significant effect was observed on erythema in dogs with non-seasonal atopic dermatitis. They were treated with EPO in a double-blind, placebo-controlled crossover study. Plasma LA and AA levels were significantly higher for the EPO group, both in the first and second phases of the study. There was also a significant treatment effect for EPO given in the second phase.[51]

CLINICAL TRIALS

Clinical trials have shown benefits in diabetic neuropathy, hypertension, mastalgia, PMS, osteoporosis and dementia. Mixed results have been obtained in trials for atopic eczema and dermatitis, rheumatoid arthritis, ulcerative colitis, diabetic lipid metabolism and alcoholism. The benefits of EPO therapy are disputed in schizophrenia and cancer. No benefit was observed in the treatment of menopausal hot flushes.

Atopic dermatitis and related skin disorders

In an open trial, 20 patients with dry skin and atopic disposition (but not actual atopic dermatitis) received 12.5% EPO cream applied to their lower right leg for 3 weeks. The other leg served as a control. The treated leg showed a significant increase in sebum content ($p<0.01$) but no change in transepidermal water loss. Transepidermal water loss was significant on the untreated side ($p<0.05$). Improvement in skin smoothness was observed on the treated side.[52] In an uncontrolled trial, infants with atopic dermatitis were treated with GLA (3 g/day) for 28 days. A gradual improvement in erythema, excoriations and lichenification was observed. Significant differences were shown for itching ($p<0.01$) and with the use of antihistamines ($p<0.01$). A significant rise in the percentage of circulating CD8 cells was found.[53] GLA reduced the requirement for topical steroids (by about 70%) and other medications such as oral steroids, antihistamines and antibiotics.[54,55] Two independent studies using different methodologies have demonstrated that skin roughness can also be significantly reduced.[56,57]

Although a number of controlled clinical trials have been conducted for EPO in the treatment of atopic dermatitis, efficacy has not been clearly demonstrated. These trials are listed below, grouped according to the positive or negative results obtained and with the most recent work listed first.

A double-blind, placebo-controlled study conducted on children with atopic dermatitis found a significant improvement in the overall severity of the condition in children treated with GLA, independent of the occurrence of IgE-mediated allergy. GLA treatment increased the amount of omega-6 fatty acids in red blood cell membranes, particularly in those treated with the highest dose. A significant increase in DGLA occurred in the high-dose group.[58] In a double-blind, placebo-controlled trial, 52 adults with atopic eczema completed 4 months' treatment with EPO. Subjects were divided into three groups: women with premenstrual exacerbation of their eczema, women without the exacerbation and men. Results for the three groups combined indicated a significant effect of EPO on erythema and surface damage compared to placebo. No significant effect was observed for lichenification. Women with premenstrual flare of their eczema showed greatest improvement with EPO treatment compared to placebo.[59]

Four weeks' treatment with EPO in children with atopic eczema resulted in significant improvement compared to those treated with an olive oil placebo. There were significant changes in plasma fatty acid composition before and after treatment and also between the placebo and EPO-treated groups.[60] Patients receiving EPO showed a significantly greater reduction in inflammation than those receiving placebo in a double-blind trial conducted over 12 weeks, although patients in the placebo group also showed a significant reduction. A statistically significant improvement was observed in the overall severity, grade of inflammation, dryness and itch and in the percentage of the body surface with eczema.[55]

A metaanalysis published in 1989 investigated nine placebo-controlled trials for the efficacy of EPO in the treatment of atopic eczema. Four of the trials were parallel and five were crossover design. Doctors and patients assessed the severity of eczema by scoring measures of inflammation, dryness, scaliness, pruritus and overall skin involvement. Individual symptom scores were combined to give a single global score at each assessment point. In the parallel studies, both patient and doctor scores showed a highly significant improvement over baseline for EPO which was also significantly better than placebo. Similar results were obtained in the crossover trials, except that the doctors' global score, although favouring EPO, did not reach significance. The effect on itch was striking, with a highly significant response to EPO occurring ($p<0.0001$) and no placebo response. A positive correlation between an improvement in clinical score and a rise in the plasma fatty acid level was observed.[61]

A review of clinical trials for the treatment of atopic eczema with EPO published in 1992 noted that placebo-controlled trials of parallel design demonstrated marked improvement for EPO. Patients treated with

EPO demonstrated less inflammation, dryness, scaling and overall severity compared to controls. Although these findings were supported by metaanalysis (see above), there was still conflicting evidence in trials based on a crossover design alone.[62] Since the publication of both the metaanalysis and the review, a number of trials with negative results have been conducted. Many of these are listed below.

In a double-blind, placebo-controlled trial, 60 children with atopic dermatitis received either EPO or placebo for 16 weeks. Improvement was observed in the eczema symptoms, although no significant difference was found between the two groups. No therapeutic effect was observed on asthma symptoms in the 22 patients who also had asthma.[63] In a double-blind, placebo-controlled, crossover trial, 24 children with atopic dermatitis received GLA (360 mg/day). After 10–14 weeks of treatment there was no improvement in the treatment compared to placebo (corn oil). Both groups improved while taking placebo.[64]

A double-blind, placebo-controlled trial for the treatment of chronic hand dermatitis in 39 patients over 24 weeks found that EPO (600 mg/day GLA equivalent) was not superior to placebo (sunflower oil 500 mg/day).[65] The choice of placebo may have masked the results, due to the linoleic acid content of the sunflower oil. In a double-blind, placebo-controlled, parallel trial, patients with atopic dermatitis were randomized to receive EPO, EPO plus fish oil or placebo for 16 weeks. One hundred and two patients completed the trial and no improvement was demonstrated by either EFA treatment.[66]

Psoriasis

A double-blind, parallel trial of a combination of EPO and fish oil in the treatment of 37 patients with chronic stable plaque psoriasis was undertaken. There was no significant improvement in clinical severity of psoriasis or change in transepidermal water loss.[67]

Female reproductive system disorders

Clinical trials conducted in the 1980s suggested that EPO demonstrated better activity than placebo in the treatment of premenstrual syndrome (PMS). Physical and psychological symptoms of PMS were significantly improved with EPO treatment, albeit slightly compared to placebo.[10] More information about several of these trials is outlined below.[68,69] However, a review of seven placebo-controlled trials of EPO in the treatment of PMS published in 1996 found inconsistent scoring and response criteria, making a rigorous metaanalysis inappropriate. The two most well-controlled trials failed to show any beneficial effects for EPO. These two trials were relatively small, however, and the authors noted that modest effects could not be ruled out.[70]

EPO treatment alleviated premenstrual symptoms and depression better than placebo in 30 women with severe PMS. The capacity of platelets to release thromboxane B_2 during spontaneous clotting was also decreased in patients receiving EPO compared to those receiving placebo.[68] Results from three double-blind, placebo-controlled studies, one large uncontrolled study on women who had failed other therapies for PMS and one large uncontrolled study on new patients all suggested EPO as an effective treatment for depression, breast pain and tenderness and fluid retention associated with PMS.[69]

Over 17 years up to 1992 at the Cardiff Mastalgia Clinic, 324 patients with cyclical and 90 with noncyclical mastalgia received a variety of drug treatments in clinical trials. In patients that responded to therapy, danazol was found to be the most effective drug (approximately 70%), with bromocriptine and EPO having equivalent efficacy (approximately 45%). Patients taking EPO reported fewer adverse events.[71,72]

A randomized, double-blind, placebo-controlled study investigated the efficacy of GLA in the treatment of menopausal hot flushes and sweating. Thirty-five women suffering hot flushes at least three times a day received either four capsules of 500 mg EPO plus 10 mg vitamin E or a placebo twice a day for 6 months. The only significant improvement for women taking GLA was a reduction in the maximum number of nighttime flushes ($p<0.05$). Overall there was no benefit over placebo in treating menopausal flushing.[73]

Diabetes

In randomized, double-blind, placebo-controlled, parallel trials conducted over seven centres in the UK and Finland, 111 patients with mild diabetic neuropathy received GLA (480 mg/day) or placebo over 1 year and were assessed by standard tests. A significant favourable change was noted in the treatment group for 13 of the 16 parameters investigated, demonstrating a clear beneficial effect on the course of mild diabetic neuropathy. Sex, age, diabetes type, age of onset or duration of diabetes did not significantly affect the result. The treatment was, however, more effective in relatively well-controlled diabetic patients.[74] Patients could continue in the trial for a further 12 months and all those who participated in this received GLA (unknowingly). Improvement continued over this period.[75]

Twenty-two patients with distal diabetic polyneuropathy who participated in a double-blind, placebo-controlled study received either 360 mg GLA per day or placebo capsules for 6 months. Patients in the treatment group showed significant improvement in the symptoms of distal diabetic polyneuropathy.[76]

Arthritis

A review of the clinical trials marked with asterisks (**) below has noted a limited applicability for their results. Overall, these studies were not well controlled (olive oil may itself produce beneficial results and may not be the best choice of placebo; the effect of vitamin E has not been completely ascertained). The trials did not run for long enough (at least 6 months is required to assess symptomatic improvement, longer than 1 year for disease-modifying potential). The concomitant use of medications was not standardized (some of the drugs may have influenced the patients' subjective assessment) and abrupt discontinuation of NSAIDs may have aggravated patients' symptoms early on, thus masking the effect of GLA. The most appropriate statistical tests were not conducted and drop-out rates were high.[77]

In a randomized, double-blind, placebo-controlled 24-week trial, 37 patients with rheumatoid arthritis and active synovitis received 1.4 g/day GLA or placebo. Treatment with GLA resulted in significant reduction in the signs and symptoms of disease activity ($p<0.05$) compared to the placebo group, which showed no change or worsened.[78]

**In a placebo-controlled clinical trial, 18 patients with rheumatoid arthritis received 20 ml/day of EPO (1500 mg GLA/day) or olive oil for 12 weeks. Plasma levels of PGE_2 decreased and thromboxane B_2 increased in both treatment groups, but no significant improvement in laboratory findings or clinical signs occurred in either group.[79] **In a double-blind, placebo-controlled clinical trial, 49 rheumatoid arthritis patients were treated with EPO (540 mg GLA/day), EPO plus fish oil (240 mg GLA + 450 mg EPA/day) or placebo, over a period of 12 months. Significant improvement was demonstrated in subjective symptoms as well as a significant reduction in NSAID therapy for those receiving EPO and EPO plus fish oil, compared to placebo. After this treatment period, placebo was given to all patients for a following 3 months. After 3 months of placebo, the condition of those originally receiving the EPO/fish oil treatment had relapsed. Despite the changes in subjective assessment of symptoms and NSAID use throughout the treatment, EPO did not alter any of the biochemical indicators of the disease.[80] **Forty patients with rheumatoid arthritis and upper gastrointestinal lesions due to NSAIDs took part in a double-blind placebo-controlled study over a 6-month period. Patients received either 6 g/day EPO or 6 g/day of olive oil. Three patients in each group also reduced their dose of NSAIDs. A significant reduction in morning stiffness occurred in the EPO group at 3 months. A significant reduction in pain and articular index occurred at 6 months for those taking olive oil.[81]

In a double-blind, placebo-controlled clinical trial, 56 patients with active rheumatoid arthritis received either GLA (2.8 g/day) or placebo (sunflower oil) over a period of 6 months. Following this, all patients received GLA for 6 months in single-blind fashion. Treatment with GLA resulted in significant reductions in the signs and symptoms of disease activity. At least 25% improvement in four measured parameters occurred for more patients in the treatment group (14 of 22) than in placebo group (four of 19). During the second 6-month period, both groups exhibited improvement in disease activity.[82] In a double-blind, placebo-controlled trial, 38 patients with psoriatic arthritis received a combination of EPO and fish oil daily for 9 months. All patients then received placebo capsules for a further 3 months. At the third month of the study, patients reduced their intake of NSAIDs and maintained the decrease, symptoms permitting. All measures of skin and joint symptoms were unchanged by the treatment. The requirement for NSAIDs was unchanged for both the treatment and placebo groups.[83]

Schizophrenia

Studies in groups of schizophrenics from England, Ireland, Scotland, Japan and the USA have indicated a lowering of linoleic acid in patients' plasma phospholipids, with variation in other EFAs.[84–86] In one study, the omega-6 EFA levels were significantly reduced, whereas the omega-3 EFA were elevated in comparison to controls.[84]

In a randomized, single-blind, placebo-controlled trial, 21 inpatients with a schizophrenic illness resistant to neuroleptic drug treatments received either neuroleptic medication and DGLA, placebo and DGLA, or two placebo medications. No marked treatment effects were noticed on ratings of the patients' behaviour or symptomatology, although some positive clinical effects were noted in dyskinetic patients.[87]

In a double-blind, placebo-controlled, crossover trial, 37 psychiatric patients, predominantly schizophrenics with tardive dyskinesia (abnormal involuntary movements), received capsules containing EPO over 16 weeks. A further 37 people in two groups, a psychiatric control group and a normal control group, were given a placebo. Although EFA supplementation did not produce improvement in abnormal movement measurements, there was significant improvement in mental state, schizophrenic symptoms and memory. In the open phase at the end of the trial, addition of co-factors (zinc, niacin and vitamins C and B_6) to EPO treatment produced an increase in omega-3 and omega-6 EFA incorporation into red cell membranes. During this phase, marked and significant clinical improvements in memory, schizophrenic symptoms and abnormal movement were observed in comparison to placebo or EPO-only treatment.[88–90]

Cardiovascular effects

In a partially double-blinded, placebo-controlled clinical trial, a combination of EPO and fish oil, magnesium oxide or a placebo were administered to pregnant women for 6 months; 21% of the women had personal or family histories of hypertension. Those taking the EPO and fish oil had significantly lower incidence of oedema (13%) compared to the control group (29%) ($p=0.004$). Significantly fewer women developed hypertension in the group receiving magnesium oxide. Three cases of eclampsia occurred, all in the control group.[91]

In an uncontrolled clinical trial, 12 hyperlipidaemic patients received 3 g/day GLA for 4 months. After treatment, plasma triglyceride levels were decreased by 48% ($p<0.001$), HDL-cholesterol levels increased by 22% ($p<0.01$) and total cholesterol and LDL-cholesterol levels were significantly decreased. Experimentally induced platelet aggregation and serum thromboxane B_2 levels decreased, with a significant increase in bleeding time.[92]

In a double-blind, placebo-controlled crossover study, 25 non-obese patients with uncomplicated essential hypertension received placebo for 4 weeks followed by EPO plus fish oil or sunflower seed and linseed oil for 12 weeks. The mean systolic blood pressure of patients receiving EPO plus fish oil was significantly lowered after 8 and 12 weeks, while those receiving sunflower/linseed oil had no significant reduction of blood pressure.[93]

In a double-blind, placebo-controlled study, 21 patients with Raynaud's phenomenon received a 2-week course of placebo, after which 11 received EPO for 8 weeks and 10 received placebo. Patients receiving EPO experienced significant improvement in symptoms, but there was no change in blood flow despite changes in platelet behaviour and thromboxane B_2 levels.[94]

Cancer therapy

EPO and vitamin C given to six patients with primary liver cell cancer demonstrated some clinical improvement and reduction in tumour size (three patients). One patient demonstrated marked reduction of liver and tumour size and liver damage.[95]

In an uncontrolled clinical trial, GLA was administered by intracerebral injection (1 mg/day for 10 days) to 15 patients with malignant gliomas. The cerebral gliomas regressed, as evidenced by computed tomography, and patients' survival was increased by 1.5–2 years.[96]

Other effects

In a clinical trial conducted in old people's homes, 40 women with confirmed osteoporosis were divided into four groups and received either fish oil, EPO, fish oil plus EPO or olive oil (control) over 16 weeks. Serum alkaline phosphatase levels dropped in both the fish oil and the combined oil groups, indicating an increase in bone mineral density. Osteocalcin levels, an indicator of bone growth, rose in the fish oil group and more significantly in the combined oil group. Although the EPO had no effect on its own, it increased the effect of the fish oil on the bone formation markers, probably due to a more balanced plasma fatty acid profile.[97]

In a randomized, placebo-controlled study, 43 patients with stable ulcerative colitis received either EPO, fish oil or olive oil (placebo) for 6 months in addition to their usual medication. Alteration of cell membrane fatty acids was observed for those taking EPO and fish oil compared to the control group. Although there was no difference in stool frequency, rectal bleeding, disease relapse, sigmoidoscopic appearance or rectal histology in the three groups, EPO significantly improved stool consistency compared to fish oil and placebo at 6 months and this difference was maintained for 3 months after treatment was discontinued ($p<0.05$).[98]

In a double-blind, placebo-controlled study, 63 patients with postviral fatigue syndrome received a preparation containing EPO (80%) and fish oil (20%) or placebo (8×500 mg capsules per day) over a 3-month period. At the end of the trial, 85% of patients in the treatment group compared to 17% in the control group assessed themselves as improved ($p<0.0001$). A normalization of essential fatty acid levels in red blood cell membranes was observed in the treatment group.[99]

In a double-blind, placebo-controlled clinical trial, the effect of EPO supplementation to alcoholics was investigated. In the early weeks of withdrawal from alcohol, EPO significantly reduced the severity of the withdrawal syndrome and improved liver function. Relapse rates over 6 and 12 months did not improve. However, in those who did not relapse, several parameters of cerebral function (such as memory and visual motor coordination) improved significantly with EPO treatment.[10] A review of the role of EFAs in alcohol dependence notes that if alcohol-induced tissue damage is associated with impaired fatty acid and phospholipid metabolism, supplements of EFAs may be beneficial in the treatment of alcoholics.[100]

In a double-blind, placebo-controlled study, 89 renal transplantation patients received either EPO or placebo, together with standard immunosuppressive medication. Graft survival was significantly better in the EPO group compared to controls during the first 3–4 months posttransplant, but not significantly different at 6 months.[101]

TOXICOLOGY

High doses of 5–10 ml/kg/day administered to several animals exhibited no toxic effects or carcinogenicity.[102]

CONTRAINDICATIONS

EPO may have potential to instigate undiagnosed temporal lobe epilepsy, especially in those receiving phenothiazines.[103] This is unlikely on current evidence but caution should apply (see Side effects below).

SPECIAL WARNINGS AND PRECAUTIONS

As listed above in Contraindications.

INTERACTIONS

Avoid concomitant use with phenothiazines.

USE IN PREGNANCY AND LACTATION

No problems anticipated; may even be beneficial.

EFFECTS ON ABILITY TO DRIVE AND USE MACHINES

None known.

SIDE EFFECTS

General

The most common adverse effects reported in trials using GLA for the treatment of the above conditions are headache and mild nausea.[77]

Arachidonate build-up

The potential risk of arachidonate build-up associated with long-term use of GLA in the treatment of rheumatoid arthritis has recently been raised. Several tests have shown GLA administration to increase arachidonate levels: 2.0 g per day of GLA given to previously obese women increased the arachidonate content of their serum phospholipids. With prolonged administration of GLA over more than a year, arachidonate could accumulate in tissue, thus possibly counteracting early therapeutic effects of GLA. Tissue build-up of arachidonate might promote subsequent inflammation, thrombosis and immunosuppression. Symptoms may rebound in patients after discontinuation of GLA.[104]

Epilepsy

In recent years there has been concern for the use of EPO in patients with a history of epilepsy. Originally this concern arose from trials in patients with schizophrenia who were being treated concomitantly with antischizophrenic drugs (phenothiazines and related compounds). Episodes of epilepsy were reported, but no definite link to EPO treatment was established. Rather, the nature of the mental illness and side effects of the orthodox medication were the more likely cause. Similar events have been reported in patients not taking EPO.[10,105] Moreover, it can be extremely difficult to distinguish between schizophrenia and temporal lobe epilepsy. Three hospitalized schizophrenics who failed to respond to conventional drug therapy became substantially worse when treated with EPO. A later diagnosis of temporal lobe epilepsy resulted in successful treatment (with conventional drugs).[106]

There have been no other reports of an epileptic attack being associated with EPO preparations other than the ones below.[107] Perhaps in response to the trials in patients with schizophrenia, the British Epilepsy Association warned those with epilepsy to avoid EPO because of a possible lowering of the threshold for seizures.[107,108] Currently the reported position of Australian doctors is that EPO should be avoided in patients with a history of epilepsy.[103,109] This position is probably excessively cautious.

A 45-year-old woman who had been taking herbal preparations containing black cohosh, chaste tree and evening primrose oil for 4 months had three seizures within a 3-month period. The herbal preparations were stopped and the patient was treated with anticonvulsants.[110] No causal link between the seizures and the herbal treatment was established.

OVERDOSE

No toxic effects reported.

CURRENT REGULATORY STATUS IN SELECTED COUNTRIES

Evening primrose oil is not covered by a Commission E monograph and is not on the UK General Sale List.

Evening primrose oil does not have GRAS status. However, it is freely available as a 'dietary supplement' in the USA under DSHEA legislation (1994 Dietary Supplement Health and Education Act).

Evening primrose oil is not included in Part 4 of Schedule 4 of the Therapeutic Goods Act Regulations of Australia.

References

1. Mabberley DJ. The plant book, 2nd edn. Cambridge University Press, Cambridge: 1997; p 499.
2. Weiss RF. Herbal medicine. Beaconsfield Publishers, Beaconsfield, 1988; p 333.
3. Grieve M. A modern herbal, vol 2. Dover Publications, New York 1971; p 657.
4. Leung AY, Foster S. Encyclopedia of common natural ingredients used in food, drugs and cosmetics, 2nd edn. John Wiley, New York, 1996; p 236.
5. Launert EL. The Hamlyn guide to edible and medicinal plants of Britain and Northern Europe. Hamlyn, London: 1981; p 86.
6. Chiej R. The Macdonald encyclopedia of medicinal plants. Macdonald, London: 1984; entry no. 208.
7. Therapeutic Goods Administration. Approved terminology for drugs. Australian Government Publishing Service, Canberra, 1995.
8. Tyler VE, Brady LR, Robbers JE. Pharmacognosy, 9th edn. Lea and Febiger, Philadelphia: 1988; p 471.
9. Redden PR, Lin X, Horrobin DF. Chem Phys Lipids 1996; 79 (1): 9–19.
10. Horrobin DF. Rev Contemp Pharmacother 1990; 1: 1–45.
11. Cameron NE, Cotter MA. Diabetes 1997; 46 (suppl 2): S31–37.
12. Jamal GA. Diabet Med 1994; 11 (2): 145–149.
13. Julu, PO. J Diabetic Complicat 1988; 2 (4): 185–188.
14. Tomlinson DR, Robinson JP, Compton AM et al. Diabetologia 1989; 32 (9): 655–659.
15. Dines KC, Cotter MA, Cameron NE. Prostagland Leukot Essent Fatty Acids 1996; 55 (3): 159–165.
16. Omawari N, Dewhurst M, Vo P et al. Br J Pharmacol 1996; 118 (1): 186–190.
17. Julu PO, Gow JW, Jamal GA. J Lipid Mediat Cell Signal 1996; 13 (2): 115–125.
18. Julu PO. J Lipid Mediat Cell Signal 1996; 13 (2): 99–113.
19. Chaintreuil J, Monnier L, Colette C et al. Hum Nutr Clin Nutr 1984; 38 (2): 121–130.
20. Karmali RA. Prostagland Leukot Med 1987; 29 (2–3): 199–204.
21. Tate GA, Mandell BF, Karmali RA et al. Arthritis Rheum 1988; 31 (12): 1543–1551.
22. Tate GA, Mandell BF, Laposata M et al. J Rheumatol 1989; 16 (6): 729–734.
23. Prichard P, Brown G, Bhaskar N et al. Aliment Pharmacol Ther 1988; 2 (2): 179–184.
24. De La Hunt MN, Hillier K, Jewell R. Prostaglandins 1988; 35 (4): 597–608.
25. Huang YS, Drummond R, Horrobin DF. Digestion 1987; 36 (1): 36–41.
26. Raederstorff D, Moser U. Lipids 1992; 27 (12): 1018–1023.
27. Johnson MM, Swan DD, Surette ME et al. J Nutr 1997; 127 (8): 1435–1444.
28. Claassen N, Coetzer H, Steinmann CM et al. Prostagland Leukot Essent Fatty Acids 1995; 53 (1): 13–19.
29. Claassen N, Potgieter HC, Seppa M et al. Bone 1995; 16 (4 suppl): 385S–392S.
30. Tauson AH, Forsberg M. Acta Vet Scand 1991; 32 (3): 345–351.
31. Tauson AH, Neil M, Forsberg M. Acta Vet Scand 1991; 32 (3): 337–344.
32. Begin ME, Ells G, Horrobin DF. J Natl Cancer Inst 1988; 80 (3): 188–194.
33. Begin ME, Ells G, Das UN. Anticancer Res 1986; 6 (2): 291–295.
34. Das UN, Begin ME, Ells G et al. Biochem Biophys Res Commun 1987; 145 (1): 15–24.
35. Pritchard GA, Jones DL, Mansel RE. Br J Surg 1989; 76 (10): 1069–1073.
36. Hoffmann P, Taube C, Bartels T et al. Biomed Biochim Acta 1984; 43 (8–9): S195–S198.
37. Hassall CH, Kirtland SJ. Lipids 1984; 19 (9): 699–703.
38. Narce M, Poisson JP. Arch Mal Coeur Vaiss 1996; 89 (8): 1025–1028.
39. Mills DE, Ward RP, Mah M et al. Lipids 1989; 24 (1): 17–24.
40. Mills DE, Summers MR, Ward RP et al. Lipids 1985; 20 (9): 573–577.
41. Mills DE, Ward RP. Lipids 1986; 21 (2): 139–142.
42. Al-Shabanah OA. Food Chem Toxicol 1997; 35 (8): 769–775.
43. Leichsenring M, Kochsiek U, Paul K. Pediatr Allergy Immunol 1995; 6 (4): 209–212.
44. Varma PK, Persaud TV. Prostagland Leukot Med 1982; 8 (6): 641–645.
45. Barcelli UO, Miyata J, Ito Y et al. Prostaglandins 1986; 32 (2): 211–219.
46. Papanikolaou N. Prostagland Leukot Med 1987; 27 (2–3): 129–149.
47. Bezard J, Blond JP, Bernard A et al. Reprod Nutr Dev 1994; 34 (6): 539–568.
48. Martens-Lobenhoffer J, Meyer FP. Int J Clin Pharmacol Ther 1998; 36 (7): 363–366.
49. Harvey RG. Vet Rec 1993; 133 (23): 571–573.
50. Harvey RG. Vet Rec 1993; 133 (9): 208–211.
51. Scarff DH, Lloyd DH. Vet Rec 1992; 131 (5): 97–99.
52. Janossy IM, Raguz JM, Rippke F et al. H & GJ 1995; 70: 498–502.
53. Fiocchi A, Sala M, Signoroni P et al. J Int Med Res 1994; 22 (1): 24–32.
54. Stewart JCM, Morse PF, Moss M et al. Cited in Horrobin DF. Rev Contemp Pharmacother 1990; 1: 1–45.
55. Schalin-Karrila M, Mattila L, Jansen CT et al. Br J Dermatol 1987; 117 (1): 11–19.
56. Marshall RJ, Evans RW. Cited in Horrobin DF (ed) Omega-6 essential fatty acids: pathophysiology and roles in clinical medicine. Wiley Liss, New York, 1990; pp 81–98.
57. Nissen HP Wehrmann W, Kvoll U et al. Fat Sci Technol 1988; 7: 247.
58. Biagi PL, Bordoni A, Hrelia S et al. Drugs Exp Clin Res 1994; 20 (2): 77–84.
59. Humphreys F, Symons JA, Brown HK et al. Eur J Dermatol 1994; 4 (8): 598–603.
60. Bordoni A, Biagi PL, Masi M et al. Drugs Exp Clin Res 1988; 14 (4): 291–297.
61. Morse PF, Horrobin DF, Manku MS et al. Br J Dermatol 1989; 121 (1): 75–90.
62. Kerscher MJ, Korting HC. Clin Invest 1992; 70 (2): 167–171.
63. Hederos CA, Berg A. Arch Dis Child 1996; 75 (6): 494–497.
64. Borrek S, Hildebrande A, Forster J. Klin Paediatr 1997; 209 (3): 100–104.

65. Whitaker DK, Cilliers J, De Beer C. Dermatology 1996; 193 (2): 115–120.
66. Berth-Jones J, Graham-Brown RA. Lancet 1993; 341 (8860): 1557–1560.
67. Oliwiecki S, Burton JL. Clin Exp Dermatol 1994; 19 (2): 127–129.
68. Puolakka J, Makarainen L, Viinikka L et al. J Reprod Med 1985; 30 (3): 149–153.
69. Horrobin DF. J Reprod Med 1983; 28 (7): 465–468.
70. Budeiri D, Li Wan Po A, Dornan JC. Control Clin Trials 1996; 17 (1): 60–68.
71. Gateley CA, Miers M, Mansel RE et al. J Roy Soc Med 1992; 85 (1): 12–15.
72. Pye JK, Mansel RE, Hughes LE. Lancet 1985; 2 (8451): 373–377.
73. Chenoy R, Hussain S, Tayob Y et al. Br Med J 1994; 308 (6927): 501–503.
74. Keen H, Payan J, Allawi J et al. Diabetes Care 1993; 16 (1): 8–15.
75. Scotia Pharmaceuticals Ltd. Pioneering research in diabetic neuropathy. The EF4 project: the role of gamma-linolenic acid. Scotia Pharmaceuticals Ltd, England, 1991: pp 11–16
76. Jamal GA, Carmichael H. Diabet Med 1990; 7 (4): 319–323.
77. Joe LA, Hart LL. Ann Pharmacother 1993; 27 (12): 1475–1477.
78. Leventhal LJ, Boyce EG, Zurier RB. Ann Intern Med 1993; 119 (9): 867–873.
79. Jantti J, Seppala E, Vapaatalo H et al. Clin Rheumatol 1989; 8 (2): 238–244.
80. Belch JJ, Ansell D, Madhok R et al. Ann Rheum Dis 1988; 47 (2): 96–104.
81. Brzeski M, Madhok R, Capell HA. Br J Rheumatol 1991; 30 (5): 370–372.
82. Zurier RB, Rossetti RG, Jacobson EW et al. Arthritis Rheum 1996; 39 (11): 1808–1817.
83. Veale DJ, Torley HI, Richards IM et al. Br J Rheumatol 1994; 33 (10): 954–958.
84. Horrobin DF, Manku MS, Morse-Fisher N et al. Biol Psychiatry 1989; 25 (5): 562–568.
85. Bates C, Horrobin DF, Ells K. Schizophr Res 1991; 6 (1): 1–7.
86. Kaiya H, Horrobin DF, Manku MS et al. Biol Psychiatry 1991; 30 (4): 357–362.
87. Vaddadi KS, Gilleard CJ, Mindham RH et al. Psychopharmacology (Berl) 1986; 88 (3): 362–367.
88. Vaddadi KS. Prostagland Leukot Essent Fatty Acids 1992; 46 (1): 67–70.
89. Vaddadi KS, Courtney P, Gilleard CJ et al. Psychiatry Res 1989; 27 (3): 313–323.
90. Vaddadi K Prostaglandins Leukot Essent Fatty Acids 1996; 55(1–2): 89–94
91. D'Almeida A, Carter JP, Anatol A et al. Women's Health 1992; 19 (2–3): 117–131.
92. Guivernau M, Meza N, Barja P et al. Prostagland Leukot Essent Fatty Acids 1994; 51 (5): 311–316.
93. Venter CP, Joubert PH, Booyens J. Prostagland Leukot Essent Fatty Acids 1988; 33 (1): 49–51.
94. Belch JJ, Shaw B, O'Dowd A et al. Thromb Haemost 1985; 54 (2): 490–494.
95. Booyens J Louwrens C, Engelbrecht P. S Afr J Sci 1984; 80: 144.
96. Das UN, Prasad VV, Reddy DR. Cancer Lett 1995; 94 (2): 147–155.
97. Van Papendorp DH Coetzer H, Kruger MC. Nutr Res 1995; 15(3): 325–334.
98. Greenfield SM, Green AT, Teare JP et al. Aliment Pharmacol Ther 1993; 7 (2): 159–166.
99. Behan PO, Behan WM, Horrobin D. Acta Neurol Scand 1990; 82 (3): 209–216.
100. Glen I, Skinner F, Glen E et al. Alcohol Clin Exp Res 1987; 11 (1): 37–41.
101. McHugh MI, Wilkinson R, Elliott RW et al. Transplantation 1977; 24 (4): 263–267.
102. Everett DJ Perry CJ, Bayliss P. Med Sci Res 1988; 16: 865–866.
103. Lin Wan Po A. Pharmaceut J 1991; 676–678
104. Phinney S. Ann Intern Med 1994; 120 (8): 692.
105. Holman CP, Bell AFJ. J Orthomolec Psychiatry 1983; 12: 302–304.
106. Vaddadi KS. Prostagland Med 1981; 6 (4): 375–379.
107. Dobbin SN. Vet Rec 1992; 131 (25–26): 591.
108. Arundel BL. Vet Rec 1992; 131 (23): 543.
109. Editorial. Curr Therapeut 1992; 67.
110. Shuster J. Hosp Pharm 1996; 31: 1553–1554.

Eyebright (*Euphrasia officinalis* L.)

SYNONYMS

E. rostkoviana Hayne (botanical synonym), Euphrasiae herba (Lat), Augentrostkraut (Ger), herbe d'euphraise officinale, casse-lunettes (Fr), eufrasia (Ital), lægeøjentrøst (Dan).

WHAT IS IT?

The name Euphrasia is derived from the Greek word *euphrosyne*, meaning gladness, due to its use in folk medicine for the treatment of eye complaints. It is this use that also gave rise to the vernacular name eyebright. Eyebright can be used topically as a poultice or eyewash for eye problems and as a nasal douche for inflamed or catarrhal mucous membranes. It can also be taken orally for these conditions.

EFFECTS

Relieves conjunctivitis, itchy, irritated eyes; reduces excessive upper respiratory secretions and catarrh.

TRADITIONAL VIEW

Eyebright was used in the 14th century as an eye medicine and was said to 'cure all evils of the eye'.[1] Eyebright was considered slightly tonic and astringent and it was employed for all mucous diseases attended with increased discharges, specifically for the nasal membranes and lacrimal apparatus (acute catarrhal diseases of the eyes, nose and ears). Catarrhal diseases of the digestive tract may also be treated with eyebright.[2]

SUMMARY OF ACTIONS

Astringent, anticatarrhal, antiinflammatory.

CAN BE USED FOR

INDICATIONS SUPPORTED BY CLINICAL TRIALS

No clinical trials have been conducted using this herb.

TRADITIONAL THERAPEUTIC USES

Eye conditions such as irritation and redness, infection, inflammation, particularly conjunctivitis and blepharitis;[2] nasal catarrh, particularly where there is profuse watery flow;[2] sinusitis, chronic sneezing, hayfever and middle ear problems; sore throat; catarrhal phase which occurs during and after measles.[3]

MAY ALSO BE USED FOR

EXTRAPOLATIONS FROM PHARMACOLOGICAL STUDIES

Because of its aucubin content, eyebright may be useful in the treatment of bacterial infections and liver toxicity. It may also possess antiviral and nerve-regenerating activity for the same reason.

PREPARATIONS

Dried or fresh herb as an infusion, poultice or liquid extract for topical use. Infusion, extract or tablets for internal use. For use in eyebaths, decoctions with greater than 10 minutes at boiling, with transfer to a sterile container, are recommended.

DOSAGE

- 2–4 g of dried herb three times per day or as an infusion.
- 2–4 ml of 1:2 liquid extract three times per day, 2–6 ml of 1:5 tincture, three times per day.

DURATION OF USE

May be taken long term.

SUMMARY ASSESSMENT OF SAFETY

No significant adverse effects from topical use or ingestion of eyebright are expected; however, the requirement for sterility of topical preparations for the eye should be observed.

TECHNICAL DATA

BOTANY

Euphrasia officinalis, in the narrow sense equivalent to *E. rostkoviana*,[4] is a small plant which grows to approximately 15 cm in height and is a member of the Scrophulariaceae (figwort) family. The leaves are

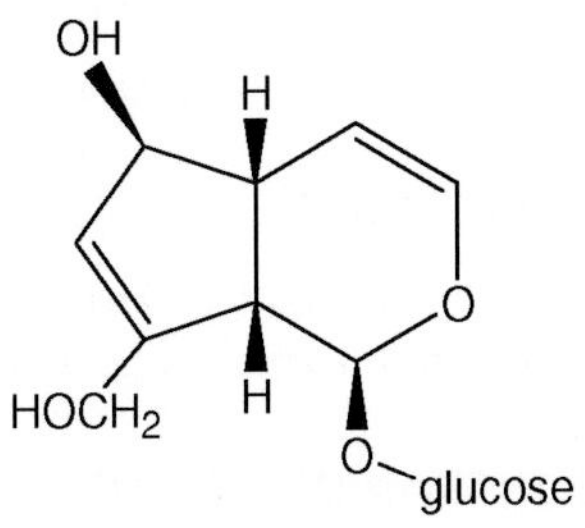

Aucubin

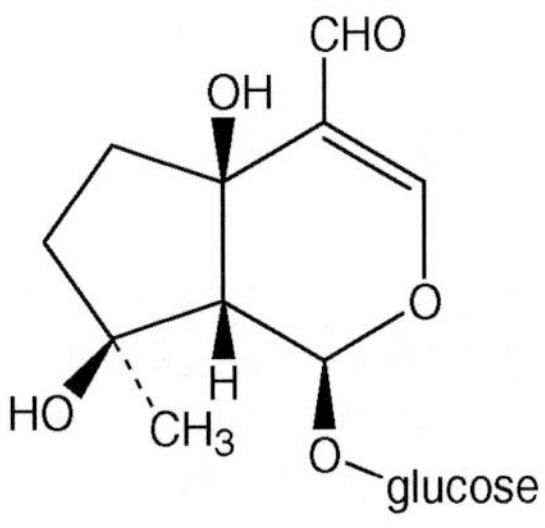

Euphroside

opposite, ovate or cordate, downy, strongly ribbed and furrowed. The inodorous flowers are axillary, solitary and very abundant. They are most commonly white, with deep purple streaks and a yellowish palate. The oblong, flattened seed pods contain numerous seeds which are oblong and grooved lengthwise.[2]

KEY CONSTITUENTS

- Iridoid glycosides, including aucubin, catalpol, euphroside, ixoroside.[5]
- Flavonoids, including quercetin and apigenin glycosides; lignans.[5]

PHARMACODYNAMICS

Most of the published pharmacodynamic papers have examined the constituent aucubin or its aglycone. Aucubin is common to many other plants, including *Plantago lanceolata*. The fact that plants containing aucubin have been used in many different traditions for the treatment of respiratory catarrh suggests that aucubin may possess chemically relevant antimicrobial and anticatarrhal activities.

Antimicrobial activity

Aucubigenin, the aglycone of aucubin, was shown to be antibacterial against organisms such as *Micrococcus aureus*, *Escherichia coli*, *Bacillus subtilis*, *Mycobacterium phlei* and to a lesser extent showed antifungal activity against a small number of fungi, with *Penicillium italicum* being the most sensitive.[6]

Aucubin alone had no antiviral activity in vitro. However, when aucubin (100–1000 μM/ml) was mixed with beta-glucosidase (an enzyme that releases the aglycone from the glycoside) it had significant antiviral activity against hepatitis B.[7]

Hepatoprotective activity

In vivo studies demonstrated that aucubin has hepatoprotective activity against such liver toxins as carbon tetrachloride,[8] alpha-amanitin[9] and an aqueous extract of amanita mushroom. Even postadministration of aucubin after amanita mushroom ingestion led to complete survival.[10]

An in vitro study demonstrated that aucubigenin inhibited cytochrome P-450 in isolated rat hepatocytes. Aucubin had no effect. The authors commented that the reported hepatoprotection of aucubin against carbon tetrachloride would appear to be due to inactivation of P-450 by the aglycone aucubigenin, which is probably formed in vivo through hydrolysis in the gut.[11]

Antitumour activity

When administered intraperitoneally at a dose of 100 mg/kg, the aglycone of aucubin was found to have antitumour activity in mice bearing the experimental tumour leukaemia P388. Aucubin, also administered intraperitoneally (100 mg/kg), showed no antitumour activity. It therefore appears that the hemiacetal aglycone structure is important for the antitumour activity.[12]

Antispasmodic activity

Peracetylated aucubin in vitro exerted a non-specific antispasmodic effect on contractions of rat uterus induced by acetylcholine and calcium chloride. In vitro antispasmodic activity was also found for rat vas deferens which was depolarized by potassium. The degree of activity was similar to papaverine.[13]

Other activity

Aucubin, administered orally at a dose of 100 mg/kg, had an antiinflammatory effect on carrageenan-induced mouse paw oedema. An antiinflammatory effect was also shown on TPA-induced mouse ear oedema with topical application of 1 mg/ear of aucubin.[14] The most important feature in neuronal cell differentiation is outgrowth of neurites and regulation of this outgrowth is considered to be one of the most basic mechanisms in the development and regeneration of the nerve tissues. Discovery of materials that increase the outgrowth of neurites could lead to the development of antidementia drugs, since dementia is characterized by progressive neuronal degeneration.[15] The aglycone of aucubin (at a dose of 1 and 10 μg/ml), but not aucubin itself, was very effective in inducing cultured cell line of paraneuron PC12h to differentiate, causing a morphological change characterized by extended neurites and promotion of neurite outgrowth.[15,16]

PHARMACOKINETICS

Anaerobic incubation of aucubin with defined strains of human intestinal bacteria and with human faeces resulted in its transformation into aucubigenin and the pyridine monoterpene alkaloids aucubinine A and aucubinine B. Among the 25 species isolated from human faeces which were examined, 21 species produced aucubinine A and a trace of aucubinine B. Aucubin may be initially hydrolysed to aucubigenin and glucose by bacterial beta-glucosidase, followed by a series of reactions, the first involving ammonia, to yield aucubinines A and B. The nitrogen atom could originate from ammonia produced by bacteria (some species such as *Klebsiella pneumoniae* have high levels of intracellular ammonia).[17] This finding suggests that, in order to convert aucubin into the active aglycone aucubigenin, there must be high levels of favourable gut bacteria.

In another pharmacokinetic study, aucubin was given intravenously, orally, intraperitoneally and hepatoportally to rats. The bioavailabilities of aucubin after administration at a dose of 100 mg/kg through hepatoportal, intraperitoneal and oral routes were 83.5%, 76.8% and 19.3% respectively. The low oral bioavailability of aucubin is probably due to its metabolism by gut flora as outlined above.[18]

TOXICOLOGY

No data available. However, toxic effects have not been noted from use of eyebright.

CONTRAINDICATIONS

None known.

SPECIAL WARNINGS AND PRECAUTIONS

None known.

INTERACTIONS

No adverse interactions known.

USE IN PREGNANCY AND LACTATION

No adverse effects expected.

EFFECTS ON ABILITY TO DRIVE AND USE MACHINES

No adverse effects.

SIDE EFFECTS

None known.

OVERDOSE

No effects known.

CURRENT REGULATORY STATUS IN SELECTED COUNTRIES

Eyebright is covered by a null Commission E monograph. The Commission E recommends that as the efficacy has not been documented, the topical application of eyebright cannot be recommended because of hygienic reasons.

Eyebright is on the UK General Sale List.

Eyebright does not have GRAS status. However, it is freely available as a 'dietary supplement' in the USA under DSHEA legislation (1994 Dietary Supplement Health and Education Act).

Eyebright is not included in Part 4 of Schedule 4 of the Therapeutic Goods Act Regulations of Australia.

References

1. Grieve M. A modern herbal, vol 1. Dover Publications, New York: 1971; pp 290–293.
2. Felter HW, Lloyd JU. King's American dispensatory, 18th edn, 3rd revision, vol 2, 1905. Reprinted by Eclectic Medical Publications, Portland: 1983; pp 751–752.
3. Bartram T. Encyclopedia of herbal medicine. Grace Publishers, Dorset: 1995; p 177.
4. Mabberley DJ. The plant book, 2nd edn. Cambridge University Press, Cambridge: 1997; p 274.
5. Wagner H, Bladt S. Plant drug analysis: a thin layer chromatography atlas, 2nd edn. Springer-Verlag, Berlin: 1996; p 75.
6. Rombouts JE, Links J. Experientia 1956; 12 (2): 78–80.
7. Chang I. Phytother Res 1997; 11: 189–192.
8. Chang IM, Ryu JC, Park YC et al. Drug Chem Toxicol 1983; 6 (5): 443–453.
9. Chang IM, Yun HS, Kim YS et al. J Toxicol Clin Toxicol 1984; 22 (1): 77–85.
10. Chang IM, Yamaura Y. Phytother Res 1993; 7: 53–56.
11. Batholomaeus A, Ahokas J. Toxicol Lett 1995; 80: 75–83.
12. Isiguro K, Yamaki M, Takagi S et al. Chem Pharm Bull 1986; 34 (6): 2375–2379.
13. Ortiz de Urbina AV, Martin ML, Fernandez B et al. Planta Med 1994; 60: 512–515.
14. Recio M, Giner RM, Manez S, Rios JL. Planta Med 1994; 60: 232–234.
15. Matsumi Y, Katsunori H, Kenzo C et al. Biol Pharm Bull 1994; 17 (12): 1604–1608.
16. Matsumi Y, Kenzo C, Tetsuro M. Biol Pharm Bull 1996; 19 (6): 791–795.
17. Hattori M, Kawata Y, Inoue K et al. Phytother Res 1990; 4 (2): 66–70.
18. Suh N, Shim C, Lee MH et al. Pharm Res 1991; 8 (8): 1059–1063.

Fennel fruit (*Foeniculum vulgare* Mill.)

SYNONYMS

Foeniculum officinale Mill. (botanical synonym), Foeniculi fructus (Lat), Fenchel, Bitterfenchel (Ger), aneth fenouil, fenouil (Fr), finocchio (Ital), fennikel frø (Dan), xian hui xiang (Chin).

WHAT IS IT?

Fennel is a well-known culinary herb or vegetable. It was cultivated by the ancient Romans for its aromatic fruit and succulent edible shoots and was frequently mentioned in Anglo-Saxon cookery and medical recipes prior to the Norman conquest. Fennel shoots, fennel seed and fennel water were all mentioned in ancient Spanish agricultural records. In medieval times, fennel, in conjunction with St John's wort and other herbs, was hung over doors on Midsummer's Eve to ward off evil spirits. Similarly, it was used as a condiment for the salt fish consumed during Lent. Fennel seeds were discovered amongst the personal chattels of Egyptian pharaohs which were salvaged from the tombs.

The fruit (often called the seed) or root are the parts most commonly used for medical purposes (although the roots are no longer used as they are considered inferior to the seed). The exact species definition varies between different authorities but it is agreed that *Foeniculum vulgare* Miller is represented by two varieties in cultivation (common names are designated bitter fennel and sweet fennel).[1,2] These different varieties of fennel are difficult to separate, mainly due to their tendency to hybridize.[3]

EFFECTS

Relaxes sphincters and decreases spasm of the gastrointestinal tract; acts as an expectorant in the respiratory tract, increases the mucociliary activity of the ciliary epithelium; exerts oestrogenic activity, increases milk flow.

TRADITIONAL VIEW

Fennel was used as a carminative to treat flatulent colic, windy colic in infants, irritable bowel syndrome and to increase appetite.[4] It had an ancient reputation for strengthening eyesight and was used topically to treat conjunctivitis and blepharitis.[5,6] The fruits are said to benefit nausea, hiccups, shortness of breath and wheezing. Syrup made from the fresh juice was used for chronic coughs. The leaves were once used by poor people to satisfy the cravings of hunger on fasting days.[5] It has also been used for the treatment of amenorrhoea and to increase milk production in nursing mothers.[7] A gargle is used to treat mouth and throat inflammation.[6] Paradoxically, fennel has been used in both anorexia[4,6] and obesity.[5,8]

In traditional Chinese medicine, fennel is used to treat *Cold* hernia-like disorders and any kind of lower abdominal pain from *Cold* and *Cold Stomach* patterns with symptoms such as abdominal pain, indigestion, decreased appetite and vomiting.[9]

SUMMARY ACTIONS

Carminative, spasmolytic, galactagogue, oestrogenic, antimicrobial, expectorant.

CAN BE USED FOR

INDICATIONS SUPPORTED BY CLINICAL TRIALS

Dyspeptic conditions of the upper GIT, including pain, nausea, belching and heartburn; chronic non-specific colitis with diarrhoea or constipation; infantile colic (all in combination with other herbs).

TRADITIONAL THERAPEUTIC USES

Digestive disorders (windy colic in infants, flatulent colic, griping pain, irritable bowel); suppressed lactation; obesity; topically for conjunctivitis, pharyngitis. Internal use and as an eyebath to strengthen eyesight and for inflammatory conditions of the external eye (such as conjunctivitis). Fennel has been added to herbal powders to allay their tendency to gripe[10] and is a constituent of 'Gripe Water',[5] a popular proprietary liquid for infants.

MAY ALSO BE USED FOR

EXTRAPOLATIONS FROM PHARMACOLOGICAL STUDIES

To reduce vaginal fragility and other symptoms in postmenopausal women.

OTHER APPLICATIONS

Fennel is also used as a flavouring agent in tea mixtures,[11] alcoholic and non-alcoholic beverages and food products.[12] Fennel oil can be used as an antiseptic ingredient in toothpastes and mouthwashes; an ingredient in antiwrinkle and antiageing skin products and cellulite products;[13] and in soaps, detergents, creams, lotions and perfumes.[12]

PREPARATIONS

Fruits as a decoction, syrup (including honey), liquid extract, essential oil and tablets for internal use. Decoction, extract or essential oil for topical use.

As with all essential oil-containing herbs, use of the fresh plant or carefully dried herb is advised. Keep covered if infusing the herb to retain the essential oil.

DOSAGE

- 900–1800 mg of the dried fruit per day or as infusion.
- 3 to 6 ml of 1:2 liquid extract per day, 7–14 ml of 1:5 tincture per day.
- 5–20 drops of the essential oil per day.

DURATION OF USE

The Commission E advises that fennel preparations should not be taken for more than several weeks without doctors' advice.[14] Despite this unexplained caution, fennel is safe for use in the long term.

SUMMARY ASSESSMENT OF SAFETY

Except in rare cases of contact allergy in susceptible patients, fennel is an extremely safe herb.

TECHNICAL DATA

BOTANY

Foeniculum vulgare, a member of the Umbelliferae (carrot) family, is a bluish green biennial or perennial herb that can grow to a height of 2 m. The leaves have a thick, fleshy edible sheath at the base, are 3–4 times pinnate, triangular and consist of thread-like segments up to 5 cm long. The flowers are 1–2 mm in diameter, have five yellow petals and are grouped in small umbels which in turn are grouped into larger umbels. The fruit consists of two prominently ribbed ovoid achenes 4–6 mm long.[15,16]

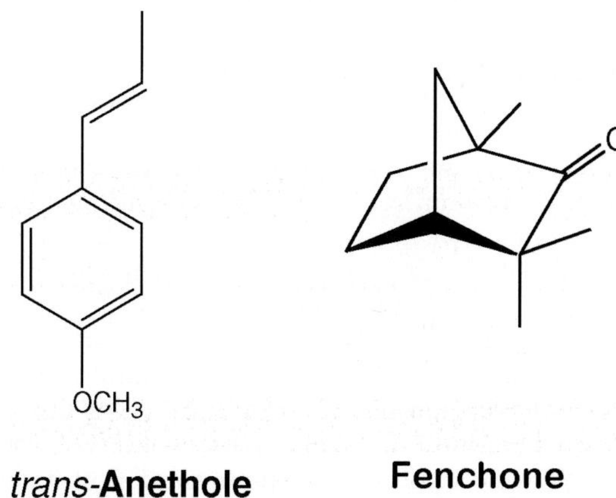

KEY CONSTITUENTS

The chemical composition differs between the two varieties and different authors report varying levels. *The European Pharmacopoeia* limits are defined here.

Foeniculum vulgare subsp. *vulgare* var. *vulgare* (bitter fennel):

- essential oil (>4%), containing >60% *trans*-anethole, >15%% fenchone, <5% estragole.[17]

Foeniculum vulgare subsp. *vulgare* var. *dulce* (sweet fennel):

- essential oil (>2%), containing >80% *trans*-anethole, <7.5% fenchone, <10% estragole.[17]

Additional constituents found in fennel are:

- fixed oil, flavonoids, organic acids,[1] stilbene trimers,[18] plant sterols, including beta-sitosterol.[19]

Note: There are only low levels of furanocoumarins in fennel fruit.[20]

The sweetness of fennel is due to the presence of *trans*-anethole and estragole, either alone or in combination. Sweet varieties of fennel taste sweeter than bitter varieties because they contain more *trans*-anethole and less fenchone.[21]

PHARMACODYNAMICS

Anethole bears a certain chemical resemblance to the catecholamines adrenaline, noradrenaline and dopamine. This structural similarity appears to be responsible for the various sympathomimetic effects exerted by fennel and anise. Like adrenaline, fennel and anise are bronchodilators and, like amphetamine, fennel is said to facilitate weight loss. Psychoactive and psychedelic effects of fennel, anise and anethole have been noted in the past.[8]

Effects on smooth muscle

Fennel oil and alcoholic extracts of fennel demonstrate significant antispasmodic activity in several in vitro models using isolated smooth muscle.[22–27] This action appears to be due to an effect on calcium metabolism in the smooth muscle cells[23] and was confirmed in an in vivo model by injection.[22] One in vitro study found that fennel oil and anethole increased smooth muscle tone under certain conditions.[24]

Tone and amplitude of peristalsis decreased in the stomach after approximately 2–8 minutes in animals receiving fennel water (5–25 ml). Thirty minutes was required to bring about a decrease in the small intestine and colon.[28] Oral administration of a combined stomachic (containing many ingredients including herbs and antacids) reduced the inhibition of stomach movement caused by sodium pentobarbitone in rabbits. The effective (stimulating) ingredients were found to be fennel, gentian and *l*-menthol. The stimulating effect of the combined stomachic was abolished by atropine sulphate or hexamethonium bromide, suggesting that the action is due to an increase in the cholinergic nerve activity, not the direct stimulation of the smooth muscle itself.[29] Thus it appears that fennel relaxes smooth muscle by direct local activity but stimulates it via the sympathetic nervous system.

Antimicrobial activity

Fennel oil demonstrated bacteriostatic activity against the following bacteria using the agar diffusion and serial dilution methods: *Aerobacter aerogenes, Bacillus subtilis, E. coli, Proteus vulgaris, Pseudomonas aeruginosa, Staph. albus, Staph aureus.*[30] Fennel oil (0.02 ml/7 mm filter) demonstrated antibacterial activity in vitro against the following organisms isolated from patients with urinary tract infections: *E. coli, Strep. pyogenes, Staph. aureus*. The antibacterial activity of fennel oil was equal to or greater than the standard antibiotics also tested (streptopenicillin, penicillin and tetracycline).[31] Rising fennel oil steam had antibacterial activity in vitro against *Mycobacterium avium*.[32] Fennel oil (0.1%) inhibited mould growth in agar for 6 days. Anethole was also effective at 0.1%.[33] The growth of *Staphylococcus aureus* and *Bacillus subtilis* was prevented by 1 mg/ml of the ethanol extract of fennel but other tested organisms were not affected at any of the concentrations used.[34] However, the chloroform extract exhibited antibacterial activity against *Bacillus subtilis* and *Proteus vulgaris*, with other bacteria unaffected.[35]

Oestrogenic and related activity

Fennel oil demonstrated a favourable influence on the total quantity of milk and its fat content in goats.[36] Lactating mice fed on fennel produced pups that ate a significantly higher quantity of fennel-containing food than controls (mothers not fed fennel during lactation).[37] This indicates that the flavour (and at least some chemical constituents) of fennel are passed in breast milk.

Injection of fennel oil triggered a mating response in sexually immature female rats and in ovariectomized mice.[38] Extracts of fennel can induce oestrus, cause growth of mammary glands and oviducts in adult ovariectomized rats and exert an antiandrogenic effect in adult male rats.[39] Fennel extract increased the organ weight of the cervix and vagina of ovariectomized rats, as well as an increase in RNA, DNA and protein concentrations. Fennel caused the growth of the cervix and vagina by inducing both hyperplasia and hypertrophy. The most potent dose was 250 μg/100 g bodyweight, which produced changes similar to oestrus-intact females.[39] Moderate doses of an acetone extract of fennel increased the weight of mammary glands, whilst higher doses increased the weight of the oviduct, endometrium, myometrium, cervix and vagina.[40] A follow-up study demonstrated that the acetone extract induced cellular growth and proliferation in the endometrium and stimulated metabolism in the myometrium in rats. Changes induced by fennel provided a more favourable environment for the survival of spermatocytes and the implantation of the zygote in the uterus.[41]

The oral administration of the acetone extract of fennel seeds to male rats for 15 days produced a significant reduction in the total protein concentration of testes and vas deferens and an increase for the seminal vesicles and prostate gland.[40]

The structural resemblance of anethole to catecholamines may have a bearing on the oestrogenic activity demonstrated by fennel. Dopamine acts to inhibit the secretion of prolactin, so anethole may influence milk secretion by competing with dopamine at appropriate receptor sites, thereby reducing the inhibition by dopamine of prolactin secretion. Moreover, dianethole and photoanethole (polymers of anethole), which resemble the oestrogenic compounds stilbene and diethylstilbestrol, demonstrate oestrogenic activity.[8]

Intragastric administration of aqueous extract of fennel seed (50 mg/day or about 2 g/kg for 25 days) significantly reduced female fertility in mice compared to controls ($p<0.025$). No effect was observed on male mice fertility.[42]

Respiratory activity

Fennel oil administered by inhalation has a mild antitussive or cough suppressant effect on coughs generated by mechanical stimulation in guinea pigs.[43] In an earlier study, the volume and thickness of expelled respiratory tract fluid (RTF) was measured after administration of anethole and fenchone in various doses to rabbits. A dose-dependent increase in RTF volume was observed for fenchone, with the maximum response at 9 mg/kg. The increase in volume for anethole was not dose dependent and the maximum response occurred at 3 mg/kg. A comparison of seasonal results indicated a strong increase in RTF volume in autumn. Thickness of RTF was reduced in a dose-dependent manner, with minima occurring at 9–27 mg/kg.[44] Bitter fennel tea (equivalent to 9.1 mg of fruit) increased mucolytic activity by 12% in isolated oesophageal mucosal membranes of frogs. The references drug bromhexine (20 µg) produced an increase of 34%.[45]

Other effects

The subcutaneous injection of fennel oil (100 mg/day or approximately 300 mg/kg) to partially hepatectomized rats for 7 days produced a significant increase ($p<0.05$) in the regeneration of liver tissue as expressed by an increase in the wet and dry liver weights in relation to total body weight.[46] Fennel reduced the toxicity of strychnine in mice, indicating that it might affect the activity of liver microsomal drug metabolizing enzyme function.[47]

Fennel oil demonstrated antioxidant activity in soybean oil.[48] Fennel inhibited lipid peroxidation (rancidity) in slated cooked ground fish. Dried fennel was a more effective antioxidant than fresh fennel.[49]

The acetone extract of fennel exhibited strong in vitro cytotoxic activity against murine leukaemia cells and human colon cancer cells.[50] Water extract of fennel inhibited the growth of mouse leukaemia cells in vitro. The ethanol extract was inactive.[42]

The aqueous extract of roasted fennel exhibited cholinomimetic activity on rabbit duodenum and guinea pig ileum. It also exhibited a nicotinic effect after the blockade of its muscarinic activity by atropine on smooth muscles. Its effect was potentiated by physostigmine and antagonized by cholinesterase or alkalinization.[51]

Fennel fruit extract caused a significant increase (33%) of collected bile when compared with control values after oral administration (500 mg/kg) to rats. The bilirubin content of the bile was similar in both treated and control groups.[34]

Ethanol extract of fennel fruit (500 mg/kg) demonstrated significant diuretic activity 5 and 24 hours after its oral administration to rats when compared to controls. The diuresis was not associated with changes in sodium and/or potassium excretion.[34] Hydroalcoholic extracts of fennel root demonstrated diuretic activity in rats, producing an increase in urinary flow and urinary sodium excretion.[52]

Ethanol extract of fennel fruit demonstrated significant but moderate analgesic activity 90 and 150 minutes after oral administration (500 mg/kg) to mice. Antipyretic activity was also evident at 30 and 90 minutes, but not at 150 minutes.[34]

PHARMACOKINETICS

Anethole was absorbed very slowly in mice after oral administration (200 mg/kg). After 30 and 120 minutes, 60% and 23% of the administered dose respectively were still present in the stomach.[53] After 72 hours, 2% of an orally administered dose was found in the faeces of rats.[54]

CLINICAL TRIALS

Effects on the gastrointestinal tract

A liquid herbal formula (25 drops three times daily) containing, in increasing proportions, wormwood, caraway, fennel and peppermint was found to be superior to the spasmolytic drug metoclopramide ($p=0.02$) in terms of relief of symptoms such as pain, nausea, belching and heartburn in a randomized double-blind clinical trial of the treatment of dyspepsia. Sixty patients took part in the trial which consisted of 2 weeks' treatment.[55] In another placebo-controlled, randomized, double-blind clinical trial, 70 patients with strongly marked chronic digestive problems such as flatulence or bloating were treated with either a herbal formula containing caraway, fennel, peppermint and gentian in tablet form or a placebo over a 14-day period. Analysis of the trial results established a significant improvement in the gastrointestinal complaint scores of the group receiving the herbal tablets compared to the placebo group ($p<0.05$). Ultrasound results evaluating the amount of gas present also demonstrated a significant benefit from the herbal formula ($p<0.05$).[56]

Twenty-four patients with chronic non-specific colitis were treated with a herb combination containing *Taraxacum officinale, Hypericum perforatum, Melissa officinalis, Calendula officinalis* and *Foeniculum vulgare*. By the 15th day of treatment, spontaneous and palpable pains along the large intestine had disappeared in 96% of the patients. Defaecation was normalized in patients with diarrhoea syndrome.[57]

The effect of a herbal instant tea preparation containing chamomile, vervain, licorice, fennel and lemon balm on infantile colic was assessed in a prospective double-blind study on babies about 3 weeks old. Tea or placebo up to 150 ml per dose was given to each infant with every episode of colic, but not more than three times a day. After the 7 days of the trial, the colic improvement scores were significantly better in the herbal tea group: 1.7 versus 0.7 for the placebo group ($p<0.05$). In addition, more babies in the treatment group had their colic eliminated: 57% compared to 26% for placebo ($p<0.01$).[58]

TOXICOLOGY

The oral LD_{50} of fennel oil in animal studies varied from 3.12 g/kg to 4.5 ml/kg.[3] Acute or chronic poisoning with fennel oil has not been reported in humans.[3] The acute oral LD_{50} for anethole in rats was found to be 2.09 g/kg.[8] No phototoxic effects were reported for undiluted bitter fennel oil on hairless mice and pigs. Bitter fennel oil (4% in petrolatum) produced no irritation in a 48-hour closed-patch test and no sensitization reactions on human subjects.[59] It is desirable to have low estragole-containing fennel. High-dosage estragole studies in rats indicate potential hepatocarcinogenicity. However, since estragole is metabolized differently in humans and with only limited absorption,[60,61] any suggested carcinogenic risk in humans is tenuous.

No toxic effects were observed in mice administered single oral doses of 0.5, 1.0 and 3.0 g/kg of fennel ethanolic extract (equivalent to 5, 10 and 30 g of fennel seed). In the chronic toxicity study, 100 mg/kg of fennel extract orally administered per day over 90 days caused no significant differences in mortality, external morphology, haematology or spermatogenesis compared to controls. After 40 days, alopecia in the snout area developed in some male animals. The average body weight of the male animals increased while that of the female mice decreased or remained the same.[62] In another study using the same dosages, only the 3 g/kg dose showed signs of reduced locomotor activity and piloerection in mice. All other parameters were negative.[34]

Methanolic and water extracts of bitter and sweet fennel were not mutagenic in the Ames test and had no DNA-damaging activity in the *Bacillus subtilis* rec-assay.[62] A fennel fruit extract prepared by percolation with 95% ethanol and concentrated by vacuum demonstrated intermediate mutagenic results in the Ames test and significant toxic activity in the brine shrimp bioassay.[63]

The mutagenic potential of fennel oil is not conclusive, as indicated by the conflicting results obtained in the following in vitro tests. Fennel oil, sweet fennel oil and estragole were negative but anethole was positive in Ames tests.[64,65] In another study, fennel oil and anethole showed weakly positive results.[66] Sweet fennel oil and anethole were negative in the *E. coli* reversion test. Sweet fennel oil but not anethole demonstrated DNA-damaging activity in the *Bacillus subtilis* rec-assay; however, the authors indicate problems with this test with respect to the testing of oils.[65] Fennel oil demonstrated negative results in the chromosomal aberration test on hamster fibroblasts.[64]

CONTRAINDICATIONS

Fennel has been categorized as a spice allergen with some publications reporting a crossreaction with fennel in the so-called 'celery-carrot-mugwort-spice' syndrome. It is therefore contraindicated in these patients. However, even in this context, allergic reactions to fennel are rare and seem to be limited to occupational exposure.[3]

SPECIAL WARNINGS AND PRECAUTIONS

Very high doses of fennel oil should be avoided in hepatic disorders. For fennel syrup and fennel honey, diabetics should be aware of the sugar content of these preparations.

INTERACTIONS

Interaction between fennel oil and other drugs in humans is not expected.[3] The dermal application of the infusion of fennel in humans results in an aggravation of inflammation caused by mustard oil, UV irradiation or the subcutaneous injection of tuberculin.[3]

USE IN PREGNANCY AND LACTATION

Fennel (especially as infusions) does not seem to represent any special risk in pregnancy and lactation and fennel has been used as a galactagogue since antiquity.[3]

EFFECTS ON ABILITY TO DRIVE AND USE MACHINES

None known.

SIDE EFFECTS

Allergic reactions in the skin and respiratory tract have been reported.[3] Despite its widespread use, the herb must have only a very limited allergic potential.[20] A percentage of patients who are allergic to celery also display allergy reactions to fennel.[67] The 'celery-carrot-mugwort-spice' syndrome is well known in Europe. People sensitized to carrot, for example, may also have allergic reactions to other vegetables or spices of the Umbelliferae family.[68,69]

OVERDOSE

No effects known.

CURRENT REGULATORY STATUS IN SELECTED COUNTRIES

Bitter and sweet fennel are official in the *European Pharmacopoeia* (1997) and the *British Pharmacopoeia* (1998). Fennel is also official in the *Pharmacopoeia of the People's Republic of China* (English edition, 1997) and fennel and its oil are official in the *Japanese Pharmacopoeia* (English edition, 1996). Fennel and fennel oil were official in the second edition of the *Indian Pharmacopoeia* (1966), but were not included in the third edition (1985).

Fennel and fennel oil are covered by positive Commission E monographs and both have the following applications:

- dyspeptic complaints, such as mild cramp-like gastrointestinal disorders, a feeling of distension, flatulence;
- catarrh of the upper respiratory tract;
- fennel syrup and fennel honey for catarrh of the upper respiratory tract in children.

Fennel is on the UK General Sale List.

Fennel and fennel oil have GRAS status. They are also freely available as a 'dietary supplement' in the USA under DSHEA legislation (1994 Dietary Supplement Health and Education Act). Fennel has been present as an ingredient in products offered over the counter (OTC) for use as an aphrodisiac. The FDA, however, advises that: 'based on evidence currently available, any OTC drug product containing ingredients for use as an aphrodisiac cannot be generally recognized as safe and effective'.

Fennel is not included in Part 4 of Schedule 4 of the Therapeutic Goods Act Regulations of Australia.

References

1. Bisset NG (ed). Herbal drugs and phytopharmaceuticals. Medpharm Scientific Publishers, Stuttgart: 1994; pp 200–202.
2. Mabberley DJ. The plant book, 2nd edn. Cambridge University Press, Cambridge 1997; p 286.
3. De Smet PAGM et al (eds). Adverse effects of herbal drugs, vol 1. Springer-Verlag, Berlin: 1992; p 135.
4. Bartram T. Encyclopedia of herbal medicine. Grace Publishers, Dorset 1995; p 181.
5. Grieve M. A modern herbal, vol 1. Dover Publications, New York, 1971; pp 293–297.
6. British Herbal Medicine Association's Scientific Committee. British herbal pharmacopoeia. BHMA, Cowling: 1983; pp 92–93.
7. Felter HW, Lloyd JU. King's American dispensatory, 18th edn, 3rd revision, vol 1, 1905. Reprinted by Eclectic Medical Publications, Portland, 1983; pp 891–892.
8. Albert-Puleo M. J Ethnopharmacol 1980; 2: 337–344.
9. Bensky D, Gamble A. Chinese herbal medicine materia medica. Eastland Press, Seattle, 1986; pp 440–441.
10. Pharmaceutical Society of Great Britain. British pharmaceutical codex 1934. Pharmaceutical Press, London 1934; p 471.
11. Weiss RF. Herbal medicine. Beaconsfield Publishers, Beaconsfield, 1988; p 68.
12. Leung AY, Foster S. Encyclopedia of common natural ingredients used in food, drugs and cosmetics, 2nd edn. John Wiley, New York, 1996; pp 240–243.
13. Smeh NJ. Creating your own cosmetics – naturally. Alliance Publishing, Garrisonville, 1995; p 88.
14. German Federal Minister of Justice. German Commission E for human medicine monograph, Bundes-Anzeiger (German Federal Gazette), no. 74, dated 18.04.1991.
15. Chiej R. The Macdonald encyclopedia of medicinal plants. Macdonald, London 1984; entry no. 133.
16. Launert EL. The Hamlyn guide to edible and medicinal plants of Britain and Northern Europe. Hamlyn, London, 1981; p 98.
17. European pharmacopoeia, 3rd edn. European Department for the Quality of Medicines within the Council of Europe, Strasbourg 1996; pp 848–850.
18. Ono M, Ito Y, Kinjo J et al. Chem Pharm Bull 1995; 43 (5): 868–871.
19. Mendez J, Castro-Poceiro J. Rev Latinoam Quim 1981; 12 (2): 91–92.
20. Hänsel R, Keller K, Rimpler H, Schneider G (eds). Foeniculum. In: Hagers Handbuch der Pharmazeutischen Praxis, 5th edn, vol 5. Drogen E-O. Springer-Verlag, Berlin, 1992; pp 156–181.
21. Hussain RA, Poveda LJ, Pezzuto JM et al. Economic Botany 1990; 44 (2): 174–182.
22. Gunn JWC. J Pharmacol Exp Ther 1921; 16: 39–47.
23. Saleh MM, Hashem FA, Grace MH. Pharm Pharmacol Lett 1996; 6 (1): 5–7.
24. Reiter M, Brandt W. Arzneim-Forsch 1985; 35 (1A): 408–414.
25. Forster HB, Niklas H, Lutz S. Planta Med 1980; 40 (4): 309–319.
26. Forster HB, Niklas H, Lutz S. Planta Med 1980; 40: 309–319.
27. Forster HB. Z Allgemeinmed 1983; 59: 1327–1333.
28. Plant OH, Miller GH. J Pharmacol Exp Ther 1926; 27: 149–164.
29. Niiho Y, Takayanagi I, Takagi K. Jpn J Pharmacol 1977; 27 (1): 177–179.
30. Kivanc M, Akgul A. Flavour Fragrance J 1986; 1: 175–179.
31. Afzal H, Akhtar MS. J Pak Med Assoc 1981; 31 (10): 230–232.
32. Maruzzella JC, Sicurella A. J Am Pharm Assoc 1960; 49: 692–694.
33. Lord CF, Husa WJ. J Am Pharm Assoc 1954; 43: 438–440.
34. Tanira MOM, Shah AH, Mohsin A et al. Phytother Res 1996; 10: 33–36.
35. Jawad ALM, Dharhir ABJ, Hussain AM et al. J Biol Sci Res 1985; 16 (2): 17–21.
36. Fingerling F. Landw Vers Sta 67: 253–289 (CAS 2: 6758).

37. Shukla HS, Upadhyay PD, Tripathi SC. Pesticides 1989; 23 (1): 33–35.
38. Zondek B, Bergmann E. Biochem J 1938; 32: 641–645.
39. Annusuya S, Vanithakumari G, Megala N et al. Ind J Med Res 1988; 87: 364–367.
40. Malini T, Vanithakumari G, Megala N et al. Ind J Physiol Pharmacol 1985; 29 (1): 21–26.
41. Mekala N, Annusuya K, Devi G et al. Ind Drugs 1989; 27 (2): 93–100.
42. Alkofahi A, Al-Hamood MH, Elbetieha AM. Arch STD/HIV Res 1996; 10 (3): 189–196.
43. Misawa M, Kizawa M. Pharmacometrics 1990; 39 (1): 81–93.
44. Boyd EM, Sheppard EP. Pharmacol 1971; 6: 65–80.
45. Muller-Limmroth W, Frohlich HH. Fortschr Med 1980; 98 (3): 95–101.
46. Gershbein LL. Food Cosmet Toxicol 1977; 15: 173–181.
47. Han YB, Shin KH, Woo WS. Annual report of natural products research institute. Seoul National University 1984; 23: 46–49.
48. Zygadlo JA, Lamarque AL, Maestri DM et al. Grasay Aceites 1995; 46 (4–5): 285–288.
49. Ramanathan L, Das NP. J Food Sci 1993; 58 (2): 318–320.
50. Kim KS, Paik JM, Hwang WI. Korean Univ Med J 1988; 25 (3): 759–770.
51. Dei S, Das BN, Devi I. Ind J Pharmacy 1976; 38 (6): 165.
52. Beaux D, Fleurentin J, Mortier F. Phytother Res 1997; 11 (4): 320–322.
53. Le Bourhis B. Ann Biol Clin 1968; 26: 711–715.
54. Sangster SA, Cladwell J, Smith RL. Food Chem Toxicol 1984; 22: 695–706.
55. Westphal J, Hörning M, Leonhardt K. Phytomedicine 1996; 2 (4): 285–291.
56. Silberhorn H, Landgrebe N, Wohling D et al. 6th Phytotherapy Conference, Berlin, October 5–7, 1995.
57. Chakurski I, Matev M, Koichev A et al. Vutr Boles 1981; 20 (6): 51–54.
58. Weizman Z, Alkrinawi S, Goldfarb D et al. J Pediatrics 1993; 122 (4): 650–652.
59. Opdyke DLJ. Food Cosmet Toxicol 1979; 17: 529.
60. Sangster SA, Caldwell J, Smith RL. Food Chem Toxicol 1984; 22: 707–713.
61. Caldwell J, Sutton JD. Food Chem Toxicol 1988; 26: 87–91.
62. Shah AH, Qureshi S, Ageel AM. J Ethnopharmacol 1991; 34 (2–3): 167–172.
63. Mahmoud I, Alkofahi A, Abdelaziz A. Int J Pharmacog 1992; 30 (2): 81–85.
64. Ishidate M Jr, Sofuni T, Yoshikawa K et al. Food Chem Toxicol 1984; 22 (8): 623–636.
65. Sekizawa J, Shibamoto T. Mutat Res 1982; 101 (2): 127–140.
66. Marcus C, Lichtenstein EP. J Agric Food Chem 1982; 30 (3): 563–568.
67. Wutherich B, Hofer T. Dtsch Med Wochenschr 1984; 109: 981–986.
68. Helbling A, Lopez M, Schwartz HJ et al. Ann Allergy 1993; 70 (6): 495–499.
69. Muhlemann RJ, Wuthrich B. Schweiz Med Wochenschr 1991; 121 (46): 1696–1700.

Feverfew (*Tanacetum parthenium* (L.) Schulz-Bip.)

SYNONYMS

Chrysanthemum parthenium (L.) Bernh., (botanical synonym), Tanaceti parthenii herba/folium (Lat), Mutterkraut (Ger), camomille grande (Fr), matrem (Dan).

WHAT IS IT?

Feverfew, a herb with long traditional use, received a lot of attention in the UK during the 1980s when it became publicized as a migraine remedy. The plant looks somewhat similar to chamomile at first glance. Feverfew has had many botanical names including *Chrysanthemum parthenium, Pyrethrum parthenium* and *Matricaria pyrethrum*. It has a strong smell, particularly disliked by bees. The common name is believed to be derived from the Latin *febris* (a fever) and *fugure* (to drive away), as it was used to cure fevers. The part used medicinally is the leaf with or without stem, collected when the plant is in flower.

EFFECTS

Antisecretory (inhibition of platelet aggregation, granule secretion from polymorphonuclear leucocytes); antiinflammatory (inhibits prostaglandin biosynthesis and arachidonic acid products).

TRADITIONAL VIEW

Warm infusions were prescribed to purge choler, to treat colds and febrile diseases, to cleanse the kidneys and to bring on menstruation and expel worms.[1] The decoction sweetened with honey or sugar was given for coughs, wheezing and difficult breathing.[2] Cold infusions were considered an excellent tonic, including for 'those who have taken Opium too liberally'.[1] This preparation was also used to relieve facial and ear pain in dyspeptic or rheumatic patients.[2] The leaves could be applied as a poultice to ease pain and swelling of the bowel and for wind or colic.[1] Eclectic physicians used feverfew as a tonic which influenced the entire intestinal tract, to increase the appetite, improve digestion, promote secretion and act upon the renal and cutaneous functions.[3] Although not widespread, there is reference to traditional use of feverfew for headache in Welsh literature.[4]

SUMMARY ACTIONS

Antiinflammatory, bitter, emmenagogue (in high doses), anthelmintic.

CAN BE USED FOR

INDICATIONS SUPPORTED BY CLINICAL TRIALS

Prophylaxis and treatment of migraine, tension headache and associated symptoms.

TRADITIONAL THERAPEUTIC USES

Coughs, colds; febrile diseases; atonic dyspepsia; nervous debility; worm infestation.

MAY ALSO BE USED FOR

EXTRAPOLATIONS FROM PHARMACOLOGICAL STUDIES

Conditions requiring antiallergic, antiinflammatory or antiplatelet activity; arthritis.[5]

OTHER APPLICATIONS

Anecdotal evidence suggests it is beneficial for psoriasis.[6]

PREPARATIONS

Although one clinical trial was conducted using freeze-dried feverfew leaf and many users take the fresh leaves, some promoters of feverfew are of the opinion that the air-dried herb is less likely to cause side effects.[7]

However, some practitioners remain convinced that only fresh or freeze-dried preparations of feverfew are effective for migraine treatment. But the results of one clinical trial clearly demonstrate an effect for conventionally dried feverfew leaves grown in Israel given as a capsule.[8] Tablets of the dried herb would also probably be effective.

DOSAGE

- 0.7–2 ml of 1:1 fresh plant tincture per day.
- 1–2 ml of 1:5 dried plant tincture per day.
- One tablet (150 mg dried herb, standardized to contain at least 0.6 mg parthenolide), 1–2 times per day.

The adequate dose varies with the quality of the herb and the severity and frequency of the migraines. In addition, it is more likely that a higher starting dose establishes the prophylactic effect more rapidly.

DURATION OF USE

There is no restriction on long-term use. Information from clinical surveys suggests treatment in excess of 4–6 months may be required to assess beneficial effect. It is advisable to reduce the dosage gradually over a month if treatment is to be ceased.

SUMMARY ASSESSMENT OF SAFETY

Except in cases of allergy in susceptible patients, feverfew is a safe herb. Some uncomfortable side effects, such as mouth ulcers, may occur in a percentage of patients, especially those who chew the fresh leaves.

TECHNICAL DATA

BOTANY

Feverfew is a perennial plant which may grow up to 70 cm. Its light green leaves (2–9 cm long) are ovate in outline, pinnate with pinnatifid lobed or toothed leaflets. The flower heads (1–2.4 cm in diameter) consist of ray florets of white, short ligules and inner, yellow disc florets. The fruit is a ribbed achene approximately 1.5 mm long.[9,10] (Tanacetum and Chrysanthemum are two separate genera of the Anthemideae tribe of the Compositae (daisy) family,[11] so *Chrysanthemum parthenium* is not technically a synonym of *Tanacetum parthenium* but a former name.)

KEY CONSTITUENTS

- Sesquiterpene lactones containing an alpha-methylene-gamma-lactone group: in particular those of the germacranolide type,[12] including parthenolide (0.06–0.6%)[13] and 3-beta-hydroxyparthenolide; the guaianolide type[12] and others containing chlorine.[14]
- Sesquiterpenes, monoterpenes, polyacetylene compounds,[15] essential oil,[16] flavonoids.[17]
- Melatonin has also been detected (1.37–2.45 μg/g) in feverfew leaf samples and in a commercial preparation.[18]

The parthenolide content of feverfew may vary. Tests conducted on Mexican- and Yugoslavian-grown plants yielded no parthenolide. The postflowering leaves can contain up to four times higher levels of parthenolide compared to preflowering.[19]

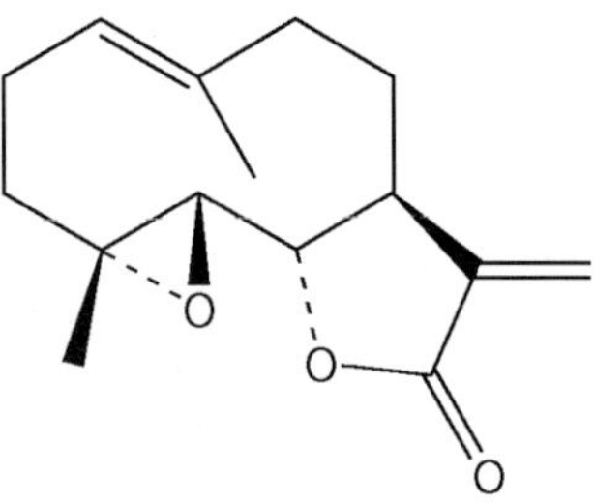

Parthenolide

PHARMACODYNAMICS

It has been proposed that a significant increase in serotonin release from platelets triggers the complex chain of events leading to a migraine attack.[20] In support of this theory, other workers have concluded that migraines are caused by abnormal platelet activity and abnormal serotonin metabolism.[21] Although one proposed mechanism of action of feverfew is the inhibition of prostaglandin production,[22,23] a more likely mechanism is that feverfew interacts with the protein kinase C pathway causing an inhibition of granule secretion from platelets (antimigraine effect) and polymorphs (antiarthritic effect).[24] It has been demonstrated that this effect is due to parthenolide and other sesquiterpene lactones in feverfew.[25] Neutralization of sulphydryl groups either inside or outside the cell is involved.[26]

The alpha-methylene-gamma-lactone group may provide much of the biological activity of feverfew. As the nucleophile in biological systems is very often a thiol (sulphydryl) group, the activity is probably due to the alpha-methylene-gamma-lactone group acting as an alkylating agent of such thiol residues[27] and thus disrupting cell function. (Thiol groups, such as cysteine residues in proteins or enzymes, are important constituents of the plasma membrane and cytoskeleton.[28] The assembly of microtubules in the latter is known to be involved in phagocytosis and degranulation of neutrophils.[29])

Antisecretory activity

A chloroform/methanol extract and an aqueous extract of feverfew inhibited the secretory activity of blood platelets and polymorphonuclear leucocytes. Release of serotonin from platelets induced by aggregating agents was inhibited. The pattern of effects of feverfew on platelets is different from that obtained with other inhibitors of platelet aggregation and the effect on polymorphs is more pronounced than that obtained by very high concentrations of NSAIDs.[24]

Aqueous extract of feverfew inhibited platelet aggregation induced by ADP, collagen or thrombin but aggregation induced by arachidonic acid was not affected. Synthesis of thromboxane B_2 from platelets incubated with arachidonic acid was also not inhibited. However, feverfew extract did inhibit platelet phospholipase A_2, suggesting its antiplatelet activities are due to a phospholipase inhibitor which prevents the release of arachidonic acid.[23]

Despite the low solubility, antisecretory activity in an aqueous medium has been demonstrated, which implies that only small amounts may be required for the biological activity. Eleven fractions obtained from chloroform extract of feverfew demonstrated antisecretory activity; two fractions were devoid of activity. All the active fractions contained compounds with an alpha-methylene-gamma-lactone group. Five such compounds were isolated.[12] Feverfew and parthenolide dramatically reduced the number of acid-soluble sulphydryl groups in platelets at concentrations similar to those that inhibited platelet secretory activity. Feverfew itself did not induce the formation of disulphide-linked protein polymers in platelets, but polymer formation occurred when aggregating agents were added to feverfew-treated platelets.[30]

In vitro studies show that there are marked similarities between the inhibitory effects of feverfew extract and of parthenolide on both serotonin secretion and platelet aggregation induced by several activating agents in human platelets. Only in one case was there any discrepancy, which may have been due to materials in the extract other than parthenolide. Both feverfew extract and parthenolide were more effective on the above parameters when induced by certain agents, which suggests an interaction with the protein kinase C pathway.[31] However, parthenolide neither activated nor inhibited protein kinase C type 1 from bovine brain preparation in concentrations up to 200 μg/ml, nor affected the activity of membrane-associated protein kinase C in isolated lymphoma cell membranes.[32]

Several feverfew extracts were tested for antisecretory activity in a bioassay of platelets and compared with parthenolide. There was a close correlation between the parthenolide content of the extracts and the antisecretory activity.[33] Other sesquiterpene lactones from feverfew were also active. The content of parthenolide and bioactivity varied enormously in feverfew plants grown under identical conditions from seeds of 10 different regions of Europe.[34] A selection of feverfew commercial preparations (leaves, tablets, drops) in the UK inhibited secretory activity in platelets, albeit at lower levels than expected (compared to freshly prepared feverfew). The tablets demonstrated activity well below that claimed.[35] Feverfew extracts modified the interaction of platelets with collagen substrates and inhibited both platelet spreading and formation of thrombus-like platelet aggregates on the collagen surface.[36] Chloroform extract of feverfew was a powerful inhibitor of platelet-collagen interaction in an in vitro model used for testing antithrombotic drugs. Feverfew also prevented endothelial cell monolayer of perfused rabbit aorta from spontaneous injury.[37]

While the platelets of patients taking feverfew aggregated normally to ADP and thrombin, the aggregation in response to serotonin was greatly reduced.[38] This implies that while normal clotting mechanisms are still intact, the biochemical chain of events leading to a migraine is broken.

Feverfew extract inhibited the activity of polymorphonuclear leucocytes (PMNL) in vitro, via blockade of cellular sulphydryl groups (as cell lysis was also ruled out).[39] Whole and fractionated acetone extracts of feverfew (and other *Tanacetum spp*) demonstrated inhibitory effects in vitro using a human polymorphonuclear leucocyte-based bioassay. Although parthenolide was clearly an important determinant of activity, it was found not to be the sole determinant of activity.[40,41] It is possible the activity of responsible compounds was a result of inhibition of protein kinase C or subsequent events in polymorphonuclear leucocyte activation in vitro.[41] Feverfew extracts markedly inhibited phagocytosis of *Candida guilliermondii* in vitro but intracellular killing was not affected. The fact that feverfew can inhibit phagocytosis as well as degranulation gives it increased potential as an antiinflammatory agent.[42]

Chloroform extract of feverfew dose dependently inhibited histamine release induced by stimulating rat peritoneal mast cells through an IgE–anti-IgE reaction. The data suggest that this action by feverfew is different from the inhibitory action on mast cells of both cromoglycate and quercetin. In addition, feverfew extract does not inhibit histamine release by interfering with oxidative phosphorylation.[43]

Inhibition of eicosanoid production

In one study parthenolide inhibited cyclooxygenase (which converts arachidonic acid to prostaglandins) in vitro.[44] Parthenolide also inhibited the expression of inducible cyclooxygenase and proinflammatory cytokines in macrophages, which correlated with the inhibition of mitogen-activated protein kinases. The alpha-methylene-gamma-lactone group conferred the inhibitory activity.[45] However, aqueous extracts of whole plant and leaf inhibited prostaglandin biosynthesis, but did not inhibit cyclooxygenase.[22] Parthenolide did not inhibit cyclooxygenase activity in vitro with enzyme derived from sheep seminal vesicles.[32] Other evidence suggests that sesquiterpene lactones, including parthenolide, inhibit the release of arachidonic acid from membrane phospholipid stores rather than its conversion into thromboxane B_2 via the cyclooxygenase pathway.[32]

Chloroform extract of feverfew evoked changes in the metabolism of arachidonic acid that were similar to those observed in glutathione-depleted platelets.[30] It also inhibited uptake and liberation of arachidonic acid into or from platelet membrane phospholipids,[46] which may be the result of altered cytoskeletal-membrane interaction.[29] SH groups (sulphydryls) are essential for phospholipase A_2 activity (and the liberation of arachidonic acid),[47] which may have been affected by feverfew.[46] Chloroform extracts of feverfew produced dose-dependent inhibition of the generation of thromboxane B_2 and leukotriene B_4 by stimulated leucocytes. The activity was due to other lactones as well as sesquiterpene lactones.[48]

At high concentrations (50–200 μg/ml), buffered aqueous feverfew extract inhibited the formation of arachidonate metabolites in rat leucocytes. Lower concentrations were ineffective.[49] Pharmacological tests indicate that tanetin, a new lipophilic flavonol isolated from feverfew, could contribute to its antiinflammatory activity by inhibiting the generation of proinflammatory eicosanoids. Given the above, it is unlikely to be the only active compound within the plant.[17]

Interaction with contractile agonists

Parthenolide had little activity at serotonin receptors.[50,51] However, parthenolide inhibited the contractile (serotonin release-mediated) responses of rat stomach fundus to two indirect-acting serotonin agonists, but not to serotonin itself.[52]

Extracts of fresh feverfew caused a dose- and time-dependent inhibition of the contractile responses of isolated smooth tissue to receptor-acting agonists such as serotonin and phenylephrine. Chloroform extracts of dried feverfew (which in this case did not contain parthenolide or other alpha-methylene-gamma-lactones) were not inhibitory, but elicited contractions.[53] Chloroform extracts of feverfew and parthenolide have inhibited smooth muscle contractility in isolated tissue, in a time-dependent, non-specific and irreversible manner. The inhibition required the presence of the alpha-methylene-gamma-lactone group.[54,55] The inhibitory effects are non-specific and may result from interference with postreceptor contractile mechanisms. The irreversible inhibition implies a long-lasting toxic effect on the tissue.[56]

Antimicrobial activity

Eudesmanolides (10 mg/ml) isolated from feverfew demonstrated antibacterial activity towards *Staph. aureus, E. coli* and *Salmonella spp.*[57] Parthenolide inhibited the growth of Gram-positive bacteria, yeasts and filamentous fungi in vitro. Species of Bacillus without endospores were particularly sensitive.[58]

Essential oil obtained from feverfew flowers showed bactericidal and fungicidal activity against most of the 27 microorganisms tested using the agar diffusion and broth dilution methods.[59] Two extracts of feverfew were tested in a similar way using many of the same test species, including *Staph. aureus, Strep. haemolyticus, Sarcina flava* and *E. coli.* The Gram-negative species were much less sensitive than Gram-positive species, fungi and dermatophytes.[60]

Other activity

Compounds containing an alpha-methylene-gamma-lactone group have inhibited tumour growth, respiration and nucleic acid synthesis in vitro[61] and ex vivo,[62] demonstrated antihyperlipidaemic activity in mice,[63] by injection inhibited carrageenan-induced oedema and chronic adjuvant-induced arthritis[64] and delayed hypersensitivity reactions in rats.[65] Several sesquiterpene lactones have been identified as important constituents of plants consumed by animals (including chimpanzees) for presumed medicinal value.[66,67] In studies conducted on a wide range of sesquiterpene lactones, there was no correlation between cytotoxicity and serotonin release inhibition.[32]

Incubation of monocytes with a feverfew extract diminished cell adherence. The activity is due to neutralization of cellular sulphydryl groups.[68] Sesquiterpene lactones containing an alpha-methylene-gamma-lactone group are potent inhibitors of macrophage adenylate cyclase activity and therefore may play a significant role in the toxicity of some sesquiterpene lactones in poisonous plants when ingested by livestock.[69]

Addition of feverfew extract protected the endothelial cell monolayer from perfusion-induced injury and led to a reversible increase in the cyclic AMP content of aorta segments. This indicates that feverfew may have a vasoprotective effect in addition to its effects on platelets.[36]

Feverfew extract inhibited mitogen-induced human peripheral blood mononuclear cell (PBMC) proliferation and cytokine-mediated responses. Both the extract and parthenolide proved cytotoxic to mitogen-induced PBMC (after incubation for 48–72 hours). If feverfew is cytotoxic in vivo to lymphocytes or macrophages which are overactive, this could possibly explain the manner in which the herb gives relief to rheumatoid arthritis sufferers.[70]

Intraperitoneal administration of feverfew extract inhibited collagen-induced bronchoconstriction in guinea pigs. The authors concluded that this was a consequence of phospholipase A_2 inhibition.[71] Similarly, parthenolide protected against experimentally induced nephrocalcinosis in rats.[72]

It has been found that a nitric oxide synthase inhibitor significantly reduces the severity of a migraine headache.[73] The sesquiterpene lactone costunolide, which is structurally close to parthenolide, exhibits strong nitric oxide synthase inhibitory activity in vivo.[74]

PHARMACOKINETICS

No data on the pharmacokinetics of feverfew or parthenolide are available. It has, however, been postulated that the actively alkylating alpha-methylene-gamma-lactone group (such as parthenolide) would be rapidly inactivated via glutathione on entering the bloodstream. This could raise doubts regarding the in vivo relevance of the above in vitro studies. However, it has been observed that sequential treatment of old samples of dried powdered feverfew leaf (which contained no 'free' parthenolide) with an oxidant and a weak base caused the regeneration of substantial amounts of parthenolide. This process may occur in vivo with cytochrome P-450 enzymes as oxidants, with conversion back into 'free' parthenolide at the cellular level.[27]

CLINICAL TRIALS

Migraine

In 1973, at the suggestion of a friend, Mrs Anne Jenkins of Wales started taking three fresh leaves of feverfew each day in an attempt to rid herself of severe and recurrent migraines. After 10 months, Mrs Jenkins' headaches had vanished and did not return so long as she kept taking feverfew. Her enthusiasm rapidly led to an epidemic of feverfew users. Dr Stewart Johnson, a migraine specialist, became interested and began a survey which was then followed up by a clinical trial. The survey revealed the following facts.[75]

1. About 72% of those surveyed (253 suffering from true migraine) found that feverfew was helpful for the prevention of their headaches; 78% of the 23 people suffering from tension headaches found that feverfew reduced headache frequency and severity. Of 242 patients who recorded the frequency, 33% no longer had attacks and 76% had fewer migraines each month compared to before taking feverfew.

2. Associated nausea and vomiting decreased or disappeared. A proportion of patients experienced the migraine aura without the attack.

3. When they did occur, attacks responded better to conventional painkillers (e.g. aspirin). Feverfew users experienced no adverse interactions with their orthodox medication.

4. Many patients also suffering from arthritis found their symptoms somewhat relieved by feverfew.

5. The onset of the effect was slow and gradual, often taking several months, and the average dose used was very low – about two and a half fresh leaves (3.8 cm long by 3.1 cm wide) per day. The average duration of treatment was 2.3 years and 2.6 years for men and women respectively. When individuals stopped taking feverfew their migraines returned soon after.

The survey also revealed some side effects in a small percentage of users. Adverse effects included mouth ulcers or inflammation. In contrast, a percentage of users experienced improved digestion, a sense of well-being and improved sleep.

This work was followed up by a double-blind, placebo-controlled clinical trial of 17 patients who had been self-medicating with raw feverfew every day for 3 months. Eight of these patients received two capsules per day containing freeze-dried feverfew powder (25 mg of leaf) and nine received placebo, for six periods of 4 weeks. Prior to the trial, the reduction in the frequency of migraines during self-treatment was significant for both groups. Compared to the migraine frequency while self-medicating, there was no change in the frequency or severity of symptoms in the feverfew treatment group during the trial. The placebo group, however, experienced a significant increase ($p<0.05$) in the frequency and severity of headaches when the results of the previous 3 months were considered. The placebo group also experienced higher incidence and severity of nausea and vomiting than the feverfew group ($p<0.05$). The authors claimed a prophylactic benefit for feverfew in preventing migraine attacks. Curiously, fewer adverse events were reported by those taking feverfew (four patients reported none), compared to all patients taking placebo reporting at least one event.[76,77] Because of ethical reasons (feverfew was considered to have unknown safety by the scientists), this trial had an unusual design. The patients were already using feverfew, so the trial therefore observed the results of patients unknowingly stopping their feverfew. As might be expected, such an abrupt discontinuance led to the recurrence of severe migraines in some patients. Perhaps more importantly, the study showed that long-term feverfew users were normal in terms of a large number of biochemical and haematological parameters.

A few years later, 59 patients with classic migraine or common migraine completed a randomized, double-blind, placebo-controlled crossover study. After a 1-month single-blind placebo run-in, patients were randomly allocated to receive either one capsule of freeze-dried powdered feverfew (averaging 82 mg and containing 2.2 μmol parthenolide, approximately two medium-sized leaves) or placebo for 4 months and then transferred to the other treatment for a further 4 months. Treatment with feverfew was associated with a 24% reduction in the mean number of attacks and a significant reduction in the degree of vomiting ($p<0.02$) in each 2-month assessment period. There was also a trend towards a reduction in severity of attacks, although the duration of individual attacks was unaltered. Significant improvement in the feverfew group was also observed in visual analogue scores ($p<0.0001$). Seventeen of these patients had previously tried feverfew and results were similar for this group. Treatment with feverfew did not produce any adverse effects. Although there was no wash-out period between feverfew and placebo treatments, patients receiving placebo after feverfew did not experience an increased deterioration compared to placebo levels.[78] No ex vivo reduction in serotonin secretion from platelets after ingestion of feverfew at 4 months could be demonstrated.[79]

A team of Dutch scientists which has been very active in the field of feverfew research tested the efficacy of a standardized extract for the prevention of migraine headaches. In a randomized, placebo-controlled, double blind, crossover design, 50 patients who had never taken feverfew before and experienced at least one migraine attack per month were followed for 4 months of active treatment and 4 months of placebo. Active treatment consisted of 143 mg per day of a granulated ethanolic extract of feverfew containing 0.5 mg of parthenolide and corresponding to about 170 mg of original dried herb. The feverfew preparation used in this study did not exert any significant preventative effect on the frequency of migraine attacks, although patients seemed to have a tendency to use fewer analgesic drugs while they were using feverfew.[80]

This result was not in accordance with the results from the above studies and the authors suggest that this might be because the previous studies were conducted in patients who had already found feverfew to be beneficial (which is not actually the case – see above). Another reason provided by the authors could be due to the dried plant preparation used or the fact that an extract was prescribed, rather than the crude leaf. (The original popularity of feverfew was based on consumption of the fresh leaves, although the two earlier clinical trials used freeze-dried leaves.) Despite the fact that the preparation contained a known dose of parthenolide, a suggested active component, perhaps other compounds are also important.

Moreover, early users of raw feverfew found that it took 6 months of use or longer to establish this benefit. It is also possible that only a subset of migraine sufferers are feverfew responders and a benefit in this subset might be missed in a randomized clinical trial. Active treatment in the above study was only for 4 months, which might be insufficient time to establish the prophylactic effect at the dosage tested.

In a double blind, placebo-controlled trial, 57 chronic migraine sufferers (43% suffered more than 10 attacks per month) were selected at random and divided into two groups. Both groups received powdered feverfew capsules (total of 100 mg per day of dried leaves containing 0.2 mg parthenolide) in the preliminary phase, which lasted 2 months. In the second and third phases, which continued for an additional 2 months, a double-blind, placebo-controlled, crossover study was conducted. The difference in pain intensity of migraines before and after treatment with feverfew (measured in phase I) was highly significant ($p<0.001$). In phase II, patients receiving feverfew continued to experience a decrease in pain intensity, while it increased in those on placebo. The difference between the two groups was significant ($p<0.01$). Moreover, a profound reduction was observed in the typical migraine symptoms such as vomiting, nausea and sensitivity to noise and light ($p<0.001$). Transferring the feverfew-treated group to placebo in phase III resulted in an increase in pain intensity and other symptoms. In contrast, shifting the placebo group to feverfew therapy resulted in an improvement in pain and other symptoms. However, no information was provided concerning the frequency of migraine attacks.[8] Rather than acting to reduce the frequency of migraines, feverfew reduced their severity. A longer treatment time or higher doses may also see an impact on migraine frequency.

Arthritis

In a randomized, double-blind, placebo-controlled trial, 40 patients with symptomatic rheumatoid arthritis received either dried, chopped feverfew (70–86 mg per day) or placebo capsules for 6 weeks. Patients continued with their NSAID and analgesic drug treatment throughout the trial. No important differences between the clinical or laboratory variables of the groups were observed during the treatment period.[81]

TOXICOLOGY

Rats fed more than 100 times the human daily dose each day for 5 weeks and guinea pigs fed 150 times the human daily dose each day for 7 weeks were identical to control animals, especially in regard to appetite and weight gain.[82]

Parthenolide at concentrations up to 800 μM was found to be non-mutagenic in a forward mutation assay using *Salmonella typhimurium*.[32] A study of chromosomal aberrations and sister chromatid exchanges in lymphocytes and urine mutagenicity was examined in 30 chronic feverfew users (use over 11 consecutive months) and compared to 30 matched non-users. The data indicated that the prophylactic use of feverfew affected neither the frequency of chromosomal aberrations nor the frequency of sister chromatid exchanges in circulating peripheral lymphocytes. The mutagenicity of urine from feverfew users was not different to urine from non-user migraine patients.[83,84]

CONTRAINDICATIONS

Individuals with a known hypersensitivity to either feverfew, parthenolide or other members of the Compositae family should not take feverfew internally.[85]

SPECIAL WARNINGS AND PRECAUTIONS

None required.

INTERACTIONS

None known.

USE IN PREGNANCY AND LACTATION

No adverse effects expected as long as the recommended dosage levels are observed. Doses during pregnancy should be kept to a minimum.

EFFECTS ON ABILITY TO DRIVE AND USE MACHINES

None known.

SIDE EFFECTS

Allergic contact dermatitis has been noted in many cases after contact with feverfew. The sesquiterpene lactones are responsible.[86,87] In the survey conducted by Johnson in the early 1980s, side effects occurred in 17.9% of 270 patients surveyed. The side effects were considered mild and included mouth ulcers/sore tongue (6.4%), abdominal pain/indigestion (3.9%), unpleasant taste (3.0%), tingling sensation (0.9%), urinary problems (0.9%), headache (0.9%), swollen lips/mouth (0.4%) and diarrhoea (0.4%). Of an additional 164 users who had stopped taking feverfew, 21% did so because of side effects.[88] The oral side effects were probably caused by chewing fresh leaves.

OVERDOSE

Not known.

CURRENT REGULATORY STATUS IN SELECTED COUNTRIES

Feverfew became official during late 1998 in the *United States Pharmacopeia-National Formulary* (USP 23-NF 18). Feverfew is not covered by a Commission E monograph. It is on the UK General Sale List.

Feverfew does not have GRAS status. However, it is freely available as a 'dietary supplement' in the USA under DSHEA legislation (1994 Dietary Supplement Health and Education Act).

Feverfew is not included in Part 4 of Schedule 4 of the Therapeutic Goods Act Regulations of Australia.

References

1. Le Strange R. A history of herbal plants. Angus and Robertson, London: 1977; p 74.
2. Grieve M. A modern herbal, vol 1. Dover Publications, New York 1971; pp 309–310.

3. Felter HW, Lloyd JU. King's American dispensatory, 18th edn, 3rd revision, vol 2, 1905. Reprinted by Eclectic Medical Publications, Portland: 1983; pp 1438–1439.
4. Johnson ES. Feverfew (overcoming common problems). Sheldon Press, London, 1984; pp 26–27.
5. Johnson ES. Feverfew (overcoming common problems). Sheldon Press, London: 1984; pp 51, 52, 56–70.
6. Hancock K. Feverfew. Your headache may be over. Keats Publishing, New Canaan: 1986; pp 36, 47–51.
7. Hancock K. Feverfew, your headache may be over, Keats Publishing, Connecticut, 1986; p23
8. Palevitch E, Earon G, Carasso R. Phytother Res 1997; 11 (7): 508–511.
9. Chiej R. The Macdonald encyclopedia of medicinal plants. Macdonald, London: 1984; entry no. 85.
10. Launert EL. The Hamlyn guide to edible and medicinal plants of Britain and Northern Europe. Hamlyn, London 1981; p 194.
11. Mabberley DJ. The plant book, 2nd edn. Cambridge University Press, Cambridge, 1997; pp 176, 699.
12. Groenewegen WA, Knight DW, Heptinstall S. J Pharm Pharmacol 1986; 38 (9): 709–712.
13. Fontanel D, Bizot S, Beaufils P. Plantes méd phytothér 1990; 24 (4): 231–237.
14. Wagner H, Fessler B, Lotter H et al. Planta Med 1988; 54 (2): 171–172.
15. Bohlmann F, Zdero C. Phytochem 1982; 21 (10): 2543–2549.
16. Hendriks H, Bos R, Woerdenbag HJ. Flavour Fragrance J 1996; 11 (6): 367–371.
17. Williams CA, Hoult JR, Harborne JB et al. Phytochem 1995; 38 (1): 267–270.
18. Murch SJ, Simmons CB, Saxena PK. Lancet 1997; 350 (9091): 1598–1599.
19. Awang DVC, Dawson BA, Kindack DG. J Nat Prod 1991; 54 (6): 1516–1521.
20. Hanington E, Jones RJ, Amess JA et al. Lancet 1981; 2 (8249): 720–723.
21. Damasio H, Beck D. Lancet 1978; 1 (8058): 240–242.
22. Collier HO, Butt NM, McDonald-Gibson WJ et al. Lancet 1980; 2 (8200): 922–923.
23. Makheja AN, Bailey JM. Prostagland Leukot Med 1982; 8 (6): 653–660.
24. Heptinstall S, White A, Williamson L et al. Lancet 1985; 1 (8437): 1071–1074.
25. Groenewegen WA, Knight DW, Heptinstall S. J Pharm Pharmacol 1986; 38 (9): 709–712.
26. Heptinstall S, Groenewegen WA, Spangenberg P et al. Folia Haematol Int Mag Klin Morphol Blutforsch 1988; 115 (4): 447–449.
27. Knight DW. Nat Prod Rep 1995; 12 (3): 271–276.
28. Abad MJ, Bermejo P, Villar A. Phytother Res 1995; 9 (2): 79–92.
29. Groenewegen WA, Knight DW, Heptinstall S. Prog Med Chem 1992; 29: 217–238.
30. Heptinstall S, Groenewegen WA, Spangenberg P et al. J Pharm Pharmacol 1987; 39 (6): 459–465.
31. Groenewegen WA, Heptinstall S. J Pharm Pharmacol 1990; 42 (8): 553–557.
32. Marles RJ, Pazos-Sanou L, Compadre CM et al. Sesquiterpene lactones revisited. In: Arnason JT et al (eds) Recent advances in phytochemistry, vol 29, phytochemistry of medicinal plants. Plenum Press, New York: 1995; pp 333–356.
33. Heptinstall S, Awang DV, Dawson BA et al. J Pharm Pharmacol 1992; 44 (5): 391–395.
34. Marles RJ, Kaminski J, Arnason JT et al. J Nat Prod 1992; 55 (8): 1044–1056.
35. Groenewegen WA, Heptinstall S. Lancet 1986; 1 (8474): 44–45.
36. Voyno-Yasenetskaya TA, Loesche W, Groenewegen WA et al. J Pharm Pharmacol 1988; 40 (7): 501–502.
37. Loesche W, Mazurov AV, Voyno-Yasenetskaya TA et al. Folia Haematol Int Mag Klin Morphol Blutforsch 1988; 115 (1–2): 181–184.
38. Biggs MJ, Johnson ES, Persaud NP et al. Lancet 1982; 2 (8301): 776.
39. Losche W, Michel E, Heptinstall S et al. Planta Med 1988; 54 (5): 381–384.
40. Brown AM, Edwards CM, Davey MR et al. J Pharm Pharmacol 1997; 49 (5): 558–561.
41. Brown AMG, Edwards CM, Davey MR et al. Phytother Res 1997; 11 (7): 479–484.
42. Williamson LM, Harvey DM, Sheppard KJ et al. Inflammation 1988; 12 (1): 11–16.
43. Hayes NA, Foreman JC. J Pharm Pharmacol 1987; 39 (6): 466–470.
44. Pugh WJ, Sambo K. J Pharm Pharmacol 1988; 40 (10): 743–745.
45. Hwang D, Fischer NH, Jang BC et al. Biochem Biophys Res Commun 1996; 226 (3): 810–818.
46. Loesche W, Groenewegen WA, Krause S et al. Biomed Biochim Acta 1988; 47 (10–11): S241–S243.
47. Silk ST, DeMarco ME. Biochem Biophys Res Commun 1987; 146 (2): 582–588.
48. Summer H, Salan U, Knight DW et al. Biochem Pharmacol 1992; 43 (11): 2313–2320.
49. Capasso F. J Pharm Pharmacol 1986; 38 (1): 71–72.
50. Weber JT, Hayataka K, O'Connor MF et al. Comp Biochem Physiol C Pharmacol Toxicol Endocrinol 1997; 117 (1): 19–24.
51. Weber JT, O'Connor MF, Hayataka K et al. J Nat Prod 1997; 60 (6): 651–653.
52. Bejar E. J Ethnopharmacol 1996; 50 (1): 1–12.
53. Barsby RW, Salan U, Knight DW et al. Planta Med 1993; 59 (1): 20–25.
54. Hay AJ, Hamburger M, Hostettmann K et al. Br J Pharmacol 1994; 112 (1): 9–12.
55. Barsby RW, Salan U, Knight DW et al. J Pharm Pharmacol 1992; 44 (9): 737–740.
56. Barsby R, Salan U, Knight DW et al. Lancet 1991; 338 (8773): 1015.
57. Stephanovic M, Ristic N, Vukmiorovic M. Sci Nat 1988; 23: 23–40.
58. Blakeman JP, Atkinson P. Physiol Plant Pathol 1979; 15 (2): 183–192.
59. Kalodera Z, Pepeljnjak S, Blazevic N et al. Pharmazie 1997; 52 (11): 885–886.
60. Kalodera Z, Pepeljnjak S, Petrak T. Pharmazie 1996; 51 (12): 995–996.
61. Hall IH, Lee KH, Starnes CO et al. J Pharm Sci 1978; 67 (9): 1235–1239.
62. Lee KH, Hall IH, Mar EC et al. Science 1977; 196 (4289): 533–536.
63. Hall IH, Lee KH, Starnes CO et al. J Pharm Sci 1980; 69 (6): 694–697.
64. Hall IH, Starnes CO Jr, Lee KH et al. J Pharm Sci 1980; 69 (5): 537–543.
65. Hall IH, Lee KH, Starnes CO et al. J Pharm Sci 1979; 68 (5): 537–542.
66. Robles M, Aregullin M, West J et al. Planta Med 1995; 61: 199–203.
67. Huffman MA, Seifu M. Primates 1989; 30 (1): 51–64.
68. Krause S, Arese P, Heptinstall S et al. Arzneim-Forsch 1990; 40 (6): 689–692.
69. Elissalde MH Jr, Ivie GW. Am J Vet Res 1987; 48 (1): 148–152.
70. O'Neill LA, Barrett ML, Lewis GP. Br J Clin Pharmacol 1987; 23 (1): 81–83.
71. Keery RJ, Lumley P. Br J Pharmacol 1986; 89: 834P.
72. Buck AC, Pugh J, Davies R et al. Abstract from Congress sur les Prostaglandines, 1986, p 53. Cited in Groenewegen WA, Knight DW, Heptinstall S. Prog Med Chem 1992; 29: 217–238.
73. Lassen LH, Ashina M, Christiansen I et al. Lancet 1997, 349(9049): 401–402.
74. Park HJ, Jung WT, Basnet P et al. J Nat Prod 1996; 59 (12): 1128–1130.
75. Johnson ES. Feverfew (overcoming common problems). Sheldon Press, London, 1984; pp 42–55.
76. Johnson ES, Kadam NP, Hylands DM et al. Br Med J (Clin Res Ed) 1985; 291 (6495): 569–573.
77. Hylands DM, Hylands PJ, Johnson ES et al. Br Med J (Clin Res Ed)1985; 291 (6502): 1128.
78. Murphy JJ, Heptinstall S, Mitchell JR. Lancet 1988; 2 (8604): 189–192.
79. Groenewegen WA. Unpublished data. Cited in Groenewegen WA, Knight DW, Heptinstall S. Prog Med Chem 1992; 29: 217–238.
80. De Weerdt CJ, Bootsma HPR, Hendriks H. Phytomed 1996; 3 (3): 225–230.

81. Pattrick M, Heptinstall S, Doherty M. Ann Rheum Dis 1989; 48 (7): 547–549.
82. Johnson ES. Feverfew (overcoming common problems). Sheldon Press, London, 1984; p 78.
83. Anderson D, Jeckinson PC, Dewdney RS et al. Hum Toxicol 1988; 7 (2): 145–152.
84. Johnson ES, Kadam NP, Anderson D et al. Hum Toxicol 1987; 6 (6): 533–534.
85. De Smet PAGM et al (eds). Adverse effects of herbal drugs, vol 1. Springer-Verlag, Berlin, 1992; p 257.
86. Lamminpaa A, Estlander T, Jolanki R et al. Contact Derm 1996; 34 (5): 330–335.
87. Arlette J, Mitchell JC. Contact Derm 1981; 7 (3): 129–136.
88. Johnson ES. Feverfew (overcoming common problems). Sheldon Press, London: 1984; pp 79–83.

Ginger
(*Zingiber officinale* Roscoe)

SYNONYMS

Zingiberis rhizoma (Lat), Ingwer (Ger), gingembre (Fr), zerzero (Ital), ingefaer (Dan), ardhrakam (Sanskrit). Dried ginger: gan jiang (Chin), kankyo (Jap). Fresh ginger: sheng jiang (Chin), shokyo (Jap).

WHAT IS IT?

Ginger root (actually the rhizome) is a familiar kitchen spice widely available either as dried root or powder or as the whole fresh root ('green ginger'). Ginger has been used as a pungent spice and medicine for thousands of years. Its use is recorded in early Sanskrit and Chinese texts and is also documented in ancient Greek, Roman and Arabic medical literature. Ginger was probably among the first vegetatively cultivated plants and is currently grown commercially in India, China, south-east Asia, West Indies, Mexico, Africa, Fiji and Australia.

EFFECTS

Reduces nausea; stimulates circulatory activity; inhibits arachidonic acid metabolism.

TRADITIONAL VIEW

In Western herbal medicine, ginger has been used for dyspepsia, flatulent colic, alcoholic gastritis and diarrhoea from relaxed bowel where there is no inflammation. As a circulatory stimulant, hot infusion of ginger was said to be beneficial for amenorrhoea due to cold. It was also used as a rubifacient.[1,2] The Eclectics used ginger particularly as a stimulating tonic, stomachic, carminative and antispasmodic. It was used to treat nausea, gastrointestinal cramping, loss of appetite and cold extremities. The hot infusion was used to 'break up' colds and to relieve painful menstruation.[3]

Ginger was also described as a diffusive stimulant.[4] The term 'stimulant' in this context means a metabolic (heating) and circulatory enhancing agent which also reinforces the therapeutic activity of other herbs. Being a diffusive stimulant, ginger was used to enhance those activities which could be classified as 'diffuse' such as expectoration, digestion and diaphoresis.

Similar uses were observed for ginger in Ayurveda. It was also topically applied for headache, toothache and to improve circulation to the limbs.[5] In Thai traditional texts the main uses described for ginger rhizome include sweetening the voice, enhancing appetite, dyspepsia, flatulence, fever, mouth ulcers and intestinal infections.[6]

In traditional Chinese medicine, distinction is made between fresh and dried ginger rhizome. Dried ginger is more effective in expelling *Interior Cold*, which is related more to the constitution of the patient, while fresh ginger promotes sweating and disperses *Exterior Cold* which is brought on by external agents. Fresh ginger is pungent and hot and is used for vomiting, cough and debilitating sweating and to reduce the poisonous effect of other herbs.[7] It is used for common colds due to pathogenic *Wind Cold*, characterized by severe intolerance to cold, slight fever, headache, general ache, nasal congestion and a runny nose.[8] Dried ginger is pungent and hot and is used for *Cold* conditions characterized by pallor, poor appetite and digestion, cold limbs, vomiting, diarrhoea, pale tongue, or thin, watery or white sputum. It is to be used cautiously during pregnancy.

SUMMARY ACTIONS

Carminative, antiemetic, peripheral circulatory stimulant, spasmolytic, antiinflammatory, antiplatelet, diaphoretic, digestive stimulant.

CAN BE USED FOR

INDICATIONS SUPPORTED BY CLINICAL TRIALS

Treatment and prophylaxis of nausea and emesis in cases of motion sickness, nausea of pregnancy and postoperative and drug-induced nausea; as an adjunct in the treatment of arthritis.

TRADITIONAL THERAPEUTIC USES

To enhance digestion, expectoration and diaphoresis; digestive problems, especially colic, flatulent dyspepsia, cramping, peptic ulcer, loss of appetite, gastrointestinal infections; fever, colds (especially the fresh rhizome); menstrual problems such as amenorrhoea and dysmenorrhoea.

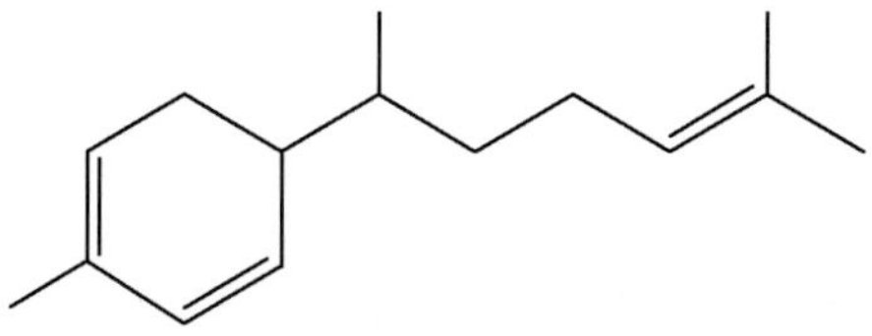

Zingiberene

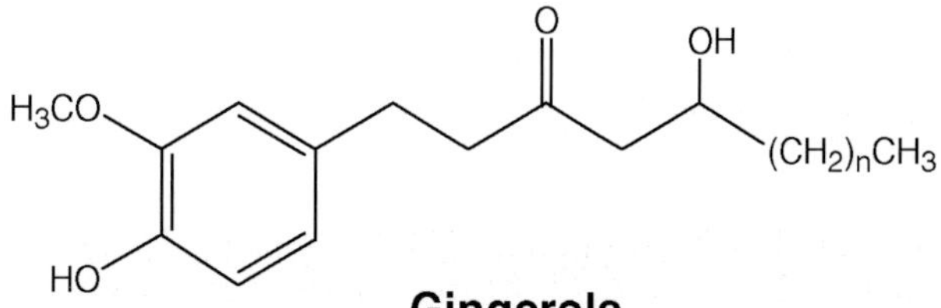

H3CO, HO, O, OH, (CH2)nCH3

Gingerols

	n
6-Gingerol	4
8-Gingerol	6
10-Gingerol	8

MAY ALSO BE USED FOR

EXTRAPOLATIONS FROM PHARMACOLOGICAL STUDIES

Treatment of peptic ulceration; inflammatory conditions; thrombocytosis; migraine headaches; to enhance the bioavailability of other treatments; as an antiplatelet agent.

PREPARATIONS

Fresh or dried root as an infusion, decoction, liquid extract, oleoresin or tablets for internal use. As with all essential oil-containing herbs, use of the fresh plant or carefully dried herb is advised. Keep covered if infusing the herb to retain the essential oil.

DOSAGE

- Fresh root equivalent 500–1000 mg three times a day; dried root equivalent 500 mg 2–4 times a day.
- Ginger tablets (500 mg): one tablet 2–4 times per day.
- 0.7–2 ml per day of 1:2 liquid extract, 1.7–5 ml per day of 1:5 tincture.

DURATION OF USE

There are no known problems with long-term consumption. However, for most purposes dosage need only be short term and directed to immediate symptom relief.

SUMMARY ASSESSMENT OF SAFETY

No problems known from ingestion in moderate doses. Ginger may enhance the bioavailability of other medications and high doses may cause heartburn and have a blood-thinning effect.

TECHNICAL DATA

BOTANY

Ginger, a member of the Zingiberaceae family, is thought to be a cultigen of Indian origin.[9] It grows with erect leafy stems 0.6–1.2 m high. The leaves are narrow, linear-lanceolate (2–3 cm long, 1–2 cm wide). The inflorescence is a terminal spike with irregular flowers, coloured yellowish-green and streaked with purple. The fruit is a capsule. It has a stout, tuberous rhizome which is branched and laterally compressed. The surface of the rhizome is greyish-white with light-brownish rings.[10] It is commonly but erroneously referred to as ginger root (instead of rhizome).

KEY CONSTITUENTS

- Essential oil (1–3%), including zingiberene, sesquiphellandrene and beta-bisabolene.[11]
- Pungent (hot) principles: 1–2.5% gingerols, shogaols.[11]

The components beta-sesquiphellandrene and (–)-zingiberene are highest in fresh ginger and decompose on drying and storage. This understanding may provide a basis for the preference in traditional Chinese medicine for the fresh rhizome in the treatment of the common cold. The gingerols gradually decompose into shogaols on storage.

PHARMACODYNAMICS

Antiemetic and antinausea activity

Early animal studies demonstrated the antiemetic property of fresh ginger.[8] Acetone and ethanolic extracts of ginger exhibited significant protection against cisplatin-induced emesis in dogs at oral doses of 25, 50, 100 and

200 mg/kg. Aqueous extract at these doses was ineffective. The extracts were less effective than the 5-HT_3 receptor antagonist granisetron and were not effective against apomorphine-induced emesis.[12]

Mowrey and Clayson compared the effects of 1.88 g of dried powdered ginger, 100 mg dimenhydrinate (Dramamine) and placebo on the symptoms of motion sickness in 36 healthy subjects who reported very high susceptibility to motion sickness. Motion sickness was induced by placing the blindfolded subject in a tilted rotating chair. Ginger was found to be superior to dimenhydrinate and placebo in preventing the gastrointestinal symptoms of motion sickness and the authors postulated a local effect in the gastrointestinal tract for ginger. This was particularly likely since it was given as a powder only 25 minutes before the test.[13] The gingerols and shogaols were subsequently identified as the main antiemetic compounds.[14]

Several subsequent clinical studies investigated the mechanism of action of ginger. A double-blind, crossover, placebo trial on healthy volunteers by Grøntved and Hentzer found that ginger significantly reduced vertigo induced by heat stimulation of the vestibular system (that is, the irrigation of the left ear with water at 44°C), but had no effect on the duration or the maximum slow-phase velocity of nystagmus (involuntary, rhythmic movement of the eyeball). In three out of 24 tests, nausea was present after placebo but it did not occur after ginger at all.[15] Currently two classes of drugs are used to treat motion sickness. Antihistamines reduce nystagmus but the second class comprising parasympatholytics and sympathomimetics (which basically reinforce the activity of the sympathetic nervous system) do not. Grøntved and Hentzer concluded that ginger root, like sympathomimetics and parasympatholytics, also dampens the induced vestibular impulses to the autonomic centres of the central nervous system (CNS).[15]

Although a second research group verified the finding that ginger had no effect on nystagmus, they disputed the interpretation of Grøntved and Hentzer and concluded that a CNS mechanism can be excluded for ginger.[16] A more accurate interpretation of their findings would be that ginger lacks central anticholinergic effects. Any reduction of motion sickness was suggested to be derived from the influence of ginger on the digestive tract.

The effect of dried ginger on the gastric emptying rate was also investigated.[17] In a randomized, double-blind, crossover trial, 16 healthy subjects received 1 g of ginger or placebo. Gastric emptying was measured using the oral paracetamol absorption model. Since ingestion of ginger had no influence on gastric emptying, it was concluded that the antiemetic effect of ginger in healthy subjects is not associated with increased gastric emptying.[17]

A team of Japanese scientists tested the hypothesis that ginger might exert its antiemetic activity by blocking serotonin receptors (5-HT_3 in particular) in the digestive tract. Ginger was found to potently inhibit the contractile response of isolated guinea pig ileum to serotonin, and 8-gingerol was more active than the control drug cocaine.[18] Subsequently 6-gingerol was observed to counter the emetic effect of the cytotoxic drug cyclophosphamide.[19] However, it is not clear how 5-HT_3 receptors are affected by cytotoxic drugs, although there is a good correlation between blocking of this receptor and antiemetic efficacy.[19,20] Galanolactone, a diterpenoid isolated from ginger, was found to be a competitive antagonist predominantly at 5-HT_3 receptors, with less effect on other 5-HT receptor subtypes.[21]

It has been suggested from these studies that ginger components could have a central antiemetic effect via 5-HT_3 antagonism.[22] In contrast, a Chinese pharmacological investigation concluded that ginger produces an antimotion sickness action possibly through central and peripheral anticholinergic and antihistaminic effects.[23]

Antiulcer activity

Ginger and 6-gingerol inhibited experimental gastric ulcers in rats.[24,25] From in vivo studies, several antiulcer compounds have been isolated from ginger including 6-gingesulfonic acid,[26] 6-shogaol and *ar*-curcumene.[27] Most notable is 6-gingesulfonic acid, which showed weaker pungency and more potent antiulcer activity than 6-gingerol and 6-shogaol.[28] Oral administration of spray-dried ginger extract (500 mg/kg), licorice extract (500 mg/kg) or the combination of the two extracts (rikkunshi-to, 1000 mg/kg) significantly prevented gastric mucosal damage induced by ethanol in rats. Pretreatment with ginger extract or rikkunshi-to inhibited the reduction in the deep corpus mucin content caused by ethanol.[29]

However, high doses of ginger probably act as a gastric irritant. Fresh ginger in quantities of 6 g or more caused a significant increase in exfoliation of gastric surface epithelial cells in human volunteers.[30]

Antiinflammatory activity

Ginger and its pungent components are dual inhibitors of arachidonic acid metabolism. That is, they inhibit both the cyclooxygenase (prostaglandin synthetase) and lipoxygenase enzymes of the prostaglandin and leukotriene biosynthetic pathways.[31–36] Gingerols were more potent inhibitors of prostaglandin biosynthesis than indomethacin[33] and are also potent inhibitors of 5-lipoxygenase.[34] However, one component of ginger actually promotes prostaglandin production. Zingerone was found to share a prostaglandin synthetase-promoting activity with a number of other emetic, purgative and irritant drugs in the digestive system.[37]

Ginger extract inhibited carrageenan-induced paw swelling and was as active as aspirin. However, ginger was devoid of analgesic activity at the doses used.[31] Essential oil of ginger inhibited chronic adjuvant arthritis in rats.[38,39]

Antiplatelet and cardiovascular activity

Srivastava and co-workers found that aqueous extract of ginger inhibited platelet aggregation induced by ADP, epinephrine, collagen and arachidonic acid in vitro.[40] Ginger acted by inhibiting thromboxane synthesis.[41,42] It also inhibited prostacyclin synthesis in rat aorta.[40] The antiplatelet action of 6-gingerol was also mainly due to the inhibition of thromboxane formation.[43]

Srivastava followed up this laboratory work with a clinical trial in healthy volunteers.[44] Danish women consumed either 70 g fresh onion or 5 g fresh ginger daily for a period of 7 days. Thromboxane was determined in serum obtained after blood clotting. Onion intake slightly increased production of thromboxane whereas ginger caused a 37% inhibition.[44] Dietary supplementation with 100 g/day of butter for 7 days in 20 healthy males was found to enhance platelet aggregation. Addition of 5 g of dried ginger to the fatty meal in two divided doses significantly inhibited platelet aggregation ($p<0.001$) compared to placebo.[45] However, in a randomized double-blind study on eight healthy male volunteers, bleeding time, platelet count and platelet aggregation were not found to be affected by a single dose of 2 g of dried ginger.[46] Given the above findings, concerns were expressed about the use of ginger for postoperative nausea until the effects of its potential antiplatelet activity were more fully investigated.[47]

One study published in 1996 has questioned the clinical antiplatelet activity of ginger. Eighteen patients consumed either 15 g of raw ginger root, 40 g of cooked stem ginger or placebo for 2 weeks in a randomized, crossover design.[48] Ginger consumption did not cause a decrease in thromboxane production by platelets ex vivo. Unfortunately, the design of this study had some problems which cast doubt on the significance of its findings. The scientists used a crossover design. This means that each participant consumed the test substances and placebo in a random order over three consecutive 2-week periods. However, there was no wash-out period between tests during which no treatment was given. It is conceivable that the effects of ginger could be sufficiently sustained to carry over into a following placebo phase. The study was concerned with dietary intake of ginger and participants received their ginger to add to vanilla custard immediately prior to consumption. Given the distinctive appearance and taste of ginger, it is unlikely that the study would have been blinded from the participant's viewpoint.

Ginger decreased serum and hepatic cholesterol in cholesterol-fed rats[49] and stimulated the conversion of cholesterol to bile acids.[50] However, ginger at five times normal human intake had no effect on serum and liver cholesterol levels in hypercholesterolaemic rats.[51] Oral administration of ginger extract reduced total cholesterol and serum LDL-cholesterol in hyperlipidaemic rabbits. Tissue lipid profiles of liver, heart and aorta showed similar changes. Ginger feeding increased the faecal excretion of cholesterol which suggests a modulation of absorption.[52]

Ginger exerted a powerful positive inotropic effect on isolated guinea pig left atria.[53] Gingerols were identified as the active components,[53,54] and later, 6- and 8-shogaol were found to show a positive inotropic activity of about the same potency as that of 8-gingerol.[55] 8-Gingerol stimulated the Ca^{2+}-pumping ATPase in skeletal and cardiac sarcoplasmic reticulum.[56] Further investigation indicated that this activity was increased in a concentration-dependent manner by 6-gingerol, 8-gingerol and 10-gingerol.[57] Zingeronolol, a substance derived from zingerone, has demonstrated beta-adrenergic blocking activity in vivo.[58] This contradicts with the cardiotonic effect demonstrated by the whole extract.

The average systolic and diastolic blood pressures of normal subjects given 1.0 g of fresh ginger to chew, without swallowing, were increased by 11.2 and 14 mmHg respectively.[8] The pressor effect may be a short-term reflex response to the pungent effect of ginger. The component 6-shogaol also shows a pressor response in pharmacological studies.[59–61]

Effects on digestive function

Early Chinese and Japanese animal research found that oral and intragastric application of fresh ginger decoction produced a stimulant action on gastric secretion.[8] Another study found that while gastric secretions, free acid and lipase activity were increased following ginger, the activity of pepsin was decreased.[8] Dietary ginger enhanced intestinal lipase activity and the disaccharidases sucrase and maltase in rats.[62]

Intraduodenal doses of ginger extract increased bile secretion in rats. Total secretion of bile solids was also increased, but not to the same extent as bile flow. 6-Gingerol and 10-gingerol were identified as the active components.[63] Fresh ginger also contains a proteolytic enzyme.[64]

Oral doses of 6-shogaol accelerated intestinal transit in rats.[65] An extract of ginger and isolated 6-shogaol and gingerols enhanced gastrointestinal motility in mice after oral doses.[66] The effects of the ginger components were comparable to the antinausea drugs metoclopramide (Maxolon) and domperidone (Motilium). Both 6-shogaol and 6-gingerol suppressed gastric contraction in rats.[65]

Acetone and ethanol extracts of ginger (oral doses: 100, 200, 500 mg/kg) and ginger juice (2 or 4 ml/kg) significantly reversed the cisplatin-induced delay in gastric emptying in rats. Ginger juice and acetone extract were more effective than the ethanol extract and the reversal produced by the acetone extract was similar to that caused by the 5-HT_3 receptor antagonist ondansetron. Ginger juice produced better reversal than ondansetron. Ginger may therefore be useful in allaying the gastrointestinal side effects of cancer chemotherapy.

Anticathartic activity is also known to be one of the effects of ginger. In a Japanese study, ginger extract significantly inhibited serotonin-induced diarrhoea in mice.[67] The pungent principles were found to be the active components.

Research suggests that ginger is one of a number of hot spices that increase bioavailability of other drugs, either by increasing their absorption rate from the gastrointestinal tract or by protecting the drug from being metabolized/oxidized in its first passage through the liver after being absorbed.[68]

German scientists found that chewing 9 g of crystallized ginger had a profound effect on saliva production in healthy volunteers.[69] Amylase activity was also increased and the saliva was not more watery, although it contained slightly less mucoprotein.

Antipyretic and thermogenic activity

A slight antipyretic activity was observed after oral administration of 6-shogaol and 6-gingerol (140 mg/kg) in rats.[65] Ginger extract given orally reduced fever in rats by 38%, while the same dose of aspirin was effective by 44%. However, ginger had no effect in normal rats.[31]

In traditional herbal therapy ginger is regarded as a warming (stimulating) medicine. This also provides the basis for its diaphoretic activity in febrile states. (This diaphoretic activity is obviously tempered by the antipyretic activity described above.) Several studies have sought to understand a possible thermogenic role for ginger. European studies proposed that the pungent principles of ginger act to stimulate thermoregulatory receptors.[63] In addition, ginger and its pungent components were thermogenic in the perfused rat hindlimb.[70]

Zingerone (like capsaicin from chillies and piperine from pepper, but unlike sulphur-containing acrid principles from garlic and mustard) increased the secretion of catecholamines, especially adrenaline, from the adrenal medulla after intravenous injection in rats, thus possibly accounting in part for the warming effect.[71]

But more sustained effects may arise from different mechanisms. Ginger extract stimulated cytokine secretion by human peripheral blood mononuclear cells.[72] A pyrogenic effect from these cytokines may play a role in any thermogenic effect of ginger. Ginger and its pungent principles significantly inhibited serotonin-induced hypothermia.[67] In contrast to chilli and mustard sauce, a ginger sauce did not increase metabolic rate in human subjects.[73]

Antimicrobial and antiparasitic activity

Some of the minor pungent components of ginger have been shown to have antifungal activity.[74] Ginger extract demonstrated mild growth inhibition of Gram-positive and Gram-negative bacteria,[31] including *E. coli, Proteus vulgaris, Salmonella typhimurium, Staph. aureus* and *Strep. viridans*.[75]

Sesquiterpenes in ginger essential oil were found to have significant antirhinoviral activity in vitro.[76] The most active components were beta-sesquiphellandrene and zingiberene and since these are highest in fresh ginger, this provides a scientific basis for the preference in traditional Chinese medicine for the fresh rhizome in the treatment of the common cold.

There are also observations of direct antiparasitic activity.[77] Gingerol completely abolished infectivity of the parasite *Schistosoma mansoni* in snails and mice.[78] An extract from ginger effectively destroyed larvae of the fish parasite Anisakis in vitro. The most active antinematodal constituent was 6-gingerol, although a synergistic action with 6-shogaol (also a potent constituent) was also observed.[79]

Other activity

Both 6-gingerol and 8-gingerol potentiated the contraction induced by prostaglandins (except PGD_2) and inhibited contraction produced by PGD_2, thromboxane A_2 and leukotrienes.[80] There is a structural requirement for this activity, as other gingerol-related derivatives do not necessarily produce the same effect.[81]

Antihepatotoxic activities of gingerols and shogaols were observed in vitro using carbon tetracholoride- and galactosamine-induced cytotoxicity in cultured rat hepatocytes.[82] 6-Shogaol, 8-shogaol and 8-gingerol showed dose-dependent inhibitory activities on experimentally induced histamine release from rat peritoneal mast cells. Other tested compounds from fresh ginger showed no inhibitory activity. In addition, 6-shogaol and 6-gingerol exhibited antiallergic activity in vivo.[55]

Ginger, ginger extract and pungent principles (gingerol and zingerone) have demonstrated antioxidant activity in vitro.[83–88] Such antioxidant activity might be expected, since many inhibitors of lipoxygenase are also strong antioxidants.

Ginger extract exhibited a prolonged hypoglycaemic activity in rabbits.[31] Injection of 6-shogaol showed an intense antitussive action in comparison with dihydrocodeine phosphate.[65]

PHARMACOKINETICS

After injection, 90% of 6-gingerol was bound to serum protein and elimination was mainly via the liver.[89] Oral or intraperitoneal dosage of zingerone resulted in the urinary excretion of metabolites within 24 hours, mainly as glucuronide and/or sulphate conjugates.[90] Appreciable biliary excretion (40% in 12 hours) also occurred.[90]

CLINICAL TRIALS

Nausea and emesis

Since the work of Mowrey and Clayson, many studies have been published which confirmed the antiemetic and antinausea effects of ginger in a clinical setting. The effect of 1 g of powdered ginger on seasickness was tested in a double-blind, randomized, placebo-controlled trial. Among 80 naval cadets, unaccustomed to sailing in heavy seas, ginger significantly reduced the tendency to vomiting and cold sweating ($p<0.05$).[91]

One thousand, four hundred and eighty-nine tourist volunteers completed a randomized, double-blind study which investigated the effects of seven antiemetic treatments on the prevention of seasickness. Ginger was found to be as effective as the antiemetic drugs tested. Nearly 80% of subjects reported no seasickness when given 250 mg of ginger 2 hours prior to departure. (In a previous study in the same setting, 80% of the passengers not receiving prophylactic drugs were seasick. For this reason the above trial was not placebo-controlled.)[92]

Twenty-four children suffering from hyperketonaemia received either ginger (average daily dose of 1.25 g in 500 mg doses) or metoclopramide in a double-blind trial. Compared to metoclopramide, ginger was significantly more effective in the opinion of the physicians ($p<0.0005$) and significantly better at preventing vomiting ($p<0.05$).[93]

Thirty women participated in a double-blind, randomized, crossover trial of the efficacy of ginger against placebo in hyperemesis gravidarum.[94] The test dose was four 250 mg capsules per day for 4 days. A significantly greater relief of symptoms such as nausea and vomiting was found after ginger treatment ($p=0.035$). One spontaneous abortion subsequently occurred, which was not considered to be a suspicious rate.[94]

The effectiveness of ginger as an antiemetic agent was compared with placebo and metoclopramide (Maxolon) in 60 women who had major gynaecological surgery in a double-blind, randomized study.[95] Patients were given 1 g of powdered ginger at the time of premedication prior to surgery. There were significantly fewer recorded incidences of nausea in the group receiving ginger compared with placebo ($p<0.05$). Incidences of nausea in the ginger and metoclopramide groups were similar.

This study, published in the journal *Anaesthesia*, prompted two letters. One letter confirmed the use of fresh ginger in Chinese medicine to reduce nausea and vomiting during pregnancy.[96] The other cautioned against wholeheartedly recommending ginger to prevent postoperative nausea until the effect on bleeding time of its pronounced antiplatelet activity was more fully investigated.[47] However, the effect of a single 1 g dose of ginger on bleeding time is unlikely to be profound.[46]

Ginger was proven as an effective antiemetic for the prevention of postoperative nausea and vomiting after laparoscopic gynaecological surgery. In a prospective, randomized double-blind trial in 120 women, 1 g of powdered ginger was as effective as 10 mg metoclopramide.[97] Since metoclopramide has extrapyramidal side effects (and can cause tardive dyskinesia) and ginger has none, ginger should be the preferred treatment.

Finally, ginger prevented psoralen-associated nausea in an open study.[98] Patients undergoing photopheresis therapy were required to ingest psoralen before each treatment. Eleven patients who regularly experienced nausea after psoralen were included in the study and acted as their own controls. When three capsules of 530 mg of ginger were taken prior to psoralen ingestion, nausea was significantly reduced.[98]

Several clinical studies on ginger have produced negative findings. In one study, 28 healthy subjects were tested with either ginger, scopolamine or a placebo in a rotating chair.[99] Dried ginger (500 or 1000 mg) or fresh ginger (1000 mg) provided no protection against motion sickness. In contrast, scopolamine was effective ($p<0.01$). Dried ginger (500 mg) also had no effect on gastric emptying in normal or motion-sick subjects. Two other studies by the same group were also negative.[100,101]

In another study conducted in South Australia, 108 patients received oral placebo or dried ginger (500 mg or 1000 mg) prior to gynaecological laparoscopic surgery in a randomized, double-blind study.[102] The incidence of nausea and vomiting increased slightly but non-significantly with increasing dose of ginger.

It is difficult to reconcile these negative findings with the nine positive studies. Perhaps the issue was one of quality, since no study attempted to chemically characterize the ginger being used.

Inflammatory conditions

In response to the pharmacological evidence and the traditional use of ginger in Ayurvedic and Tibb medicine, Srivastava and Mustafa proposed that ginger may be an effective treatment for rheumatic disorders.[103] They cite case histories for seven patients with rheumatoid arthritis living in Canada and Denmark, aged between 50 and 67 years. All patients received additional relief from their symptoms by including ginger with their conventional treatment. A larger study by these scientists reported results for 56 patients (28 with rheumatoid arthritis, 18 with osteoarthritis and 10 with muscular discomfort) who used dried ginger.[104] More than 75% of the arthritis patients experienced relief in pain and swelling and all the patients with muscular discomfort experienced relief of pain. No patients reported adverse effects during the period of ginger consumption, which ranged from 3 months to 2.5 years.[104]

The same scientists have also suggested the use of ginger for the treatment of migraine headaches.[105] They describe a case history of a 42-year-old female who experienced an abortive effect on a migraine headache by taking 1.5–2.0 g per day of powdered ginger. She then included ginger in her diet and experienced a marked reduction in migraine frequency. The authors proposed a number of possible mechanisms for ginger's activity against migraines, but the inhibition of thromboxane and other prostaglandins may be paramount.[105] In contrast to feverfew (*Tanacetum parthenium*), ginger did not inhibit serotonin release from bovine platelets.[106]

Antiplatelet activity

Backon and co-workers claim extensive therapeutic experience with ginger.[47] They believe that as it is a very powerful thromboxane synthetase inhibitor and prostacyclin agonist, ginger has therapeutic potential in alcohol withdrawal and the complications of liver damage,[107] in recovery from serious burns,[108] in treating peptic ulceration,[109] as an antidepressant,[110] in preventing ageing penile vascular changes and impotence[111] and as an analgesic in dysmenorrhoea.[112]

One interesting use for ginger postulated by Backon is for the treatment of Kawasaki disease. This syndrome, mainly prevalent in children, presents with coronary artery aneurysms and thrombocytosis. In Kawasaki disease, hypersensitivity reactions due to antigen-antibody complexes may damage the blood vessel wall and induce arteritis. Antigens may be of microbial or viral origin. Since thromboxane has been implicated in the pathogenesis of Kawasaki disease, Backon suggests ginger and carbon dioxide (in the form of soda water) as thromboxane synthetase inhibitors. A case history of thrombocytosis in a 78-year-old male, due to a myeloproliferative disorder (not Kawasaki disease), is described. Ginger (about 2 g) plus soda water dropped his platelet count from 1.8 million to 240 000 in one day. This fall was subsequently clearly associated with the treatment since platelet count plummeted while the patient was taking the ginger and rose to over 1.5 million when not.[113]

Powdered ginger given at a dose of 4 g daily to 30 patients with coronary artery disease (CAD) did not affect platelet aggregation measured after 1.5 and 3 months of administration. In addition, no change in fibrinolytic activity and fibrinogen level was observed. No information was provided for controls. However, a single dose of 10 g ginger to each of 10 CAD patients produced a significant reduction in platelet aggregation after 4 hours ($p<0.05$). There was a small non-significant rise in platelet aggregation for the placebo group. Ginger did not affect blood lipids and blood sugar when administered at a 4 g daily dose for 3 months. The doses used in these studies were relatively high and lower doses are probably unlikely to offer any significant risk protection.[114]

TOXICOLOGY

The acute oral LD_{50} for ginger oil in rats and the acute dermal LD_{50} value in rabbits both exceeded 5 g/kg.[115] Ginger extract caused no mortality at doses of up to 2.5 g/kg in mice (equivalent to about 75 g/kg of fresh rhizome).[31] This low acute toxicity was confirmed in a separate study, which also found that ginger extract at 100 mg/kg per day for 3 months caused no signs of chronic toxicity.[116]

Chemical components of ginger have both mutagenic[117] and antimutagenic activity.[118,119] Depending on the test model, ginger extract has also shown mutagenic[6,120] and antimutagenic[121] and anticarcinogenic effects.[122]

CONTRAINDICATIONS

According to the Commission E, use of ginger is contraindicated in patients with gallstones, except under close supervision, and should *not* be administered for morning sickness during pregnancy.[123]

However, the dictate from traditional Chinese medicine that dried ginger should be used cautiously during pregnancy is probably a more rational approach.[124] A daily dose of 2 g of dried ginger should not be exceeded in pregnancy.

SPECIAL WARNINGS AND PRECAUTIONS

Proceed with caution in cases of peptic ulceration or other gastric diseases. Any exacerbation in such cases should, however, be immediately apparent and transient.

INTERACTIONS

Ginger may increase the absorption of pharmaceutical drugs.[68,125] Although no problems have been reported in humans, ginger may increase the chance of bleeding.[126] Daily doses of ginger in excess of 4 g should particularly be prescribed with caution in patients who are already taking blood-thinning drugs such as warfarin or aspirin or who have increased risk of haemorrhage.[114]

USE IN PREGNANCY AND LACTATION

No adverse effects are expected. Ginger has been utilized in clinical trials of the treatment of pregnant women with nausea.[94]

EFFECTS ON ABILITY TO DRIVE AND USE MACHINES

None known.

SIDE EFFECTS

At higher doses a blood-thinning effect and an increase in gastric secretory activity leading to heartburn is possible. Topical application of ginger may cause contact dermatitis in sensitive patients.[127]

Occupational allergic contact dermatitis from spices including ginger has been reported.[128]

OVERDOSE

No effects known.

CURRENT REGULATORY STATUS IN SELECTED COUNTRIES

Ginger is official in the *British Pharmacopoeia* (1998), the *United States Pharmacopeia-National Formulary* (USP23–NF18, 1995-June 1998), the *Pharmacopoeia of the People's Republic of China* (English edition, 1997) and the *Japanese Pharmacopoeia* (English edition, 1996). It was official in the second edition of the *Indian Pharmacopoeia* (1966) but was not included in the third edition (1985).

Ginger is covered by a positive Commission E monograph and can be used for dyspepsia and the prevention of motion sickness.

Ginger is on the UK General Sale List.

Ginger and ginger oil have GRAS status. Ginger is also freely available as a 'dietary supplement' in the USA under DSHEA legislation (1994 Dietary Supplement Health and Education Act). It has been present in the following OTC drug products: digestive aid drug products and as an ingredient in products offered for use as a smoking deterrent. The FDA, however, advises: 'that based on evidence currently available, there is inadequate data to establish general recognition of the safety and effectiveness of these ingredients for the specified uses'.

Ginger is not included in Part 4 of Schedule 4 of the Therapeutic Goods Act Regulations of Australia. However, products containing ginger with an equivalent dry weight per dosage unit of 2 g and above are required to carry warnings regarding concomitant use with anticoagulants and advising those with bleeding problems to seek medical advice.

References

1. Grieve M. A modern herbal, vol 1. Dover Publications, New York, 1971, pp 353–354.
2. British Herbal Medicine Association's Scientific Committee. British herbal pharmacopoeia. BHMA, Cowling, 1983, pp 239–240.
3. Felter HW, Lloyd JU. King's American dispensatory, 18th edn, 3rd revision, vol 2, 1905. Reprinted by Eclectic Medical Publications, Portland, 1983, pp 2109–2112.
4. Lyle TJ. Physio-medical therapeutics, materia medica and pharmacy, 1897. Reprinted by the National Association of Medical Herbalists of Great Britain, London, 1932, p 343.
5. Thakur RS, Puri HS, Husain A. Major medicinal plants of India. Central Institute of Medicinal and Aromatic Plants, Lucknow, 1989, pp 540–546.
6. Farnsworth NR, Bunyapraphatsara N (eds). Thai medicinal plants. Medicinal Plant Information Center, Bangkok, 1992, pp 253–260.
7. Bensky D, Gamble A. Chinese herbal medicine materia medica. Eastland Press, Seattle, 1986, pp 46–47, 431–432.
8. Chang HM, But PP. Pharmacology and applications of Chinese materia medica, vol 1. World Scientific, Singapore, 1987, pp 366–369.
9. Mabberley DJ. The plant book, 2nd edn. Cambridge University Cambridge Press, 1997, p 767.
10. World Health Organization. Medicinal plants in China. World Health Organization, Regional Office for the Western Pacific, Manilla, 1989, p 297.
11. Wagner H, Bladt S. Plant drug analysis: a thin layer chromatography atlas, 2nd edn. Springer-Verlag, Berlin, 1996, p 293.
12. Sharma SS, Kochupillai V, Gupta SK et al. J Ethnopharmacol 1997; 57 (2): 93–96.
13. Mowrey DB, Clayson DE. Lancet 1982; 1 (8273): 655–657.
14. Kawai T, Kinoshita K, Koyama K et al. Planta Med 1994; 60 (1): 17–20.
15. Grontved A, Hentzer E. ORL J Otorhinolaryngol Relat Spec 1986; 48 (5): 282–286.
16. Holtmann S, Clarke AH, Scherer H et al. Acta Otolaryngol 1989; 108 (3/4): 168–174.
17. Phillips S, Hutchinson S, Ruggier R. Anaesthesia 1993; 48 (5): 393–395.
18. Yamahara J, Huang QR, Iwamoto M et al. Phytother Res 1989; 3 (2): 70–71.
19. Yamahara J, Rong HQ, Naitoh Y et al. J Ethnopharmacol 1989; 27 (3): 353–355.
20. Fozard JR. Trends Pharmacol Sci 1987; 8: 44–46.
21. Huang QR, Iwamoto M, Aoki S et al. Chem Pharm Bull 1991; 39 (2): 397–399.
22. Lumb AB. Anaesthesia 1993; 48 (12): 1118.
23. Qian DS, Liu ZS. Chung-Kuo Chung Hsi I Chieh Ho Tsa Chih 1992; 12 (2): 95–8, 70.
24. Yamahara J, Mochizuki M, Rong HQ et al. J Ethnopharmacol 1988; 23 (2–3): 299–304.
25. Al-Yahya MA, Rafatullah S, Mossa JS et al. Am J Chin Med 1989; 17 (1–2): 51–56.
26. Yoshikawa M, Hatakeyama S, Taniguchi K et al. Chem Pharm Bull 1992; 40 (8): 2239–2241.
27. Yamahara J, Hatakeyama S, Taniguchi K et al. Yakugaku Zasshi 1992; 112 (9): 645–655.
28. Yoshikawa M, Yamaguchi S, Kunimi K et al. Chem Pharm Bull 1994; 42 (6): 1226–1230.
29. Goso Y, Ogata Y, Ishihara K et al. Comp Biochem Physiol C Pharmacol Toxicol Endocrinol 1996; 113 (1): 17–21.
30. Yamahara J, Huang QR, Li YH et al. Chem Pharm Bull 1990; 38 (2): 430–431.
31. Mascolo N, Jain R, Jain SC et al. J Ethnopharmacol 1989; 27 (1–2): 129–140.
32. Flynn DL, Rafferty MF, Boctor AM et al. Prostagland Leukot Med 1986; 24 (2–3): 195–198.
33. Kiuchi F, Shibuya M, Sankawa U. Chem Pharm Bull 1982; 30 (2): 754–757.
34. Iwakami S, Shibuya M, Tseng CF et al. Chem Pharm Bull 1986; 34 (9): 3960–3963.
35. Kiuchi F, Iwakami S, Shibuya M et al. Chem Pharm Bull 1992; 40 (2): 387–391.
36. Suekawa M, Yuasa K, Isono M et al. Nippon Yakurigaku Zasshi 1986; 88 (4): 263–269.
37. Collier HO, McDonald-Gibson WJ, Saeed SA. Br J Pharmacol 1976; 58 (2): 193–199.
38. Sharma JN, Srivastava KC, Gan EK. Pharmacology 1994; 49 (5): 314–318.
39. Sharma JN, Ishak FI, Yusof APM et al. Asia Pac J Pharmacol 1997; 12 (1–2): 9–14.
40. Srivastava KC. Prostagland Leukot Med 1984; 13: 227–235.
41. Srivastava KC. Biomed Biochim Acta 1984; 43 (8–9): S335–346.
42. Srivastava KC. Prostagland Leukot Med 1986; 25 (2–3): 187–198.
43. Guh JH, Ko FN, Jong TT et al. J Pharm Pharmacol 1995; 47 (4): 329–332.
44. Srivastava KC. Prostagland Leukot Essent Fatty Acids 1989; 35 (3): 183–185.
45. Verma SK, Singh J, Khamesra R et al. Ind J Med Res [B] 1993; 98: 240–242.
46. Lumb AB. Thromb Haemost 1994; 71 (1): 110–111.
47. Backon J. Anaesthesia 1991; 46 (8): 705–706.
48. Janssen PL, Meyboom S, Van Staveren WA et al. Eur J Clin Nutr 1996; 50 (11): 772–774.
49. Giri J, Sakthidevi TK, Meerarani S. Ind J Nutr Diet 1984; 21 (12): 433–436.
50. Srinivasan K, Sambaiah K. Int J Vitam Nutr Res 1991; 61 (4): 364–369.
51. Sambaiah K, Srinivasan K. Nahrung 1991; 35 (1): 47–51.
52. Sharma I, Gusain D, Dixit VP. Phytother Res 1996; 10 (6): 517–518.
53. Shoji N, Iwasa A, Takemoto T et al. J Pharm Sci 1982; 71 (10): 1174–1175.
54. Kobayashi M, Ishida Y, Shoji N et al. J Pharmacol Exp Ther 1988; 246 (2): 667–673.
55. Yamahara J, Matsuda H, Yamaguchi S et al. Nat Med 1995; 49 (1): 76–83.
56. Kobayashi M, Shoji N, Ohizumi Y. Biochim Biophys Acta 1987; 903 (1): 96–102.
57. Ohizumi Y, Sasaki S, Shibusawa K et al. Biol Pharm Bull 1996; 19 (10): 1377–1379.
58. Wu BN, Ho WC, Chiang LC et al. Asia Pac J Pharmacol 1996; 11 (1): 5–12.
59. Suekawa M, Aburada M, Hosoya E. J Pharmacobiodyn 1986; 9 (10): 853–860.
60. Suekawa M, Aburada M, Hosoya E. J Pharmacobiodyn 1986; 9 (10): 842–852.
61. Suekawa M, Sone H, Sakakibara I et al. Nippon Yakurigaku Zasshi 1986; 88 (5): 339–347.
62. Platel K, Srinivasan K. Int J Food Sci Nutr 1996; 47 (1): 55–59.
63. Yamahara J, Miki K, Chisaka T et al. J Ethnopharmacol 1985; 13 (2): 217–225.
64. Thompson EH, Wolf ID, Allen CE. J Food Sci 1973; 38: 652–655.
65. Suekawa M, Ishige A, Yuasa K et al. J Pharmacobiodyn 1984; 7 (11): 836–848.

66. Desai HG, Kalro RH, Choksi AP. Ind J Med Res 1990; 92: 139–141.
67. Huang Q, Matsuda H, Sakai K et al. Yakugaku Zasshi 1990; 110 (12): 936–942.
68. Atal CK, Zutshi U, Rao PG et al. J Ethnopharmacol 1981; 4 (2): 229–232.
69. Blumberger W, Glatzel H. Nutr Dieta 1964; 6: 181–192.
70. Eldershaw TP, Colquhoun EQ, Dora KA et al. Int J Obes Relat Metab Disord 1992; 16 (10): 755–763.
71. Kawada T, Sakabe SI, Watanabe T et al. Proc Soc Exp Biol Med 1988; 188 (2): 229–233.
72. Chang CP, Chang JY, Wang FY et al. J Ethnopharmacol 1995; 48 (1): 13–19.
73. Henry CJ, Piggott SM. Hum Nutr Clin Nutr 1987; 41 (1): 89–92.
74. Endo K, Kanno E, Oshima Y. Phytochem 1990; 29 (3): 797–799.
75. Gugnani HC, Ezenwanze EC. J Commun Dis 1985; 17 (3): 233–236.
76. Denyer CV, Jackson P, Loakes DM et al. J Nat Prod 1994; 57 (5): 658–662.
77. Guerin JC, Reveillere HP. Ann Pharm Fr 1984; 42 (6): 553–559.
78. Adewunmi CO, Oguntimein BO, Furu P. Planta Med 1990; 56 (4): 374–376.
79. Goto C, Kasuya S, Koga K et al. Parasitol Res 1990; 76 (8): 653–656.
80. Kimura I, Kimura M, Pancho LR. Jpn J Pharmacol 1989; 50 (3): 253–261.
81. Kimura I, Pancho LR, Koizumi T et al. J Pharmacobiodyn 1989; 12 (4): 220–227.
82. Hikino H, Kiso Y, Kato N et al. J Ethnopharmacol 1985; 14 (1): 31–39.
83. Govindarajan VS. Crit Rev Food Sci Nutr 1982; 17 (3): 189–258.
84. Aeschbach R, Loliger J, Scott BC et al. Food Chem Toxicol 1994; 32 (1): 31–36.
85. Krishnakantha TP, Lokesh BR. Ind J Biochem Biophys 1993; 30 (2): 133–134.
86. Reddy AC, Lokesh BR. Mol Cell Biochem 1992; 111 (1–2): 117–124.
87. Cao ZF, Chen ZG, Guo P et al. Chung Kuo Chung Yao Tsa Chih 1993; 18 (12): 750–751, 764.
88. Zhou Y, Xu R. Chung Kuo Chung Yao Tsa Chih 1992; 17 (6): 368–369, 373.
89. Naora K, Ding G, Hayashibara M et al. Chem Pharm Bull 1992; 40 (5): 1295–1298.
90. Monge P, Scheline R, Solheim E. Xenobiotica 1976; 6 (7): 411–423.
91. Grontved A, Brask T, Kambskard J et al. Acta Otolaryngol 1988; 105 (1–2): 45–49.
92. Schmid R, Schick T, Steffen R et al. J Travel Med 1994; 1: 203–206.
93. Careddu P. Unpublished Pharmaton report 1986. Cited in Scientific Committee of ESCOP. ESCOP monographs: Zingiberis rhizoma. European Scientific Cooperative on Phytotherapy, Exeter, March 1996.
94. Fischer-Rasmussen W, Kjaer SK, Dahl C et al. Eur J Obstet Gynecol Reprod Biol 1990; 38 (1): 19–24.
95. Bone ME, Wilkinson DJ, Young JR et al. Anaesthesia 1990; 45 (8): 669–671.
96. Liu WH. Anaesthesia 1990; 45 (12): 1085.
97. Phillips S, Ruggier R, Hutchinson SE. Anaesthesia 1993; 48 (8): 715–717.
98. Meyer K, Schwartz J, Crater D et al. Dermatol Nurs 1995; 7 (4): 242–244.
99. Stewart JJ, Wood MJ, Wood CD et al. Pharmacology 1991; 42 (2): 111–120.
100. Wood DC, Manno JE, Wood MJ et al. Clin Res Pract Drug Regul Affairs 1988; 6 (2): 129–136.
101. Stewart JJ, Wood MJ, Wood CD et al. Aviat Space Environ Med 1991; 62 (5): 465.
102. Arfeen Z, Owen H, Plummer JL et al. Anaesth Intensive Care 1995; 23 (4): 449–452.
103. Srivastava KC, Mustafa T. Med Hypotheses 1989; 29 (1): 25–28.
104. Srivastava KC, Mustafa T. Med Hypotheses 1992; 39 (4): 342–348.
105. Mustafa T, Srivastava KC. J Ethnopharmacol 1990; 29 (3): 267–273.
106. Marles RJ, Kaminski J, Arnason JT et al. J Nat Prod 1992; 55 (8): 1044–1056.
107. Backon J. Alcohol Alcohol 1986; 21 (4): 403–404.
108. Backon J. Burns Incl Therm Inj 1987; 13 (3): 252.
109. Backon J. Gut 1987; 28: 1323.
110. Backon J. Med Sci Res 1987; 15: 1078.
111. Backon J. Arch Androl 1988; 20 (1): 101–102.
112. Backon J. Med Hypotheses 1991; 36 (3): 223–224.
113. Backon J. Med Hypotheses 1991; 34 (3): 230–231.
114. Bordia A Verma SK, Srivastava KC Prostagland Leukot Essent Fatty Acids 1997; 56 (5): 379–384.
115. Opdyke DLJ. Food Cosmet Toxicol 1974; 12: 901–902.
116. Qureshi S, Shah AH, Tariq M et al. Am J Chin Med 1989; 17 (1–2): 57–63.
117. Nakamura H, Yamamoto T. Mutat Res 1983; 122 (2): 87–94.
118. Nagabhushan M, Amonkar AJ, Bhide SV. Cancer Lett 1987; 36 (2): 221–233.
119. Nakamura H, Yamamoto T. Mutat Res 1982; 103 (2): 119–126.
120. Mahmoud I, Alkofahi A, Abdelaziz A. Int J Pharmacog 1992; 30 (2): 81–85.
121. Soudamini KK, Unnikrishnan MC, Sukumaran K et al. Ind J Physiol Pharmacol 1995; 39 (4): 347–353.
122. Tarjan V, Csukas I. Mutat Res 1989; 216: 297.
123. German Federal Minister of Justice. German Commission E for human medicine monograph, Bundes-Anzeiger (German Federal Gazette) no. 85, dated 05.05.1988, no. 50, dated 13.03.1990, no. 164, dated 01.09.1990.
124. Bensky D, Gamble A. Chinese herbal medicine materia medica. Eastland Press, Seattle, 1986, pp 431–432.
125. Sakai K, Oshima N, Kutsuna T et al. Yakugaku Zasshi 1986; 106 (10): 947–950.
126. USP Drug Information, US Pharmacopeia patient leaflet, ginger (oral). United States Pharmacopeial Convention, Rockville, 1998.
127. Futrell JM, Rietschel RL. Cutis 1993; 52 (5): 288–290.
128. Kanerva L, Estlander T, Jolanki R. Contact Derm 1996; 35 (3): 157–162.

Ginkgo
(*Ginkgo biloba* L.)

SYNONYMS

Maidenhair tree (Engl), Ginkgoblätter (Ger), arbre aux quarante écus (forty coin tree) (Fr), Ginkgo (Ital), tempeltrae (Dan).

WHAT IS IT?

Ginkgo biloba is a deciduous tree which has survived unchanged for about 150 million years. This living fossil may have been saved from extinction by the Chinese who revered the tree and planted it around their temples. In the 1960s a group of German scientists were investigating the effects of exotic herbs on circulation and found that the leaves of Ginkgo were particularly active. A special, highly concentrated extract standardized for flavonoid content was patented soon after. In the years that followed, standardized extracts of Ginkgo leaves became widely used in Europe.

EFFECTS

Increases blood flow, tissue oxygenation and tissue nutrition; platelet-activating factor (PAF) antagonism; prevention of membrane damage caused by free radicals; enhances memory and cognitive function, especially in the elderly.

TRADITIONAL VIEW

Only Ginkgo nuts were widely used in traditional Chinese medicine. The nuts are used as an antiasthmatic and against polyuria.[1] The only information on Ginkgo leaves for use as a circulatory stimulant comes from clinical trials on the standardized extract conducted in the past three decades. However, the Chinese have now incorporated the use of Ginkgo leaves into their materia medica.

SUMMARY ACTIONS

Anti-PAF activity, antioxidant, tissue perfusion enhancer, circulatory stimulant, nootropic.

CAN BE USED FOR

INDICATIONS SUPPORTED BY CLINICAL TRIALS

Disorders and symptoms due to restricted cerebral blood flow (memory and/or cognitive impairment, dizziness, tinnitus, headaches, anxiety/depression, fatigue, stroke); vertigo, acute cochlear deafness; peripheral arterial disease (particularly intermittent claudication); early stages of primary degenerative dementia (Alzheimer-type); multiinfarct dementia; disorders due to reduced retinal blood flow, senile macular degeneration; congestive dysmenorrhoea; effects of high altitude or hypoxia.

TRADITIONAL THERAPEUTIC USES

Ginkgo leaf does not have well-documented traditional use.

MAY ALSO BE USED FOR

EXTRAPOLATIONS FROM PHARMACOLOGICAL STUDIES

Disorders due to restricted peripheral blood flow (including diabetic vascular disease, atherosclerosis, Raynaud's syndrome); anti-PAF activity (useful in the treatment of asthma, allergic reactions, immunological reactions, shock, ischaemia, thrombosis); antioxidant activity, protection against ischaemia and reperfusion injury. New uses may follow from the anti-PAF activity, e.g. prevention of migraine headaches.

PREPARATIONS

Standardized extract for internal and topical application.

DOSAGE

The dose of liquid extracts is uncertain if they have not been standardized for major active constituents.

Usually the daily dose is 120 mg of a 50:1 Ginkgo standardized extract equivalent to 27–30 mg Ginkgo flavone glycosides and about 10 mg terpenoids per day (this corresponds to 4–8 g of leaf, depending on the quality). This can be incorporated into liquids or tablets at 40 mg per ml or 40 mg per tablet, making the daily dose 3 ml or three tablets. Recent clinical trials have used twice this dose for some applications.

DURATION OF USE

There is no restriction on the long-term use of Ginkgo. However, it should be given to patients for at least 6 weeks before any clinical benefit is assessed.

SUMMARY ASSESSMENT OF SAFETY

There is very low risk associated with the administration of Ginkgo.

TECHNICAL DATA

BOTANY

Ginkgo biloba is a member of the Ginkgoaceae family, a gymnosperm which has survived unchanged from the Triassic period. It can grow to a height of over 100 m, living for 1000 years. Ginkgo is dioecious (possessing male and female flowers on separate trees) and its leaves have open dichotomous venation and a characteristic fan-like appearance with two lobes (hence the species name, *biloba*). The naked seed (or nut) is oily and edible but the seed coat and embryo are bitter.[2,3]

KEY CONSTITUENTS

- 0.5–1% mono-, di- and triglycosides of the flavones: quercetin, kaempferol and isorhamnetin,[4] including coumaric acid esters of flavonoids.
- Terpene lactones (terpenoids), including bilobalide and ginkgolides A, B, C, J.[5]
- Biflavonoids, ginkgolic acids, sterols, procyanidins, polysaccharides.[5]

The majority of the pharmacological studies and clinical trials have been conducted using a special concentrated standardized extract which is chemically complex, containing at least 26 identified components and standardized to contain 24% flavonoid glycosides (Ginkgo flavone glycosides) and 6% terpenoids (ginkgolides and bilobalide). The standardized extract allows the concentration of active constituents and elimination of undesirable substances. For this reason many of the known constituents of Ginkgo leaves are present only in minute amounts or absent from these extracts, including ginkgolic acids, biflavonoids and sterols.

Pharmacodynamics

The considerable number of pharmacological studies on *Ginkgo biloba* extract have not been comprehensively reviewed in this monograph. Rather, the results from important, unique or representative studies have been included. For an extensive review, see the book by DeFeudis.[6]

PAF antagonism

Platelet-activating factor (PAF) is an ether-linked phospholipid which is formed by platelets, basophils, neutrophils, monocytes and macrophages. It is a potent platelet-aggregating agent and inducer of systemic anaphylactic symptoms. The ginkgolides are potent and specific PAF antagonists.[7,8] Their effects are long-lived and are rapidly established after oral doses.[9] No side effects were recorded, even when given in high doses (120 mg of a ginkgolide mixture) to healthy human subjects.[7]

High doses of ginkgolides control mast cell degranulation,[10] and have been used to treat systemic mastocytosis (high levels of mast cells).[11] Ginkgolides partially countered PAF-induced and antigen-induced bronchoconstriction[12,13] and inhibited the induction of airways hyperreactivity by PAF in vivo.[14] Ginkgolides inhibit the response of eosinophils to PAF[15] and decrease the IgE-mediated cytotoxicity of eosinophils.[8] Ginkgolides and the standardized extract of Ginkgo have demonstrated a potent thrombolytic effect on PAF-induced thrombus.[16,17] Standardized Ginkgo extract has improved peak flow rates in asthmatic children and caused significant clinical improvement in adults.[17]

Effects on ischaemia and blood flow

Ginkgolides prevent the metabolic damage caused by experimental cerebral ischaemia and even have a normalizing effect when given 1 hour after the event. They reduce the infarct size in experimental myocardial occlusion. Arrhythmias induced by experimental myocardial ischaemia are significantly countered by the prior administration of ginkgolides.[18] Bilobalide has demonstrated a potent neuroprotective effect against ischaemic damage, which is stronger than ginkgolide B.[19]

There is much experimental evidence to support the view that Ginkgo extracts have neuroprotective properties under conditions such as hypoxia/ischaemia, seizure activity and peripheral nerve damage, although on a mg/kg basis, the effective doses of Ginkgo extract in animal studies are often at least 10 times larger than those used in human studies.[20] Standardized Ginkgo extract, as well as its non-flavone fraction (probably the ginkgolides), but not the flavone glycosides, conferred protection in mice against brain damage caused by hypoxia and retarded the breakdown of brain energy metabolism.[21] Oral administration of Ginkgo extract produced slight to moderate changes in glucose utilization in the brain structures of rats. Glucose utilization was significantly decreased in the frontoparietal somatosensory cortex, nucleus accumbens, cerebellar cortex and pons when 50 mg/kg dose of extract was administered. This may help explain the clinical effectiveness of Ginkgo extract in

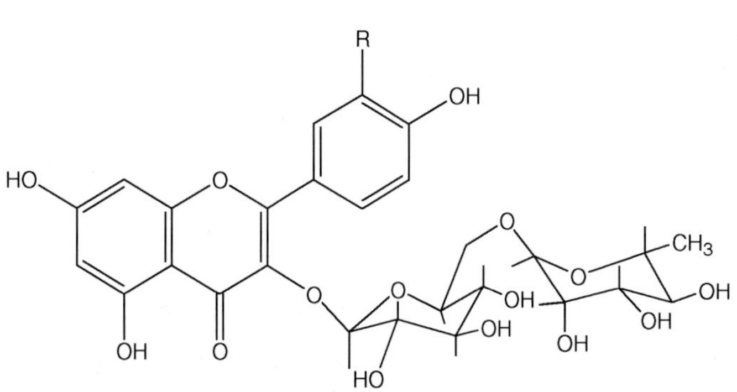

Flavonol diglycosides

	R
kaempferol-3-*O*-rutinoside	H
quercetin-3-*O*-rutinoside	OH
isorhamnetin-3-*O*-rutinoside	OCH_3

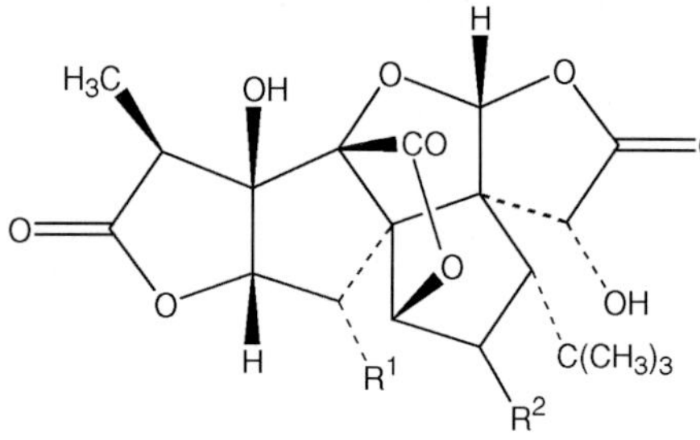

Ginkgolides

	R^1	R^2
Ginkgolide A	H	H
Ginkgolide B	OH	H
Ginkgolide C	OH	OH
Ginkgolide J	H	OH

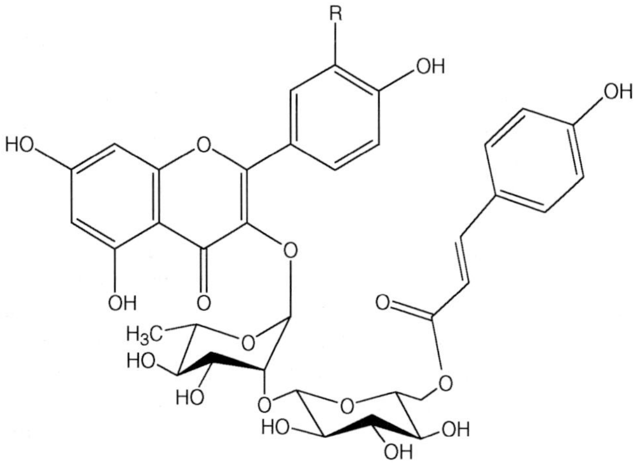

Bilobalide

Coumaric esters of flavonoids

	R
kaempferol-3-*O*-α-(6'''-*trans*-p-coumaroylglucosyl)-β-1,2-rhamnoside	H
quercetin-3-*O*-α-(6'''-*trans*-p-coumaroylglucosyl)-β-1,2-rhamnoside	OH

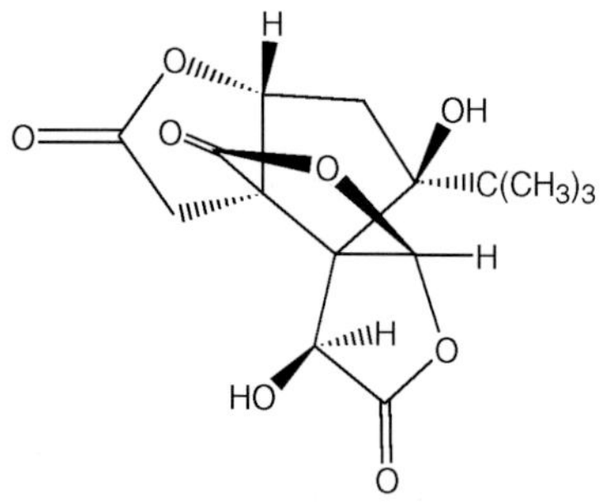

treating problems associated with deficient somatosensory processing (e.g. impairment of vigilance) and vestibular mechanisms (e.g. vertiginous syndromes).[22]

Ginkgo has favourably influenced a number of the metabolic events which accompany cerebral ischaemia, including a preventative effect on ischaemia by inhibiting vasospasm and thrombus formation and improving cerebral blood flow to underperfused areas without robbing adjacent areas. It has increased cerebral perfusion after oral administration[23] and increased hypoxia tolerance[24] in humans. Also, Ginkgo has inhibited thrombus formation,[25] promoted prostacyclin synthesis,[26] reduced cerebral oedema,[27–29] normalized brain ATP and glucose following ischaemia,[28,30] improved neuronal function following infarction[27] and inhibited arteriolar spasm[31] in animals. Ginkgo inhibited thromboxane synthesis[26] and free radical production[32,33] in vitro.

Standardized Ginkgo extract and bilobalide inhibited the hypoxia-induced decrease in ATP content in endothelial cells in vitro. After oral administration in an in vivo model of hypoxia, both compounds increased the respiratory control ratio of mitochondria isolated from rat hepatocytes. The authors concluded that these agents retained the ability to form ATP, thereby reducing the cell's need to induce glycolysis, probably by preserving ATP regeneration by mitochondria as long as oxygen was available.[34] A protective effect of standardized Ginkgo extract on the hypoxic myocardium was demonstrated by the changes in enzyme activities in rat myocardium after pretreatment with Ginkgo for 3 months.[35]

In a comparative study on stroke victims, intravenous standardized Ginkgo extract was more active at improving cerebral blood flow compared to 28 orthodox drugs.[36] In a randomized placebo-controlled cross-over study of 10 healthy subjects, Ginkgo markedly decreased erythrocyte aggregation and increased the blood flow in nail-fold capillaries.[37]

Antioxidant activity

Flavonoids from Ginkgo extract scavenged free radicals and antagonized lipid peroxidation and cell necrosis of rat hepatocytes more potently than the terpene lactones (ginkgolides, bilobalide) in vitro.[38] Ginkgo extract scavenges various reactive oxygen species, such as hydroxyl and superoxide radicals, and also peroxyl radicals, which are involved in the propagation step of lipid peroxidation.[39] Standardized Ginkgo extract, due to its antioxidant activity, protects against postischaemic injury[40] and apoptosis (programmed cell death) in rat cerebellar neuronal cells[41] and inhibits or reduces functional and morphological retinal impairments observed after lipoperoxide release.[42] The extract has demonstrated powerful antioxidant effects on copper-mediated human low density lipoprotein oxidation in vitro.[43]

Standardized Ginkgo extract demonstrated a protective effect on hydrogen peroxide-induced oxidative damage of red blood cells in vitro. Subjects given standardized Ginkgo extract (200 mg per day) for 1 week also exhibited red blood cells which were more resistant to oxidative damage.[44] Ginkgo extract decreased the clastogenic activity (a marker of oxidative stress) of blood taken from salvage personnel working on the Chernobyl reactor accident.[45] In a further study, 30 recovery workers were treated with standardized Ginkgo extract (120 mg per day) for 2 months. The clastogenic activity of their plasma was reduced to control levels at the end of the treatment period and persisted for at least 7 months thereafter.[46]

Effect on memory and/or learning

The evidence supporting the view that Ginkgo extracts have memory-enhancing properties in healthy animals and humans is currently considered inconclusive, as relatively few well-controlled studies have been conducted.[20] In a well-controlled animal study, Ginkgo treatment (100 mg/kg/day, 4–8 weeks prior to training and 10 weeks prior to testing) enhanced performance on the tested task, indicating improved retrieval of the learned response.[47] However, it did not affect performance in a passive avoidance test.[48] Oral administration of standardized Ginkgo extract to young and old rats facilitated behavioural adaptation despite adverse environmental influences. Stress-induced detrimental changes in both discrimination learning and plasma hormones became significant after the third day of learning. Ginkgo was more effective in decreasing the number of inefficient lever presses and reaction time in the older animals.[49]

In eight healthy subjects, a double-blind, placebo-controlled, crossover study found that a single dose of standardized Ginkgo extract administered 1 hour before testing significantly improved short-term memory, but only when the dose was five times that normally prescribed (600 mg). No significant difference from placebo was observed in other psychological tests. The response time in the memory scanning test was significantly improved, indicating that Ginkgo affected central cognitive function.[50] This was an acute dose study but long-term intake of lower doses may have a similar effect.

To elucidate the mechanism of clinical benefit of Ginkgo in the treatment of symptoms of impaired brain functions in advanced age, its effect on cognitive information processing was investigated by means of long-latency auditory event-related potentials (P300). In a double-blind, placebo-controlled study, 48 elderly patients with age-associated memory impairment received 120 mg of Ginkgo extract or placebo per day for 57 days. P300 latency was shortened in the Ginkgo group and this may reflect shorter stimulus-evaluation time.[51]

The effect on psychomotor and memory performances was investigated in a double-blind, placebo-controlled crossover study of 12 young healthy subjects, who received either a single oral dose of placebo, standardized Ginkgo extract or non-standardized Ginkgo extract. No significant differences from placebo were observed with regard to tests evaluating vigilance and recognition of numbers and images. The score obtained for free recall of image 1 hour after administration of standardized Ginkgo extract remained identical to that observed before treatment, whereas it decreased for placebo and non-standardized Ginkgo extract. The authors suggested that the effect might be one of reduced deterioration ('antideficit') rather than of memory enhancement.[52]

Adult volunteers (28) who participated in a 30-day double-blind study received either placebo or 100 mg/day of Ginkgo extract.[53] In order to assess a wide range of cognitive abilities, the Multidimensional Aptitude Battery (MAB) was administered before and after treatment. Results indicated that Ginkgo significantly enhanced MAB subtests which tap long-term memory and abstract reasoning.

Other activity

Ginkgo extract inhibited rat brain monoamine (MAO-A, MAO-B) in vitro. The active compound(s) were present in dried or fresh Ginkgo leaves, were heat stable and of low molecular weight.[54]

Bilobalide inhibited *Pneumocystis carinii* growth in vitro and reduced the number of organisms in rats.[55]

The effects of various fractions of Ginkgo extract on human (obtained from impotent men) and rabbit penis corpus cavernosal tissue in vitro were investigated.[56] One fraction was particularly active at relaxing corpus cavernosal tissues.

Oral administration of standardized Ginkgo extract (10 mg/kg per day, for 12 weeks in conjunction with a high-fat diet) reduced disturbances of lipid metabolism and the severity of plaque formation in rabbits, when compared to placebo and rutin. In addition to hypolipidaemic and antioxidant (antiatherosclerotic) activities, Ginkgo also affected metabolic processes in the liver and may modify lipid deposition in major arteries.[57]

Intragastric administration of a preparation containing standardized extracts of Ginkgo and ginger demonstrated anxiolytic effects comparable to diazepam (by injection) in vivo. However, the herbal preparation demonstrated anxiety-promoting effects at a high dosage (100 mg/kg).[58]

Standardized Ginkgo extract showed a promoting effect on hair regrowth after cutaneous administration to shaved mice.[59]

Oral administration of standardized Ginkgo extract inhibited the development of stress-induced polydipsia (excessive thirst) in rats.[60] Chronic administration of Ginkgo extract to rats inhibited stress-induced corticosterone hyposecretion through a reduction in the number of adrenal peripheral benzodiazepine receptors.[61] Ginkgo extract and ginkgolide B were also found to act at the hypothalamic level and were able to reduce corticotrophin-releasing hormone expression and secretion.

Standardized Ginkgo extract demonstrated an anti-inflammatory activity with a potency comparable to that of indomethacin after topical application in the croton oil test in mice.[62] Unilateral vestibular deafferentation (UVD) causes ocular motor and postural disorders, some of which disappear over time in a process of behavioural recovery known as vestibular compensation. Vestibular compensation may be enhanced either by reducing the initial symptoms of UVD or by accelerating the compensation process. The demonstrated efficacy of Ginkgo extract in treating UVD in vivo by the intraperitoneal route was suggested to be due to acceleration of compensation.[63]

PHARMACOKINETICS

No flavonoid glycosides or aglycones were detected in urine, faeces or blood within 24 hours of intragastric administration of Ginkgo extract to rats. Seven metabolites of flavonoid degradation were found.[64]

Data obtained from human studies, suggest that ginkgolide A and B and bilobalide are excreted unchanged in the urine (70%, 50%, 30%, respectively of the administered dose) and have relatively high bioavailability after oral ingestion (>80%, >80%, 70%, respectively).[65] High bioavailability was observed from a single oral dose of ginkgolides A and B and bilobalide to healthy human subjects. Elimination half-lives (after oral dosing while fasting) of 4.5, 10.6 and 3.2 hours were measured for the three compounds respectively.[66]

CLINICAL TRIALS

Cerebral insufficiency and stroke

Cerebral (not cerebrovascular) insufficiency is not strictly a medical condition and it is not accepted as being associated with any pathological change. Rather, it is a collection of symptoms associated with mental deterioration from ageing which affects many elderly people who do not necessarily have dementia or a history of strokes.

Cerebral insufficiency manifests as the following 12 symptoms in elderly people: difficulties in concentration and memory, absentmindedness, confusion, lack of energy, tiredness, decreased physical performance, depressive mood, anxiety, dizziness, tinnitus and headaches. These symptoms can also be associated with the early stages of dementia, of either the Alzheimer (degenerative) or multiinfarct (circulatory) types.

The concentration of clinical trials with Ginkgo on cerebral insufficiency has been a barrier to its acceptance in orthodox circles as a treatment for the elderly. Trials (such as the one listed below[67]) which clearly demonstrate the benefit of Ginkgo in dementia should break down this resistance to its value which exists among English-speaking scientists. But there is another development in the field of pathology which could lead to wider use and acceptance of Ginkgo. This is the concept of 'white matter ischaemia'. After computed tomography was introduced in clinical practice, it was realized that rarefaction or low attenuation of the white matter of the brain (the axons) was much more common than previously thought. Although this can occur for several reasons, for example after head injury, age and ischaemia to the white matter are regarded as the commonest causes.[68]

The vulnerability of the white matter to ischaemia is due to the fact that it is supplied by long penetrating end arterioles from the surface and base of the brain that travel for a long distance with very few interconnections. Computed tomography of the brain shows that 30% of subjects aged 85 years have evidence of low attenuation of the white matter. Magnetic resonance imaging shows the incidence approaching 100% at age 85. Studies show that normal subjects with white matter ischaemia could have subtle neuropsychological deficits such as slower rate of mental processing and impaired attention and concentration. Hence a tentative link between white matter ischaemia and cerebral insufficiency has been established. Since Ginkgo has antiischaemic activity, it could prevent or ameliorate symptoms associated with white matter ischaemia. White matter ischaemia is also closely associated with vascular or so-called multiinfarct dementia. The key development is that a patient need not show a history of strokes to have a cognitive impairment brought about by ischaemia. A recent review has concluded that abnormalities in the small vessels caused by ageing and hypertension, together with systemic circulatory disturbances such as heart diseases or abrupt variations in blood pressure, may lead to selective white matter injury. The damage is structurally characterized by incomplete infarction or selective cellular injury.[69]

A critical review of 40 clinical trials conducted from 1975 to 1991 on Ginkgo and cerebral insufficiency and other conditions found eight to be well conducted with a score greater than 65 points (these trials are listed in Table 1).[72] Trials under this general heading of cerebral insufficiency also included the following conditions: primary degenerative dementia, dizziness associated with labyrinth and/or vestibular disorders, acute cochlear deafness, senile cognitive decline; vertigo, hearing loss or tinnitus.

The trials included Ginkgo versus placebo or registered drug, mostly by oral route, and in one case combined with physical training. Shortcomings of the 40 trials included limited numbers of patients and incomplete description of randomization procedures, patient characteristics, effect measurement and data presentation. All except one of the 40 trials showed positive results, 26 trials with significant results. The inconclusive result was obtained for a trial on senile dementia of vascular origin.[70] In most trials the dosage was 120–160 mg Ginkgo extract per day, given for at least 4–6 weeks. No serious side effects were reported in any trial and those that were reported were not different from those observed in placebo-treated patients. An assessment of published clinical trials using the registered drug Co-dergocrine (dihydroergotoxine) yielded similar scores on the methodological assessment to that of the Ginkgo trials. Moreover, a clinical trial of direct comparison between Ginkgo extract and Co-dergocrine indicated similar efficacy between the two treatments (120 mg/day Ginkgo extract, 4.5 mg/day Co-dergocrine, 6 weeks[71]).

Metaanalysis is a statistical tool for quantitatively summarizing the results of clinical trials with comparable treatments and designs. Eleven double-blind, placebo-controlled trials using, in most cases, 150 mg per day of standardized Ginkgo extract over 12 weeks were evaluated by metaanalysis. Global effectiveness was confirmed in five studies compared to one study which was not conclusive.[70] Three studies were excluded on the basis of methodological or objective reasons and two were excluded as the assessment by physician or patients was missing. The analysis of the total score of clinical symptoms from eight of the 11 studies indicated similar results (seven studies demonstrated Ginkgo significantly better than placebo, one study was inconclusive.[70] It was concluded that treatment with Ginkgo extract provides a better therapeutic effect compared to placebo in the treatment of cerebral insufficiency.[81] Four of the trials included in this metaanalysis are listed in the above table (references [73,74,78,79]); the other four trials comprise references [70,82,83] and [84].

In early trials (uncontrolled, double-blind, placebo and comparative), standardized Ginkgo extract was found to be of benefit in the treatment of recent

Table 1 Placebo-controlled clinical trials with Ginkgo extract for cerebral insufficiency

Indication	Total no. of patients analysed	Type of study	Dose of Ginkgo extract (mg/day)	Duration of treatment	Results	Ref
Cerebral insufficiency	99	Double-blind vs placebo	150	12 weeks	Significant difference found for eight of 12 symptoms. Assessment by doctors showing improvement in 72% of Ginkgo-treated patients compared to 8% of patients on placebo.	73
Cerebral insufficiency	209	Multicentre double-blind vs placebo	150	12 weeks	Significant difference found for eight of 12 symptoms. Assessment by doctors showing improvement in 71% of patients treated with Ginkgo compared with 32% of patients on placebo.	74
Tinnitus, dizziness, hearing impairment	100	Multicentre double-blind vs placebo	160	3 months; follow-up at 13 months	Overall evolution and intensity of tinnitus was statistically better in the Ginkgo group. Improvement or cure in 50% of patients was found after an average of 70 days for patients treated with Ginkgo and an average of 119 days in patients on placebo.	75
Cerebral insufficiency	166	Double-blind vs placebo	160	12 months	Significant result obtained: the difference from baseline in the 7-point clinical scale measured at 3, 6, 9 and 12 months (10% vs 4%, 15% vs 4%, 15% vs 8%, 17% vs 8% for Ginkgo and placebo-treated patients respectively).	76
Vertiginous syndrome and associated symptoms	670	Multicentre double-blind vs placebo	160	3 months	End of treatment period: 47% of Ginkgo-treated patients were symptom free, compared to 18% for placebo-treated patients; the number of patients recovered or much improved was twice as great as in the placebo group. Significant result obtained for Ginkgo on the intensity, frequency and duration of the vertigo.	77
Cerebral insufficiency	96	Double-blind vs placebo	112	12 weeks	Significant result observed: improvement from baseline for difficulties of concentration (54% vs 19%), memory (52% vs 17%), anxiety (48% vs 17%), dizziness (61% vs 23%), headaches (65% vs 24%) and tinnitus (37% vs 12%) for Ginkgo and placebo-treated patients respectively.	78
Cerebral insufficiency	58	Double-blind vs placebo	160	6 weeks	Significant differences for 11 of 12 symptoms after 4 and 6 weeks.	79

Table 1 Placebo-controlled clinical trials with Ginkgo extract for cerebral insufficiency

Indication	Total no. of patients analysed	Type of study	Dose of Ginkgo extract (mg/day)	Duration of treatment	Results	Ref
Mild idiopathic cognitive impairment	54	Double-blind vs placebo	120	12 weeks	Significant differences for combined scores on the cognitive test battery but no differences were observed for behavioural rating scale and VAS mood. Overall assessment by doctors and patients showed no significant differences, nearly all patients improved.	80

stroke victims. Improvement was observed in cerebral blood flow, motor recovery, intellectual performance, memory, mood and behaviour.[85–88] In a recent double-blind, placebo-controlled trial, 47 patients with acute ischaemic stroke received either Ginkgo extract (40 mg) or placebo at 6-hourly intervals along with routine management over 4 weeks. Both groups showed significant improvement, with negligible difference in degree of change in either group. The study group did, however, consist of patients who were treated more than 48 hours after stroke, and the treatment time was relatively short (4 weeks).[89]

In other recent double-blind, placebo-controlled trials investigating cerebral insufficiency:

- significant improvement in mental speed, concentration and memory were observed after the sixth week of Ginkgo treatment (150 mg per day, 12 weeks),[82]
- improvement in short-term memory and learning rate became significant in the 24th week (160 mg per day, 24 weeks).[90]

In other related placebo-controlled clinical trials, Ginkgo treatment demonstrated significant improvement in:

- dizziness and general subjective symptoms in dizziness of central origin, after treatment over 6 months,[91]
- retinal sensitivity in chronic cerebral retinal insufficiency syndrome at the higher dosage regime (160 mg per day, 4 weeks).[92]

Eighteen subjects with slight age-related memory impairment participated in a double-blind, placebo-controlled crossover trial. Subjects received placebo or one of two doses of standardized Ginkgo extract (320 mg or 600 mg) 1 hour before performing a dual-coding test. After each dose of the Ginkgo extract, the point between coding verbal material and images was significantly shifted towards a shorter presentation time, indicating an improvement in the speed of information processing.[93] Short-term memory (attention, perception) and verbal fluidity in patients with age-related memory impairment benefited from the combination of Ginkgo treatment (160 mg per day, 24 weeks) and mental exercises, suggesting a positive synergy between the two treatments.[94] The best results were obtained in subjects combining Ginkgo with mental exercises, followed by subjects undertaking exercises alone, followed by subjects receiving Ginkgo alone, then the placebo group.[95]

Primary degenerative dementia

Ginkgo has been used successfully in the treatment of senile dementia of the Alzheimer type. In a randomized, double-blind, placebo-controlled trial, 40 patients with early-to-moderate senile dementia of the Alzheimer-type received 240 mg per day of Ginkgo extract or placebo for 3 months. Memory and attention improved significantly in the Ginkgo group after 1 month, as did psychopathology, psychomotor performance, functional dynamics and neurophysiology.[96] Standardized Ginkgo extract may benefit primary degenerative dementia via its antioxidant activity by preventing neuronal damage, cellular degeneration and cellular damage.[97]

In a prospective, randomized, double-blind,placebo-controlled multicentre study, 216 outpatients with presenile and senile dementia of Alzheimer type and multiinfarct dementia received either standardized Ginkgo extract (240 mg per day) or placebo for 24 weeks. The data from the 156 patients who com-pleted psychopathological, attention, memory and behavioural assessment indicated that the groups differed significantly in favour of Ginkgo.[98] In a representative survey of 145 physicians and 14 neuropsychiatrists in Germany, practitioners were randomly assigned a case history typical of either senile dementia of Alzheimer type or vascular dementia and asked which drugs would be chosen to treat the patient's cognitive disorders. Piracetam, Ginkgo and nimodipine were considered most frequently. Physicians considered Ginkgo more often than nimodipine or Co-dergocrine.[99]

The efficacy and safety of extract of Ginkgo biloba in the treatment of patients with mild to severe Alzheimer disease or multiinfarct dementia were assessed in a 52-week, randomized, double-blind, placebo-controlled clinical trial.[67] Patients received either 120 mg per day of the concentrated standardized 50:1 extract or placebo. Primary outcome measures were the Alzheimer's Disease Assessment Scale (ADAS), Geriatric Evaluation by Relative's Rating Instrument (GERRI) and Clinical Global Impression of Change (CGIC). Of the 309 patients who began the trial, 202 provided useful data for the endpoint analysis, with 27% of patients treated with Ginkgo achieving at least a four-point improvement on the ADAS compared with 14% taking placebo ($p=0.005$); on the GERRI, 37% were considered improved with Ginkgo, compared with 23% taking placebo ($p=0.003$). No difference was seen in the CGIC and no significant difference compared with placebo was observed in the number of patients reporting adverse events or in the incidence and severity of these events. The authors concluded that *Ginkgo biloba* extract was safe and appears capable of stabilizing and, in a substantial number of cases, improving the cognitive performance and the social function of patients with dementia.

This is a highly significant study for several reasons. Most notably, it was conducted by psychiatrists in the USA and accepted for publication in the prestigious *Journal of the American Medical Association*. Other reasons for the importance of this study include:

- the size and duration of the study;
- the rigorous execution of a good experimental protocol;
- it was a positive study on the treatment of dementia, a highly problematic medical condition.

This clinical trial has already had a substantial impact on the use of *Ginkgo biloba* in the USA.

The influence of oral treatment with 240 mg/day of Ginkgo extract on the clinical course of Alzheimer-type dementia was investigated over 3 months in a double-blind, randomized, placebo-controlled design in 20 outpatients.[100] There was a significant improvement in patients receiving Ginkgo ($p<0.013$) as assessed by a psychometric test.

A metaanalysis of the four studies (summarized above) which met inclusion criteria (of more than 50 articles identified on Ginkgo and cognitive impairment) found that there was a small but significant effect for 3–6 month treatment with 120–240 mg of Ginkgo extract on objective measures of cognitive function in Alzheimer's disease.[101]

Peripheral arterial disease

Five placebo-controlled trials (references[102–106]) were included in a metaanalysis of nine controlled clinical trials of standardized Ginkgo extract in patients with peripheral arterial disease. Included were trials with similar criteria regarding dosage (120–160 mg per day), length of study (4–6 weeks), treatment and targets. Patients in these trials had Fontaine stage II or stage III peripheral arterial disease and the treatment was quantified by the increase of walking distance, measured by standardized treadmill. The metaanalysis found the increase in walking distance achieved by Ginkgo was 0.75 times the standard deviation higher than that of placebo. This indicates a real and highly significant therapeutic effect over placebo for standardized Ginkgo extract for the treatment of peripheral arterial disease.[107]

An analysis of randomized, placebo-controlled, double-blind clinical trials of the efficacy of standardized Ginkgo extract and pentoxifylline (a vasodilating drug) in the treatment of intermittent claudication found the studies on both active substances to be similar in methodological quality and clinical outcomes.[108] In the studies reviewed, the median treatment periods differed with Ginkgo at 20 weeks and pentoxifylline at 11 weeks. The increase in the target objective (pain-free walking distance) was highly variable, especially in the pentoxifylline studies. On average, an increase in walking distance of 45% was found for standardized Ginkgo extract versus placebo (five trials, 120–160 mg per day) compared to 57% for pentoxifylline versus placebo (nine trials, 600–1200 mg per day). (Three of the Ginkgo trials included in this analysis were analysed in the above metaanalysis – these are references [104,105,106] – and the other two trials are references [109,110].)

In subsequent randomized, double-blind, placebo-controlled trials in patients with intermittent claudication, treatment with Ginkgo extract yielded the following results:

- significantly improved walking performance in trained patients (120 mg per day, 24 weeks, $p<0.0001$);[111]
- improved cognitive function but it did not change signs and symptoms of vascular disease in patients with moderate arterial insufficiency (120 mg per day, 3 months);[112]
- a rapid antiischaemic activity, as evidenced by a 38% decrease in ischaemic area in the Ginkgo group (320 mg per day, 4 weeks);[113]
- improved walking distance and reduced pain severity but there was no evidence of any gross improvement in the perfusion of the ischaemic leg (120 mg per day, 24 weeks).[114]

Ear, nose, throat problems

In a randomized comparative study, 80 patients with idiopathic sudden hearing loss existing no longer than 10 days were treated with either standardized Ginkgo extract or naftidrofuryl (a vasodilator). After 1 week, 40% of patients in each group experienced a complete remission. After 3 weeks there was a significant borderline benefit for Ginkgo over naftidrofuryl. Ginkgo treatment was preferred due to a lack of side effects, unlike the naftidrofuryl.[115] Standardized Ginkgo extract (intravenous 200 mg/day for 9 days, followed by oral 160 mg/day for 6 weeks) was found to be superior to the drug piracetam for the treatment of sudden deafness.[116]

Studies have shown contradictory results of Ginkgo extract treatment of tinnitus: some uncontrolled and/or comparative trials have shown significant results, others (including placebo-controlled trials) have shown no significant results or no effect demonstrated. Twenty patients reporting a positive effect on persistent severe tinnitus in an open study of 80 patients were included in a double-blind, placebo-controlled, crossover study.[117] They received either Ginkgo extract (29.2 mg per day, 2 weeks) or placebo. The success of the treatment was based on patient preference (as there is no objective measurement) and on this basis Ginkgo did not demonstrate a significant effect. However, the dosage of Ginkgo extract used was probably subtherapeutic.

Other conditions

Standardized Ginkgo extract has improved peak flow rates in asthmatic children and caused significant clinical improvement in adults.[17]

In a randomized, placebo-controlled trial to study the preventative effect of Ginkgo during a Himalayan expedition, 44 subjects received either standardized Ginkgo extract (160 mg per day) or placebo. Ginkgo significantly prevented acute mountain sickness for moderate altitude (5400 m) and decreased vasomotor disorders of the extremities.[118]

In a double-blind, placebo-controlled trial, 15 patients undergoing aortic valve replacement (in cardiopulmonary bypass) received either standardized Ginkgo extract (320 mg per day) or placebo for 5 days before surgical intervention. Plasma samples taken at crucial stages of the operation indicated that Ginkgo limited the free radical-induced oxidative stress generated throughout the surgery. Recovery of the Ginkgo patients was improved (but not significantly) compared to placebo but Ginkgo was considered useful in limiting oxidative stress. The protective activity was attributed to a membrane-protective mechanism rather than a direct scavenging effect.[119] (Earlier in vitro and in vivo studies suggest the cardioprotective effects of the Ginkgo terpenoids involve an inhibition of free radical formation rather than direct free radical scavenging.)[120]

In a controlled, multicentre, double-blind study of 165 women with congestive symptoms of premenstrual syndrome, patients received either 160 mg per day of standardized Ginkgo extract or placebo. The medication was taken from day 16 of the menstrual cycle to day 5 of the following cycle. Ginkgo significantly improved breast tenderness. There were marked improvements in other symptoms for the Ginkgo group including oedema, anxiety, depression and headaches.[121]

In an uncontrolled trial, 20 outpatients with a long history of elevated plasma viscosity and fibrinogen levels and a variety of underlying diseases received 240 mg per day standardized Ginkgo extract for 12 weeks. Steady and significant reductions in fibrinogen levels and blood viscosity were observed over the treatment period.[122]

In 24 patients suffering from blockage of veins in the retina, Ginkgo extract produced improvement in blood vessels, visual acuity and in the field of vision in a double-blind, placebo-controlled trial. Where the blood supply to the retina was deficient, Ginkgo improved many aspects of vision such as near and far vision, colour recognition and field of vision.[123] In an uncontrolled trial, 35 patients with poor blood supply to the retina, or to those parts of the brain which interpret the signals from the eyes, were treated with Ginkgo extract (120 mg/day) over a 3-month period; 86% of patients with reduced vision improved markedly. Symptoms of cerebral insufficiency also improved.[124] Ginkgo treatment (160 mg/day) for 6 months improved visual acuity compared to placebo in a double-blind, placebo-controlled trial in 10 patients with senile macular degeneration.[125]

After limited success in an open trial using intravenous ginkgolide B with multiple sclerosis patients in acute relapse, a double-blind, placebo-controlled study was undertaken with 104 patients. There was no significant difference between placebo and the low or high-dose ginkgolide B groups.[126,127]

In an uncontrolled trial, Ginkgo extract (average dose 207 mg/day) was found to be 84% effective in alleviating sexual dysfunction secondary to antidepressant drug use in 33 female and 30 male patients.[128] No adverse effects were reported.

TOXICOLOGY

Standardized Ginkgo extract had an LD_{50} value of 7.7 g/kg in mice (oral). Chronic toxicity studies over 27 weeks, at an initial dose of 20 and 100 mg/kg/day gradually increasing to 400 and 500 mg/kg/day, showed no evidence of organ damage and no impairment of hepatic or renal function. Oral administration of up to 900 and 1600 mg/kg/day to rabbits and rats respectively did not elicit teratogenic effects or affect reproduction.[123]

Both in vitro and in vivo assays showed that Ginkgo extract does not possess mutagenic activity.[123]

The seeds, stems and leaves of Ginkgo contain 4′-O-methylpyroxidine, which can cause vitamin B_6 deficiency symptoms, including convulsions. Poisoning has occurred in China and Japan (prior to 1960) where the stems are eaten as a luxury food or in times of food shortage. This toxin has been measured at levels of 42 μg per gram fresh weight of Ginkgo stem. Of the medicinal preparations tested, the highest concentration of 4′-O-methylpyroxidine conferred a daily dose of 60 μg of the toxin. In contrast, the acute oral toxic dose was measured at 11 mg/kg in guinea pigs. The ingestion of Ginkgo extracts and of boiled Ginkgo seeds (eaten in Japan) is not expected to cause detrimental effects, although ingestion of seed should be limited, particularly for children. Furthermore, the presence of bilobalide decreases the severity of convulsions.[129,130]

CONTRAINDICATIONS

None.

SPECIAL WARNINGS AND PRECAUTIONS

Caution in patients on anticoagulant or antiplatelet medication.

INTERACTIONS

Caution should be exercised when prescribing Ginkgo with warfarin and aspirin.

USE IN PREGNANCY AND LACTATION

No adverse effects expected.

EFFECTS ON ABILITY TO DRIVE AND USE MACHINES

Possible improvement of these functions, especially in older subjects.

SIDE EFFECTS

In clinical trials, standardized Ginkgo extract was associated with a remarkably low incidence of side effects. Only two adverse events were reported in 314 000 patient-years of use in 1988.[131] (A 'patient-year' is a measurement of the number of patients under treatment and is based on the number of units sold and the recommended daily dosage, assuming an average duration of therapy of 1 year/patient.) An analysis of double-blind clinical trials (932 Ginkgo-treated patients, 919 placebo) found a similar number of adverse events were reported by Ginkgo-treated patients (16) as by placebo-treated patients (14).[123] In one clinical trial, patients suffering from chronic cerebral insufficiency received 120 mg per day standardized Ginkgo extract for 1 year. Slight gastric symptoms occurred at the start of the trial but did not continue as the trial proceeded. The cardiovascular parameters measured (heart rate, blood pressure, blood lipids) remained practically unchanged.[132] In recent clinical trials, Ginkgo has continued to be well tolerated.[89,98,111]

Three independent reports which have attributed episodes of spontaneous bleeding to intake of *Ginkgo biloba* have appeared in the medical literature. The first case report described a 33-year-old Korean woman with no significant medical history who noted the onset of diffuse headaches which increased in severity over a 3-month period.[133] Her headaches were accompanied by diplopia, nausea and vomiting. Her physician prescribed ergotamine/caffeine tablets. MRI of her brain revealed bilateral subdural haematomas. These were evacuated by a neurosurgeon, which resulted in considerable symptom improvement. However, a mild chronic headache persisted. At this point 4 months later, the patient's consumption of *Ginkgo biloba* at 120 mg per day of standardized extract was revealed. She had been taking the Ginkgo for 2 years. Her only other medication consumption was paracetamol and the ergotamine/caffeine tablets. Her neurological examination was normal. MRI of the brain showed only postoperative changes, without reaccumulation of subdural fluid. Coagulation parameters were normal but bleeding time was slightly prolonged at 15.0 and 9.5 minutes (normal range 3.0–9.0 minutes). When the patient stopped Ginkgo, bleeding times were 6.5 and 6.5 minutes 35 days later. On follow-up 15 months later, the patient was doing well without further headache or neurological symptoms.

The second case report described recurrent spontaneous bleeding from the iris into the anterior chamber of the eye.[134] This is a rare problem which developed in a 70-year-old man. One week earlier he began ingestion of 80 mg per day of standardized *Ginkgo biloba* extract. The patient's other medication was 325 mg of aspirin per day, which he had taken for 3 years after coronary artery bypass surgery. There was no history of eye trauma, ischaemia or vascular occlusion.

A 61-year-old man was diagnosed with mild subarachnoid haemorrhage, which was attributed to the patient's intake of 120–160 mg/day of Ginkgo extract.[135] While the author does state that it is not proven that the subarachnoid haemorrhage was caused by the *Ginkgo biloba*, the increased bleeding time of the patient to 6 minutes (normal is 1–3 minutes according to the author) appeared to be associated with the patient's use of this herb. The author of this case report bases his conclusion on the fact that Ginkgo appeared to increase the patient's bleeding time. However, a bleeding time of 6 minutes can hardly be taken as pathogenic and it is in fact widely considered to be in the normal range.

OVERDOSE

Not known.

CURRENT REGULATORY STATUS IN SELECTED COUNTRIES

A draft monograph of Ginkgo is being prepared and may appear in the *European Pharmacopoeia* subsequent to the 1997 edition. Ginkgo became official in the *United States Pharmacopeia-National Formulary* (USP 23-NF 18).

Ginkgo leaf is covered by a null Commission E monograph.

As the efficacy of crude Ginkgo leaf has not been documented, no therapeutic application can be recommended. Due to the content of ginkgolic acids, which are contact allergens, an allergic risk is not ruled out.

In contrast, the standardized Ginkgo extract is covered by a positive Commission E monograph and has the following applications:

- symptomatic treatment of demential syndromes (including primary degenerative dementia, vascular dementia and mixed forms of both) characterized by the following symptoms: memory deficit, disturbances in concentration, depression, dizziness, tinnitus and headache.
- improvement in pain-free walking distance in peripheral arterial occlusive disease in intermittent claudication in a regimen of physical therapeutic measures;
- vertigo and tinnitus of vascular and involutional origin.

The Commission E recommends that the standardized extract of Ginkgo should be low in ginkgolic acids.

Ginkgo biloba is an approved medicine in Germany and prescriptions from medical practitioners are reimbursed by health schemes.

Ginkgo is not on the UK General Sale List.

Ginkgo does not have GRAS status. However, it is freely available as a 'dietary supplement' in the USA under DSHEA legislation (1994 Dietary Supplement Health and Education Act).

Ginkgo is not included in Part 4 of Schedule 4 of the Therapeutic Goods Act Regulations of Australia.

References

1. Bensky D, Gamble A. Chinese herbal medicine materia medica. Eastland Press, Seattle, 1986, pp 560–561.
2. Allaby M (ed). The concise Oxford dictionary of botany. Oxford University Press, Oxford, 1992, p 177.
3. Willard T. The Wild Rose scientific herbal. Wild Rose College of Natural Healing Ltd, Calgary, 1991, p 142.
4. Wagner H, Bladt S. Plant drug analysis: a thin layer chromatography atlas, 2nd edn. Springer-Verlag, Berlin, 1996, p 237.
5. DeFeudis FV. Ginkgo biloba extract (EGb 761): pharmacological activities and clinical applications. Elsevier, Amsterdam, 1991, pp 10–13.
6. DeFeudis FV. Ginkgo biloba extract (EGb 761): pharmacological activities and clinical applications. Elsevier, Amsterdam, 1991.
7. Chung KF, Dent G, McCusker M et al. Lancet 1987; 1 (8527): 248–251.
8. Braquet P Touqui L, Shen TY et al. Pharmacol Rev 1987; 39: 97–145.

9. Lane HC, Fauci AS. Ann Intern Med 1985; 103 (5): 714–718.
10. Stanworth DR, Griffiths HR, Braquet P. New Trends Lipid Mediat Res 1988; 2: 18–25.
11. Guinot P, Summerhayes C, Berdah L et al. Lancet 1988; 2 (8602): 114.
12. Roberts NM, McCusker M, Chung KF et al. Br J Clin Pharmacol 1988; 26: 65–72.
13. Braquet P, Etienne A, Touvay C et al. Lancet 1985; 1: 1501.
14. Vilain B, Lagente V, Touvay C et al. Pharmacol Res Commun 1986; 18 (suppl): 119–126.
15. Barnes PJ, Chung KF, Page CP. Pharmacol Rev 1988; 40 (1): 49–84.
16. Bourgain RH, Maes L, Andries R et al. Prostaglandins 1986; 32(1): 142–144.
17. Braquet P. Adv Prostagland Thromboxane Leukot Res 1986; 16: 179–198.
18. Braquet P, Paubert-Braquet M, Koltai M et al. Trends Pharmacol Sci 1989; 10 (1): 23–30.
19. Krieglstein J, Ausmeier F. International Congress on Phytotherapy, Munich, September 10–13, 1992.
20. Smith PF, Maclennan K, Darlington CL. J Ethnopharmacol 1996; 50: 131–139.
21. Oberpichler H, Beck T, Abdel-Rahman MM et al. Pharmacol Res Commun 1988; 20 (5): 349–368.
22. Duverger D, DeFeudis FV, Drieu K. Gen Pharmacol 1995; 26 (6): 1375–1383.
23. Safi N, Galley P. Bordeaux Med 1977; 10: 171–176.
24. Schaffler K, Reeh PW. Arzneim-Forsch 1985; 35: 1283–1286.
25. Borzeix MG, Labos M, Hartl C et al. Sem Hop (Paris) 1980; 56: 393–398.
26. Hansel R, Haas H. Therapie mit Phytopharmaka. Springer-Verlag, Berlin, 1984, p 76.
27. Spinnewyn B, Blavet N, Clostre F. Presse Med 1896; 15: 1511–1515.
28. Le Poncin-Laffitte M, Rapin J, Rapin JR. Arch Int Pharmacodyn 1980; 243: 236–244.
29. Gabard B, Chatterjee SS. Naunyn Schmiedeberg's Arch Pharmacol 1980; 321: R68; 311 (suppl) abstr 271.
30. Hansel R, Haas H. Therapie mit Phytopharmaka. Springer-Verlag, Berlin, 1984, p 68–69.
31. Reuse-Blom S, Drieu K. Presse Med 1986; 15: 1520–1523.
32. Pincemail J, Deby C. Presse Med 1986; 15: 1475–1479.
33. Pincemail J, Thirion A, Dupuis M et al. Experientia 1987; 43 (2): 181–184.
34. Janssens D, Michiels C, Delaive E et al. Biochem Pharmacol 1995; 50 (7): 991–999.
35. Punkt K, Welt K, Schaffranietz L. Acta Histochem 1995; 97 (1): 67–79.
36. Heiss WD, Zeiler K. Pharmakother 1978; 1: 137–144.
37. Jung F, Mrowietz C, Kiesewetter H et al. Arzneim-Forsch 1990; 40 (5): 589–598.
38. Joyeux M, Lobstein A, Anton R et al. Planta Med 1995; 61 (2): 126–129.
39. Maitra I, Marcocci L, Droy-Lefaix MT et al. Biochem Pharmacol 1995; 49 (11): 1649–1655.
40. Seif-El-Nasr M, El-Fattah AA. Pharmacol Res 1995; 32 (5): 273–278.
41. Ni Y, Zhao B, Hou J et al. Neurosci Lett 1996; 214 (2–3): 115–118.
42. Hasenohrl RU, Nichau CH, Frisch CH et al. Pharmacol Biochem Behav 1996; 53 (2): 271–275.
43. Yan LJ, Droy-Lefaix MT, Packer L. Biochem Biophys Res Commun 1995; 212 (2): 360–366.
44. Artmann GM, Schikarski, C. Clin Haem 1993; 13 (4): 529–539.
45. Emerit I, Arutyunyan R, Oganesian N et al. Free Radic Biol Med 1995; 18 (6): 985–991.
46. Emerit I, Oganesian N, Sarkisian T et al. Radiat Res 1995; 144 (2): 198–205.
47. Winter E. Pharmacol Biochem Behav 1991; 38 (1): 109–114.
48. Porsolt RD, Martin P, Lenegre A et al. Pharmacol Biochem Behav 1990; 36 (4): 963–971.
49. Rapin JR, Lamproglou I, Drieu K et al. Gen Pharmacol 1994; 25 (5): 1009–1016.
50. Subhan Z, Hindmarch I. Int J Clin Pharmacol Res 1986; 4 (2) 89–93.
51. Semlitsch HV, Anderer P, Saletu B et al. Pharmacopsychiatry 1995; 28 (4): 134–142.
52. Warot D, Lacomblez L, Danjou P et al. Therapie 1991; 46 (1): 33–36.
53. Stough C, Bonyhai A. Proceedings of the 3rd Pan Pacific Brain Topography Conference, 21.1.98, no. 31.
54. White HL, Scates PW, Cooper BR et al. Life Sci 1996; 58 (16): 1315–1321.
55. Atzori C, Bruno A, Chichino G et al. Antimicrob Agents Chemother 1993; 37 (7): 1492–1496.
56. JaeSeung P, JinHaeng L. J Urol 1996; 156 (5): 1876–1880.
57. Wojcicki J, Samochowiec L, Juzwiak S et al. Phytomed 1994; 1: 33–38.
58. Droy-Lefaix MT, Cluzel J, Menerath JM et al. Int J Tissue React 1995; 17 (3): 93–100.
59. Kobayashi N, Suzuki R, Koide C et al. Yakugaku Zasshi 1993; 113 (10): 718–724.
60. Rodriguez de Turco EB, Droy-Lefaix MT, Bazan NG. Physiol Behav 1993; 53 (5): 1001–1002.
61. Marcilhac A, Dakine N, Bourhim N et al. Life Sci 1998; 62 (25): 2329–2340.
62. Della Loggia R, Sosa S, Tubaro A et al. Fitoterapia 1996; 67 (3): 257–264.
63. Smith PF, Darlington CL. J Vestib Res 1994; 4 (3): 169–179.
64. Pietta PG, Gardana C, Mauri PL et al. J Chromatog B Biomed Appl 1995; 673 (1): 75–80.
65. Kleijnen J, Knipschild P. Lancet 1992; 340 (8828): 1136–1139.
66. Fourtillan JB, Brisson AM, Girault J et al. Therapie 1995; 50 (2): 137–144.
67. Le Bars PL, Katz MM, Berman N et al. JAMA 1997; 278 (16): 1327–1332.
68. Amar K, Wilcock G. Br Med J 1996; 312 (7025): 227–231.
69. Pantoni L, Garcia JH. Ann NY Acad Sci 1997; 826: 92–102.
70. Hartmann A, Frick M. MMW 1991; 133 (suppl): S23–S25.
71. Gerhardt G, Rogalla K, Jaeger J. Fortschr Med 1990; 108 (19): 384–388.
72. Kleijnen J, Knipschild P. Br J Clin Pharmacol 1992; 34 (4): 352–358.
73. Schmidt U, Rabinovici K, Lande S. Munch Med Wochenschr 1991; 133 (suppl 1): S15–S18.
74. Bruchert E, Heinrich SE, Ruf-Kohler P. Munch Med Wochenschr 1991; 133 (suppl 1): S9–S14.
75. Meyer B. Presse Med 1986; 15: 1562–1564.
76. Taillandier J, Ammar A, Rabourdin JP et al. Presse Med 1986; 15: 1583–1587.
77. Haguenauer JP, Cantenot F, Koskas H et al. Presse Med 1986; 15: 1569–1572.
78. Vorberg G, Schenk N, Schmidt U. Herz Gefasse 1989; 9: 936–941.
79. Eckmann F. Fortschr Med 1990; 108: 557–560.
80. Wesnes K, Simmons D, Rook M et al. Hum Psychopharmacol 1987; 2: 159–169.
81. Hopfenmuller W. Arzneim-Forsch 1994; 44 (9): 1005–1013.
82. Vesper J, Hansgen KD. Phytomed 1994; 1: 9–16.
83. Hofferberth B. MMW 1991; 133 (suppl 1): 30–33.
84. Halama P. MMW 1990; 133 (suppl 1): 190–194.
85. Eckmann F, Schlag H. Fortschr Med 1982; 100 (31–32): 1474–1478.
86. Leroy H, Salaun P, Chovelon R et al. Vie Medicale 1978; 28: 2513–2519.
87. Boudouresques C, Vigouroux R, Boudouresques J. Med Pract 1975; 598: 75–78.
88. Tea S, Celsis P, Clanet M et al. Gaz Med Fr 1979; 86 (35): 4149–4152.
89. Garg RK, Nag D, Agrawal A. J Assoc Physicians India 1995; 43 (11): 760–763.
90. Grassel E. Fortschr Med 1992; 110 (5): 73–76.
91. Kim JS, Lee SH, Kim JM et al. J Korean Soc Clin Pharmacol Therapeut 1995; 3 (2): 187–195.
92. Raabe A, Raabe M, Ihm P. Klin Monatsbl Augenheilkd 1991; 199 (66): 432–438.

93. Allain H, Raoul P, Lieury A et al. Clin Ther 1993; 15 (3): 549–558.
94. Pietri S, Maurelli E, Drieu K et al. J Mol Cell Cardiol 1997; 29 (2): 733–742.
95. Deberdt W. Life Sci 1994; 55 (25–26): 2057–2066.
96. Hofferberth B. Human Psychopharmacol 1994; 9: 215–222.
97. Warburton DM. Br J Clin Pharmacol 1993; 36 (2): 137.
98. Kanowski S, Herrmann WM, Stephan K et al. Pharmacopsychiatry 1996; 29 (2): 47–56.
99. Stoppe G, Sandholzer H, Staedt J et al. Pharmacopsychiatry 1996; 29 (4): 150–155.
100. Maurer K, Ihl R, Dierks T et al. J Psychiat Res 1997; 31 (6): 645–655.
101. Oken BS, Storzbach DM, Kaye JA. Arch Neurol 1998; 55: 1409–1415.
102. Ambrosi C, Bourde C. Gaz Med Fr 1975; 82 (6): 628–633.
103. Courbier R, Jausseran JM, Reggi M. Mediterr Med 1977; 126: 61–64.
104. Salz H. Ther Gegenw 1980; 119: 1345–1356.
105. Bauer U. Arzneim-Forsch 1984; 34 (6): 716–720.
106. Natali J et al. Unpublished results, 1985. Cited in Schneider B. Arzneim-Forsch 1992; 42 (4): 428–436.
107. Schneider B. Arzneim Forsch 1992; 42 (4): 428–436.
108. Letzel H, Schoop W. Vasa 1992; 21 (4): 403–410.
109. Bulling B, Von Bary S. Med Welt 1991; 42 (8): 702–708.
110. Diehm C, Heinrich F, Morl H. Internal Report, Dr Willmar Schwabe Arzneimittel, Clinical Research, Karlsruhe, 1990. Cited in Letzel H, Schoop W. Vasa 1992; 21 (4): 403–410.
111. Blume J, Kieser M, Holscher U et al. Vasa 1996; 25 (3): 265–274.
112. Drabaek H, Petersen JR, Wiinberg N et al. Ugeskr Laeger 1996; 158: 3928–3931.
113. Mouren X, Caillard P, Schwartz F. Angiology 1994; 45 (6): 413–417.
114. Thomson GJ, Vohra RK, Carr MH et al. Int Angiol 1990; 9 (2): 75–78.
115. Hoffmann F, Beck C, Schutz A et al. Laryngorhinootologie 1994; 73 (3): 149–152.
116. Baschek V, Steinert W. Vertigo, nausea, tinnitus and hypoacusia. In: Claussen, CF, Kirtane MV, Schlitter K (eds). Metabolic disorders. Elsevier, Amsterdam, 1988, p 575–582.
117. Holgers KM, Azelsson A, Pringle I. Audiology 1994; 33 (2): 85–92.
118. Roncin JP, Schwartz F, D'Arbigny P. Aviat Space Environ Med 1996; 65 (5): 445–452.
119. Pietri S, Seguin JR, D'Arbigny P et al. Cardiovasc Drugs Ther 1997; 11 (2): 121–131.
120. Israel L, Della' Accio E, Martin G et al. Psychol Med 1987; 19: 1431–1439.
121. Tamborini A, Taurelle R. Rev Fr Gynecol Obstet 1993; 88 (7–9): 447–457.
122. Witte S, Anadere I, Walitza E. Fortschr Med 1992; 110 (13): 247–250.
123. DeFeudis FV. Ginkgo biloba extract (EGb 761): pharmacological activities and clinical applications. Elsevier, Amsterdam, 1991, pp 133–134.
124. Lagatz WH, Fies AM, Bartsch G. Z Allg Med 1990; 66: 573–578.
125. Lebuisson DA, Leroy L, Rigal G. Presse Med 1986; 15: 1556–1558.
126. Brochet B, Orgogozo JM, Guinot P et al. Rev Neurol (Paris) 1992; 148 (4): 299–301.
127. Brochet B, Guinot P, Orgogozo JM et al. J Neurol Neurosurg Psychiatry 1995; 58 (3): 360–362.
128. Cohen AJ, Bartlik B. J Sex Marital Therapy 1998; 24: 139–145.
129. Leistner E, Arenz A. Z Phytother 1997; 18: 230–231.
130. Arenz A, Klein M, Fiehe K et al. Planta Med 1996; 62: 548–551.
131. DeFeudis FV. Ginkgo biloba extract (EGb 761): pharmacological activities and clinical applications. Elsevier, Amsterdam, 1991, pp 143–144.
132. Vorberg G. Clin Trials J 1985; 22: 149–157.
133. Rowin J, Lewis SL. Neurology 1996; 46: 1775–1776.
134. Rosenblatt M, Mindel J. N Engl J Med 1997; 336 (15): 1108.
135. Vale S. Lancet 1998; 352 (9121): 36.

Ginseng
(*Panax ginseng* C. Meyer)

SYNONYMS

Korean ginseng, panax, man root (Engl), Ginseng radix (Lat), Ginsengwurzel, Kraftwurzel (Ger), racine de ginseng (Fr), ginseng (Dan), ren shen (Chin), ninjin (Jap), insam (Kor).

WHAT IS IT?

Ginseng (*Panax ginseng*) is one of the most valued (and expensive) medicinal plants. Originally part of traditional Chinese medicine, the root is now widely consumed in the West. Panax is derived from the Greek word for panacea and it is said to 'cure all'. According to the Chinese sages, ginseng replenished the vital energy, increased the production of body fluids and promoted health and longevity. Since the 1960s, ginseng has been the subject of numerous scientific investigations. The great diversity of pharmacological properties now attributed to ginseng suggest that it might act in a unique and fundamental way on the body. In fact, its activity often appears to be based on whole-body effects, rather than particular organs or systems. This is notwithstanding the fact that ginseng can profoundly influence the metabolism of the individual cell. These outcomes lend weight to the traditional view that ginseng is above all a tonic herb which can revitalize the functioning of the organism as a whole. There is no equivalent concept or treatment in contemporary conventional medicine.

Medicinal ginseng consists of the main and lateral roots. The smaller root hairs, which are widely used in the West, should be regarded as an inferior substitution. Most of the available root is from cultivated sources but roots sourced from the wild are superior in quality and attract a premium price. Two forms of the root are available in commerce: red ginseng where the root is steamed before drying and white ginseng which is dried by normal processes.

EFFECTS

Increases vitality and the ability to withstand stress by acting on the hypothalamus-pituitary-adrenal cortex axis; restores and strengthens the body's immune response; promotes longevity, metabolism and growth of normal cells.

TRADITIONAL VIEW

In traditional Chinese medicine ginseng is classified as a herb that tonifies the *Qi* (energy); hence it is used for severe collapsed *Qi* conditions (shallow respiration and shortness of breath). It benefits *Yin* and generates *Fluids* (so is used in profuse sweating), tonifies the *Lungs*, the *Stomach* and strengthens the *Spleen* (so is used for laboured breathing, lethargy, chest and abdominal distension and prolapse). Ginseng also benefits the *Heart Qi* and calms the *Spirit* (so is used for palpitations with anxiety, insomnia and restlessness). Traditionally ginseng would be taken as the powdered, dried root or as a decoction.[1,2]

Western herbalists have used ginseng traditionally as a mild stomachic, tonic and stimulant for anorexia and digestive complaints arising from mental and nervous exhaustion.[3] The BHP recommends its use in the treatment of neurasthenia, neuralgia and for depressive states associated with sexual inadequacy.[4] In addition to the above conditions, the Eclectics used ginseng for cerebral anaemia, asthma, convulsions, paralysis and urinary gravel.[5]

SUMMARY ACTIONS

Adaptogenic, tonic, immunomodulator, cardiotonic, cancer preventative.

CAN BE USED FOR

INDICATIONS SUPPORTED BY CLINICAL TRIALS

To improve performance and well-being; to improve general performance under stress; as a tonic for the elderly; congestive heart failure, elevates HDL-cholesterol, improves cerebrovascular deficit; selected extracts decrease the risk of developing certain types of cancer (excluding cancers of the female breast, cervix, bladder and thyroid) when consumed for extended periods; protective effect on depressed bone marrow in cervical cancer patients undergoing radiation therapy; impotence, male fertility problems; non-insulin dependent diabetes.

TRADITIONAL THERAPEUTIC USES

Prostration, heart failure, dyspnoea, asthma, organ prolapse, spontaneous sweating, cold limbs, digestive complaints, palpitations, neuralgia, convulsions, neurosis, anxiety, long-term debility, sexual inadequacy.

MAY ALSO BE USED FOR

EXTRAPOLATIONS FROM PHARMACOLOGICAL STUDIES

To improve resistance to a wide variety of stressors; to counter some effects of ageing; to improve learning and memory; to improve ethanol clearance which may be beneficial in alcoholism; may be useful in drug-dependent states.

OTHER APPLICATIONS

As a constituent of antiwrinkle and antiageing creams and lotions.[6]

PREPARATIONS

Dried root for decoction, liquid extract and tablets; powdered root.

DOSAGE

The traditional dried dosage is 1–10 g per day of the dried root by decoction. Larger doses up to 30 g may be used to treat haemorrhagic shock.[2]

The adult dose used in the West is from 0.5 to 3.0 g per day of the dried main or lateral roots (depending on the quality of the root and the application) or 1–6 ml per day of the 1:2 liquid extract. Preparations from the root hairs are therapeutically inferior and should be avoided. Many clinical trials have been conducted using a dose of 200 mg of a 5:1 standardized extract.

A study of commercial ginseng products in the USA published in 1978 found a wide variation in quality in the marketplace, with several products containing no detectable levels of ginsenosides.[7] A similar variation in quality is still likely to exist today in many countries.

DURATION OF USE

Generally up to 3 months, with a repeated course.[8] Continuous use in the unwell and elderly is appropriate.

SUMMARY ASSESSMENT OF SAFETY

No adverse effects are expected if used as recommended. Overstimulation may occur in susceptible individuals or at excessive doses.

TECHNICAL DATA

BOTANY

Panax ginseng, a member of the Araliaceae (ginseng) family, is a perennial slow-growing herb native to the mountainous regions of China, Japan, Korea and the Soviet Union. The stem is erect, simple not branching, the leaves are verticillate and compound with five leaflets; the three terminal leaflets are larger than the lateral ones. The inflorescence is a small terminal, hemispherical umbel consisting of pink, polygamous flowers containing five petals. The fruit is a small berry which is red in colour when ripe. The root produces a branch root from its middle.[9]

KEY CONSTITUENTS

- A complex mixture of dammarane saponins (2–3%), called ginsenosides, and an oleanolic saponin.[10] The ginsenosides can be divided into two classes: the protopanaxatriol class, consisting mainly of Rg_1, Rg_2, Rf and Re, and the protopanaxadiol class, consisting mainly of Rc, Rd, Rb_1 and Rb_2.[11]
- Polysaccharides and essential oil.[1]
- Polyacetylenes, peptides and trilinolein and other lipids.[12–14]

It can be seen from Table 1 that the total level of ginsenosides is not the sole determinant of quality, otherwise the leaves and root hairs would be preferred. Clearly, the activity of ginseng must be attributable to the particular combination of ginsenosides found in the main and lateral roots. In particular, the ratio of Rg_1 to Rb_1 being greater than 0.5 is now accepted as a marker of ginseng quality. However, it is also likely that other components found in the main root contribute significantly to the therapeutic activity of ginseng.

PHARMACODYNAMICS

More than 500 studies have been published on the pharmacological activity of ginseng. Since it is beyond the scope of this review to cover these in detail, the following information provides a broad but not comprehensive review of the literature, with an emphasis on review papers and recent or more interesting studies.

One interpretative caution which should be observed for the in vivo pharmacological studies is that in many cases the ginseng or ginsenosides were administered by injection. Since the ginsenosides are probably not the active forms which reach the bloodstream after oral doses of ginseng, more weight should be given to the oral pharmacological studies. The same

Table 1 Distribution of ginsenosides in *Panax ginseng*[15]

	% Content								
	Rg_1	Re	Rf	Rg_2	Rb_1	Re	Rb_2	Rd	Total
Leaves	1.078	1.524	–	–	0.184	0.736	0.553	1.113	5.188
Leafstalks	0.327	0.141	–	–	–	0.190	–	0.107	0.765
Stem	0.292	0.070	–	–	–	–	0.397	–	0.759
Main root	0.379	0.153	0.092	0.023	0.342	0.190	0.131	0.038	1.348
Lateral roots	0.406	0.668	0.203	0.090	0.850	0.738	0.434	0.143	3.532
Root hairs	0.376	1.512	0.150	0.249	1.351	1.349	0.780	0.381	6.148

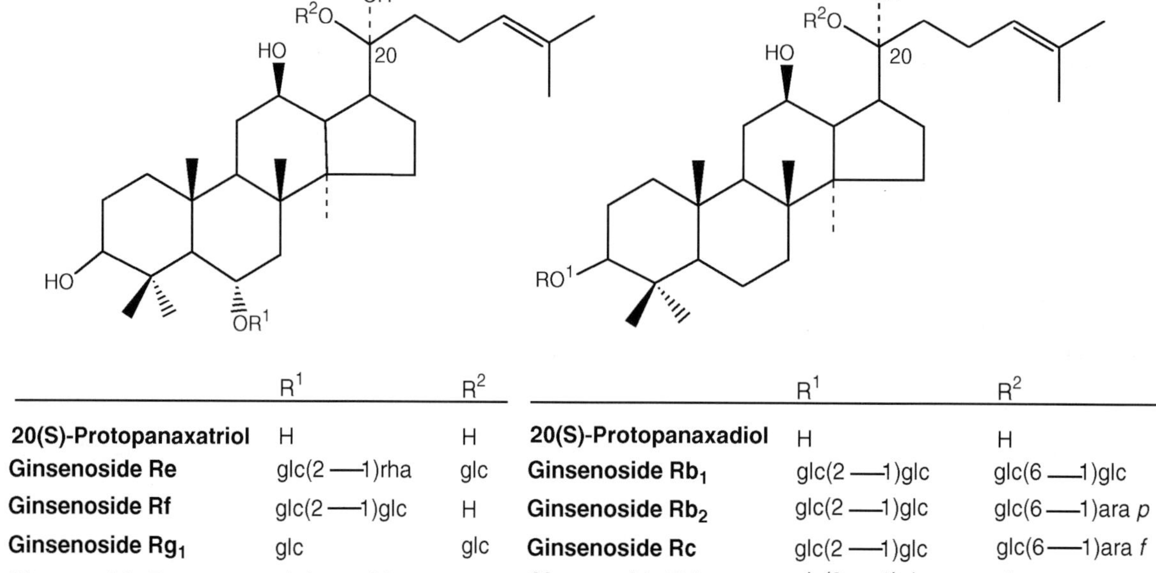

Protopanaxatriol Class **Protopanaxadiol Class**

glc = β-D-glucose
rha= α-L-rhamnose
ara= α-L-arabinose
p = pyranose
f = furanose

caution also applies to the interpretation of in vitro investigations.

Adaptogenic and related activities

Ginseng appears to act mainly on the hypothalamus and has a sparing action on the adrenal cortex, mediated through the anterior pituitary and ACTH release.[1] It appears to tune the adrenal cortex so that phase 1 of the general adaptation syndrome (GAS) is more efficient. Response is stronger and quicker and feedback control is more effective so that when stress decreases, glucocorticoid levels fall more rapidly to normal.[16,17] During prolonged stress (or phase 2 of GAS) glucocorticoid production is reduced by ginseng (a sparing effect), while at the same time adrenal capacity is increased (a trophic effect).[16,17] Ginseng also raises plasma ACTH and cortisone in the relaxed (non-stressed) state when given by injection (thereby possibly generating a sense of alertness and well-being).[18]

In countless animal experiments, ginseng has increased resistance to a wide variety of physical, chemical and biological stressors. Some of these studies are reviewed below.

- Oral administration of ginseng root saponins or ginsenoside Rb_1 antagonized the immunosuppression induced by cold-water swim stress in mice and rats. Conflicting results were obtained for serum corticosterone levels. The increase in serum corticosterone was inhibited in stressed rats but accentuated in stressed mice.[19]
- Ginseng or its components countered stress-induced changes from heat stress,[20–22] cold stress[23,24] and forced exercise.[22,25,26]
- Other models where ginseng or its components demonstrated improved adaptation to stress included food deprivation,[27] the cold hypoxia restraint model,[28] radiation exposure,[29,30] electroshock[22] and emotional stress (open field test).[31]
- There has been one negative study published, where ginseng infusion did not counter cold-water swim stress.[32] This may reflect on the poor activity of this form of aqueous extract of ginseng.

Other studies which may reflect on tonic and adaptogenic properties for ginseng include the following.

- Inclusion of red ginseng in the water offered to growing rabbits significantly increased the relative weights of digestive organs.[33]
- Oral doses of 100 mg/kg of ginseng (in a comparison with Withania, which was also active) significantly increased wet and dry weights of levator ani muscles in rats.[34]
- The effects of ginseng extract administered by injection prior to exercise in rats suggested that it could exert an antifatigue effect by increasing the biochemical capability of working skeletal muscle to better utilize free fatty acids, thus sparing body carbohydrate stores.[35,36]
- In rats fed a low-carbohydrate diet, injected ginsenosides increased pyruvate kinase activity in the liver but decreased it in rats fed high carbohydrate.[37] Such normalizing activity is said to be a characteristic of adaptogens.
- Ginseng extract (oral doses, 33 mg/kg) produced an increase in adrenal zona fasciculata cell size compared to controls. In mice treated with ginsenoside Rb_1 or Rg_1 (oral doses), the mean cell areas were unchanged but the distribution of cell sizes differed from controls.[38]
- Ginsenosides administered by injection to rats decreased thymus weight and increased the size of the adrenal cortex. These effects were not evident in rats without a pituitary gland.[39]

Consistent with the understanding that it is a tonic herb, ginseng administration countered some effects of ageing in animal models. For example, ginseng extract at an oral dose of 600 mg/kg significantly stimulated granuloma collagen synthesis in an aged rat model and restored this parameter to near levels seen in young rats.[40] Repeated intraperitoneal injections of ginsenoside Rg_1improved the performance of aged rats in the radial-arm maze, possibly through an increase of choline acetyltransferase activity in the brain.[41] Daily oral administration of ginseng extract (8 g/kg/day for 12–33 days) ameliorated the impaired learning performance of aged rats in a radial maze.[42] Oral intake of a water extract of ginseng for 4 weeks produced an increase in spontaneous motor activity during the dark period in old rats, while it caused a decrease in the activity of young rats (rats are nocturnal animals).[43]

Mental function and performance

The total effect of the root is stimulatory but the diols such as Rb_1 are sedative and the triols such as Rg_1 are stimulatory.[44] Standardized ginseng extract was administered orally at doses of 3, 10, 30, 100 and 300 mg/kg for 10 days as 10 rats were used with each dose. With the 'shuttle-box' method for active avoidance, the most pronounced effect on learning and memory was obtained by the dose of 10 mg/kg. With the 'step-down' method for passive avoidance, the dose of 30 mg/kg significantly improved retention. In the staircase maze training with positive (alimentary) reinforcement, only the dose of 10 mg/kg significantly improved learning and memory. The dose of 100 mg/kg greatly increased the locomotor activity of mice. These results show that ginseng at appropriate doses improves learning, memory and physical capabilities.[45] Standardized ginseng extract, administered at a dose of 30 mg/kg orally for 10 days, markedly countered the memory-impairing effect of electric shock.[46]

Oral doses of ginsenosides Rb_1 and Rg_1 (each at about 50 mg/kg) accelerated brain and body development in young mice and facilitated memory acquisition in two models.[47] Oral administration of ginseng ethanol extract 90 minutes before testing dose dependently improved the maze performance of rats after disruption by scopolamine.[48]

The effect of oral doses of standardized extracts of ginseng (17, 50 and 150 mg/kg), Ginkgo and their combination were investigated on young and old rats in a series of behavioural tests. The effects varied with the dose and the test used, but both ginseng and Ginkgo extracts demonstrated properties similar to nootropic drugs (drugs that affect neurons favourably). The two extracts and their combination improved the retention of learned behaviour.[49]

Immune system effects

Immune system effects attributed to ginseng have been reviewed.[50] However, the majority of the studies included in that review and subsequent investigations have employed in vitro tests or in vivo models where ginseng or ginsenosides were given by injection.

Oral administration of ginseng extract:

- was found to be effective against experimental Semliki forest viral infection in mice (the dose was 5.4 g/kg ginseng over 9 days before viral challenge);[51]
- enhanced B and T-lymphocyte and natural killer cell activities in mice and increased production of interferon following an interferon inducer (the dose was 10 mg/mouse/day of ginseng for 4 consecutive days);[52]
- increased natural killer cell activity and dose dependently enhanced antibody formation in mice (in vitro it inhibited lymphocyte proliferation);[53]
- protected one particular mouse strain against *Candida albicans* infection.[54]

One study observed a particular immunosuppressive effect. Saponins from ginseng, when injected into mice at approximately 10 mg/kg, had no significant effect on lymphocyte responses to a subsequent influenza virus infection. However, the saponins selectively suppressed delayed-type hypersensitivity to the virus when administered before, but not after, virus sensitization. The authors suggested that this effect may be related to the steroid-like structure of the saponins (ginsenosides).[55]

Effects on cellular function

The effects of ginseng and its components on cultures of normal cells have been the subject of several studies, although recent attention has focused on ginseng's influence on abnormal cells. The positive effects of ginseng in promoting the longevity, metabolism and growth of normal cells are seen by many investigating scientists as confirmation of its tonic activity.

As early as 1969, aqueous extract of ginseng was found to delay degeneration of human amnion cells in vitro, an activity also exhibited by hydrocortisone and some of its analogues.[56] Fulder confirmed this observation using cell cultures of human fibroblasts. Ginseng promoted growth and delayed cellular necrosis, as did hydrocortisone.[57]

Subsequent in vitro studies have demonstrated the effects of ginseng or its components on the metabolism of a variety of cell types. These included the stimulation of DNA and protein synthesis in testes,[58] an increase in lactate levels[59] and a decrease in intracellular protein degradation in human fibroblasts.[60] Ginseng total saponins stimulated haematopoietic progenitor cell growth of cells taken from normal subjects and from 14 of 29 patients with aplastic anaemia.[61] Ginsenoside Rg_1 stimulated activity of tyrosine aminotransferase in hepatocytes.[62]

A tetrapeptide isolated from ginseng root stimulated the growth of several cell lines.[13,63] Based on immunoreactivity, a basic fibroblast growth factor-like molecule was identified in ginseng root.[64]

Ginseng or its components administered orally or by injection have also been found to stimulate cellular metabolism. Of a number of herbs tested, only injection of ginseng stimulated nuclear RNA synthesis in the liver cells of rats.[65] Injection of various components of ginseng root stimulated activities of nuclear RNA polymerase[66] and cytoplasmic RNA in rat liver cells,[67] increased RNA, protein and lipid synthesis in rat bone marrow cells[68] and stimulated rat renal nuclear RNA synthesis.[69]

Oral doses of various ginseng components substantially increased rough endoplasmic reticulum and RNA synthesis in rat hepatocytes,[70] stimulated DNA, protein and lipid synthesis in rat bone marrow cells[71] and increased hepatic lactate dehydrogenase activity in mice.[72] This last finding, according to the authors of the study, could provide one explanation for the putative antifatigue properties of ginseng.[72]

Anticancer activity

Considerable interest has been shown by researchers in the ways that ginseng might prevent or assist in the treatment of cancer. It has been implied that the tonic and adaptogenic effects of ginseng could lead to improved natural resistance against malignant tumours.[73] However, the research summarized below suggests that more specific mechanisms could apply.

Ginseng extract, ginsenosides and other components in the root such as the polyacetylenic alcohols have inhibited the growth of various tumour cell lines in several test tube experiments.[74–79] Moreover, diol-type prosapogenins and sapogenins (which are likely to be among the active forms of ginsenosides after oral ingestion) were also active against several cancer cell lines.[80] Various molecular mechanisms behind this antiproliferative activity have been studied.[81–84]

One interesting property of the ginsenosides is their ability to induce differentiation in cancer cell cultures. (Differentiation means that a tumour cell divides into daughter cells which show normal behaviour.) This has been demonstrated for cultures of Morris hepatoma cells,[85] mouse melanoma cells[86] and teratocarcinoma cells.[87] This activity may involve interaction of the ginsenoside with a glucocorticoid receptor in the cell.[87]

Ginseng extract[88] and ginsenosides Rb_1[89] and Rh_2[90] have exhibited antimutagenic activity against genotoxic agents in various in vitro models. One mechanism of action could involve enhanced DNA repair.[88,89]

Early animal experiments on the antitumour activity of ginseng yielded mainly inconclusive or negative results.[91] One group of scientists focused on the activity of ginsenoside Rh_2, finding that that oral doses prolonged survival of mice bearing human ovarian cancer cells[92] and acted synergistically with the anticancer drug cisplatin.[75] Another component of ginseng root, panaxytriol (a polyacetylenic alcohol), produced significant tumour growth delays ($p<0.01$) at an injected dose of 40 mg/kg in mice transplanted with B16 melanoma cells.[93] The most positive study on ginseng extract suggests that it acts best in conjunction with other anticancer treatments. Oral administration of ginseng extract, radiation treatment and the combination of both increased the survival of intrahepatic sarcoma-180 tumour-bearing mice to 20.4%, 16.9% and 82.1% respectively. Radiation treatment destroyed both cancer and liver cells but ginseng extract seemed to help recovery of healthy liver cells from radiation treatment and inhibited the infiltration of cancer cells.[94]

More conclusive results have been reached in anticarcinogenicity experiments where ginseng was co-administered with a known cancer-causing agent. For example, prolonged administration of red ginseng extract (1 mg/ml in drinking water) to mice significantly inhibited the incidence and proliferation of tumours produced by 9,10-dimethyl-1,2-benz(alpha)anthracene (DMBA), urethane and aflatoxin B1, but not N-2-fluorenylacetamide (FAA) and tobacco smoke condensate.[95] The same authors found that red ginseng had more activity than white ginseng (although both have good cancer-preventing activity) and that activity increased with the age of the root.[95] Ginseng prevented cancer caused by benzo(alpha)pyrene[95] and may do so by altering its metabolism.[96]

Some ginsenosides appear to inhibit metastasis. Injection of ginsenoside Rg_3 in rats significantly decreased the incidence of cancer metastases induced by the chemicals azoxymethane and bombesin[97] and in other in vivo models.[98] Ginsenoside Rg_3 was also found to be a potent inhibitor of invasion by various tumour cell lines when tested in a cell monolayer invasion model.[98] However, other ginsenosides were inactive in this model.[98] Ginsenoside Rb_2 inhibited tumour angiogenesis and metastasis produced by melanoma cells in mice. Intravenous administration of ginsenoside Rb_2 after tumour inoculation achieved a remarkable reduction in the number of blood vessels oriented towards the tumour mass but did not cause a significant inhibition of tumour growth. In contrast, intratumoral or oral administration caused a marked inhibition of both neovascularization and tumour growth.[99]

As alluded to above, ginseng extract or its components can potentiate the activity of cytotoxic drugs. This has additionally been demonstrated for the drug mitomycin C in both in vitro[100] and in vivo experiments.[101] The in vivo results suggest that this effect happens without an increase in toxicity to the host.[102]

Ginseng may also prevent cancer through effects on the immune system. The effects of long-term oral administration of ginseng extract (30 and 150 mg/kg per day) on levels of immunoglobulin types were studied in mice. Serum levels of gamma-globulin fell dose dependently ($p<0.05$) after ginseng. Among the immunoglobulin isotypes, only serum IgG_1 was decreased ($p<0.05$). The authors suggested that since IgG_1 is rarely involved in killing cancer cells and can act as a blocking antibody, this effect of ginseng may be beneficial for the prevention and inhibition of cancer.[103] Experiments have also shown that the anticarcinogenic activity of ginseng may be related to the augmentation of natural killer cell activity.[104]

Other activity

Ginseng extract or total saponins administered by injection countered the deleterious effects of repeated administration of narcotic drugs such as morphine,[105] cocaine,[106] methamphetamine and apomorphine[107] in animal models. Ginseng total saponins may inhibit the dopaminergic activation induced by morphine[108] and ginseng extract inhibited the development of tolerance to the analgesic and hyperthermic effects of morphine, depending on the administered doses of ginseng and morphine.[109] It is encouraging that oral doses of ginseng extract (ranging from 50 to 400 mg/kg) also significantly inhibited the development of morphine-induced tolerance and physical dependence, as well as inhibiting the decrease in hepatic glutathione induced by morphine multiple injections.[110]

Recent studies have been reviewed which suggest that the antioxidant and organ-protective actions of ginseng are linked to enhanced nitric oxide synthesis in the endothelium of the lung, heart and kidney and in the corpus cavernosum.[111] It was suggested that enhanced nitric oxide synthesis could contribute to ginseng-associated vasodilation and perhaps also to an aphrodisiac action. However, these findings are largely based on in vitro tests. Enhanced nitric oxide synthesis could be linked to the antiischaemic and other cardiovascular activities of ginseng.

Oral doses of 30 mg/kg of ginseng extract for 5 days significantly accelerated ethanol clearance from blood but not the brain of experimental rats.[112] This finding was confirmed in a Korean study which found that red ginseng (a single dose of 200 mg/kg orally) increased ethanol clearance in rats.[113] Fourteen healthy male volunteers were studied to assess the effects of ginseng on blood alcohol clearance, using each subject as his own control. Subjects received 72 g of 25% ethanol and at another time 3 g of ginseng extract (about 6 g of root) and the ethanol, all doses per 65 kg of body weight. At 40 minutes after the last drink, the average blood alcohol level after ginseng and ethanol consumption was 35% lower than after ethanol alone.[114]

Despite considerable research interest in the antidiabetic activity of ginseng, results to date are unconvincing. Potential hypoglycaemic constituents identified in ginseng have been reviewed.[115] These components consisted of glycans, which are called panaxans (more have subsequently been identified[116]), adenosine and unidentified large molecules with insulin-like activity. However, hypoglycaemic activity has only been established after injection and it is unlikely that any of these compounds would confer significant hypoglycaemic activity to oral doses of ginseng. These reservations would also apply to a polypeptide which was isolated from ginseng root and found to have hypoglycaemic activity.[117] Perhaps of greater interest are results for injection of ginsenoside Rb_2, which countered some of the unfavourable metabolic changes observed in diabetic rats. In particular, it boosted intracellular ATP and decreased cyclic AMP[118] and improved protein biosynthesis[119] and nitrogen balance.[120] Body weight was improved and diabetic symptoms such as polyuria were decreased.[121]

PHARMACOKINETICS

The pharmacokinetics of ginsenosides Rg_1, Rb_1 and Rb_2 in rats have been reviewed. Rg_1 was easily decomposed to its prosapogenin in both rat stomach and dilute hydrochloric acid, whereas Rb_1 and Rb_2 were little decomposed in rat stomach but were easily converted to their prosapogenins by dilute hydrochloric acid. The ginsenosides were also metabolized to several prosapogenins by gut bacteria and enteric enzymes. The amount of Rg_1, Rb_1 and Rb_2 absorbed from the gastrointestinal tract of the rat were 1.9%, 0.1% and 3.7% respectively of the administered dose. Rb_1 and Rb_2 were mainly excreted in the urine, whereas Rg_1 was excreted in the urine and bile in a 2:5 ratio. Unabsorbed saponins were metabolized by gut flora.[122]

Studies on humans tend to support the above picture that the ginsenosides have low bioavailability as such, but their decomposition products after the action of digestion and bowel flora are absorbed and may be the true active forms of the ginsenosides. Analysis of urine samples from 60 Swedish athletes who had consumed various ginseng preparations within 10 days before urine collection revealed that samples contained significant quantities of the sapogenin 20(s)-protopanaxatriol.[123] The results after intake of single oral doses of ginseng preparations demonstrated a linear relationship between the amounts of ginsenosides consumed and the 20(s)-protopanaxatriol glycosides excreted in the urine. Only about 1.2% of the dose was recovered in the glycosidic (ginsenoside) form over 5 days.[124] The main metabolites of ginsenosides after incubation with human faecal flora were identified as prosapogenins and sapogenins and these were also detected in the blood and urine of humans after oral administration of high doses of ginseng extract.[125] One organism implicated in hydrolysing ginsenosides was *Prevotella oris*.[126]

CLINICAL TRIALS

More than 60 clinical studies have been published on ginseng. The majority of studies have been on two preparations. The first is a 5:1 extract standardized for ginsenoside levels so that 200 mg of extract (the typical dose used) corresponds to about 1 g of root. The second preparation involves the combination of this standardized extract with vitamins and minerals. All the clinical studies on ginseng have not been included in this review and because of the potentially uncertain effect of adding vitamins and minerals to ginseng, only some of the studies on this second product have been reviewed.

Effect on performance

If ginseng has tonic and adaptogenic properties, it can be expected to improve human performance and well-being in a variety of circumstances. Clinical studies tend to support this hypothesis, although some have produced negative findings.

In particular, recent studies on the effect of ginseng on physical performance have been negative. A randomized, double-blind, placebo-controlled study was used to examine a group of 19 healthy adult females who took 200 mg per day of ginseng extract or placebo for 8 weeks. The ginseng extract had no effect on maximal work performance using a cycle ergometry test and on resting, exercise and recovery oxygen uptake. Other parameters such as heart rate and blood lactic acid were also not influenced by ginseng.[127] A follow-up study on 36 healthy men given 200–400 mg per day of ginseng extract or placebo over 8 weeks again failed to show any favourable influence of ginseng intake on the same parameters during graded maximal aerobic exercise.[128] Another small study (eight participants) by a different research team found that 1 week of ginseng intake had no effect on maximal work performance.[129] This last study is of doubtful significance because of the small number of participants and the short duration of administration of the ginseng. The same reservations also apply to a study involving 11 military cadets which found that 2 g of ginseng for 4 weeks did not alter performance during heavy, prolonged exercise.[130]

Despite these negative findings, the balance of evidence is that ginseng does increase physical performance and recovery (at least in male athletes), although well-designed trials involving larger numbers of participants are required to conclusively resolve this issue.

In a randomized, double-blind, placebo-controlled trial on 60 people aged between 22 and 80 years, ginseng treatment (200 mg extract, about 1 g of root) for 12 weeks caused a significant improvement in visual and auditory reaction times and recovery from physical exercise (stair climbing).[131] The same research group then tested the effect of 9 weeks' intake of 200 mg of ginseng extract (about 1 g of root) on the performance of 20 elite athletes in an open study using a graded ergometric test. Aerobic capacity was significantly increased and blood lactate levels and heart rate were significantly reduced.[132] A subsequent open study on 30 participants yielded similar results and there was no significant difference between the two doses tested (200 or 400 mg of ginseng extract per day).[133] These initial findings were then put to the test of a double-blind, placebo-controlled trial on 30 elite male athletes (19–31 years of age) subjected to a graded ergometric test. Ten athletes in each of three groups received either 200 mg of ginseng extract, 200 mg ginseng extract and 400 mg vitamin E, or placebo for 9 weeks. While there was no statistically significant difference between the groups receiving ginseng or ginseng plus vitamin E, there was a clear benefit of these two treatments over placebo for heart rate ($p<0.001$), blood lactate ($p<0.01$) and maximal oxygen uptake ($p<0.01$).[134]

In an attempt to quantify the duration of these observed benefits of ginseng intake, the same research team conducted a randomized, placebo-controlled, double-blind study on 28 male athletes where ginseng extract (200 mg per day) or placebo was administered for 9 weeks and effects were monitored for up to 11 weeks thereafter. Following 9 weeks of treatment there were significant increases in oxygen uptake, forced expiratory volume at 1 s, vital capacity and visual reaction time and a significant decrease in exercise heart rate. However, only a few of these differences persisted 3 weeks after treatment and none existed after 11 weeks.[135]

In a small, single-blind, placebo-controlled crossover trial, eight male participants received 100 mg of ginseng extract per day before testing or 200 mg per day during testing. A placebo was supplied in the second phase of the trial with an identical routine. All tested parameters were identical in the ginseng or placebo phases during which participants were at rest or subjected to an intermittent exercise load. However, when tested for exercise to exhaustion, results showed that ginseng produced a 64% increase in endurance accompanied generally by lower blood pressure readings ($p<0.01$). Mechanical efficiency was better for ginseng which results in a better running style.[136]

Ginseng in conjunction with vitamins and minerals improved parameters such as total workload, maximal oxygen uptake, heart rate and blood lactate levels in a randomized, double-blind, placebo-controlled trial on 50 male sports teachers. The authors suggested that their results indicate that the ginseng preparation increased work capacity by improving muscular oxygen utilization.[137]

In a double-blind, placebo-controlled, crossover trial, 43 male triathletes received either 200 mg of ginseng extract (about 1 g of root) or placebo for two consecutive training periods of 10 weeks. Although there were no significant changes in physical fitness during the first period, ginseng retarded the loss of fitness during the second 10-week period.[138]

A few studies have examined the influence of ginseng on psychomotor performance and overall results to date indicate ginseng appears to be of limited value. The effect of ginseng (200 mg per day, about 1 g of root) or placebo on reaction time to auditory and visual stimuli was investigated in a double-blind study. Significant decreases in reaction times ($p<0.01$) were seen only in older participants (40–60 years). In addition, significant improvements in subjective feelings related to well-being ($p<0.01$) were observed in both older males and all females.[139] Various tests of psychomotor performance were carried out in a group of 16 healthy male volunteers given a ginseng extract (200 mg per day, about 1 g of root) for 12 weeks and in a similar group given an identical placebo under double-blind conditions. Ginseng was only statistically superior to placebo for the mental arithmetic test and did not enhance pure motor function, recognition and visual reaction time. No adverse effects were reported.[140] The effects of ginseng extract (400 mg per day, about 2 g of root) on a variety of cognitive functions were compared with those of placebo in a double-blind, randomized test-retest design. Trial participants (112) were healthy volunteers older than 40 years of age and the treatment duration was 8–9 weeks. The ginseng group showed a tendency to faster simple reaction times (not significant) and significantly better abstract thinking than controls ($p=0.02$, Wisconsin Card Sorting Test). However, baseline values were not established for this test and it is conceivable that the significant difference was inherent between the two groups, rather than caused by the ginseng treatment. There was no significant difference between ginseng or placebo for concentration or memory.[141]

Ginseng has shown benefit in a variety of trials assessing quality of life or general performance under stress. In a randomized, double-blind trial, 501 participants received either ginseng extract with vitamins and minerals or a preparation containing only vitamins and minerals. After 4 months, the group receiving ginseng showed highly significant improvements ($p<0.0001$) in all of the 11 quality-of-life questionnaire items, whereas the group receiving only vitamins and minerals showed no significant improvement in any of these items. Adverse effects were minimal in both groups.[142] The effect on quality of life of ginseng extract in conjunction with vitamins and minerals was compared with placebo in a randomized, 12-week double-blind study on 390 participants. Healthy employed volunteers older than 25 years were included. Significant improvements above placebo were noted for alertness ($p<0.05$), relaxation ($p=0.02$), appetite ($p=0.04$) and overall score on 18 quality-of-life factors ($p=0.03$). Among the subgroup with the 20% lowest score at baseline, the active treatment improved both vitality ($p=0.03$) and depressed mood ($p=0.05$).[143]

In a randomized, double-blind trial on the treatment of fatigue, 232 patients between the ages of 25 and 60 years received either ginseng extract (80 mg/day, approximately 0.4 g of root) with vitamins and minerals or placebo over a period of 6 weeks. Patients were allowed to choose the five items that best described their condition from a preestablished list of 20 items. Analysis of these scores of fatigue levels at the end of the study indicated a statistically greater improvement for the active treatment. Side effects were minimal with only two patients withdrawing from active treatment.[144]

In a randomized, double-blind study on 83 participants (average age 38 years) the effect of ginseng extract (200 mg per day, approximately 1 g of root) or placebo on several parameters related to well-being were assessed. After 4 months of treatment the following significant changes were observed for the ginseng group when compared to the placebo group: fall in systolic blood pressure ($p<0.01$), improvements in colds ($p<0.005$) and bronchitis ($p<0.05$) (whether this was frequency, severity or both was not specified), improvement in appetite ($p<0.01$) and improvements in sleep ($p<0.025$), well-being ($p<0.005$) and performance ($p<0.005$).[145]

The effects of ginseng (1.2 g per day) on 12 fatigued night nurses were assessed by self-rating scales in a double-blind, placebo-controlled, crossover design. Shifts consisted of three or four consecutive nights followed by 3 days of rest and participants received treatment for the first three consecutive nights of work.

According to the crossover design, each subject was tested after ginseng, placebo or a good night's sleep. Although ginseng improved 11 of the 16 mood variables and eight of the 14 somatic symptoms compared with placebo, none of the differences were statistically significant. This may reflect on the short duration of ginseng use. Participants slept less and rated sleep quality as worse during ginseng use.[146]

Ginseng is particularly valued in China as a tonic for the elderly and a number of studies have examined the benefits of ginseng use in elderly people. Ginseng extract with vitamins and minerals (dose not specified) caused a significant increase ($p<0.05$) in REM sleep compared to placebo in a 10-week double-blind trial on 20 elderly subjects. Other treatment effects were noted which suggest a positive effect on sleep quality.[147] In a double-blind crossover trial to test whether ginseng improved depression and impaired performance associated with old age, 49 participants were given 1500 mg Korean red ginseng root or an identical placebo each for 10 days, with a washout period between dosages. The major result was a highly significant improvement in reaction time and decision making, as assessed by the tapping test and the reaction timer. Participants felt slightly more alert and energetic when taking ginseng but were also less happy. No major side effects were recorded and the treatment did not influence blood pressure.[148] One study produced negative results. Ginseng extract (80 mg per day, about 0.4 g of root) with vitamin and minerals for 8 weeks did not improve rehabilitation of geriatric patients in a randomized, placebo-controlled, double-blind design involving 49 patients.[149]

Infection and immunity

Groups of Korean scientists have examined the effects of Korean red ginseng in patients with HIV infection in a series of open trials.[150–153] These trials suffer from poor experimental design but they do suggest that the value of ginseng in this disorder should be examined further. In one of these studies, the influence of a daily intake of 5.4 g of red ginseng powder on prognostic markers was assessed in 23 patients after 3 and 6 months. The following significant changes were noted at 6 months: decreased lymphocyte percentage ($p<0.05$), mean CD4+ T-cell percentage increased from $16.3 \pm 5.2\%$ at baseline to $20.1 \pm 9.0\%$ ($p<0.05$), CD8+ T-cell percentage increased ($p<0.01$), and two patients with measurable serum p24 antigen levels seemed to have these suppressed during treatment.[151] These beneficial results were reflected in a second trial where ginseng therapy was compared with zidovudine.[152]

The effects of ginseng on cell-mediated immune function were studied in 60 healthy volunteers. Three groups received either placebo, 200 mg/day standardized ginseng extract (about 1 g of root) or 200 mg/day of ginseng aqueous extract. Significant improvements after 8 weeks were noted in both ginseng groups for chemotaxis, phagocytic activity and intracellular killing, whereas only the last parameter increased in the placebo group. Results tended to be better for the standardized ginseng extract.[154]

The same research team examined the effect of ginseng extract (200 mg/day, about 1 g of root) on the function of alveolar macrophages in 40 patients with chronic bronchitis in a placebo-controlled single-blind trial. The ginseng extract was able to improve the immune response of alveolar macrophages collected by bronchoalveolar lavage.[155] In a subsequent randomized double-blind study, 227 volunteers (average age 48 years) received either ginseng extract (200 mg per day, about 1 g of root) or placebo for a period of 12 weeks during which they also received an antiinfluenza polyvalent vaccination at week 4. As a result, while the incidence of influenza or common cold between weeks 4 and 12 was 42 cases in the placebo group, it was only 15 cases in the ginseng group ($p<0.0001$). Also antibody titres ($p<0.0001$) and natural killer cell activity ($p<0.0001$) were significantly higher in the ginseng group. There were nine adverse events: two cases of nausea, one of epigastralgia, one of anxiety and four of insomnia in the ginseng group, compared to one case of insomnia in the placebo group.[156]

Cardiovascular effects

Forty-five patients with advanced congestive heart failure were divided into three groups and received either digoxin, red ginseng or both treatments in an open design. The group receiving ginseng and digoxin showed the best results in terms of biochemical and haemodynamic parameters, followed by the group receiving ginseng. There were no adverse effects.[157]

The effect of Korean red ginseng on sexual dysfunction and serum lipid profile was investigated in 35 elderly men with psychogenic impotence in a controlled study. Treatment was with 2.7 g or 1.8 g of ginseng root or placebo for 2 months. The overall therapeutic effect on erectile function was 67% for ginseng versus 28% for placebo ($p<0.05$) and results tended to be better in the higher dose ginseng group. HDL-cholesterol was significantly elevated by ginseng ($p<0.05$) but there was no other effect on serum lipids.[158] However, an open study on 15 postmenopausal women found that 500 mg of ginseng root per day for 12 weeks had no effect on serum lipid profile.[159] Therefore the effect on HDL-cholesterol may be dose related.

The effect of ginseng extract (200 mg per day) on mainly moderate cerebrovascular deficit in 45 patients (average age 58 years) was compared to the drug hydergine (3 mg per day) or placebo under double-blind conditions over 3 months. Significantly, improved cerebrovascular circulation was noted in both active treatment groups.[160] A combined Ginkgo and ginseng formula improved circulation and lowered blood pressure in a controlled single-dose study on 10 healthy young volunteers.[161]

Cancer prevention and therapy

South Korea is in a unique position. As the socioeconomic status of Korea began to improve about 15–20 years ago and Koreans began to prefer their traditional herbal teas, many Koreans started to drink ginseng tea. Nowadays in Korea, ginseng (*Panax ginseng*) tea is served as often as coffee and the use of other forms of this herb is equally as widespread. This provides an opportunity to observe the effects of the large-scale consumption of what is a powerful medicinal plant. A group of Korean clinicians and epidemiologists have taken advantage of this opportunity. In their first study, they found an inverse association between ginseng intake and cancer incidence.[162] The scientists have now extended this initial study to a case-controlled study on 1987 pairs.[163]

The cancer sites studied were all primary tumours classified according to WHO guidelines. All cases were confirmed by cytological and/or histopathological examination and were admitted to the Korea Cancer Centre Hospital. Controls were selected from a pool of patients diagnosed as having other diseases. Each cancer case was matched with one control, based on year of birth, sex and admission date. The types of diseases in controls were mainly acute diseases. Cases and controls were interviewed personally by trained interviewers who were unaware of the category of their interviewees. Standard questionnaires were checked for consistency, completeness and accuracy. To evaluate the accuracy of the answers, 10% of subjects were reinterviewed 1 year later. Agreement between these and the initial interviews was found to be excellent. Corrections for confounding factors such as age, sex, education, marital status, smoking and alcohol consumption were performed during the statistical analysis of results.

Overall, the relative risk of cancer for ginseng users was 50% lower than for ginseng non-users. Concerning the type of ginseng, the relative risk of cancer was 37% for fresh ginseng extract users, 57% for white ginseng extract users, 30% for white ginseng powder users and a remarkable 20% for red ginseng users. However, users of fresh ginseng slice, fresh ginseng juice and white ginseng tea showed no reduction in cancer risk. There was a decrease in risk with rising frequency and duration of ginseng intake, showing a clear dose–response relationship. Not all cancers were affected by ginseng. For cancers of the female breast, cervix, bladder and thyroid gland there was no association (positive or negative) with ginseng intake. Smokers particularly benefited from ginseng intake, with incidences of cancers of the lung, lip, oral cavity and pharynx substantially lower in smokers who were ginseng users compared to smokers who were not. There was no significant difference in cancer risk between those who began to use ginseng between the ages of 30–39 and after age 60. In both groups the preventative effect appeared 1 year after the first ginseng intake and increased with duration of consumption. The authors concede that the greatest weakness of their study was the inability to adjust for diet for cancers of the digestive organs and sexual behaviour for reproductive cancers.

The same authors conducted a cohort study in a ginseng-growing area of Korea on 4634 adults over 40 years of age.[164] There were 79 deaths from cancer over 5 years. Ginseng users had only a 48% chance of contracting cancer when compared with non-users.

The effect of ginseng (5 g per day) was assessed in 50 cervical cancer patients undergoing radiation therapy in a double-blind, placebo-controlled study. After 5 weeks, a number of haematological parameters were tested. Results suggested that ginseng had a protective effect on depressed bone marrow only in terms of platelet count, which was significantly elevated in the ginseng group ($p<0.05$). A longer and more detailed study was suggested by the authors.[165]

Reproductive function

A common misconception is that ginseng (*Panax ginseng*) is a treatment which is exclusive for males. However, two recent clinical trials have confirmed that ginseng does have a significant role to play in the treatment of male sexual and fertility problems. In an open study, 66 male patients were treated with ginseng extract, of whom 20 were controls, 30 had an idiopathic low sperm count and 16 had a low sperm count associated with varicocoele.[166] All received 4 g of ginseng extract per day for 3 months. Sperm count, total testosterone, sperm motility, free testosterone and dihydrotestosterone (DHT) rose in all groups after 3 months of ginseng treatment. Normal control subjects only showed small increases whereas increases in the low sperm count groups were substantial for these parameters (although only in the case of free testosterone did levels approach those of the control group). In contrast, prolactin levels, which were elevated in the low sperm count groups, fell in all groups. Gonadotrophins showed a progressive increase in the low sperm count groups but in the control group a moderate decrease was observed, probably due to the corresponding increase in androgens. It was suggested that the ginseng, and specifically ginsenosides, may have an effect at different levels of the hypothalamus-pituitary-testes axis to improve male fertility.

In a second clinical trial conducted in Korea, the effect of red ginseng on impotence was compared to placebo and the drug trazodone.[167] A total of 90 patients were closely followed, with 30 patients in each group. The overall therapeutic efficacy on erectile dysfunction as evaluated by the patient was 60% for the ginseng group and 30% for the placebo- and trazodone-treated groups ($p<0.05$). In particular, ginseng significantly improved libido. The ginseng dose used was 1.8 g of extract per day. (Also, note the study on erectile function reviewed above under Cardiovascular effects.)

The designs of both the above studies were lacking. In particular, there was no placebo control group in the first study and neither study was conducted under double-blind conditions. Nonetheless, as preliminary results they do suggest that ginseng is valuable in the management of male disorders and further well-designed studies are warranted.

Ginseng consumption during pregnancy is popular in Hong Kong. Eighty-eight patients taking ginseng during their pregnancy were matched with control patients with similar characteristics who delivered within the same period but were not taking ginseng. Eight patients in the control group had preeclampsia, but only one patient in the ginseng group suffered this condition ($p<0.02$). The control group also had higher mean blood pressures in the second and third trimesters but the differences were not statistically significant. The authors suggested that further studies are necessary to clarify this possible benefit of ginseng during pregnancy.[168]

Other conditions

In a double-blind, placebo-controlled study, 30 patients with non-insulin dependent diabetes were treated for 8 weeks with ginseng extract (100 mg or 200 mg) or placebo. Ginseng improved patients' mood, vigour, well-being and psychomotor performance. Results were more significant for the higher dose. Both doses of ginseng caused a small but significant fall in fasting blood glucose ($p<0.05$).[169]

A case history was described where a patient with severe postpartum hypopituitarism (Sheehan's syndrome) was successfully treated with high doses of ginseng and licorice over 50 days.[170]

TOXICOLOGY

Ginseng root has very low toxicity. A 5:1 extract of ginseng root was found to be safe up to 6 g/kg in mice when administered intraperitoneally and up to 30 g/kg given by the oral route in a single dose.[51] Subacute toxicity studies at 1.5–15 mg/kg per day of the same extract revealed no treatment-related effects on body weight, food consumption, haematology, biochemical parameters and histopathological findings.[171]

The effect of the above extract on reproductive performance was studied in rats at oral doses of 1.5, 5 and 15 mg/kg per day in males and females. No adverse effects were seen in two generations of offspring.[172]

CONTRAINDICATIONS

Signs of heat, acute infections, acute asthma, hypertension, excessive menstruation or nose bleeds.

SPECIAL WARNINGS AND PRECAUTIONS

Concurrent use with stimulants such as caffeine and amphetamines should be avoided.

INTERACTIONS

May interact with the monoamine oxidase inhibitor phenelzine and also with warfarin.

USE IN PREGNANCY AND LACTATION

No adverse effects expected.

EFFECTS ON ABILITY TO DRIVE AND USE MACHINES

No negative influence is expected.

SIDE EFFECTS

Results from controlled clinical trials using a daily dose of 1 g indicate that ginseng is generally safe and well tolerated. However, higher doses may cause side effects and ginseng abuse syndrome (GAS) has been described.[173] GAS is defined as hypertension, together with nervousness, euphoria, insomnia, skin eruptions and morning diarrhoea and is thought to be related to ginseng's interaction with glucocorticoid production in the body. However, since this particular study did not differentiate the species of ginseng used, its reliability can be questioned. Moreover, a follow-up study found that many subjects with reported GAS were actually taking *Eleutherococcus senticosus* (Siberian ginseng).[174] Nonetheless, it is likely that high doses of ginseng can cause overstimulation and symptoms of GAS have been reported in independent studies.[175,176]

Ginseng may cause side effects related to an oestrogen-like activity in women.[177] Cases of mastalgia[178] and vaginal bleeding in a 72-year-old woman[179] have been reported. A case of postmenopausal bleeding attributed to the use of a ginseng face cream has also been published.[180]

Ginseng is widely used and several other adverse reactions have been reported which are at best possibly related to ginseng or may otherwise reflect on contamination, adulteration or coincidence. These include Stevens–Johnson syndrome,[181,182] diuretic resistance,[183] cerebral arthritis,[184] mania[185] and mydriasis.[186,187]

Two independent reports of a possible interaction of the monoamine oxidase inhibitor phenelzine with ginseng have been published.[188,189] A case of a possible interaction between warfarin and ginseng has been described. Ginseng intake appeared to reduce the anticoagulant activity of the warfarin but the mode of action was unclear.[190]

OVERDOSE

Has not been reported.

CURRENT REGULATORY STATUS IN SELECTED COUNTRIES

Ginseng is official in the *Pharmacopoeia of the People's Republic of China* (English edition, 1997) and the *Japanese Pharmacopoeia* (English edition, 1996). Ginseng became the *United States Pharmacopeia-National Formulary* (USP 23–NF 18) in late 1998.

Ginseng is covered by a positive Commission E monograph and can be used as a tonic to combat feelings of lassitude and debility, lack of energy and ability to concentrate and during convalescence.

Ginseng is on the UK General Sale List.

Ginseng does not have GRAS status. However, it is freely available as a 'dietary supplement' in the USA under DSHEA legislation (1994 Dietary Supplement Health and Education Act). Korean ginseng has been present as an ingredient in products offered OTC for use as an aphrodisiac. The FDA, however, advises that: 'based on evidence currently available, any OTC drug product containing ingredients for use as an aphrodisiac cannot be generally recognized as safe and effective'.

Ginseng is not included in Part 4 of Schedule 4 of the Therapeutic Goods Act Regulations of Australia.

References

1. Chang HM, But PP. Pharmacology and applications of Chinese materia medica, vol 1. World Scientific, Singapore, 1986, pp 17–31.
2. Bensky D, Gamble A. Chinese herbal medicine materia medica. Eastland Press, Seattle, 1986, pp 450–454.
3. Grieve M. A modern herbal, vol 1. Dover Publications, New York, 1971, pp 354–357.
4. British Herbal Medicine Association's Scientific Committee. British herbal pharmacopoeia. BHMA, Cowling, 1983, p 152.
5. Felter HW. The eclectic materia medica, pharmacology and therapeutics, 1922. Reprinted by Eclectic Medical Publications, Portland, 1983, pp 1429–1430.
6. Smeh NJ. Creating your own cosmetics – naturally. Alliance Publishing, Garrisonville, 1995, p 82.
7. Liberti LE, Der Marderosian A. J Pharm Sci 1978; 67 (10): 1487–1489.
8. German Federal Minister of Justice. German Commission E for human medicine monograph, Bundes-Anzeiger (German Federal Gazette), no. 11, dated 17.01.1991.
9. World Health Organization. Medicinal plants in China. World Health Organization, Regional Office for the Western Pacific. Manilla, 1989, pp 194–195.
10. Wagner H, Bladt S. Plant drug analysis: a thin layer chromatography atlas, 2nd edn. Springer-Verlag, Berlin, 1996, p 307.
11. Tang W, Eisenbrand G. Chinese drugs of plant origin. Springer Verlag, Berlin, 1992, pp 711–737.
12. Kwon BM, Nam JY, Lee SH et al. Chem Pharm Bull 1996; 44 (2): 444–445.
13. Yagi A, Ishizu T, Okamura N et al. Planta Med 1996; 62 (2): 115–118.
14. Wang YH, Hong CY, Chen CF et al. J Liq Chromatograph Relat Tech 1997; 20 (6): 899–905.
15. Soldati F, Sticher O. Planta Med 1980; 39 (4): 348–357.
16. Fulder S. The root of being: ginseng and the pharmacology of harmony. Hutchinson, London, 1980.
17. Fulder SJ. Am J Chin Med 1981; 9 (2): 112–118.
18. Hiai S, Yokoyama H, Oura H et al. Endocrinol Jpn 1979; 26 (6): 661–665.
19. Luo YM, Cheng XJ, Yuan WX. Chung Kuo Yao Li Hsueh Pao 1993; 14 (5): 401–404.
20. Yoshimatsu H, Sakata T, Machidori H et al. Physiol Behav 1993; 53 (1): 1–4.
21. Yuan Wx, Wu XJ, Yang FX et al. Chung Kuo Yao Li Hsueh Pao 1989; 10 (6): 492–496.
22. Banerjee U, Izquierdo JA. Acta Physiol Lat Am 1982; 32 (4): 277–285.
23. Kita T, Hata T, Kawashima Y et al. J Pharmacobiodyn 1981; 4 (6): 381–393.

24. Hata T, Kita T, Kawabata A et al. J Pharmacobiodyn 1985; 8 (12): 1068–1072.
25. Saito H, Yoshida Y, Takagi K. Jpn J Pharmacol 1974; 24 (1): 119–127.
26. Filaretov AA, Bogdanova TS, Podivigina TT et al. Exp Clin Endocrinol 1988; 92 (2): 129–136.
27. Lee SP, Honda K, Rhee YH et al. Neurosci Lett 1990; 111 (1–2): 217–221.
28. Ramachandran U, Divekar HM, Grover SK et al. J Ethnopharmacol 1990; 29 (3): 275–281.
29. Takeda A, Yonezawa M, Katoh N. J Radiat Res 1981; 22: 323–335.
30. Yonezawa M, Katoh N, Takeda A. J Radiat Res 1981; 22: 336–343.
31. Bittles AH, Fulder SJ, Grant EC et al. Gerontology 1979; 25 (3): 125–131.
32. Lewis WH, Zenger VE, Lynch RG. J Ethnopharmacol 183; 8 (2): 209–214.
33. King JO. Vet Rec 1983; 112 (6): 127.
34. Grandhi A Mujumdar AM, Patwardhan B. J Ethnopharmacol 1994; 44 (3): 131–135.
35. Avakian EV, Sugimoto RB, Taguchi S et al. Planta Med 1984; 50 (2): 151–154.
36. Avakian EV Jr, Evonuk E. Planta Med 1979; 36 (1): 43–48.
37. Yokozawa T, Kitahara N, Okuda S et al. Chem Pharm Bull 1979; 27 (2): 419–423.
38. Buffi O, Ciaroni S, Guidi L et al. Boll Soc Ital Biol Sper 1993; 69 (12): 791–797.
39. Hiai S, Sasayama Y, Oguro C. Chem Pharm Bull 1987; 35 (1): 241–248.
40. Metori K, Furutsu M, Takahashi S. Biol Pharm Bull 1997; 20 (3): 237–242.
41. Yamaguchi Y, Higashi M, Kobayashi H. Eur J Pharmacol 1997; 329 (1): 37–41.
42. Nitta H, Matsumoto K, Shimizu M et al. Biol Pharm Bull 1995; 18 (9): 1286–1288.
43. Watanabe H, Ohta H, Imamura L et al. Jpn J Pharmacol 1991; 55 (1): 51–56.
44. Shibata S, Tanaka O, Shoji J et al. Chemistry and pharmacology of panax. In: Farnsworth NR et al (eds) Economic and medicinal plant research, vol 1. Academic Press, London, 1985 pp 265, 266, 268
45. Petkov VD, Mosharrof AH. Am J Chin Med 1987; 15 (1–2): 19–29.
46. Lasarova MB, Mosharrof AH, Petkov VD et al. Acta Physiol Pharmacol Bulg 1987; 13 (2): 11–17.
47. Ying Y, Zhang JT, Shi CZ et al. Yao Hsueh Pao 1994; 29 (4): 241–245.
48. Nitta H, Matsumoto K, Shimizu M et al. Biol Pharm Bull 1995; 18 (10): 1439–1442.
49. Petkov VD, Kehayov R, Belcheva S et al. Planta Med 1993; 59 (2): 106–114.
50. Zee-Cheng RK. Methods Find Exp Clin Pharmacol 1992; 14 (9): 725–736.
51. Singh VK, George CX, Singh N et al. Planta Med 1983; 47 (4): 234–236.
52. Singh VK, Agarwal SS, Gupta BM. Planta Med 1984; 50 (6): 462–465.
53. Jie YH, Cammisuli S, Baggiolini M. Agents Actions 1984; 15 (3–4): 386–391.
54. Akagawa G, Abe S, Tansho S et al. Immunopharmacol Immunotoxicol 1996; 18 (1): 73–89.
55. Yeung HW, Cheung K, Leung KN. Am J Chin Med 1982; 10 (1–4): 44–54.
56. Yuan GC, Chang RS. J Gerontol 1969; 24 (1): 82–85.
57. Fulder SJ. Exp Geront 1977; 12: 125–131.
58. Yamamoto M, Kumagai A, Yamamura Y. Arzneim-Forsch 1977; 27 (7): 1404–1405.
59. Shia GT, Ali S, Bittles AH. Gerontology 1982; 28 (2): 121–124.
60. Lu ZQ, Dice JF. Biochem Biophys Res Commun 1985; 126 (1): 636–640.
61. Gao RL, Xu CL, Jin JM. Chung Kuo Chung Hsi I Chieh Ho Tsa Chih 1992; 12 (5): 285–287.
62. Kang SY, Lee KY, Lee SK. Biochem Biophys Res Commun 1994; 205 (3): 1696–1701.
63. Yagi A, Akita K, Ueda T et al. Planta Med 1994; 60 (2): 171–173.
64. Takei Y, Yamamoto T, Higashira H et al. Biosci Biotechnol Biochem 1996; 60 (4): 584–588.
65. Oura H, Hiai S, Nakashima S et al. Chem Pharm Bull 1971; 19 (3): 453–459.
66. Hiai S, Oura H, Tsukada K et al. Chem Pharm Bull 1971; 19 (8): 1656–1663.
67. Oura H, Tsukada K, Nakagawa H. Chem Pharm Bull 1972; 20 (2): 219–225.
68. Yamamoto M, Masaka M, Yamada Y et al. Arzneim-Forsch 1978; 28 (12): 2238–2241.
69. Nagasawa T, Oura H, Hiai S et al. Chem Pharm Bull 1977; 25 (7): 1665–1670.
70. Oura H, Hiai S, Nabetani S et al. Planta Med 1975; 28 (1): 76–88.
71. Yamamoto M, Takeuchi N, Kumagai A et al. Arzneim-Forsch 1977; 27 (6): 1169–1173.
72. Harper N, Osborne AJ, Makov VE et al. Biochem Pharmacol 1984; 33 (9): 1571–1573.
73. Han R. Stem Cells 1994; 12 (1): 53–63.
74. Kikuchi Y, Sasa H, Kita T et al. Anticancer Drugs 1991; 2 (1): 63–67.
75. Tode T, Kikuchi Y, Sasa H et al. Nippon Sanka Fujinka Gakkai Zasshi 1992; 44 (5): 589–594.
76. Yokozawa T, Iwano M, Dohi K et al. Nippon Jinzo Gakkai Shi 1994; 36 (1): 13–18.
77. Motoo Y, Sawabu N. Cancer Lett 1994; 86 (1): 91–95.
78. Saita T, Katano M, Matsunaga H et al. Biol Pharm Bull 1995; 18 (7): 933–937.
79. Matsunaga H, Saita T, Nagumo F et al. Cancer Chemother Pharmacol 1995; 35 (4): 291–296.
80. Baek NI, Kim DS, Lee YH et al. Arch Pharmacol Res 1995; 18 (3): 164–168.
81. Lee KY, Lee YH, Kim SI et al. Anticancer Res 1997; 17 (2A): 1067–1072.
82. Ota T, Maeda M, Odashima S et al. Life Sci 1997; 60 (2): PL39–44.
83. Abdrasilov BS, Kim Yu A, Nurieva RI et al. Biochem Mol Biol Int 1996; 38 (3): 519–526.
84. Byun BH, Shin I, Yoon YS et al. Planta Med 1997; 63 (5): 389–392.
85. Abe H, Arichi S, Hayashi T et al. Experientia 1979; 35 (12): 1647–1649.
86. Ota T, Fujikawa-yamamoto K, Zong ZP et al. Cancer Res 1987; 47 (14): 3863–3867.
87. Lee YN, Lee HY, Chung HY et al. Eur J Cancer 1996; 32A (8): 1420–1428.
88. Rhee YH, Ahn JH, Choe J et al. Planta Med 1991; 57 (2): 125–128.
89. Park HJ, Rhee MH, Park KM et al. J Ethnopharmacol 1995; 49 (3): 157–162.
90. Zhu JH, Takeshita T, Kitagawa I et al. Cancer Res 1995; 55 (6): 1221–1223.
91. Lee KD, Huemer RP. Jpn J Pharmacol 1971; 21 (3): 299–320.
92. Tode T, Kikuchi Y, Hirata J et al. Nippon Sanka Fujinka Gakkai Zasshi 1993; 45 (11): 1275–1282.
93. Katano M, Yamamoto H, Matsunaga H et al. Gan To Kagaku Ryoho 1990; 17 (5): 1045–1049.
94. You J-S, Hau D-M, Chen K-T et al. Phytother Res 1995; 9 (5): 331–335.
95. Yun TK. Nutr Rev 1996; 54 (11 pt 2): S71–81.
96. Lee FC, Park JK, Ko JH et al. Drug Chem Toxicol 1987; 10 (3–4): 227–236.
97. Ishi H, Tatsuta M, Baba M et al. Clin Exp Metastasis 1997; 15 (6): 603–611.
98. Shinkai K, Akedo H, Mukai M et al. Jpn J Cancer Res 1996; 87 (4): 357–362.
99. Sato K, Mochizuki M, Saiki I et al. Biol Pharm Bull 1994; 17 (5): 635–639.
100. Tong CN, Matsuda H, Kubo M. Yakugaku 1992; 112 (11): 856–865.
101. Matsuda H, Tong CN, Kubo M. Yakugaku 1992; 112 (11): 846–855.
102. Kubo M, Chun-ning T, Matsuda H. Planta Med 1992; 58: 424–428.

103. Kim YW, Song DK, Kim WH et al. J Ethnopharmacol 1997; 58 (1): 55–58.
104. Yun YS, Moon HS, Oh YR et al. Cancer Detect Prev Suppl 1987; 1: 301–309.
105. Kim HS, Kang JG, Oh KW. Gen Pharmacol 1995; 26 (5): 1071–1076.
106. Kim HS, Kang JG, Seong YH et al. Pharmacol Biochem Behav 1995; 50 (1): 23–27.
107. Kim HS, Kang JG, Rheu HM et al. Planta Med 1995; 61 (1): 22–25.
108. Kim HS, Jang CC, Oh KW et al. J Ethnopharmacol 1998; 60: 33–42.
109. Bhargava HN, Ramarao P. Gen Pharmacol 1991; 22 (3): 521–525.
110. Kim HS, Jang CG, Lee MK. Planta Med 1990; 56 (2): 158–163.
111. Gillis CN. Biochem Pharmacol 1997; 54 (1): 1–8.
112. Petkov V, Koushev V, Panova Y. Acta Physiol Pharmacol Bulg 1977; 3 (1): 46–50.
113. Lee YJ, Pantuck CB, Pantuck EJ. Planta Med 1993; 59 (1): 17–19.
114. Lee FC, Ko JH, Park JK et al. Clin Exp Pharmacol Physiol 1987; 14 (6): 543–546.
115. Ng TB, Yeung HW. Gen Pharmacol 1985; 16 (6): 549–552.
116. Oshima Y, Konno C, Hikino H. J Ethnopharmacol 1985; 14 (2–3): 255–259.
117. Wang BX, Yang M, Jin YL et al. Yao Hsueh Pao 1990; 25 (6): 401–405.
118. Yokozawa T, Fujitsuka N, Yasui T et al. J Pharm Pharmacol 1991; 43 (4): 290–291.
119. Yokozawa T, Oura H. J Nat Prod 1990; 53 (6): 1514–1518.
120. Yokozawa T, Oura H, Kawashima Y. J Nat Prod 1989; 52 (6): 1350–1352.
121. Yokozawa T, Kobayashi T, Oura H et al. Chem Pharm Bull 1987; 35 (10): 4208–4214.
122. Takino Y. Yakugaku Zasshi 1994; 114 (8): 550–564.
123. Gui JF, Garle M, Bjorkhem I et al. Scand J Clin Lab Invest 1996; 56(2): 151–161.
124. Cui JF, Bjorkem I, Eneroth P. J Chromatogr B Biomed Appl 1997; 689 (2): 349–355.
125. Hasegawa H, Sung JH, Matsumiya S et al. Planta Med 1996; 62 (5): 453–457.
126. Hasegawa H, Sung JH, Benno Y. Planta Med 1997; 63: 436–440.
127. Engels H-J, Said JM, Wirth JC. Nutr Res 1996; 16 (8): 1295–1305.
128. Engels HJ, Wirth JC. J Am Diet Assn 1997; 97 (10): 1110–1115.
129. Morris AC, Jacobs I, McLellan TM et al. Int J Sport Nutr 1996; 6 (3): 263–271.
130. Knapik JJ, Wright JE, Welch MJ et al. Fed Proc 1983; 42 (3): 336.
131. Dorling E, Kirchdorfer AM, Ruckert KH. Notabene Med 1980; 10 (5): 241–246.
132. Forgo I, Anton M, Kirchdorfer AM. Arztliche Praxis 1981; 44 (2): 1784–1786.
133. Forgo I, Kirchdorfer AM. Notabene Med 1982; 12 (9): 721–727.
134. Forgo I. Munch Med Wochenschr 1983; 125 (38): 822–824.
135. Forgo I, Schimert G. Notabene Med 1985; 15 (9): 636–640.
136. Wyss V, Ganzit GP, Rienzi A et al. Medicina Dello Sport 1987; 40 (1): 7–16.
137. Pieralisi G, Ripari P, Vecchiet L. Clin Therapeut 1991; 13 (3): 373–382.
138. Van Schepdael P. Acta Ther 1993; 19: 338–347.
139. Forgo I, Kayasseh L, Staub JJ. Med Welt 1981; 32 (19): 751–756.
140. D'Angelo L, Grimaldi R, Caravaggi M et al. J Ethnopharmacol 1986; 16 (1): 15–22.
141. Sorensen H, Sonne J. Curr Therapeut Res 1996; 57 (12): 959–968.
142. Caso Marasco A, Vargas Ruiz R, Salas Villagomez A et al. Drugs Exp Clin Res 1996; 22 (6): 323–329.
143. Wiklund I, Karlberg J, Lund B. Curr Therapeut Res 1994; 55 (1): 32–42.
144. Le Gal M, Cathebras P, Struby K. Phytother Res 1996; 10: 49–53.
145. Gianoli AC, Riebenfeld D. Cytobiologische Revue 1984; 8 (3): 177–186.
146. Hallstrom C, Fulder S, Carruthers M. Comparative Med East West 1982; 6 (4): 277–282.
147. Kerkhof GA, Middlekoop HAM, Van Der Hoeve R et al. J Interdisciplinary Cycle Res 1989; 20 (1): 57–64.
148. Fulder S, Mohan K, Gethyn-Smith B. Proceedings of the 4th International Ginseng Symposium, Daejon Korea, Seoul, Korean Ginseng and Tobacco Research Institute, 1984, pp 215–223.
149. Thommessen B, Laake K. Aging (Milano) 1996; 8 (6): 417–420.
150. Cho YK, Kim YB, Choi BS et al. J Korean Soc Microbiol 1993; 28 (5): 409–417.
151. Cho YK, Kim YB, Choi BS et al. J Korean Soc Microbiol 1994; 29 (4): 371–379.
152. Cho YK, Kim YB, Lee I et al. J Korean Soc Microbiol 1996; 31 (3): 353–360.
153. Cho YK, Lee HJ, Kim YB et al. J Korean Soc Microbiol 1997; 32 (5): 611–623.
154. Scaglione F, Ferrara F, Dugnani S et al. Drugs Exp Clin Res 1990; 16 (10): 537–542.
155. Scaglione F, Cogo R, Cocuzza C et al. Int J Immunother 1994; 10 (1): 21–24.
156. Scaglione F, Cattaneo G, Alessandria M et al. Drugs Exp Clin Res 1996; 22 (2): 65–72.
157. Ding DZ, Shen TK, Cui YZ. Chung Kuo Chung Hsi I Chieh Ho Tsa Chih 1995; 15 (6): 325–327.
158. Kim YC, Hong YK, Shin JS et al. Korean J Ginseng Sci 1996; 20 (2): 125–132.
159. Punnonen R, Lukola A. Asia Oceania J Obstet Gynaecol 1984; 10 (3): 399–401.
160. Quiroga H. Orientacion Med 1982; 31 (1281): 201–202.
161. Kiesewetter H, Jung F, Mrowietz C et al. Int J Clin Pharmacol Ther Toxicol 1992; 30 (3): 97–102.
162. Yun TK, Choi SY. Int J Epidemiol 1990; 19: 871–876.
163. Yun TK, Choi SY. Cancer Epidemiol Biomarkers Prev 1995; 4 (4): 401–408.
164. Yun TK, Choi SY. Korean J Ginseng Sci 1995; 19: 87–92.
165. Chang YS, Park CI. Seoul J Med 1980; 21 (2): 187–193.
166. Salvati G, Genovesi G, Marcellini L et al. Panminerva Med 1996; 38 (4): 249–254.
167. Choi HK, Seong DH, Rha KH. Int J Impotence Res 1995; 7 (3): 181–186.
168. Chin RK. Asia Oceania J Obstet Gynaecol 1991; 17 (4): 379–380.
169. Sotaniemi EA, Haapakoski E, Rautio A. Diabetes Care 1995; 18 (10): 1373–1375.
170. Cheng-chia L, Ching-ch'u T. Chin Med J 1973; 11: 156.
171. Hess FG Jr, Parent RA, Stevens KR et al. Food Chem Toxicol 1983; 21 (1): 95–97.
172. Hess FG Jr, Parent RA, Cox GE et al. Food Chem Toxicol 1982; 20 (2): 189–192.
173. Siegel RK. JAMA 1979; 241 (15): 1614–1615.
174. Siegel RK. JAMA 1980; 243 (1): 32.
175. Chen KJ. J Trad Chin Med 1981; 1 (1): 69–72.
176. Hammond TG, Whitworth JA. Med J Aust 1981; 1 (9): 492.
177. Punnonen R, Lukola A. Br Med J 1980; 281 (6248): 1110.
178. Palmer BV, Montgomery ACV, Monteiro JCMP. Br Med J 1978; 1 (6122): 1284.
179. Greenspan EM. JAMA 1983; 249 (15): 2018.
180. Hopkins MP, Androff L, Benninghoff AS. Am J Obstet Gynecol 1988; 159 (5): 1121–1122.
181. Faleni R, Soldati F. Lancet 1996; 348 (9022): 267.
182. Dega H, Laporte JL, Frances C et al. Lancet 1996; 347 (9011): 1344.
183. Becker BN, Greene J, Evanson J et al. JAMA 1996; 276 (8): 606–607.
184. Ryu SJ, Chien YY. Neurology 1995; 45: 829–830.
185. Gonzalez-Seijo JC, Ramos YM, Lastra I. J Clin Psychopharmacol 1995; 15 (6): 447–448.
186. Chan TY. Vet Hum Toxicol 1995; 37 (2): 156–157.
187. Lou BY, Li CF, Li PY et al. Yen Ko Hsueh Pao 1989; 5 (3–4): 96–97.
188. Jones BD, Runikis AM. J Clin Psychopharmacol 1987; 7 (3): 201–202.
189. Shader RI, Greenblatt DJ. J Clin Psychopharmacol 1988; 8 (4): 235.
190. Janetzky K, Morreale AP. Am J Health-Syst Pharm 1997; 54: 692–693.

Globe artichoke (*Cynara scolymus* L.)

SYNONYMS

French artichoke, Cynara (Engl), Cynarae folium (Lat), Artischocke (Ger), artichaut (Fr), artichiocco, carciofo (Ital), artiskok (Dan).

WHAT IS IT?

The use of the immature flower of the globe artichoke as a vegetable is widely appreciated. (It should not be confused with another edible plant: the tuber of Jerusalem artichoke or *Helianthus tuberosus*, a species of sunflower.) However, herbalists also value other parts of the plant for their medicinal properties. In particular, the leaves have a well-established reputation for stimulating bile and urine flow, restoring the liver and lowering cholesterol. Much attention has been centred on the active component cynarin which is found mainly in the leaves. However, it is likely that many other compounds, some related to cynarin, contribute to the observed therapeutic effects. In recent studies, clinical attention has centred on the globe artichoke extract and its value in non-ulcer dyspepsia. Additionally, one reviewer has suggested that the combination of antioxidant and unique cholesterol-lowering properties makes this herb a prime candidate for the natural prevention of atherosclerosis.

The medicinal properties of Cynara have been known since antiquity. It was particularly prized in the 16th to 19th centuries but was out of favour between 1870 to about 1925. *Cynara scolymus* is actually a variety of thistle and some writers believe that it was never found in the wild state, being a product of cultivation and selection from *Cynara carduncul us* L. (wild thistle, cardoon). The flower of *C. carduncul us* is used in South America to curdle milk; *C. scolymus* has also been used for this purpose.

EFFECTS

Stimulates hepatorenal function; stimulates bile flow from the liver; reduces blood lipids, inhibits cholesterol biosynthesis; protects liver cells against toxins via antioxidative processes, promotes regeneration of liver cells; prevents cholestasis; reduces nausea of various origins.

TRADITIONAL VIEW

The leaves of Cynara were used traditionally by the Eclectic physicians as a diuretic and depurative, for the treatment of rheumatism, gout, jaundice and especially for dropsies.[1] In Europe, Cynara is considered to have choleretic, cholagogue, laxative and diuretic activities. It has been used to clear the complexion, stimulate appetite, to alleviate the symptoms of arthritis, uraemia and hypercholesterolaemia. According to Leclerc, the activity of Cynara depends on tonifying the liver, in particular 'wringing out of the hepatic sponge',[2] and thus has an antitoxic (hepatoprotective) action. Cynara was also traditionally used to treat nephrosclerosis, urinary stones, oliguria of toxic or infectious origin, hepatic insufficiency and as a depurative for simple itch in children. Taken internally, it was said to produce a deodorant activity.[3]

SUMMARY ACTIONS

Hepatoprotective, hepatic trophorestorative, choleretic, cholagogue, bitter, hypocholesterolaemic, anticholestatic, antiemetic, diuretic; the combination of choleretic and diuretic activities makes it an ideal depurative.

CAN BE USED FOR

INDICATIONS SUPPORTED BY CLINICAL TRIALS

Hyperlipidaemia; non-ulcer dyspepsia; conditions requiring an increase in choleresis and antiemetic activity (functional bowel disorders, constipation, dyspepsia, functional gallbladder conditions, nausea, vomiting, flatulence).

TRADITIONAL THERAPEUTIC USES

Rheumatism, arthritis, gout, uraemia, jaundice, oedema, nephrosclerosis, urinary stones, gallstones, oliguria, hepatic insufficiency and conditions requiring a depurative action (such as skin itch).

MAY ALSO BE USED FOR

EXTRAPOLATIONS FROM PHARMACOLOGICAL STUDIES

Prevention and treatment of toxic conditions, particularly those involving the liver; long-term prevention

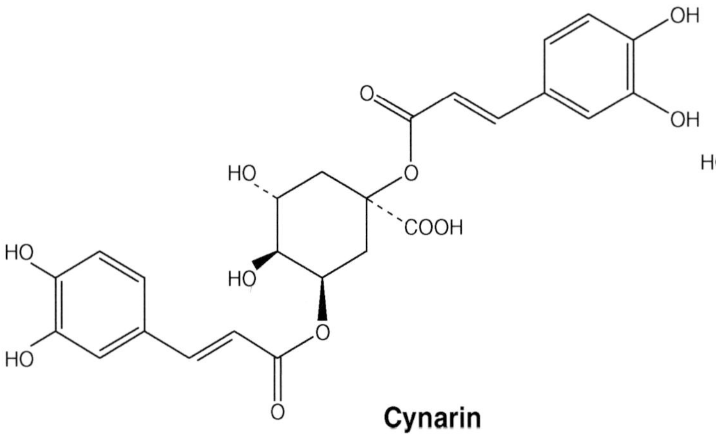

Cynarin

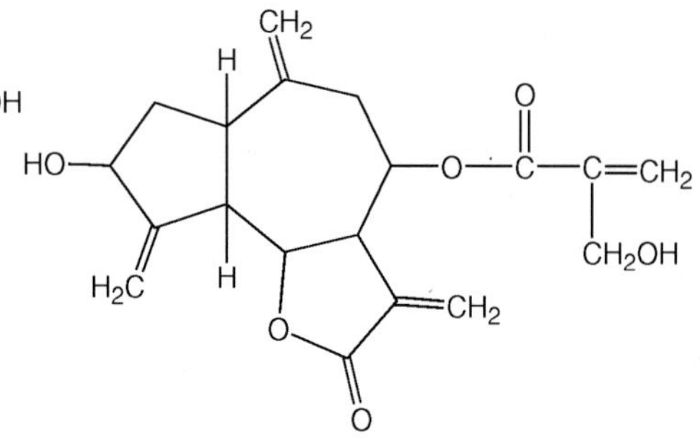

Cynaropicrin

and treatment of cardiovascular disease; to improve and regenerate hepatic function; as an antioxidant.

PREPARATIONS

Dried herb, liquid extract or pressed juice for internal use.

DOSAGE

3–8 ml of 1:2 liquid extract per day.

The clinical studies indicate that doses need to be relatively high, especially to achieve a clinically relevant reduction in cholesterol levels (in the range of the equivalent of 4–9 g of dried leaves per day). However, doses for the other therapeutic applications can be about 1.5–4 g per day. It is unlikely that drop doses of tinctures will achieve the effects described below.

DURATION OF USE

No restriction on long-term use.

SUMMARY ASSESSMENT OF SAFETY

No adverse effects from ingestion of Cynara are expected.

TECHNICAL DATA

BOTANY

Cynara is a member of the Compositae (daisy) family and in the same tribe as *Silybum marianum. Cynara scolymus* is a cultigen, probably a form of *Cynara cardunculus* L.[4] It is a herbaceous plant which produces stems of 1 m or more in length. The basal, lobate-bipinnatisect leaves are very large, the stem leaves may be pinnatisect or entire. (These leaves are eaten as a vegetable.) The inflorescence is formed of purplish-blue flowers grouped in heads which have an involucre of several long bracts which may be spiny. The fruit is an oval achene with a plumed pappus (tuft of bristles).[5]

KEY CONSTITUENTS

- Sesquiterpene lactones (0.5–6%), including cynaropicrin (40–80% of the total).[6]
- Caffeic acid derivatives (polyphenols): chlorogenic acid (3-caffeoylquinic acid), cynarin (1,3-dicaffeoyl quinic acid),[6] and many other dicaffeoylquinic acid derivatives.[7,8]
- Flavonoids (mainly derivatives of luteolin).[8]

Phenolic acids (such as the caffeic acid derivatives) are potentially unstable but careful drying of the leaves ensures that losses are minimal.[9,10]

PHARMACODYNAMICS

The most important active components in Cynara are probably the dicaffeoylquinic acids as a group and not just cynarin, although cynarin probably well represents the pharmacological activity of this group. In addition, it is quite possible that the 'cynarin' used in early clinical and pharmacological studies was not pure and included these related compounds.

In the 1930s to 1950s several scientific investigations were conducted by French and Italian scientists.[3] Although there was much debate about active components, these studies confirmed the choleretic (increased bile flow from the liver) and diuretic activity of Cynara leaves. Extensive clinical and pharmacological research in the 1930s confirmed that Cynara was choleretic, lowered cholesterol and caused diuresis in conjunction with an increase in urea and other nitrogen-containing substances in the urine.[11] This last activity is of particular interest and was confirmed by other researchers.[3] Cynara also stimulated the antitoxic (hepatoprotective) activity of the liver in chronic arsenic poisoning and eliminated the signs of arsenobenzol poisoning in patients treated for syphilis.[3]

Choleretic activity

Experiments in the 1950s found that cynarin given by intraperitoneal injection produced a marked choleretic activity of longer duration than sodium dehydrocholate (a bile salt), with an increase in the excretion of cholesterol and solids in the bile.[12] In contradiction to other conventional choleretics such as bile salts, cynarin administered by intravenous injection to rats stimulated bile production without later impairing the excretory function of the liver.[13] In recent experiments, Cynara extract increased the secretion of bile in liver cell cultures and from isolated perfused rat liver.[14]

Cynarin caused an increase of faecal bile acid excretion in seven healthy individuals and four patients with fatty liver.[15] Total extract of Cynara (containing 19% caffeoylquinic acids; 25 mg/kg) and purified extract (containing 46% caffeoylquinic acids; 200 mg/kg) demonstrated a marked choleretic effect in rats when administered by intraperitoneal injection. The choleretic activity mostly influenced bile salt secretion.[16] In an early study on 24 healthy subjects, Cynara extract caused stimulation of choleresis.[17]

Hepatoprotective and hepatorestorative activity

Several studies have investigated the protective effect of cynarin against damage to isolated liver cells in vitro. One study found that cynarin afforded significant protection against the toxin galactosamine and was more active than silybin from *Silybum marianum*.[18] However, it was less active than silybin against carbon tetrachloride (CCl_4) damage.[19] Caffeic acid was found to be much less active than cynarin against CCl_4 toxicity.[20] However, cynarin and caffeic acid both showed significant hepatoprotective activity against CCl_4 in vivo.[21] This protective activity has also been demonstrated for Cynara extract and is related to its antioxidant properties.[22]

Water-soluble extracts of Cynara demonstrated a marked antioxidative and protective activity against hydroperoxide-induced oxidative stress in cultured rat hepatocytes. Chlorogenic acid and cynarin accounted for only part of the antioxidative principle of the extracts, which was resistant against tryptic digestion, boiling, acidification and other treatments but was slightly sensitive to alkalinization.[23] In an earlier study using the same model, standardized Cynara extract offered similar protective activity and strong antioxidant activity.[24]

Oral doses of an aqueous extract of Cynara leaves stimulated liver repair and regeneration in rats.[25] This was confirmed in a follow-up study which found that Cynara leaves were more active than roots.[26]

Hypolipidaemic activity

Cynarin (400 mg/kg, IP injection) was also found to inhibit the hepatic synthesis of cholesterol and was of low toxicity.[12] Injection of cynarin in rats prevented the ethanol-induced increase in total esterified fatty acids ($p<0.001$). The administration of cynarin was followed by levels that were approximately 28% lower than those observed in the control group. Total serum lipids were also lower.[27] Oral cynarin (6 g/kg per day for 3 days) administered simultaneously with ethanol produced a distinct reduction of serum and hepatic cholesterol levels.[28] In rats receiving ethanol and cynarin simultaneously, a distinct reduction of serum and hepatic triglyceride levels occurred.[29]

Injection of Cynara extracts reduced plasma cholesterol in hyperlipidaemic rats. Oral administration of purified extract of Cynara (containing 46% caffeoylquinic acids; 100 mg/kg) decreased plasma cholesterol levels in ethanol-fed rats.[16] Cynara extract inhibited the increase in serum lipids and the manifestation of atherosclerotic plaques induced by an atherogenic diet in rats.[30,31]

The results of in vitro tests suggests that standardized Cynara extract produces its antiatherosclerotic activity via a dual mechanism: an inhibition of cholesterol synthesis and as a free radical scavenger which inhibits LDL oxidation.[32] Standardized Cynara extract significantly inhibited cholesterol biosynthesis in primary cultures of rat hepatocytes ($p<0.001$). The inhibition of the de novo synthesis was not due to cytotoxic effects.[33] Luteolin has been identified as a possible key component involved in this process.[14] Globe artichoke contains glycosidic derivatives of luteolin, which are probably converted to free luteolin by the action of bowel flora. Whether clinically significant quantities of luteolin are absorbed is not known. Cynara extract in vitro inhibited cholesterol synthesis at several levels in the biosynthetic sequence and therefore, unlike modern cholesterol drugs (the HMG-CoA reducatase inhibitors), might not result in the accumulation of potentially undesirable intermediate metabolites.[14]

Other activity

Two dicaffeoylquinic acid derivatives (3,5-dicaffeoylquinic acid, 4,5-dicaffeoylquinic acid) demonstrated antiinflammatory activity in vitro.[34] Dicaffeoylquinic acids also exhibited activity against human immunodeficiency virus (HIV) integrase in vitro and prevent HIV replication in tissue culture.[35] These compounds are found in Cynara.[7,8]

Cynarin (50–125 mg/kg, IP injection) also stimulated spontaneous diuresis and enhanced the excretion of a water or saline load. It antagonized the antidiuretic action of posterior pituitary extract (which contains antidiuretic hormone).[12]

No stimulatory effect on acid secretion was exerted by Cynara extract in cultured cells from rat gastric mucosa.[36] Aqueous extract of Cynara (35.7 and 150 mg/kg) administered to sexually mature male rats five times per week for 75 days did not lead to any significant change in the structure of the semen.[37]

Oral administration of the total extract of Cynara (containing 19% caffeoylquinic acids; 400 mg/kg) or purified extract (containing 46% caffeoylquinic acids; 200 mg/kg) increased the small intestinal transit of rats by 11% and 14% respectively.[16]

PHARMACOKINETICS

No data available.

CLINICAL TRIALS

Hypolipidaemic activity

Many earlier clinical studies investigated cynarin, rather than extracts of Cynara. However, it is worth reviewing these briefly since they probably also reflect on the activity of the leaf extract. Uncontrolled studies found that cynarin in oral doses of 750 mg to 1500 mg per day substantially reduced levels of total serum cholesterol.[38,39] A significant decrease (15%) was observed in 17 patients who received cynarin at the dose of 1000 mg per day over 4 weeks ($p<0.005$).[40]

Double-blind, placebo-controlled clinical trials also demonstrated significant reductions in serum cholesterol.[41–43] For example, 60 patients with elevated serum lipids were treated for 50 days with cynarin (500 mg) or placebo. Total cholesterol was lowered significantly by about 20% ($p<0.001$). Surprisingly, there was also a significant reduction in average body weight in the treated group of about 5 kg.[42] The reason for the weight loss is unknown but may be related to the influence of Cynara on liver metabolism.

In a double-blind, placebo-controlled study, cynarin at 500 mg per day also significantly lowered triglyceride levels in elderly patients with hypertriglyceridaemia.[44] Not all clinical studies on cynarin have been positive. An uncontrolled study on 17 patients with type II familial hyperlipoproteinaemia found that cynarin had no effect over 3–6 months.[45]

Clinical studies of Cynara in the 1930s established its value in lowering serum levels of cholesterol, urea and other nitrogen metabolites.[3] Cynara extract brought about a decrease of serum cholesterol and of triglycerides in an uncontrolled trial on 132 patients. The decrease was 59% and 82% respectively for 25 of these patients with type II hyperlipoproteinaemia.[46] A review of the clinical data from 1936 to 1994 indicated that Cynara extract lowered lipid levels (cholesterol and/or triglyceride) from between just below 5% to approximately 45%. However, this does not take into consideration the differences between experimental conditions in the various studies.[14] Several of these trials are outlined below. A decrease in serum cholesterol of 12–25% followed administration of Cynara extract (900 mg per day, about 5 g of leaf) for 6 weeks.[47,48] A reduction of about 15% was observed in a large group of hyperlipidaemic patients from general practice treated with a herbal formula containing Cynara and rhubarb root.[49] A decrease in serum lipid levels in 84 patients with secondary hyperlipidaemia was observed in three connected uncontrolled clinical trials. Patients were treated for 6–12 weeks with the pressed juice of fresh leaves and flower buds (10 ml, three times per day). Reductions in triglycerides of 4.7%, 12.9% and 4.4% were observed in the three trials and a reduction of 15.5% in LDL cholesterol was found in the second trial. High doses of fibrates generally led to a reduction of between 10% and 15%.[50]

In a conference report which has not been published, Cynara leaf extract or placebo were administered to 44 healthy volunteers under double-blind conditions. Total cholesterol was significantly decreased and HDL-cholesterol tended to rise. There were no significant differences between the two treatment groups with respect to side effects.[51]

Choleretic activity

In an early, open clinical study of 198 patients with biliary fistula, Cynara extract demonstrated choleretic and cholagogic effects and clinical improvement.[52] The increase in choleresis after intraduodenal administration of standardized Cynara extract was investigated in a randomized, placebo-controlled, monocentre, double-blind pilot study using a crossover design. Twenty healthy male volunteers were given a single dose of six capsules, each of which contained 320 mg of 4.5–5:1 Cynara extract equivalent to 1.5 g of leaf or 0.2 mg of cynarin per capsule. The amount of bile in the duodenum was defined as the primary variable. A maximum effect from the Cynara extract was achieved after 1 hour ($p<0.01$). Significant and clinically relevant differences were still apparent 3 hours after the Cynara was administered ($p<0.05$), whereas secretion fell after 3 hours in the placebo group. An effective period of approximately 120–150 minutes was regarded as satisfactory to favourably influence enzymatic digestion and the motor function of the intestine when Cynara is given postprandially. No side effects were observed.[53]

In another randomized, placebo-controlled, double-blind study, 60 patients with non-ulcer dyspepsia were treated with placebo or a herbal formula containing Cynara extract. Bile secretion measured with a duodenal probe increased significantly and there was also a significant improvement in symptoms such as bloating, nausea and heartburn. The herbal formula contained extracts of Cynara (50%), *Peumus boldus* (30%) and *Chelidonium majus* (20%).[54]

Dyspepsia

The above studies confirm a commonly held opinion in Germany that the choleretic and possibly antiemetic properties of Cynara mean that it is a valuable treatment for a range of functional bowel disorders. This has been supported by two postmarketing surveillance studies. In a multicentre trial, patients with symptoms such as nausea, constipation, dyspepsia and functional gallbladder conditions were treated with a Cynara extract (standardized for caffeoylquinic acids). The average dose corresponded to about 7 g of leaf per day. After 6 weeks of treatment, results for 170 patients were analysed. Improvements in symptoms were most marked for nausea and vomiting (improvement in 95% of cases), nausea (85%), abdominal pain (75%) and cramping right-sided pain (25%). In addition, symptoms such as flatulence and fat intolerance were favourably influenced. There was also a significant reduction in mean total cholesterol from 267 mg/dl to 228 mg/dl. Patient assessment of the treatment differed only slightly from that of the physicians (22% excellent, 67% good) and mild side effects were noted in only 1.2% of cases.[32]

A study on 553 dyspeptic patients (related to the above study) also found that symptoms improved in a clinically impressive and statistically significant ($p<0.001$) manner after 6 weeks of treatment with an average dose of about 7 g of leaf per day. The therapeutic efficacy of the standardized Cynara extract was rated by physicians as excellent or good in 87% of patients. Substantial improvement was recorded for the following symptoms: vomiting, nausea, abdominal pain, constipation, flatulence, belching and fat intolerance. Mean cholesterol values were lowered from 264 to 215 mg/dl ($p<0.001$) and triglycerides fell from 234 to 188 mg/dl ($p<0.001$). Tolerability of the Cynara extract was good, with only 1.3% of patients experiencing mild adverse reactions including flatulence, feeling of weakness and hunger.[55,56] These open surveillance reports need to be followed by well-designed clinical trials to confirm the dramatic benefits of Cynara in functional dyspepsia.

Other conditions

In an early trial, clinical application of Cynara extract in patients with ascites caused by portal stasis resulted in stimulation of diuresis.[57]

Sixty-two workers chronically exposed to carbon disulphide experienced a favourable outcome from prophylactic treatment with a Cynara preparation over 2 years. The treatment significantly reduced their platelet aggregation.[58] (One of the many symptoms of exposure to carbon disulphide is increased platelet adhesiveness, possibly resulting from lipid metabolism disturbances.)

TOXICOLOGY

The following acute LD_{50} values were recorded in rats: 1000 mg/kg (IP injection) for total extract of Cynara (containing 19% caffeoylquinic acids); 265 mg/kg (IP injection) for purified Cynara extract (containing 46% caffeoylquinic acids) and greater than 2000 mg/kg for purified Cynara extract by oral administration.[16]

CONTRAINDICATIONS

Closure of the gallbladder.[59]

SPECIAL WARNINGS AND PRECAUTIONS

Patients with known allergies to artichoke and similar plants (Compositae family). Use only with professional supervision in cholelithiasis.[59]

INTERACTIONS

None known.

USE IN PREGNANCY AND LACTATION

No adverse effects expected.

EFFECTS ON ABILITY TO DRIVE AND USE MACHINES

No negative influence is expected.

SIDE EFFECTS

The safety and tolerability of Cynara recorded in clinical studies are good to very good. However, as with other members of the Compositae family, contact with the fresh plant can cause contact dermatitis.[60] No cases of allergic reaction after oral intake have been reported.

OVERDOSE

Not known.

CURRENT REGULATORY STATUS IN SELECTED COUNTRIES

Cynara is covered by a positive Commission E monograph and is used for the treatment of dyspeptic disorders.

Cynara is on the UK General Sale List. Cynara does not have GRAS status. However, it is freely available as a 'dietary supplement' in the USA under DSHEA legislation (1994 Dietary Supplement Health and Education Act).

Cynara is not included in Part 4 of Schedule 4 of the Therapeutic Goods Act Regulations of Australia.

References

1. Felter HW, Lloyd JU. King's American dispensatory, 18th edn, 3rd revision, vol 1, 1905. Reprinted by Eclectic Medical Publications, Portland, 1983, p 641.
2. Leclerc H. Précis de phytothérapie, 5th edn. Masson, Paris, 1983, pp 143–144.
3. Rocchietta S. Minerva Med 1959; 50: 612–618.
4. Mabberley DJ. The plant book, 2nd edn. Cambridge University Press, Cambridge, 1997, p 175.
5. Chiej R. The Macdonald encyclopedia of medicinal plants. Macdonald, London, 1984, entry no. 107.
6. Wagner H, Bladt S. Plant drug analysis: a thin layer chromatography atlas, 2nd edn. Springer-Verlag, Berlin, 1996, p 77.
7. Puigmacia M, Adzet T, Ruviralta M et al. Planta Med 1986; 52: 529–530.
8. Hammouda FM, Seif El-Nasr MM, Ismail SI et al. Int J Pharmacog 1993; 31 (4): 299–304.
9. Nichiforesco E. Ann Pharm Fr 1967; 25 (4): 285–290.
10. Nichiforesco E, Coucou V. Ann Pharm Fr 1966; 24 (2): 127–132.
11. Tixier L. Presse Med 1939; 44: 880–883.
12. Preziosi P, Loscalzo B. Arch Int Pharmacodyn 1958; 117: 63–80.
13. Preziosi P, Loscalzo B, Marmo E. Experientia 1989; 15: 135–138.
14. Kraft K. Phytomed 1997; 4 (4): 369–378.
15. Schreiber J, Erb W, Wildgrube J et al. Z Gastroenterologie 1970; 8: 230–239.
16. Lietti A. Fitoterapia 1977; 48: 153–158.
17. Struppler A, Rossler H. Med Mschr 1957; 11: 221–223.
18. Kiso Y, Tohkin M, Hikino H. J Nat Prod 1983; 46 (6): 841–847.
19. Kiso Y, Tohkin M, Hikino H. Planta Med 1983; 49 (4): 222–225.
20. Adzet T, Camarasa J, Laguna JC. J Nat Prod 1987; 50 (4): 612–617.
21. Camarasa J, Laguna JC, Gaspar A et al. Med Sci Res 1987; 15: 91–92.
22. Gebhardt R. Pharm Ztg 1995; 140 (43): 3858–3861.
23. Gebhardt R. Toxicol Appl Pharmacol 1997; 144 (2): 279–286.
24. Gebhardt R. Med Welt 1995; 46 (7): 393–395.
25. Maros T, Racz G, Katonai B et al. Arzneim-Forsch 1966; 16 (2): 127–129.
26. Maros T, Seres-Sturm L, Racz G et al. Arzneim-Forsch 1968; 18 (7): 884–886.
27. Samochowiec L, Wojcicki J, Kadykow M. Pan Med 1971; 13: 87–88.
28. Wojcicki J. Drug Alcohol Depend 1978; 3 (2): 143–145.
29. Wojcicki J. Arzneim-Forsch 1976; 26 (11): 2047–2048.
30. Samochowiec L. Diss Pharm 1959; 11: 99–112.
31. Samochowiec L. Fol Biol 1962; 10: 75–83.
32. Wegener T. Z Phytother 1995; 16: 81.
33. Gebhardt R. Med Welt 1995; 46 (6): 348–350.
34. De Feo V, De Simone R, Bresciano E et al. J Nat Prod 1995; 58 (5): 639–646.
35. McDougall B, King PJ, Wu BW et al. Antimicrob Agents Chemother 1998; 42 (1): 140–146.
36. Gebhardt R. Pharm Pharmacol Lett 1997; 7 (2–3): 106–108.
37. Ilieva P, Khalkova Zh, Zaikov Kh et al. Probl Khig 1994; 19: 105–111.
38. Cima G, Bonora R. Minerva Med 1959; 50: 2288–2291.
39. Mancini M, Oriente P, D'Andrea L. Minerva Med 1960; 51: 2460–2463.
40. Adam G, Kluthe R. Therapiewoche 1979; 29: 5637–5640.
41. Cairella M, Volpari B. Clin Ter 1971; 57 (6): 541–552.
42. Montini M, Levoni P, Ongaro A et al. Arzneim-Forsch 1975; 25: 1311–1314.
43. Eberhardt G. Z Gastroenterologie 1973; 11 (3): 183–186.
44. Mars G, Brambilla G. Med Welt 1974; 25 (39): 1572–1574.
45. Heckers H, Dittmar K, Schmahl FW et al. Atherosclerosis 1977; 26 (2): 249–253.
46. Hammerl H, Kindler K, Kranzl C et al. Wien Med Wochenschr 1973; 123: 601–605.
47. Wojcicki J, Samochowiec K, Kosmider K. Herba Pol 1981; 27(3): 265–268.
48. Wojcicki J, Winter S. Med Pracy 1975; 26: 213–217.
49. Vorberg G. Z Allg Med 1980; 56 (25): 1598–1602.
50. Dorn M. Br J Phytother 1995/1996; 4 (1): 21–26.
51. Petrowicz O, Gebhardt R, Donner M et al. 67th meeting of the European Atherosclerosis Society, München, 1996.
52. Hammerl H, Pichler O. Wien Med Wochenschr 1957; 107 (25/26): 545–546.
53. Kirchhoff R, Beckers Ch, Kirchhoff GM et al. Phytomed 1994; 1 (2): 107–115.
54. Kupke D, Sanden HV, Trinzcej-Gartner H et al. Z Allg Med 1991; 67 (16): 1046–1058.
55. Fintelmann V. Z Allg Med 1996; 72 (suppl 2): 3–19.
56. Fintelmann V, Menβen HG. Dtsch Apoth Ztg 1996; 136 (17): 63–74.
57. Beggi D, Dettori L. Policlin Sez Prat 1931; 41: 489–490.
58. Woyke M, Cwajda H, Wojcicki J et al. Med Pr 1981; 32 (4): 261–264.
59. German Federal Minister of Justice. German Commission E for human medicine monograph, Bundes-Anzeiger (German Federal Gazette), no. 122, dated 06.07.1988, no. 164, dated 01.09.1990.
60. Meding B. Contact Derm 1983; 9 (4): 314.

Hawthorn (*Crataegus spp*)

SYNONYMS

Crataegi (Lat), Weiβdorn (Ger), aubépine (Fr), biancospino (Ital), alm. hvidtjørn (Dan).

WHAT IS IT?

The leaf, flower and berry of several species of hawthorn are used medicinally, most often: *Crataegus laevigata* (Poiret) DC (synonyms: *C. oxyacantha* auct., *C. oxyacanthoides* Thuill.) and *C. monogyna* Jacq. The Greek meaning of *Crataegus oxyacantha* refers to hard (wood) and sharp thorn. References to hawthorn are extensive throughout history and the shrub has been utilized in many ways including for wood, cultivation as a hedge and flavouring of liquor by the berries. Although the berries were traditionally used as medicine, modern research has tended to focus on preparations from the leaves or leaves and flowers.

The first use of hawthorn in cardiac therapy is attributed to Dr Green, an Irish doctor who used a tincture of the fresh berries. With the increasing incidence of heart disease in the Western world, its use rapidly spread to other countries, notably France, the United States, England and Germany. In Western herbal medicine hawthorn is now considered to be the most significant herb for ischaemic heart disease and there is considerable objective evidence to support its status.

EFFECTS

Increases force of myocardial contraction, increases coronary blood flow, reduces myocardial oxygen demand, protects against myocardial damage, hypotensive, improves heart rate variability, antiarrhythmic.

TRADITIONAL VIEW

Hawthorn berries have been traditionally used to treat heart problems, including hypertension with myocardial weakness, angina pectoris and tachycardia and other circulatory disorders (arteriosclerosis, Buerger's disease). The flowers and berries were also used as an astringent for sore throats and as a diuretic for kidney problems and dropsy.[1,2] The fruit and bark were used by the Eclectics as a heart remedy for indications such as pain, praecordial oppression, dyspnoea, cardiac hypertrophy, valvular insufficiency and anaemia.[3] The fruit of other *Crataegus species* (*C. pinnatifida, C. cuneata*) have been used in traditional Chinese medicine to improve digestion, stimulate circulation and remove blood stasis.[4]

SUMMARY OF ACTIONS

Cardiotonic (mild), cardioprotective, antioxidant, collagen stabilizing, mild astringent, hypotensive, antiarrhythmic.

CAN BE USED FOR

INDICATIONS SUPPORTED BY CLINICAL TRIALS

Congestive heart disease due to ischaemia or hypertension; cardiac insufficiency (particularly corresponding to NYHA stages I and II); topically for acne (uncontrolled trial).

TRADITIONAL THERAPEUTIC USES

Used as a treatment for mild heart conditions (angina pectoris, coronary artery disease, cardiac arrhythmias, hypertension, myocardial weakness) and for prevention of arterial degeneration caused by atherosclerosis.

MAY ALSO BE USED FOR

EXTRAPOLATIONS FROM PHARMACOLOGICAL STUDIES

Antioxidant activity; co-factor for vitamin C intake; stabilization of connective tissue tone; reduction of cholesterol.

OTHER APPLICATIONS

Cosmetics and hair care products for antiseborrhoeic, antiinflammatory activity and to increase hydration and elasticity of the skin.[5]

PREPARATIONS

Dried or fresh leaf, flower or fruit for infusion or decoction, liquid extract and tablets for internal use. Decoction or extract for topical use.

DOSAGE

- 1.5–3.5 g of dried flower, leaf or berry per day, as infusion or decoction.
- Hawthorn tablets (1 g leaves and flowers, standardized to 15–20 mg oligomeric procyanidins and 6–7 mg flavonoids) 2–3 times per day.
- 3–6 ml of 1:2 liquid extract of hawthorn leaf per day, 3–7 ml of 1:2 liquid extract of hawthorn berry per day, 7.5–15 ml of 1:5 tincture of hawthorn leaf per day, 7.5–17.5 ml of 1:5 tincture of hawthorn berry per day. Higher doses than these may be necessary for effective control of hypertension.
- Other concentrated extracts and powders (4:1 or 5:1), standardized to various levels of flavonoid and/or oligomeric procyanidins (OPC) content are also available in solid dosage form.

DURATION OF USE

There is no restriction on the long-term use of hawthorn and, if used to treat heart conditions, it should be prescribed over a period of at least 2 months.

SUMMARY ASSESSMENT OF SAFETY

No adverse effects from ingestion of hawthorn are expected. Hawthorn may act in synergy with digitalis glycosides and beta-blockers. Modification of drug dosage may be required. However, adverse effects are not generally anticipated from this interaction.

TECHNICAL DATA

BOTANY

Hawthorn, a member of the Rosaceae (rose) family, is a deciduous, thorny shrub or small tree up to 10 m tall. The leaves are broader than long and have 3–5 lobes. The white flowers, with their red anthers, are arranged in groups of 5–10 at the apex of small branches. The dark red, false fruits are oval and contain a small kernel which is the true fruit.[6,7]

Note: There has been confusion and debate over the nomenclature of *Crataegus species*. It was suggested in 1975 that the name *C. oxyacantha* L. should be rejected since it is a source of confusion[8] and *C. laevigata* used in preference.[9] In addition, extensive hybridization has occurred between *C. monogyna* and *C. laevigata*.[10–12]

KEY CONSTITUENTS

- Oligomeric procyanidins, mainly procyanidin B-2.[13] Epicatechin and catechin are present which are generally included in chemical tests for OPC levels.

	OPC%	Major flavonoids%
Leaves with flowers (average of 7 samples)	2.50	0.92
Flowers (average of 4 samples)	2.67	1.31
Leaves (spring, flowers open)	3.02	0.53
Leaves (summer, berries green)	2.71	0.74
Leaves (autumn, berries ripe)	2.06	0.76
Berries (summer, green)	3.18	0.15
Berries (autumn, ripe)	1.74	0.13

- Flavonoids, including quercetin glycosides (hyperoside, rutin) and particularly flavone-C-glycosides (vitexin and related compounds).[13]
- Amines, catechols, carboxylic and triterpene acids.[14]

The flowers contain the highest levels of flavonoids and the leaves contain the highest levels of OPC. The main active constituents of *Crataegus monogyna*, with variations with plant part and time of harvest, are outlined above.[15]

The relative astringency of OPC increases with the degree of polymerization. OPC from *Crataegus oxyacantha* berries, with an average number of monomers of 4, have an astringency relative to tannic acid of 0.73.[16]

PHARMACODYNAMICS

The therapeutic value of hawthorn may extend beyond its cardiovascular applications, largely due to a significant OPC content. Although most of the research was not specifically on the OPC found in hawthorn, it is likely that the hawthorn OPC will share many of the described pharmacological properties. In 1966 the French scientist Masquelier and his co-workers analysed the bark of several conifers from Quebec. Some species, especially *Tsuga canadensis* (previously known as *Pinus canadensis*), were rich in OPC. However, Masquelier's interest in this tree was based on the accounts of the French explorer Jacques Cartier.[17] During the winter of 1534 Cartier's group in Canada was afflicted by scurvy, which was cured on the advice of a native who directed that the sailors use a decoction of the bark and leaves of the 'Anneda' tree. The liquid was consumed and the solid residue applied as a poultice to the swollen joints. On the basis of Cartier's description, Masquelier postulated that 'Anneda' was *Tsuga canadensis*. He further speculated that the leaves provided a source of vitamin C and the bark, by providing OPC, acted as a vitamin C synergist, perhaps in a similar manner to the chemically related flavonoids.

Masquelier's original interest in OPC was for their 'vitamin P-like' activity.[18] He later postulated

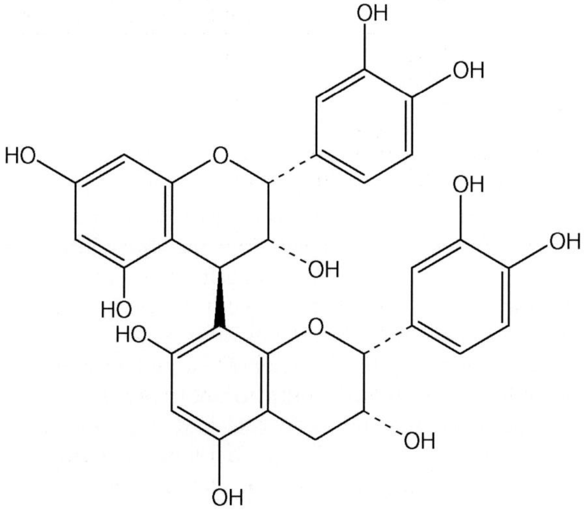

Procyanidin B-2

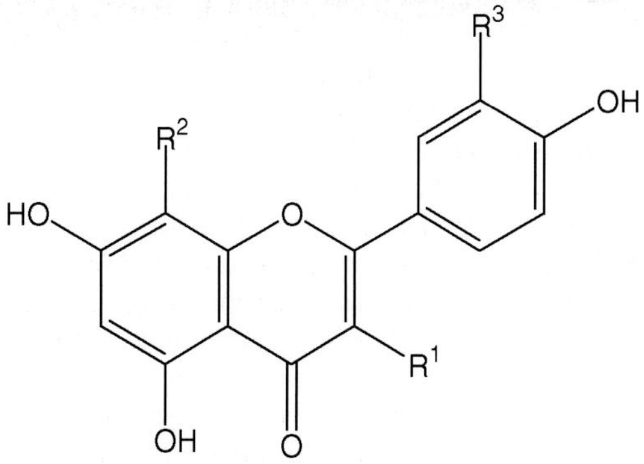

	R^1	R^2	R^3
Quercetin	OH	H	OH
Hyperoside	*O*-β-galactosyl	H	OH
Vitexin	H	glucosyl	H

Flavonoids

that they may be important in the prevention of atheroma.[19] In 1987, he drew attention to the potent antioxidant properties of OPC and proposed that they may help to prevent any illness related to free radical damage or lipid peroxidation. This could include cancer, atheroma and any cell damage occurring under hypoxic conditions. Other French research groups have studied OPC from *Vitis vinifera* (also found in red wine) and *Cupressus sempervirens* for their angioprotective properties.[20]

Effect on the cardiovascular system

Crataegus acids increased coronary blood flow in vitro and decreased blood pressure in vivo;[21–23] crataegolic and ursolic acid increased coronary flow in vitro and crataegolic acid was also positively inotropic.[24] Epicatechin increased coronary blood flow and was positively inotropic and chronotropic in vitro.[24–26]

The total flavonoids from hawthorn have a phosphodiesterase inhibitory activity in vitro.[27] Hawthorn extract exhibited a positive inotropic effect on the contraction amplitude accompanied by a moderate increase of energy turnover in cardiac myocytes in vitro. In comparison with other positive inotropic procedures, the effects of hawthorn extract were significantly more economical with respect to the energetics of the myocytes. Hawthorn also prolonged the apparent refractory period in the presence and absence of isoprenaline (beta-adrenergic agonist), indicating an antiarrhythmic potential.[28]

Two flavonoid fractions of hawthorn were positively inotropic (increasing the force of contraction) in isolated heart. One fraction had an effect on frequency, being negatively chronotropic (decreasing the heart rate). In isolated hearts vitexin-4′-*O*-rhamnoside was positively inotropic and negatively chronotropic at higher doses while flavonoid aglycones were inactive.[24]

The main flavonoids of hawthorn (*O*-glycosides: luteolin-*O*-glucoside, hyperoside, rutin; and *C*-glycosides: vitexin, vitexin-rhamnoside and monoacetyl vitexin-rhamnoside) increased coronary flow, demonstrated slight positive inotropic effects and raised heart rate in isolated hearts. An inhibition of cAMP phosphodiesterase was also observed.[29] The purified flavonoids from hawthorn leaves administered to rats with myocardial infarction caused a smaller necrotic focus and improved revascularization of finer vessels when compared to controls.[30]

Oligomeric procyanidin subfractions were more positively inotropic in isolated heart than flavonoid fractions but had no effect on frequency.[31] In another study, hawthorn OPCs had a mild negative chronotropic effect in isolated heart but caused a marked increase in contraction and blood flow. Procyanidin dimers were more active than oligomers, with 3–4 units, and the OPC fraction from hawthorn leaves was more active than that from the berries. In general, the effects of the OPC are similar to those of flavonoids but are elicited at lower doses.[24] Crataegus OPC increased coronary blood flow in dogs after oral administration.[32]

The cardioprotective effect of several fractions of standardized hawthorn leaf and flower extract (containing 18.75% OPC) were investigated in vitro and in vivo. The lipophilic fraction containing flavonoids was as active as the whole extract in inhibiting human neutrophil elastase, but only half as active as a radical scavenger. The water-soluble fraction was weak in both in vitro systems. In contrast, the inhibiting potencies of the OPC-rich (and flavonoid-free) fraction were significantly higher than the extract. Oral administration of the OPC-rich fraction (20 mg/kg per day) to rats afforded similar protection against ischaemia-reperfusion-induced pathologies to treatment with a higher dose of the standardized extract (100 mg/kg per day).[33]

Hawthorn improves myocardial performance and myocardial tolerance in oxygen deficiency, decreases peripheral vascular resistance, has an antiarrhythmic and partial beta-antagonistic effect.[34] It reinforced the positive inotropic action of cardiac glycosides without an increase in glycoside toxicity and increased coronary blood flow, even after experimental damage in vitro.[35] Compared with a digoxin preparation, hawthorn extract increased the erythrocyte flow rate in all the vascular networks examined and reduced both leucocyte endothelial adhesion and diapedesis in the venular network in rat mesenteric vessels.[36]

The water-soluble fraction of hawthorn extract demonstrated a cardioprotective effect on the ischaemic-reperfused heart (which mimics myocardial infarction). The cardioprotective effect was not accompanied by an increase in coronary flow.[37]

Hawthorn may exert its activity in vitro in a similar way to phosphodiesterase inhibitors, raising cAMP levels in cardiac muscle cells. Hawthorn extract prolonged the effective refractory period in isolated heart, in comparison to four other inotropic drugs (including adrenalin and digoxin) which shortened it. Thus, hawthorn has a relatively lower risk of causing arrhythamias and may in fact have antiarrhythmic activity.[38] Multielectrode techniques have demonstrated that hawthorn extract prolonged the action potential duration and delayed recovery of the maximum upstroke velocity of guinea pig papillary muscle.[39]

Hawthorn extracts increased coronary blood flow after oral administration.[40] Oral administration of hawthorn extract to rats for 3 months resulted in myocardial protection, as evidenced by attenuation of levels of lactase dehydrogenase (LDH) release after induced ischaemia and reperfusion in the isolated hearts. Hawthorn pretreatment suggests a preservation of the cell membrane and a protection from myocardial damage.[41]

Pretreatment with hawthorn or garlic extract, but particularly the combination of both extracts, resulted in protective effects on induced heart, liver and pancreas damage in rats.[42] Oral administration of hawthorn reduced the deleterious metabolic influence of hypoxia on ventricular muscle fibres in rabbits. Hawthorn may protect the sodium pump against anoxia.[43] Vitexin-4′-*O*-rhamnoside increased coronary blood flow by up to 64% after intracoronary administration.[44] Intravenous or intracoronary administration of hawthorn flavonoids in cats and dogs increased coronary blood flow, decreased blood pressure and increased heart contractility. No change was observed in heart rate.[45–47]

Intravenous administration of hawthorn extract decreased blood pressure, decreased experimental arrhythmia and increased peripheral blood flow to skeletal muscle.[48–50]

Administration of hawthorn to volunteers improved the anoxic symptoms produced by inhalation of an 8% oxygen gas mixture.[51] In patients with ischaemic heart disease, hawthorn decreased the signs of ischaemia as assessed by an exercise ECG test.[52]

In a placebo-controlled, crossover study, the effect of a single dose of 900 mg of concentrated hawthorn extract (3:1, standardized to 2.2% flavonoids) on the cutaneous microcirculation was compared to 0.3 mg medigoxin. Six hours after taking hawthorn, the haematocrit had dropped by a mean of 3.2%, whereas erythrocyte aggregation increased significantly by a mean of 19% 3 hours after taking the digoxin. No significant changes were recorded for the other measured parameters (plasma viscosity, flow rate in nail bed capillaries, heart rate, blood pressure).[53]

Hypocholesterolaemic activity

A protective action against diet-induced hypercholesterolaemia was demonstrated by hawthorn extracts in vivo.[54] Hawthorn berry tincture administered simultaneously to rats fed an atherogenic diet significantly increased the binding of LDL to the liver plasma membranes in vitro, increased bile acid excretion and depressed hepatic cholesterol synthesis.[55]

Antioxidant activity

Hawthorn extracts obtained using acetone, methanol and water demonstrated antioxidant activity on hepatic microsomal preparations in vitro. A correlation was demonstrated between the total phenolic content (mainly flavonoids and OPC) and antioxidant activity for leaf, flower and berry at all stages of growth. The most active individual components were (–)-epi-catechin and procyanidin B-2.[56] Similar hawthorn extracts exhibited in vitro antioxidant activities in three different models of generation of reactive oxygen species.[57]

Chinese research found that the Chinese hawthorn berry (*Crataegus pinnatifida*) was a potent inducer of superoxide dismutase (SOD) activity in mice.[58] Oral doses of aqueous extracts were used and the SOD activity was measured in red blood cells. SOD is the enzyme which combats the harmful effects of the superoxide radical.

Collagen stabilization

Oligomeric procyanidins (OPC) demonstrated highly effective activity in stabilizing collagen in vitro. OPC may create stabilizing crosslinks between the polypeptide chains of collagen, thus strengthening connective tissue.[59] Common flavonoids were found to be completely inactive in stabilizing collagen compared to OPC, which had maximum activity.[60] Collagen fibres from rat tails treated with (+)-catechin and epicatechin-2-sulphate showed an increase in stability (in terms of denaturation temperature, energy during shrinkage and amount of solubilized collagen).[61]

Other activity

Induction of epidermal ornithine decarboxylase (ODC) activity, stimulation of hydroperoxide production and increased DNA synthesis are three biochemical effects linked to skin tumour promotion by the tumour promoter 12-O-tetradecanoylphorbol 13-acetate (TPA). Topical applications of procyanidins to mouse epidermis prior to administration of TPA resulted in inhibition of ODC activity. The inhibition of ODC activity increased with the degree of polymerization of the procyanidins (trimer (procyanidin C-1) > dimer (procyanidin B-2) > monomer (epicatechin)).[62]

Hawthorn flower extract inhibited thromboxane A_2 biosynthesis in vitro.[63]

PHARMACOKINETICS

The pharmacokinetics of oral doses of OPC given to mice have been studied using an isotopic labelling technique.[64] OPC showed rapid absorption and preferential localization in tissues rich in glycosaminoglycans. The plasma half-life was about 5 hours, indicating a prolonged presence in the bloodstream. In contrast, the flavonoid glycoside rutin showed poor absorption, the bulk of the radioactivity residing with the contents of the digestive tract. This work and that of other reviewed by Middleton[65] suggests that OPC or OPC fragments resulting from bacterial activity in the gut are more bioavailable than flavonoids. (For more details on the pharmacokinetics of flavonoids and OPC, see Ch. 2.)

CLINICAL TRIALS

The New York Heart Association (NYHA) classifies loss of cardiac output: for stage I the patient is symptom-free when at rest and on treatment; stage II patients have loss of capacity with medium effort; for stage III even minor effort results in dyspnoea, with no symptoms at rest; in stage IV symptoms are present when at rest.

Heart disease

In a placebo-controlled, double-blind trial conducted in Japan the effect of a combination of hawthorn leaves and berries on heart disease was studied over a 6-week period.[66] Eighty patients suffering from mild congestive heart disease due to ischaemia or hypertension took part in the trial, 35 in the treated group (180 mg/day of 5:1 hawthorn extract) and 45 in the placebo group. Most patients were already receiving a variety of drugs including diuretics, antihypertensive agents and cardiac glycosides and their medication was maintained throughout the trial.

As shown below, patients receiving hawthorn showed a significant benefit as assessed by a number of parameters. The high values for placebo reflect the benefits of bed rest and hospital care. Results are presented only for patients assigned to NYHA stage II. There were insufficient numbers in the other NYHA stages for statistical significance. Blood pressure was also slightly but significantly lowered. More importantly, heart rate times middle blood pressure was significantly reduced with $p<0.05$, indicating a reduced workload for the heart. No adverse interactions with conventional medication were observed and hawthorn was well tolerated, with minor side effects in only one patient. The authors concluded that hawthorn unmistakably surpasses placebo in its effect on subjective symptoms and objective parameters (see Table below).

A metaanalysis reviewing eight clinical trials from 1989 to 1994 found standardized hawthorn extract to be effective over the entire daily dosage range of 160–900 mg. A total of 323 patients with heart failure (mostly of NYHA stage II) were treated from 4 to

Parameter	Improvement % Active	Placebo	Statistical significance
Overall improvement	80.8	48.7	p<0.001
Subjective symptoms	84.6	56.4	p<0.001
Heart function	76.9	46.2	p<0.01
Dyspnoea	76.5	43.9	p<0.01
Palpitations	75.9	41.2	p<0.01
Cardiac oedema	83.3	45.5	p<0.05
Pulmonary congestion	81.8	45.0	p<0.05

8 weeks with hawthorn leaf and flower extract standardized to either 2.2% flavonoids or 18.75% OPC. Two trials were open, five were double-blind and one was a comparative trial with the drug captopril. A significant effect was observed for subjective findings in all but one trial, for pressure-rate product in four trials and for work tolerance in three trials.[67] The internal cardiac work performed is represented by the heart rate-blood pressure product. When the pressure-rate product is reduced there is decreased workload for the heart. Six of these trials are outlined below (references [68–73]).

In an open trial, seven patients received a concentrated extract of hawthorn (240 mg per day (5:1)) over 4 weeks. Left ventricular ejection fraction increased in five patients and subjective complaints decreased in six patients. Systolic and diastolic volumes, blood pressure and heart rate did not change significantly.[68] In a randomized, double-blind, placebo-controlled trial of 30 patients with NYHA stage II cardiac disease, patients treated with two tablets per day of concentrated hawthorn extract (5:1, equivalent to 30 mg OPC) for 8 weeks showed significant advantage over placebo in terms of reduced workload for the heart and improvement in subjective symptoms. Systolic and diastolic blood pressures were mildly reduced.[69]

In a multicentre, double-blind comparative study, 132 patients with NYHA stage II stable heart disease were treated with 900 mg of concentrated hawthorn extract (3:1, standardized to 2.2% flavonoids) or 37.5 mg captopril for 8 weeks. None of the measured parameters (exercise tolerance, pressure-rate product and five typical symptoms) showed any significant difference between the two treatments. One patient treated with captopril had to discontinue therapy due to adverse effects; no patients withdrew from the hawthorn treatment.[70]

In a randomized, double-blind, placebo-controlled trial, 72 patients received concentrated hawthorn extract (900 mg per day, 3:1) or placebo over 8 weeks. Exercise time taken to reach the anaerobic threshold was longer in the treated group when compared to placebo. Significant improvement in terms of subjective assessment of symptoms was also observed in those treated with hawthorn.[71] In a randomized, double-blind, placebo-controlled trial, 78 patients with NYHA stage II heart disease received a daily dose of 600 mg of concentrated hawthorn extract (3:1, standardized to 2.2% flavonoids) or placebo for 8 weeks. A significant increase was observed in patients' work capacity (measured by a bicycle ergometry exercise) for the hawthorn group. Significant reductions in systolic blood pressure, heart rate and pressure-rate product were observed. Clinical symptoms also decreased in the treated group.[72]

One trial failed to demonstrate a positive effect. In a randomized, double-blind, placebo-controlled trial, 85 patients with NYHA stage II heart disease received a daily dose of 300 mg of concentrated hawthorn extract (3:1, standardized to 2.2% flavonoids) or placebo for 4 weeks. Exercise tolerance, pressure-rate product and clinical symptomatology all showed a trend toward superiority of hawthorn over placebo but were not statistically significant.[73] Since the preparation used in this study is normally given in doses of 600–900 mg/day, this lack of effect may reflect the lower dosage used.

The effect of an extract of *Crataegus oxyacantha* on heart rate variability (HRV) was studied in 20 geriatric patients over 6 weeks in a randomized, double-blind, placebo-controlled trial.[74] Low HRV has been shown to be associated with a high mortality in patients who have already experienced a heart attack. Patients with a coefficient of variation (CV) in heart rate of less than 5% were chosen for the study. Those with frequent ectopic beats and diabetes were excluded. The average age of patients was about 80 years. A small but statistically significant positive trend was seen in the hawthorn group. The CV of heart rate rose steadily over the 6-week treatment period from 1.9% to 2.5%. There was no change in the placebo group. The authors postulated that this effect may become more marked over longer treatment periods. In some patients given hawthorn, the improvement in HRV was dramatic. The sinus activity of the heart undergoes a natural fluctuation. Short-term fluctuations occur with inhalation and exhalation (sinus arrhythmia) but there are also second-grade variations associated with blood pressure rhythm. With age, diabetes and damage to the heart, this variability of heart rate decreases. Recently it was shown that low HRV is a risk factor in coronary heart disease and that there is a positive correlation between HRV and life expectancy.[75]

In a randomized, double-blind, placebo-controlled trial, 60 patients with mild, stable angina pectoris (NYHA stage I and II) received either concentrated hawthorn extract (5:1, 180 mg per day) or placebo over 3 weeks. For the treated group, pathological ECG changes under exertion improved significantly and load tolerance showed a strong trend towards significance in treated versus control groups. Blood pressure or pulse rate did not differ between the two groups.[76] In a multicentre, double-blind, placebo-controlled trial, 136 patients with NYHA stage II cardiac insufficiency were treated with two tablets of concentrated hawthorn extract per day (each tablet containing 80 mg hawthorn leaf and flower extract (5:1), standardized to 15 mg OPC) or placebo over 8 weeks. A significant improvement in the performance of the heart was observed in the group receiving hawthorn, in particular, improvement in the main symptoms (such as reduced performance, shortness of breath and ankle oedema, $p<0.05$) and a better quality of life for the patient with respect to mental well-being.[77]

Hawthorn was also effective in combination with passionflower. In a randomized, double-blind, placebo-controlled study, 40 patients with dyspnoea commensurate with NYHA stage II received either hawthorn and passionflower extracts or placebo over 6 weeks. Exercise capacity, measured in terms of a walking test, increased significantly in those patients receiving the herbal preparation. A slight but significant decrease in heart rate at rest and in mean diastolic blood pressure during exercise and a decrease in total plasma cholesterol levels in the group receiving the extract was observed.[19] The two groups did not differ significantly in other tests: maximum exercise capacity measured during a bicycle ergometer test, subjective assessment of breathlessness or blood lactate levels, although the trend favoured the treated group.

A postmarketing surveillance study gathered data for 3664 patients with heart disease stages I and II according to the NYHA classification.[78] The hawthorn extract (900 mg of 3:1 extract) was shown to be well tolerated. Of the 48 patients (1.3%) who reported 72 adverse reactions, a causal relationship with the treatment was confirmed in 22 cases and considered probable in another four (a total of 0.7%). Seven patients reported minor gastrointestinal effects, three complained of palpitations, two of headache and dizziness; circulatory disturbances, sleeplessness and inner agitation were each reported once. The efficacy of the hawthorn treatment was evaluated on data from 1476 patients who received only the hawthorn treatment.[78] After 8 weeks of treatment the symptom score had improved on average by 66.6%. In particular, the NYHA stage I patients were largely symptom free by this time. Evaluation by clinicians assessed the treatment as very good for 61.2% of patients and good for 34.3%, giving an overall efficacy rate of better than 90%. Striking results were achieved in the subgroup of patients exhibiting symptoms of borderline hypertension, tachycardia and cardiac arrhythmias. (These patients were classified by the authors as having a stimulated sympathoadrenergic system.) Average systolic blood pressure for this subgroup fell from 160 to 150 mmHg and average diastolic dropped from 89 to 84 mmHg. Average heart rate was reduced from 89 to 79 beats per minute and the incidence of arrhythmias was considerably reduced. In contrast, patients with normal or even low blood pressure or heart rates showed no further mean reduction in these parameters.

A large number of patients, previously unsuccessfully treated with digoxin alone, were compensated for rest and slight stress with relatively low oral doses of the glycoside in combination with hawthorn.[79,80]

Blood pressure

In an uncontrolled trial, mean systolic pressure fell from 205 mmHg to 148 mmHg and mean diastolic pressure fell from 112 mmHg to 83 mmHg in hypertensive patients receiving hawthorn berry tincture. When treatment was stopped, blood pressures returned to their initial values over a 2-week period. There was only a slight effect on subjects with normal blood pressure.[81] Other clinical studies (see above) have shown that hawthorn extract causes a slight reduction in blood pressure in patients with heart conditions.

Other conditions

In an uncontrolled, multicentre trial, 50 patients with and without acne in various stages of development uniformly applied 1–2 ampoules of liposome-containing hawthorn extract to the most affected areas of the skin each day for at least 30 days. Hawthorn extract demonstrated a general capillary-protective activity which resulted in the reduction or disappearance of capillary congestion. A mild antiinflammatory activity was demonstrated by a significant reduction in acne and erythema. (The improvement in stratum corneum hydration and roughness of skin and the antiseborrhoeic effect were attributed to the phosphatidylcholine liposomes.)[5]

TOXICOLOGY

The acute oral toxicity of hawthorn is 6 g/kg (animal undefined). No target organ toxicity was defined at 100 times the human dose of concentrated hawthorn extract (standardized to 18.75% OPC). Standard mutagenic and clastogenic tests were also negative.[82]

Schimmer and co-workers found that an ethanolic extract of crataegus was weakly mutagenic in the Salmonella test, a finding which they attributed to the quercetin content of the extract.[83] Popp and co-workers found a DNA-damaging potency of commercial Crataegus preparations in human lymphocyte cultures.[84] The active principles were not identified but were probably flavonoids. Several procyanidins with different degrees of polymerization (dimers, a trimer and a polymer) were found to be non-mutagenic in the Salmonella mutagenesis assay system.[85]

CONTRAINDICATIONS

None known.

SPECIAL WARNINGS AND PRECAUTIONS

None known.

INTERACTIONS

Hawthorn may act in synergy with digitalis, glycosides, beta-blockers and other hypotensive drugs. Modification of drug dosage may be required.

USE IN PREGNANCY AND LACTATION

No adverse effects expected.

EFFECTS ON ABILITY TO DRIVE AND USE MACHINES

No adverse effects expected.

SIDE EFFECTS

No significant adverse events have been reported in clinical trials.

OVERDOSE

Not known.

CURRENT REGULATORY STATUS IN SELECTED COUNTRIES

Hawthorn berries are official in the *British Pharmacopoeia* (1998). A draft monograph of hawthorn is being prepared and may appear in *European Pharmacopoeia* subsequent to the 1997 edition. A draft monograph of hawthorn leaf with flower is being prepared and may become official in the *United States Pharmacopeia-National Formulary* subsequent to June 1999.

Hawthorn berry, hawthorn leaf and hawthorn flower are covered by null Commission E monographs. The Commission E suggests that as the efficacy of hawthorn berry, leaf or flower has not been documented, no therapeutic application can be recommended. Hawthorn leaf with flower is covered by a positive Commission E monograph and can be used to treat decreased cardiac output as described in functional stage II of NYHA.

Hawthorn is not on the UK General Sale List.

Hawthorn does not have GRAS status. However, it is freely available as a 'dietary supplement' in the USA under DSHEA legislation (1994 Dietary Supplement Health and Education Act).

Hawthorn is not included in Part 4 of Schedule 4 of the Therapeutic Goods Act Regulations of Australia.

References

1. Grieve M. A modern herbal, vol 1. Dover Publications, New York, 1971, p 385.
2. British Herbal Medicine Association's Scientific Committee. British herbal pharmacopoeia. BHMA, Cowling, 1983, pp 74–75.
3. Felter HW, Lloyd JU. King's American dispensatory, 18th edn, 3rd revision, vol 2, 1905. Reprinted by Eclectic Medical Publications, Portland, 1983, p 1613.
4. Chang HM, But PP. Pharmacology and applications of Chinese materia medica, vol 1. World Scientific, Singapore, 1987, pp 100–107.
5. Longhi MG, Rocchi P, Gezzi A et al. Fitoterapia 1984; 55 (2): 87–99.
6. Launert EL. The Hamlyn guide to edible and medicinal plants of Britain and Northern Europe. Hamlyn, London, 1981, p 76.
7. Chiej R. The Macdonald encyclopedia of medicinal plants. Macdonald, London, 1984, entry no. 99.
8. Byatt JI. Bot J Linn Soc 1974; 69: 15–21.
9. Mabberley DJ. The plant book, 2nd edn. Cambridge University Press, Cambridge, 1997, p 190.
10. Byatt JI. Watsonia 1975; 10: 253–264.
11. Bevan J. Watsonia 1980; 13 (2): 119–121.
12. Christensen KI. Acta Universitatis Upsaliensis Symb Bot Ups 1996; 31 (3): 211–220.
13. Wagner H, Bladt S. Plant drug analysis: a thin layer chromatography atlas, 2nd edn. Springer-Verlag, Berlin, 1996, p 198.
14. Bisset NG (ed) Herbal drugs and phytopharmaceuticals. Medpharm Scientific Publishers, Stuttgast, 1994, p 162.
15. Kartnig T, Hiermann A, Azzam S. Sci Pharm 1987; 55 (2): 95–100.
16. Porter LJ, Woodruffe J. Phytochem 1984; 23 (6): 1255–1256.
17. Masquellier J. Pycnogenols: recent advances in the therapeutic activity of procyanidins. In: Beal JL, Reinhard E (eds) Natural products as medicinal agents. Hippokrates-Verlag, Stuttgart, 1981, pp 243–256.
18. Michaud J, Masquellier J. Prod Probl Pharm 1973; 28 (7): 499–520.
19. Von Eiff M, Brunner H, Haegeli A et al. Acta Therapeut 1994; 20 (1–2): 47–66.
20. Wegrowski J, Robert AM, Moczar M. Biochem Pharmacol 1984; 33 (21): 3491–3497.
21. Ammon HPT, Handel M. Planta Med 1981; 43 (2): 105–120.
22. Ammon HPT, Handel M. Planta Med 1981; 43 (3): 209–239.
23. Ammon HPT, Handel M. Planta Med 1981; 43 (4): 313–322.

24. Occhiuto F, Circosta C, Costa R et al. Plantes méd phytothér 1986; 20 (1): 52–63.
25. Rewerski W, Piechocki T, Rylski M et al. Arzneim Forsch 1971; 21 (6): 886–888.
26. Schwabe W, Neu R. Arzneim Forsch 1960; 10: 60–61.
27. Petkov E, Nikdov N, Uzunov P. Planta Med 1981; 43 (2): 183–186.
28. Popping S, Rose H, Ionescu I et al. Arzneim-Forsch 1995; 45 (11): 1157–1161.
29. Schussler M, Holzl J, Fricke U. Arzneim-Forsch 1995; 45 (8): 842–845.
30. Guendjev Z. Arzneim Forsch 1977; 27 (8): 1576–1579.
31. Leukel A, Fricke U, Holzl J. Planta Med 1986; 52: 545–546.
32. Roddewig C, Hensel H, Arzneim Forsch 1977; 27 (7): 1407–1410.
33. Chatterjee SS, Koch E, Jaggy H et al. Arzneim-Forsch 1997; 47 (7): 821–825.
34. Loew D. ESCOP 3rd International Symposium: European Harmony in Phytotherapy, Scheveningen, The Hague, 18th March 1994; cited in Br J Phytother 1993/1994; 3(3): 140.
35. Trunzler G, Schuler E. Arzneim Forsch 1962; 12: 198–202.
36. Ernst F-D, Reuther G, Walper A. Munch Med Wochenschr 1994; 136 (suppl 1): S57–S59.
37. Nasa Y, Hashizume H, Hoque AN et al. Arzneim-Forsch 1993; 43 (9): 945–949.
38. Joseph G, Zhao Y, Klaus W. Arzneim-Forsch 1995; 45 (12): 1261–1265.
39. Muller A, Linke W, Zhao Y et al. Phytomed 1996; 3 (3): 257–261.
40. Mävers H, Hensel H. Arzneim-Forsch 1974; 24 (5): 783–785.
41. Al Makdessi S, Sweidan H, Mullner S et al. Arzneim Forsch 1996; 46 (1): 25–27.
42. Ciplea AG, Richter KD. Arzneim-Forsch 1988; 38 (11): 1583–1592.
43. Kanno T, Toshihiro S, Yamamoto M. Jpn Heart J 1976; 17: 512–520.
44. Manalov P, Daleva L. Farmatsiya (Sofia) 1969; 19 (3): 38–44.
45. Manalov P. Suvrem Med 1971; 22: 20–23.
46. Petrov L, Gagov S, Popova A. Acta Physiol Pharmacol Bulg 1974; 2: 82–89.
47. Liévre M, Andrieu JL, Baconin A. Ann Pharm Franc 1985; 43 (5): 471–477.
48. Stepka W, Winters AD. Lloydia 1973; 36: 436.
49. Thompson EB, Aynilian GH, Gora P et al. J Pharm Sci 1974; 63 (12): 1936–1937.
50. Braasch W, Bienroth W. Arzneim-Forsch 1960; 10: 127–129.
51. Frank E, Heymanns E. Arztl Forsch 1956; 10: 248–254.
52. Kandziora J. MMW 1969; 111: 295–298.
53. Fischer K, Jung F, Koscielny J et al. Munch Med Wochenschr 1994; 136 (suppl 1): S35–S38.
54. Gusseinow DJ. Farmakoli Toksikol 1963; 26 (4): 435–439.
55. Rajendran S, Deepalakshmi PD, Parasakthy K et al. Atherosclerosis 1996; 123 (1–2): 235–241.
56. Bahorun T, Trotin F, Pommery J et al. Planta Med 1994; 60 (4): 323–328.
57. Bahorun T, Gressier B, Trotin F et al. Arzneim-Forsch 1996; 46 (11): 1086–1090.
58. Dai Y, Gao CM, Tian QL et al. Planta Med 1987; 53 (3): 309–310.
59. Masquellier J. Pycnogenols: recent advances in the therapeutic activity of procyanidins. In: Beal JL, Reinhard E (eds) Natural products as medicinal agents. Hippokrates-Verlag, Stuttgart, 1981, pp 247–249.
60. Masquellier J, Dumon MC, Dumas J. Acta Therapeut 1981; 7: 101–105.
61. Schlebusch H, Kern D. Angiologica 1972; 9: 248–256.
62. Gali HU, Perchellet EM, Gao XM et al. Planta Med 1994; 60 (3): 235–239.
63. Vibes J, Lasserre B, Gleye J et al. Prostagland Leukot Essent Fatty Acids 1994; 50 (4): 173–175.
64. Laparra J, Michaud J, Masquelier J. Plantes méd phytothér 1977; 11: 133.
65. Middleton E Jr. Trends Pharmacol Sci 1984; 5(8): 335–338.
66. Iwamoto M, Ishizaki T, Sato T. Planta Med 1981; 42 (1): 1–16.
67. Loew D. Der Kassenarzt 1994; 15: 43–52.
68. Weikl A, Noh HS. Herz Gefabe 1993; 11: 516–524.
69. Leuchtgens H. Fortschr Med 1993; 111 (20–21): 352–354.
70. Tauchert M, Ploch M, Hubner WD et al. Munch Med Wochenschr 1994; 136 (suppl 1): S27–S33.
71. Forster A, Forster K, Buhring M et al. Munch Med Wochenschr 1994; 136 (suppl 1): S21–S26.
72. Schmidt U, Kuhn M, Ploch M et al. Phytomed 1994; 1: 17–24.
73. Bodigheimer K, Chase D. Munch Med Wochenschr 1994; 136 (suppl 1): S7–S11.
74. Rudolph HT, Erben C, Buhring M. International Congress on Phytotherapy, Munich, September 10–13, 1992.
75. Kleiger RE, Miller JP, Bigger JT Jr et al. Am J Cardiol 1987; 59(4): 256–262..
76. Hanack T, Bruckel MH. Therapiewoche 1983; 33: 4331–4333.
77. Weikl A, Assmus KD, Neukum-Schmidt A et al. Fortschr Med 1996; 114 (24): 291–296.
78. Schmidt U, Albrecht M, Podzuweit H et al. Z Phytother 1998; 19: 22–30.
79. Wolkerstorfer H. MMW 1966; 108: 438–441.
80. Jaursch U, Landers E, Schmidt R et al. Med Welt 1969; 27: 1547–1552.
81. Graham JDP. Br Med J 1939; 951–953.
82. Schlegelmilch R, Heywood R. J Am Coll Toxicol 1994; 13 (2): 103–111.
83. Schimmer O, Hafele F, Kruger A. Mutat Res 1988; 206 (2): 201–208.
84. Popp R, Paulini H, Volkl S et al. Planta Med 1989; 55: 644–645.
85. Yu CL, Swaminathan B. Food Chem Toxicol 1987; 25(2): 135–140.

Horsechestnut seed (*Aesculus hippocastanum* L.)

SYNONYMS

Hippocastani semen (Lat), Roßkastaniensamen (Ger), graine de marronier d'Inde, aescule (Fr), eschilo (Ital), hestekastanje (Dan).

WHAT IS IT?

The horsechestnut tree (*Aesculus hippocastanum* L.) is mainly grown as an ornamental in parks and gardens in Europe, although it is in fact a native of Asia minor. Horsechestnut seeds and bark have been extensively used in European traditional medicine since the 16th century and a wine based on the flowers was imbibed for neuralgia and arthritis. The flowers and flower buds are now used to make two of the Bach Flower Remedies. However, this monograph will only describe the herbal use of the seed. Unlike true chestnuts, the seeds of the horsechestnut are not edible, although a specially prepared seed meal has been used as fodder.

EFFECTS

Increases venous tone, increases capillary resistance, decreases capillary permeability, improves circulation by toning veins; decreases oedema from lymphatic congestion or of inflammatory origin.

TRADITIONAL VIEW

Horsechestnut seed (hereafter referred to as horsechestnut) was traditionally used in the treatment of rheumatism and neuralgia and conditions of venous congestion, particularly with dull, aching pain and fullness. Other major uses include rectal complaints (particularly haemorrhoids, rectal neuralgia and proctitis) and reflex conditions attributed to rectal involvement (including headache, spasmodic asthma, dizziness, disturbed digestion). It was regarded as a remedy for congestion and engorgement. Uneasy and throbbing sensations, with dull aching pain in any part of the body, but especially in the hepatic region, was one specific indication.[1,2]

SUMMARY ACTIONS

Venotonic, antioedematous, antiinflammatory.

CAN BE USED FOR

INDICATIONS SUPPORTED BY CLINICAL TRIALS

Chronic venous insufficiency, varicose veins, oedema of the lower limbs. Prophylactic use to decrease the incidence of deep venous thrombosis following surgery. Topically for haematoma, contusions, non-penetrating wounds and sports injuries involving oedema.

TRADITIONAL THERAPEUTIC USES

Venous insufficiency (especially varicose veins, haemorrhoids); rheumatism; neuralgia; rectal complaints; disease states associated with inflammatory congestion.

MAY ALSO BE USED FOR

EXTRAPOLATIONS FROM PHARMACOLOGICAL STUDIES

To improve circulation by improving venous tone (peripheral vascular disorders, slow-healing leg ulcers); disorders where local tissue oedema may be involved (e.g. carpal tunnel syndrome, Bell's palsy, dysmenorrhoea, intervertebral disc lesions); conditions requiring treatment of the early phase of inflammation such as soft tissue injuries, swelling, minor surgery.

OTHER APPLICATIONS

Skin care products: for normal skin, baby skin, sensitive skin; to tone the skin; as an antiinflammatory; to treat fragile capillaries, pimples, sunburn or cellulite.[3]

PREPARATIONS

Decoction of dried or fresh seeds, liquid extract and tablets for internal use. Decoction, extract, cream, gel or ointment for topical use.

DOSAGE

- 1–2 g of dried seed per day.
- Horsechestnut tablets (200 mg of 5:1 concentrated extract, standardized to contain 40 mg escin): 2–3 tablets per day.

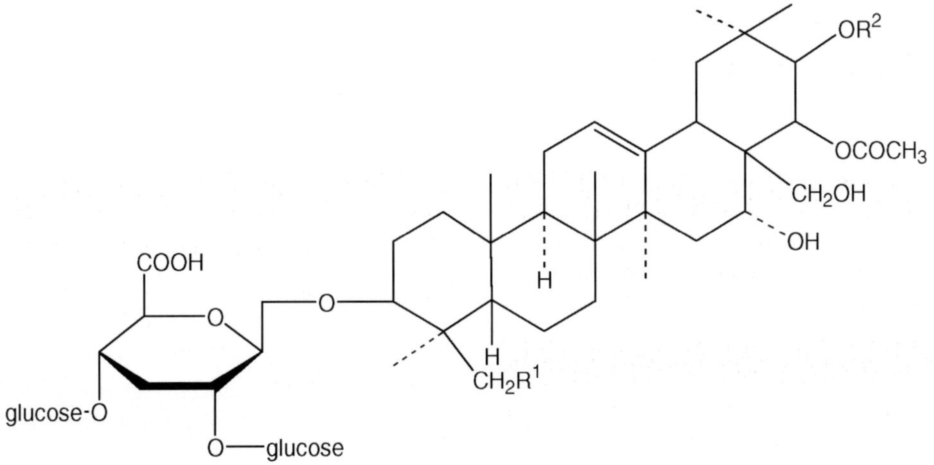

R^1 = OH (aglycone: barringtogenol C)
R^1 = H (aglycone: protoaescigenin)
R^2 = tigloyl, angelicoyl, 2-methylbutyryl, or isobutyryl

Escin (aescin)

β-aescin: major glycosides consist of aglycones protoaescigenin or barringtogenol C esterified with tiglic acid, angelic acid, 2-methylbutyric acid or isobutyric acid

- 2–6 ml of 1:2 liquid extract, 5–15 ml of 1:5 tincture per day.
- Preparations containing 100 mg of escin per day.

DURATION OF USE

There is no suggestion that the long-term use of horsechestnut should be restricted.

SUMMARY ASSESSMENT OF SAFETY

Despite its inclusion in texts on poisonous plants, there is a very low risk associated with the oral or topical administration of horsechestnut seed.[4]

TECHNICAL DATA

BOTANY

The horsechestnut, a member of the Hippocastanaceae (buckeye family), is a deciduous tree with grey bark which grows to 25 m. The leaves are opposite and palmate with 5–7 strongly ribbed leaflets. The flowers are white with yellow to pink spots, contain five petals and are arranged in noticeable panicles up to 30 cm long. The fruit has a leathery, prickly capsule and contains 1–2 brown seeds with large whitish scar.[5,6]

KEY CONSTITUENTS

- Saponins (3–6%), referred to as escin (which is a complex mixture of over 30 individual pentacyclic triterpene diester glycosides).[7]
- Flavonoids, lipids, sterols.[8,9]

PHARMACODYNAMICS

Escin (also spelt 'aescin') is a registered drug in Germany and is the active ingredient in a number of preparations used either topically or orally for the treatment of peripheral vascular disease, in particular that related to altered capillary permeability and resistance. But it is mainly used by injection for conditions associated with oedema.

Venotonic, vascular protective and antioedema activity

Escin reduces the localized oedema associated with inflammation[10] and acts by reducing capillary permeability to water, thus decreasing exudation into intercellular spaces.[11] Escin induced contraction of isolated portal vein and stimulated the generation and release of prostaglandin F_2-alpha in vitro. Thus the antiexudative activity of escin may be mediated by prostaglandin F_2-alpha.[12] Escin administered by injection has inhibited oedema induced by several agents in rat paw, but was not effective in models representing the late reparative phase of inflammation.[13,14] This suggests that it acts on the initial stages of inflammation. Parenteral administration of escin to rats indicated the antiexudative activity to be the result of an influence on the small pores of the capillary wall through which fluid is exchanged.[15] Tests conducted on adrenalectomized and hypophysectomized animals indicate that normal production of corticosteroids is necessary for its antioedema activity. Escin thus mimics and relies upon the activity of corticosteroids.[16–18] Oral administration of escin has demonstrated antiexudative and antiinflammatory activity in vivo. The activity occurred in both prophylaxis and treatment and was due to a beneficial effect on permeability and diuresis.[19] Topical application of escin significantly inhibited exudation in vivo.[20]

In a randomized, double-blind, placebo-controlled crossover study, the influence of oral doses of escin on capillary resistance was tested on 12 healthy subjects. After 7 days of treatment with escin, capillary resistance was significantly improved as measured by the petechiae test. There was no effect from the placebo.[21]

The whole extract of the horsechestnut also shares these properties of escin. In fact, some writers suggest that the combination of escin with flavonoids, as found in the natural plant extract, is a superior treatment to escin alone. Horsechestnut extract demonstrated venotonic activity in vitro by inducing contraction of isolated vein preparations. Perfusion with horsechestnut extract increased the venous pressure of normal veins and, with prior administration, pathological veins also. During perfusion in inverse direction to the bloodstream, a clear contracting effect on the valves was obtained. Horsechestnut extract (2.5, 5.0 mg/kg IV) increased femoral venous pressure and flow, as well as thoracic lymphatic flow, with no change in arterial parameters.[22]

Oral administration of a standardized horsechestnut extract (50–400 mg/kg, containing 70% escin) reduced the cutaneous capillary hyperpermeability induced in rat and rabbit. It also increased skin capillary resistance in guinea pigs fed a vitamin C-deficient diet, as measured by the petechiae method. The extract (200–400 mg/kg) decreased the formation of oedema of lymphatic or inflammatory origin induced in rat hind paw. The horsechestnut extract suppressed plasmatic extravasation and leucocyte emigration into the pleural cavity in experimental pleurisy (200–400 mg/kg oral and 1–10 mg/kg IV) and decreased connective tissue formation in subchronic inflammatory granuloma (400 mg/kg oral and 5–10 mg/kg SC).[22]

Pharmacological and clinical studies indicate that oral administration of horsechestnut extract improved the tone of connective tissue and improved circulation by toning the veins. In a double-blind, placebo-controlled study, a decrease in the vascular capacity (i.e. increased flow) and in filtration coefficients was observed in volunteers with healthy circulation treated with standardized horsechestnut extract (600 mg per day, containing 100 mg escin).[23,24] The antioedematous activity demonstrated by standardized horse-chestnut extract in chronic venous insufficiency was mainly dependent on the inhibition of proteoglycan degradation and lysosomal enzyme activity.[25]

The effect of oral administration of horsechestnut extract (total of 360 mg, containing 90 mg escin) to 14 healthy volunteers on the venous tone of a segment of the lower leg was compared to placebo controls. Horsechestnut resulted in significant reduction of the pressure-dependent vein capacity ($p<0.02$), which is an indication of reduced deformation of the veins and an increase in vein tonus. An intravenous infusion of escin did not result in a noticeable change.[26]

In a double-blind, placebo-controlled trial on 20 healthy volunteers, 100 mg of horsechestnut extract (containing 16% or 70% escin) demonstrated similar venotonic activity on peripheral venous pressure-volume curves as placebo.[27] The lack of a positive effect may reflect on inadequate dosage.

In an uncontrolled trial, the velocity of blood in varicose veins of the lower extremities of patients was assessed after patients received horsechestnut extract for 12 days. Blood viscosity was significantly lowered and correlated to subjective improvement in 73% of cases.[28] A single dose of standardized horsechestnut extract (600 mg containing 100 mg escin) prevented or significantly reduced the increase in ankle and foot oedema ($p<0.05$) in healthy humans during a 15-hour air flight. The study was of randomized, double-blind design and the oedema was compared to the preflight circumference.[29]

Antioxidant activity

Horsechestnut extract demonstrated strong active oxygen-scavenging activity and protective activity in vitro against cell damage induced by active oxygen.[30] Standardized horsechestnut extract (containing 70% escin) inhibited enzymatic and non-enzymatic lipid peroxidation in vitro and counteracted the deleterious effects of free radical oxidative stress in mice and rats (200–400 mg/kg oral, 25 mg/kg IV, respectively).[22]

Other activity

The inhibitory effects of plant constituents on the activity of the connective tissue enzymes elastase and hyaluronidase was investigated in vitro. Saponin constituents from horsechestnut showed inhibitory effects on hyaluronidase. The activity was mainly linked to escin and, to a lesser extent, its genin, escinol.[31]

Triterpene oligoglycosides from horsechestnut (escin Ia, Ib, IIa and IIb) exhibited an inhibitory effect on ethanol absorption and hypoglycaemic activity on oral glucose tolerance test in rats.[32] Saponins can inhibit absorption of small molecules (see Ch. 2).

The saponin components hippocaesulin and barringtogenol-C 21-angelate have demonstrated cytotoxic activity in vitro.[33] For an aqueous-alcoholic extract of horsechestnut (5% w/w), an antiirritant effect was observed in a cosmetic test for irritancy.[34]

PHARMACOKINETICS

Very high concentrations of escin were measured in skin and muscle tissue underlying the site of topical application of radiolabelled sodium escinate. Low values were measured in internal organs, blood, urine, skin and musculature from other parts of the body. A range of 0.5–1% of the applied dose was excreted in urine within 24 hours of administration. The total elimination (bile and urine) was calculated at 1–2.5% of the dose. Less than one half is excreted as escin, the remainder as metabolites.[35] However, the availability of escin to skin and muscle tissue may not be as high as reported in this study, since the radioactivity detected may have been carried by the metabolites of escin as well as by escin itself.

Studies indicate that escin is eliminated quickly following intravenous injection, with two-thirds excreted via the bile and one-third by renal elimination.[36] Two recent studies of the bioavailability of beta-escin following oral doses of various horsechestnut preparations have been conducted using healthy volunteers. Validated radioimmunosorbent assay (RIA) was used to determine levels of beta-escin in plasma. One study in 18 subjects on two solid-dose preparations found a large variation in absorption parameters for beta-escin. Maximum concentration (C_{max}) after a dose containing 50 mg escin varied from 0.19 to 45.1 ng/ml, time for maximum concentration (T_{max}) varied from 0.73 to 8.5 hours and the area under the curve (AUC, an assessment of concentration over time) varied from 24.6 to 389 ng/h/ml.[37] The second study, also on two solid-dose preparations (one sustained-release), and using 24 volunteers found more consistent results. This may have been because horsechestnut extract containing a defined dose of escin was used, rather than just escin alone. Parameters for the sustained-release tablet were superior. For example, after a dose containing 50 mg escin, C_{max} for the sustained-release tablet was 9.81 ± 8.9 ng/ml, T_{max} was 2.23 ± 0.9 h and AUC averaged 187.1 ng/h/ml.[38] The half-life for both preparations was about 20 hours.

Saponins are large molecules containing highly polar groups and their intact bioavailability can be expected to be low after oral doses. This was confirmed in the above studies, since the pharmacokinetic parameters indicate an absorption of less than 1% of the administered dose. However, saponins can be hydrolysed by intestinal flora, leaving the less polar aglycone or sapogenin available for absorption. These sapogenins, or their hepatic metabolites, may in fact be the main active form of escin following oral doses. More studies are needed to clarify this issue.

CLINICAL TRIALS WITH ESCIN

In a placebo-controlled trial in patients undergoing surgery of the hand, intravenous administration of escin produced a fast reduction in postoperative inflammation and oedema.[39] Escin is mainly used by injection; for example, to treat road accident victims with severe head injury, where it reduced the dangerous rise in intracranial pressure, leading to a more favourable prognosis.[40] Escin has been effective in the treatment of cerebral oedemas following cranial fractures and cranial traumas with or without retrograde amnesia, cerebral tumours, intracranial aneurysms, cerebral sclerosis, subdural haematomas, encephalitis, meningitis and cerebral abscesses. Depending on the seriousness of the condition, disappearance of cephalgia, vertigo and general discomfort were observed within 3–16 days. Cerebral oedemas due to acute vasomotor insufficiency were resolved quickly, while in chronic diseases remission occurred slowly over a long period of administration.[41]

Topical preparations of escin have been successfully used for a variety of applications: treatment of oedema and haematoma in surgical practice,[42] the prevention and treatment of sports injuries, including acute injuries, blunt injuries (non-penetrating wounds) and oedema.[43–48] It has been used alone and in combination with heparin, buphenin, salicylate or polyunsaturated phosphatidylcholine in venous disorders (inflammation of veins, venous insufficiency, varicose veins);[49–52] in combination with *l*-thyroxine for the treatment of hypertrophic scars, keloid scars, stretch marks and lymphoedema after mastectomy,[53–55] in combination with heparin and phospholipids for the treatment of joint and venous diseases,[56,57] anorectal varicose pathologies, particularly in gynaecology and obstetrics,[58–60] postoperative treatment of episiotomies[61] and in oral and periodontal surgery.[62]

In a randomized, double-blind trial, 81 patients with contused traumas following limb injuries received treatment with an escin gel or placebo gel for 9 days. Compared to placebo, the mobility of the injured extremity increased significantly in comparison to the uninjured extremity in those treated with escin ($p<0.02$). The circumferences of the lower extremities returned to almost normal (compared to the uninjured leg) in the treatment group but remained unchanged in the placebo group. Escin treatment was also superior for reduction in lower leg swelling, subjective complaints and remission frequencies ($p<0.05$).[63]

Topically applied 2% escin gel was compared to placebo in experimentally induced haematoma in a randomized, double-blind trial. Efficacy was measured over 9 hours after a single application of gel. The escin gel significantly reduced tenderness to pressure within 1 hour and then at all other times during the trial.[64]

CLINICAL TRIALS WITH HORSECHESTNUT

Venous insufficiency

Chronic venous insufficiency is an imprecise term which is frequently referred to and not easily defined. It refers to the impairment of venous return usually from the legs, often with oedema and sometimes with stasis ulcers at the ankle. Other terms used are chronic deep vein incompetence and peripheral venous incompetence. In an uncontrolled trial on 35 patients with chronic venous insufficiency, standardized horsechestnut extract was effective against foot oedema. Haematocrit, body weight and serum potassium were unchanged.[65] In another uncontrolled trial on healthy volunteers and patients with varicose veins, administration of standardized horsechestnut extract demonstrated an increase in venous tone (as measured by plethysmography and radioactive blood flow rate) without arterial constriction or change in blood pressure.[66]

Standardized horsechestnut extract (600 mg per day, containing 100 mg escin, for 3 weeks) significantly reduced the subjective symptoms of patients with varicose veins ($p<0.001$) in a double-blind, placebo-controlled trial.[67] In another double-blind, placebo-controlled trial, 40 patients with leg oedema caused by chronic deep venous incompetence received either standardized horsechestnut extract (738–824 mg per day, containing 150 mg escin) or placebo over 7 weeks. Significant reduction in average leg volume was observed for the treated group compared to placebo, both before and after an oedema provocation test ($p<0.01$). Leg pressure at rest was decreased (indicating better venous tone) and pronounced alleviation of symptoms occurred in the treated group.[68]

The efficacy of standardized horsechestnut extract was investigated in a randomized, double-blind, placebo-controlled trial on 22 patients with proven chronic venous insufficiency. Three hours after taking 600 mg of horsechestnut extract (containing 100 mg escin), a significant decrease in the capillary filtration coefficient (22%) was observed in the treated group.[69] In a randomized, double-blind, placebo-controlled trial, treatment with standardized horsechestnut extract (600 mg per day, containing 100 mg escin) in 20 patients over a 4-week period resulted in significant improvement in volume changes of the foot and ankle ($p<0.001$), compared to the 20 patients treated with placebo. Symptoms such as oedema, pain, fatigue, feeling of tension and itching were also significantly improved ($p<0.05$). There were, however, no changes in venous capacity or calf muscle spasm.[70]

Seventy-four patients with chronic venous insufficiency and lower leg oedema participated in a randomized, double-blind, placebo-controlled trial. An antioedema effect was observed for those treated with standardized horsechestnut extract (600 mg per day, containing 100 mg escin) for 8 weeks. Leg volume was reduced, while in the placebo group it was increased. The progress of the oedema was slowed in the treatment group, as were the subjective symptoms.[71] In a randomized, double-blind, placebo-controlled, crossover trial on 20 women with pregnancy-induced varicose veins or chronic venous insufficiency, treatment with standardized horsechestnut extract for 4 weeks resulted in significant reduction in leg volume ($p<0.01$).[72] The influence of standardized horsechestnut extract (approximately 600 mg per day, standardized to 100 mg escin for 4 weeks) was tested in a randomized, placebo-controlled trial involving 30 patients with peripheral venous incompetence. Horsechestnut effected a reduction in leg circumference and improvement in subjective symptoms.[73] In a double-blind trial using the same dosage over 20 days involving 30 outdoor patients suffering from chronic venous incompetence, a significant reduction of leg circumference was shown ($p<0.05$).[74]

One hundred and eighteen patients with varicose veins or chronic venous insufficiency were treated for 40 days with 60 mg per day of standardized horsechestnut extract (containing 70% escin) or placebo. The trial was double-blinded. Significant improvement in symptoms (oedema, cramps, pain, fatigue, sensation of heaviness) was observed in the treated group ($p<0.05$).[75] The dosage quoted for this trial is a low dose in comparison to the majority of trials conducted. Similar results were observed in a double-blind, placebo-controlled, crossover trial for those treated with horsechestnut. Improvement was observed for: oedema and pain ($p<0.01$), itchiness, fatigue and sensation of heaviness ($p<0.05$). Calf cramping, however, was not significantly improved.[76]

Treatment with standardized horsechestnut extract (600 mg per day, containing 100 mg escin) for 2 weeks was superior to placebo in pregnant women with oedema due to venous insufficiency. Reduction in oedema and symptoms such as pain, fatigue and itching were observed in the treatment group and these patients also showed a greater resistance to oedema provocation. The trial was double-blinded and crossover in design.[77]

In a randomized, partially blinded, placebo-controlled parallel study published in *The Lancet*, 240 patients with chronic venous insufficiency took part in a comparison of the efficacy of compression stockings class II and standardized horsechestnut extract (600 mg per day, containing 100 mg escin) over 12 weeks. Lower leg volume decreased by a similar amount (43–47 ml) for both horsechestnut and compression therapy compared to placebo. A significant reduction in oedema was observed for horsechestnut ($p=0.005$) and compression ($p=0.002$) compared to placebo and the two therapies were shown to be equivalent ($p=0.001$). Compression achieved high oedema reductions at the beginning of the study, while horsechestnut gradually decreased oedema volume, reaching a maximum by the end of the trial. (Patients allocated to compression treatment received a diuretic once daily during the first week of the trial to ensure the best possible stocking fit. Class II stockings provide a certain pressure.) Compliance was better for the herbal therapy.[78]

In a case observation study involving more than 800 German general practitioners, more than 5000 patients with chronic venous insufficiency were treated with standardized horsechestnut extract and followed up at regular intervals. All the symptoms investigated (pain, tiredness, tension, swelling in the leg, itching, tendency towards oedema) improved markedly or completely disappeared. Horsechestnut extract was considered an economical, practice-relevant therapeutic tool which, in comparison with compression therapy, has the additional advantage of better compliance.[79] In a postmarketing surveillance study, 1183 patients with chronic venous insufficiency received the recommended dosage of horsechestnut extract over a 5-month period. A clear reduction in the objective and subjective symptoms was proven.[80]

A review of oedema-protective agents (diosmin, beta-hydroxyethyl rutosides and horsechestnut extract) used in double-blind, placebo-controlled clinical trials for the treatment of chronic venous insufficiency indicates they combine proven therapeutic efficacy with excellent safety of use and have a favourable benefit:risk ratio. The extent of oedema reduction in patients is equivalent to that achieved by compression therapy with elastic stockings. Combined treatment with oedema-protective agents and compression therapy has a better clinical benefit compared to either treatment alone.[81] A review of medicines used in the treatment of chronic venous diseases of the lower limb found horsechestnut extract moderates the development of tissue oedema.[36]

Both standardized horsechestnut extract (720–824 mg per day, containing 150 mg escin) and beta-hydroxyethyl rutosides (2000 mg per day) demonstrated an oedema-protective effect in a randomized, double-blind trial on 40 patients with chronic venous insufficiency and peripheral venous oedema.[82] In a multicentre, randomized, double-blind trial, the comparative efficacy of oxerutins (hydroxylethyl derivatives of rutin) and horsechestnut extract was investigated in 137 postmenopausal patients with grade II chronic venous insufficiency. Patients received either 600 mg per day of standardized horsechestnut extract (containing 100 mg escin), 1000 mg per day of oxerutins for 12 weeks or 1000 mg per day of oxerutins for 4 weeks followed by 500 mg per day (of oxerutins) for 8 weeks. All treatments achieved a mean leg volume reduction of about 100 ml after 12 weeks of treatment, comparable to that achieved in compression therapy. The 6-week follow-up period without treatment indicated that both treatments also exhibit a substantial carry-over effect.[83]

Deep vein thrombosis

Over a 3-year period, a controlled trial of 4176 patients with thrombosis, lung infarction or lung embolism investigated prophylactic treatment for thrombosis and embolism arising from surgery. Patients received an intravenous injection of horsechestnut extract (10 ml per day), strophanthin or digitalis, vitamin B complex and vitamin C or a similar injection without the horsechestnut extract for 4 days prior to surgery and continuing for up to 7 days after the operation. Horsechestnut significantly reduced the incidence of deep venous thrombosis following surgery compared to the control group (lung embolism patients: $p<0.01$; other patients: $p<0.001$).[84]

Topical use

A gel containing horsechestnut extract and heparin was found to be effective in the treatment of acute and chronic traumas and venopathies in an uncontrolled study. In particular, the gel quickly broke down haematomas.[85] The tolerance and efficacy of a topical horsechestnut preparation were assessed in 15 patients with first and second-degree chronic venous insufficiency. The horsechestnut preparation contained 1.4% triterpene glycosides calculated as escin and was compared with a preparation containing heparin. Efficacy was assessed via the change in circumference of the lower, middle and upper leg and by changes in symptoms. Both treatments were well tolerated and the horsechestnut preparation showed a higher tendency to improvement than the heparin.[86]

TOXICOLOGY

Oral administration of sodium salt of escin to rats (10 mg/kg, 70 mg/kg) did not induce any substantial changes in carbohydrate and lipid metabolism and steatosis did not develop.[87] Intraperitoneal administration of 10 mg/kg escin to juvenile male rats did not affect fertility or produce any nephrotoxic activity.[88]

Horsechestnut seeds have low acute and chronic toxicities and the therapeutic index is high.[4] Escin also has a high therapeutic index.[89] The LD_{50} of the water-soluble portion of horsechestnut extract after single oral dose in chicks was 10.6 g/kg body weight and for dried, powdered seed after two consecutive daily doses was 6.5 g/kg.[90] The LD_{50} of horsechestnut seed by oral administration was 990 mg/kg in mice, 2150 mg/kg in rats, 1530 mg/kg in rabbits and 130 mg/kg in dogs. No toxicity was observed in rats administered oral doses of 400 mg/kg of horsechestnut.[91]

CONTRAINDICATIONS

Horsechestnut should not be applied to broken or ulcerated skin.

SPECIAL WARNINGS AND PRECAUTIONS

None required.

INTERACTIONS

None known.

USE IN PREGNANCY AND LACTATION

No adverse effects expected.

EFFECTS ON ABILITY TO DRIVE AND USE MACHINES

No adverse effects expected.

SIDE EFFECTS

As with all saponin-containing herbs, oral use may cause irritation of the gastric mucous membranes and reflux. However, the gastric irritation and reflux can be avoided by the use of enteric-coated preparations. Because of the irritant effect of the saponins, horsechestnut should not be applied to broken or ulcerated skin. Saponins and sapogenins in the bloodstream cause haemolysis but this effect is negligible at the oral doses used. From 1968 until 1989 nearly 900 million individual doses of one brand of standardized horsechestnut extract (Venostasin) were prescribed. In that time, only 15 patients reported significant side effects.[92]

OVERDOSE

Very high doses will result in gastrointestinal irritation. If sufficient quantities of escin are absorbed through damaged or irritated gastrointestinal mucous membranes, haemolysis with associated kidney damage could result.

CURRENT REGULATORY STATUS IN SELECTED COUNTRIES

A draft monograph of horsechestnut is being prepared and may appear in the *European Pharmacopoeia* subsequent to the 1997 edition.

Horsechestnut seed is covered by a positive Commission E monograph and can be used to treat symptoms of venous disorders and chronic venous insufficiency, such as pain and a feeling of heaviness in the legs, night cramps, itching and swelling.

Horsechestnut (unspecified) is on the UK General Sale List.

Horsechestnut does not have GRAS status. However, it is freely available as a 'dietary supplement' in the USA under DSHEA legislation (1994 Dietary Supplement Health and Education Act).

Horsechestnut is not included in Part 4 of Schedule 4 of the Therapeutic Goods Act Regulations of Australia.

References

1. Grieve M. A modern herbal, vol 1. Dover Publications, New York, 1971, p 193.
2. Felter HW. The eclectic materia medica, pharmacology and therapeutics, 1922, Reprinted by Eclectic Medical Publications, Portland, 1983, p 406.
3. Smeh NJ. Creating your own cosmetics – naturally. Alliance Publishing, Garrisonville, 1995, pp 83, 134, 136, 139, 141, 142.
4. Liehn HD. Franco PA, Hampel H et al. Pan Med 1972; 14: 84–91.
5. Launert EL. The Hamlyn guide to edible and medicinal plants of Britain and Northern Europe. Hamlyn, London, 1981, p 57.
6. Fitter R, Fitter A, Blamey M. The wild flowers of Britain and Northern Europe, 2nd edn. Collins, London, 1974, p 36.
7. Hostettmann K, Marston A. Chemistry and pharmacology of natural products: saponins. Cambridge University Press, Cambridge, 1995, p 318.
8. Wagner H, Bladt S. Plant drug analysis: a thin layer chromatography atlas, 2nd edn. Springer-Verlag, Berlin, 1996, p 308.
9. Leung AY, Foster S. Encyclopedia of common natural ingredients used in food, drugs and cosmetics, 2nd edn. John Wiley, New York, 1996, pp 304–306.
10. Vogel G, Marek ML. Arzneim-Forsch 1962; 12: 815–825.
11. Vogel G, Marek ML. Oertner R. Arzneim-Forsch 1970; 20(5): 699–703.
12. Berti F, Omini C, Longiave D. Prostaglandins 1977; 14 (2): 241–249.
13. Lorenz D, Marek ML. Arzneim-Forsch 1960; 10: 263–272.
14. Vogel G et al. Arztliche Forsch 1965; 19: 98.
15. Vogel G, Strocker H. Arzneim-Forsch 1966; 16 (12): 1630–1634.
16. Preziosi P, Manca P. Folia Endocrinol 1964; 17: 527–555.
17. Preziosi P, Manca P. Arzneim-Forsch 1965; 15 (4): 404–413.
18. Preziosi P, Manca P. Arzneim-Forsch 1965; 15 (4): 413–415.
19. Eisenburger R, Hofrichter G, Liehn HD et al. Arzneim-Forsch 1976; 26 (5): 821–824.
20. Przerwa M, Arnold M. Arzneim-Forsch 1975; 25 (7): 1048–1053.
21. Wienert V. Int J Angiol 1997; 6 (2): 115–117.
22. Guillaume M, Padioleau F. Arzneim-Forsch 1994; 44 (1): 25–35.
23. Pauschinger P, Piechowiak, Schnizer W et al. Med Welt 1974; 25 (14): 603–607.
24. Pauschinger P. Ergebnisse Angiolog 1984; 30: 129–137.
25. Enghofer E Seibel K, Hammersen F. Therapiewoche 1984; 34(27): 4130–4144.
26. Ehringer H. Arzneim-Forsch 1968; 18 (4): 432–434.
27. Lochs H Baumgartner H, Honzatt H. Arzneim-Forsch 1974; 24(9): 1347–1350.
28. Klemm J. Munch Med Wochenschr 1982; 124: 579–582.
29. Marshall M, Dormandy JA. Phlebology 1987; 2: 123–124.
30. Masaki H, Sakaki S, Atsumi T et al. Biol Pharm Bull 1995; 18 (1): 162–166.
31. Facino R M, Carini M, Stefani R et al. Arch Pharm 1995; 328(10): 720–724.
32. Yoshikawa M, Murakami T, Matsuda H et al. Chem Pharm Bull 1996; 44 (8): 1454–1464.
33. Konoshima T, Lee KH. J Nat Prod 1986; 49 (4): 650–656.
34. Guillot JP Martini MC, Giaoffert JY et al. Int J Cosmet Sci 1983; 5: 255–265.
35. Lang W. Res Exp Med (Berl) 1977; 169(3): 175–187.
36. Markwardt F. Phlebology 1996; 11: 10–15.
37. Schrader E, Schwankl W, Sieder C et al. Pharmazie 1995; 50 (9): 623–627.
38. Oschmann R, Biber A, Lang F et al. Pharmazie 1996; 51: 577–581.
39. Wilhelm K, Feldmeier C. Med Klin 1977; 72 (4): 128–134.
40. Put TR. Munch Med Wochenschr 1979; 121 (31): 1019–1022.
41. Heppner F, Ascher WP, Argyropoulos G. Wien Med Wochenschr 1967; 117(29): 706–709.
42. Isbary JW. Z Allgemeinmed 1975; 51(14): 684–686.
43. Rothhaar J, Thiel W. Med Welt 1982; 33(27): 1006–1010.
44. Crielaard JM, Franchimont P. Acta Bel Med Phys 1986; 9(4): 287–298.
45. Pabst H, Kleine MW. Fortschr Med 1986; 104(3): 44–46.
46. Arslanagic I, Brkic N. Med Arh 1982; 36(4): 205–208.
47. Zuinen C. Rev Med Liege 1976; 31(5): 169–174.
48. Anonymous. Munch Med Wochenschr 1992; 134: 70, 73.
49. Rocco P. Minerva Med 1980; 71(29): 2071–2078.
50. Scremin S, Piccinni P, Potenza A. Eur Rev Med Pharmacol Sci 1986; 8: 219–224.
51. Paciaroni E, Marini M. Policlin 1982; 89(3): 255–264.
52. Pozza E Menghi R, Pansini GC et al. Acta Chir Ital 1980; 36: 157–166.
53. Baruffaldi M, Turchi G. Gazzetta Med Ital 1982; 141(5): 251–256.
54. Agostini F, Califano L. Clin Eur 1979; 18(6): 1008–1012.
55. Dini D, Bianchini M, Massa T et al. Minerva Med 1981; 72 (35): 2319–2322.
56. Tozzi E, Scatena M, Castellacci E. Clin Ter 1981; 98 (5): 517–524.
57. Wojcicki J, Samochowiec L, Lawczynski L et al. Arch Immunol Ther Exp (Warsz) 1976; 24 (6): 807–810.
58. Tolino A. Minerva Ginecol 1979; 31(3): 169–174.
59. Malin L, Pollinzi V. G Clin Med 1978; 59(11): 521–529.
60. Nappi R. Clin Ter 1978; 86(3): 219–223.
61. Lapas K, Todorov I. Akush Ginekol (Sofiia) 1987; 26(4): 88–89.
62. Bertrand GL. Rev Odontostomatol Midi Fr 1981; 39(4): 211–216.
63. Rothhaar J, Thiel W. Med Welt 1982; 33 (27): 1006–1010.
64. Calabrese C, Preston P. Planta Med 1993; 59 (5): 394–397.
65. Dustman HO, Godolias G, Seibel K. Therapiewoche 1984; 34: 5077–5088.
66. Enghofer E, Seibel K, Hammersen F. Therapiewoche 1984; 34(29): 4360–4372.
67. Alter H. Z Allge Med 1973; 49 (27): 1301–1304.
68. Diehm C, Vollbrecht D, Amendt K et al. Vasa 1992; 21 (2): 188–191.
69. Bisler H, Pfeifer R, Kluken N et al. Dtsch Med Wochenschr 1986; 111 (35): 1321–1329.
70. Rudofsky G, Neiss A, Otto K et al. Phlebol Proktol 1986; 15: 47–54.
71. Lohr E, Garanin G, Jesau P et al. Munch Med Wochenschr 1986; 128: 579–581.
72. Steiner M, Hillemanns HG. Munch Med Wochenschr 1986; 128 (31): 551–552.
73. Erdlen F. Med Welt 1989; 40: 994–996.
74. Pilz E. Med Welt 1990; 41: 1143–1144.
75. Friedrich HC, Vogelsang H, Neiss A. Z Hautkr 1978; 53: 369–374.
76. Neiss A, Bohm C. Munch Med Wochenschr 1976; 118 (7): 213–216.
77. Steiner M, Hillemanns HG. Phlebology 1990; 5: 41–44.
78. Diehm C, Trampisch HJ, Lange S et al. Lancet 1996; 347 (8997): 292–294.
79. Greeske K, Pohlmann BK. Fortschr Med 1996; 114 (15): 196–200.
80. Leskow P. Therapiewoche 1996; 46: 874–877.
81. Diehm C. Phlebology 1996; 11 (1): 23–29.
82. Erler M. Med Welt 1991; 42: 593–596.
83. Rehn R, Unkauf M, Klein P et al. Arzneim-Forsch 1996; 46 (5): 483–487.
84. Kronberger L, Gölles J. Med Klin 1969; 64: 1207–1209.
85. Saffar H. Therapiewoche 1981; 31 (36): 5666–5667.
86. Buchherger, Metzner. 2nd International Congress on Phytomedicine, Munich, September 11–14, 1996.
87. Ulicna O, Volmut J, Kupcova V et al. Bratisl Lek Listy 1993; 94 (3): 158–161.
88. Von Kreybig T, Prechtel K. Arzneim-Forsch 1977; 27: 1465.
89. Hostettmann K, Marston A. Chemistry and pharmacology of natural products: saponins. Cambridge University Press, Cambridge, 1995, p 273.
90. Williams M, Olsen JD. Am J Vet Res 1984; 45 (3): 539–542.
91. German Federal Minister of Justice. German Commission E for human medicine monograph, Bundes-Anzeiger (German Federal Gazette), no. 71, dated 15.04.94.
92. Hitzenberger G. Wien Med Wochenschr 1989; 139 (17): 385–389

Kava
(*Piper methysticum* Forst. f.)

SYNONYMS

Kava, kava kava, intoxicating pepper (Engl), Piperis methystici rhizoma (Lat), Kawa Pfeffer, Rauschpfeffer (Ger), kawa (Fr), pepe kava (Ital), kavarod (Dan), kava, kawa, kava kava (Polynesian), yaqona (Fiji).

WHAT IS IT?

Captain James Cook, in the account of his voyage to the South Seas in 1768, first described for the Western world the ceremonial use of an intoxicating drink prepared from the root of *Piper methysticum*, better known as kava. The kava beverage first causes a numbing and astringent effect in the mouth. This is followed by a relaxed, sociable state where fatigue and anxiety are lessened. Eventually a deep restful sleep ensues from which the user awakens the next morning refreshed and without a hangover. Excessive consumption can lead to dizziness and stupefaction and a syndrome of kava abuse has been described. For this reason some practitioners have been reluctant to use kava therapeutically. However, recent clinical studies from Germany have demonstrated the important value of kava as a safe, non-addictive anxiolytic with an efficacy comparable to benzodiazepines (such as Valium).

Kava is found and used in nearly all the Pacific islands except New Zealand, New Caledonia and most of the Solomon Islands. Use in Hawaii was once common but has now practically disappeared.[1] Potent kava beverages were prepared by first chewing or grinding with a pestle to produce a cloudy, milky mash. Saliva breaks down the starch and facilitates the suspension of the resin. Its cultural role in Pacific societies is compared with the role of wine in southern Europe.

EFFECTS

Decreases anxiety and relaxes the body without loss of mental acuity; a mild analgesic with a local anaesthetic effect on mucous membranes.

TRADITIONAL VIEW

Apart from its ceremonial use, kava has been used medicinally in the Pacific region. In Fiji, it is used to treat kidney and bladder troubles, as a diuretic, for filariasis and as a panacea for a variety of common complaints including coughs, colds and sore throat. A decoction of the pounded roots is reputed to be used as a contraceptive by women who have recently given birth.[2,3] In Samoa the root is used to treat gonorrhoea.[2] At one time, kava was used in Hawaii to treat skin disorders,[4] to soothe nerves, induce relaxation and sleep and to treat general debility, colds and chills.[5] Topical application in Polynesian medicine included skin diseases, leprosy, to prevent suppuration and for vaginal prolapse.[3] In Western herbal medicine, kava was recommended for acute and chronic gonorrhoea, vaginitis (topically), leucorrhoea (topically), nocturnal incontinence (particularly when due to muscular weakness) and other ailments of the genitourinary tract. In addition to these applications, the Eclectics recommended kava for the treatment of neuralgia, toothache, earache, ocular pain, dizziness, despondency, anorexia, dyspepsia, intestinal catarrh, haemorrhoids and renal colic.[6,7]

SUMMARY ACTIONS

Anxiolytic, hypnotic, mild sedative, skeletal muscle relaxant, local anaesthetic, mild analgesic.

CAN BE USED FOR

INDICATIONS SUPPORTED BY CLINICAL TRIALS

Anxiety, nervous tension, restlessness or mild depression of non-psychotic origin; menopausal symptoms.

TRADITIONAL THERAPEUTIC USES

For inflammations and infections of the genitourinary tract of both men and women; pain of muscular and nervous origin; insomnia. Topically for toothache and vaginitis.

MAY ALSO BE USED FOR

EXTRAPOLATIONS FROM PHARMACOLOGICAL STUDIES

Improvement of cognitive performance; relaxes skeletal muscles (and may therefore be of benefit in treating conditions associated with skeletal muscle spasm and tension, such as headaches due to neck tension); treatment of insomnia; to assist in withdrawal from benzodiazepine drugs; pain relief as an analgesic and/or local anaesthetic.

PREPARATIONS

Decoction of dried root; tablets or liquid extract for internal use; liquid extract for external use or as an ingredient in ointments and creams.

DOSAGE

For anxiolytic activity the following doses are recommended:

- 1.5–3 g per day of dried root or in decoction;
- 3–6 ml per day of 1:2 liquid extract;
- standardized preparations containing 100–200 mg of kava lactones per day;
- kava tablets (1.2–1.8 g, standardized to contain 60 mg kava lactones): one tablet 2–4 times per day.

The daily dose should be divided throughout the day. Clinical trials on the standardized extract employed doses at the higher end of this range. For hypnotic activity the same daily quantity can be taken as a single dose 1 hour before bed. For the other effects of kava, similar or higher doses may be required.

DURATION OF USE

Has been used for 6 months in a clinical trial at a dose equivalent to 210 mg lactones/day without adverse effects. Long-term use of a dose equivalent to 400 mg or more of kava lactones per day is likely to cause a scaly skin rash in some subjects.

SUMMARY ASSESSMENT OF SAFETY

Adverse effects from ingestion of kava are not generally expected when used within the recommended dosage. Skin reactions and dopamine antagonism have, however, been reported.

TECHNICAL DATA

BOTANY

Piper methysticum is a cultigen derived from *P. wichmannii*. It is indigenous from New Guinea to Vanuatu and is a member of the Piperaceae (pepper) family. Kava is a dioecious shrub growing up to 3 m in height which is particularly cultivated in Fiji and the western Pacific.[8,9] Kava has pale green to yellowish leaf blades up to 28 cm long, with up to 13 veins spreading from the base. The flower spikes are up to 9 cm long and are borne in the leaf axils.[2] The rootstock (also referred to as stump) has been erroneously called a rhizome by botanists. Kava has no rhizome. From the pithy rootstock extends a fringe of lateral roots up to 3 m long. Rootstock colour varies from white to dark yellow, depending upon the amount of kava lactones present in a lemon-yellow resin. The first inflorescence appears at 2–3 years of age.[10]

KEY CONSTITUENTS

- Resin containing 6-stytyl-4-methoxy-alpha-pyrone derivatives, known as kava pyrones or kava lactones (5–9%, depending on geographical location),[11] including kavain (or kawain), dihydrokavain (DHK), methysticin, dihydromethysticin (DHM), yangonin and desmethoxyyangonin.[12,11]
- Flavonoids (flavokavains).[13]

PHARMACODYNAMICS

Sedative and hypnotic activity

Kava resin and kava lactones had no interaction with GABA (gamma-aminobutyric acid) or benzodiazepine-binding sites in the brain.[14] Later studies, however, suggest that the kava lactones do have an effect on GABA-A receptor binding.[15]

Studies using isolated hippocampal tissue of guinea pigs suggest that kavain and dihydromethysticin may have additive actions and they may enhance the effects of the anxiolytic serotonin-1A agonist ipsapirone. The activation of NMDA receptors and/or voltage-dependent calcium channels may be involved in the elementary mechanism of action.[16,17] (NMDA receptors are a class of glutamate receptors characterized by affinity for N-methyl-D-aspartate.)

Kava extracts or purified lactones demonstrated sedative effects and induced sleep in a variety of in vivo experimental models.[18,19] In one study the total extract of the rootstock was more active than any of the isolated kava lactones.[20] Dihydrokavain (DHK) and dihydromethysticin (DHM) produced sedation and hypothermia in mice[21] and kava lactones given to rabbits produced EEG (electroencephalogram) changes similar to sedative drugs.[22] Kava resin inhibited experimentally induced hypermotility and conditioned avoidance responses in mice. The effect was mild compared to antipsychotic drugs. Higher doses of kava caused marked sedation.[23]

Testing of lactone-free (aqueous) kava extract and kava resin by injection in mice indicated that the major pharmacological effects of reduced motor control and sleep induction are due to the components in the resin.[24] Sedative effects have also been observed from the injection of the aqueous extract of kava.[25]

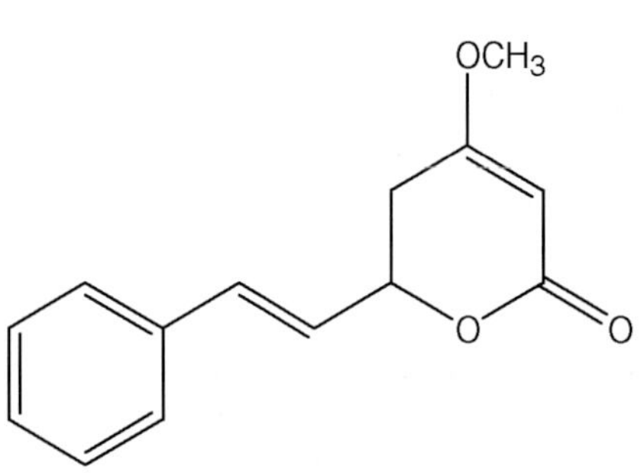

OCH_3 O O

Kavain

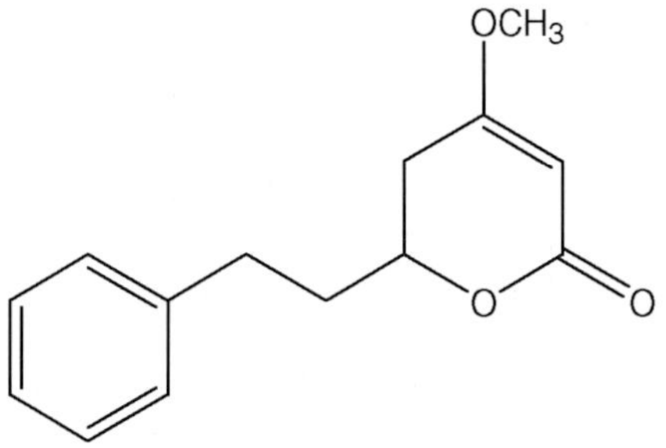

OCH_3 O O

Dihydrokavain

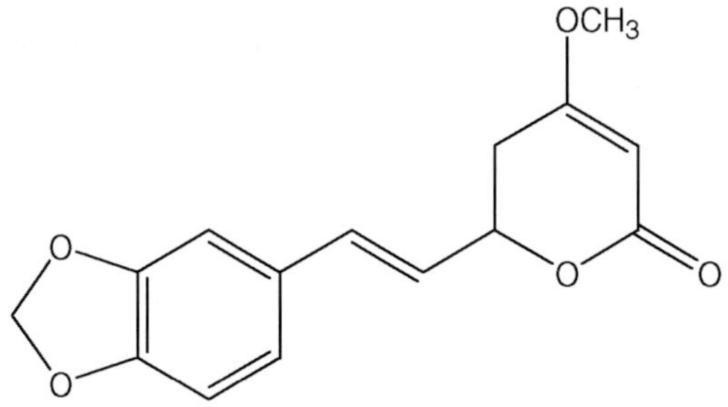

OCH_3 O O O O

Methysticin

Modifications to EEG patterns observed in an experimental model suggest that kava and kavain induce sleep by acting on the limbic system, in particular the amygdala complex. Hence sleep may be promoted by modulation of emotional processes. The effect of kava on the brain is different from that of benzodiazepines or tricyclic antidepressants.[26]

Kava extract and Passiflora extract were tested individually and in combination in a controlled pharmacological study on hypermotility and sleeping time in mice. Both of the herbal extracts exerted statistically significant but different sedative effects. Kava reduced the induced hypermotility to a greater extent than Passiflora, while Passiflora prolonged barbiturate sleeping time to a greater extent than kava. Synergism between the two extracts was observed when they were administered simultaneously.[27]

The efficacy of standardized kava extract was investigated in a placebo-controlled trial with 12 healthy volunteers over 4 days. Placebo was taken for 3 days and followed the next day by three divided doses totalling either 150 mg kava extract (containing 105 mg kava lactones) or 300 mg extract (containing 210 mg kava lactones). With kava administration the lability to fall asleep and the light sleep phase were shortened, the deep sleep phase was lengthened, the duration of REM sleep was not influenced and the duration of wakeful phases in sleep EEG recordings was decreased. These effects were viewed as being favourable, in comparison with orthodox sedatives such as benzodiazepines and barbiturates which depress both REM and deep sleep. Kava administration also increased the density of sleep spindles, an effect which is comparable to orthodox sedatives.[28]

Anxiolytic activity

In a single-blind study with placebo employing six healthy volunteers, a standardized extract of kava improved cognitive performance and stabilized emotional disposition without causing sedation. EEG measurements indicate that an antianxiety activity was produced without sedation or hypnotic effects.[29]

Muscle relaxant, spasmolytic and anticonvulsant activities

Kava extract and lactones have produced relaxation of skeletal muscle in vitro and in vivo, respectively.[30,31] The anticonvulsant activity of kavain was investigated on stimulated synaptosomes and sodium channel receptor sites. The results suggest an interaction of kavain with voltage-dependent sodium and calcium channels, thereby suppressing an induced increase in cytosolic concentrations of sodium and calcium and the release of endogenous glutamate.[32] Further in vitro tests with kavain and its racemate indicate that kavain inhibits veratridine-activated sodium channels non-stereospecifically.[33] Kavain potently inhibited the uptake of labelled noradrenaline from synaptosomes. This non-selective inhibition may be responsible for or contribute to the psychotropic properties of kava lactones.[34]

Kava lactones have demonstrated anticonvulsant activity in several experimental models.[35,36] They were up to 10 times more effective than mephenesin against the convulsant effect of strychnine.[35] A mixture of the lactones (similar to that found in the root) demonstrated a synergistic effect against strychnine-induced convulsions. The potency of the mixture was comparable to the most potent lactone (DHM), which was only 5% of the mixture.[20] When injected intravenously, the differences in the anticonvulsant activity of the lactones are only small.[37] The synergistic effect was more marked when administered orally, due to enhanced absorption of the lactone mixture. (Despite these in vivo results, kava has not proven suitable for treatment of epilepsy in clinical trials.)

Kava lactones have demonstrated spasmolytic activity on smooth muscle similar to papaverine, in vitro.[1] Studies using isolated guinea pig ileum suggest that kavain may exhibit a general inhibitory effect on contractile activity. It may act in a non-specific musculotropic way on the lipid bilayer of the membrane.[38]

Local anaesthetic and analgesic activities

Kava lactones have potencies similar to cocaine and procaine as local anaesthetics[39] and have demonstrated analgesic activity in several experimental models.[24,40,41] As an analgesic, DHK was superior to aspirin but considerably less potent than morphine. Combined administration of DHK with aspirin indicated an additive synergism between the two compounds. Caffeine diminished the duration but not the intensity of the analgesic effects of DHK and DHM.[40] Kava resin, kava lactones and a lactone-free (aqueous) extract of kava all demonstrated analgesic properties in experimental models when given by injection. The analgesia produced by kava occurs via non-opiate pathways.[41]

Effect on performance and vision

Ingestion of 500 ml of traditionally prepared kava beverage by one subject caused changes in visual function. A reduced near-point of accommodation and convergence, an increase in pupil diameter and disturbance of the ocular muscle balance were noted. Maximum changes occurred 30–40 minutes after taking the kava drink.[42] In a double-blind study, 40 healthy subjects received standardized kava extract to assess the effect on performance capability relevant to operating machines and driving. No significant changes were found.[43]

In a double-blind, crossover study to study the effect on event-related potentials in a word recognition task, 12 healthy volunteers received the benzodiazepine drug oxazepam (3 days of placebo, 15 mg on the day before testing, 75 mg on the morning of testing) and standardized kava extract (600 mg per day for 5 days). While there was a significant decrease in the quality and speed of responses with oxazepam in several psychometric tests, no changes were observed with kava treatment. In a memory test using word recognition, there was a tendency for kava to improve reaction time and correct answers which was not statistically significant, whereas oxazepam significantly slowed reaction time and reduced the number of correct answers. The changes in event-related potentials induced by kava during the word recognition task were quite different to changes caused by oxazepam.[44] In another trial of similar design, 12 healthy men were tested in a visual search paradigm assessed by event-related potentials. The results indicate kava had a positive effect on the allocation of attention and processing capacity, while oxazepam reduced the capacity to allocate focal attention and reduced processing capacity.[45]

In a placebo-controlled, double-blind study of 40 healthy volunteers, the effect of a standardized kava extract combined with ethanol (0.05% blood alcohol concentration) on safety-relevant performance parameters was investigated. No negative effects were caused by the kava extract; in fact, it tended to counter the adverse effect of alcohol on mental concentration.[46]

In a randomized, double-blind, crossover clinical study, 12 healthy volunteers received single doses of the following tablets: standardized kava extract (120 mg kava lactones), diazepam (10 mg) or placebo. Neurophysiological and psychophysiological tests were conducted immediately before and 2 and 6 hours after administration of the preparations in order to compare mental alertness. Results for both test groups (kava, diazepam) differed significantly from the placebo group. Differences were also apparent between diazepam and kava. The increase in beta-activity, specific to benzodiazepines, did not occur with kava. In addition, the action of kava was undiminished even 6 hours after application. In one of the psychophysiological tests, performance of complex challenges was better than placebo or diazepam, despite the relaxing properties of kava. The apparently contradictory combination of properties (increased relaxation and increased performance) was confirmed for kava.[47]

The objective of the following study was to evaluate whether simultaneous administration of bromazepam (4.5 mg twice daily) and kava extract (containing 120 mg of kava lactones twice daily) would produce an effect on safety-related performance over and above those anticipated by the single treatment.[48] A double-blind, randomized, three-way cross-over design was used with 18 healthy volunteers. During the course of the study, subjects received either kava, bromazepam or a combination of these. Performance was measured at 0, 1, 2 and 14 days after each treatment, with a 7-day wash-out between treatment periods. Seven computer-assisted mental performance tests were used to assess cognitive performance. These comprised visual orientation, extended concentration, acoustic reaction time, discriminative reaction time, stress tolerance, vigilance and motor coordination. Three of the seven tests showed significant between-treatment differences. Vigilance, stress tolerance and motor coordination worsened with bromazepam and the combination but remained unchanged with kava. Overall, bromazepam and the combination produced the most pronounced impairment of well-being (mainly fatigue). The authors concluded that kava extract plus a benzodiazepine is unlikely to produce greater effects on general well-being and mental performance aspects required for safety than the benzodiazepine alone. Patients are not exposed to additional side effects or risks while taking both treatments at the same time.

Other activity

Kava has been traditionally used as an antibacterial agent, especially for urinary tract infections, but in vitro studies failed to establish significant antibacterial activity.[49,50] Some of the kava lactones exhibited potent fungistatic activity against a wide variety of pathogenic fungi, excluding species of *Candida*.[50] It is possible that the reputed effectiveness of kava in bacterial urinary tract infections is for different reasons. The lactones can undergo chemical changes before being excreted in the urine which may affect antibacterial activity.[51,52]

Kava extract, methysticin and dihydrokavain protected brain tissue against ischaemic damage in experimental models. The results were similar to those produced by the anticonvulsant compound memantine.[53]

In an experimental model, high doses of ethanol potentiated the sedative and hypnotic activity of kava resin and markedly increased the toxicity.[54]

Kava resin did not produce physiological tolerance or learned tolerance in mice when administered at a minimally effective daily dose for 7 weeks or 3 weeks respectively. A considerably higher dose caused partial physiological tolerance.[55]

Antithrombotic activity observed for kavain in vitro is likely to be due to inhibition of cyclooxygenase which suppresses the generation of thromboxane A_2.[56]

PHARMACOKINETICS

After oral doses of kava lactones in rats, approximately half the dose of dihydrokavain was found in the urine within 48 hours, of which two-thirds was hydroxylated metabolites. Lower amounts of urinary metabolites were recorded for the other major lactones.[52] Kava lactones are more rapidly absorbed when given orally as an extract of the root than when given as single compounds. The bioavailability of lactones is up to 3–5 times higher for the extract than when given as single substances.[57]

Kava lactones showed a range of uptake rates into brain tissue when administered as single compounds by intraperitoneal injection to mice. However, when crude kava resin was administered the same way, the concentrations of two lactones were markedly increased (2–20 times), while the others remained at the level of incorporation established for their individual injection.[58]

These results indicate that kava lactones are more bioactive and bioavailable when administered as the root extract rather than as isolated compounds.

CLINICAL TRIALS

Anxiety

Earlier trials used purified kavain at a dose of 400 mg per day. In a placebo-controlled, double-blind study of 84 patients with anxiety symptoms, kavain improved vigilance, memory and reaction time.[59] In comparison with an antianxiety drug (oxazepam) in a placebo-controlled, double-blind trial of 38 patients with anxiety associated with neurotic disturbances, kavain demonstrated equivalent activity.[60] The substances proved to be equivalent in the nature and the potency of their anxiolytic action. Both treatments caused progressive improvement in two different anxiety scores over a 4-week period.

In a randomized, placebo-controlled, double-blind study of 58 patients with anxiety not caused by psychotic disorders, a standardized kava extract significantly improved measures of anxiety and depression.[61,62] Patients received standardized kava extract (300 mg per day, containing 210 mg kava lactones) or placebo over a 4-week period. For patients receiving the kava extract, there was a significant reduction of anxiety as measured by the Hamilton Anxiety Scale (total score, $p<0.02$). The difference in anxiety between kava and placebo began in the first week and increased during the course of treatment. There were no adverse effects reported for the kava extract.

A standardized extract of kava was compared to the benzodiazepine drugs bromazepam and oxazepam in a randomized, controlled, double-blind study. One hundred and seventy-six outpatients were divided into three approximately equal groups. One group received kava extract equivalent to 210 mg of kava lactones per day, the second group received 15 mg of oxazepam per day and the third group received 9 mg of bromazepam. The total Hamilton Anxiety Score was reduced from 27.3 to 15.6 after 6 weeks of kava treatment, compared to 27.3 down to 13.4 for bromazepam and 27.7 down to 16.6 for oxazepam. Statistical analysis showed that kava treatment was equivalent to the benzodiazepine drugs. Side effects were higher in the conventional drug groups.[63]

Although there have been positive outcomes for the use of kava demonstrated in the above controlled trials, none of the trials lasted for more than 6 weeks, the inclusion criteria were insufficiently defined and patient numbers were relatively small. These issues were addressed in a subsequent study. In a randomized, placebo-controlled, double-blind, multicentre study, 100 patients presenting with nervous anxiety, tension and restlessness of non-psychotic origin (DSM-III-R) were followed over a period of 6 months. Patients were randomized to receive either 300 mg per day of a concentrated kava extract containing 210 mg of kava lactones (equivalent to about 4 g of dried root) or placebo. Assessment was based on changes in the cumulative Hamilton Anxiety Score (HAMA) in addition to other assessments. Comparison of the pre- and posttherapy HAMA scores revealed a significant ($p=0.0015$) superiority of the kava treatment as against placebo. The difference between the two treatment groups was even apparent at 8 weeks ($p=0.055$). Kava treatment led to a marked reduction in the symptoms of anxiety, together with its physical and psychic manifestations. In addition, the accompanying depressive component was positively influenced by kava. During the study, six adverse events in five patients were reported in the kava group. Four of these were rated by the investigator as not being related to the treatment, two (in both cases stomach upset) were rated as 'possibly related'. Fifteen adverse events from nine patients were reported in the placebo group. Seven patients dropped out under placebo and three under kava (two of these three were due to improvement of symptoms). There was no significant change in biochemical parameters during the study period and the overall tolerability of kava was rated as excellent. The authors concluded that their results support kava as a treatment alternative to tricyclic antidepressants and benzodiazepines in anxiety, with proven long-term efficacy and none of the tolerance problems associated with these drugs.[64,65]

A number of observational studies have been reported. Treatment of 3029 patients with standardized kava extract (800 mg per day, containing 240 mg kava pyrones) over a minimum of 4 weeks resulted in improvement of primary symptoms such as nervousness, restlessness and anger. Other indications including sleep disturbances, menopausal complaints, muscle tension and sexual disturbances were also improved. Sixty-nine patients recorded undesirable side effects, including allergic reaction, gastrointestinal complaints, headache or dizziness.[66] At the end of almost 5 weeks of treatment with standardized kava extract, symptoms of nervousness, restlessness and fear were reduced in 1673 patients. Mild adverse effects were experienced in 1.7% of patients.[67] Similar improvement in symptoms and a similar percentage of mild adverse reactions were observed in 4049 patients treated with standardized kava extract (150 mg per day, containing 105 mg kava pyrones) for 7 weeks.[68]

Other conditions

Past and recent clinical trials indicate kava extract and kava pyrones (especially dihydromethysticin) are not suitable for the treatment of epilepsy. Although effective in grand mal seizures, the trials were abandoned due to incidence of side effects (mainly skin problems) when used long term and in high doses. No efficacy was observed with petit mal.[69,70]

In a randomized, placebo-controlled, double-blind trial of 40 patients with neurovegetative symptoms associated with menopause, standardized kava extract

(210 mg kava lactones per day for 8 weeks) produced a significant reduction in anxiety ($p<0.01$), depression, severity of symptoms and menopausal symptoms. The subjective well-being of patients improved with kava and the treatment was well tolerated.[71]

TOXICOLOGY

In mice the LD_{50} for oral administration of dihydrokavain was 920 mg/kg and for dihydromethysticin was 1050 mg/kg.[21] Doses of 50 mg/kg of dihydrokavain three times a week for 3 months to rats produced no evidence of chronic toxicity.[72] The following LD_{50} values of standardized kava extract (containing 70% kava lactones) have been recorded: 16 g/kg (oral, rats), 1.8 g/kg (oral, mice), 370 mg/kg (intraperitoneal, rats) and 380 mg/kg (IP, mice).[73]

CONTRAINDICATIONS

The Commission E lists the following contraindications: pregnancy, nursing, endogenous depression.[74] However, these have resulted from a lack of data, rather than any direct concerns.

SPECIAL WARNINGS AND PRECAUTIONS

Due to possible dopamine antagonism, kava should be used cautiously in elderly patients, especially those with Parkinson's disease (refer to Side effects section).

INTERACTIONS

According to the Commission E, a synergistic effect is possible for substances acting on the central nervous system, such as alcohol, barbiturates and psychopharmacological agents.[74]

USE IN PREGNANCY AND LACTATION

No adverse effects expected, despite the caution from the Commission E.

EFFECTS ON ABILITY TO DRIVE AND USE MACHINES

No negative influence is expected at normal therapeutic doses.

SIDE EFFECTS

Skin reactions

A dry, scaly, pigmented skin condition known as kava dermopathy is a well-known side effect of excessive and chronic use of kava.[75] The cutaneous effects were first reported by members of Captain James Cook's Pacific expeditions. The cause may relate to interference with cholesterol metabolism[76] and is unlikely to occur after normal therapeutic use. It has also been suggested that this rash may be due to a deficiency of one of the B vitamins, but a clinical trial of 100 mg of nicotinamide per day failed to have a significant effect.[77] The rash quickly regresses if kava intake is ceased. A clinical pharmacological evaluation of DHM found that doses of 300–800 mg per day produced a scaly skin rash in a high percentage of subjects.[18]

The adverse effects of heavy kava usage in an Australian aboriginal community have been reported.[78] Kava users were more likely to have adverse biochemical and haematological changes and the typical scaly rash. However, the kava consumption was extremely high, more than 310 g per week for 35 of the 39 kava users. Also, it has been questioned whether all the adverse effects reported were only due to kava consumption,[79] since ethanol in large doses can potentiate the toxicity of kava.[54] (The difference in exhibited behaviour between kava and alcohol intoxication has also been noted: stupor or sleep after kava, aggression or fighting after alcohol.[80])

A case of systemic contact-type dermatitis occurred after oral administration of kava extract.[75] Two cases of a drug eruption in sebaceous gland-rich areas, induced by 3 weeks of systemic kava administration, have been reported. No other cause for the reaction, including reactions from ingestion of orthodox drugs, could be found. In one case, a diagnostic allergy test revealed significant proliferation of peripheral blood lymphocytes in response to kava extract and the second patient had a strongly positive patch test to kava extract after 24 hours. The authors suggest the skin reactions observed from kava ingestion may relate to interference with cholesterol metabolism.[81] Patients sometimes comment that the condition of their hair is poorer while taking kava.

Other reactions

A group of German neurologists have described four cases of patients who developed clinical signs suggestive of dopamine antagonism after taking kava. A 28-year-old man who had a history of acute dystonic reactions after taking anxiolytic drugs also developed involuntary neck extension with forceful upward deviation of his eyes 90 minutes after taking kava for the first time. A 22-year-old woman experienced involuntary oral and lingual dyskinesia, tonic rotation of the head and painful twisting movements of the trunk 4 hours after her first dose of kava. A similar reaction was experienced by a 63-year-old woman after taking kava for 4 days and aggravation of Parkinson's disease occurred in a 76-year-old woman. The authors concluded that the sedative effects of kava might result from dopamine antagonistic properties, which is supported by reports of beneficial effects of kava on schizophrenic symptoms.[82]

A case of possible interaction between kava and a benzodiazepine drug (alprazolam) has been reported. The 54-year-old man was hospitalized in a lethargic and disoriented state. His medications included alprazolam, cimetidine and terazosin. He had not consumed alcohol or any of the medications in excess.[83]

Recent research on abuse in Australian aboriginal communities has revealed links between chronic excessive kava use and increased susceptibility to serious infectious disease; the development of neurological abnormalities; pulmonary hypotension; haematuria, suggesting effects on the kidneys and renal system; ischaemic heart disease and sudden cardiac deaths. In addition to the effect on skin, there have been reports of thrombotic effects, liver damage and effects on eyes and vision.[84] However, many of these effects might also be due to associated heavy alcohol consumption. A case of an acute neurological syndrome associated with heavy kava consumption was reported. The 27-year-old Australian Aboriginal man presented three times with generalized choreoathetosis secondary to kava bingeing. During the episodes he had severe choreoathetosis involving his limbs, trunk, neck and facial musculature, with marked athetosis of the tongue. Other possible medical causes were excluded.[85]

Kava was falsely implicated in health complications in a group of people believed to have consumed a product containing kava at a 'rave' party in Los Angeles on New Year's Eve, 1996. The label of the product included kava as well as two other herbs. Samples tested initially by Los Angeles Police Department and subsequently by the American Botanical Council showed no kava lactones present. The product was found to contain caffeine and 1,4-butanediol (an industrial solvent which is metabolized to gamma-hydroxybutyrate) which were not listed on the label.[86] (Analysis conducted on behalf of the FDA confirmed the presence of the industrial solvent.) A Californian chiropractor was sentenced in February 1998 after pleading guilty to misbranding the product. The industrial solvent was deliberately substituted because he could not obtain the kava/kavain in time.[87]

OVERDOSE

There is no documented evidence of overdose but information from chronic usage and adverse reactions suggest that skin rash, shortness of breath, liver damage[78] and neurological manifestations[85] may occur.

CURRENT REGULATORY STATUS IN SELECTED COUNTRIES

Development of a monograph of kava is pending and it may appear in the *United States Pharmacopeia-National Formulary* subsequent to June 1999.

Kava is covered by a positive Commission E monograph and can be used for anxiety and nervous tension.

Kava is on the UK General Sale List.

Kava does not have GRAS status. However, it is freely available as a 'dietary supplement' in the USA under DSHEA legislation (1994 Dietary Supplement Health and Education Act).

Kava is not listed in State (excluding Western Australia) or Commonwealth government legislation which restricts the use of herbs or herbal material by herbal practitioners in Australia. In early 1998, the relevant Commonwealth department began the process of assessing the scheduling status of preparations containing kava for therapeutic use. Later that year an expert committee agreed that scheduling need not be progressed but required that kava products contain a warning for pregnant and lactating women and a caution for prolonged use. In Western Australia the sale and supply of kava ('traditional substance subject to abuse') is prohibited except with the consent of the relevant government department. Consent could only be given 'to people who use the substance for ceremonial purpose in accordance with their tradition, or for the purpose of medical or scientific research, including clinical trials'. The Therapeutic Goods Administration of the Australian government monitors the importation of kava into Australia and obligates importers of kava to hold a licence. These restrictions regulate the activity of importers and do not directly affect practitioners of herbal medicine.

References

1. Singh YN. J Ethnopharmacol 1992; 37 (1): 13–45.
2. Cambie RC, Ash J. Fijian medicinal plants. CSIRO Australia, 1994, pp 239–240.
3. Lebot V, Merlin M, Lindstrom L. Kava – the Pacific elixir: the definitive guide to its ethnobotany, history and chemistry. Yale University Press, New Haven, 1992, pp 112– 117.

4. Norton SA. Hawaii Med J 1998; 57 (1): 382–386.
5. Titcomb M. J Polynes Soc 1948; 57: 105–171.
6. Grieve M. A modern herbal, vol 2. Dover Publications New York, 1971, pp 454–455.
7. Felter HW, Lloyd JU. King's American dispensatory, 18th edn, 3rd revision, vol 2, 1905, Reprinted by Eclectic Medical Publications, Portland, 1983, pp 1505–1507.
8. Mabberley DJ. The plant book, 2nd edn. Cambridge University Press, Cambridge, 1997, p 560.
9. Leung AY, Foster S. Encyclopedia of common natural ingredients used in food, drugs and cosmetics, 2nd edn. John Wiley, New York, 1996, pp 330–331.
10. Lebot V, Merlin M, Lindstrom L. Kava – the Pacific elixir: the definitive guide to its ethnobotany, history and chemistry. Yale University Press, New Haven, 1992, pp 10–13.
11. Wagner H, Bladt S. Plant drug analysis: a thin layer chromatography atlas, 2nd edn. Springer-Verlag, Berlin, 1996, pp 258–259.
12. Smith RM, Thakrar H, Arowolo TA et al. J Chromatog 1984; 283: 303–308.
13. Lebot V, Merlin M, Lindstrom L. Kava – the Pacific elixir: the definitive guide to its ethnobotany, history and chemistry. Yale University Press, New Haven, 1992, pp 68–69.
14. Davies LP, Drew CA, Duffield P et al. Pharmacol Toxicol 1992; 71 (2): 120–126.
15. Jussofie A, Schmiz A, Hiemke C. Psychopharmacol 1994; 116 (4): 469–474.
16. Walden J, Von Wegerer J, Winter U et al. Prog Neuropsychopharmacol Biol Psychiatry 1997; 21 (4): 697–706.
17. Walden J, Von Wegerer J, Winter U et al. Human Psychopharmacol 1997; 12 (3): 265– 270.
18. Keller F, Klohs MW. Lloydia 1963; 26 (1): 1–15.
19. Hänsel R, Beiersdorff HV. Arzneim-Forsch 1959; 9: 581–585.
20. Klohs MW, Keller WF, Williams RE et al. J Med Pharm Chem 1959; 1 (1): 95–103.
21. Meyer HJ. Arch Int Pharmacodyn 1962; 138 (3–4): 505–535.
22. Kretzschmar R, Teschendorf HJ. Chemtg Z 1974; 98: 24–28.
23. Duffield PH, Jamieson DD, Duffield AM. Arch Int Pharmacodyn Ther 1989; 301: 81–90.
24. Jamieson DD, Duffield PH, Cheng D et al. Arch Int Pharmacodyn Ther 1989; 301: 66–80.
25. Furgiuele AR, Kinnard WJ, Aceto MD et al. J Pharm Sci 1965; 54: 247–252.
26. Holm E, Staedt U, Heep J et al. Arzneim-Forsch 1991; 41 (7): 673–683.
27. Capasso A, Pinto A. Acta Therapeut 1995; 21 (2): 127–140.
28. Emser W, Bartylla K. TW Neurologie Psychiatrie 1991; 5: 636–642.
29. Johnson D, Frauendorf A, Stecker K et al. TW Neurologie Psychiatrie 1991; 5: 349.
30. Meyer HJ, Kretzschmar R. Klin Wochenschr 1966; 44 (15): 902–903.
31. Singh YN. J Ethnopharmacol 1983; 7 (3): 267–276.
32. Gleitz J, Friese J, Beile A et al. Eur J Pharmacol 1996; 315 (1): 89–97.
33. Gleitz J, Gottner N, Ames A et al. Planta Med 1996; 62: 580–581.
34. Seitz U, Schule A, Gleitz J. Planta Med 1997; 63 (6): 548–549.
35. Kretzschmar R, Meyer HJ, Teschendorf HJ. Experientia 1970; 26 (3): 283–284.
36. Kretzschmar R, Meyer HJ. Arch Int Pharmacodyn Ther 1969; 177 (2): 261–267.
37. Meyer HJ, Kretzschmar R. Arzneim-Forsch 1969; 19 (4): 617–623.
38. Seitz U, Ameri A, Pelzer H et al. Planta Med 1997; 63 (4): 303–306.
39. Meyer HJ, May HU. Klin Wochenschr 1964; 42 (8): 407.
40. Bruggenmann F, Meyer HJ. Arzneim Forsch 1963; 13: 407–409.
41. Jamieson DD, Duffield PH. Clin Exp Pharmacol Physiol 1990; 17 (7): 495–507.
42. Garner LF, Klinger JD. J Ethnopharmacol 1985; 13 (3): 307–311.
43. Herberg KW. Z Allg Med 1991; 67: 842–846.
44. Munte TF, Heinze HJ, Matzke M et al. Neuropsychobiol 1993; 27 (1): 46–53.
45. Heinze HJ, Munthe TF, Steitz J et al. Pharmacopsychiatry 1994; 27 (6): 224–230.
46. Herberg KW. Blutalkohol 1993; 30 (2): 96–105.
47. Gessner B, Cnota P. Z Phytother 1994; 15 (1): 30–37.
48. Herberg KW, Winter U. 2nd International Congress on Phytomedicine Munich, September 11–14, 1996.
49. Hansel R. Pacific Sci 1966; 22: 293–313.
50. Hänsel R, Weiss D, Schmidt B. Planta Med 1966; 14: 1–9.
51. Duffield AM, Jamieson DD, Lidgard RO et al. J Chromatogr 1989; 475: 273–281.
52. Rasmussen AK, Scheline RR, Solheim E et al. Xenobiotica 1979; 9 (1): 1–16.
53. Backhauss C, Krieglstein J. Eur J Pharmacol 1992; 215: 265–269.
54. Jamieson DD, Duffield PH. Clin Exp Path Physiol 1990; 17: 509–514.
55. Duffield PH, Jamieson D. Clin Exp Path Physiol 1991; 18: 571–578.
56. Gleitz J, Beile Z, Wilkens P et al. Planta Med 1997; 63 (1): 27–30.
57. Biber A. Internal publications of Dr Willmar Schwabe GmbH & Co, Karlsruhe 1989.
58. Keledjian J, Duffield PH, Jamieson DD et al. J Pharm Sci 1988; 77 (12): 1003–1006.
59. Scholing WE, Clausen HD. Med Klin 1977; 72 (32–33): 1301–1306.
60. Lindenberg D, Pitule-Schodel H. Fortschr Med 1990; 108 (2): 49–50, 53–54.
61. Kinzler E, Kromer J, Lehmann E. Arzneim-Forsch 1991; 41 (6): 584–588.
62. Lehmann E, Kinzler E, Friedemann J. Phytomed 1996; 3 (2): 113–119.
63. Woelk H, Kapoula O, Lehrl S et al. Z Allg Med 1993; 69 (10): 271–277.
64. Volz HP. 6th Phytotherapy Conference, Berlin, October 5–7, 1995.
65. Volz HP, Kieser M. Pharmacopsychiatry 1997; 30: 1–5.
66. Hofmann R, Winter U. 5th Phytotherapy Congress, Bonn, November 3–5, 1993.
67. Spree MH, Croy HH. Der Kassenarzt 1992; 17: 44–51.
68. Siegers CP, Honold E, Krall B et al. Arztl Forsch 1992; 39: 7–11.
69. Kretzschmar R. Pharmakologische Untersuchungen zur zentralnervoses Wirkung und zum Wirkungsmechanismus der Kava-Droge (*Piper methysticum*) und ihrer kristallinen Inhaltsstoffe. In: Loew D, Rietbrock N (eds) Phytopharmaka in Forschung und klinischer Anwendung. Steinkoff (Verlag), Darmstadt, 1995, pp 29–38.
70. Hansel R. Z Phytother 1996; 17: 180–195.
71. Warnecke G. Fortschr Med 1991; 109: 119–122.
72. Meyer HJ. Postdoctoral thesis: Pharmakologie der Kawa-Droge. Pharmakologie Institut der Albert-Ludwig Universität, Freiburg, 1966.
73. Hansel R, Woelk H. Spektrum Kava-Kava (Arzneimitteltherapie heute: Phytopharmaka; Bd. 6). Aesopus Verlag, Basel, 1994, p 40.
74. German Federal Minister of Justice. German Commission E for human medicine monograph, Bundes-Anzeiger (German Federal Gazette) no. 101, dated 01.06.1990.
75. Suss R, Lehmann P. Hautarzt 1996; 47 (6): 459–461.
76. Norton SA, Ruze P. J Am Acad Dermatol 1994; 31 (1): 89–97.
77. Ruze P. Lancet 1990; 335 (8703): 1442–1445.
78. Mathews JD, Riley MD, Fejo L et al. Med J Aust 1988; 148 (11): 548–555.
79. Douglas W. Med J Aust 1988; 149 (6): 341–342.
80. Cantor C. Med J Aust 1997; 167 (10): 560.
81. Jappe U, Franke I, Reinhold D et al. J Am Acad Dermatol 1998; 38 (1): 104–106.
82. Schelosky L, Raffauf C, Jendroska K et al. J Neurol Neurosurg Psychiatry 1995; 58 (5): 639–640.
83. Almeida JC, Grimsley EW. Ann Intern Med 1996; 125 (11): 940–941.
84. D'Abbs P, Burns C. Report on inquiry into the issue of kava regulation. Prepared for the Sessional Committee on the Use and Abuse of Alcohol by the Community, Legislative Assembly of the Northern Territory. Menzies School of Health Research, Darwin, 1997.
85. Spillane PK, Fisher DA, Currie BJ. Med J Aust 1997; 167 (3): 172–173.
86. Blumenthal M. Natural Pharmacy, April 1997, pp 12–15.
87. Nordenberg T. FDA consumer. FDA investigators' reports – July/August 1998 Vol 32, No. 4. FDA, Washington DC, 1998.

Licorice (*Glycyrrhiza glabra* L.)

SYNONYMS

Liquiritia officinalis (botanical synonym), liquorice, sweet root (Engl), Liquiritiae radix, Radix glycyrrhizae (Lat), Suβholzwurzel, Lakritzenwurzel (Ger), réglisse, bois doux (Fr), liquirizia (Ital), Lakrids (Dan), yashimadhu (Sanskrit), gancao (Chin), kanzo (Jap), kamcho (Kor).

WHAT IS IT?

Licorice is one of the herbs most widely used by practitioners of Western herbal medicine and is also a major herb of the Chinese, Kampo and Ayurvedic traditions. It has a long history and was used by the ancient Chinese, Egyptians and Greeks. The generic name Glycyrrhiza is derived from the Greek meaning 'sweet root'. The dried root and stolons are used medicinally. Licorice is also used extensively in food (especially confectionery) and tobacco products. In traditional Chinese medicine, radix glycyrrhizae is defined as *Glycyrrhiza uralensis, G. glabra* or *G. inflata*. (Although they are treated as similar, minor constituents such as the phenolics differ between the species.)

Since the 1950s, scientific investigation into the pharmacological properties of licorice has revealed a wide variety of activities and even resulted in the development of a major antiulcer drug. In this decade, research on licorice and its well-documented side effects has shed new light on the biochemistry of steroid hormones. The informed use of licorice is a powerful aspect of phytotherapy but a full understanding of its side effects is also necessary for safe and effective use.

EFFECTS

Eases inflammation and tissue damage in the upper digestive tract; potentiates the antiinflammatory effect of glucocorticoids; mimics aldosterone (by potentiation of cortisol); facilitates movement of mucus from the respiratory tract.

TRADITIONAL VIEW

Licorice has been used extensively for the treatment of cough, consumption, chest complaints (especially bronchitis) and as a soothing ingredient in cough medicines.[1] The Eclectics used it to reduce irritation of mucous surfaces of the urinary, respiratory and digestive tracts.[2] Licorice was also used for chronic gastritis, peptic ulcer and adrenocortical insufficiency (specifically Addison's disease).[3] In traditional Chinese medicine, licorice tonifies the *Spleen*, benefits the *Qi*, moistens the *Lungs* and stops coughing, clears *Heat* and detoxifies *Fire Poison* (boils, sore throat) and soothes spasms. It moderates and harmonizes the characteristics of other herbs and is also used as an antidote to a variety of toxic substances.[4] In Ayurveda, licorice is used as a tonic and to treat eye diseases, throat infections, peptic ulcer, catarrh of the genitourinary tract, constipation and arthritis.[5,6]

SUMMARY ACTIONS

Antiinflammatory, mucoprotective, adrenal tonic, expectorant, demulcent, mild laxative, anticariogenic.

CAN BE USED FOR

INDICATIONS SUPPORTED BY CLINICAL TRIALS

Indications supported by trials using glycyrrhizin, carbenoxolone or deglycyrrhizinized licorice: gastric and duodenal ulceration; topical use for recurrent mouth ulcers.

Indications supported by trials using licorice: gastric and duodenal ulceration; polycystic ovarian syndrome (uncontrolled trials).

TRADITIONAL THERAPEUTIC USES

Bronchitis, cough; peptic ulcer, gastritis; adrenal insufficiency, Addison's disease; urinary tract inflammation.

MAY ALSO BE USED FOR

EXTRAPOLATIONS FROM PHARMACOLOGICAL STUDIES

Treatment of corticosteroid dependency (to aid the withdrawal of corticosteroid drugs) and to extend the pharmacological effects of steroid drugs; hyperkalaemia (resulting from low aldosterone) associated with NIDDM; inflammatory conditions, such as rheumatoid arthritis; to protect against ulcer-forming medications; liver damage; depression; prevention of carcinogenesis; HIV/AIDS; to prevent bacterial adherence in bladder infections; topical use as an antiviral and antiinflammatory agent.

OTHER APPLICATIONS

As a flavouring agent to disguise the taste of nauseous medicines and senna extract; a component of cough lozenges; as an absorbent excipient in pill manufacture;[7] as a solubilizing agent for aqueous extracts of herb mixtures.

PREPARATIONS

Dried root as a decoction, liquid extract or tablet for internal use. Decoction or liquid extract for external use or as an ingredient in mouthwash, gargle, cream or ointment.

DOSAGE

- 2–6 ml per day of 1:1 liquid extract.
- 1.2–4.6 g per day of deglycyrrhizinized licorice extract BP.

The Commission E indicates that when licorice is used as a flavouring component, a maximum daily dosage of less than 100 mg glycyrrhizin is acceptable.[8]

DURATION OF USE

Higher doses of licorice should not be consumed long term. The Commission E advises that licorice should not be taken for longer than 6–8 weeks without professional supervision.[8] (This relatively short time restriction is probably related to the high dose of licorice recommended by the Commission E: 5–15 g of root, equivalent to 200–600 mg of glycyrrhizia. Using the lower doses recommended above, licorice may be administered for a longer time period without risk of side effects.)

SUMMARY ASSESSMENT OF SAFETY

Since higher doses can cause an aldosterone-like side effect, licorice must be taken within the recommended therapeutic range. Careful assessment of the patient's blood pressure and other medications is required before prescribing licorice. A high potassium intake will minimize the risk of this adverse reaction.

TECHNICAL DATA

BOTANY

Glycyrrhiza glabra is a member of the Leguminosae (pea) family, the Papilionoideae subfamily and grouped in the same tribe as the Astragalus genus.[9] It is a perennial herb with a thick rhizome of dark, reddish-brown colour outside and yellowish inside, from which its stolons and long rootlets spring. The oval-elliptic leaves are opposite, in pairs and contain oil glands. The almost sessile, violet flowers are arranged in a raceme, the tubular calyx has five pointed teeth and the corolla is five-petalled. The fruit is a pod.[10]

KEY CONSTITUENTS

- Triterpenoid saponins: glycyrrhizin,[11] present in the form of potassium and calcium salts;[12] other saponins are also present.[13] The concentration of glycyrrhizin in the root depends on the source and the method of assay[14] and is typically 2–6%.[15,16]
- Glycyrrhetinic acid (18-beta-glycyrrhetinic acid, GA), the aglycone of glycyrrhizin (GL) is also present in the root (0.5–0.9%).[17]
- A wide range of flavonoids (1–1.5%) which impart a yellow colour to the root: flavanones, mainly liquiritin,[11] chalcones and isoflavonoids.[18]
- Sterols.[13]

The *European Pharmacopoeia* recommends that *G. glabra* contain not less than 4% glycyrrhizin.[19] Glycyrrhizin has an intense sweet taste (between 50 and 170 times sweeter than sugar)[20,21] but glycyrrhetinic acid does not. It is also referred to as glycyrrhizic acid or glycyrrhizinic acid.

PHARMACODYNAMICS

The immunostimulating, antiviral, antitumour, antiinflammatory, hepatoprotective and choleretic activity of licorice could possibly be interpreted as correlated to the induction of the glutathione-dependent adenosyl methionine transferase and resultant methylation processes such as those of viral and human DNA and RNA.[22] However, given the chemical complexity of the herb, other underlying mechanisms could also apply.

Antiulcer activity

In the late 1940s a Dutch doctor named Revers noticed that patients with gastric ulcers were being cured by high doses of a licorice extract dispensed by a local pharmacist. Revers conducted a clinical trial on

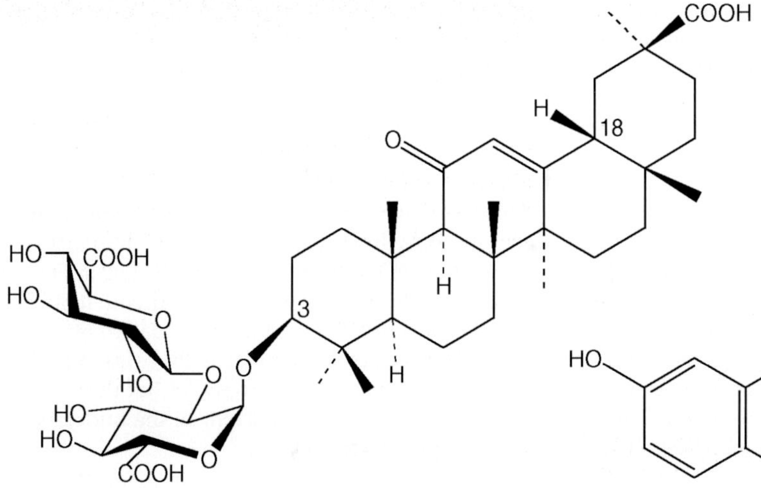

Glycyrrhizic acid

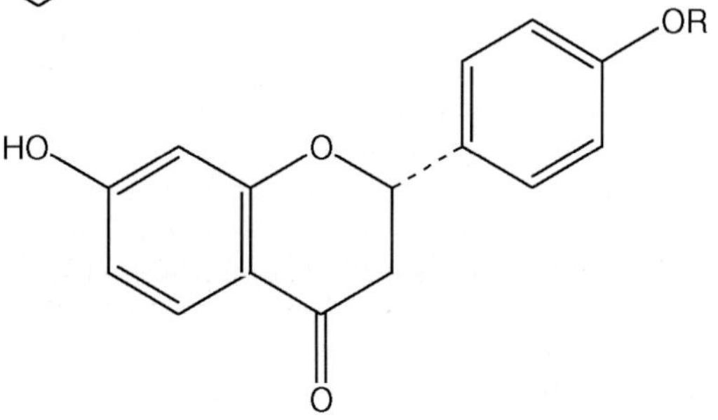

	R
Liquiritigenin	H
Liquiritin	glucosyl

licorice and found it to be effective but he also observed a significant incidence of side effects, mainly fluid retention and hypertension.[23] Revers' study led to the investigation of glycyrrhizin (GL) and glycyrrhetinic acid (GA) as the constituents responsible for ulcer healing and it was found that these compounds, especially GA, also exhibited significant local antiinflammatory activity. However, the relatively poor water solubility of GA prohibited the use of high doses in pharmacological experiments, so English scientists developed a semisynthetic derivative and named it carbenoxolone. Although carbenoxolone was developed with a view to its antiinflammatory properties, it was soon discovered that it was very effective at healing gastric ulcers and it became the major antiulcer drug of the 1960s. It was also shown to heal duodenal ulcers, although this application was more controversial. Unfortunately, carbenoxolone also caused the same side effects as licorice and GL and its use rapidly diminished when cimetidine, the first of the acid inhibitors, became available.

Some investigators were not satisfied that the antiulcer activity of licorice was entirely due to GL. Moreover, GL was responsible for the undesired side effects. This led to the investigation of deglycyrrhinized licorice (DGL), which ironically was a byproduct of the manufacture of carbenoxolone. DGL has been shown to be an effective treatment for both gastric and duodenal ulcers, although its use has always been controversial in medical circles. If GL and carbenoxolone are the factors which increase gastric mucosal resistance, what are the factors in deglycyrrhinized licorice (DGL) which also confer ulcer-healing properties? Is DGL effective? These questions were the subject of much debate in the 1970s. In fact, DGL is not completely free of GL: it is a concentrated extract of licorice (a soft extract) with a GL content not exceeding 3%.[24] It contains a high level of flavonoids.

In 1986 Japanese workers 'rediscovered' the value of using a whole licorice extract for peptic ulcers. This is reasonable given the desirable properties of both GL and DGL. In fact, the evidence casts doubt on the logic of any other approach.

Carbenoxolone is chemically and pharmacologically similar to GL and most of the effects attributed to carbenoxolone would also apply to GL. Carbenoxolone was the first successful modern drug for the treatment of gastric ulcers and acts by restoring gastric physiology to normal.[25] It improves the protective qualities of the gastric mucosal barrier[25] and recent research suggests that these effects may involve the mediation of prostaglandins,[26] specifically the inhibition of 15-hydroxyprostaglandin dehydrogenase and delta-13-prostaglandin reductase. Thus, licorice-derived compounds have the effect of raising the local concentration of those prostaglandins that promote mucus secretion and cell proliferation in the stomach, leading to healing of ulcers.[27] Carbenoxolone was also effective for the treatment of duodenal ulcers[25] but there was debate as to whether this was a local or a systemic effect.

The use of carbenoxolone has largely been supplanted by modern acid-inhibiting drugs. However, there is increasing documentation that the suppression of gastric acid by long-term use of cimetidine may cause detrimental changes in the gastrointestinal epithelium.[28] Moreover, one study found that cimetidine and ranitidine are less effective at healing ulcers than other drug treatments and have a three times higher rate of ulcer recurrence.[29] It can be concluded that licorice might still have an important role in the treatment of peptic ulcers.

In animal studies DGL prevents ulcer development,[30] inhibits gastric acid secretion[31] and protects the gastric mucosa against damage from aspirin and bile.[32] Licorice and licorice derivatives protected against gastric ulcer induced by aspirin[33] or ibuprofen[34] in rats. Deglycyrrhinized licorice and GA also reduced the number and size of ulcers.[34] Licorice (500 mg/kg) was effective in preventing gastric mucosal damage by ethanol in rats. It affected surface mucin production, which was increased to 146% of the control value with pretreatment.[35]

Japanese workers have demonstrated a number of effects for Fm100, a semipurified methanol extract of licorice which contains about 19% GL and 13% flavonoids.[36] As might be expected, Fm100 has shown a marked antiulcer activity.[37,38,39] More surprisingly, both Fm100 and an aqueous extract of licorice were found to directly stimulate exocrine secretion from the pancreas but this effect was not due to GL or flavonoids.[36] However, total enzyme release from the pancreas was not increased. The authors found a correlation between the gastric antisecretory activity and the pancreatic stimulation, which implies that an unidentified constituent may be responsible for both effects.[36] A study in normal human volunteers showed that Fm100 increased both plasma secretin concentration and pancreatic bicarbonate output.[40] Fm100 also increased the content of endogenous prostaglandins in the gastric mucosa. The ability to release endogenous secretin in humans as well as animals may explain the antiulcer effect.[41]

Antiinflammatory activity

In the 1950s, GA and GL were investigated as antiinflammatory agents because of their ulcer-healing properties. Antiinflammatory effects were demonstrated in a number of animal models.[42,43,44] The mechanism is not understood and GA and GL have no intrinsic glucocorticoid action, although they do potentiate the action of hydrocortisone. Oral doses of GL were antiinflammatory in adrenalectomized rats, which implies an intrinsic antiinflammatory activity.[45] Also GA was found to have similar antiinflammatory activity to hydrocortisone in experimental arthritis in normal rats.[44] These studies led to the use in France of GA and licorice for the treatment of rheumatoid arthritis.[46] The fact that GA uncouples oxidative phosphorylation aroused speculation that this was responsible for its antiinflammatory activity[47,48] but this particular mechanism is no longer current in the understanding of antiinflammatory effects.[49]

Recently, several possible mechanisms behind the antiinflammatory activity have been proposed. Glycyrrhizin has been identified as a thrombin inhibitor by in vitro studies.[50] An earlier in vitro study demonstrated that GL exerts antiinflammatory activity by inhibiting the generation of reactive oxygen species by neutrophils.[51] An animal study demonstrated moderate antiinflammatory activity for oral doses of GA but, unlike many other antiinflammatory agents, GA did not inhibit prostaglandin synthesis.[52] It was proposed that GA may inhibit the migration of white cells into sites of inflammation.[52] However, in vitro studies have shown that GL inhibits prostaglandin production and phospholipase A_2.[53] The significance of many of these findings can be questioned since GL is probably converted to GA in vivo.[54]

Topical antiinflammatory activity

In early studies, GA caused considerable interest as a topical treatment for inflammatory skin disorders.[55] However, there were a number of negative findings, possibly due to inactive isomers of GA being produced by incorrect extraction procedures.[56] Antiinflammatory activity was demonstrated on guinea pig skin for a licorice extract liniment which had similar activity to a 0.5% prednisolone preparation.[57] In the skin vasoconstrictor assay, GA potentiated the action of hydrocortisone on human skin.[58] Glycyrrhetinic acid is only present in low levels in licorice; it is mainly formed from GL after oral ingestion, therefore this particular research may be not be relevant to the topical use of licorice.

Using the conjunctival inflammation method for the quantitative evaluation of topically applied antiinflammatory agents, a 5% solution of glycyrrhizin demonstrated comparable antiinflammatory activity to a 1% solution of the steroidal antiinflammatory drug dexamethasone.[59] Topical application of licochalcone A demonstrated antiinflammatory activity in experimentally induced mouse ear oedema.[60]

Influence on steroid metabolism

There is no doubt that GL and GA exert a powerful influence on human steroid hormone function. However, their intrinsic glucocorticoid, mineralocorticoid and oestrogenic activities are extremely low.[47–49,52,55–57,61–64] There is instead strong evidence to suggest that GA and GL act by altering the way that certain steroid hormones are metabolized.

In an early clinical study it was found that GL inhibits the metabolism of corticosteroids and thereby potentiates the effect of cortisone and ACTH.[65] In vitro studies on rat liver preparations have shown that both GA and GL inhibit 5-beta-reductase and probably inhibit the breakdown of corticosteroids by the liver.[66] While GL has been shown to increase the antiinflammatory action of cortisol,[67] it also antagonizes some of its less desirable effects such as its antigranulomatous action[68] and its suppressive effect on ACTH synthesis and secretion and on adrenal weight.[69] These findings have important clinical significance for the use of licorice to aid the withdrawal of steroidal antiinflammatory drugs. GA also antagonizes some of the effects of exogenously administered oestrogen, but has no action on the effects of natural levels of oestrogen.[70]

The aldosterone-like effects of licorice and carbenoxolone are well documented and these effects can also be produced by both GA and GL.[71] Research has shown that this effect occurs in the kidney and this curious action of licorice has been a valuable tool in increasing the understanding of kidney physiology. Briefly put, GA inhibits the enzyme which inactivates cortisol (to cortisone), leading to a high level of cortisol in the kidney, which in turn activates type 1 mineralocorticoid receptors to cause sodium retention.[72,73] The fact that licorice or GA potentiates the effect of cortisol, and not aldosterone, to cause sodium and fluid retention would explain why cortisone and licorice can control sodium balance in Addison's disease without the need for a mineralocorticoid.[74]

The interaction of GL with steroid hormone receptors has been confirmed. One study revealed that GA (the likely active metabolite from oral doses of GL) potentiated the activity of the glucocorticoid hormone cortisol.[75] In previously published studies, this potentiation has been recognized via an inhibition of liver breakdown of cortisol but in the above study the potentiation found was more direct. The enzyme 11-beta-hydroxysteroid hydrogenase (11-beta-HSD) converts cortisol, the active form, into its inactive metabolites. Oral doses of GL to rats, and GA in vitro, inhibit 11-beta-HSD activity and decrease the production of 11-beta-HSD. This leads to significantly increased levels of cortisol and thereby greater stimulation of the glucocorticoid receptor as well as the mineralocorticoid effect in the kidney. As further confirmation of this mechanism, pure GA (500 mg/day) administered orally to 10 healthy, normotensive young volunteers resulted in an elevated urinary excretion of free cortisol and unchanged plasma cortisol levels in the presence of markedly decreased levels of both plasma cortisone and urinary free cortisone.[76]

Licorice inhibits corticoid, progesterone and prostaglandin dehydrogenases. The mechanism for conferring cellular specificity on mineralocorticoid action thus appears to share a common ancestor with a mechanism for regulating prostaglandin action.[77] Licorice also inhibits 3-alpha,20-beta-hydroxysteroid dehydrogenase, an enzyme derived from a certain species of bacteria, which is homologous to both 11-beta-HSD and 15-hydroxyprostaglandin dehydrogenase. (These enzymes diverged at least 2 billion years ago from a common ancestor. It is therefore likely that other oxidoreductases will be inhibited by licorice-derived compounds.)[27]

No difference in blood levels of GA was observed between patients with and without licorice-induced pseudoaldosteronism. Further testing suggested that licorice-induced pseudoaldosteronism is due to an increased concentration of 3-beta-D-(monoglucuronyl)-18-beta-glycyrrhetinic acid (another metabolite of GL), but not GA.[78] This liver metabolite of GA is probably the active form of GL in the bloodstream with aldosterone-like activity. The mechanism behind the mineralocorticoid activity of licorice in humans was further evaluated in six male volunteers who received 7 g per day of licorice preparation (containing 500 mg per day of GL) for 7 days. Pseudoaldosteronism was evident during the treatment as expressed by increased body weight, suppression of plasma renin activity and plasma aldosterone and reduced serum potassium. The study concluded that the pseudoaldosteronism is initially related to decreased activity of 11-beta-HSD, but afterwards also to a direct effect of licorice derivatives on mineralocorticoid receptors which becomes evident in some cases. In other cases, the effect on the enzyme is prevailing, probably as a result of individual factors.[79]

Immunomodulatory activity

GA demonstrated potent inhibition of the classic complement pathway but no activity towards the alternative pathway. The anticomplementary activity was dependent on its conformation, since the alpha-form was not active. GA acts at the level of the complement component C2.[80]

The daily consecutive oral administration of *Glycyrrhiza uralensis* decoction at a dosage of 2 g/kg per day to mice countered the carrageenan-induced decrease in immune complex clearance. However, oral administration to normal mice did not reduce immune complex clearance. This effect of licorice decoction could not be explained by the action of GL.[81] Licorice (oral, 50 mg/kg per day) and GA (intraperitoneal, 5 mg/kg per day) helped the recovery of total leucocyte count, lymphocyte count and cellular immunity in irradiated mice.[82]

Antitumour activity

Tumour promotion is considered to be an important factor in the chemical induction of cancers. GA but not GL exhibits a significant and specific antitumour-promoting activity[83,84] by inhibiting the binding of tumour promoters to test cells.[85] The mechanism may involve inhibition of protein kinase C.[86]

GA inhibits the growth of cultured mouse melanoma cells but is cytostatic and not cytotoxic.[87] It also induces phenotypic reversion – that is, the cancer cell becomes more like a normal cell.[87] GA inhibited ear oedema and ornithine decarboxylase activity induced by croton oil in mice. It also protected rapid DNA damage and decreased the experimentally induced, unscheduled DNA synthesis, which demonstrates a potential chemopreventive activity. (Although not stated, it is likely that GA was administered by injection.)[88] Oral administration of 1% water extract of licorice to mice protected against lung and forestomach tumorigenesis induced by chemical carcinogens.[89] Chronic oral feeding of GL to mice also resulted in substantial protection against skin tumorigenesis.[90] Topical application of GA affected decreases in skin tumour-initiating and promoting activities in mice.[91]

Licorice extract showed antimutagenic activity against ethyl methanesulphonate and ribose-lysine in the Salmonella/microsome reversion assay.[92] Licorice extract decreased the mutation frequencies induced by a series of well-known mutagens and carcinogens in vitro over a range of concentrations well below the toxic level.[93] GA inhibited mutagenicity in the Salmonella assay.

Hepatoprotective activity

It has been proposed that GL is only active by injection as a protective agent for the liver.[94] However, in vitro studies on hepatocytes have shown that both GL and GA, the oral metabolite of GL, are equally hepatoprotective.[95,96] The clinical significance of oral doses of GL or licorice in liver disease remains to be established. (See Clinical trials section for studies on injected GL.)

Oral administration of licorice root (1 g/kg) or GL (23 mg/kg) activated glucuronidation in a study investigating the metabolism of acetaminophen (paracetamol). This result suggests that licorice may influence detoxification of drugs in rat liver.[97] Very high oral doses of licorice or GL induced cytochrome P-450-dependent enzyme activities in mice.[98]

In an experimental hepatotoxicity model, oral administration of GA reduced the increase of serum transaminase activities, whereas GL did not. In vitro studies suggest that the potency of the hepatoprotective compounds parallels their absorption by hepatocytes.[99]

Antiviral activity

GL but not GA inhibits virus growth and in some instances inactivates virus particles. It has been shown to be particularly active against herpes simplex virus,[100,101] varicella-zoster virus,[102] human herpesvirus[28,103] and human immunodeficiency virus.[104,105] Glycyrrhizin also induces interferon production in vivo and in vitro but GA has only weak activity.[106] Indigenous GL (isolated from licorice) was a more potent antiviral agent than licorice and synthetic GL (ammonium salt of glycyrrhizic acid) for Japanese encephalitis virus in vitro.[107] Intraperitoneal administration of GL reduced morbidity and mortality of mice infected with lethal doses of influenza virus.[108]

With oral ingestion, GL is converted to GA,[109] therefore oral doses of GL (or licorice) will not have systemic antiviral effects. Glycyrrhizin exerts systemic antiviral effects after injection but this mode of application is not relevant to herbal medicine. However, both GL and licorice will be active as topical antiviral agents, especially for herpes simplex and shingles.

In vitro studies have indicated that the antiviral agent idoxuridine (IDU) penetrates skin more effectively when incorporated in a glycyrrhizin gel than a commercial IDU ointment.[110]

Antimicrobial activity

The following isoflavonoids and related substances isolated from licorice demonstrated significant antimicrobial activity in vitro: hispaglabridin A, hispaglabridin B, 4′-*O*-methylglabridin, glabridin, glabrol, 3-hydroxyglabrol.[111] Licochalcone A inhibited the growth of both chloroquine-susceptible and chloroquine-resistant *Plasmodium falciparum* strains in vitro and protected mice from *P. yoelii* infection when administered either orally or intraperitoneally for 3–6 days.[112] Licochalcone A inhibited the growth of *Leishmania major* and *L. donovani* promastigotes and amastigotes in concentrations that are non-toxic to host cells.[113]

Neither licorice nor GL promoted growth of *Streptococcus mutans* or induced plaque formation (measured by adherence of *S. mutans* to the surface) in vitro. In the presence of sucrose, GL did not affect bacterial growth but plaque formation was markedly inhibited. GL at 0.5–1% caused almost complete inhibition.[114]

Antioxidant activity

Six constituents isolated from licorice demonstrated very potent antioxidant activity toward LDL-cholesterol in vitro. The constituents were four isoflavans (including glabridin which was the most abundant and most potent antioxidant) and two chalcones. The isoflavone formononetin was inactive.[115]

Both licorice extract and glabridin protected LDL-cholesterol against peroxidation in vitro and ex vivo in humans and in atherosclerotic apolipoprotein E-deficient mice. In the ex vivo study, LDL-cholesterol isolated from the plasma of 10 normolipidaemic subjects orally supplemented for 2 weeks with 100 mg of licorice per day was more resistant to oxidation than LDL-cholesterol isolated before licorice administration.[116]

Other activity

Carbenoxolone enhances the defence mechanism of the bladder[117] and inhibits bacterial adherence to the injured urothelium.[118] Glycyrrhetinic acid demonstrated a strong, dose-dependent inhibitory effect on histamine synthesis and release in cultured mast cells. It also inhibited the transdifferentiation of the cells.[119]

Oral doses of GA have an antitussive effect similar to codeine.[120] In Chinese medicine, licorice is considered to have an antitoxic activity and the protective effect of GL against saponin toxicity has been demonstrated.[121]

Liquiritin, the glycoside mainly present in licorice root, is inactive as a spasmolytic.[122] However, on hydrolysis, which occurs with the application of heat, it is converted to isoliquiritigenin which has strong spasmolytic activity.[122] Isoliquiritigenin was strongly active as an inhibitor of monoamine oxidase, which may have implications for use of licorice in depression.[123] Licorice extract inhibited both xanthine oxidase and monoamine oxidase in vitro.[124]

Isoliquiritigenin inhibited platelet aggregation in vitro with activity comparable to that of aspirin. It also showed antiplatelet activity in vivo. Isoliquiritigenin appears to be the only aldose reductase inhibitor with a significant antiplatelet activity, which may be of benefit in prophylaxis of diabetic complications.[125] Oral administration of licorice extract (7.5 mg/kg per day, 7 days) dramatically reduced sorbitol levels in red blood cells of diabetic rats without affecting blood glucose levels significantly. Licorice therefore inhibits aldose reductase after oral doses.[126] Oral administration of licorice reduced hyperphagia and polydipsia in diabetic mice compared to controls. There was no effect observed on hyperglycaemia or hypoinsulinaemia.[127] Licorice extract, administered by mouth or intravenous injection, caused choleretic activity in rats.[128]

PHARMACOKINETICS

A number of pharmacokinetic studies of GA and GL in animals and humans have been conducted but the results obtained are not consistent. The disagreement appears to be due to difficulties with analytical methods.[129,130] A more complete review of the pharmacokinetic literature indicates that the pharmacokinetics of GL and GA are characterized by a biphasic elimination from the central compartment with a dose-dependent second elimination phase. Depending on the dose, the second elimination phase in humans has a half-life of 3.5 hours for GL and between 10 and 30 hours for GA. The major part of both GA and GL is eliminated via the bile. While GL can be eliminated unmetabolized and undergoes enterohepatic cycling, GA is conjugated to glucuronide or sulphate prior to biliary excretion. Orally administered GL is almost completely hydrolysed by intestinal bacteria and reaches the systemic circulation as GA.[131]

Results obtained for oral administration in both rats and humans indicate that GL and GA were consistently 2–3 times more bioavailable from pure GL than from aqueous licorice extract (containing 7.6% w/w GL). The authors attributed this to the interaction during intestinal absorption between GL and several components in the aqueous extract. The modified bioavailability could explain the adverse clinical effects resulting from chronic oral administration of GL as opposed to aqueous licorice extract.[132,133]

From studies in rats, it has been found that the intestinal absorption of GA was larger than that of GL and the absorption of GA was larger in the small intestine than in the large intestine. Although GL was poorly absorbable, both GL and GA were detected in rat plasma after oral administration of GL, suggesting that GL can be absorbed in both parent and metabolite forms, although their bioavailabilities were low.[134]

In vitro studies using rat liver homogenate indicate GL is first hydrolysed to 18-beta-glycyrrhetinic acid mono-beta-D-glucuronide, which is successively hydrolysed slowly to GA.[135] This suggests that even if GL is absorbed after oral ingestion it is still broken down by the liver.

Based on the single-dose kinetics in volunteers given oral GL, after multiple doses of 1.5 g GL per day 11-beta-HSD might be constantly inhibited, whereas at daily doses of 500 mg or less such an inhibition might occur only transiently.[136] Maximum levels of GA of 6.3 mg/l were reached 2–4 hours after ingestion of 500 mg GA in 10 healthy young volunteers. Twenty-four hours after ingestion GA levels could still be detected in seven subjects.[137]

CLINICAL TRIALS

Gastric and duodenal ulcer

Despite showing early promise, there were several trials on DGL which gave negative findings,[138–140] although some of these may have been due to poor product formulation.[141] More recently, in well-controlled clinical trials DGL has been shown to be as effective in healing gastric and duodenal ulcers as carbenoxolone, cimetidine and ranitidine.[142–144] DGL was widely used in the UK, in combination with conventional antacids, which may also contribute to the observed clinical effects.[141]

Revers successfully treated patients with peptic ulcer using about 7 g of licorice juice per day but he also found that about 70% of his patients developed oedema.[145–147] The curative effects of licorice extract on peptic ulcer and the unfortunate side effects were confirmed by many other workers, some using up to 40 g of licorice extract per day.[148–150] Side effects could be countered by a low sodium diet[151,152] but daily doses of 40 g still caused side effects even with restricted sodium intake.[153] Unfortunately, the quantities of GL corresponding to these doses of licorice were not assayed and variations in GL content could explain discrepancies as to what was a safe dose of extract.

Addison's disease

A craving for licorice sweets was found in 25% of patients with Addison's disease, a phenomenon known as 'glycyrrhizophilia'.[154] Dutch workers in the early 1950s found that licorice extract alone had a dramatic effect in maintaining electrolyte equilibrium in patients with Addison's disease.[155] If adrenal cortex function was severely impaired, licorice alone was not a suitable treatment. However, a synergistic action was demonstrated for licorice and cortisone prescribed together.[155]

Topical applications

In a pilot trial, 40 volunteers brushed their teeth twice daily with a toothpaste containing 0.25% and 0.05% GL or a control toothpaste for 6 weeks. The GL toothpastes did not induce significant changes in plaque, gingival or bleeding parameters compared to controls. The authors note that the lack of efficacy may have been due to insufficient GL concentration or chemical incompatibility with the toothpaste itself.[156] An open, controlled clinical trial was conducted on 21 dental students, using a split-mouth technique for GL application. After 3 days, a reduction in plaque was detected in the experimental sides relative to the control sides of students' mouths.[157]

A carbenoxolone mouthwash was used in a double-blind, crossover trial for the treatment of recurrent mouth ulcers. The mouthwash significantly reduced the average number of ulcers per day, the number of new ulcers developing and the discomfort associated with the lesions.[158]

Twenty patients with mouth ulcers were treated with deglycyrrhinized licorice for 2 weeks in an uncontrolled trial. Fifteen of the patients experienced improvement within one day followed by complete healing of the ulcers by the third day.[159]

An ointment containing crude licorice powder gave good results for the treatment of chronic eczema.[160] Appreciable activity without side effects was demonstrated for topical application of licorice extract in patients with melasma (increased melanin pigmentation).[161]

The efficacy of a formulation which incorporates the antiviral drug idoxuridine (0.2%) in glycyrrhizin gel was tested on patients suffering from herpes of the lips and nose. The preparation was significantly more effective than a 0.5% idoxuridine ointment in reducing the healing time and providing almost instantaneous pain relief. The higher efficacy of the new preparation is believed to be due to the antiinflammatory and antiviral activities of GL combined with enhanced skin penetration of the idoxuridine.[162] Carbenoxolone cream showed some beneficial effect (although not significant) compared with placebo in the treatment of initial and recurrent herpes genitalis under double-blind conditions.[163]

Polycystic ovarian syndrome

Eight infertile, hyperandrogenic and oligomenorrhoeic women were investigated for the lowering of serum testosterone levels and the induction of regular ovulation by a formula comprising *Paeonia lactiflora* and licorice in an uncontrolled trial.[164] The formula was prescribed for 2–8 weeks at doses of 5–10 g per day. After the treatment period, serum testosterone levels had normalized in seven patients and six patients were ovulating regularly. Two of these six patients subsequently became pregnant. A later pharmacological study found that paeoniflorin (from Paeonia) and glycyrrhetinic acid significantly decreased testosterone production from ovaries.[165]

A recent study specifically examined the effect of a Paeonia-licorice combination in polycystic ovarian syndrome (PCOS). Thirty-four Japanese women with PCOS were treated daily with 7.5 g of the combination for 24 weeks in an uncontrolled trial.[166] Serum testosterone and free testosterone levels were significantly decreased after 4 weeks. However, after 12 weeks testosterone was only lower in the patients who became pregnant. After 24 weeks the LH to FSH ratio was significantly lower.

Miscellaneous

The successful treatment of chronic fatigue syndrome (CFS) by licorice has been reported in a case study. Although the pathogenesis of CFS is unknown, the symptoms (such as hypocortisolism) may reflect a mild glucocorticoid insufficiency in patients who fail to show the symptoms of classic Addison's disease and hence may respond to treatment with licorice.[167]

Ingestion of a commercial licorice preparation, calculated at 3 g per day of GL, ameliorated postural hypotension caused by diabetic autonomic neuropathy in a 63-year-old type II diabetes patient.[168]

In a study of eight subjects, GL (150 mg per day) was observed to be a safe treatment for hyperkalaemia due to selective hypoaldosteronism in diabetes mellitus. The mean serum potassium concentration decreased significantly after the addition of GL to therapy.[169] The dose of GL used in this study correlates to about 3 g of licorice per day. This study demonstrates the potential danger of even normal doses of licorice to cause hypokalaemia where potassium intake is compromised, since elevated potassium levels were reduced.

HIV/AIDS

One hundred and twelve HIV patients (72 of whom had AIDS) received oral doses of 120 mg of Glyke for 3–6 months in an uncontrolled study. The total effective rate was 46.4%; 30% of patients improved immunologically (as measured by T4:T8 ratio and T4 counts). Three patients showed seronegative conversion after treatment but tests confirmed the virus was still present.[170] Glyke is a patent preparation made from *G. uralensis* by the Chinese Academy of Traditional Medicine.

A group of 16 asymptomatic HIV-positive haemophiliacs were treated with daily oral doses of GL ranging from 150 to 225 mg for 3–7 years in an open study.[171] There was no change in the treated group, whereas untreated controls showed decreases in T-lymphocyte counts. A follow-up study revealed similar results.[172] Results of a clinical trial in which GL was administered intravenously to haemophiliacs with AIDS suggests that GL might inhibit HIV-1 replication in vivo.[173]

Viral hepatitis

Intravenous administration of GL has been beneficial in the treatment of chronic viral hepatitis.[174] In Japan, a preparation of GL, cysteine and glycine known as SNMC is administered by injection for the treatment of acute hepatitis, chronic hepatitis (including hepatitis C) and subacute hepatic failure due to viral hepatitis.[175–178] Intravenous GL was significantly effective in the treatment of oral lichen planus in 67% of patients with hepatitis C virus infection, compared to controls.[179]

TOXICOLOGY

Long-term administration of GL to mice did not induce tumours.[180] Oral consumption of GA by rats (0.1 mg/ml and 1.0 mg/ml) caused an increase in right atrial pressure and thickening of the pulmonary vessels, suggesting pulmonary hypertension.[181]

At doses of 100–1000 mg/kg per day (intragastric route, for a 1-year period) no significant changes were observed in rats. Dogs given the highest dose displayed decreased body weight gain and increased transaminase levels. The MTD (maximum tolerated dose) is 300 mg/kg per day for dogs. (MTD is the highest dose of a chemical that does not alter the lifespan or severely affect the health of an animal.)[182]

In the single-dose portion of a phase I clinical trial, patients with previous breast cancer received oral doses of GA (0.02–0.04 mmol/kg) without evidence of significant toxicity. In the multidose study, patients receiving 0.02 and 0.03 mmol/kg GA experienced hypertension or hypokalaemia which necessitated dose reduction or discontinuance.[183]

CONTRAINDICATIONS

Contraindications listed by the Commission E include: cholestatic liver disorders, liver cirrhosis, hypertension, hypokalaemia, severe kidney insufficiency and pregnancy.[8] Licorice is also contraindicated if there is oedema or congestive heart failure.

SPECIAL WARNINGS AND PRECAUTIONS

Patients who are prescribed licorice preparations high in GL for prolonged periods should be placed on a high-potassium, low-sodium diet. They should be closely monitored for blood pressure increases and weight gain. Hypokalaemia is the greatest threat and can occur at relatively low doses. Special precautions should be taken with elderly patients and patients with hypertension or cardiac, renal or hepatic disease. They should not receive licorice preparations high in GL for prolonged periods.

INTERACTIONS

There is a slight chance that GL or GA may counteract the contraceptive pill and prolonged use of high doses of licorice is best avoided in this circumstance.

Potassium loss may be severe if taken in conjunction with potassium-depleting drugs (such as thiazides or slimming diuretics or laxatives), leading to side effects. With potassium loss, sensitivity to cardioactive glycosides increases. The intake of licorice may exaggerate the effects of a high-salt diet.

The pharmacokinetics of prednisolone with or without pretreatment with oral GL (four doses of 50 mg) was investigated in six healthy men. The results suggest that oral administration of GL increases plasma prednisolone concentrations and influences its pharmacokinetics by inhibiting its metabolism but not by affecting its distribution. It thereby potentiates the pharmacological effects of prednisolone.[184,185]

USE IN PREGNANCY AND LACTATION

The Commission E advises that licorice is contraindicated in pregnancy[8] but doses up to 3 g per day are likely to be safe.[3]

EFFECTS ON ABILITY TO DRIVE AND USE MACHINES

No negative influence is expected.

SIDE EFFECTS

Licorice has been known to cause hypertension, sodium and water retention and hypokalaemia through the mineralocorticoid effect of GL. There have been a number of accounts of side effects due to licorice consumption.[186–188] However, these usually resulted from its use as a food or flavouring agent.

In order to provide a safety assessment of GL in licorice sweets, a review of literature to 1993 indicated that it is not possible to determine precisely the minimum level of GL required to produce side effects. There is a great deal of individual variation in the susceptibility to GL: in the most sensitive individuals a regular daily intake (several weeks) of no more than 100 mg GL (corresponding to about 50 g of sweets) can produce symptoms; most individuals who consume 400 mg GL daily experience side effects.[189]

Three cases of congestive heart failure after high intake of licorice sweets have been reported. In one of these cases, ingestion of 700 g of licorice candy over 9 days occurred prior to the development of pulmonary oedema. In the other two cases, there were additional complications. A case of pulmonary oedema following licorice sweet consumption (1020 g over 3 days) has recently been reported in which a significant structural heart abnormality was ruled out.[190]

Licorice-induced myopathy may also occur. In one case a patient had been consuming about 1 kg of licorice sweets per week.[191] A case has been reported of a child with pseudoaldosteronism secondary to prolonged licorice ingestion, associated with haemorrhagic gastritis.[192] Hypokalaemic rhabdomyolysis secondary to chronic glycyrrhizic acid intoxication has also been reported.[193] A 38-year-old male developed the following symptoms after ingesting 200 g of licorice sweets daily for 10 weeks, together with a thiazide diuretic for 2 weeks: somnolence, flaccid paralysis of the extremities, arterial hypertension, oedema, severe hypokalaemia and rhabdomyolysis.[194] Serious side effects resulted from the prescription of a potassium-depleting diuretic to a patient who had a fondness for licorice sweets.[188]

Acute generalized oedema was reported in three people who had consumed a moderate daily dose of licorice sweets (10–26 g per day, 4–21 days). Severe acute generalized oedema is not a common side effect of licorice abuse but slight oedema is usual. The authors suggested that licorice constituents could increase capillary permeability and in combination with the mineralocorticoid effect, precipitate the severe and fast onset of oedema.[195]

In a trial to study the effect of prolonged ingestion, graded doses of dried, aqueous extract of licorice root were administered to four groups of six healthy volunteers of both sexes for 4 weeks. The graded daily doses contained 108, 217, 380 and 814 mg of GL. In healthy subjects, only the highest doses of licorice led to adverse effects and these were favoured by subclinical disease or oral contraceptive use. The adverse effects were less common and less pronounced than those previously reported after the intake of GL alone, including reports for confectionery products.[133]

The amount of licorice ingested (as confectionery) by several patients presenting with licorice-induced hypertension to Icelandic doctors in 1993 was quite variable and not grossly excessive.[196] This led to an investigation of whether a relatively normal intake of licorice induces hypertension or if an altered function of the 11-beta-HSD enzyme system is responsible for making part of the population sensitive to licorice ingestion. A pilot study confirmed that 200 g of licorice sweets daily elevated blood pressure and lowered plasma potassium impressively. In a prospective trial, 30 healthy, normotensive volunteers received 100 g of licorice confectionery (containing 270 mg GL) per day for 4 weeks. Blood pressure was significantly raised in the whole group but the response varied among individuals, with the highest rise being 19 mmHg for systolic blood pressure. Plasma potassium levels were also lowered. A subgroup of 13 women who had participated in the study and showed some elevation in blood pressure consumed 50 g of licorice daily for 4 weeks. A smaller, but significant rise in systolic blood pressure was observed. The study indicates that moderate licorice consumption raises blood pressure but the effect varies between individuals. The authors concluded that licorice-induced hypertension might be more common than previously appreciated and that clinicians should be alert to this effect in the prevention and treatment of hypertension.[197]

OVERDOSE

Overdose with licorice is likely to cause pseudoaldosteronism, hypokalaemia, hypertension, oedema, inhibition of the renin-angiotensin system, myopathy and rhabdomyolysis.[198]

CURRENT REGULATORY STATUS IN SELECTED COUNTRIES

Licorice is official in the *European Pharmacopoeia* (1997), the *British Pharmacopoeia* (1998), the *Chinese Pharmacopoeia of the People's Republic of China* (English edition, 1997) and the *Japanese Pharmacopoeia* (English edition, 1996). Development of a monograph of licorice is pending and may appear in the *United States Pharmacopeia-National Formulary* subsequent to June 1999. It was official in the second edition of the *Indian Pharmacopoeia* (1996) but was not included in the third edition (1985).

Licorice is covered by a positive Commission E monograph and can be used for catarrh of the upper respiratory tract and gastric and duodenal ulcers.

Licorice is on the UK General Sale List.

Licorice natural extractive and ammoniated glycyrrhizin have GRAS status. Licorice is also freely available as a 'dietary supplement' in the USA under DSHEA legislation (1994 Dietary Supplement Health and Education Act). Licorice has been present in the following OTC drug products: orally administered menstrual drug products and as an ingredient in products offered for use as an aphrodisiac and as a smoking deterrent. The FDA, however, advises that: 'based on evidence currently available, there is inadequate data to establish general recognition of the safety and effectiveness of these ingredients for the specified uses'.

Licorice is not included in Part 4 of Schedule 4 of the Therapeutic Goods Act Regulations of Australia.

References

1. Grieve M. A modern herbal, vol 2. Dover Publications, New York, 1971, pp 487–492.
2. Felter HW, Lloyd JU. King's American Dispensatory, 18th edn, 3rd revision, vol 2, 1905. Reprinted by Eclectic Medical Publications, Portland, 1983, pp 946–948.
3. British Herbal Medicine Association's Scientific Committee. British herbal pharmacopoeia. BHMA, Cowling, 1983, pp 104–105.
4. Bensky D, Gamble A. Chinese herbal medicine materia medica. Eastland Press, Seattle, 1986, pp 463–466.
5. Swami Prakashananda Ayurveda Research Centre. Selected medicinal plants of India Chemexcil, Bombay, 1992, pp 171–173.
6. Chopra RN, Chopra IC, Handa KL et al. Chopra's indigenous drugs of India, 2nd edn 1958, Reprinted by Academic Publishers, Calcutta, 1982, pp 183–187.
7. Pharmaceutical Society of Great Britain. British pharmaceutical codex 1934. Pharmaceutical Press, London, 1941, pp 487–488.
8. German Federal Minister of Justice. German Commission E for human medicine monograph, Bundes-Anzeiger (German Federal Gazette), no. 90, dated 15.05.1985, no. 50, dated 13.03.1990, no. 74, dated 19.04.1991 and no. 178, dated 21.09.1991
9. Mabberley DJ. The plant book, 2nd edn. Cambridge University Press, Cambridge, 1997, pp 64, 396–398.

10. Chiej R. The Macdonald encyclopedia of medicinal plants. Macdonald, London, 1984, Entry no. 145.
11. Wagner H, Bladt S. Plant drug analysis: a thin layer chromatography atlas, 2nd edn. Springer-Verlag, Berlin, 1996, p 308
12. Hostettmann K, Marston A. Chemistry and pharmacology of natural products: saponins. Cambridge University Press, Cambridge, 1995, pp 312–318.
13. Bisset NG (ed). Herbal drugs and phytopharmaceuticals Medpharm Scientific Publishers, Stuttgart, 1994, p 302.
14. De Smet PAGM et al (eds). Adverse effects of herbal drugs, vol 3. Springer-Verlag, Berlin, 1997, p 67.
15. Sticher O, Soldati F. Pharm Acta Helv 1978; 53 (2): 46–52.
16. Takino Y, Koshioka M, Shiokawa M et al. Planta Med 1979; 36: 74–78.
17. Killacky J, Ross MS, Turner TD et al. Planta Med 1976; 30 (4): 310–316.
18. British Herbal Medicine Association. British herbal compendium, vol 1. BHMA, Bournemouth, 1992, pp 145–148.
19. European pharmacopoeia, 3rd edn. European Department for the Quality of Medicines within the Council of Europe, Strasbourg, 1996, pp 1103–1105.
20. Mizutani K, Kuramoto T, Tamura Y et al. Biosci Biotechnol Biochem 1994; 58 (3): 554–555.
21. Newbrun E. Int Dent J 1973; 23 (2): 328–345.
22. Bielenberg J. Z Phytother 1998; 19: 197–208.
23. Doll R, Hill ID, Hutton C et al. Lancet 1962; 793–796.
24. Anon. Br Med J 1970; 1 (5689): 159–160.
25. Jones FA, Langman MJS, Mann RD (eds). Peptic ulcer healing: recent studies on carbenoxolone. MTP Press, Lancaster, 1978, p 1.
26. Wan BY, Gottfried S. J Pharm Pharmacol 1985; 37 (10): 739–741.
27. Baker ME. Steroids 1994; 59 (2): 136–141.
28. Lojda Z, Maratka Z. Hepatogastroenterol 1982; 29: 88–89.
29. McLean AJ, Harcourt DM, McCarthy PG et al. Med J Aust 1987; 146 (8): 431–433, 436–438, 442.
30. Andersson S, Barany F, Caboclo JL et al. Scand J Gastroenterol 1971; 6 (8): 683–686.
31. Hakanson R, Liedberg G, Oscarson J et al. Experientia 1973; 29 (5): 570–571.
32. Russell RI, Morgan RJ, Nelson LM. Scand J Gastroenterol 1984; 92 (suppl): 97–100.
33. Dehpour AR, Zolfaghari ME, Samadian T et al. J Pharm Pharmacol 1994; 46 (2): 148–149.
34. Dehpour AR, Zolfaghari ME, Samadian T et al. Int J Pharm 1995; 119 (2): 133–138.
35 Goso Y, Ogata Y, Ishihara K et al. Comp Biochem Physiol C Pharmacol Toxicol Endocrinol 1996; 113 (1): 17–21.
36. Ishii Y, Terada M. Jpn J Pharmacol 1979; 29 (4): 664–666.
37. Takagi K, Ishii Y. Arzneim-Forsch 1967; 17 (12): 1544–1547.
38. Ishii Y. Arzneim Forsch 1968; 18: 53–56.
39. Takagi K, Okabe S, Kawashima K et al. Jpn J Pharmacol 1971; 21 (6): 832–833.
40. Shiratori K, Watanabe S, Takeuchi T. Pancreas 1986; 1 (6): 483–487.
41. Takeuchi T, Shiratori K, Watanabe S et al. J Clin Gastroenterol 1991; 13 (suppl 1): S83–S87.
42. Finney RSH, Somers GF, Wilkinson JH. J Pharm Pharmacol 1958; 10: 687–695.
43. Finney RSH, Somers CF. J Pharm Pharmacol 1958; 10: 613–620.
44. Tangri KK, Seth PK, Parmar SS et al. Biochem Pharmacol 1965; 14 (8): 1277–1281.
45. Gujral ML, Sareen K, Phukan DP et al. Ind J Med Sci 1961; 15: 624–629.
46. Trease GE, Evans WC. Pharmacognosy, 13th edn. Baillière Tindall, London, 1983, p 493.
47. Whitehouse MW, Haslam JM. Nature 1962; 196 (4861): 1323–1324.
48. Whitehouse MW, Dean PD, Halsall TG. J Pharm Pharmacol 1967; 19 (8): 533–544.
49. Crossland J. Lewis's pharmacology, 5th edn. Churchill Livingstone, London, 1980.
50. Francischetti IM, Monteiro RQ, Guimaraes JA et al. Biochem Biophys Res Commun 1997; 235 (1): 259–263.
51. Akamatsu H, Komura J, Asada Y et al. Planta Med 1991; 57 (2): 119–121.
52. Capasso F, Mascolo N, Autore G et al. J Pharm Pharmacol 1983; 35 (5): 332–335.
53. Ohuchi K, Kamada Y, Levine L et al. Prostagland Med 1981; 7: 457–463.
54. Hattori M, Sakamoto T, Kobashi K et al. Planta Med 1983; 48 (1): 38–42.
55. Evans Q. Br Med J 1956; 1239.
56. Jorgensen BB. Acta Derm-Venereol 1958; 38: 189–193.
57. Murav'ev IA, Mar'iasis ED, Krasova TG et al. Farmakol Toksikol 1983; 46 (1): 59–62.
58. Teelucksingh S, Mackie AD, Burt D et al. Lancet 1990; 335 (8697): 1060–1063.
59. Tanaka H, Hasegawa T, Matsushita M et al. Ophthalmic Res 1987; 19 (4): 213–220.
60. Shibata S, Inoue H, Iwata S et al. Planta Med 1991; 57 (3): 221–224.
61. Ohuchi K, Kamada Y, Levine L et al. Prostagland Med 1981; 7 (5): 457–463.
62. Armanini D, Karbowiak I, Funder JW. Clin Endocrinol (Oxf) 1983; 19 (5): 609–612.
63. Takeda R, Miyamori I, Soma R et al. J Steroid Biochem 1987; 27 (4–6): 845–849.
64. Tamaya T, Sato S, Okada H. Acta Obstet Gynecol Scand 1986; 65 (8): 839–842.
65. Kumagai A, Yano S, Otomo M et al. Endocrinol Jpn 1957; 4 (1): 17–27.
66. Tamura Y. Folia Endocrinol Jpn 1975; 51: 589–600.
67. Suzuki H, Ohta Y, Takino T et al. Asian Med J 1984; 26: 423–438.
68. Kumagai A, Yano S, Takeuchi K et al. Endocrinology 1964; 74: 145–148.
69. Kumagai A, Asanuma Y, Yano S et al. Endocrinol Jpn 1966; 13 (3): 234–244.
70. Kraus SD, Kaminskis A. Exp Med Surg 1969; 27 (4): 411–420.
71. Takeda R, Morimoto S, Uchida K et al. Endocrinol Jpn 1979; 26 (5): 541–547.
72. Stewart PM, Wallace AM. Lancet 1987; 2 (8563): 821–824.
73. Edwards CR, Stewart PM, Burt D et al. Lancet 1988; 2 (8618): 986–989.
74. Pelser HE, Willebrands AF, Frenkel M et al. Metabolism 1953; 2: 322–334.
75. Whorwood CB, Sheppard MC, Stewart PM. Endocrinology 1993; 132 (6): 2287–2292.
76. MacKenzie MA, Hoefnagels WH, Jansen RW et al. J Clin Endocrinol Metab 1990; 70 (6): 1637–1643.
77. Baker ME, Fanestil DD. Mol Cell Endocrinol 1991; 78 (1–2): C99–C102.
78. Kato H, Kanaoka M, Yano S et al. J Clin Endocrinol Metab 1995; 80 (6): 1929–1933.
79. Armanini D, Lewicka S, Pratesi C et al. J Endocrinol Invest 1996; 19 (10): 1387–1389.
80. Kroes BH, Beukelman CJ, Van Den Berg AJ et al. Immunology 1997; 90 (1): 115–120.
81. Matsumoto T, Tanaka M, Yamada H et al. J Ethnopharmacol 1996; 53 (1): 1–4.
82. Lin IH, Hau DM, Chen KT et al. Chin Med J (Engl) 1996; 109 (2): 138–142.
83. Okamoto H, Yoshida D, Saito Y et al. Cancer Lett 1983; 21 (1): 29–35.
84. Okamoto H, Yoshida D, Mizusaki S. Cancer Lett 1983; 19 (1): 47–53.
85. Kitagawa K, Nishino H, Iwashima A. Oncology 1986; 43 (2): 127–130.
86. O'Brian CA, Ward NE, Vogel VG. Cancer Lett 1990; 49 (1): 9–12.
87. Abe H, Ohya N, Yamamoto KF et al. Eur J Cancer Clin Oncol 1987; 23 (10): 1549–1555.
88. Chen X, Han R. Chin Med Sci J 1995; 10 (1): 16–19.
89. Wang ZY, Agarwal R, Khan WA et al. Carcinogenesis 1992; 13 (8): 1491–1494.
90. Agarwal R, Wang ZY, Mukhtar H. Nutr Cancer 1991; 15 (3–4): 187–193.
91. Wang ZY, Agarwal R, Zhou ZC et al. Carcinogenesis 1991; 12 (2): 187–192.

92. Zani F, Cuzzoni MT, Daglia M et al. Planta Med 1993; 59 (6): 502–507.
93. Hrelia P, Fimognari C, Maffei F et al. Phytother Res 1996; 10: S101–S103.
94. Hikino H. Recent research on Oriental medicinal plants. In: Farnsworth NR (eds) Economic and medicinal plant research, vol 1. Academic Press, London, 1985, p 58.
95. Kiso Y, Tohkin M, Hikino H. Planta Med 1983; 49 (4): 222–225.
96. Kiso Y, Tohkin M, Hikino H et al. Planta Med 1984; 50 (4): 298–302.
97. Moon A, Kim SH. Planta Med 1997; 63 (2): 115–119.
98. Paolini M, Pozzetti L, Sapone A et al. Life Sci 1998; 62 (6): 571–582.
99. Nose M, Ito M, Kamimura K et al. Planta Med 1994; 60 (2): 136–139.
100. Pompei R, Flore O, Marccialis MA et al. Nature 1979; 281 (5733): 689–690.
101. Pompei R, Pani A, Flore O et al. Experientia 1980; 36(3): 304.
102. Baba M, Shigeta S. Antiviral Res 1987; 7 (2): 99–107.
103. Cermelli C, Portolani B, Colombari B et al. Phytother Res 1996: 10: S27–S28.
104. Nakashima H, Matsui T, Yoshida O et al. Jpn J Cancer Res 1987; 78 (8): 767–771.
105. Ito M, Nakashima H, Baba M et al. Antiviral Res 1987; 7: 127–137.
106. Abe N, Ebina T, Ishida N. Microbiol Immunol 1982; 26 (6): 535–539.
107. Badam L. J Commun Dis 1997; 29 (2): 91–99.
108. Utsunomiya T, Kobayashi M, Pollard RB et al. Antimicrob Agents Chemother 1997; 41 (3): 551–556.
109. Hattori M, Sakamoto T, Kobashi K et al. Planta Med 1983; 48 (1): 38–42.
110. Touitou E, Segal R, Pisanty S et al. Drug Des Deliv 1988; 3 (3): 267–272.
111. Mitscher LA, Park YH, Clark D et al. J Nat Prod 1980; 43 (2): 259–269.
112. Chen M, Theander TG, Christensen SB et al. Antimicrob Agents Chemother 1994; 38 (7): 1470–1475.
113. Chen M, Christensen SB, Blom J et al. Antimicrob Agents Chemother 1993; 37 (12): 2550–2556.
114. Segal R, Pisanty S, Wormser R et al. J Pharm Sci 1985; 74 (1): 79–81.
115. Vaya J, Belinky PA, Aviram M. Free Radic Biol Med 1997; 23 (2): 302–313.
116. Fuhrman B, Buch S, Vaya J et al. Am J Clin Nutr 1997; 66 (2): 267–275.
117. Mooreville M, Fritz RW, Mulholland SG. J Urol 1983; 130 (3): 607–609.
118. Pantazopoulos D, Legakis N, Antonakopoulos G et al. Br J Urol 1987; 59 (5): 423–426.
119. Lee YM, Kim YC, Kim HM. Arch Pharmacol Res 1996; 19 (1): 36–40.
120. Anderson DM, Smith WG. J Pharm Pharmacol 1961; 13: 396–404.
121. Segal R, Milo-Goldzweig I, Kaplan G et al. Biochem Pharmacol 1977; 26 (7): 643–645.
122. Wagner H. Phenolic compounds in plants of pharmaceutical interest. In: Swain T, Harborne JB, Van Sumere CF (eds) Biochemistry of plant phenolics. Plenum Press, New York, 1979; pp 604–605.
123. Tanaka S, Kuwai Y, Tabata M. Planta Med 1987; 53 (1): 5–8.
124. Hatano T, Fukuda T, Liu YZ et al. Yakugaku Zasshi 1991; 111 (6): 311–321.
125. Tawata M, Aida K, Noguchi T et al. Eur J Pharmacol 1992; 212 (1): 87–92.
126. Zhou Y, Zhang J. Chung Kuo Chung Yao Tsa Chih 1990; 15 (7): 433–435.
127. Swanston-Flatt SK, Day C, Bailey CJ et al. Diabetologia 1990; 33 (8): 462–464.
128. Raggi MA, Bugamelli F, Nobile L et al. Boll Chim Farm 1995; 134 (11): 634–638.
129. Cantelli-Forti G, Raggi MA, Bugamelli F et al. Pharmacol Res 1997; 35 (5): 463–470.
130. Yamamura Y, Kawakami J, Santa T et al. J Chromatogr 1991; 567: 151–160.
131. Krahenbuhl S, Hasler F, Krapf R. Steroids 1994; 59 (2): 121–126.
132. Cantelli-Forti G, Maffei F, Hrelia P et al. Environ Health Perspect 1994; 102 (suppl 9): 65–68.
133. Bernardi M, d-Intimo PE, Trevisani F et al. Life Sci 1994; 55 (11): 863–872.
134. Wang Z, Kurosaki Y, Nakayama T et al. Biol Pharma Bull 1994; 17 (10): 1399–1403.
135. Akao T, Akao T, Hattori M et al. Biochem Pharmacol 1991; 41 (6–7): 1025–1029.
136. Krahenbuhl S, Hasler F, Frey BM et al. J Clin Endocrinol Metab 1994; 78 (3): 581–585.
137. Heilmann P, Heide J, Schoneshofer M. Eur J Clin Chem Clin Biochem 1997; 35 (7): 539–543.
138. Anon. Br Med J 1971; 3 (773): 501–503.
139. Feldman H, Gilat, T. Gut 1971; 12 (6): 449–451.
140. Bardhan KD, Cumberland DC, Dixon RA et al. Gut 1978; 19 (9): 779–782.
141. Glick L. Lancet 1982; 2 (8302): 817.
142. Larkworthy W, Holgate PF. Practitioner 1975; 215 (1290): 787–792.
143. Gutz HJ, Berndt H, Jackson D. Practitioner 1979; 222 (1332): 849–853.
144. Morgan AG, McAdam WA, Pacsoo C et al. Gut 1982; 23 (6): 545–551.
145. Revers FE. Ned Tijdschr Geneeskd 1946; 90: 135–137.
146. Revers FE. Ned Tijdschr Geneeskd 1948; 92: 2968–2973.
147. Revers FE. Ned Tijdschr Geneeskd 1948; 92: 3567–3569.
148. Schulze E, Franke R. Dtsch Med Wochenschr 1951; 76: 988–990.
149. Argelander H. Arztl Wochenschr 1952; 7: 35.
150. Hensel O. Pharmazie 1955; 10: 60.
151. Wilde G. Arztl Wochenschr 1952; 7: 1058–1061.
152. Schulze E, Franke R, Keller N. Dtsch Med Wochenschr 1954; 79: 716–719.
153. Klimpel W, Finkenauer H. Therapiewoche 1952; 2: 520–523.
154. Knowles JP. Proc R Soc Med 1958; 51: 178.
155. Borst JGG de Vries LA, Holt SP et al. Lancet 1953; 657–663.
156. Goultschin J, Palmon S, Shapira L et al. J Clin Periodontol 1991; 18 (3): 210–212.
157. Steinberg D, Sgan-Cohen HD, Stabholz A et al. Isr J Dent Sci 1989; 2 (3): 153–157.
158. Poswillo D, Partridge M. Br Dent J 1984; 157 (2): 55–57.
159. Das SK, Das V, Gulati AK et al. J Assoc Physicians Ind 1989; 37 (10): 647.
160. Loewy E. Ars Medici 1956; 46(1): 483.
161. Iurassich S, Bianco P, Rossi E. Chron Dermatol 1996; 6 (5): 653–658.
162. Segal R, Pisanty S. J Clin Pharm Ther 1987; 12 (3): 165–175.
163. Csonka GW, Tyrrell DA. Br J Vener Dis 1984; 60 (3): 178–181.
164. Yaginuma T, Izumi R, Yasui H et al. Nippon Sanka Fujinka Gakkai Zasshi 1982; 34 (7): 939–944.
165. Takeuchi T, Nishii O, Okamura T et al. Am J Chin Med 1991; 19 (1): 73–78.
166. Takahashi K, Kitao M. Int J Fertil Menopausal Stud 1994; 39 (2): 69–76.
167. Baschetti R. NZ Med J 1995; 108 (1002): 259.
168. Basso A, Dalla Paola L, Erle G et al. Diabetes Care 1994; 17 (11): 1356.
169. Murakami T, Uchikawa T. Life Sci 1993; 53 (5): PL63–68.
170. Lu W. Int Conf AIDS 1994 Aug 7–12; 10 (2): 214 (abstract no. PB0868).
171. Ikegami N, Akatani K, Imai M et al. Int Conf AIDS 1993 Jun 6–11; 9 (1): 234 (abstract no. PO-A25–0596).
172. Kinoshita S, Tsujino G, Yoshioka K et al. Int Conf AIDS 1994 Aug 7–12; 10 (1): 222 (abstract no. PB0317).
173. Hattori T, Ikematsu S, Koito A et al. Antiviral Res 1989; 11 (5–6): 255–261.
174. Eisenburg J. Fortschr Med 1992; 110 (21): 395–398.
175. Fujisawa K, Watanabe Y, Kimura K. Asian Med J 1980; 23(10): 745–756.
176. Matsunami H, Lynch SV, Balderson GA et al. Am J Gastroenterol 1993; 88 (1): 152–153.
177. Arase Y, Ikeda K, Murashima N et al. Cancer 1997; 79 (8): 1494–1500.

178. Acharya SK, Dasarathy S, Tandon A et al. Ind J Med Res 1993; 98: 69–74.
179. Da Nagao Y, Sata M, Suzuki H et al. J Gastroenterol 1996; 31 (5): 691–695.
180. Kobuke K, Inai K, Nambu S et al. Food Chem Toxicol 1985; 23: 979–983.
181. Ruszymah BH, Nabishah BM, Aminuddin S et al. Clin Exp Hypertens 1995; 17 (3): 575–591.
182. Kelloff GJ, Crowell JA, Boone CW et al. J Cell Biochem Suppl 1994; 20: 166–175.
183. Vogel VG, Newman RZ, Ainslie N et al. Proc Am Assoc Cancer Res 1992; 33: A1245.
184. Chen MF, Shimada F, Kato H et al. Endocrinol Jpn 1991; 38 (2): 167–174.
185. Chen MF, Shimada F, Kato H et al. Endocrinol Jpn 1990; 37 (3): 331–341.
186. Epstein MT, Espiner EA, Donald RA et al. Br Med J 1977; 1 (6059): 488–490.
187. Bannister B, Ginsburg R, Shneerson J. Br Med J 1977; 2 (6089): 738–739.
188. Heidemann HT, Kreuzfelder E. Klin Wochenschr 1983; 61 (6): 303–305.
189. Stormer FC, Reistad R, Alexander J. Food Chem Toxicol 1993; 31 (4): 303–312.
190. Chamberlain JJ, Ablonik IZ. West J Med 1997; 167 (3): 184–185.
191. Chataway SJ, Mumford CJ, Ironside JW. Postgrad Med J 1997; 73 (863): 593–594.
192. Cataldo F, Di Stefano P, Violante M et al. Pediatr Med Chir 1997; 19 (3): 219–221.
193. Barrella M, Lautria G, Quatrale R et al. Ital J Neurol Sci 1997; 18 (4): 217–220.
194. Folkersen L, Knudsen NA, Teglbjaerg PS. Ugeskr Laeger 1996; 158 (51): 7420–7421.
195. Sailler L, Juchet H, Ollier S et al. Eur J Intern Med 1995; 6 (1): 51–52.
196. Sigurjonsdottir HA, Ragnarsson J. Laeknabladid 1993; 79: 87–91.
197. Sigurjonsdottir HA, Ragnarsson J, Franzson L et al. J Hum Hypertens 1995; 9 (5): 345–348.
198. Saito T, Tsuboi Y, Fujisawa G et al. Nippon Jinzo Gakkai Shi 1994; 36 (11): 1308–1314.

Meadowsweet (*Filipendula ulmaria* L.)

SYNONYMS

Spiraea ulmaria L. (botanical synonym), filipendula, queen of the meadow (Engl), Spiraeae flos, flores ulmariae (Lat), Mädesüssblüten, Spierblumen (Ger), fleur d'ulmaire, reine des prés, ulmaire (Fr), ulmaria (Ital), almindelig mjødurt (Dan).

WHAT IS IT?

Meadowsweet was one of three herbs held most sacred by the Druids. It was one of 50 ingredients in a drink called 'Save', mentioned in Chaucer's *Knight's Tale* of the 14th century. It was then known as medwort or meadwort, the mead or honey-wine herb, and the flowers were often ingredients of wine or beers.

Meadowsweet played an important role in the development of the drug aspirin. In 1839 salicylic acid was first isolated from the flowerbuds. It was later synthesized and became an important drug in the 19th century. Unfortunately, unlike the herb, salicylic acid caused so much gastric discomfort and nausea in users that the pain was preferable to the cure. In an effort to overcome this problem, the drug acetylsalicylic acid was developed and named aspirin, from the combination of 'a' for 'acetyl' and 'spirin' from 'Spirae', the generic name of the plant at that time.

EFFECTS

Reduces excess stomach acidity; protects and heals the mucosa of the upper gastrointestinal tract; reduces fever; antiinflammatory for joint and rheumatic pain; thins the blood; protects the cells of the cervix and vagina.

TRADITIONAL VIEW

Meadowsweet is used to treat conditions of the gastrointestinal tract associated with flatulence and hyperacidity, including indigestion, gastric reflux, gastric ulceration and foul breath.[1] Its astringent property is valuable for the treatment of diarrhoea[2] and it is almost a specific for children's diarrhoea.[3] It has also been used for the treatment of arthritis and rheumatism, oedema, cellulitis, liver disorders, kidney disorders, cystitis, urinary stones and red sandy deposits in the urine with an oily film on the surface.[1] King reports that it is effective in passive haemorrhages, menorrhagia and leucorrhoea and is a good tonic in cases of debility and convalescence from diarrhoea.[2] The leaves were traditionally used to ease cramps and to promote sweating and as a diuretic. Wizenman considered it good for fevers and Künzle recommended it for puerperal fever.[4] Meadowsweet is also used as a homoeopathic remedy for rheumatism and gout, rheumatic heart problems, acne, headaches with dizziness and congestion, stomach pains and stomach catarrh.[4]

SUMMARY ACTIONS

Antiulcerogenic, antacid, antiinflammatory, possibly diuretic, mild urinary antiseptic, astringent.

CAN BE USED FOR

INDICATIONS SUPPORTED BY CLINICAL TRIALS

Cervical dysplasia (topical application in an uncontrolled trial).

TRADITIONAL THERAPEUTIC USES

Disorders of the GIT associated with flatulence and hyperactivity (indigestion, gastric reflux, gastric ulcers); diarrhoea (particularly in children); urinary disorders (cystitis, kidney stones), gout and rheumatic disease; fevers.

MAY ALSO BE USED FOR

EXTRAPOLATIONS FROM PHARMACOLOGICAL STUDIES

Gastric disorders requiring repair or protection of the gastric mucosa (ulceration, gastritis); as an antithrombotic agent; as a topical antibacterial agent to aid wound healing; topically to protect and repair the mucosa of the vagina and cervix.

OTHER APPLICATIONS

Included as a food additive in many herb beers and wines.[3]

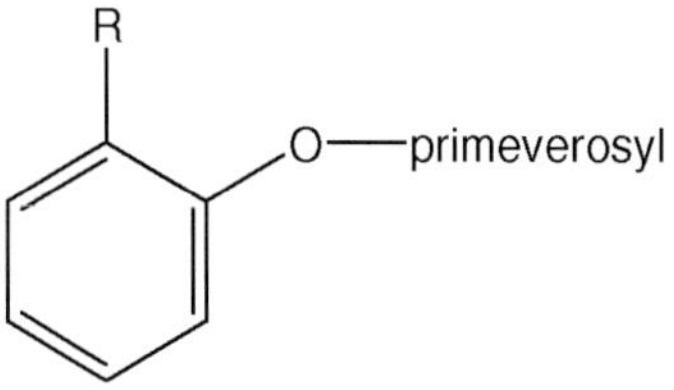

	R
Spiraein	CHO
Monotropitin	$COOCH_3$

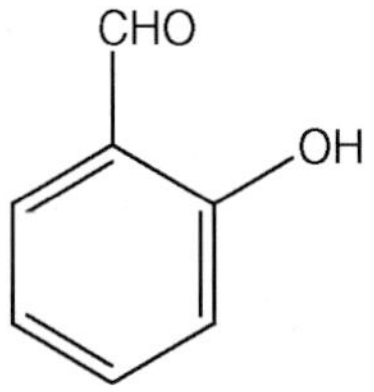

Salicylaldehyde

PREPARATIONS

Dried flowers and herb as a powder, decoction and liquid extract for internal use. Decoction or extract for topical use.

DOSAGE

- 2.5–3.5 g flowers or 4–5 g of the herb per day.
- 3–6 ml of 1:2 liquid extract per day, 7.5–15 ml of 1:5 tincture per day.

DURATION OF USE

May be taken long term for most applications.

SUMMARY ASSESSMENT OF SAFETY

No significant adverse effects from the ingestion of meadowsweet are expected but caution should be observed in cases of salicylate sensitivity and in patients taking warfarin.

TECHNICAL DATA

BOTANY

Filipendula ulmaria, a member of the Rosaceae (rose) family, is a perennial herb up to 120 cm tall, with long petioled leaves up to 65 cm long and composed of 2–5 pairs of 8 cm-long ovate leaflets with double-toothed margins and a tomentose underside. The small creamy white flowers are arranged in dense, many flowered, cymose panicles with many protruding stamens.[5]

KEY CONSTITUENTS

- Flavonoids (3–5%) consisting primarily of rutin and other glycosides of quercetin; kaempferol glycosides.[6,7]
- Phenolic glycosides, including spiraein (salicylaldehyde primveroside) in the flowers, monotropitin (methyl salicylate primveroside) in the flowers and leaves and isosalicin, a glucoside of salicyl alcohol.[6]
- Essential oil (0.2% from the flowers) contains salicylaldehyde (75%), phenylethyl alcohol (3%), benzyl alcohol (2%), methylsalicylate (1.3%) and others.[6]
- Tannins (10–15%), the major one being rugosin-D.[6]

PHARMACODYNAMICS

Antiulcerogenic activity

Decoctions (1:10, 1:20) of the flowers of meadowsweet reduced the ulcerogenic effect of procedures such as ligation of the pylorus in rats and reduced the formation of experimental lesions of the glandular part of the stomach after reserpine injections in rats and mice and phenylbutazone injections in rats. The decoctions were also effective in preventing acetylsalicylic acid-induced lesions of the stomach in rats and promoted healing of stomach lesions induced by ethanol in rats. However, the decoction did not protect rats from the ulcerogenic action of cinchophen and increased the bronchospastic and ulcerogenic properties of histamine in guinea pigs.[8] (Cinchophen increases gastric secretion and reduces gastric mucosal microcirculation.)[9] Alcohol extracts and water decoctions of the flowers decreased the development of experimental erosion and ulcers in vivo.[10]

Immunomodulatory activity

An in vitro study demonstrated that the ethylacetate extract of the flowers strongly inhibited the classic pathway of complement activation. The observed inhibitory action could not be attributed to the presence of salicylates, flavonoids or tannins.[11] In the same model, strong inhibitory activity was also observed using methanol extracts of herb and flower. Further testing indicated that only the ethyl-acetate extract of the flowers retained this activity, supporting the conclusion that complement inhibitory activity could be attributed to compounds other than tannins.

Except for the light-petroleum extracts, all other fractions (ethyl acetate, diethyl ether, methanol, freeze-dried aqueous extracts of flowers and of herb) inhibited the production of reactive oxygen species by human polymorphonuclear leucocytes in vitro. The inhibitory activity and the total flavonoid content of fractions did not correlate, suggesting that other constituents may be involved in the immunomodulatory activity. The authors suggested that this activity may explain the effective use of meadowsweet preparations in inflammatory diseases.[12]

Antimicrobial activity

In vitro studies have demonstrated antimicrobial activity of extracts from the rhizomes, leaves, flowers and upper stems against *Staphylococcus aureus haemolyticus, Streptococcus pyogenes haemolyticus, Escherichia coli, Shigella flexneri, Klebsiella pneumoniae* and *Bacillus subtilis*.[13] Another study suggested that water extracts of various parts of meadowsweet showed high antibacterial activity and can be used on wounds.[14]

Other activity

Both in vivo and in vitro studies have demonstrated that extracts of the flowers and seeds show a high level of anticoagulant activity.[15] This action is thought to be due to a heparin-like anticoagulant found in the flowers.[16]

In an investigation of 42 Rosaceae species, only species from the Rosoideae subfamily, including meadowsweet, exhibited high tannin content and elastase-inhibiting activity.[17]

Local administration of a decoction of the flowers resulted in a 39% drop in the frequency of squamous cell carcinoma of the cervix and vagina induced in mice by carcinogen administration.[18]

A study on the neurotrophic properties demonstrated a moderate inhibitory effect on CNS activity.[19] Ethanol extracts and water decoctions of the flowers depressed the CNS in vivo as exhibited by decreased motor activity and rectal temperature, induced myo-relaxation and increased effects of narcotic toxins. Preparations also decreased vascular permeability.[10]

PHARMACOKINETICS

No data available.

CLINICAL TRIALS

Cervical dysplasia

In 48 cases of cervical dysplasia treated with an ointment containing meadowsweet, a positive result was recorded in 32 patients and complete remission in 25 cases. No recurrence was observed in 10 of the completely cured patients within 12 months.[18]

TOXICOLOGY

Animal studies on the flowers and the alcoholic and aqueous extracts have suggested that meadowsweet is without toxic effects.[20]

CONTRAINDICATIONS

None known.

SPECIAL WARNINGS AND PRECAUTIONS

Meadowsweet contains salicylates and should be avoided or used with caution by subjects with salicylate sensitivity.

INTERACTIONS

None known. Given the experimental anticoagulant effect, it should be used with caution if patients are taking warfarin.

USE IN PREGNANCY AND LACTATION

No adverse effects expected.

EFFECTS ON ABILITY TO DRIVE AND USE MACHINES

No adverse effects.

SIDE EFFECTS

None known.

OVERDOSE

No effects known.

CURRENT REGULATORY STATUS IN SELECTED COUNTRIES

Meadowsweet is covered by a positive Commission E monograph and has the following applications:

- supportive treatment for chills, colds, etc.;

- externally: rheumatic conditions affecting muscles and joints, blunt traumas such as contusions, strains, sprains, bruises, haematomas, etc.

Meadowsweet is on the UK General Sale list.

Meadowsweet does not have GRAS status. However, it is freely available as a 'dietary supplement' in the USA under DSHEA legislation (1994 Dietary Supplement Health and Education Act).

Meadowsweet is not included in Part 4 of Schedule 4 of the Therapeutic Goods Act Regulations of Australia.

References

1. Bartram T. Encyclopedia of herbal medicine. Grace Publishers, Dorset, 1995, p 287.
2. Felter HW, Lloyd JU. King's American dispensatory, 18th edn, 3rd revision, vol 2, 1905. Reprinted by Eclectic Medical Publications, Portland, 1983, p 1809.
3. Grieve M. A modern herbal, vol 1. Dover Publications, New York, 1971, pp 524–525.
4. Madaus G. Lehrbuch der biologischen Heilmittel, Band III und Register. Georg Olms Verlag, Hildesheim, 1976, pp 2592–2596.
5. Launert EL. The Hamlyn guide to edible and medicinal plants of Britain and Northern Europe. Hamlyn, London, 1981, p 66.
6. British Herbal Medicine Association. British herbal compendium, vol 1. BHMA, Bournemouth, 1992, p 158.
7. Wagner H, Bladt S. Plant drug analysis: a thin layer chromatography atlas, 2nd edn. Springer-Verlag, Berlin, 1996, p 199.
8. Barnaulov OD, Denisenko PP. Farmakol Toksikol 1980; 43 (6): 700–705.
9. Nagamachi Y, Nishida Y, Akiyama N. Gastroenterol Jpn 1979; 14 (2): 95–102.
10. Barnaulov OD, Kumkov AV, Khalikova NA et al. Rastitel'Nye Resursy 1977; 13 (4): 661–669.
11. Halkes SBA, Beukelman CJ, Kroes BH et al. Pharm Pharmacol Lett 1997; 7 (2–3): 79–82.
12. Halkes SBA, Beukelman CJ, Kroes BH et al. Phytother Res 1998; 11: 518–520.
13. Csedo K, Monea M, Sabau M et al. Planta Med 1993; 59 (suppl 7): A675.
14. Kallman S. Svensk Botanisk Tidskrift 1994; 88 (2): 97–101.
15. Liapina LA, Koval'chuk GA. Izv Akad Nauk Ser Biol 1993; (4): 625–628.
16. Kudryashov BA, Lyapina LA, Kondashevskaya VM et al. Vestn Moskovskogo Universiteta Seriya Xvi Biologiya 1994; (3): 15–17.
17. Lamaison JL, Carnat A, Petitjean-Freytet C. Ann Pharm Fr 1990; 48 (6): 335–340.
18. Peresun'ko AP, Bespalov VG, Limarenko AI et al. Vopr Onkol 1993; 39 (7–12): 291–295.
19. Lymarenko AY, Barnaulov OD, Yanutsh AY et al. Farmatsevtychnyi Zhurnal 1984; (4): 57–59.
20. Barnaulov OD, Boldina IG, Galushko VV et al. Rastitel'Nye Resursy 1979; 15 (3): 399–407.

Melilotus (*Melilotus officinalis* L.)

SYNONYMS

Sweet clover, melilot (Engl), Meliloti herba (Lat), Gelber Steinklee, Honigklee (Ger), couronne royale (Fr), meliloto (Ital), mark-stenkløver (Dan).

WHAT IS IT?

Melilotus officinalis, when in flower, has a characteristic fragrant odour (similar to newly mown hay) which intensifies upon drying. This is due to the formation of coumarin (benzo-alpha pyrone). The flowers have been used to perfume snuff and pipe tobacco and to give an aromatic quality to tisanes and herbal medicines.

In Europe, Melilotus is highly regarded as an important and safe herb for the circulatory system, particularly the venous and lymphatic circulation. Over the past 50 years coumarin, its major constituent, has been responsible for some important pharmacological advances. Most notably, the discovery of dicoumarol (a bacterial metabolite of coumarin) in spoiled Melilotus hay resulted in the development of modern anticoagulant drugs such as warfarin.

EFFECTS

Reduces inflammatory and congestive oedema by breaking down accumulated protein; increases venous return and improves lymph flow.

TRADITIONAL VIEW

Melilotus was much esteemed in medicine as an emollient and digestive[1] and the Eclectics favoured its use in neuralgic conditions.[2] It was recommended for many external applications including the juice or infusion as an eyewash and plasters and ointments for abdominal and rheumatic pains and for application to veins and ulcers.[1]

SUMMARY ACTIONS

Antioedematous, antiinflammatory, possibly antitumour, possibly immune enhancing.

CAN BE USED FOR

INDICATIONS SUPPORTED BY CLINICAL TRIALS

Clinical indications supported by Melilotus/coumarin with rutin trials: lymphoedema; venous insufficiency, haemorrhoids, varicose veins; episiotomy, posttraumatic inflammation.

Clinical indications supported by coumarin trials: filaritic lymphoedema and elephantiasis; cancer (malignant melanoma, renal cell carcinoma, prostatic carcinoma), particularly to prevent recurrence or metastases.

TRADITIONAL THERAPEUTIC USES

Internally to relieve flatulence, colic and diarrhoea. For neuralgia affecting many areas (headaches, ovarian, stomach) and particularly for conditions marked by pain with cold, soreness or tenderness; externally for ulcers, veins, abdominal and rheumatic pains.[1,2]

MAY ALSO BE USED FOR

EXTRAPOLATIONS FROM PHARMACOLOGICAL STUDIES

High-protein oedemas including burns; thrombophlebitis; to reduce vascular damage such as endothelaemia, for the prevention of ischaemic heart disease; for conditions requiring enhanced peripheral blood mononuclear cell activity.

OTHER POSSIBLE APPLICATIONS

Coumarin has also been used to treat brucellosis in humans and other chronic infections including mononucleosis, mycoplasmosis, toxoplasmosis, Q fever and psittacosis.[3] This may reflect on immune-enhancing activity.

The dried plant has been used to scent linen and protect it from moths and used to scent snuff and smoking tobacco.[1] Melilotus has been included in oral preparations to reduce cellulite but its efficacy is unproven.

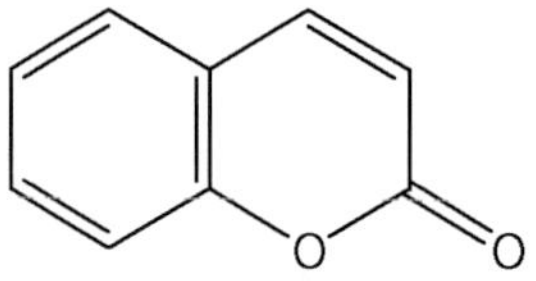

Coumarin

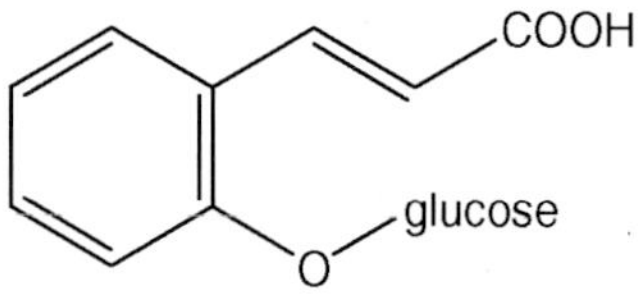

Melilotoside

PREPARATIONS

Dried or fresh aerial parts for infusion, liquid extract for internal or external use.

DOSAGE

The therapeutic dose of coumarin has been established at around 1 mg/kg per day,[4] although higher doses have been recommended.[5] This probably corresponds to about 10 ml/day of a Melilotus 1:2 extract, which for best results can be divided into 5–6 doses taken at regular intervals throughout the day.

Melilotus is best used in combination with herbs having a vitamin P-like activity such as horsechestnut, hawthorn flower, lime flowers and other herbs containing flavone glycosides.

DURATION OF USE

May be used in the long term if prescribed within the recommended therapeutic range.

SUMMARY ASSESSMENT OF SAFETY

No adverse effects from ingestion of Melilotus are expected when consumed within the recommended dosage. Coumarin use has been associated with hepatotoxicity.

TECHNICAL DATA

BOTANY

Melilotus officinalis is a member of the Leguminosae (pea) family and of the subfamily Papilionoideae.[6] It is a trailing to erect branched herb reaching up to 120 cm tall. The leaves consist of three oblong-elliptic leaflets, 1.5–3 cm long with finely toothed margins. The flowers are borne in slender racemes, are yellow and up to 6 mm long. The fruit is a pod containing greenish seeds.[7,8]

KEY CONSTITUENTS

- Coumarin (0.2–0.45%) and its precursor melilotoside and substituted coumarins: umbelliferone, scopoletin.[9]
- Flavonoids, caffeic acid and derivatives.[9]

PHARMACODYNAMICS

Historical background

'Sweet clover disease' was a bleeding disorder first noted in cattle fed spoiled Melilotus. Although it was first described in the 1920s it was not until 1941 that the causative factor was identified as dicoumarol.[10] Dicoumarol is formed from coumarin by bacterial action in damaged hay and was subsequently developed as the first oral anticoagulant. However, its anticoagulant action is slow in onset and difficult to terminate and this led to the use of synthetic analogues, the most widely used of which is warfarin. Properly dried Melilotus does not contain dicoumarol and has no anticoagulant activity under normal circumstances. Coumarin has an anticoagulant activity which is 1000 times less than dicoumarol because it lacks a 4-hydroxy group.[11] However, one case of excessive bleeding due to a large consumption of coumarin-containing herbs has been recorded[12] but the possibility exists that the herbs were not properly dried and contained some dicoumarol. Other factors also contributed to the anticoagulant effect.[12]

In the 1960s research conducted in Germany demonstrated the beneficial effects of a Melilotus extract on circulatory problems. This led to the development of a synthetic drug consisting of coumarin and a rutin derivative (troxerutin). Several other research groups followed up this work, including workers at Flinders University in Adelaide. The Australian scientists discovered the potential value of coumarin for the treatment of lymphoedema and elephantiasis, disorders which affect more than 140 million people. Large-scale clinical trials were conducted in China and India.

Most of the research has been conducted on isolated coumarin or a mixture of coumarin and troxerutin (a flavone glycoside). Since Melilotus contains both coumarin and flavone glycosides, this research can probably be extrapolated to the use of the herb. The other coumarin-related compounds in Melilotus also appear to have an activity similar to coumarin.[13]

PHARMACODYNAMICS OF COUMARIN

Antioedema and antiinflammatory activities

Coumarin possesses unique antioedema and antiinflammatory activities[14] which make it particularly effective for the treatment of high-protein oedemas such as burn injury and lymphoedema.[15,16] It enhances the breakdown by macrophages of protein accumulated in the extracellular spaces.[14] Coumarin also has other important actions on the vascular system. It causes constriction of the precapillary sphincters and dilation of arteriovenous junctions,[17] which can result in an improved blood flow to injured tissue. Thoracic duct and lymph flow are increased by coumarin,[18] hence it aids lymphatic drainage.

Coumarin improves the course of experimental thrombophlebitis,[19] reduces postoperative oedema[20] and improves venous return.[21] Coumarin slows the onset of blood coagulation but this is *not* an anticoagulant effect since bleeding and prothrombin times are not changed.[22]

Coumarin and 7-hydroxycoumarin successfully corrected lymphoedema in an experimental model ($p<0.01$). These compounds may activate the production of proteinases by mononuclear phagocytes.[23] (7-Hydroxycoumarin, also known as umbelliferone, the major human metabolite of coumarin, may be the active form of the drug.)[24]

The administration of coumarin in lymphoedema stimulates macrophage activity and numbers. The reasons for stimulation are uncertain but alterations in the fine structure of the proteins and complement which make these more attractive for phagocytosis seem the most likely. The end result is a rapid, enhanced break-up of excess interstitial protein and the removal of the osmotically attracted fluid together with a more gradual removal of the deposits of fibrotic tissue by the non-stimulated macrophage. Clinically, this manifests itself as a softening of the tissues, a reduction in circumference of the lymphoedematous extremity, a return to normal tissue remodelling processes and a range of subjective improvements for the patient.[25]

Cardiovascular activity

Endothelaemia, the presence of vascular endothelial cells in the blood, is an indication of vascular damage.[26] Low doses of coumarin reduce the endothelaemia caused by various chemicals, as does aspirin.[26] This effect may be partly responsible for the beneficial effect of low-dose aspirin on the course of ischaemic heart disease. Given that coumarin also inhibits prostaglandin formation in a similar manner to aspirin[27] and has a favourable effect on myocardial ischaemia,[13] it may also prove useful in the management of ischaemic heart disease.

Immunomodulatory and anticancer activity

Both HLA-DR and HLA-DQ antigen expression by peripheral blood mononuclear cells were enhanced in vitro over controls after 48 hours of exposure to coumarin. Enhanced expression is consistent with an activated state. This supports the hypothesis that coumarin acts, at least in part, through immune augmentation. Coumarin therapy resulted in augmented HLA-DR antigen expression by peripheral blood monocytes in cancer patients.[28]

The action of coumarin is dose dependent and a doubling of the dose can produce inhibition instead of activation of cellular immunity. As well as acting in low doses through the cellular immune system and the macrophages, coumarin appears to act by inhibition of oncogene activity, while high doses have a direct action on the tumour.[29]

PHARMACOKINETICS

The pharmacokinetics of coumarin are well studied. Human metabolism of coumarin is unique[30] and results in quick conversion of coumarin to umbelliferone.[31] Umbelliferone (7-hydroxycoumarin) does not possess all the activities of coumarin,[32] implying that best results from coumarin therapy are obtained with frequent dosing or slow-release preparations, especially for acute treatment. In a crossover study with a healthy volunteer, grapefruit juice given at the high dose of 1 litre with coumarin (10 mg) retarded the appearance of umbelliferone.[33]

CLINICAL TRIALS WITH COUMARIN

Most clinical trials were conducted using oral doses of a combination of coumarin and troxerutin. These trials have shown beneficial effects in haemorrhoids,[34] acute pancreatitis[35] and the complications of varicose veins, particularly varicose ulcers, oedema and subjective symptoms.[17] A beneficial effect from oral doses in the postoperative treatment of episiotomy was demonstrated in a double-blind trial.[4] This study would also indicate the value of coumarin and troxerutin for the general treatment of posttraumatic inflammation. A similar preparation was effective in the treatment of long-standing lymphoedema. After more than 24 months, all patients experienced subjective improvement and 53% also showed objective improvement.[36]

Lymphoedema

Benzopyrones including coumarin and oxerutins have been used in high doses in many clinical trials on a variety of high-protein oedemas. The results of four such trials (lymphoedema from many causes in Australia and filaritic lymphoedema and elephantiasis in India and China) are summarized here. Coumarin (400 mg per day) was administered over 6 months to patients in the Australian trial and for 1–2 years in India. In China, oxerutin (3 g per day) was administered for 6 months. The drugs reduced these conditions much more slowly than adequate physical therapy, but did reduce them. About half the excess volume was removed over 6 months in the Australian trials. In India and China similar rates were achieved with lymphoedema but elephantiasis reduced at a slower rate. The benzopyrones convert a slowly worsening condition into a slowly improving one. In these trials, compression garments were not necessary. The drugs considerably reduce the number of attacks of secondary acute infection, reduce the deformities of elephantiasis and improve patients' comfort and mobility. Taken orally or topically, they have very low toxicities and only few, minor side effects. The drugs act by increasing the numbers of macrophages and their normal proteolysis.[37]

In addition to the trials described above, a randomized double-blind, placebo-controlled trial investigated the use of coumarin (400 mg per day) and diethylcarbamazine (6 mg/kg per day) on patients with filaritic lymphoedema and elephantiasis over 2 years. In 169 patients there were significant reductions ($p<0.01$) in the amount of oedema for the patients taking coumarin. The excess limb volumes were reduced from 40% to 25%. A similar but less significant improvement ($p<0.05$) was found for circumference measurements. The rate of reduction was increased when the initial amount of oedema was greater. This therapy, while much slower than many other methods of treatment, does convert a slowly worsening condition into a slowly improving one. There were no significant reductions from the use of diethylcarbamazine.[38]

Cancer

Activity of coumarin in cancer is believed to be due to enhanced cellular immunity.[3] Coumarin (50 mg per day) was evaluated in a multicentre, prospectively randomized, double-blind, placebo-controlled trial to prevent early recurrence of malignant melanoma TNM stage IB and stage II. Intake began in 1984 and was stopped prematurely in 1987. There were two recurrences in 13 treated patients and 10 in 14 controls, which was significant ($p=0.01$). The sites of the metastases differed in each group, being local and in bone in the treated group and in lymph nodes, skin and lung in the control group. No toxic effects were observed with coumarin treatment.[39] On subsequent publication in 1994, there were four recurrences in the coumarin-treated group and 10 recurrences in the placebo group.[29]

Twenty-two patients with advanced melanoma received coumarin (100 mg/day) for 14 days; on day 15 cimetidine (300 mg, four times per day) was added. Both drugs were continued until progression of disease. No response was observed in 19 patients, two patients with a low tumour burden achieved a partial response and a third of patients showed a minor response. No toxicity was observed.[40] Earlier it was observed that the combination of coumarin and cimetidine yielded objective tumour regression in patients with metastatic renal cell carcinoma and malignant melanoma. Coumarin appears to have direct effects on tumour cells as well as immunomodulatory activity while cimetidine appears to be immunomodulatory.[12]

Patients with advanced malignancies received coumarin (100 mg/day) for 14 days; on day 15 cimetidine (300 mg four times per day) was added. The following laboratory tests were performed at pretreatment and at 2, 4 and 8 weeks on therapy: monoclonal antibody labelling techniques to monitor peripheral blood lymphocytes and natural killer cell and monocyte phenotypes. There were no alterations in T-cells, helper/inducer T-cells, cytotoxic/suppressor T-cells, B-cells, Ia+ lymphocytes or natural killer cells. An increase was, however, noted after 2 weeks in the percentage of monocytes and the percentage of DR+ monocytes and this occurred in the presence of coumarin alone, before the addition of cimetidine.[41] The same design was used in an earlier pilot study involving 45 patients with metastatic renal cell carcinoma. Objective responses (greater than or equal to 50% reduction in measurable disease) occurred in 14 of 42 evaluable patients, with three complete responses and 11 partial responses. There was no toxicity observed amongst these patients.[42]

The same design was used more recently in a phase I trial of 54 patients with advanced malignancies,

37 having renal cell carcinoma. The dose of coumarin was escalated (400–7000 mg/day) while the cimetidine dose was held constant. Responses occurred over a wide range of doses (600–5000 mg/day), giving no hint of a dose–response relationship. Objective tumour regressions were observed in six patients.[43] Preliminary results of ongoing multicentre clinical trials of metastatic prostatic carcinoma patients treated with coumarin (1 g per day) suggest that patients with normal performance status and small tumour volumes are the most likely to respond.[44]

CLINICAL TRIALS WITH MELILOTUS

In an uncontrolled trial, 76 patients with lymphoedema of the lower limbs at the IId stage of surgical classification received the following preparation at the indicated oral dosage for 6–8 months: Melilotus extract (40 mg per day), Ginkgo extract (40 mg per day) and coumarin (60 mg per day). The preparation induced a very significant improvement in lymphoedema (centimetre aspect) both in functional symptoms (pain and heaviness in affected limbs) and physical signs (oedema, episodes of infection). Tolerance was good and improvement was observed from the third month of treatment.[45]

Many trials have been conducted using a proprietary preparation containing Melilotus and rutin. In an uncontrolled trial on 385 patients with venous insufficiency, oral administration of the preparation (600 mg Melilotus extract per day) over 45 days resulted in 90% improvement. Marked reduction of oedema in both legs was also noted. (In some acute cases, intramuscular injections were also given for approximately 1 week.)[46] Twenty-five pregnant women received a Melilotus/rutin preparation containing 400 mg of Melilotus extract and 150 mg of rutin per day for at least 20 days in an uncontrolled trial. Symptoms such as heavy legs disappeared completely in 68% of cases.[47]

TOXICOLOGY

Coumarin (0.8 and 1.71 mmol/kg) produced dose-related acute hepatic necrosis in rats.[48] In contrast, none of the coumarin derivatives examined produced either hepatic necrosis or elevated plasma transaminase activities. A no-effect dose of 8 mg/kg coumarin was established.[49] The rat is particularly sensitive to hepatotoxic effects from coumarin.[50]

Although some early chronic toxicology research with high doses implicated coumarin as a carcinogen,[51] subsequent work has demonstrated a low toxicity and absence of carcinogenicity,[52] absence of teratogenicity[53] and even an anticarcinogenic effect.[54] Tumour formation in the rat appears due to chronic hepatotoxicity with sustained regenerative hyperplasia.[50] Recently it has been shown that an oral dose of 200 mg/kg of coumarin increased the incidence of alveolar/bronchiolar adenomas and carcinomas in mice in a chronic bioassay.[55] Acute administration caused selective lung cell injury in mice.

CONTRAINDICATIONS

Avoid in patients with impaired liver function or elevated liver enzymes.

SPECIAL WARNINGS AND PRECAUTIONS

Watch for hepatotoxicity. Contrary to popular writings, properly dried Melilotus does not have anticoagulant activity. One case report linked a haemorrhagic diathesis to a herbal tea intake, which included coumarin-containing herbs such as Melilotus.[56] However, there were many confounding factors in this case. In contrast, a double-blind, comparative study in 41 patients suffering from chronic venous insufficiency found that an oral coumarin/troxerutin preparation over 6 weeks did not cause anticoagulant effects.[57] There were no significant changes in coagulation, clotting factors or fibrinolysis over the treatment period.

INTERACTIONS

Caution is advised in the prescribing of Melilotus with warfarin and aspirin.[58]

USE IN PREGNANCY AND LACTATION

No adverse effects expected.

EFFECTS ON ABILITY TO DRIVE AND USE MACHINES

No adverse effects expected.

SIDE EFFECTS

There are no data available for Melilotus.

In the phase I trial outlined above in which the dose of coumarin was escalated (400–7000 mg/day) in combination with cimetidine, renal cell carcinoma patients experienced a few, mild symptomatic side effects (insomnia, nausea, vomiting, diarrhoea, dizziness). Of the 44 patients, two withdrew because of these side effects. In most patients, these side effects abated spontaneously with continuation of therapy. No significant haematological or renal toxicity occurred. Hepatotoxicity occurred in only one patient and was manifested by asymptomatic abnormal elevations of serum hepatic transaminases, which were reversible upon interruption of therapy.[43]

Treatment of 2173 patients with cancer or chronic infections with coumarin in a clinical trial resulted in an incidence of hepatotoxicity in only eight patients.[59] The authors suggested that this hepatitis was probably a form of idiosyncratic hepatotoxicity and may have been immune in origin.

OVERDOSE

No toxic effects reported.

CURRENT REGULATORY STATUS IN SELECTED COUNTRIES

Melilotus is covered by a positive Commission E monograph with the following internal applications:

- disorders arising from chronic venous insufficiency, such as pains and heaviness in the legs, night cramps in the legs, itching and swellings;
- in supportive treatment of thrombophlebitis, postthrombotic syndrome, haemorrhoids and lymphatic congestion;

and can be used for the following external applications:

- contusions, sprains and superficial effusion of blood.

Melilotus is not on the UK General Sale List.

Melilotus does not have GRAS status. However, it is freely available as a 'dietary supplement' in the USA under DSHEA legislation (1994 Dietary Supplement Health and Education Act).

Melilotus is not included in Part 4 of Schedule 4 of the Therapeutic Goods Act Regulations of Australia. Coumarin is listed in the SUSDP (Standard for the Uniform Scheduling of Drugs and Poisons) with a Schedule 4 rating. Such substances are available from a pharmacist on presentation of a prescription by a medical practitioner (doctor, dentist or veterinarian). This restriction also now applies to Melilotus because of its coumarin content.

References

1. Grieve M. A modern herbal, vol 2. Dover Publications, New York, 1971, p 527.
2. Felter HW, Lloyd JU. King's American dispensatory, 18th edn, 3rd revision, vol 2, 1905. Reprinted by Eclectic Medical Publications, Portland, 1983, p 1251.
3. Egan D, O'Kennedy R, Moran E et al. Drug Metab Rev 1990; 53 (suppl): 209–218.
4. Pethö A. Arzneim-Forsch 1981; 31: 1303–1307.
5. Piller NB. Arzneim-Forsch 1977; 27 (6): 1135–1138.
6. Mabberley DJ. The plant book, 2nd edn. Cambridge University Press, Cambridge, 1997, pp 396–397, 468.
7. Launert EL. The Hamlyn guide to edible and medicinal plants of Britain and Northern Europe. Hamlyn, London, 1981, p 62.
8. Chiej R. The Macdonald encyclopedia of medicinal plants. Macdonald, London, 1984, entry no. 192.
9. Wagner H, Bladt S. Plant drug analysis: a thin layer chromatography atlas, 2nd edn. Springer-Verlag, Berlin, 1996, p 127.
10. Stahmann MA, Huebner CF, Link KP. J Biol Chem 1941; 138: 513–527.
11. Sione TO. J Pharm Sci 1964; 53: 231–264.
12. Hogan RP. JAMA 1983; 249 (19): 2679–2680.
13. Kovách AG, Hamar J, Dora O et al. Arzneim-Forsch 1970; 20 (11 suppl 11A): 1630.
14. Piller NB. Arzneim-Forsch 1977; 27 (6): 1135–1138.
15. Casley-Smith JR, Foldi-Borcsok E, Foldi M. Br J Exp Pathol 1974; 55 (1): 88–93.
16. Piller NB. Br J Exp Pathol 1975; 56 (1): 83–91.
17. Casley-Smith JR. Folia Angiol 1976; 24: 7–22.
18. Bartós V, Brzék V. Med Klin 1970; 65 (39): 1701–1703.
19. Piukovich I Zoltan OT, Traub A et al. Arzneim-Forsch 1966; 16 (1): 94–95.
20. Hopf G, Kaeffmann HJ, Pekker I et al. Arzneim Forsch 1971; 21 (6): 854–855.
21. Aso K, Hishida Y. Arztl Prax 1965; 17: 2463.
22. Shimamoto K, Takaori S. Arzneim-Forsch 1965; 15 (8): 897–899.
23. Knight KR, Khazanchi RK, Pedersen WC et al. Clin Sci 1989; 77 (1): 69–76.
24. Marshall ME, Mohler JL, Edmonds K et al. J Cancer Res Clin Oncol 1994; 120 (suppl): S39–42.
25. Pillar NB. Arch Histol Cytol 1990; 53 (suppl): 209–218.
26. Hladovec J. Arzneim-Forsch 1977; 27 (5): 1073–1076.
27. Lee RE, Bykadi G, Ritschel WA. Arzneim-Forsch 1981; 31 (4): 640–642.
28. Marshall ME, Rhoades JL, Mattingly C et al. Mol Biother 1991; 3 (4): 204–206.
29. Thornes D, Daly L, Lynch G et al. J Cancer Res Clin Oncol 1994; 120 (suppl): S32–34.
30. Shilling WH, Crampton RF, Longland RC. Nature 1969; 221 (5181): 664–665.
31. Ritschel WA, Brady ME, Tan HSI et al. Int J Clin Pharmacol Biopharm 1979; 17 (3): 99–103.
32. Hardt TJ, Ritschel WA. Arzneim-Forsch 1983; 33 (12): 1662–1666.
33. Runkel M, Tegtmeier M, Legrum W. Eur J Clin Pharmacol 1996; 50 (3): 225–230.
34. Florian A. Med Mschr 1972; 26 (3): 135–136.
35. Vida S. Therapiewoche 1977; 27: 5476–5483.
36. Piller NB, Clodius L. Lymphology 1976; 9 (4): 127–132.
37. Casley-Smith JR, Casley-Smith JR. Australas J Dermatol 1992; 33 (2): 69–74.
38. Jamal S, Casley-Smith JR, Casley-Smith JR. Ann Trop Med Parasitol 1989; 83 (3): 287–290.
39. Thornes D, Daly L, Lynch G et al. Eur J Surg Oncol 1989; 15 (5): 431–435.
40. Marshall ME, Butler K, Cantrell J et al. Cancer Chemother Pharmacol 1989; 24 (1): 65–66.
41. Marshall ME, Riley LK, Rhoades J et al. J Biol Response Mod 1989; 8 (1): 62–69.
42. Marshall ME, Mendelsohn L, Butler K et al. J Clin Oncol 1987; 5 (6): 862–866.
43. Marshall ME, Butler K, Fried A. Mol Biother 1991; 3 (3): 170–178.
44. Mohler JL, Williams BT, Thompson IM et al. J Cancer Res Clin Oncol 1994; 120 (suppl): S35–38.
45. Vettorello G, Cerrata G, Derwish A et al. Minerva Cardioangiol 1996; 44 (9): 447–455.
46. Babilliot J. Gaz Med Fr 1980; 87: 3242–3246.

47. Leng JJ, Heugas-Darraspen JP, Fernon MJ. Bordeaux Med 1974; 7: 2755–2756.
48. Lake BG, Evans JG, Lewis DFV et al. Food Chem Toxicol 1994; 32 (4): 357–363.
49. Preuss-Ueberschar C, Ueberschar S. Arzneim-Forsch 1988; 38 (9): 1318–1326.
50. Lake BG, Grasso P. Fundam Appl Toxicol 1996; 34 (1): 105–117.
51. Bar F, Griepentrog F. Medizin Ernähr 1967; 8: 244–251.
52. Cohen AJ. Food Cosmet Toxicol 1979; 17 (3): 277–289.
53. Grote W, Sudeck M. Arzneim Forsch 1973; 23 (9): 1319–1320.
54. Wattenberg LW, Lam LKT, Fladmore AV. Cancer Res 1979; 39 (5): 1651–1654.
55. Born SL, Fix AS, Caudill D et al. Toxicol Appl Pharmacol 1998; 151 (1): 45–56.
56. Hogan RP. JAMA 1983; 249 (19): 2679–2680.
57. Kostering VH, Bandura B, Merten HA et al. Arzneim-Forsch 1985; 35 (2): 1303–1306.
58. Harder S, Thurmann P. Clin Pharmacokinet 1996; 30 (6): 415–444.
59. Cox D, O'Kennedy R, Thornes RD. Hum Toxicol 1989; 8 (6): 501–506.

Nettle
(*Urtica dioica* L., *Urtica urens* L.)

SYNONYMS

Nettles, stinging nettle (Engl), Urtica herba, Urtica radix (Lat), Brennesselkraut, Haarnesselkraut, Brennesselwurzel, Haarnesselwurzel (Ger), herbe d'ortie, racine d'ortie (Fr), ortica (Ital), brændenælde (Dan).

Urtica dioica: Stinging nettle, common nettle (Engl), Grosse Brennessel (Ger), grande ortie (Fr).

Urtica urens: Small nettle (Engl), Kleine Brennessel (Ger), ortie bûrlante, petite ortie (Fr).

WHAT IS IT?

Nettle is generally regarded as a weed. It grows throughout the temperate regions of the world, particularly on nitrate-rich soil in waste places. The plant has been used extensively throughout history for a variety of uses. It provided a source of fibre before the general introduction of flax. It had an old reputation as a spring vegetable, the young shoots being cooked and eaten like spinach (and as a remedy for scurvy). The leaf was used as livestock fodder and the oil from nettle seed has been used as a burning oil in Egypt. Nettle is also used as a commercial source of chlorophyll. The leaf, root and seeds are used medicinally. The BHC recommends nettle leaf to comprise the dried leaf or aerial parts collected during the flowering period.[1] Nettle root includes the root and rhizome.

EFFECTS

- *Nettle leaf*: decreases inflammation; assists eliminative function.
- *Nettle root*: inhibits cellular proliferation in benign prostatic hyperplastic tissue; inhibits binding activity of sex hormone-binding globulin.

TRADITIONAL VIEW

Nettle was traditionally considered to be a blood purifier, styptic (stops bleeding), stimulating tonic and diuretic used to treat diarrhoea, dysentery, discharges, chronic diseases of the colon and chronic skin eruptions. (The Eclectics used leaf and root for these applications.)[2,3] A syrup made from the juice of root or leaves was said to relieve bronchial and asthmatic troubles. Nettle infusion or fresh plant tincture has been used topically for nosebleed, as a lotion for burns, as an astringent gargle and as a hair lotion. The beating of nettle leaves on afflicted joints was considered a remedy for arthritis, chronic rheumatism and loss of muscular power.[2] A poultice was also used to relieve gout, sciatica or joint pain.[4] The seeds were used in cases of consumption and goitre and combined with flowers for ague.[2,3] *U. urens* was considered very efficient in uterine haemorrhage, reputedly eased urethral and cystic irritation and had galactagogic activity.[3] Oral intake of nettle leaves was used to treat eczema, nettle rash and other skin conditions.[5]

SUMMARY ACTIONS

- *Nettle leaf*: antirheumatic, antiallergic, depurative, styptic (haemostatic).
- *Nettle root*: antiprostatic.

CAN BE USED FOR

INDICATIONS SUPPORTED BY CLINICAL TRIALS

- *Nettle leaf*: oral and topical application of leaf for relief of osteoarthritis; allergic rhinitis.
- *Nettle root*: improvement of urological symptoms in benign prostatic hyperplasia.

TRADITIONAL THERAPEUTIC USES

- *Nettle leaf or root*: diarrhoea, dysentery, internal bleeding, chronic diseases of the colon, chronic skin eruptions, bladder irritations, bronchial or asthmatic conditions.
- *Nettle leaf*: topically for burns, wounds, nosebleeds, inflammation of the mouth or throat, joint pain (via the stinging of the skin around the joint); orally for skin rashes.

MAY ALSO BE USED FOR

EXTRAPOLATIONS FROM PHARMACOLOGICAL STUDIES

Nettle leaf: as an antiinflammatory with broad activity including inhibition of cytokines.

OTHER APPLICATIONS

Nettle leaf: topically for treatment of insect bites in combination with other herbs. Nettle leaf may also provide a source of absorbable silica. The silicon in nettle is more rapidly extracted than horsetail (*Equisetum arvense*). A 1:100 decoction of the dried leaves simmered for 30 minutes yields about 5 mg of soluble silicon for every 1 g of nettle used. This is only about half as much silicon as that obtained from the same quantity of horsetail decocted for 3 hours.[6]

PREPARATIONS

Liquid and solid dosage forms as normal.

DOSAGE

- 8–12 g of dried herb per day; 4–6 g of dried root per day.
- *Nettle herb*: 3–6 ml per day of 1:2 liquid extract, 7–14 ml per day of 1:5 tincture.
- *Nettle root*: 4–9 ml per day of 1:2 liquid extract.

Doses mainly used in clinical trials are as follows.

- *Nettle root and BPH*: 600–1200 mg of a 5:1 extract per day (3–6 g).
- *Nettle leaf and arthritis*: extract equivalent to about 9 g per day.

DURATION OF USE

No restriction on long-term use.

SUMMARY ASSESSMENT OF SAFETY

Except in rare cases of contact allergy following topical use of leaf in susceptible patients, nettle is a safe herb.

TECHNICAL DATA

BOTANY

Nettle is a member of the Urticaceae family. *U. dioica* is a perennial herb, 25–150 cm in height and covered all over with brittle stinging hairs. The leaves are opposite, 3.5–8.5 cm long, ovate from a usually heart-shaped base with toothed margins. The small flowers are green, unisexual and arranged in axillary inflorescences up to 10 cm long. The fruit is an achene (1–1.25 mm long), enclosed by large perianth segments. *U. urens* can be distinguished by its annual habit, smaller size, smaller leaves[7] and is monoecious (containing male and female flowers in separate clusters).[8] The root and rhizome are long, creeping and yellowish in colour.[9]

KEY CONSTITUENTS

Nettle leaf

- Flavonol glycosides, sterols, scopoletin (isolated from the flowers),[10] chlorophyll, carotenoids, vitamins (including C, B group, K_1), minerals, plant phenolic acids. The stinging hairs contain amines, including histamine, serotonin[11] and acetylcholine.[12] The vitamin K content may be responsible for the styptic action associated with nettle leaf.[13]
- Nettle leaf is also a rich source of silicon. Much of this silicon occurs in the stinging hairs which are effectively fine silica glass needles.[6]

Nettle root

- Sterols and steryl glycosides (including sitosterol),[14] lignans (including (–)-secoisolariciresinol),[15] a small, single-chain lectin (UDA, *Urtica dioica* agglutinin).[16]
- Phenylpropanes, polyphenols, polysaccharides.[17]
- The coumarin scopoletin.[18]

PHARMACODYNAMICS

Nettle root and benign prostatic hyperplasia (BPH)

Several lignans from nettle root including secoisolariciresinol reduced binding activity of human sex hormone-binding globulin (SHBG) in vitro.[19] Additional lignans from nettle root except (–)-pinoresinol developed a binding affinity to SHBG in vitro. The affinity of (–)-3,4-divanillyltetrahydrofuran was outstandingly high. Metabolites of secoisolariciresinol (enterodiol, enterolactone) displayed binding affinities for SHBG and a higher binding affinity was observed with the metabolite of (–)-3,4-divanillyltetrahydrofuran (enterofuran).[15] From assays using a number of lignans, including those found in nettle root, lignans may also produce a competitive inhibition of the SHBG-5-alpha-dihydrotestosterone interaction.[20] Aqueous extract of nettle root demonstrated dose-dependent (0.6–10 mg/ml) inhibition of SHBG interaction with its receptor on human prostatic membranes. Alcoholic extract, *Urtica dioica* agglutinin (UDA) and stigmasta-4-en-3-one were all inactive.[21] Other studies indicate that nettle root extract (20% methanol) inhibited the binding capacity of SHBG after preincubation in human serum.[22] Morphological studies of BPH cells were conducted in 31 patients orally treated with nettle root extract (1200 mg (5:1 extract) per day) for 20 weeks. Relevant changes were observed in the nucleus and cytoplasm of prostate cells taken at the end of treatment. These cellular changes may be due to inhibition of the binding capacity of SHBG.[23]

Five subfractions of an aqueous methanol extract of nettle root inhibited cellular proliferation in BPH tissue in concentrations ranging from 10 to 1500 μg/ml.[24] A reduction in cellular proliferation of BPH tissue was observed ex vivo after treatment of patients with an aqueous-methanol nettle root extract.[25]

Organic solvent extracts of nettle root (0.1 mg/ml) caused inhibition (27–82%) of Na^+,K^+-ATPase from BPH tissue. Hydrophobic constituents of the root, especially stigmasta-4-en-3-one, also inhibited this enzyme activity.[26] (The enzyme is believed to be responsible for androgen control (as an androgen receptor).[27])

Pygeum extract (0.1 mg/ml) was shown to be an inhibitor of 5-alpha-reductase (which converts testosterone into 5-alpha-dihydrotestosterone (DHT) in vitro, and nettle root (>12 mg/ml), a very weak inhibitor. The combined Pygeum/nettle root extract had an activity similar to the nettle root. Both extracts also inhibited aromatase, which converts testosterone into oestradiol.[28] Another study found that inhibitory effects on aromatase were only detected after the separation of a methanolic extract of nettle root into constituents. Weak to moderate activity was observed for some of the isolated compounds including secoisolariciresinol, oleanolic acid, ursolic acid and 13-hydroxy-9,11-octadecadienoic acid.[29] In contrast, aqueous ethanol nettle root extract inhibited aromatase in vitro. Active constituents included fatty acids and 9-hydroxy-10,12-octadecadienoic acid. Although nettle extracts are weak inhibitors of aromatase compared to synthetic preparations, a pharmacological effect might be expected from the lipophilic compounds in nettle in fatty tissues where androgens are aromatized.[30,31] Evaluation of the combined activity of nettle root and saw palmetto extracts indicated that they each inhibit aromatase by a different mechanism.[32,33]

Nettle root extract at concentrations up to 0.5 mg/ml did not inhibit 5-alpha-reductase in vitro or the binding of dihydrotestosterone to the rat prostatic androgen receptor. It also did not inhibit testosterone- or dihydrotestosterone-stimulated prostate growth in castrated rats.[34] A mild inhibition of DHT binding to cytosolic androgen receptors in the prostate was observed.[22]

Nettle root extract demonstrated a specific and dose-dependent inhibition of human leucocyte elastase (HLE) in vitro.[35] (The presence of the proteolytic enzyme HLE in seminal plasma is an important marker in clinically silent genitourinary tract infection/inflammation.[36]) Nettle root extract inhibited the alternative and the classic complement pathways with a half maximum inhibition concentration of <50 μg/ml.[37] Five differently prepared nettle root extracts were tested in experimentally induced BPH in mice. The methanolic extract was the most effective and demonstrated significant inhibition of prostate growth compared to controls (51%, $p<0.003$). The aqueous extract also inhibited growth, although not significantly. There was no correlation between the amounts of sitosterin and scopoletin with the growth-inhibiting effect.[38] After 100 days of oral treatment with 90 mg/kg nettle root extract (5:1), an average decrease of 30% in prostatic volume and a slight lowering of plasma testosterone was observed in animals suffering from BPH.[39]

A decrease in biological activity was observed for prostate cells removed from 33 BPH patients given 1200 mg of 5:1 nettle root extract for 20 weeks. The morphological changes were associated with a decrease in secretory granules.[40] Ultrastructural changes in the smooth muscle cells of the BPH tissue were observed before and after therapy with nettle root extract.[41]

Fluorescence measurements indicated that a specific reaction occurred in BPH tissue after administration of nettle root extract both in vitro and in vivo.[42] This phenomenon may have been due to the presence of the fluorescent compound scopoletin.[18] UDA has been demonstrated to bind to cell membranes of smooth muscle and epithelial cell within BPH tissue.[43]

Antiinflammatory activity (nettle leaf)

In order to understand the antiinflammatory potential of nettle leaves, a group of German scientists carried out a series of in vitro tests. In their first published study, the effect of a nettle leaf extract on biosynthesis of arachidonic acid metabolites was evaluated in vitro. The nettle leaf extract and caffeic malic acid (the major phenolic component of the extract) showed partial, concentration-dependent inhibition of both cyclooxygenase and 5-lipoxygenase-derived reactions. Caffeic malic acid was suggested as a possible (but not the only) ingredient of the nettle extract responsible for this activity.[44]

In the second published series of experiments, the effects of a nettle leaf extract and possible active components on the in vitro release of proinflammatory cytokines were examined. Lipopolysaccharide (LPS) stimulation of cytokine release from the whole blood of healthy human volunteers was adopted as the experimental model. In this assay system, LPS stimulation causes an increase of tumour necrosis factor-alpha (TNF-alpha) and interleukin-1-beta (IL-1-beta) secretion, which is correlated with the number of monocytes/macrophages in the blood of each volunteer. In confirmation of possible antiinflammatory activity, nettle leaf extract significantly reduced this release of cytokines in a concentration-dependent manner. The nettle leaf extract also independently stimulated the secretion of interleukin-6 (IL-6). Since IL-6 acts antagonistically to IL-1-beta in decreasing prostaglandin E_2 synthesis and also induces inhibitors of proteinases, this finding might also reflect a favourable antiinflammatory result. Phenolic acid derivatives and flavonoids showed no activity in this assay, so the cytokine inhibitory components are currently unknown.[45]

Conflicting results have been reported using the carrageenan rat paw oedema model of inflammation. No activity was detected using an ethanol extract of nettle.[46] Prolonged activity for 22 hours (of similar efficacy to indomethacin) began 5 hours after the oral administration of the crude polysaccharide fraction of nettle. Some polysaccharides isolated from nettle stimulated T-lymphocytes in vitro, others influenced the complement system or triggered the release of TNF-alpha.[47]

Twenty healthy volunteers ingested 1.34 g per day of a nettle leaf extract for 21 days. This dosage was probably equivalent to about 9 g per day of dried nettle leaf. Although the nettle leaf had no effect on basal levels of cytokines, it did significantly decrease the release of TNF-alpha and IL-1-beta after LPS stimulation ex vivo. However, an increase in IL-6 was not observed after oral ingestion, confirming that in vitro results are not necessarily translatable into clinical findings. This is probably because some compounds in the plant exhibit poor bioavailabilities after oral doses.[48]

In their discussion of their findings, the authors highlighted some of the inadequacies of current treatments for arthritis. In particular, drugs reducing only the inflammatory process, especially those which inhibit prostaglandin synthesis, do not affect the progression of either rheumatoid arthritis or osteoarthritis. They suggest that the pathogenesis of both types of arthritis is similar, with the exception that the initial insult is different and the cells responding to these insults are different. However, in both diseases the responding cell populations react to cytokines such as TNF-alpha and IL-1-beta produced by activated monocytes/macrophages. These cytokines perpetuate the inflammatory destruction of cartilage and bone. Thus the inhibition of these cytokines offers a powerful approach for inhibiting joint and bone destruction and in this way slowing the progression of the disease.

Nettle leaf urticaria

Studies involving six people up to 12 hours after nettle contact suggest that part of the immediate reaction to nettle stings is due to histamine introduced by the nettle. However, the persistence of the stinging sensation might be due to the presence of substances in nettle fluid directly toxic to nerves or capable of secondary release of other mediators.[49] Acetylcholine is present in the hairs and contributes to the stinging reaction. The sting produced by the hairs can be imitated by the intradermal injection of a mixture of acetylcholine and histamine but not by either given separately. The high concentrations of acetylcholine in nettle hairs may be comparable to the concentrations in stores of cholinergic nerve endings in animals. Extracts of acetone-dried nettle leaf powder catalysed the synthesis of acetylcholine in vitro, indicating the presence of choline acetyltransferase. Synthesis of acetylcholine is not restricted to the younger leaves but continues in older plants.[12]

In another study, nettle hairs and whole plant extract were found to contain high levels of the leukotrienes (LB_4, LC_4) as well as histamine. Nettle hairs therefore could resemble insect venoms and cutaneous mast cells with regard to their spectrum of mediators.[50]

A phospholipid isolated from nettle leaf which induced rabbit platelet aggregation was identified as platelet-activating factor (PAF). The urtication caused by nettle could be partly due to the presence of PAF.[51]

Other activity

UDA demonstrates potent inhibition of chitin-containing fungal growth in vitro (*Trichoderma hamatum, Phycomyces blakesleeanus, Botrytis cinerea*) and exhibits binding specificity toward chitin. The antifungal activity of UDA differs from the action of chitinases and acts synergistically with these in inhibiting fungal growth.[52,53] This activity by UDA may be applicable to topical application. The nettle lectin UDA has also demonstrated antiviral,[54] cytotoxic,[55] immunomodulatory[56,57] and anticancer activities,[58,59] mainly in vitro. However, such activities are uncertain for normal oral doses of nettle root preparations due to the poor bioavailability of UDA (see the Pharmacokinetics section).

The aqueous alkaline extract of nettle leaf demonstrated antibacterial activity in vitro. It depressed the growth of staphylococci (500 μg/ml) and Sporozoa (62.5 μg/ml).[60]

Nettle infusion administered via the diet of experimentally induced diabetic mice aggravated the diabetic condition, as measured by parameters of glucose homoeostasis. It did not affect these parameters in normal mice.[61] Aqueous decoction of nettle or aqueous ethanol extract of nettle orally administered 2 hours prior to glucose load improved glucose tolerance in mice. The dose was equivalent to 25 g herb per kilogram body weight.[62]

No significant diuretic effect was observed in rats after oral treatment with nettle leaf extract (1 g/kg) during a 2-hour observation period but urinary (and potassium ion) excretion increased after intraperitoneal injection (500 mg/kg). No analgesic activity was observed in the hot plate test after intraperitoneal or oral administration but nettle reduced the writhing response at the above doses. The transitory hypotension and arrhythmias observed at high doses were attributed to the high potassium ion concentration of the extract.[46]

PHARMACOKINETICS

Oral administration of radiolabelled UDA indicates excretion occurred via the gut and kidneys.[63] Oral administration of 20 mg UDA to volunteers and patients indicated it was excreted with the faeces (30–50%) and via urine (<1%).[64] This indicates that the bioavailability of UDA is low, with a significant proportion excreted unchanged from the digestive tract.

CLINICAL TRIALS

Benign prostatic hyperplasia (BPH)

In a number of uncontrolled clinical trials conducted from 1979 to 1988, nettle root extract demonstrated improvement of urological symptomatology in BPH patients. The dosage ranged from 600 to 1200 mg per day of nettle root extract (5:1) over 3 weeks to 20 months.[65–74] In a large multicentre observational trial conducted on 4051 patients with BPH at various stages, a reduction in nocturia (by 50%) was observed after 8–9 weeks.[68] In another similar multicentre trial, results for 4396 patients indicated improvement in 78% of patients after 3 months and in 91% of patients after 6 months. Urinary frequency and mean urinary flow were significantly improved. Patients received 1200 mg of nettle root extract (5:1) daily for 3 months and 500 mg per day for the remaining period.[69]

In an uncontrolled study on 253 patients who received nettle root extract (1200 mg (5:1) per day for 12 weeks), significant decreases ($p<0.05$) of SHBG, oestradiol and oestrone as well as a decrease of prostate volume and residual urine were observed.[73] Long-term treatment over 8–10 years of 226 BPH patients found that therapy with nettle root extract could maintain more than 50% of patients without the need for surgery. Using long-term treatment, the usual enlargement of the prostate was not evident.[75]

Nettle root extract (1200 mg (5:1) per day) demonstrated a significant decrease in urinary frequency ($p<0.05$) and serum levels of SHBG in a double-blind, placebo-controlled trial with 40 patients.[76] In a randomized, controlled, open trial, the zinc, calcium and sodium levels in prostatic secretions from patients with BPH were investigated. The treated group of 20 patients received 1800 mg of nettle root extract (5:1) daily for 7 days. Both treated and control patients had samples taken on the first day (prior to treatment) and the seventh day. The 7-day specimens from treated patients revealed a significant drop in the zinc level and a correlation was found to exist between the zinc and calcium levels. No difference was observed between the first-day and seventh-day samples in the control group. The authors concluded that nettle root extract may alter the zinc-testosterone metabolism and lower the zinc secretion in adenomatous tissue.[77]

Liquid preparations of nettle root have also been successfully utilized in uncontrolled trials.[78,79] Sixty-seven patients experienced a reduction of nocturnal micturition frequency after 6 months of treatment with nettle root tincture (5 ml of 1:5 per day). In those with a mild condition, symptoms could be relieved within about 3 weeks.[79]

In a placebo-controlled clinical trial involving 79 BPH patients, nettle root extract (600 mg (5:1) per day, for 6–8 weeks) was superior to placebo in all parameters measured (urinary flow, urinary volume, residual urine).[80] In a similar trial design, 50 patients (BPH stages I and II) treated with nettle root extract (600 mg (5:1) per day for 9 weeks) demonstrated a significant decrease in sex hormone-binding globulin ($p<0.0005$) and significant improvement of micturition volume and maximum urinary flow. There was also improvement in average flow for the herbal treatment group. The authors suggested that the length and dosage of therapy were probably not sufficiently adjusted.[81]

Combination therapy for BPH

In an uncontrolled, prospective, multicentre observational study, the efficacy and tolerability of combined nettle root and saw palmetto extract in 2080 patients with BPH stage I–II were rated as 'very good' or 'good' by physicians. An improvement in pathological findings and in obstructive and irritative symptoms was observed. Fifteen patients (0.7%) were suspected of developing mild side effects.[82]

In a placebo-controlled clinical trial, 40 patients with BPH were treated with combined nettle and saw palmetto extract (240 mg 10:1 extract of nettle root, 320 mg liposterolic extract of saw palmetto) or placebo over 24 weeks. Significant improvement was observed in the herbal treatment group, with peak flow 23% compared to 4% in placebo ($p<0.05$) and IPSS (International Prostate Symptom Score) down by 40% compared to 7% ($p<0.05$). PVR (postvoid residual) was also better compared to placebo (–33%, –13%). A curious aspect of this study is the marked placebo effect which developed in a 24-week unblinded phase which followed the placebo phase. Nonetheless, active treatment remained significantly superior to placebo.[83]

In a randomized, double-blind, multicentre clinical trial, the efficacy of combined nettle and saw palmetto extract was compared to the drug finasteride in the treatment of BPH stages I–II. Five hundred and sixteen patients completed a 48-week treatment with the herbal combination (240 mg) extract of nettle root (10:1) and 320 mg liposterolic extract of saw palmetto per day) or finasteride (5 mg per day). Both treatments significantly improved urinary flow and IPSS. There was no significant difference between the two treatments. Fewer adverse events were reported for the herbal combination, especially diminished ejaculation volume, erectile dysfunction and headache. Economic evaluation revealed that the herbal treatment was also more cost-effective.[84]

In a randomized, double-blind clinical trial, 134 patients received either two capsules of a nettle/Pygeum preparation (each capsule containing 300 mg of nettle root extract (5:1) and 25 mg of Pygeum bark extract (200:1)) or two capsules containing half this dosage, twice daily for 8 weeks. The lower dosage was found to be effective since urinary flow, nocturia and residual volume improved equally with both dosages. Five patients reported adverse effects.[85] In a randomized, double-blind clinical trial on 63 patients, a nettle/Pygeum combination (one capsule: 300 mg of nettle root extract (5:1) and 25 mg of Pygeum bark extract (200:1)) was therapeutically superior to Pygeum extract alone, particularly in reducing urine flow and residual urine volume. The two preparations were equally effective in the control of nocturia. Both treatments were equally well tolerated.[86]

Arthritis

A case has been reported of a man with osteoarthritis and joint narrowing in the left hip who self-prescribed nettle leaves to the region after NSAID therapy did not ease the pain. Counterirritation with fresh nettle leaves over several weeks produced a remarkable improvement and reduction of pain. He was able to decrease the application of nettle to once every few days.[87]

In an open, multicentre comparative trial with NSAID therapy, nettle leaf extract exhibited a comparable efficacy in reduction of pain and improvement of motility, with a very good tolerability, over 3 weeks in 219 patients with rheumatic articular complaints.[88] Thirty-seven patients with acute arthritis completed an open, randomized trial comparing the effects of nettle leaf (50 g stewed fresh young leaf) and 50 mg diclofenac per day with 200 mg diclofenac over 2 weeks. C-reactive protein and total joint scores improved significantly in both groups, with a median score change of about 70% relative to the initial value. The authors concluded that stewed nettle leaf may enhance the antirheumatic effectiveness of NSAID. (A 50 mg daily dose of diclofenac is below the therapeutic level.)[89]

In an open pilot study, patients suffering from painful osteoarthrosis and arthritis of the knee achieved a dose reduction of NSAID of 50% by consuming a proprietary nettle leaf preparation (1.3 g per day of a 6–8:1 extract).[90] A multicentre, uncontrolled, postmarketing surveillance study was undertaken over a 3-week period to research the safety and efficacy of a nettle leaf preparation in 8955 patients with arthritis (7935 had osteoarthritis, the remainder suffered rheumatoid arthritis).[91] Results from a 12-point self-rating scale indicated that 82% of patients felt that the treatment had relieved their symptoms. Also, 38% could have their NSAID therapy reduced and 26% no longer required NSAID therapy. Only 1.2% of patients showed minor side effects such as unspecified gastrointestinal problems.

Other conditions

In a randomized, double-blind, placebo-controlled clinical trial, the efficacy of a homoeopathic combination gel (homoeopathic mother tinctures of nettle, Echinacea, *Ledum palustre* and witchhazel extract) was compared to placebo in the treatment of insect bites. Although the homoeopathic gel reduced erythema development ($p=0.098$), there was no difference between the itch relief, even though a reduction in erythema may relieve itching.[92]

Sixty-nine volunteers completed a randomized, double-blind, placebo-controlled study investigating the effect of a freeze-dried preparation of nettle leaf on allergic rhinitis. Subjects were advised to take two capsules of nettle (300 mg per capsule) or placebo at the onset of symptoms. Assessment was based on daily symptom diaries and global response recorded after 1 week of therapy. In the global assessment, participants were asked to compare the medicines to previous medications and whether they would buy the medicine for future use. Nettle was rated higher than placebo in the global assessments (58% compared to 37% rating the respective medicine as effective or better) but was only slightly higher in diary data.[93]

TOXICOLOGY

The LD_{50} values for nettle leaf infusion and nettle leaf decoction administered intravenously to mice were 1.92 g/kg and 1.72 g/kg respectively. The LD_{50} in chronic experiments with rats given the nettle leaf infusion by gavage was 1.31 g/kg.[94]

Nettle leaf did not demonstrate any antifertility activity when administered orally to rats.[95] Nettle leaf tea demonstrated weak genotoxic activity in a somatic assay. Quercetin and rutin also exhibited weak activity.[96]

CONTRAINDICATIONS

Patients who are allergic to nettle stings should not apply the fresh or unprocessed dried leaves topically.

SPECIAL WARNINGS AND PRECAUTIONS

The Commission E advises that nettle root is useful for the problems associated with an enlarged prostate. However, they advise that its use for BPH should occur under professional supervision.[97]

INTERACTIONS

None known.

USE IN PREGNANCY AND LACTATION

No adverse effects expected.

EFFECTS ON ABILITY TO DRIVE AND USE MACHINES

No negative influence is expected.

SIDE EFFECTS

Occasional, mild gastrointestinal trouble may occur from ingestion of nettle root.[98] In a multicentre trial of 4051 BPH patients, mild side effects affecting the gastrointestinal tract were experienced in 0.7% of cases.[68]

A woman showing the symptoms of atropine poisoning after drinking nettle tea was found to have consumed a tea mixture containing belladonna (*Atropa belladonna*) among other contaminants.[99]

Both an immediate and delayed hypersensitivity reaction was exhibited in a child after falling into a nettle patch.[100] A man who had developed a contact dermatitis after treating his eczema with a poultice of herbs including chamomile also manifested a diffuse oedematous gingivostomatitis. He regularly drank nettle tea. This reaction was believed to be an allergic contact reaction to the chamomile and also the nettle (and not an irritant reaction).[101]

OVERDOSE

Not known.

CURRENT REGULATORY STATUS IN SELECTED COUNTRIES

Development of a monograph of nettle root is pending and may appear in the *United States Pharmacopeia-National Formulary* subsequent to June 1999. Nettle leaf is covered by a positive Commission E monograph and has the following applications:

- internally and externally: only as supportive treatment for rheumatic complaints;
- internally: for irrigation in inflammation of the urinary tract and in the prevention and treatment of kidney gravel. The following warning is advised: in irrigation therapy, care must be taken to ensure an abundant fluid intake.

Nettle root may be used for difficulties in urination associated with stages I and II prostate adenoma. The following warning is advised: this remedy only improves the problems associated with an enlarged prostate without reducing the actual enlargement itself. A doctor should be consulted at regular intervals.

Nettle is on the UK General Sale List.

Nettle does not have GRAS status. However, it is freely available as a 'dietary supplement' in the USA under DSHEA legislation (1994 Dietary Supplement Health and Education Act). Nettle has been present in OTC digestive aid drug products. The FDA, however, advises that: 'based on evidence currently available, there is inadequate data to establish general recognition of the safety and effectiveness of these ingredients for the specified uses'.

Nettle is not included in Part 4 of Schedule 4 of the Therapeutic Goods Act Regulations of Australia.

References

1. British Herbal Medicine Association. British herbal compendium, vol 1. BHMA Bournemouth, 1992, pp 166–167.
2. Grieve M. A modern herbal, vol 2. Dover Publications, New York, 1971, pp 574–579.
3. Felter HW, Lloyd JU. King's American dispensatory, 18th edn, 3rd revision, vol 2, 1905. Reprinted by Eclectic Medical Publications, Portland, 1983, pp 2032–2034.
4. Sales H. Culpeper's complete herbal and English physician. Reproduced from an original edition published in 1826. Pitman Press, Bath, 1981, p 106.
5. British Herbal Medicine Association's Scientific Committee. British herbal pharmacopoeia. BHMA, Cowling, 1983, pp 224–225.
6. Piekos R, Paslawaska S. Planta Med 1976; 30 (4): 331–336.
7. Launert EL. The Hamlyn guide to edible and medicinal plants of Britain and Northern Europe. Hamlyn, London, 1981, p 118.
8. Chiej R. The Macdonald encyclopedia of medicinal plants. Macdonald, London, 1984, entry no. 319.
9. Bruneton J. Pharmacognosy, phytochemistry, medicinal plants. Lavoisier Publishing, Paris, 1995, pp 603–605.
10. Chaurasia N, Wichtl M. Planta Med 1987; 53: 432–433.
11. Lutomski J, Speichert H. Pharm Unserer Zeit 1983; 12 (6): 181–186.
12. Barlow RB, Dixon RO. Biochem J 1973; 132 (1): 15–18.
13. Sapronova NN, Grinkevich NI, Orlova LP et al. Rastitel'nye-Resursy 1989; 25 (2): 243–247.
14. Chaurasia N, Wichtl M. J Nat Prod 1987; 50 (5): 881–885.
15. Schottner M, Gansser D, Spiteller G. Planta Med 1997; 63: 529–532.
16. Peumans WJ, De Ley M, Broekaert WF. FEBS Lett 1984; 177 (1): 99–103.
17. Bisset NG (ed). Herbal drugs and phytopharmaceuticals. Medpharm Scientific Publishers, Stuttgart, 1994, pp 508–509.
18. Schilcher H. Phytotherapie in der Urologie. Hippokrates, Stuttgart, 1992, pp 84–88.
19. Gansser D, Spiteller G. Z Naturforsch [C] 1995; 50 (1–2): 98–104.
20. Schottner M, Spiteller G, Gansser D. J Nat Prod 1998; 61 (1): 119–121.
21. Hryb DJ, Khan MS, Romas NA et al. Planta Med 1995; 61 (1): 31–32.
22. Schmidt K. Fortschr Med 1983; 101 (15): 713–716.
23. Ziegler H. Fortschr Med 1982; 100 (39): 1832–1834.
24. Enderle-Schmidt U, Gutschank WM, Aumuller G. Wachstumskinetik von Zellkulturen aus BPH unter Einflüβ von Extractum radicis urticae (ERU). In: Bauer HW (ed) Benigne Prostatahyperplasie II. Zuckschwerdt, München, 1988, pp 56–61.
25. Rausch U, Aumuller G, Eicheler W et al. Der Einfluβ von Phytopharmaka auf BPH-Gewebe und Explantatkulturen in vitro. In: Rutishauser G (ed) Benigne Prostatahyperplasie III. Zuckschwerdt, München, 1992, pp 117–124.
26. Hirano T, Homma M, Oka K. Planta Med 1994; 60 (1): 30–33.
27. Farnsworth WE. Med Hypotheses 1993; 41 (4): 358–362.
28. Hartmann RW, Mark M, Soldati F. Phytomed 1996; 3 (2): 121–128.
29. Gansser D, Spiteller G. Planta Med 1995; 61 (2): 138–140.
30. Koch E. Extrakte aus Brennesselwurzeln (Urticae radix). In: Loew D, Rietbrock N (eds) Phytopharmaka in Forschung und klinischer Anwendung. Steinkopff Verlag, Darmstadt, 1995, p 69.
31. Kraus R, Spiteller G, Bartsch W. Liebigs Ann Chem 1991; 4: 335–339.
32. Koch E, Biber A. Urologe B 1994; 34: 90–95.
33. Koch E, Biber A. Cited in Koch E. Extrakte aus Brennesselwurzeln (Urticae radix). In: Loew D, Rietbrock N (eds) Phytopharmaka in Forschung und klinischer Anwendung. Steinkopff Verlag, Darmstadt, 1995, p 69.
34. Rhodes L, Primka RL, Berman C et al. Prostate 1993; 22 (1): 43–51.
35. Koch E, Jaggy H, Chatterjee SS. Naunyn-Schmiedeberg's Arch Pharmacol 1995; 351: R57.
36. Wolff H, Bezold G, Zebhauser M et al. J Androl 1991; 12 (5): 331–334.
37. Koch E. Extrakte aus Brennesselwurzeln (Urticae radix). In: Loew D, Rietbrock N (eds) Phytopharmaka in Forschung und klinischer Anwendung. Steinkopff Verlag, Darmstadt, 1995, p 70.
38. Lichius JJ, Muth C. Planta Med 1997; 63 (4): 307–310.
39. Daube G. Pilotstudie zur Behandlung der benignen Prostatahyperplasie bei Hunden mit extractum radicis urticae (ERU). In: Bauer HW (ed) Benigne Prostatahyperplasie II. Zuckschwerdt, München 1988, pp 63–66.
40. Ziegler H. Fortschr Med 1983; 101 (45): 2112–2114.
41. Oberholzer M, Schambock A, Rugendorff EW et al. Elektronen mikroskopische Ergebnisse bei medikamentos behandelter benigner Prostatahyperplasie. In: Bauer HW (ed) Benigne Prostatahyperplasie. Zuckschwerdt, München, 1986, pp 13–17.
42. Dunzendorfer U. Z Phytother 1984; 5: 800–804.
43. Sinowatz F, Amselgruber W, Boos G et al. Zur parakrinen Regulation des Prostatawachstums: Besteht eine Wechselwirkung zwischen dem basischen Fibroblasten-Wachstumsfaktor und dem Lektin UDA? In: Boos G (ed) Benigne Prostatahyperplasie. PMI, Frankfurt, 1994, pp 79–86.
44. Obertreis B, Giller K, Teucher T et al. Arzneim Forsch 1996; 46 (1): 52–56.
45. Obertreis B, Ruttkowski T, Teucher T et al. Arzneim Forsch 1996; 46 (4): 389–394.
46. Tita B, Faccendini P, Bello U et al. Pharmacol Res 1993; 27 (suppl 1): 21–22.
47. Wagner H, Willer F, Samtleben R et al. Phytomed 1994; 1: 213–224.
48. Teucher T, Obertreis B, Ruttkowski T et al. Arzneim Forsch 1996; 46 (9): 906–910.
49. Oliver F, Amon EU, Breathnach A et al. Clin Exp Dermatol 1991; 16 (1): 1–7.
50. Czarnetzki BM, Thiele T, Rosenbach T. Int Arch Allergy Appl Immunol 1990; 91 (1): 43–46.
51. Antonopoulou S, Demopoulos CA, Andrikopoulos NK. J Agric Food Chem 1996; 44 (10): 3052–3056.
52. Van Parijs J, Broekaert WF, Peumans WJ et al. Arch Int Physiol Biochim 1988; 96 (1): 31.
53. Broekaert WF, Van Parijs J, Leyns F et al. Science 1989; 245 (4922): 1100–1102.
54. Balzarini J, Neyts J, Schols D et al. Antiviral Res 1992; 18 (2): 191–207.
55. Wagner H, Willer F. Neue chemische und pharmakologische Untersuchungen des Radix-urticae-Extraktes (ERU). In: Bauer HW (ed) Benigne Prostatahyperplasie II. Zuckschwerdt, München, 1988, pp 51–54.
56. Musette P, Galelli A, Chabre H et al. Eur J Immunol 1996; 26 (8): 1707–1711.
57. Koch E. Extrakte aus Brennesselwurzeln (Urticae radix). In: Loew D, Rietbrock N (eds) Phytopharmaka in Forschung und klinischer Anwendung. Steinkopff Verlag, Darmstadt, 1995, p 71.
58. Wagner H, Geiger WN, Boos G et al. Phytomed 1995; 1: 287–290.
59. Suh N, Luyengi L, Fong HH et al. Anticancer Res 1995; 15 (2): 233–239.
60. Lezhneva LP, Murav'ev IA, Cherevatyi VS. Rastilel'nye-Resursy 1986; 22 (2): 255–257.
61. Swanston-Flatt SK, Day C, Flatt PR et al. Diabetes Res. 1989; 10 (2): 69–73.
62. Neef H, Declercq P, Laekeman G. Phytother Res 1995; 9 (1): 45–48.
63. Geiger WN, Haak C, Wagner H. 2nd International Congress on Phytomedicine, Munich, September 11–14, 1996.
64. Samtleben R, Boos G, Wagner H. 2nd International Congress on Phytomedicine, Munich, September 11–14, 1996.
65. Barsom S, Bettermann AA. Z Allg Med 1979; 55 (33): 1947–1950.
66. Djulepa J. Arztl Praxis 1982; 63: 2199–2202.
67. Tosch U. Euromed 1983; 6: 1–3.
68. Stahl HP. Z Allg Med 1984; 60 (3): 128–132.
69. Friesen A. Statistische Analyse einer Multizenter-Langzeitstudie mit ERU. In: Bauer HW (ed) Benigne Prostatahyperplasie II. Zuckschwerdt, München, 1988, pp 121–130.

70. Feiber H. Sonographische Verlaufsbeobachtungen zum Einfluβ der medikamentösen Therapie der benignen Prostatahyperplasie (BPH). In: Bauer HW (ed) Benigne Prostatahyperplasie II. Zuckschwerdt, München, 1988, pp 75–82.
71. Romics I. Int Urol Nephrol 1987; 19 (3): 293–297.
72. Maar K. Fortschr Med 1987; 105 (1): 50–52.
73. Bauer HW, Sudhoff F, Dressler S. Endokrine Parameter während der Behandlung der benignen Prostatahyperplasie mit ERU. In: Bauer HW (ed) Benigne Prostatahyperplasie II. Zuckschwerdt, München, 1988, pp 44–49.
74. Vandierendounck EJ, Burkhardt P. Therapiewoche Schweiz 1986; 2: 892–895.
75. Ziegler H. 6th Phytotherapy Conference, Berlin, October 5–7, 1995.
76. Fischer M, Wilbert D. Wirkprüfung eines Phytopharmakons zur Behandlung der benignen Prostatahyperplasie (BHP). In: Rutishauser G (ed) Benigne Prostatahyperplasie III. Zuckschwerdt, München, 1992, pp 79–84.
77. Romics I, Bach D. Int Urol Nephrol 1991; 23 (1): 45–49.
78. Goetz P. Z Phytother 1989; 10: 175–178.
79. Belaiche P, Lievoux O. Phytother Res 1991; 5: 267–269.
80. Dathe G, Schmid H. Urologe B 1987; 27: 223–226.
81. Vontobel HP, Herzog R, Rutishauser G et al. Urologe A 1985; 24 (1): 49–51.
82. Schneider HJ, Honold E, Masuhr T. Fortschr Med 1995; 113 (3): 37–40.
83. Metzker H, Kieser M, Holscher U. Urologe A 1996; 36 (4): 292–300.
84. Sokeland J, Albrecht J. Urologe A 1997; 36 (4): 327–333.
85. Krzeski T, Kazon M, Borkowski A et al. Clin Ther 1993; 15 (6): 1011–1020.
86. Montanari E, Mandressi A, Magri V et al. Der Informierte Arzt 1991; 6A: 593–598.
87. Randall CF. Br J Gen Pract 1994; 44 (388): 533–534.
88. Sommer RG, Sinner B. Therapiewoche 1996; 46 (1): 44–49.
89. Chrubasik S, Enderlein W, Bauer R et al. Phytomed 1997; 4 (2): 105–108.
90. Ramm S, Hansen C. Therapiewoche 1996; 28: 3–6.
91. Buck G. Z Phytother 1998; 19 (4): 216.
92. Hill N, Stam C, Van Haselen RA. Pharm World Sci 1996; 18 (1): 35–41.
93. Mittman P. Planta Med 1990; 56 (1): 44–47.
94. Baraibar C, Broncano FJ, Lazaro-Carrasco MJ et al. An Bromatol 1984; 35 (1): 99–103.
95. Sharma BB, Varshney MD, Gupta DN et al. Int J Crude Drug Res 1983; 21 (4): 183–187.
96. Graf U, Moraga AA, Castro R et al. Food Chem Toxicol 1994; 32 (5): 423–430.
97. German Federal Minister of Justice. German Commission E for human medicine monograph, Bundes-Anzeiger (German Federal Gazette), no. 173, dated 18.09.1986; no. 11, dated 17.01.1991.
98. German Federal Minister of Justice. German Commission E for human medicine monograph, Bundes-Anzeiger (German Federal Gazette), no. 173, dated 18.09.1986; no. 43, dated 02.03.1989.
99. Scholz H, Kascha S, Zingerle H. Fortschr Med 1980; 98 (39): 1525–1526.
100. Edwards EK Jr, Edwards EK Sr. Contact Derm 1992; 27 (4): 264–265.
101. Bossuyt L, Dooms-Goossens A. Contact Derm 1994; 31 (2): 131–132.

Pau d'arco (*Tabebuia spp*. Gomes ex DC.)

SYNONYMS

Lapacho (Engl, Span), ipe roxo, peuva, taheebo, pau d'arco, lapacho (Sth Amer).

WHAT IS IT?

Pau d'arco has been used for at least 1000 years by the Brazilian Indians from where its use gradually spread to other parts of South America. These large timber trees with spectacular tubular flowers originate mostly in Brazil and Argentina, although they are widely planted throughout the South American tropics. They are renowned for their durable timber and resistance to insect and fungal attack. The most widely used species in western countries are *Tabebuia impetiginosa (T. avellanedae)* and *T. ipe*. Other species used include *Tabebuia rosea (T. pentaphylla), T. chrysantha, T. cassinoides* and *T. serratifolia*.

Pau d'arco was first used in Western medicine in Sao Paulo, Brazil, in 1960 where physicians prescribed decoctions of the inner bark for terminal cancer patients at the Santo Andre hospital. According to reports, most patients showed no symptoms after 30 days of commencing treatment. Subsequently, the hospital also used the unapproved medicine for viral-linked diseases, including leukaemia. One of the doctors, Professor Accorsi, stated that pau d'arco eliminates the pain (of cancer) and increases the amount of red corpuscles. Knowledge of the herb became more widespread following a number of 'miraculous' cancer cures, including three successful leukaemia treatments by Dr Ruiz at the Concepcion hospital.

Dr Theodore Meyer, a leading South American botanist born in Argentina, was the first scientist on record to analyse pau d'arco's chemical composition, discovering xyloidone, an antibiotic and virucidal agent. Meyer supplied medicinal herbs, including pau d'arco, to pharmaceutical companies but is also credited with beginning the effort to save the tree from destruction. More recently, pau d'arco has attained almost fad status in the West, particularly as an anti-fungal agent in chronic candidiasis. While its use has faded slightly as other treatments have become available, it is still valued for its benefit to those with weakened immunity. Few side effects have been recorded despite its widespread usage, often self administered, and the potential toxicity of its active components.

The inner bark is the main part of the tree used in medicine but the outer bark and wood contain, to a lesser or greater degree, the same constituents, depending on the species of tree and part used.

EFFECTS

Cytotoxic (via induction of cellular and immune factors); active against certain species of parasites, antimicrobial; immune enhancing.

TRADITIONAL VIEW

The Incas used pau d'arco to cure many diseases, including even degenerative disorders. The Brazilian Indians used the bark as a poultice or decoction for treating skin diseases such as eczema, psoriasis, fungal infections and skin cancers. A tea from the bark is used as a blood purifier, while the inner bark has been favoured for dysentery, fever, sore throat, wounds, snakebites and carcinomas.[1]

Inhabitants of the Rio Vaupés believe the decoction of the bark of *T. insignis* var. *monophylla* to be an excellent treatment for stomach ulcers. The Tikunas use *T. neochrysantha* to treat malaria, chronic anaemia and ulcers. The bark of *T. obscura* is used as an antirheumatic by the Boras of Peru.[2]

SUMMARY ACTIONS

Immunostimulant, antitumour, antimicrobial, antiparasitic, depurative.

CAN BE USED FOR

INDICATIONS SUPPORTED BY CLINICAL TRIALS

Clinical trials using lapachol: carcinoma and leukaemia. Use as an adjuvant complementary therapy in cancer (all studies uncontrolled).

TRADITIONAL THERAPEUTIC USES

Internally for dysentery, fever, malaria, sore throat, wounds, carcinomas, stomach ulcers, anaemia, degenerative disorders. Topically for skin diseases, fungal infections, skin cancers. Used as a depurative and antirheumatic.

MAY ALSO BE USED FOR

EXTRAPOLATIONS FROM PHARMACOLOGICAL STUDIES

As an adjunctive treatment for bacterial, fungal and protozoal infections; to enhance immune function. The immune-enhancing activity may explain the anticancer activity. Topical application for fungal infections, scabies, ulcers and wounds.

PREPARATIONS

Decoction of dried inner bark or liquid extract for internal use; decoction of dried inner bark or liquid extract for external use.

DOSAGE

1.5–3.5 g/day or 3 to 7 ml per day of a 1:2 extract, 45% ethanol. In cancer therapy, pau d'arco is often administered in higher doses both as an ethanolic extract and as a decoction. Alcohol is a better solvent than water for the naphthoquinones. For a decoction, simmer 10 g of bark in 600 ml of water for 15 minutes. Strain and drink throughout the day.

DURATION OF USE

May be used long term if prescribed within the recommended therapeutic range.

SUMMARY ASSESSMENT OF SAFETY

No adverse effects from ingestion of pau d'arco are expected when consumed within the recommended dosage.

TECHNICAL DATA

BOTANY

Pau d'arco refers to several trees in the Bignoniaceae (jacaranda) family which are indigenous to South America. They belong to the genera Tabebuia (100 species) and Tecoma (13 species). Pau d'arco is a tropical tree growing up to 38 metres high, with opposite, long-petiolate leaves with entire or toothed leaflets. The flower is large in terminal cymes or panicles, with tubular or campanulate calyx, four stamens, corolla tube ampiate. The capsule is slender-cylindric and the seeds are broadly winged.[2-4]

Species identification is determined by leaf configuration and flower colour; the red, violet and pink-flowering species are preferred as medicines while the yellow flower species are considered inferior.[5]

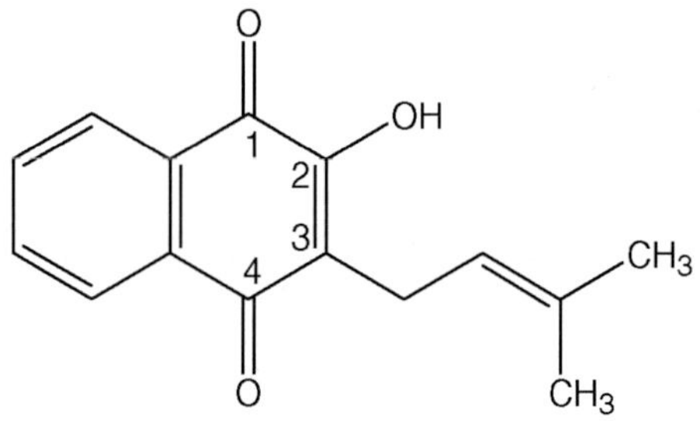

O
OH
1
2
3
4
CH_3
O
CH_3

Lapachol

KEY CONSTITUENTS

Tabebuia impetiginosa

- Naphthoquinones of the 1,4 type (including lapachol, beta-lapachone, xyloidone, deoxylapachol, alpha-lapachone, and dehydro-alpha-lapachone),[1,6] naphthofurandiones (or furonaphthoquinones) which are naphthoquinones with a furan ring attached to carbons at the 2 and 3 positions.[7-10]
- Anthraquinones (which rarely occur in plants containing naphthoquinones).[1,6]
- Benzoic acid derivatives, benzaldehyde derivatives, iridoids, coumarins, flavonoids and carnosol.

A review of pau d'arco products on the Canadian market found no or low levels of lapachol in all of the products. In contrast, two Brazilian products contained relatively high amounts of lapachol.[11] While poor quality of products is probably one reason for this finding, levels of lapachol also depend on whether the inner bark or the wood is used. Typical levels of total naphthoquinones expressed as lapachol are 1–2% for the inner bark, but lapachol itself is likely to be only a minor constituent of this plant part.

PHARMACODYNAMICS

Lapachol has been identified as the 'signature' compound in pau d'arco and much of the pharmacological research is based on it, though more recently its significance has been questioned.[12] Particularly, the furonaphthoquinones may possess significant immune-enhancing and antitumour activities.

Quinones form an important component of the electron-transport system in plants and mammals. Ubiquinol, the reduced form of co-enzyme Q_{10}, and menaquinone (a vitamin K) have significant antioxidant properties and play a major role in protecting cells from free radical damage. Redox reactions are inherent features of quinones and are recognized as 'the basis for their functional roles and cytotoxic and chemotherapeutic actions'.[13] While much active component research for pau d'arco has concentrated on lapachol, other naphthoquinones and their furano derivatives probably contribute significantly to any therapeutic activity of the inner bark. Hence quality assessment should involve an understanding of the total naphthoquinone content of the bark, rather than just lapachol. The corollary is that more information is needed about the relative levels of naphthoquinones in the various species which are used as medicines.

Antitumour and immune-enhancing activity

Following the clinical use of pau d'arco for cancer in Brazilian hospitals, studies in 1968 identified lapachol as an antitumour agent. In vivo tests showed lapachol to have significant activity against Walker 256 carcinosarcoma, particularly following twice daily oral administration.[14] This result was confirmed in studies by De Santana and co-workers, who found lapachol inhibited Yoshida's sarcoma (82%) and Walker 256 carcinosarcoma (50%) at a dose of 100 mg/kg. Beta-lapachone also inhibited Yoshida's sarcoma (16%) and Walker 256 carcinosarcoma (33.5%) at a dose of 7 mg/kg. However, alpha-lapachone and xyloidone showed no inhibition of Walker 256 carcinosarcoma at a dose of 200 mg/kg.[15] Lapachol was compared with lawsone, another 1,4 naphthoquinone, and found to have stronger inhibitory effects than the latter compound, especially against Yoshida's sarcoma.[16] Aqueous extracts of pau d'arco also inhibited Walker carcinoma (44%) when administered by injection to rats.[15]

Lapachol was also shown to be active against Murphy-Sturm lymphosarcoma but was inactive in the mice neoplasias sarcoma 180, adenocarcinoma 775, Lewis lung carcinoma (LLC), lymphocytic leukaemia P-388 and leukaemia L1210. However, in confirmation of previous results, it was found to be active against Walker 256 with a therapeutic index of 6.[17] Under different experimental conditions, twelve 1,4 naphthoquinones prolonged the life of mice bearing ascitic sarcoma 180 tumours. Statistical analysis revealed a link between the redox potentials of various compounds and their antitumour activity.[18] Later studies evaluated inhibitory effects of 1,4 naphthoquinones on beef heart mitochondrial succinoxidase and NADH-oxidase enzyme systems and found a strong relationship between succinoxidase inhibition, redox potential and antitumour activity. However, NADH-oxidase inhibition per se did not appear to influence the incidence of tumours.[19]

Lapachol has demonstrated significant antitumour activity in vitro as well as in vivo.[20] Lapachol and other naphthoquinones showed growth inhibition activity on KB cells (cultured tumour cells) at doses less than 4 μg/ml.[21] More recently, lapachol showed significant dose-dependent inhibition of four human melanoma cell lines and a human renal cell carcinoma line, though only after continual exposure.[22]

In the 1960s lapachol was positively identified as an uncoupling agent of mitochondrial respiration which mimics the behaviour of the classic uncoupling agent 2,4-dinitrophenol (DNP). This phenomenon occurs because of the structural similarity between lapachol and the endogenous hydroxyquinone, with which it competes for a position in the respiration chain. According to the hypothesis, lapachol exposes a mitochondrial thiol group which occupies a pivotal position between the respiration cycles.[23] This mechanism may explain its apparent cytotoxic activity.

However, other mechanisms may apply. Studies with quinone anticancer agents including lapachol using microsomal systems in normal and malignant tissues found that quinones are converted intracellularly to site-specific free radical intermediaries producing cytotoxic activity. The intermediaries bind to DNA or RNA resulting in chromosome damage, while also having potential to generate superoxide or hydroxyl radicals.[24] In a separate study using aqueous extracts of Tabebuia on LLC in mice, stimulation of superoxide ions in mouse macrophages was observed, with a maximum stimulation of superoxide at 5 mg/ml of the extract. The extract 'killed' LLC cells in vitro and in vivo and, by inhibiting DNA synthesis, protected against metastases.[25]

Lapachol also inhibits de novo pyrimidine synthesis by inhibition of dihydroorotate, resulting in depletion of nucleotide pools. Depletion of uridine triphosphate and cytidine triphosphate in hepatoma cells leads to their death. Hence lapachol may be combined with other antipyrimidines in tumour chemotherapy.[26] Vitamin K3 and other quinones including lapachol were also found to alter the affinity of receptors for epidermal growth factor, a potent mitogen capable of stimulating growth of human fibroblasts and other cells.[27]

Another potential mode of lapachol's cytotoxicity may be inhibition of glyoxalase I, which may lead to a lethal build-up of alpha-ketoaldehydes. In vitro studies showed lapachol to be a linear competitive inhibitor of yeast glyoxalase I.[28,29] Later studies examined glyoxalase inhibition in terms of tumour selectivity, that is, the relative inhibition between normal and tumour cells. However, it was found that lapachol was far less inhibitory of tumour than normal cells.[30] Lapachol was also found to be an inhibitor of ribonucleotide reductase, an enzyme involved in DNA replication which occurs at much higher levels in malignant cells than in non-proliferating cells.[31]

Pau d'arco extracts and other components have also demonstrated antitumour effects in vivo (see above and below). A methanolic extract of the inner bark of *T. avellanedae* reduced the number of papillomas in mice with induced skin carcinogenesis.[20] An alcoholic extract of stem bark from *Tabebuia cassinoides* showed slight, reproducible activity against leukaemia P-388 in vivo. Further investigations identified the active constituents as three previously unknown furonaphthoquinones.[32] In a separate study, two furonaphthoquinones from *T. impetiginosa* cell cultures showed significant dose-dependent antitumour activity.[33]

Wagner and co-workers proposed that lapachol and other naphthoquinones such as furonaphthoquinones exert cytotoxic or immunosuppressive effects, while in low concentrations they have immunostimulating properties.[34] They conclude the cytotoxic effect of the extracts may arise by induction of cellular and immune factors. Later in vitro investigations of compounds isolated from *T. impetiginosa* confirmed dose-dependent immune-modulating effects on human granulocytes and lymphocytes.[35]

Studies conducted at Harvard Medical School showed that beta-lapachone sensitized X-ray-resistant human melanoma cell lines when administered following X-radiation. The mechanism is thought to involve the inactivation of eukaryotic topoisomerase I, which is involved in DNA repair mechanisms following X-ray damage. Lapachol and other related compounds were inactive in this model.[36]

The furonaphthoquinone compound 5-hydroxy-2-(1-hydroxyethyl)-naptho[2,3-b]furan-4,9-dione (NFD), recently isolated from *T. impetiginosa*, has been patented by a Japanese pharmaceutical company as an antitumour agent, based on the new NCI screening protocols utilizing human cancer cell lines. NFD, administered in 100 mg tablets containing 1.5 mg active ingredient, was found to be an excellent antitumour agent against a wide range of cancers with minimal side effects.[37]

Other investigations into naphthoquinones were carried out in Japan by Hakura and co-workers. Most naphthoquinones tested, with the exceptions of lapachol and lawsone, showed mutagenicity and cytotoxicity for Ames Salmonella tester strains. The magnitude of naphthoquinone mutagenicity was much lower than for cytotoxicity and in both cases also depended on the structure of substituents in the molecules. The results on bacterial cytotoxicity support the oxidative stress theory, in which quinones are reduced to oxygen radical-activating semiquinones.[38]

Antiparasitic activity

Pau d'arco and some of its constituents, including lapachol, are active against various tropical parasites. Wendel carried out original work on naphthoquinones and malarial parasites in ducks, concluding the compounds inhibit oxygen uptake of parasitized cells at more than 100 times the concentration required to inhibit respiration in normal cells.[39] Further studies at Harvard Medical School confirmed these results and proposed that lapachol and other naphthoquinones act like cyanide in inhibiting the main respiration pathway, but leaving certain secondary and minor respiratory processes untouched. The authors concluded that naphthoquinones act below cytochrome c and above cytochrome b in the main chain of respiratory enzymes.[40] Willard suggests respiratory inhibition may apply to the more general antimicrobial actions of lapachol and its relatives.[6] In more recent research, naphthoquinones tested against drug-resistant strains of *Plasmodium falciparum* were superior to the controls chloroquine and quinine. Eight compounds related to lapachol, all isolated from plants in the Bignoniaceae family, showed this activity. However, despite its reputed antimalarial action, lapachol showed borderline activity only.[41]

Lapachol has been used as a chemoprophylactic against *Schistosoma mansoni* (a tropical fluke) cercarial penetration and infection. Studies by Austin showed that 0.9% lapachol in the diet of mice reduced infections by 97% after 3 days' feeding. The study further demonstrated that lapachol is secreted onto the skin where it forms a barrier to penetration.[42] Lapachol and other naphthoquinones derived from lapachol were also shown to work as topical applications.[43]

Trypanosoma cruzi is a parasite responsible for American trypanosomiasis or Chagas' disease, which is particularly common in Brazil.[44] Lapachol and several derivatives are toxic to *T. cruzi* in vitro but the toxic effect is nullified in the presence of blood. Hence, in vivo tests do not confirm in vitro studies. However, a synthetic beta-lapachone derivative, allyl-beta-lapachone, is not inactivated by blood and retains potent suppressive activity on trypomastigote infectivity.[45,46]

Antibacterial and antifungal activity

De Lima and co-workers in the 1950s first demonstrated antibacterial activity for lapachol, alpha- and beta-lapachone and xyloidone, as well as antifungal activity for alpha- and beta-lapachone and xyloidone. Naphthoquinones from pau d'arco, especially xyloidone, were effective against *Candida albicans* and Trichophyton, the fungus responsible for ringworm.[16] Pau d'arco tea is used as a topical application (via tampon) for vaginal candidiasis and taken internally for systemic infections.[1] The wide range of organisms that are susceptible to compounds from pau d'arco are summarized by Willard.[6] These include pathogenic species of Brucella, Staphylococcus and Candida.

In more recent studies, aqueous extracts of *T. heptaphylla* and *T. impetiginosa* showed no antibacterial activity against *Pseudomonas aeruginosa* in in vitro studies.[47] In a separate study, *T. impetiginosa* extract inhibited a penicillin-resistant strain of *Staph. aureus* but was inactive against *E. coli* and *Aspergillus niger*.[48]

Campos-Takaki and co-workers studied the influence of culture medium composition on the antifungal activity of lapachol and beta-lapachone from *T. avellanedae* and four synthetic hydroxynaphthoquinones. Lapachol demonstrated some activity against Candida and Cryptococcus fungi, contradicting previous results obtained by De Lima.[16] Of the six compounds tested, beta-lapachone and two synthetic naphthoquinones showed the best overall activity.[49] French workers also found beta-lapachone was more efficient than lapachol at inhibiting both bacteria and fungi. The antibacterial action showed a narrow spectrum, consisting mainly of Gram-positive strains and the Gram-negative Brucella. Beta-lapachone was more effective as an antifungal agent than ketoconazole, the standard used. The mechanism of the antimicrobial action may involve uncoupling of oxidative phosphorylation or electron transfer inhibition.[50]

Antiviral activity

Studies in 1975 by Linhares and De Santa showed that lapachol inhibited a number of viral strains including herpes virus hominis types I and II.[6] In separate studies, beta-lapachone was shown to be a potent inhibitor of reverse transcriptase from the retroviruses avian myeloblastosis virus and Rauscher murine leukaemia virus. It also inhibited eukaryotic DNA-dependent DNA polymerase. It is possible other retroviruses such as HIV are also susceptible. In this study, the enzyme inhibition was found to occur only in the presence of the reagent dithiothereitol. The antiviral mechanism involved is thought to involve redox reactions.[51]

In 1983, Lagrota and co-workers tested lapachol for activity against a range of viruses in vitro. Lapachol demonstrated significant inhibition of poliovirus and vesicular stomatitis virus. It also significantly inhibited haemagglutinating titres of influenza viral strains.[52] Three years later, the same team found several 1,4-naphthoquinone derivatives to be inactive against viral cell cultures, while 1,2-naphthoquinone derivatives inhibited echovirus.[53] Only one of these, beta-nor-lapachone, is a natural compound. However, the antiviral action could only be shown in vitro and no virucidal action against viral particles was observed. The authors suggest this antiviral action occurs through either interferon production or enzyme inhibition.[54,55]

Extracts of the inner bark of *T. avellanedae* were found to inhibit induction of Epstein–Barr virus (EBV)-associated early antigen in EBV genome-carrying human lymphoblastic cell lines. The aqueous extract was found to be less active than the methanolic extract, while lapachol caused viral inhibition at the lowest concentrations.[20]

Other activity

Lapachol and related naphthoquinones are known to be anticoagulants in rats and humans. Using animal models, Pruesch and Suttie found the anticoagulant activity to occur as a result of potent inhibition of vitamin K quinone and epoxide reductases. This action of lapachol appears similar to that of 4-hydroxycoumarin anticoagulants – they bind to the oxidized form of the vitamin K reductases.[56] Further studies by Preusch on rat liver microsomes showed lapachol inhibits another enzyme linked to blood coagulation.[57] Some writers link this anticoagulant activity to the anticancer applications of pau d'arco.

Lapachol has been found to have antiulcerogenic effects in experimental animals.[58] In a Brazilian study, lapachol demonstrated antiinflammatory effects, producing significant inhibition of carrageenan-induced paw oedema comparable to phenylbutazone.[59] An ethanolic extract of *Tabebuia chrysotricha*, and lapachol isolated from this species, showed significant analgesic activity in vivo.[60]

Lapachol has been found to possess both oestrogenic and antioestrogenic activity in mice. Lapachol from *Tectona grandis* demonstrated significant uterotrophic effects following intramuscular injection, though its oestrogenic activity was weak. Administration post-coitum resulted in inhibition of pregnancy and embryo resorption.[61]

PHARMACOKINETICS

No pharmacokinetic data are available for pau d'arco. Studies with lapachol in humans indicated that intestinal absorption was considerably less than that determined for the rat.[62]

CLINICAL TRIALS

Although pau d'arco contains potentially toxic active components which can generate free radicals and interfere with mitochondrial respiration and blood coagulation, there is no evidence that the long-term use of the inner bark is unsafe, provided certain precautions are observed (the dosage should not be too high and it should not be taken by patients on anticoagulant therapy).

However, it also follows that the therapeutic effects of the inner bark are likely to be mild and the herb should not be relied upon as a sole treatment for cancer or infections. One qualification of this is the immune-enhancing potential of pau d'arco, which could lead to a reevaluation of its therapeutic potential. This property requires more investigation in well-designed clinical studies.

Cancer

A phase I clinical trial of lapachol was initiated in 1967 at the Baltimore Cancer Research Center. The trial involved 21 leukaemia patients, each of whom was initially given capsules containing 0.25 or 0.5 g lapachol and later switched to a syrup formulation. The trial was stopped prematurely because prolonged prothrombin times were observed at the high oral doses required to test for antitumour activity. The high oral doses also resulted in nausea and vomiting, while measurements of plasma lapachol showed intestinal absorption of lapachol to be considerably less than previously determined for rats.[62] However, lapachol may be much better absorbed from its natural plant matrix.

In a more recent study, prescription of lapachol (daily dose 20–30 mg/kg) caused shrinkage of tumours and reduction in pain for nine cancer patients partaking in a small clinical trial. Three patients ceased the treatment due to experiences of nausea and vomiting, the other patients had no significant side effects. Three patients had complete remissions.[63]

TOXICOLOGY

Despite the widespread use of pau d'arco preparations, often for lengthy periods, there is no evidence of toxicity in humans. Some toxicity studies have been carried out on isolated constituents. De Santana and co-workers reported intraperitoneal LD_{50} values for lapachol in white mice at 1600 mg/kg, for xyloidone 600 mg/kg and beta-lapachone 80 mg/kg.[15] Lapachol has a relatively high therapeutic index of nearly 20. In 1970 the toxic effects of lapachol were studied in rodents and other animals. The LD_{50} for mice was 621 mg/kg and for albino rats over 2.4 g/kg. The following signs of toxicity were recorded: moderate to severe anaemia, reticulocytosis, normoblastosis, transient thrombocytosis and leucocytosis and elevated serum alkaline phosphatase activity and prothrombin times.[64]

In order to investigate the potential abortive and teratogenic action of lapachol, a study was carried out on pregnant albino rats. At a dose of 100 mg/kg, abortive activity was reported in some groups and malformations in others. While these results do not relate to bark extracts, they indicate that a degree of caution should be adopted in using pau d'arco during pregnancy.[65]

Mild contact sensitivity has been demonstrated with lapachol and other naphthoquinones. However, this is mainly a problem related to exposure of timber workers rather than use of oral medicines.[66,67]

CONTRAINDICATIONS

Patients on anticoagulant therapy should not be prescribed pau d'arco due to the warfarin-like action of naphthoquinones at high doses.

SPECIAL WARNINGS AND PRECAUTIONS

None required.

INTERACTIONS

The prescribing of pau d'arco with anticoagulants is contraindicated.

USE IN PREGNANCY AND LACTATION

Caution in pregnancy due to possible abortive and teratogenic actions.

EFFECTS ON ABILITY TO DRIVE AND USE MACHINES

None known.

SIDE EFFECTS

Adverse effects have been recorded during clinical trials of lapachol but there is no evidence to suggest that pau d'arco would cause similar effects.

OVERDOSE

No toxic effects reported.

CURRENT REGULATORY STATUS IN SELECTED COUNTRIES

Pau d'arco is not covered by a Commission E monograph and it is not on the UK General Sale List.

Pau d'arco does not have GRAS status. However, it is freely available as a 'dietary supplement' in the USA under DSHEA legislation (1994 Dietary Supplement Health and Education Act).

Pau d'arco is not included in Part 4 of Schedule 4 of the Therapeutic Goods Act Regulations of Australia.

References

1. Oswald EH. Br J Phytother 1993/1994; 3 (3): 112–117.
2. Evans Schultes R, Raffauf RF. The healing forest: medicinal and toxic plants of the northwest Amazonia. Dioscorides Press, Portland, 1990, pp 107–108.
3. Mabberley DJ. The plant book, 2nd edn. Cambridge University Press, Cambridge, 1997, pp 696, 702.
4. Willard T. Textbook of advanced herbology. Wild Rose College of Natural Healing, Calgary, 1992, pp 198–203.
5. Pederson M. Nutritional herbology. Pederson Publishing, Utah, 1987, p 206.
6. Willard T. *Tabebuia avellanedae*. In: Pizzorno JE, Murray MT (eds) A textbook of natural medicine, vol 1. John Bastyr College Publications, Seattle, 1987, V:Tabeb-1–8.
7. Girard M, Kindack D, Dawson BA et al. J Nat Prod 1988; 51 (5): 1023–1024.
8. Wagner H, Kreher B, Lotter H et al. Helv Chim Acta 1989; 72: 659–667.
9. Fujimoto Y, Eguchi T, Murasaki C et al. J Chem Soc Perkin Trans 1991; 1: 2323–2327.
10. Steinert J, Khalaf H, Rimpler M. J Chromatogr A 1995; 693: 281–287.
11. Awang DVC, Dawson BA, Ethier JC et al. J Herbs Spices Med Plants 1994; 2: 27–43.
12. Houghton PJ, Kahdra J, Theobald AE. J Pharm Pharmacol 1992; 44 (suppl): 1081.
13. Cadenas E, Hochstein P. Adv Enzymol Relat Areas Mol Biol 1992; 65: 97–146.
14. Rao KV, McBride TJ, Oleson JJ. Cancer Res 1968; 28: 1952–1954.
15. De Santana CF, De Lima OG, D'Albuquerque IL et al. Rev Inst Antibiot (Recife) 1968; 8 (1–2): 89–94.
16. De Lima OG, De Barros Coelho JS, D'Albuquerque IL et al. Rev Inst Antibiot (Recife) 1971; 11 (1): 21–26.
17. Da Consolacao M, Linardi F, De Oliveira MM et al. J Med Chem 1975; 18 (11): 1159–1161.
18. Hodnett E Wongwiechintana C, Dun WJ 3rd et al. J Med Chem 1983; 26 (4): 570–574.
19. Pisani DE, Elliott AJ, Hinman DR et al. Biochem Pharmacol 1986; 35 (21): 3791–3798.
20. Ueda S, Tokuda H. Planta Med 1990; 56: 669–670.
21. Favaro OCN, De Oliveira MM, Rossini MAA et al. An Acad Bras Cienc 1990; 62 (3): 217–224.
22. Houghton PJ, Photiou A, Uddin S et al. Planta Med 1994; 60 (5): 430–433.
23. Hadler H, Moreau T. J Antibiot 1969; 22 (11): 513–520.
24. Bachur NR, Gordon SL, Gee MV. Cancer Res 1978; 38: 1745–1750.
25. Moikeha Jr DH, Hokama Y. Unpublished results. Department of Pathology, John A Burns School of Medicine, University of Hawaii, Honolulu, Hawaii.
26. Keppler D, Fauler J, Gasser T et al. Adv Enzyme Regul 1985; 23: 61–79.
27. Shoyab M, Todaro G. J Biol Chem 1980; 255 (18): 8735–8739.
28. Douglas KT, Nadvi IN, Thakrar N. IRCS Med Sci 1982; 10: 683.
29. Douglas KT, Gohel DI, Nadvi IN et al. Biochim Biophys Acta 1985; 829 (1): 109–118.
30. Douglas KT, Keyworth LTA. Med Sci Res 1994; 22: 641–642.
31. Smith S, Douglas K. IRCS Med Sci 1986; 14: 541–542.
32. Rao MM, Kingston DGI. J Nat Prod 1982; 45: 600–604.
33. Ueda S, Umemura T, Dohguchi K et al. Phytochem 1994; 36 (2): 323–325.
34. Wagner H, Knaus U. Planta Med 1986; 52: 550A (P99).
35. Kreher B, Lotter H, Cordell GA et al. Planta Med 1988; K1-11: 562–563.
36. Boothman DA, Trask DK, Pardee AB. Cancer Res 1989; 49 (3): 605–612.
37. International Patent 9406786-A1, March 1994. 2-(1-Hydroxyethyl)-5-hydroxynaphtho[2,3-b]furan-4,9-dione and antitumour agents comprising this compound. Taheebo Japan Co Ltd.
38. Hakura A, Mochida H, Tsutsui Y et al. Chem Res Toxicol 1994; 7 (4): 559–567.
39. Wendel WB. Fed Proc 1946; 5: 406–407.
40. Ball E, Anfinsen CB, Cooper O. J Biol Chem 1947; 168: 257–270.
41. Carvalho LH, Rocha EM, Raslan DS et al. Braz J Med Biol Res 1988; 21 (3): 485–487.
42. Austin F. Am J Trop Med Hyg 1974; 23 (3): 412–419.
43. Pinto AV, Pinto MD, Gilbert B et al. Trans R Soc Trop Med Hyg 1977; 71 (2): 133–135.
44. Chiari E, De Oliveira AB, Raslan DS et al. Trans R Soc Trop Med Hyg 1991; 85 (3): 372–374.
45. Lopes JN, Cruz FS, Docampo R et al. Ann Trop Med Parasitol 1978; 72 (6): 523–531.
46. Sepulveda-Boza S, Cassels B. Planta Med 1996; 62: 98–105.
47. Perez C, Anesini C. Fitoterapia 1994; 65 (2): 169–172.
48. Anesini C, Perez C. J Ethnopharmacol 1993; 39 (2): 119–128.
49. Campos-Takaki G, Steiman R, Seigile-Murandi F et al. Rev Latinoam Microbiol 1992; 23 (2): 106–111.
50. Guiraud P, Steiman R, Campos-Takaki GM et al. Planta Med 1994; 60 (4): 373–374.
51. Schuerch AR, Wehrli W. Eur J Biochem 1978; 84 (1): 197–205.
52. Do Carmo Lagrota MM, Wigg MD, Pereira LOB et al. Rev Latinoam Microbiol 1983; 14 (1): 21–26.
53. Preusch PC, Hazelett SE, Lemasters KK. Arch Biochem Biophys 1989; 269 (1): 18–24.
54. Do Carmo Lagrota MM, Wigg MD, Aguiar ANS et al. Rev Latinoam Microbiol 1986; 28: 221–225.
55. Pinto AV, Pinto M de C, Lagrota MH et al. Rev Latinoam Microbiol 1987; 29 (1): 15–20.
56. Preusch PC, Suttie JW. Arch Biochem Biophys 1984; 234 (2): 405–412.
57. Preusch PC. Biochem Biophys Res Commun 1986; 137 (2): 781–787.
58. Goel RK, Pathak NK, Biswas M et al. J Pharm Pharmacol 1987; 39 (2): 138–140.
59. De Almeida ER, Da Silva Filho AA, Dos Santos ER et al. J Ethnopharmacol 1990; 29 (2): 239–241.
60. Grazziotin JD, Schapoval EE, Chaves CG et al. J Ethnopharmacol 1992; 36 (3): 249–251.
61. Sareen V, Jain S, Narula A. Phytother Res 1995; 9: 139–141.
62. Block JB, Serpick AA, Miller W et al. Cancer Chemother Rep [2] 1974; 4 (4): 27–28.
63. De Santana CF Pessoalins LJ, Asfora JJ et al. Rev Inst Antibiot (Recife) 1980/1981; 20: 61.

64. Morrison RK, Brown DE, Oleson JJ et al. Toxicol Appl Pharmacol 1970; 17 (1): 1–11.
65. De Almeida ER, De Mello AC, De Santana CF et al. Rev Port Farm 1988; 38 (3): 21–23.
66. Schultz K, Garbe I, Hausen BM et al. Arch Derm Res 1977; 258: 41–52.
67. Sigman CC, Helmes CT, Fay JR et al. J Environ Sci Health 1984; A19 (5): 533–577.

Peppermint (*Mentha* x *piperita* L.)

SYNONYMS

Pfefferminze, Katzenkraut (Ger), menthe anglaise, menthe poivrée, feuilles de menthe (Fr), menta prima (Ital), pebermynte (Dan).

WHAT IS IT?

The mints, including peppermint, are amongst the oldest European herbs used for both culinary and medicinal purposes. The Greeks and Romans crowned themselves with peppermint at their feasts and adorned their tables with its sprays. Their cooks flavoured both their sauces and their wines with its essence. Peppermint was cultivated by the Egyptians and is mentioned in the Icelandic pharmacopoeias of the 13th century but only came into general use in the medicine of Western Europe in the 18th century. Mints are used in both home remedies and pharmaceutical preparations to relieve the stomach of intestinal gas associated with the consumption of certain foods; hence the many different varieties of after-dinner mints. Menthol, a compound of peppermint, has been used as an inhalant for upper respiratory ailments and as an ingredient in many liniments and rubs for sore muscles.

EFFECTS

Gastrointestinal spasmolytic, carminative; increases bile production; reduces cough frequency; sedative to the central nervous system; local anaesthetic.

TRADITIONAL VIEW

Peppermint was used to treat flatulent colic, digestive pain, cramps and spasms of the stomach, dyspepsia, nausea and vomiting, morning sickness and dysmenorrhoea. As an inhalant it was used to relieve the cough of bronchitis and pneumonia and to induce perspiration in the early phase of a cold. The bruised fresh herb was applied over the bowel to allay a sick stomach and the same kind of application was also used to relieve headaches.[1,2] An infusion of peppermint in combination with wood betony and caraway was used in the treatment of nervous disorders and hysteria and in combination with elderflowers, yarrow or boneset for the treatment of colds and mild cases of influenza.[3]

SUMMARY ACTIONS

Spasmolytic, carminative, cholagogue, antiemetic, antitussive, antimicrobial, sedative, diaphoretic. Locally: antiseptic, analgesic, antipruritic.

CAN BE USED FOR

INDICATIONS SUPPORTED BY CLINICAL TRIALS

Indications supported by trials using menthol: to reduce airway hyperresponsiveness in asthma (by inhalation).

Indications supported by trials using peppermint oil: symptoms of irritable bowel syndrome; nonulcer dyspepsia; postoperative nausea; topically: as an analgesic for headaches.

Indications supported by trials using peppermint leaf in combination with other herbs: for the treatment of dyspepsia.

TRADITIONAL THERAPEUTIC USES

Digestive disorders (dyspepsia, flatulence, colic, cramps, vomiting, nausea); inhalation and oral doses for respiratory disorders (bronchitis, cough, colds, influenza); headaches (topically) and nervous disorders.

MAY ALSO BE USED FOR

EXTRAPOLATIONS FROM PHARMACOLOGICAL STUDIES

Inhibition of muscular contraction induced by serotonin and substance P; reduction in pain sensitivity by activating the endogenous opiate systems; increased bronchial secretion and inhibition of cough; as a mild central nervous system sedative.

OTHER APPLICATIONS

Peppermint leaf or oil are widely used as flavourings in medicinal teas, cough preparations, food products and beverages.[4] Peppermint leaf has also been used as a carminative in antacid products.[5]

PREPARATIONS

As with all essential oil-containing herbs, use of the fresh plant or carefully dried herb is advised.

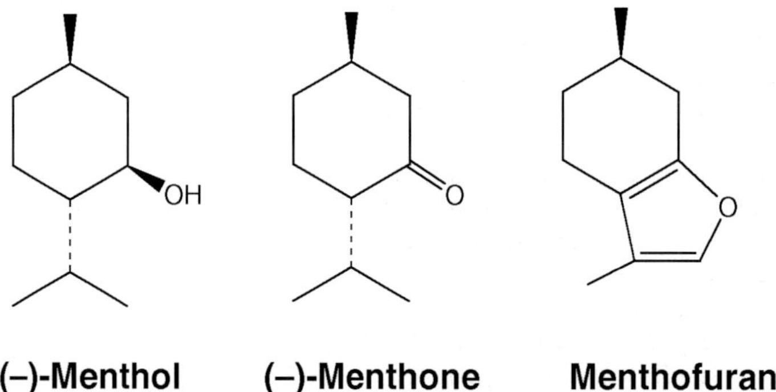

Keep covered if infusing the herb to retain the essential oil.

Dried leaf as an infusion, liquid extract, tincture or essential oil for internal use. The essential oil dissolved in alcohol works well for topical use.

DOSAGE

- 6–9 g of the dried leaf per day or as infusion.
- 1.5–4 ml of 1:2 liquid extract per day, 3.5–11 ml of 1:5 tincture per day.
- 0.15–0.6 ml (approximately 3–12 drops) of the essential oil per day.

DURATION OF USE

May be taken long term for most applications.

SUMMARY ASSESSMENT OF SAFETY

No significant adverse effects from the ingestion of peppermint leaf are expected but higher doses of the essential oil can produce a variety of adverse reactions including skin rashes, headaches, bradycardia, muscle tremor, heartburn and ataxia.

TECHNICAL DATA

BOTANY

Mentha x *piperita*, a member of the Labiatae (mint) family, is a perennial plant approximately 50 cm in height with quadrangular stems terminated with a flower spike consisting of numerous congested whorls. The leaves have very short petioles, are opposed, ovate-lanceolate from a wedge shape to an almost heart-shaped base. They have a venation that gives them a rough-textured appearance, are dark green on the upper surface and slightly paler on the lower. The pinkish mauve flowers are tubular with four lobes, one of which is normally larger than the others, contained within a calyx with five pointed lobes. The fruits are dark, four-sectioned, glossy ovoidal cremocarps. The plant is always sterile and has a pungent peppermint scent.[6,7] Peppermint is a hybrid species from two parents: *Mentha spicata* (spearmint) and *Mentha aquatica* (water mint).[8]

KEY CONSTITUENTS

- Essential oil (0.5–4%), consisting predominantly of menthol (35–45%) and (–)-menthone (10–30%).[9]
- Flavonoids, tannins (6–12%), triterpenes and bitter substances.[10]

The *European Pharmacopoeia* recommends that whole peppermint leaf contain not less than 12 ml/kg and the cut leaf not less than 9 ml/kg of essential oil.[11] Peppermint oil is obtained by steam distillation from the fresh aerial parts of flowering *Mentha* x *piperita*.[12]

PHARMACODYNAMICS

Gastrointestinal effects

The in vitro effects of peppermint oil on the gastrointestinal smooth muscles of guinea pigs and rabbits resemble those of calcium antagonist drugs. Peppermint oil markedly attenuated contractile responses in guinea pig taenia coli to acetylcholine, histamine, serotonin and substance P. It also reduced contractions evoked by potassium depolarization and inhibited potential-dependent calcium currents in rabbit jejunum smooth muscle cells in a dose-dependent manner.[13] Intravenous administration of an aqueous solution of peppermint oil reduced morphine-induced spasm in Oddi's sphincter in guinea pigs.[14]

Peppermint leaf extract demonstrated spasmolytic activity on acetylcholine- and histamine-induced contractions in isolated guinea pig ileum.[15,16] An aqueous solution of flavonoids isolated from peppermint inhibited barium chloride-induced contractions.[17]

The intraluminal administration of peppermint oil (0.1–20 ml saline) to the sigmoid colon of five normal humans produced increased intraluminal pressure, abdominal cramps and the urge to defaecate and micturate, which suggested a widespread stimulation of smooth muscle.[18] This might reflect a local irritant effect of the peppermint oil, since in another study examining the effect of peppermint oil on colonic spasm during colonoscopy, the opposite effect was observed. Peppermint oil injected along the biopsy channel of the colonoscope in 20 patients relieved colonic spasm within 30 seconds, allowing easier passage of the instrument or assisting in polypectomy. Due to the potential irritant effect of peppermint oil, a diluted suspension is now used with equally good effects.[19]

The direct administration of 15 drops of peppermint oil in 30 ml of water into the stomachs of 27 subjects caused relaxation of the lower oesophageal sphincter and equalization of intragastric and intra-oesophageal pressures (carminative activity). Reflux occurred in 25 out of 27 patients within 1–7 minutes of administration. The sphincter relaxation lasted approximately 30 seconds and was terminated by an oesophageal peristaltic wave.[20]

Single oral doses of menthol (468 mg/kg) or cineole (262 mg/kg) inhibited the HMG-CoA reductase activity in rats by up to 70%. The effect was specific and not due to generalized hepatotoxicity.[21,22]

Peppermint oil in the intestinal lumen at concentrations varying from 1 to 5 mg/ml inhibited enterocyte glucose uptake via a direct action at the brush border membrane in vitro. This effect was thought to be due to changes in the charge on tight junctions between cells and to an inhibition of sodium-linked active transport. The standard bolus dose of peppermint oil for humans is about 400 mg and this could achieve a local concentration in this range in the intestinal lumen during the fasting state.[23]

Antimicrobial effects

Peppermint oil has shown significant antibacterial and antifungal effects in several studies.[24,25,26] Samples of 18 different commercial peppermint oils were obtained from a wide range of suppliers and tested for antibacterial activity against 25 different species of bacteria and 20 different strains of *Listeria monocy-togenes* isolated from different food sources. Antifungal activity was assessed against *Aspergillus nigra, Aspergillus ochraceus* and *Fusarium culmorum*. The chemical composition of the oils was variable with menthone ranging from 16.7% to 31.4%, menthol 32.1% to 49% and menthofuran 5.1% to 12%. Most of the species of bacteria tested, with the exception of *Acaligenes faecalis, Flavobacterium suaveolens, Leuconostoc cremoris, Pseudomonas aeruginosa* and *Streptococcus faecalis*, were inhibited by some of the peppermint oils, with nine species being inhibited by all of the oils. All the strains of *Listeria monocytogenes* were inhibited by some peppermint oils, nine strains by all of the oils and one strain by only three of the oils. The three filamentous fungi were inhibited by all peppermint oils but three oils showed a low activity against *Fusarium culmorum*. The oils showing the most potent antibacterial activity were amongst the most ineffectual oils against one of the fungal species and there appeared to be an inverse relationship between antibacterial and antifungal activity.[24] Another study found that peppermint oil (0.1%) was more inhibitory towards Gram-negative than Gram-positive bacteria.[27]

Respiratory effects

Volatile aromatics such as menthol exhibit a surfactant-like effect in vitro. In vivo it decreased surface tension between water and air and therefore improved lung compliance values.[28] Menthol inhalation produced a significant reduction in cough frequency and an increase in cough latency in guinea pigs challenged with aerosolized citric acid for 2 minutes, thus demonstrating the efficacy of menthol as an antitussive in chemically induced cough.[29]

In several studies on healthy volunteers (by inhalation of menthol vapour)[30,31] and those with nasal congestion associated with common cold infection (by oral administration of a menthol lozenge),[32] menthol brought about a change in the nasal sensation of airflow with a subjective sensation of nasal decongestion but had no effect on nasal resistance to airflow. This finding is due to a significant pharmacological action on nasal sensory nerve endings and is unrelated to the peppermint smell.[33]

The spasmolytic and secretolytic effects of an ointment containing menthol, camphor and essential oils were tested in animals. Acetylcholine-induced bronchospasm was reduced by 50% when the ointment was insufflated through the respiratory tract, whereas the epicutaneous application of the ointment only produced a slight reduction. Significant secretolytic effects were demonstrated after insufflation and topical administration.[34]

Analgesic effects

The topical application of menthol (at concentrations of 1–30% in ethanol) showed a major antinociceptive effect in the early phase of pain response of the formalin test in mice. Menthol-induced analgesia was blocked by naloxone and potentiated by bestatin. Menthol also produced antinociceptive effects in the hot plate test of mice and hind paw pressure test in rats but did not inhibit carrageenan-induced paw oedema in rats and the synthesis of prostaglandin E_2 in vitro. These results suggest that menthol produces antinociceptive effects by activation of the endogenous opioid system and/or partially by local anaesthetic actions without antiinflammatory effects.[35]

The long-lasting cooling effect produced by topical application of peppermint oil is caused by a steric alteration of the calcium channels of cold receptors.[36,37] In a double-blind, crossover study with 15 healthy subjects, the analgesic activity of peppermint oil was differentiated from the physical effect resulting from heat of evaporation and appeared to be based on central inhibitory effects mediated by cold-sensitive A delta nerve fibres.[38]

Other effects

Peppermint oil induced a significant increase in the skin blood flow of capillaries of the forehead in healthy subjects and migraine patients after local application, as measured by laser Doppler.[39]

A dried aqueous extract of peppermint containing approximately 3.3% flavonoids, 18.4% tannins and 1.2% essential oil produced an initial excitatory effect followed by a sedative action on mice at a dose of 1000 mg/kg. The initial excitation is thought to be due to a stimulation of the sensorial system. The same extract also showed a mild diuretic effect.[40]

Dietary additions of menthol and limonene resulted in a significant inhibition of DMBA-initiated rat mammary tumours.[41]

PHARMACOKINETICS

Pharmacokinetic studies demonstrate that peppermint oil in normal capsules gives higher peak excretion levels of menthol (as glucuronide) than enteric-coated capsules. This suggests that peppermint oil is mainly absorbed in the upper gastrointestinal tract unless enterically coated and should be taken in this form for effects in the lower gastrointestinal tract.[42]

CLINICAL TRIALS

Gallstones

In a controlled, double-blind trial, the addition of menthol to ursodeoxycholic acid significantly reduced the size of gallstones by dissolution and reduced the incidence of stone calcification.[43] Rowachol, a proprietary choleretic containing menthol 32%, pinene 17%, menthone 6%, borneol 5%, camphene 5% and cineole 2% dissolved in olive oil, significantly lowers the cholesterol saturation index of human bile. Twenty-four patients with radiolucent gallstones were given two capsules three times daily for periods in excess of 6 months in an uncontrolled study. At 6 months the gallstones had disappeared in two patients and were significantly fewer or smaller in a further three patients. The remaining 19 patients' stones were unchanged but one of these showed evidence of a reduction of stone size after 1 year.[44]

Irritable bowel syndrome

Clinical trials suggest that peppermint oil may be beneficial in the treatment of some symptoms of irritable bowel syndrome (IBS), although the evidence is not strong. The peppermint oil capsules are usually enteric coated to prevent the side effect of gastric reflux, which such high doses will inevitably cause.

In an uncontrolled trial, 40 patients received effective treatment for irritable bowel syndrome after a 14-day course of enteric-coated peppermint oil capsules. Intestinal transit time was prolonged and subjective improvement was observed in the rating scores for fullness, bloating, bowel noises and abdominal pain.[45] This was followed by a double-blind trial in 18 patients with active symptoms of IBS who were given 1–2 enteric-coated capsules (containing 0.2 ml peppermint oil or placebo) three times daily. Patients felt significantly better while taking peppermint oil capsules compared to the peanut oil placebo ($p<0.01$) and considered peppermint oil to be better than placebo in relieving abdominal symptoms ($p<0.05$). Analysis of the symptom grades showed a lower total and mean daily score with peppermint oil treatment but the values were not significantly different to placebo.[46] A second similar double-blind crossover study conducted in the same centre with 29 patients yielded similar results. Patients taking peppermint oil had a lower daily symptom score ($p<0.01$) but there was no effect on the number of bowel actions per day.[47]

However, these two studies have been criticized for faulty design and inappropriate statistical analysis and a later trial with a more robust design showed no superiority over placebo. In this double-blind trial, 41 patients were given two capsules containing 0.2 ml peppermint oil or a peanut oil placebo three times daily before food. The patients' assessment of progress at the end of the second and fourth weeks showed no significant difference between peppermint oil and placebo in terms of overall symptoms and pain. There was no difference in weekly stool frequency during either treatment.[48] Peppermint oil (0.6 ml per day over 4 weeks) demonstrated a small significant increase in frequency of defaecation in irritable bowel patients compared to placebo in a double-blind trial. But there was no significant change in scores for global severity of symptoms or for scores of specific symptoms.[49]

In a prospective, randomized, double-blind, placebo-controlled clinical trial, 110 outpatients with irritable bowel syndrome received an enteric-coated capsule containing 187 mg peppermint oil or placebo, 3–4 times per day, 15–30 minutes before meals for 1 month. Symptom improvements (abdominal pain, abdominal distension, stool frequency, borborygmi, flatulence) after peppermint oil treatment were significantly better than after placebo ($p<0.05$). There was no adverse effect on upper digestive tract symptoms. One patient developed a mild skin rash over both forearms.[50]

Other gastrointestinal disorders

Fifty-four patients with non-ulcer dyspepsia were given one enteric-coated capsule containing 90 mg of peppermint oil and 50 mg of caraway oil in a double-blind, placebo-controlled, multicentre trial. After 4 weeks of treatment the intensity of pain ($p=0.015$) and global clinical impressions ($p=0.008$) were significantly improved for the active group compared to the placebo group. Before treatment commenced, all active patients reported moderate to severe pain, whilst by the end of the study 63.2% of these patients were pain free and 26.3% reported a reduction of their pain.[51]

Peppermint oil accelerated the gastric emptying rate in both dyspeptic patients and controls. The gastric emptying rate of dyspeptic patients became comparable to that of aged match controls after administration of 0.2 ml peppermint oil in 25 ml of water ($p<0.001$).[52] The incidence of postoperative nausea in gynaecological patients was significantly reduced ($p=0.02$) in an active group that inhaled peppermint oil in a placebo-controlled trial involving 18 patients.[53]

A liquid herbal formula (25 drops three times daily) containing, in increasing proportions, wormwood, caraway, fennel and peppermint was found to be superior to the spasmolytic drug metoclopramide in terms of relief of symptoms such as pain, nausea, belching and heartburn in a randomized, double-blind clinical trial on the treatment of dyspepsia ($p=0.02$).[54] In another placebo-controlled, randomized, double-blind clinical trial, 70 patients with marked chronic digestive problems such as flatulence or bloating were treated with either a herbal formula containing caraway, fennel, peppermint and gentian in tablet form or a placebo over a 14-day period. Analysis of the trial results established a significant improvement in the gastrointestinal complaint scores of the group receiving herbal tablets compared to the placebo group ($p<0.05$). Ultrasound results evaluating the amount of gas present in the bowel also demonstrated a significant benefit from the herbal formula ($p<0.05$).[55]

Headaches

The topical application of peppermint oil in ethanol solution has proven to be a well-tolerated and cost-effective treatment for tension headache. In a randomized, placebo-controlled, double-blind, crossover study, 10 g of peppermint oil in a 90% ethanol solution was compared to acetaminophen (1 g) and placebo in the treatment of 164 chronic tension headaches in 41 patients of both sexes. Headache episodes were treated with the following: placebo capsule and peppermint oil, acetaminophen (paracetamol) and placebo solution, acetaminophen and peppermint oil, or placebo capsule and placebo solution. Peppermint oil solution was spread across the forehead and temples and the application was repeated after 15 and 30 minutes. Peppermint oil solution significantly reduced headache intensity after 15 minutes compared to placebo ($p<0.01$). Acetaminophen was effective relative to placebo ($p<0.01$) but did not differ significantly from treatment with peppermint oil. The simultaneous administration of the peppermint oil solution with acetaminophen produced an additive effect ($p<0.001$). The authors concluded that peppermint oil is an acceptable and cost-effective alternative to oral analgesics in the treatment of tension headache.[56]

In a randomized, double-blind, placebo-controlled crossover study, topical application of peppermint and eucalyptus oil preparations on headache parameters were investigated in 32 healthy men. The combination of peppermint oil, eucalyptus oil and ethanol increased cognitive performance while having muscle-relaxing and mentally relaxing effects but had no significant effect on pain sensitivity. The peppermint oil and ethanol preparation produced a significant analgesic effect with reduction in sensitivity to headache ($p<0.01$ for experimental ischaemia, $p<0.001$ for experimental heat stimuli). These pharmacological and clinical results indicate that peppermint oil has both central and peripheral activity.[57,58]

Other conditions

The effect of inhaled menthol on asthma was studied in a placebo-controlled trial with 23 patients. The menthol vapour did not produce acute bronchodilatory effects but long-term inhalation over 4 weeks produced an improvement of airway hyperresponsiveness without altering the magnitude of airflow limitation. There was a decreased diurnal variation in peak expiratory flow rate ($p<0.05$), a value that reflects airway hyperresponsiveness, but no significant effects on the forced expiratory volume in 1 second. The number of metered dose inhaler inhalations were also significantly reduced in the menthol group ($p<0.01$).[59]

TOXICOLOGY

The acute oral LD_{50} of menthol was reported to be 3.3 g/kg in the rat.[60] The estimated lethal dose for menthol in humans may be as low as 2 g but there are reports of individuals surviving doses as high as 9 g.[61] Histopathological changes consisting of cyst-like spaces scattered in the white matter of the cerebellum and nephropathy were seen in male rats given a daily oral dose of 100 mg/kg of peppermint oil for 90 days. No adverse effects were seen at doses below 40 mg/kg.[62]

Oral administration of a spray-dried infusion of peppermint (4 g/kg) did not result in any macroscopic signs of toxicity or death in mice over a 7-day period.[40]

CONTRAINDICATIONS

Patients with oesophageal reflux symptoms should eliminate substances which decrease lower oesophageal sphincter pressure, including peppermint.[63] The Commission E suggests that peppermint oil is contraindicated for internal use in occlusion of the gallbladder passages, cholecystitis and severe liver disease. Peppermint oil should not be applied to the facial areas of babies and small children and especially not around the nose.[64]

SPECIAL WARNINGS AND PRECAUTIONS

Use with care in patients with salicylate sensitivity and aspirin-induced asthma. Care should be taken in patients with gallstones.[10] Oral intake of peppermint oil should be used with caution in patients with preexisting heartburn and enteric-coated capsules may produce anal burning in patients with diarrhoea due to excreted peppermint oil.[61]

INTERACTIONS

None known with peppermint leaf.

USE IN PREGNANCY AND LACTATION

No adverse effects expected.

EFFECTS ON ABILITY TO DRIVE AND USE MACHINES

No adverse effects expected.

SIDE EFFECTS

Nasal preparations containing menthol may cause spasm of the glottis in young children.[61] Skin rashes, headache, bradycardia, muscle tremor, heartburn and ataxia are rarely reported side effects associated with enteric-coated capsules of peppermint oil.[48,61] Bradycardia has been reported in a patient addicted to menthol cigarettes and fibrillation has been associated with the excessive consumption of peppermint-flavoured confectionery. Mild dermatological reactions on the skin and mucous membranes have been described and neat peppermint oil can produce chemical burns. Reports of gastrointestinal irritation or aggravation of gastrointestinal complaints including stomatitis, severe oesophagitis, gastritis, unexplained diarrhoea and pancreatitis have been associated with the use of peppermint preparations including confectionery.[61] Allergic reactions to peppermint appear to be rare or of a relatively minor nature.[61]

OVERDOSE

No effects known for peppermint leaf but see above for peppermint oil.

CURRENT REGULATORY STATUS IN SELECTED COUNTRIES

Both peppermint leaf and peppermint oil are official in the *European Pharmacopoeia* (1997), the *British Pharmacopoeia* (1998) and the *United States Pharmacopeia-National Formulary* (USP23–NF18, 1995 – June 1999).

Peppermint leaf and peppermint oil are covered by positive Commission E monographs and can be used for the following applications.

Peppermint leaf:

- cramp-like complaints in the gastrointestinal tract and the gallbladder and biliary tract.

Peppermint oil:

- internal: spastic discomfort of the upper gastrointestinal tract and bile ducts, irritable colon, catarrh of the respiratory tract, inflammation of the oral mucosa.
- external: myalgia and neuralgia.

Peppermint is on the UK General Sale List.

Peppermint, peppermint oil and menthol have GRAS status. Peppermint is also freely available as a 'dietary supplement' in the USA under DSHEA legislation (1994 Dietary Supplement Health and Education Act). Peppermint has been present in OTC digestive aid drug products. Peppermint oil has been present in OTC nasal decongestant drug products (mouthwash), expectorant drug products, digestive aid drug products, insect bite and sting drug products and astringent drug products. The FDA, however, advises that: 'based on evidence currently available, there is inadequate data to establish general recognition of the safety and effectiveness of these ingredients for the specified uses'.

Peppermint is not included in Part 4 of Schedule 4 of the Therapeutic Goods Act Regulations of Australia.

References

1. Felter HW, Lloyd JU. King's American dispensatory, 18th edn, 3rd revision, vol 1, 1905. Reprinted by Eclectic Medical Publications, Portland, 1983, pp 1254–1255.
2. British Herbal Medicine Association's Scientific Committee. British herbal pharmacopoeia. BHMA, Cowling, 1983, p 142.
3. Grieve M. A modern herbal, vol 2. Dover Publications, New York, 1971, pp 537–543.
4. Leung AY, Foster S. Encyclopedia of common natural ingredients used in food, drugs and cosmetics, 2nd edn. John Wiley, New York, 1996, pp 368–372.
5. Robson NJ. Anaesthesia 1987; 42 (7): 776–777.
6. Chiej R. The Macdonald encyclopedia of medicinal plants. Macdonald, London 1984, entry no. 195.
7. Launert EL. The Hamlyn guide to edible and medicinal plants of Britain and Northern Europe. Hamlyn, London, 1981, p 156.
8. Evans WC. Trease and Evans' pharmacognosy, 14th edn. WB Saunders, London, 1996, pp 259–261.
9. Wagner H, Bladt S. Plant drug analysis: a thin layer chromatography atlas, 2nd edn. Springer-Verlag, Berlin, 1996, p 156.
10. Bisset NG (ed). Herbal drugs and phytopharmaceuticals Medpharm Scientific Publishers, Stuttgart, 1994, pp 336–338.
11. European pharmacopoeia, 3rd edn. European Department for the Quality of Medicines within the Council of Europe, Strasbourg, 1996, p 1298.
12. European pharmacopoeia, 3rd edn. European Department for the Quality of Medicines within the Council of Europe, Strasbourg, 1996, p 1299.
13. Hills JM, Aaronson PI. Gastroenterology 1991; 101 (1): 55–65.
14. Giachetti D, Taddei E, Taddei I. Planta Med 1988; 54 (5): 389–392.
15. Forster HB, Niklas H, Lutz S. Planta Med 1980; 40 (4): 309–319.
16. Forster H. Z Allg Med 1983; 59 (24): 1327–1333.
17. Lallement-Guilbert N, Bezanger-Bearuquesne L. Plant Med Phytother 1970; 4: 92–107.
18. Rogers J, Tay HH, Misiewicz JJ. Lancet 1988; 2 (8602): 99.
19. Leicester RJ, Hunt RH. Lancet 1982; 2 (8305): 989.
20. Sigmund CJ, McNally EF. Gastroenterology 1969; 56 (1): 13–18.
21. Clegg RJ, Middleton B, Bell GD et al. J Biol Chem 1982; 257 (5): 2294–2299.
22. Clegg RJ, Middleton B, Bell GD et al. Biochem Pharmacol 1980; 29 (15): 2125–2128.
23. Beesley A, Hardcastle J, Hardcastle PT et al. Gut 1996; 39 (2): 214–219.
24. Lis-Balchin M, Deans SG, Hart S. Med Sci Res 1997; 25: 151–152.
25. El-Naghy MA, Maghazy SN, Fadl-Allah EM et al. Zentralbl Mikrobiol 1992; 147 (3–4): 214–220.
26. Maiti D, Kole CR, Sen C. Pfl Krankh 1985; 92 (1): 64–68.
27. Shapiro S, Meier A, Guggenheim B. Oral Microbiol Immunol 1994; 9: 202–208.
28. Zanker KS, Tolle W, Blumel G et al. Respiration 1980; 39 (3): 150–157.
29. Laude EA, Morice AH, Grattan TJ. Pulmon Pharmacol 1994; 7 (3): 179–184.
30. Eccles R, Jones AS. J Laryngol Otol 1983; 97 (8): 705–709.
31. Burrow A, Eccles R, Jones AS. Acta Otolaryngol 1983; 96 (1–2): 157–161.
32. Eccles R, Jawad MS, Morris S. J Pharm Pharmacol 1990; 42 (9): 652–654.
33. Eccles R, Griffiths DH, Newton CG et al. Clin Otolaryngol 1988; 13 (1): 25–29.
34. Rai MK, Upadhyay S. Arzneim-Forsch 1981; 31 (1): 82–86.
35. Taniguchi Y, Deguchi Y, Saita M et al. Nippon Yakurigaku Zasshi 1994; 104 (6): 433–446.
36. Watson HR, Hems R, Rowsell DG et al. J Soc Cosmet Chem 1978; 29 (4): 185–200.
37. Eccles R. J Pharm Pharmacol 1994; 46: 618–630.
38. Bromm B, Scharein E, Darsow U et al. Neurosci Lett 1995; 187: 157–160.
39. Gobel H, Dworschak M, Ardabili S et al. The 7th International Headache Congress, Toronto, September 16–20, 1995.
40. Della Loggia R, Tubaro A. Fitoterapia 1990; 61 (3): 215–221.
41. Russin WA, Hoesly JD, Elson CE et al. Carcinogenesis 1989; 10 (11): 2161–2164.
42. Somerville KW, Richmond CR, Bell GD. Br J Clin Pharmacol 1984; 18: 638–640.
43. Leuschner M, Leuschner U, Lazarovici D et al. Gut 1988; 29 (4): 428–432.
44. Bell CD, Doran J, Middleton A et al. Br J Clin Pharmacol 1978; 6 (5): 454P.
45. Wildgrube HJ. Natur Heilpraxis 1988; 41: 2–5.
46. Rees WD, Evans BK, Rhodes J. Br Med J 1979; 2 (6194): 835–836.
47. Dew MJ, Evans BK, Rhodes J. Br J Clin Pract 1984; 38: 394–398.

48. Nash P, Gould SR, Barnardo DE. Br J Clin Pract 1986; 40 (7): 292–293.
49. Lawson MJ, Knight RE, Tran K et al. J Gastroenterol Hepatol 1988; 3: 235–238.
50. Liu JH, Chen GH, Yeh HZ et al. J Gastroenterol 1997; 32 (6): 765–768.
51. May B, Kuntz HD, Kieser M et al. Arzneim-Forsch 1996; 46 (12): 1149–1153.
52. Dalvi SS, Nadkarni PM, Pardesi R et al. Ind J Physiol Pharmacol 1991; 35 (3): 212–214.
53. Tate S. J Adv Nurs 1997; 26 (3): 543–549.
54. Westphal J, Hörning M, Leonhardt K. Phytomed 1996; 2 (4): 285–291.
55. Silberhorn H, Landgrebe N, Wohling D et al. 6th Phytotherapy Conference, Berlin, October 5–7, 1995.
56. Gobel H, Fresenius J, Heinze A et al. Nervenarzt 1996; 67 (8): 672–681.
57. Gobel H, Schmidt G, Soyka D. Cephalalgia 1994; 14 (3): 228–234.
58. Gobel H, Schmidt G, Dworschak M et al. Phytomed 1995; 2 (2): 93–102.
59. Tamaoki J, Chiyotani A, Sakai A et al. Respir Med 1995; 89 (7): 503–504.
60. Opdyke DLJ. Food Cosmet Toxicol 1976; 14: 471–472.
61. De Smet PAGM, Keller K, Hansel R et al (eds). Adverse effects of herbal drugs, vol 1. Springer-Verlag, Berlin, 1992, pp 171–176.
62. Spindler P, Madsen C. Toxicol Lett 1992; 62 (2–3): 215–220.
63. Friedman G. Gastroenterol Clin North Am 1991; 20 (2): 313–324.
64. German Federal Minister of Justice. German Commission E for human medicine monograph, Bundes-Anzeiger (German Federal Gazette), no. 50, dated 13.03.1986.

Poke root (*Phytolacca decandra* L.)

SYNONYMS

Phytolacca americana L. (botanical synonym), poke weed (Engl), Phytolaccae radix (Lat), Kermesbeere (Ger), herbe de la laque (Fr), fitolacca (Ital), kermesbær (Dan).

WHAT IS IT?

Phytolacca decandra is a striking plant with large leaves, clusters of purple berries, often on the same branch with green unripe fruit and flowers still in bloom. It is indigenous to the United States of America and has the following common names: poke root, poke weed. Its common name derives from the indigenous word *pocon* meaning a plant with red or yellow dye (referring to the juice of the ripe berries). The genus name Phytolacca is from the Greek *phuton* meaning plant and from the Latin *lacca* meaning milky lac. Many parts have been used medicinally, including the berries, leaves and roots. This monograph focuses on the therapeutic use of the dried root, which is toxic in overdose.

'Poke weed' occurs extensively in medical literature due to the use of poke weed mitogens (PWM) to investigate cellular immune response and a poke weed antiviral protein which inhibits viral protein synthesis. These are unlikely to be significantly absorbed into the bloodstream after oral doses except when the gastrointestinal tract is damaged.

EFFECTS

An antiinflammatory remedy with action on the lymphatics and respiratory system. Potentially immune stimulating but caution is required with dosage.

TRADITIONAL VIEW

Poke root has been used traditionally for the treatment of inflammatory conditions of the upper respiratory tract (such as laryngitis, tonsillitis); lymphadenitis, mumps and chronic rheumatism. Topically it has been used for the treatment of skin and glandular disorders, such as scabies, tinea, acne, mastitis and mammary abscess.[1] The Eclectic physicians favoured poke root to act upon the skin and the glandular structures, particularly of the mouth, throat or reproductive tract (tonsillitis, ulceration, ovaritis, glandular swellings) and to act markedly upon the mammary glands. It was used as an emetic and depurative.[2] Traditional texts record its application in breast cancer (oral use) and topically for uterine cancer.[3]

Radix Phytolaccae, or shang lu in traditional Chinese medicine, refers to *Phytolacca acinosa* or *P. americana* which has been used to treat oedema, oliguria and ascites and externally for trauma, haemorrhage and pyogenic infections of the skin.[4]

SUMMARY ACTIONS

Antiinflammatory, lymphatic, depurative, immunostimulant, expectorant.

CAN BE USED FOR

INDICATIONS SUPPORTED BY CLINICAL TRIALS

No clinical trials have been conducted using poke root.

TRADITIONAL THERAPEUTIC USES

As a depurative for skin conditions acting primarily via the lymphatic system; treatment of inflammatory conditions or infections, especially of the respiratory tract and reproductive systems. Topically for treatment of skin irritation/infection/infestation and female reproductive system disorders (mastitis, mammary abscess, possibly uterine cancer). This is a valuable herb which must be treated with respect.

PREPARATIONS

Only the dried root should be used for making decoctions (the fresh root should not be used). Tincture can also be used for internal or external use.

DOSAGE

- 0.2–1 g of dried root per day for adults.
- 0.15–0.7 ml of 1:5 tincture per day for adults. Avoid the use of liquid extracts and fresh plant tinctures because of potential toxic effects.

DURATION OF USE

In light of the potential risks, medium-term use of poke root up to 6 months is advised.

SUMMARY ASSESSMENT OF SAFETY

Poke root tinctures may be safely prescribed if the recommended dosage is not exceeded. Liquid extracts and fresh plant tinctures have the potential to cause poisoning, because they are more active and may contain higher levels of PWM.

TECHNICAL DATA

BOTANY

Poke root, a member of the Phytolaccaceae family, is a herbaceous perennial which grows up to 3 m. The stem divides into two, with the alternate leaves borne on a very short petiole. The flowers, carried on short pedicles, have a bract and no petals but five greenish-white tepals (combined calyx and corolla). The fruit consists of dark, fleshy berries with raised ribs on the surface.[5] The large root is tuberous, with an outer colouring of yellowish-, reddish- or greyish-brown.[6] The plant is striking as its large leaves and beautiful clusters of purple berries often mingle upon the same branch with the green unripe fruit and flowers.[7]

KEY CONSTITUENTS

- Triterpenoid saponins (phytolaccosides).[8]
- Sterols, mitogens and antiviral proteins.[8]

PHARMACODYNAMICS

The immunological activity of poke root may be due to the presence of traces of lectins which, although too large to be absorbed through the gut wall, may interact with gut-associated lymphoid tissue and may even be absorbed in small quantities. In situations of overdosage the saponins may facilitate the bioavailability of the lectins via their detergent activity and their irritating effects on the gastrointestinal mucosa.

Immunological activity

Poke weed mitogen (PWM) possesses three distinct biological activities: haemagglutination, leucagglutination and mitogenicity (stimulates the production of lymphocytes in vitro).[9] The studies on or using the mitogenic activity of PWM are extensive. Peripheral blood plasmacytosis (increase in the number of plasma cells) occurred in children resulting from systemic exposure to poke root mitogen from *P. decandra* berries. Exposure occurred through oral ingestion of large amounts of berries or by exposure of fresh cuts and abrasions to berry juice.[10]

Lymphocyte-stimulating factors (LSF) were isolated from cultures of murine spleen or thymus cells to which poke root mitogen was added. LSF induced cultured lymphocytes to differentiate into IgM-secreting cells and to proliferate without the addition of mitogen. LSF also stimulated polyclonal B-cell differentiation into IgM-secreting cells.[11]

Poke root antiviral protein (PAP, isolated from the leaves and seeds) is a ribosome-inactivating protein which acts on eukaryotic and prokaryotic ribosomes.[12] PAP has potent antiviral activity against many plant and animal viruses in vitro, including HIV,[13] and has demonstrated immunological activity in vivo by injection.[14]

Antiinflammatory activity

Crude saponins isolated from poke root exhibited potent inhibitory activity on acute oedema in rats and mice when given by intraperitoneal injection. A 50% inhibition of carrageenan-induced paw oedema in rats was demonstrated at 15–30 mg/kg.[15,16]

PHARMACOKINETICS

No data available.

CLINICAL TRIALS

No clinical trials have been conducted using poke root.

TOXICOLOGY

Saline suspensions of poke root extract produced high intraperitoneal lethality in mice, rats and guinea pigs. Intravenous injection into anaesthetized cats markedly depressed respiratory and circulatory functions. Intragastric administration of dilute poke root extract produced violent vomiting in cats. Large oral doses of liquid extracts markedly impaired liver function, but not kidney function, in rabbits.[17] An acidic steroidal saponin obtained from poke root had an LD_{50} of 0.065 mg/kg by the intraperitoneal route in mice, which indicates high toxicity by this route.[18]

Human ingestion of a quantity of fresh root sufficient to cause a severe toxic reaction (including cardiac complications) also caused a nearly fourfold increase in lymphocyte count within 1 week of intoxication.[19] Intoxication occurred after ingestion of one cup of infused, powdered poke root. The indicative severe gastrointestinal symptoms of nausea, diarrhoea and vomiting occurred followed by prostration, hypotension and tachycardia.[20]

A person who ingested raw and/or cooked leaves of *P. americana* developed a Moritz type I heart block (a type of arrhythmia). Cardiac effects of poke root may be secondary to the increased vagal tone which accompanies the usually severe gastrointestinal colic.[21] Other cases of poisoning (including fatality) resulted from ingestion of raw root and tea prepared from leaf and stem, powdered root and berries.[22]

There has been a widespread belief (which is historically documented) that the young green leaves of the plant gathered in spring can be safely eaten as a vegetable (similar to asparagus) provided they are boiled twice. This is called poke salad and tinned poke salad is sold as a vegetable in the USA. An outbreak of 21 cases of poisoning occurred in a group of campers who had reputedly prepared poke salad properly.[22]

Poke root intoxication involves an initial burning sensation in the mouth and throat. A few hours later nausea and repeated vomiting with salivation and profuse sweating take hold. Sometimes there is blood in the vomit. Severe abdominal cramps and pain with watery or bloody diarrhoea accompany the nausea and vomiting. Other symptoms commonly include generalized weakness, headaches, dizziness, hypotension and tachycardia. Urinary incontinence, confusion, unconsciousness and tremors may also occur. The onset of symptoms usually occurs 2–4 hours after ingestion.[19,22] Non-fatal cases usually recover within 24–48 hours with medical treatment. Deaths have been reported.[19]

Although tachycardias, arrhythmias and ischaemia may occur as a result of poke root intoxication, the saponins are not considered to be cardiotoxic.[19] From the literature, it is apparent that there is considerable variability in the toxicity of various Phytolacca preparations. The main toxic components are the saponins but the immunological changes which usually accompany poisoning are probably due to the lectins. To date, there have been no studies which correlate toxic effects with levels of particular saponins.

CONTRAINDICATIONS

Pregnancy, lactation, lymphocytic leukaemia and gastrointestinal irritation.

SPECIAL WARNINGS AND PRECAUTIONS

The recommended dosage of poke root has been exceeded in some cases (see section on Side effects) due to variation in the potency of the root. Fresh plant tinctures should be used with extreme caution, if at all. Accurate measurement of tinctures is vital to ensure the safe dosage is not exceeded.

INTERACTIONS

None known.

USE IN PREGNANCY AND LACTATION

Contraindicated.

EFFECTS ON ABILITY TO DRIVE AND USE MACHINES

None known.

SIDE EFFECTS

Poisonings were widespread in North America during the 19th century, due to overdose of tinctures, ingestion of berries or roots mistaken for other vegetables.[20]

A number of adverse events related to the use of poke root have occurred in Australia. These have all been caused by excessive intake. In some cases hospitalization was required and in one case a shock reaction with pronounced hypotension and tachycardia occurred.

Topical application of preparations derived from the green plant and root have produced inflammation of the skin.[23] Reddening and irritation of the conjunctivae occurred after instillation of saline suspension of poke root extract into rabbit eyes.[17] Topical application of poke root should be restricted to tinctures and the eyes should be avoided.

OVERDOSE

Toxic effects are possible from overdose with poke root. Medical advice should be sought immediately.

CURRENT REGULATORY STATUS IN SELECTED COUNTRIES

Poke root is official in the *Pharmacopoeia of the People's Republic of China* (English edition, 1997). It is not covered by a Commission E monograph but it is on the UK General Sale List.

Poke root does not have GRAS status. However, it is freely available as a 'dietary supplement' in the USA under DSHEA legislation (1994 Dietary Supplement Health and Education Act).

Poke root is included in Part 4 of Schedule 4 of the Therapeutic Goods Act Regulations of Australia. This means that OTC products containing poke root need to undergo a full evaluation by a committee for quality, safety and efficacy. This restriction regulates the activity of suppliers of OTC products but does not directly affect practitioners of herbal medicine.

References

1. British Herbal Medicine Association's Scientific Committee. British herbal pharmacopoeia. BHMA, Cowling, 1983, pp 156–157.
2. Felter HW, Lloyd JU. King's American dispensatory, 18th edn, 3rd revision, vol 2, 1905. Reprinted by Eclectic Medical Publications, Portland, 1983, pp 1471–1475.
3. Grieve M. A modern herbal, vol 2. Dover Publications, New York, 1971, pp 648–649.
4. Chang HM, But PP. Pharmacology and applications of Chinese materia medica, vol 2. World Scientific Publishing, Singapore, 1987, pp 1131–1134.
5. Chiej R. The Macdonald encyclopedia of medicinal plants. Macdonald, London, 1984, entry no. 229.
6. British Herbal Medicine Association's Scientific Committee. British herbal pharmacopoeia, 4th edn. BHMA, Bournemouth, 1996, pp 151–152.
7. Osol A, Farrar GE et al. The dispensatory of the United States of America, 24th edn. JB Lippincott, Philadelphia, 1947, p 1551.
8. Tang W, Eisenbrand G. Chinese drugs of plant origin. Springer Verlag, Berlin, 1992, pp 763–775.
9. Reisfeld RA, Börjeson J, Chessin LN et al. Biochem 1967; 58: 2020–2027.
10. Barker BE, Farnes P, LaMarche PH. Pediatrics 1966; 38 (3): 490–493.
11. Basham TY, Toyoshima S, Finkelman F et al. Cell Immunol 1981; 63 (1): 118–133.
12. Cenini P, Bolognesi A, Stirpe F. J Protozool 1998; 35 (3): 384–387.
13. Tumer NE, Hwang DJ, Bonness M. Proc Natl Acad Sci USA 1997; 94 (8): 3866–3871.
14. Spreafico F, Malfiore C, Moras ML et al. Int J Immunopharmacol 1983; 5 (4): 335–343.
15. Woo WS, Shin KH, Kang SS. Soul Tachakkyo Saengyak Yonguso Opjukjip 1976; 15: 103–106.
16. Woo WS, Shin KH. Soul Tachakkyo Saengyak Yonguso Opjukjip 1976; 15: 90–96.
17. Macht DI. J Am Pharm Assoc Sci Ed 1937; 26: 594–599.
18. Ahmed ZF, Zufall CJ, Jenkins GL. J Am Pharm Assoc 1949; 38: 443–448.
19. Roberge R, Brader E, Martin ML et al. Ann Emerg Med 1986; 15 (4): 470–473.
20. Lewis WH, Smith PR. JAMA 1979; 242 (25): 2759–2760.
21. Hamilton RJ, Shih RD, Hoffman RS. Vet Human Toxicol 1995; 37 (1): 66–67.
22. De Smet PAGM, Keller K, Hansel R et al (eds). Adverse effects of herbal drugs, vol 2. Springer-Verlag, Berlin, 1993, p 253.
23. Mitchell J, Rook A. Botanical dermatology: plants and plant products injurious to the skin. Greengrass, Vancouver, 1979, p 513.

Rehmannia (*Rehmannia glutinosa* (Gaertn.) Libosch.)

SYNONYMS

Glutinous Rehmannia, Chinese foxglove (Engl), Rehmanniae radix (Lat), di huang (Chin), shojio (Jap), saengjihwang (Kor).

WHAT IS IT?

The root of *Rehmannia glutinosa* (Gaertn.) Libosch., *R. glutinosa* var. *hueichingensis* (Chao et Schih) Hsiae., *R. glutinosa* var. *purpurea* Makino or *R. glutinosa* var. *lutea* Makino has been used extensively in traditional Chinese medicine. Rehmannia can be used fresh, dried or after processing (curing) and has various Chinese names depending on its form: shen di huang (uncured), shu di hung (cured).

EFFECTS

Antiinflammatory in autoimmune disease and allergies and to support the adrenal cortex; may protect against the suppressive effects of corticosteroid therapy and chemotherapy.

TRADITIONAL VIEW

Uncured Rehmannia is described as sweet, slightly bitter and cold; cured Rehmannia is sweet and slightly warm. The former clears *Heat* and cools the *Blood* (i.e. used in *Warm*-febrile diseases causing high fever, thirst and a scarlet tongue, haemorrhage due to *Heat* entering the *Blood* level), nourishes *Yin* and *Blood* and generates *Fluids* (used in some cases of dry mouth, low-grade fever, constipation), cools the upward blazing of *Heart Fire* (mouth sores, insomnia, low-grade fevers, constipation) and is used for *Wasting* and *Thirsting* syndrome (including diabetes).[1]

SUMMARY ACTIONS (UNCURED REHMANNIA)

Antipyretic, adrenal trophorestorative, antihaemorrhagic, antiinflammatory, mild laxative.

CAN BE USED FOR

INDICATIONS SUPPORTED BY CLINICAL TRIALS

Although thorough clinical trial data on Rehmannia are lacking, the following conditions have been successfully treated in Chinese studies: rheumatoid arthritis, asthma, urticaria and chronic nephritis.

TRADITIONAL THERAPEUTIC USE

Uncured Rehmannia: antipyretic, haemostatic and removes latent heat from the blood; used for skin rashes, diabetes, low-grade fevers and bleeding.

Cured Rehmannia: regulates menstruation and promotes blood production; used for anaemia, dizziness, weakness, tinnitus; amenorrhoea and metrorrhagia.

MAY ALSO BE USED FOR

EXTRAPOLATIONS FROM PHARMACOLOGICAL STUDIES

To prevent the suppressive effects of corticosteroid drugs on endogenous levels of corticosteroids. Rehmannia gives support to adrenal function but, unlike licorice, is not hypertensive.

PREPARATIONS

Dried or fresh root, decoction and liquid extract for internal use.

To prepare cured Rehmannia, fresh roots are washed in millet wine, steamed and dried with resteaming and redrying several times.

DOSAGE

- 10–30 g per day of the dried (uncured) root in decoction.
- 4–12 ml per day of the 1:2 liquid extract.

DURATION OF USE

May be used long term.

SUMMARY ASSESSMENT OF SAFETY

No adverse effects are expected.

TECHNICAL DATA

BOTANY

Rehmannia glutinosa, a member of the Scrophulariaceae (foxglove) family, is a perennial herb growing to 40 cm.

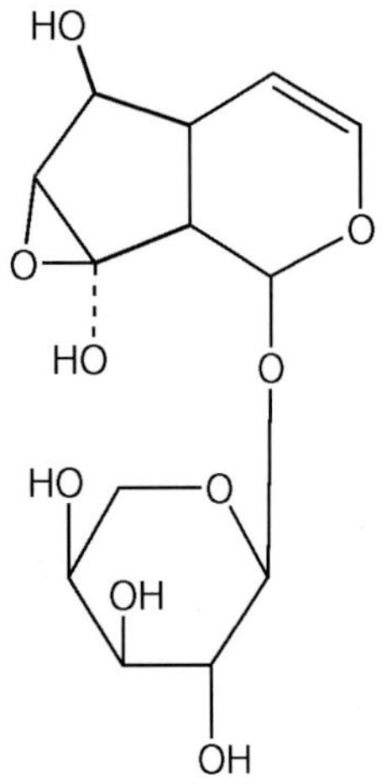

Jioglutoside A

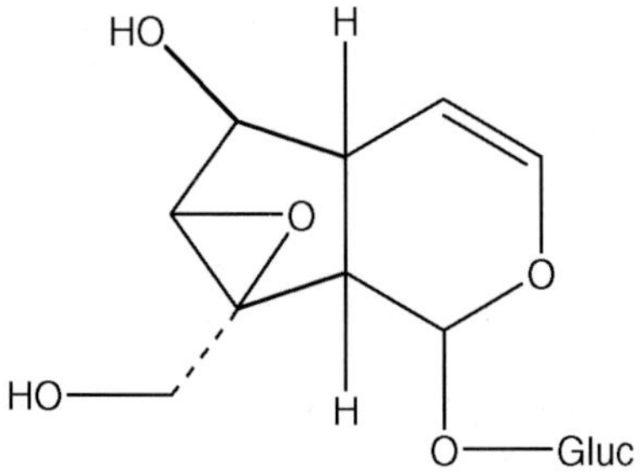

Catalpol

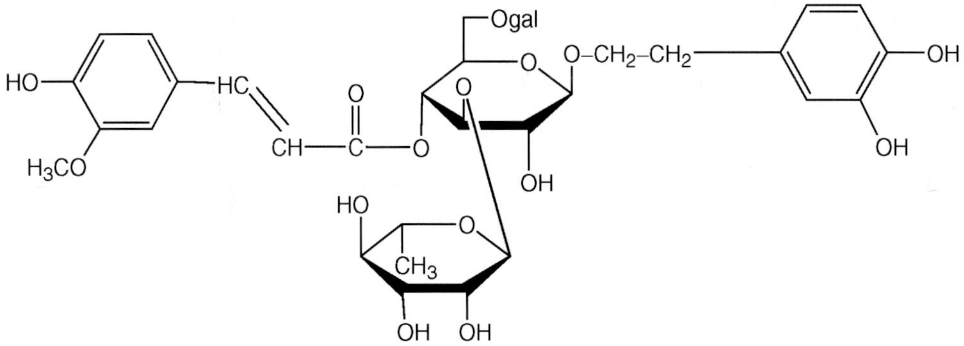

gal = β– D –galactopyranose

Jionoside A_1

The plant bears light reddish-purple tubular flowers and has a thick orange tuberous root approximately 3–6 cm in diameter.[2]

KEY CONSTITUENTS

- Iridoid glycosides, including aucubin, catalpol (0.3–0.5%), ajugol, rehmanniosides A–D,[3] jioglutosides and rehmaglutins A–D.[4]
- Other glycosides, including the phenethyl alcohol glycosides (jionosides).[5]

PHARMACODYNAMICS

Immune and adrenal cortex function

Uncured Rehmannia inhibited the metabolism of cortisol by hepatocytes in vitro. Simultaneous administration of exogenous adrenocortical hormones resulted in cortisol levels remaining close to normal. The authors believed the mechanism to be a competitive effect at the hepatocellular receptor which affected the uptake of corticosteroid hormone, thereby slowing the catabolism of cortisol.[6]

Oral administration of uncured Rehmannia (3 g/kg) for 2 weeks to rabbits chronically treated with a glucocorticoid (dexamethasone) significantly raised serum corticosterone levels ($p<0.001$). Continuation of treatment resulted in further increases. Rehmannia treatment also prevented or reversed morphological changes in the pituitary and adrenal cortex, appearing to antagonize the suppressive effect of glucocorticoids on the hypothalamic-pituitary-adrenal axis.[7]

Oral administration (10–500 mg/kg) of several fractions from the ethanol extract of Rehmannia suppressed the induction of haemolytic plaque-forming cells in mice. Further fractionation yielded the following immunosuppressive phenolic glycosides: jionoside A_1, jionoside B_1, acetoside, isoacetoside, purpureaside C, cistanoside A and cistanoside F.[5]

Oral administration of cured Rehmannia to mice abolished the suppressive effects of cyclophosphamide and dexamethasone on immunity. Parameters measured included spleen and thymus indices, serum haemolysin, lymphocyte transformation rate, phagocytic activity of peritoneal macrophages and numbers of peritoneal T-lymphocytes.[8]

Oral administration of a herbal preparation containing Rehmannia demonstrated protective effects on haematopoiesis, immunity, heart, liver and kidney functions during chemotherapy in tumour-bearing mice.[9]

Other activity

An in vitro study has found that three compounds of Rehmannia (acetylacteoside, jionoside C and jionoside D) demonstrated aldose reductase inhibitory activity.[10]

Orally administered uncured Rehmannia demonstrated improvement in haemorrheology in arthritic and thrombotic rats.[11]

Ethanol extract of cured Rehmannia increased erythrocyte deformability and erythrocyte ATP contents, reduced erythrocyte aggregation and promoted activity of the fibrinolytic system in vivo. Extracts of uncured Rehmannia had weak or no activity.[12]

Intraperitoneal administration of a polysaccharide isolated from Rehmannia to mice bearing sarcoma improved production of the suppressor T-lymphocyte subset.[13] Two acidic polysaccharides isolated from raw Rehmannia showed remarkable reticuloendothelial system-potentiating activity in a carbon clearance test.[14] Although polysaccharides may show considerable immune-enhancing activity in vitro or by injection, this activity may not be relevant to the oral use of Rehmannia.

PHARMACOKINETICS

No data available.

CLINICAL TRIALS

Uncured Rehmannia produced therapeutic effects in uncontrolled trials of rheumatoid arthritis, asthma and urticaria.[15]

Oral administration of a herbal preparation including Rehmannia and Astragalus demonstrated therapeutic effects on chronic nephritis. Significant improvement was observed in 91% of the treatment group compared to 67% in the control group ($p<0.001$). The preparation also demonstrated antiallergic effects and promotion and modulation of immunity.[16] The design of this clinical research was not rigorous and results should be interpreted with caution.

TOXICOLOGY

The mutagenic potential of Rehmannia was tested with the Ames test and in vivo. Uncured Rehmannia showed no mutagenic activity, whereas cured Rehmannia was mutagenic in the in vivo mammalian (mice) assay when given by intraperitoneal injection.[17]

Oral administration of Rehmannia tended to increase the levels of urea nitrogen, creatinine, methylguanidine and guanidinosuccinic acid in rats with renal failure.[18]

CONTRAINDICATIONS

None known.

SPECIAL WARNINGS AND PRECAUTIONS

None.

INTERACTIONS

None known.

USE IN PREGNANCY AND LACTATION

No adverse effects expected.

EFFECTS ON ABILITY TO DRIVE AND USE MACHINES

No adverse effects.

SIDE EFFECTS

In a small open trial of rheumatoid arthritis, intermittent treatment with Rehmannia decoction elicited mild oedema in a minority of patients.[14] Excessive doses can cause diarrhoea.

OVERDOSE

None known.

CURRENT REGULATORY STATUS IN SELECTED COUNTRIES

Rehmannia is official in the *Pharmacopoeia of the People's Republic of China* (English edition, 1997). Rehmannia is not covered by a Commission E monograph and is not on the UK General Sale List.

Rehmannia does not have GRAS status. However, it is freely available as a 'dietary supplement' in the USA under DSHEA legislation (1994 Dietary Supplement Health and Education Act).

Rehmannia is not included in Part 4 of Schedule 4 of the Therapeutic Goods Act Regulations of Australia.

References

1. Bensky D, Gamble A. Chinese herbal medicine materia medica. Eastland Press, Seattle, 1986, p 96.
2. World Health Organization. Medicinal plants in China. World Health Organization, Regional Office for the Western Pacific, Manila, 1989, p 247.
3. Wagner H, Bladt S. Plant drug analysis: a thin layer chromatography atlas, 2nd edn. Springer-Verlag, Berlin, 1996, p 76.
4. Tang W, Eisenbrand G. Chinese drugs of plant origin. Springer Verlag, Berlin, 1992, pp 849–852.
5. Sasaki H, Nishimura H, Morota T et al. Planta Med 1989; 55: 458–462.
6. Zhang LL et al. Acta Academiae Medicinae Primae Shanghai 1980; 7 (1): 37–42.
7. Cha LL, Shen ZY, Zhang XF et al. Chin J Integr Trad West Med 1988; 8 (2): 95–97.
8. Li P, Shi XH, Wang FL. Chin J Immunol 1987; 3 (5): 296–298, 320.
9. Xu JP. Chung Kuo Chung Hsi I Chieh Ho Tsa Chih 1992; 12 (12): 734–737, 709–710.
10. Nishimura H, Yamaguchi T, Sasaki H et al. Planta Med 1990; 56: 684.
11. Kubo M, Asano T, Shiomoto H et al. Biol Pharm Bull 1994; 17 (9): 1282–1286.
12. Kubo M, Asano T, Matsuda H et al. Yakugaku Zasshi 1996; 116 (2): 158–168.
13. Chen LZ, Feng XW, Zhou JH. Chung Kuo Yao Li Hsueh Pao 1995; 16 (4): 337–340.
14. Tomoda MI, Miyamoto H, Shimizu N et al. Biol Pharm Bull 1994; 17 (11): 1456–1459.
15. Hu CS. Chin Med J 1965; 51: 290.
16. Su ZZ, He YY, Chen G. Chung Kuo Chung Hsi I Chieh Ho Tsa Chih 1993; 13 (5): 259–260, 269–272.
17. Yin XJ, Liu DX, Wang HC et al. Mutat Res 1991; 260 (1): 73–82.
18. Yokozawa T, Fujioka K, Oura H et al. Phytother Res 1995; 9 (1): 1–5.

Saw palmetto (*Serenoa repens* (Bartram) Small)

SYNONYMS

Serenoa serrulata (Michaux) Nutall ex Schultes, *Sabal serrulata* R. et Sch. (botanical synonyms), sabal (Engl), Sabal fructus (Lat), Zwegpalme, Sabalfrüchte (Ger), palmier de l'Amérique du Nord (Fr), savpalme (Dan).

WHAT IS IT?

Saw palmetto has traditionally been associated with therapy for the prostate gland. Earlier this century entries could be found in many pharmacopoeias testifying to its use for benign prostatic hyperplasia. The petiole has a sharp spiny edge which can cut the clothing or legs of those unfortunate enough to come in contact with it, hence the common name of saw palmetto (literally a small saw-like palm). The fruit, which is a one-seeded dark brown to black drupe (known as the berry), is the part used in medicine. In recent times a more sophisticated pharmaceutical form of saw palmetto has been developed, known as the liposterolic extract (containing lipids and sterols). The liposterolic extract has been the subject of many open and double-blind clinical trials. Although these trials have resulted in increased use of the liposterolic extract, especially in Europe where it is widely prescribed by medical practitioners for benign prostatic hyperplasia, the strong traditional use information suggests that the use of galenical forms of saw palmetto such as extracts and tinctures should not be discounted.

EFFECTS

Reduces inflammation and oedema; reduces smooth muscle spasm; decreases androgen activity.

TRADITIONAL VIEW

The dried berries, liquid extract or pressed oil of saw palmetto were used for respiratory complaints, particularly those accompanied by chronic catarrh, and conditions of the genitourinary tract, especially to reduce irritation (for all forms of cystitis) and for prostatic hypertrophy. It was considered to build tissues.[1,2]

The eclectics used saw palmetto for upper and lower respiratory problems, atrophy of the breast, ovaries and testes and for benign prostatic hyperplasia (BPH). It was described as the 'old man's friend' and, with amazing accuracy, as 'a remedy for prostatic irritation and relaxation of tissue (rather) than for a hypertrophied prostate'. It was also used for inflamed gonads in the male or female and as an aphrodisiac. One interesting application was uterine hypertrophy.[3]

SUMMARY ACTIONS

Antiinflammatory, endocrine agent, spasmolytic, possibly antiandrogenic.

CAN BE USED FOR

INDICATIONS SUPPORTED BY CLINICAL TRIALS

Mild to moderate benign prostatic hyperplasia.

TRADITIONAL THERAPEUTIC USES

Inflammation of the respiratory tract; inflammation of the genitourinary tract, especially cystitis, prostatic hypertrophy; atrophy of sexual tissues; as an aphrodisiac.

MAY ALSO BE USED FOR

EXTRAPOLATIONS FROM PHARMACOLOGICAL STUDIES

Non-infectious prostatitis; reduction of inflammation and oedema.

OTHER APPLICATIONS

As a topical application for male-pattern baldness.

PREPARATIONS

Decoction of dried berries, tablets or liquid extract for internal use.

The liposterolic extract is mentioned often in this monograph. According to the Commission E, this can be prepared by extraction of dried saw palmetto berries with either hexane or 90% ethanol. More recently, extracts prepared using supercritical carbon dioxide have become available. Although various manufacturers might claim that one type of liposterolic extract is superior to another, they are very similar chemically and there is little clinical evidence to suggest the superiority of a particular extract. However, the hexane extract probably has been the subject of more clinical trials than the others.

The liposterolic extract contains 85–95% fatty acids and 0.2–0.4% total sterols (with 0.1–0.3% beta-sitosterol). Flavonoids are unlikely to be present, except in the extract prepared using 90% ethanol.

DOSAGE

The accepted dose is 160 mg twice a day of the liposterolic extract. This extract is about an 8:1–10:1 concentrate compared to the original dried berries. Hence this dose corresponds to about 2–4 g of dried berries per day. Otherwise, 2–4 ml per day of a 1:2 extract prepared using 45–90% ethanol can be used. The higher ethanol percentages will better extract the liposterolic components. Saw palmetto combines well with pumpkin seed oil or extract and with extract of nettle root.

DURATION OF USE

No restriction on long-term use.

SUMMARY ASSESSMENT OF SAFETY

No adverse effects are expected if used as recommended.

TECHNICAL DATA

BOTANY

Serenoa repens, a member of the Palmae (palm) family, is a small shrub native to the south-eastern region of North America.[4,5] The leaves are palmate, without continuing rib, divided into lance-shaped linear-lanceolate leaflets, the petioles armed with spiny teeth. The inflorescence is many-branched, less than 1 m, with white flowers. The fruit is a prominent olive-like mesocarp, 16–25 mm long, with a single large oblong seed.[5]

KEY CONSTITUENTS

- Lipid content: free fatty acids (including lauric, myristic and oleic acids) together with triglycerides, diglycerides and monoglycerides, phytosterols (mainly beta-sitosterol) and fatty alcohols.[6]
- A particularly active lipase which splits the triglycerides into free fatty acids during ripening and drying.[6]
- Flavonoids and polysaccharides.[6]

The action of the lipase gives the fruit its characteristic rancid odour and taste due to the free fatty acids formed. This 'rancidity' can cause digestive upsets in some people. Methyl and ethyl esters of fatty acids also form in the fruit and contribute to the characteristic aroma.[6]

PHARMACODYNAMICS

Benign prostatic hyperplasia (BPH) is a slow, progressive enlargement of the fibromuscular and epithelial structures within the prostate gland. There is no direct correlation between histologic and macroscopic BPH and symptoms. Histologic evidence of BPH is found in more than 50% of men aged 60 and this increases to 90% at age 85. Yet of men with histologic changes, only 50% will have clinical enlargement of the prostate or macroscopic changes and of these individuals, only 50% will develop symptoms. Symptoms can be due to obstruction or irritation or both. The clinical course of BPH is variable. Not every man with symptomatic BPH worsens clinically with time and symptom severity does not correlate well with prostate size or urinary outlet obstruction.[7] Although BPH is a common problem, the pathogenesis of the disease is poorly understood. Many factors are thought to be involved including sex hormones, stem cells, growth factors, insulin and prolactin. Irritation and associated spasm of smooth muscle tissue, inflammation and oedema may also contribute to the development of symptoms.

Inhibition of 5-alpha-reductase

Testosterone is the major circulating androgen in humans. Most of the testosterone circulating in the bloodstream is bound to sex hormone-binding globulin (SHBG). The remaining unbound or free testosterone exerts the biological effects. Synthesis of SHBG is controlled by the ratio of oestradiol to testosterone. In many androgen target tissues, including the prostate, testosterone is converted by the enzyme 5-alpha-reductase into 5-alpha-dihydrotestosterone (DHT), which is about five times more potent than testosterone. There are two isoforms of 5-alpha-reductase: type 1 and type 2. Studies suggest that mainly type 2 is found in the prostate gland.

There is now substantial evidence that androgen deprivation can decrease the obstructive symptoms of BPH.[7] Also 5-alpha-reductase activity appears to be higher in cells obtained from BPH tissue than from normal prostate tissue. Inhibitors of 5-alpha-reductase, such as the drug finasteride (Proscar), block the conversion of testosterone to DHT and have been found to reduce the size of the prostate and lead to an increase in peak urinary flow rate and a reduction in symptoms.[8] In various reviews, much has been made of the observation that saw palmetto extracts also inhibit 5-alpha-reductase. This, together with inhibition of androgen binding, is often given as an explanation for the pharmacological activity of saw palmetto in BPH.

In 1984 it was shown that the liposterolic extract of saw palmetto (LESP – see above in the Preparations section) inhibited 5-alpha-reductase-mediated intracellular conversion of testosterone to DHT in human foreskin fibroblasts.[9] This property was also demonstrated in vitro for an alcoholic extract.[10] In vitro studies using a eukaryotic (baculovirus-directed insect cell) expression system found that LESP inhibits activity of both isoenzymes of 5-alpha-reductase, whereas finasteride selectively inhibits type 2.[11,12] Moreover, finasteride is a competitive inhibitor, whereas LESP displayed non-competitive inhibition of the type 1 isoenzyme and uncompetitive inhibition of the type 2 isoenzyme.[13] These observations suggest that the lipid components of LESP might be responsible for its inhibitory effect by modulating the membrane environment of 5-alpha-reductase. In vitro studies have confirmed that this inhibitory activity is mainly due to the free fatty acids found in LESP.[14,15]

However, these interesting in vitro results appear to have doubtful clinical significance. The in vitro inhibitory effects of various saw palmetto extracts on 5-alpha-reductase activity were measured to be 5600–40 000 times weaker than finasteride.[16] However, LESP is usually administered at about 100 times the dose of finasteride, which makes its clinical potency about 60 times weaker in terms of 5-alpha-reductase inhibition. In a 7-day human trial only finasteride and not LESP or placebo decreased serum DHT in men.[16] This latter finding was confirmed by a larger double-blind randomized study in 32 healthy male volunteers.

Normal doses of LESP (320 mg/day) had no effect above placebo on serum DHT levels.[17] But there could be an effect in prostate tissue. A German group studied 18 patients in a randomized, placebo-controlled, double-blind trial. Patients with BPH received six times the normal dose of LESP (eight cases) or placebo (10 cases) daily for 3 months. Following prostatectomy, prostatic epithelia and stroma were examined for enzyme activities. While these high doses of LESP caused some moderate biochemical changes, including a small reduction in 5-alpha-reductase activity in prostatic epithelium, the authors volunteered that the significance of their results in understanding the effects of LESP in BPH were uncertain.[18]

Spasmolytic activity

Antiadrenergic agents are used in BPH to decrease dynamically caused obstruction associated with increased smooth muscle tone. In particular, selective alpha$_1$-blockers are preferred such as terazosin, doxazosin and alfuzosin, which have been recently released as prescription drugs. This has stimulated an interest among scientists as to whether saw palmetto extracts might act in a similar way.

An ethanolic liposterolic extract from saw palmetto and a saponifiable extract produced a spasmolytic effect on isolated rat uterus, bladder and aorta.[19] This effect appeared to be related to inhibition of calcium influx and intracellular effects. Follow-up research suggested that cyclic AMP may be a possible mediator, together with the involvement of protein synthesis.[20] Additional research on the above liposterolic extract of saw palmetto found spasmolytic effects which were attributed to alpha-adrenoceptor and calcium-blocking activities.[21]

Inhibition of androgen binding and antiandrogenic activity

Androgens exert their effects by binding to an intracellular cytoplasmic receptor, forming a hormone–receptor complex which is transferred to the cell nucleus, binds to DNA and can activate and modulate protein transcription. Androgen potency is determined by the binding affinity to the receptor. Another important component of the mechanism of LESP might be an inhibitory effect on the binding of DHT to androgen receptors in the cytosolic component of prostate cells.

This inhibitory effect has been demonstrated for LESP prepared using n-hexane in two in vitro models[9,22] but not for an ethanolic LESP.[10] Subsequent in vitro research found that LESP inhibited testosterone and DHT binding in several tissue specimens including vaginal skin and prepuce.[23] However, the most recent study found that LESP did not inhibit binding of DHT to the rat prostatic androgen receptor at LESP concentrations up to 100 μg/ml.[16]

The effects of LESP on two prostatic cancer cell lines differing in androgen responsiveness were investigated.[24] LESP had a proliferative effect on androgen-responsive cells at low concentrations (≤10 μg/ml) and a cytotoxic effect at higher concentrations (≥25 μg/ml). At 25 μg/ml, LESP antagonized androgen-stimulated cell growth. In cells unresponsive to androgen stimulation, LESP had a concentration-dependent antiproliferative action. When these cells were co-transfected with wild-type androgen receptors, LESP inhibited androgen-induced effects. The authors concluded that their findings support a clear antiandrogenic action of LESP. This antiandrogenic activity was confirmed for LESP in several animal models.[25,26]

Other hormonal activity

Addition of LESP at concentrations ranging from 1 to 10 μg/ml to Chinese hamster ovary cells completely inhibited the effects of prolactin, suggesting that the extract may inhibit prolactin-induced prostate growth.[27] The authors suggested that LESP may also be useful for other diseases implicating prolactin.

Early in vivo experiments suggested that saw palmetto had oestrogenic activity.[28] However, recent evidence suggests that LESP has in fact antioestrogenic activity in patients with BPH.[29] In a double-blind, placebo-controlled study, 35 patients received either LESP at 320 mg/day (18 cases) or placebo (17 cases) for 3 months. Following prostatectomy, steroid receptors were evaluated in the nuclear and cytosolic fractions of prostate cells. Oestrogen receptors in the nuclear fraction were significantly lower in the group receiving LESP, as determined by three different tests. Single-point assay found that androgen receptors in the nuclear fraction were also reduced by treatment with LESP. These results suggest that LESP has an antioestrogenic effect, possibly by competitively blocking translocation of cytosolic oestrogen receptors to the nucleus. It may even be that the inactivation of androgen receptors is secondary to oestrogen blockade and that the antioestrogenic effect may potentiate other actions of LESP.

Twenty men with BPH were treated with 320 mg/day of LESP for 30 days.[30] No changes in plasma levels of testosterone, follicle-stimulating hormone and luteinizing hormone occurred as a result of treatment.

Antiinflammatory activity

As a result of secretory stagnation, BPH is associated with congestion and non-infectious prostatitis which is evidenced by white cell infiltration of the prostate. For this reason, agents with antiinflammatory and oedema-protective activities may improve the clinical picture of BPH.

A group of French scientists reported on the antioedematous activity of LESP.[25,31] Various experimental models were used to test the influence of LESP on cutaneous permeability. Interestingly, an antagonistic effect of the extract was observed whenever histamine was involved, either directly through injection or indirectly via mast cell degranulation. An oral dose of 5–10 ml/kg produced a significant effect. However, this is a very high dose. LESP showed no action on serotonin- or bradykinin-induced weals in rats. Since the antioedematous effect was also demonstrable in adrenalectomized rats, the participation of glucocorticoids is definitely excluded.

In contrast to the above, a pronounced antioedematous effect was observed for oral doses of an alcoholic extract of saw palmetto in carrageenan-induced oedema of rat paw.[32] A water-based preparation had no effect and polysaccharides, beta-sitosterol derivatives and flavonoids were not responsible for the antiinflammatory effect. Another group of scientists reported on the isolation of an acidic polysaccharide with antiinflammatory effects (after intravenous injection) from a water-based extract of saw palmetto.[33,34] Since this polysaccharide could be expected to have poor oral bioavailability and would not occur in LESP, the clinical significance of this finding is doubtful.

The most important proinflammatory metabolites of arachidonic acid are prostaglandins and leukotrienes and their production is respectively mediated by the enzymes cyclooxygenase and 5-lipoxygenase. LESP prepared by supercritical liquid extraction with carbon dioxide was found in vitro to be a dual inhibitor of cyclooxygenase (IC_{50} 28.1 μg/ml) and 5-lipoxygenase (IC_{50} 18.0 μg/ml).[35] Activity was found to reside in the acidic lipophilic fraction; fatty alcohols and sterols were inactive. It is possible that this inhibition of the arachidonic acid cascade causes the observed antioedematous effect of LESP. The potent inhibition of the production of 5-lipoxygenase metabolites (especially leukotriene B4) by LESP has been confirmed in a recent in vitro study.[36]

Experimental models of BPH

High oral doses of LESP (300 mg/day for 12 days) inhibited prostatic growth in castrated mice given testosterone and 200 mg/day for 6 days achieved a similar outcome in a rat model.[25] The increase of prostate weight induced by oestradiol/testosterone treatment in castrated rats was countered by oral administration of LESP at 50 mg/kg/day.[37] In contrast, high oral doses of LESP (180 mg/day and 1800 mg/day) did not influence prostatic growth induced by testosterone and DHT in castrated rats.[16]

One model of BPH uses transplants of human prostate tissue into hairless mice. Growth of this tissue is then stimulated by the administration of DHT and oestradiol. Using this model, high oral doses of LESP (6 ml/kg) were observed to reverse the hormonal stimulation of prostate growth.[38]

PHARMACOKINETICS

A study carried out on rats given oral doses of LESP supplemented with ^{14}C-labelled oleic or lauric acids or beta-sitosterol demonstrated that radioactivity uptake in prostatic tissue was highest after administration of LESP supplemented with ^{14}C-labelled oleic acid.[39] This was clearly demonstrated on a rat with experimentally induced BPH. Uptake of radioactivity in the prostate was greater than other organs.

Human pharmacokinetic data on LESP can be gleaned from a bioequivalence study on two different dosage forms.[40] Twelve healthy male subjects each received a single oral dose of 320 mg of LESP. Since LESP is a complex mixture of several components, one component was chosen for the study. This component was not identified but was defined by a validated HPLC method and referred to as *Serenoa repens* second component. Based on analysis of this component, a mean peak plasma concentration of 2.6 μg/ml was reached after 1.5 hours. The mean elimination half-life was 1.9 hours. Given this half-life, administration of LESP twice daily is probably preferable.

CLINICAL TRIALS

The mechanism of action of saw palmetto in the treatment of benign prostatic hyperplasia is inconclusive. This is perhaps understandable since the exact cause of BPH is still unknown. As with many other medicinal plants, the therapeutic benefit probably derives from a combination of pharmacodynamic activities. These could include spasmolytic activity, inhibition of androgen activity, effects on other hormones and antiinflammatory and oedema-reducing properties. However, the current balance of evidence leads to the conclusion that saw palmetto does not possess clinically significant activity as an inhibitor of 5-alpha-reductase.

Saw palmetto has been used for the treatment of BPH for hundreds of years. The modern clinical evidence supporting the efficacy of its liposterolic extract for this disorder is compelling. While this evidence is not yet incontrovertible, it is sufficient to justify the use of this plant for the treatment of mild to moderate BPH in circumstances where conventional therapy is either not wanted or inadvisable. The safety profile of this herbal preparation is very good.

Benign prostatic hyperplasia

Evaluation of treatments for BPH is mainly determined on the basis of reduced symptoms and increased peak urinary flow rates. Additional parameters such as residual urinary volume after voiding (PVR – postvoid residual) are also reported in many clinical trials. Changes in prostate size are sometimes reported in trials with saw palmetto although, unlike finasteride, its effect on this parameter is doubtful.

Seven randomized, double-blind, placebo-controlled trials of the efficacy of LESP in BPH are summarized in Table 1. An additional open, placebo-controlled trial is also included in the table.[41] All except one trial had a positive outcome. In that trial, patients' symptoms improved with LESP treatment, but there was equal improvement in the placebo group.

The validity of the second to fifth studies in the table has been questioned because they failed to demonstrate a substantial placebo effect for urodynamic parameters.[51] The authors of this review suggest that the results of the negative study by Reece Smith and co-workers[47] are more believable because they observed the greatest placebo effect, a phenomenon which is well described in BPH studies. But Reece Smith and co-workers did not assess PVR, unlike most of the other trials, and when urinary frequency (shown in the table) is considered, a consistent placebo effect *is* demonstrated for these earlier trials.

However, this criticism of the LESP trials is addressed in the recent study by Descotes and co-workers.[50] In this trial, only non-responders to placebo were selected for the trial. The study is also significant because it was a large-scale multicentre trial. Improvement in dysuria was seen in a significantly greater proportion of LESP recipients (31.3%) than placebo recipients (16.1%). Daytime urinary frequency fell significantly in the LESP group (11.3% reduction) but was unchanged in the placebo group. Nocturnal urinary frequency fell to a significantly greater extent with LESP than placebo and LESP produced a significantly greater increase in peak urinary flow rate than did placebo (28.9 vs 8.5%). However, there was no significant difference for global efficacy as judged by patients or therapists. The main drawback of this trial is the relatively short assessment period (30 days).

The First International Consultation on BPH in 1991 set the basic criteria for assessing the pharmacological treatment of BPH.[52] All clinical trials were expected to be randomized, placebo controlled and double-blind and to include a follow-up period of at least 1 year. All trials should assess several independent parameters for treatment outcome and should include an analysis of the tolerability of the treatment. To date, no clinical trials of LESP in BPH have completely satisfied these criteria.

With the development and acceptance of conventional drug therapy for BPH, a number of double-blind,

Table 1 Placebo-controlled clinical trials of LESP in BPH

Reference	Year	Daily dose (mg)	Patient number	Study duration (days)	Symptom evaluation	Nocturnal frequency change (days)	Change in flow rate (ml/sec)	Change in PVR (ml)	Tolerability
Boccafoschi and Annoscia[42]	1983	320	22	60	Decreased	−2.2* A −1.0 P	4.1* A 1.9 P	−48 A −29.2 P	Excellent
Emile et al[43]	1983	320	30	30	Decreased	−1.65 A −0.35 P	3.4* A 0.2 P	−36 A −12 P	Excellent
Champault et al[44,45]	1984	320	88	28	Decreased **	−1.43** A −0.50 P	2.7** A 0.3 P	−42** A 9 P	Excellent
Cukier et al[41]	1985	320	146	60 to 90	Decreased **	−1.1** A −0.5 P	NA	−16* A 55 P	Good
Tasca et al[46]	1985	320	30	31 to 90	Decreased	−2.6 A −1.2 P	3.3* A 0.6 P	NA	Excellent
Reece Smith et al[47]	1986	320	80	84	Not changed	−1.06 A −1.05 P	2.15 A 2.15 P	NA	Good
Mattei et al[48,49]	1990	320	40	90	Decreased *	−2.9 A −0.1 P	NA	−55* A 8 P	Excellent
Descote et al[50]	1995	320	176	30	Decreased *	−0.7* A −0.3 P	3.4* A 1.1 P	NA	Good

*$p<0.05$ A = active treatment
**$p<0.001$ P = placebo
NA = not assessed

comparative studies involving LESP have been completed. These trials are summarized in Table 2 together with an earlier trial comparing LESP with the herb *Pygeum africanum*.

The most significant of these comparative trials is the large-scale comparison with finasteride.[53] Patients were recruited from a number of urology centres in nine European countries and the study is the largest international comparative trial for the treatment of BPH. The trial data clearly support the therapeutic value of LESP in BPH. However, this study did have some problems with its design. Most notable of these were the absence of a placebo group or placebo run-in period (which would have afforded a three-way comparison) and the insufficient duration of the trial (minimum 1 year). This latter point is particularly relevant to comparisons using finasteride, since this agent can show increasing efficacy up to 1 year after initiation of therapy.[52]

An important outcome of the study was the observation that LESP does not significantly influence prostate volume or serum PSA, whereas finasteride does. This is clear and significant clinical evidence that LESP does not act primarily as a 5-alpha-reductase inhibitor. Since PSA is used as a marker of prostate cancer and 5-alpha-reductase inhibitors can decrease PSA, there is a concern that these agents could mask the detection of prostate cancer. On the basis of the data provided by this large trial, it can be confidently concluded that this concern does not apply to LESP. This is particularly reassuring since LESP is often self-prescribed and an investigating urologist may be unaware of its use by a particular patient.

It should not be concluded from the study of Grasso and co-workers[54] that alfuzosin is clearly superior to LESP. This study was of extremely short duration and alpha$_1$-blocking agents such as alfuzosin are known to be fast acting. Similarly, with respect to the trial by Duvia and co-workers,[57] it should not be concluded that LESP is a superior phytotherapeutic agent to pygeum. This trial was of short duration and involved small patient numbers. Moreover, the trial was unblinded, a condition which would raise questions about the results of any comparative trial.

Since the development of the liposterolic extract of saw palmetto, there have been more than 20 uncontrolled clinical trials on its use for the treatment of BPH. The value of the information from these trials must be questioned. The placebo effect in the treatment of BPH is well documented and extends to urodynamic parameters as well as symptoms.[52] However, the placebo effect in BPH, as in most cases, decreases with time. Hence results from long-term open studies may have some informative value. The results of some of the larger or longer trials are summarized in Table 3. Some of these trials could be better regarded as post-marketing surveillance studies and have provided valuable information about the tolerability and safety of LESP.

Table 2 Recent comparative clinical trials of LESP

Reference	Year	Daily dose of LESP	Trial design	Comparative treatment and daily dose	Relative results			Relative tolerability
Carraro et al[53]	1996	320 mg	Double-blind, over 26 weeks on 1098 patients with moderate BPH	Finasteride 5 mg (5α-reductase inhibitor)	 IPSS Quality of life (improvement) Peak flow rate Prostate volume PSA	LESP –37% +38% +25% –6% No change	Finasteride –39% +41% +30%* –18%** –41%**	LESP showed a small advantage over finasteride in a sexual function score** and gave rise to fewer complaints of decreased libido and impotence
Grasso et al[54]	1995	320 mg	Double-blind over 3 weeks on 63 patients	Alfuzosin 7.5 mg (α_1-blocker)	 Boyarsky score Obstructive score Peak flow responders No significant difference between mean PVR, peak urinary flow and between the two groups.	LESP –26.9% –23.1% 48.4%	Alfuzosin –38.8%* –37.8%* 71.8%	Both treatments were well tolerated
Adriazola Semino et al[55]	1992	320 mg	Double-blind over 12 weeks on 41 patients	Prazosin 4 mg (α_1-blocker)	Improvements in urinary frequency, mean urinary flow rate and PVR slightly favoured prazosin. No statistical analysis was conducted.			NA
Comar and Di Rienzo[56]	1986	320 mg	Double-blind on 19 patients (duration of study not specified)	Mepartricin (100,000 U) (cholesterol-lowering agent)	Both substances caused improvements in parameters such as nocturnal frequency, dysuria and PVR. Mepartricin was superior although results as provided make quantitative assessment difficult and statistical analysis was not conducted.			NA
Duvia et al[57]	1983	320 mg	Controlled over 30 days on 30 patients	*Pygeum africanum* liposterolic extract (100 mg)	Global evaluation by patients was positive for 80% of cases in both groups. Individual symptom results favoured LESP, but only reached statistical significance for voiding rate.			Both treatments were well tolerated – two patients receiving pygeum complained of heartburn vs none for LESP.

**p<0.05* *PVR = postvoid residual*
***p<0.001* *NA = not assessed*
IPSS = international prostate symptom score
PSA = prostate-specific antigen

Of the uncontrolled trials, the study by Bach and Ebeling[58] is most useful in that it demonstrates a therapeutic effect for LESP in BPH which was maintained for 3 years. For the parameters of peak urinary flow and PVR, the therapeutic effect was fully established after about 12 months and was then maintained (with only slight deterioration) in the ensuing 24 months. These results suggest the observed efficacy of LESP was not due to a placebo effect. One drawback of the trial was that a statistical evaluation of the results was not provided. Not included in Table 3 was a 6-month open, dose-finding study in which 49 patients with BPH were randomized to receive either 320 or 960 mg per day.[59] Similar efficacy was demonstrated between the two treatment groups. Results of this trial would have been more significant if a placebo control group was used.

LESP is often used in combination with other phytotherapeutic agents. The results of three double-blind,

Table 3 Uncontrolled clinical trials of LESP for BPH

Reference	Year	Daily dose (mg)	Patient number	Study duration	Results (decrease from baseline)	Tolerability
Romics et al[61]	1993	320	42	12 months	PVR (–80%)*, peak flow (+38%)*	Excellent
Vahlensieck et al[62]	1993	320	578	84 days	PVR (–48%)**, peak flow (+52%)** Efficacy rated good to very good in 80% of cases.	Rated as good to very good in 95% of cases.
Vahlensieck et al[63]	1993	320	1334	84 days	PVR (–50%)**, dysuria score (–44%)** Nocturia (–54%)**, no data for peak flow Efficacy rated good to very good in 80% of cases.	Rated as good to very good in 95% of cases.
Braeckman[64]	1994	320	505	90 days	PVR (–20%)**, peak flow (+25%)** Prostate volume (–11%)**, PSA – no change IPSS (–35%)**	Very good. Side effects stopped treatment in only 2% of patients.
Bach and Ebeling[58,65]	1995/6	320	435	3 years	PVR(–50%), peak flow (+46%) Nocturia improved in 73.3% of cases. Efficacy rated as good to very good in 90% of cases.	Rated as good to very good in 98% of cases.
Kondas et al[66]	1996	320	38	12 months	PVR decreased by 47 ml**, peak flow (+39%)** Prostate volume (–11%)* 74% of patients showed improvement in IPSS.	Excellent

*$p<0.05$ PVR = postvoid residual
**$p<0.001$ PSA = prostate-specific antigen
IPSS = international prostate symptom score

controlled trials of combination therapy with LESP are summarized in Table 4. While the comparative trial of combination therapy vs finasteride by Sokeland and Albrecht[60] was not as comprehensive in its assessment of urodynamic parameters, prostate volume and PSA as the study of Carraro and co-workers,[53] it does satisfy the issue of adequate study duration. It is therefore an important finding that there was no significant difference between phytotherapy and finasteride.

TOXICOLOGY

Published toxicological data on saw palmetto and LESP is limited. Brine shrimp lethality-directed fractionation of an ethanolic LESP led to the isolation of two monoacylglycerides.[69] These compounds showed moderate biological activities in the brine shrimp lethality test and against renal and pancreatic human tumour cells in vitro; borderline cytotoxicity was exhibited against human prostatic cells.

The company Madaus has released toxicological data on their ethanolic LESP.[70] The LD_{50} in the rat, mouse and guinea pig is greater than 10 g/kg. High doses given to rats over 6 weeks (360 times the human therapeutic dose of about 5 mg/kg) did not cause adverse haematologic, histologic or biochemical changes. A long-term study over 6 months in rats at 80 times the human dose again found no negative influences. The same dose administered to rats had no influence on fertility.

CONTRAINDICATIONS

None known.

SPECIAL WARNINGS AND PRECAUTIONS

None required.

INTERACTIONS

None known.

USE IN PREGNANCY AND LACTATION

No adverse effects expected.

EFFECTS ON ABILITY TO DRIVE AND USE MACHINES

No adverse effects are expected.

Table 4 Double-blind, controlled clinical studies of combination therapy for BPH

Reference	Year	Treatment per day	Comparison treatment	Patient number	Study duration	Results			Tolerability
Carbin et al[67]	1996	Saw palmetto extract 480 mg Pumpkin seed	Placebo	53	90 days		Active	Placebo	No untoward side effects reported.
						Urinary flow	+45%**	+5%	
						PVR	–31%*	–6%	
						Nocturnal frequency	–32%*	–5%	
						Improvement of dysuria symptoms and patient evaluation of therapy were significantly better for active treatment.**			
Metzker et al[68]	1996	LESP 320 mg Nettle root (*Urtica dioica*) 10:1 extract 240 mg	Placebo	40	24 weeks		Active	Placebo	Good
						Peak flow	+23%*	+4%	
						PVR	–33%	–13%	
						IPSS	–40%*	–7%	
						See footnote			
Sokel and Albrecht[60]	1997	LESP 320 mg Nettle root (*Urtica dioica*) 10:1 extract 240 mg	Finasteride 5 mg/day	543	48 weeks	Both treatments significantly improved urinary flow and IPSS. There was no significant difference between the two treatments.			Fewer adverse events reported for the herbal combination.

$p<0.05$ PVR = postvoid residual
$**p<0.001$ PSA = prostate-specific antigen
IPSS = international prostate symptom score
Footnote: A curious aspect of this study is the marked placebo effect which developed in a 24-week unblinded phase which followed the placebo phase. Nonetheless, active treatment remained significantly superior to placebo.

SIDE EFFECTS

The clinical information in Tables 1–3 suggests that LESP is well tolerated by most patients and causes relatively few side effects. No serious side effects can be conclusively attributed to therapy with LESP.

In the long-term uncontrolled study by Bach and Ebeling[58] a total of 46 adverse events were documented in 34 patients (8%); 30% of these were gastrointestinal disturbances. However, the withdrawal rate from the study due to adverse events was a low 1.8%, mostly due to digestive disturbances (three patients) and tumours (three patients), as opposed to 11% with finasteride and 10% with terazosin.[58] Carcinoma of the prostate was diagnosed in four patients during the 3-year follow-up period. These tumours are unlikely to be related to the treatment. About 2% of patients reported adverse events in a French uncontrolled trial of 500 men receiving 320 mg of LESP for 3 months.[71] A majority of complaints were minor gastrointestinal problems such as nausea which resolved when the LESP was taken with meals.

In the double-blind study of Descotes and co-workers[72] there was no significant difference between the tolerability of active and placebo treatments. Only one patient discontinued active treatment with complaints of fatigue, depression and stomach upset.

The large comparative study of Carraro and co-workers[53] found that gastrointestinal complaints were the most frequently reported adverse events with both therapies and tended to occur more frequently with finasteride. As might be expected, decreased libido and impotence were also more common with finasteride treatment. Two deaths occurred during the trial (one in each group) and three serious adverse events occurred (two with LESP, one with finasteride). None of these were deemed to be related to treatment. The German Commission E lists stomach upsets as the only side effect from treatment with LESP.

OVERDOSE

Not known.

CURRENT REGULATORY STATUS IN SELECTED COUNTRIES

Saw palmetto became official during late 1998 in the *United States Pharmacopeia-National Formulary* (USP23–NF18, 1995–June 1999).

Saw palmetto is covered by a positive Commission E monograph and has the following application: urination problems in benign prostatic hyperplasia stages I and II.

Saw palmetto is on the UK General Sale List.

Saw palmetto does not have GRAS status. However, it is freely available as a 'dietary supplement' in the USA under DSHEA legislation (1994 Dietary Supplement Health and Education Act). Saw palmetto has been present in OTC drug products to relieve the symptoms of benign prostatic hypertrophy. The FDA, however, advises that: 'based on evidence currently available, there is inadequate data to establish general recognition of the safety and effectiveness of these ingredients for the specified uses, and ... there is no definitive evidence that any drug product offered for the relief of the symptoms of benign prostatic hypertrophy would alter the obstructive or inflammatory signs and symptoms of this condition'. Saw palmetto is not included in Part 4 of Schedule 4 of the Therapeutic Goods Act Regulations of Australia.

References

1. Grieve M. A modern herbal, vol 2. Dover Publications, New York, 1971, pp 719–720.
2. British Herbal Medicine Association's Scientific Committee. British herbal pharmacopoeia. BHMA, Cowling, 1983, pp 196–197.
3. Felter HW, Lloyd JU. King's American dispensatory, 18th edn, 3rd revision, vol 2, 1905. Reprinted by Eclectic Medical Publications, Portland, 1983, pp 1750–1752.
4. Mabberley DJ. The plant book, 2nd edn. Cambridge University Press, Cambridge, 1997, p 657
5. Leung AY, Foster S. Encyclopedia of common natural ingredients used in food, drugs and cosmetics, 2nd edn. John Wiley, New York, 1996, p 467.
6. Bombardelli E, Morazzoni P. Fitoterapia 1997; 68 (2): 99–113.
7. Tenover JS. Endocrinol Metab Clin North Am 1991; 20 (4): 893–909.
8. Farmer A, Nobel J. Br Med J 1997; 314 (7089): 1215–1216.
9. Sultan C, Terraza A, Devillier C et al. J Steroid Biochem 1984; 20 (1): 515–519.
10. Düker EM, Kopanski L, Schweikert HU. Planta Med 1989; 55: 587.
11. Delos S, Iehle C, Martin P-M et al. J Steroid Biochem Mol Biol 1994; 48 (4): 347–352.
12. Delos S, Carsol JL, Ghazararossian E et al. J Steroid Biochem Mol Biol 1995; 55 (34): 375–383.
13. Iehle C, Delos S, Guirou O et al. J Steroid Biochem Mol Biol 1995; 54 (5–6): 273–279.
14. Niederprüm HJ, Schweikert HU, Zanker KS. Phytomed 1994; 1: 127–133.
15. Weisser H, Tunn S, Behnke B et al. Prostate 1996; 28 (5): 300–306.
16. Rhodes L, Primka RL, Berman C et al. Prostate 1993; 22 (1): 43–51.
17. Strauch G, Perles P, Vergult G et al. Eur Urol 1994; 26 (3): 247–252.
18. Weisser H, Behnke B, Helpap B et al. Eur Urol 1997; 31 (1): 91–101.
19. Gutierrez M, Garcia de Boto MJ, Cantabrana B et al. Gen Pharmacol 1996; 27 (1): 171–176.
20. Gutierrez M, Hidalgo A, Cantabrana B. Planta Med 1996; 62 (6): 507–511.
21. Odenthal KP. Phytother Res 1996; 10: S141–S143.
22. Carilla E, Briley M, Fauran F et al. J Steroid Biochem 1984; 20 (1): 521–523.
23. El Sheikh MM, Dakkak MR, Saddique A. Acta Obstet Gynecol Scand 1988; 67 (5): 397–399.
24. Ravenna L, Di Silverio F, Russo MA et al. Prostate 1996; 29 (4): 219–230.
25. Stenger A, Tarayre JP, Carilla E et al. Gaz Med de France 1982; 89 (17): 2041–2048.
26. Cristoni A, Morazzoni P, Bombardelli E. Fitoterapia 1997; 68 (4): 355–358.
27. Vacher P, Prevarskaya N, Skryma R et al. J Biomed Sci 1995; 2 (4): 357–365.
28. Elghamry MI, Hansel R. Experientia 1969; 25 (8): 828–829.
29. Di Silverio F, D'Eramo G, Lubrano C et al. Eur Urol 1992; 21 (4): 209–314.
30. Casarosa C, Cosci di Coscio M, Fratta M. Clin Ther 1988; 10 (5): 585–588.
31. Tarayre JP, Delhon A, Lauressergues H et al. Ann Pharm Fr 1983; 41 (6): 559–570.
32. Hiermann A. Archiv der Pharmazie 1989; 322 (2): 111–114.
33. Wagner H, Flachsbarth H. Planta Med 1981; 41 (3): 244–251.
34. Wagner H, Flachsbarth H, Vogel G. Planta Med 1981; 41 (3): 252–258.
35. Breu W, Hagenlocher M, Redl K et al. Arzneim Forsch 1992; 42 (4): 547–551.
36. Paubert-Braquet M, Mencia Huerta J-M, Cousse H et al. Prostagland Leukot Essent Fatty Acids 1997; 57 (3): 299–304.
37. Paubert-Braquet M, Richardson FO, Servent-Saez N et al. Pharmacol Res 1996; 34 (3–4): 171–179.
38. Otto U, Wagner B, Becker H et al. Urol Int 1992; 48: 167–170.
39. Chevalier G, Benard P, Cousse H et al. Eur J Drug Metab Pharmacokinet 1997; 22 (1): 73–83.
40. De Bernardi Di Valserra M, Tripodi AS, Contos S et al. Acta Toxicol Ther 1994; 15 (1): 21–39.
41. Cukier, Ducassou, Le Guillou et al. C R Ther Pharmacol Clin 1985; 4 (25): 15–21.
42. Boccafoschi C, Annoscia S. Urology 1983; 50: 1257.
43. Emili E, Lo Cigno M, Petrone U. Urology 1983; 50: 1042.
44. Champault G, Bonnard AM, Cauquil J et al. Ann Urol 1984; 18 (6): 407–410.
45. Champault G, Patel JC, Bonnard AM. Br J Clin Pharmacol 1984; 18 (3): 461–462.
46. Tasca A, Barulli M, Cavazzana A et al. Minerva Urol Nefrol 1985; 37 (1): 87–91.
47. Reece Smith H, Memon A, Smart CJ et al. Br J Urol 1986; 58 (1): 36–40.
48. Mattei FM, Capone M, Acconcia A. Urology 1988; 55 (5): 547–552.
49. Mattei FM, Capone M, Acconcia A. Tw Urol Nephrol 1990; 2 (5): 346–350.
50. Descotes JL, Rambeaud JJ, Deschaseaux P et al. Clin Drug Invest 1995; 9 (5): 291–297.
51. Lowe FC, Ku JC. Urology 1996; 48 (1): 12–18.
52. Denis LJ. Prostate 1996; 29: 241–242.
53. Carraro J-C, Raynaud J-P, Koch G et al. Prostate 1996; 29 (4): 231–240.
54. Grasso M, Montesano A, Buonaguidi A et al. Arch Esp Urol 1995; 48 (1): 97–103.

55. Adriazola Semino M, Lozano Ortega JL, Garcia Cobo E et al. Arch Esp Urol 1995; 45 (3): 211–213.
56. Comar OB, Di Rienzo A. Riv Ital Biol Med 1986; 6 (2): 122–125.
57. Duvia R, Radice GP, Galdini R. Med Praxis 1983; 4: 143.
58. Bach D, Ebeling L. Phytomed 1996; 3 (2): 105–111.
59. Dathe G, Schmid H. Urologe Ausg B 1991; 31 (5): 220–223.
60. Sokeland J, Albrecht J. Urologe Ausg B 1997; 36 (4): 327–333.
61. Romics I, Schmitz H, Frang D. Magyar Urol 1993; 5 (4): 343–347.
62. Vahlensieck W Jr, Volp A, Kuntze M et al. Urologe Ausg B 1993; 33 (6): 380–383.
63. Vahlensieck W Jr, Volp A, Lubos W et al. Fortschr Med 1993; 111 (18): 323–326.
64. Braeckman J. Cur Ther Res Clin Exp 1994; 55 (7): 776–785.
65. Bach D. Urologe Ausg B 1995; 35 (3): 178–183.
66. Kondás J, Philipp V, Diószeghy G. Int Urol Nephrol 1996; 28: 767–772.
67. Carbin BE, Larsson B, Lindahl O. Br J Urol 1990; 66 (6): 639–641.
68. Metzker H, Kieser M, Holscher U. Urologe Ausg B 1996; 36 (4): 292–300.
69. Kondás J, Philipp V, Diószeghy G. Orv Hetil 1997; 138 (7): 419–421.
70. Prosta Urgenin® Uno, Zur Behandlung der BPH. Madaus AG, Koln, 1996, p 33.
71. Authie D, Cauquil J. CR Ther Pharmacol Clin 1987; 5 (56): 3–13.
72. Descotes JL, Rambeaud JJ, Deschaseaux P et al. Clin Drug Invest 1995; 9 (5): 291–297.

Siberian ginseng (*Eleutherococcus senticosus* (Rupr. & Maxim.) Maxim.)

SYNONYMS

Acanthopanax senticosus (botanical synonym), Eleutherococcus (Engl), Eleutherococci radix (Lat), Taigawurzel (Ger), éleuthérocoque (Fr), wu jia pi, cu wu jia (Chin), gokahi (Jap), ogap'I (Kor), Russisk rod (Dan), eleuterokokka (Russ).

WHAT IS IT?

For reasons more related to marketing than botany, the root of *Eleutherococcus senticosus* is known in the West as Siberian ginseng. Although the use of Eleutherococcus is important to traditional Chinese medicine (where it is known by its synonym *Acanthopanax senticosus*), its potential as an adaptogen was demonstrated by Russian scientists. Their work from the 1950s onwards led to the inclusion of Eleutherococcus in the *Soviet Pharmacopoeia* and by 1976 it was estimated that more than 3 million people were using the extract regularly. It was used by Russian athletes to prepare for the Olympic Games in the late 1970s and early 1980s and was included in the Russian space programme for cosmonauts in 1977. Use of Siberian ginseng was not, however, recorded in Russian folk medicine. A survey conducted in the early 1980s of products sold as 'Siberian ginseng' in the United States revealed that many products were not authentic, being derived from related species or adulterants.

The problem may have originated from companies importing 'jia pi' and not distinguishing between the various forms, which includes species of Eleutherococcus and species of Periploca.[1]

EFFECTS

Assists the body to counteract and adapt to stress of many origins; restores and strengthens the body's immune response; increases vitality.

TRADITIONAL VIEW

In Chinese medicine the root barks of several species of Eleutherococcus (including *E. senticosus, E. gracilistylus* and *E. sessiliflorus*) are used to expel Wind Dampness, to strengthen the sinews and bones, transform Dampness and reduce swelling. It is especially useful when the smooth flow of Qi and Blood is obstructed and is particularly used for treating the elderly. These properties mean that it is used to treat oedema, joint pain, muscular spasm, difficult urination and, in combination with other herbs, to assist muscular development in children.[2] It has Spleen-invigorative, Kidney-tonifying and tranquillizing actions and is also used for back pain, insomnia and anorexia.[3]

SUMMARY ACTIONS

Adaptogen, immunomodulator, tonic.

CAN BE USED FOR

INDICATIONS SUPPORTED BY CLINICAL TRIALS

To improve mental and physical performance; to minimize the effects of stress in those subject to chronic illness or to environmental or occupational stress; to improve performance and minimize the effects of stress in athletes; enhancement of immune function, especially natural killer cells and T-helper cells; adjuvant treatment in dysentery; cancer (especially to improve immune function and decrease side effects from orthodox therapy); convalescence after antibiotic therapy (mainly uncontrolled trials).

TRADITIONAL THERAPEUTIC USES

Oedema, joint pain, muscular spasm, difficult urination. Used as tonic, particularly in the elderly, and to treat fatigue, stress and lowered immunity. These applications apply for the root bark.

MAY ALSO BE USED FOR

EXTRAPOLATIONS FROM PHARMACOLOGICAL STUDIES

To treat the effects of prolonged stress or overwork such as exhaustion, chronic fatigue syndrome, irritability, insomnia and mild depression; assist recovery from acute or chronic diseases, trauma, surgery and other stressful episodes.

PREPARATIONS

Dried root for decoction, liquid extract, tablets or powdered root for internal use.

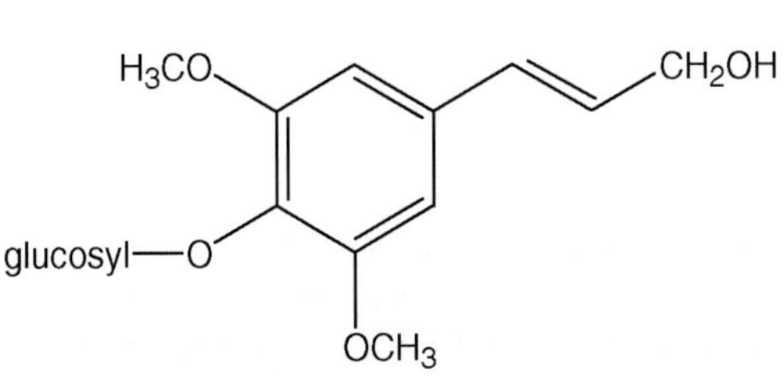

H3CO, CH2OH, glucosyl—O, OCH3

Eleutheroside B

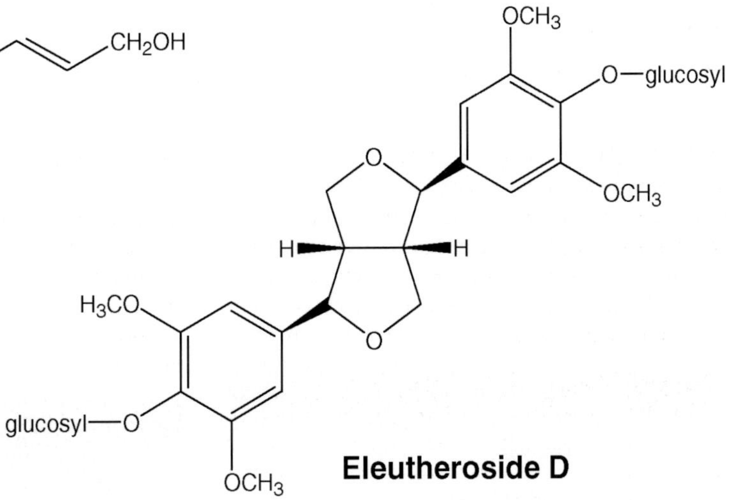

OCH3, O—glucosyl, O, H, H, OCH3, H3CO, O, glucosyl—O, OCH3

Eleutheroside D

DOSAGE

Adult doses used in most studies were in the range of 1–4 g daily, which corresponds to 2–8 ml/day of a 1:2 extract. Maintenance doses for healthy individuals should be toward the lower end of the dosage range but higher doses should be used for the treatment of illnesses and for high-stress situations including athletic training. Eleutherococcus tablets, for example 1.25 g standardized to contain 0.7 mg eleutheroside E, can be taken 1–3 times per day.

DURATION OF USE

The recommended regime for healthy people is for a course of 6 weeks followed by a 2-week break. This regime can be repeated for as long as is necessary. For the treatment of specific illnesses, continuous use is preferable.

The Commission E and BHC take a more cautious stance, recommending the following.

- Generally no longer than 3 months; use again at a later time.[4]
- Eleutherococcus should not be taken continuously for long periods. Occasional use or courses of 1 month followed by a 2-month interval are preferable.[5]

However, there appears to be little reason to support these dosage approaches.

SUMMARY ASSESSMENT OF SAFETY

No adverse effects are expected if used as recommended. It is advisable to discontinue use during acute infections, unless used in conjunction with powerful antimicrobial therapy.

TECHNICAL DATA

BOTANY

Eleutherococcus senticosus, a member of the Araliaceae (ginseng, ivy) family, is a hardy, wild shrub which grows abundantly in parts of the Soviet Far East, Korea, China and Japan, north of latitude 38. It usually grows to about 2 metres, with grey-brown coloured branches covered with thin, downward-pointing spikes. The bright green leaves (12–15 cm long) are divided into 3–5 leaflets. It produces three types of flowers (male, female, bisexual) which are branched together in umbrella-shaped clusters. The flowers vary in colour, depending on type: light violet or yellow. The fruits are oval and berry-like. The rhizome lies shallow in the ground and is 1.5 cm in diameter. The roots are long, woody and pliable, spreading beneath the surface in massive webs and thickets.[6]

KEY CONSTITUENTS

- Eleutherosides (0.6–0.9%): eleutherosides A, B, B_1, C, D, E.[7]
- Triterpenoid saponins (glycosides of protoprimulagenin A).[8]
- Glycans (eleutherans A, B, C, D, E, F and G).[9]

The eleutherosides are not unique to Eleutherococcus, although eleutherosides D and E are not common and are probably pharmacologically important. The eleutherosides are a chemically diverse group and are quite different from the steroidal saponins found in Panax (the ginsenosides).

PHARMACODYNAMICS

In the 1950s, Russian scientists became interested in substances which could improve general health and performance under stress. In their systematic search for a cheaper and more abundant alternative to panax, they discovered that Eleutherococcus was an almost ideal herbal adaptogen. The term 'adaptogen' was first coined by Lazarev and was elaborated by Brekhman.[10] According to Brekhman, an adaptogen is a substance which can effect a non-specific increase in the resistance of an organism to noxious influences. Ideally it has the following properties.

- It is non-toxic and relatively free from side effects.
- It is non-specific and can increase resistance to a wide range of physical, chemical and biological stressors.
- It may have a normalizing action irrespective of whether the pathological state is hypo- or hyperfunctional.

Since most of the original research on Eleutherococcus is in Russian, this monograph has been partly compiled from several English language reviews. The observed activity of Eleutherococcus may be due to the combined effect of all its constituents or could even be due to undiscovered compounds. Several polysaccharides found in the root, such as the glycans mentioned above, have demonstrated immunostimulant[11] and hypoglycaemic effects[9] when administered by injection. However, the importance of these types of compounds to the oral activity of Eleutherococcus is questionable. The exact mechanism of action of Eleutherococcus and the significance of each of its various constituents is not yet fully understood. One study has concluded that eleutheroside E, a major constituent, was mainly responsible for increasing resistance to stress and fatigue.[12] It is therefore pertinent that a chromatographic study of Eleutherococcus roots indicated that Russian and Korean Eleutherococcus are chemically different to Chinese Eleutherococcus and contain higher levels of eleutheroside E.[13] Hence, Eleutherococcus sourced from China may not have the same therapeutic activity as the widely studied Russian variety.

Adaptation to stress

The majority of animal studies have demonstrated adaptogenic activity for Eleutherococcus under a wide variety of stressful conditions. Most of these studies have been conducted in the Far East and Eastern Europe. In his original work with mice, Brekhman found that Eleutherococcus increased stamina by up to 70%.[14] Stressed rats show enlarged adrenal glands, reduced thymus and spleen size and damage to the gastric mucosa.[15] Eleutherococcus significantly reduced this adrenal hypertrophy and adrenal ascorbic acid depletion.[10] These and other effects indicate that Eleutherococcus modifies the physiological response to stress (general adaptation syndrome). The sparing effect on the adrenal cortex by Eleutherococcus allows the organism to better withstand prolonged stress.

Additional research has found that Eleutherococcus can increase the resistance of animals to stressors such as heat, cold, immobilization, trauma, surgery, blood loss, increased or decreased barometric pressure, narcotics, toxins and bacteria.[10,16,17] Eleutherococcus also appears to exert an immune-enhancing action in immune-compromised mice.[18] Oral administration of water extract of Eleutherococcus and its components eleutheroside B and E demonstrated protective effects on behavioural, functional and biochemical changes in mice subjected to acute or chronic stress (exhaustion).[19] Oral administration of this extract (500 mg/kg per day) for 7 weeks led to improvement in learning and memory in rats in the active avoidance model.[20]

Addition of aqueous extract of Eleutherococcus (0.1 mg/ml) caused significant liberation of ACTH and luteinizing hormone from isolated rat pituitary glands. In vivo experiments indicate that a single intraperitoneal dose of standardized aqueous extract (3 mg/ml) enhanced the liberation of corticosterone, while subchronic administration (3 mg/ml IP or 500 mg/kg oral) did not alter ACTH or corticosterone levels, body or organ weight after 7 weeks. Elevations of corticosterone serum levels induced by mild stress were significantly suppressed in animals treated subchronically either by oral administration or by intraperitoneal injection of standardized Eleutherococcus extract.[21]

Not all the studies have been positive. An American investigation of the adaptogenic effects of Eleutherococcus in stressed mice did not confirm improved stamina and instead demonstrated aggressive behaviour for mice given unlimited quantities of the root.[22] Rats given Eleutherococcus show increased levels of noradrenaline and serotonin in the brain and adrenaline in the adrenal glands and this may explain the increased aggressive behaviour observed above.[23]

It has been proposed that Eleutherococcus exerts its adaptogenic effect by inducing enzyme activity. The stress of swimming for 15 minutes inhibited RNA polymerase in the liver and skeletal muscle of rats.

Prior injection of eleutherosides delayed the RNA polymerase inhibition and accelerated its restoration during rest.[24] However, in another study using mice injected with Eleutherococcus and a sedative drug, Eleutherococcus caused an inhibition of enzyme activity. The action of the drug (hexobarbitol sodium) was enhanced by Eleutherococcus to produce a longer sleep period, while its metabolism was inhibited by up to 66%.[25]

Resistance to radiation and chemical carcinogens

Eleutherococcus given to mice by injection prior to radiation treatment showed a promotion of the self-repair mechanism rather than a direct protective effect, thereby confirming its non-specific activity.[26] The survival rate of mice given Eleutherococcus both before and after irradiation was increased.[27] A maximum of 80% of mice given Eleutherococcus beforehand survived a lethal dose of radiation. When Eleutherococcus was administered as late as 12 hours after irradiation, the survival rate was 30%. The stimulation of red blood cell production by the spleen was considered to be responsible for this sustained effect of Eleutherococcus.[27] An in vitro study using isolated mammalian cells exposed to gamma radiation found that *Panax ginseng* increased their resistance to irradiation whereas Eleutherococcus did not.[28] It can be concluded from the above studies that panax confers a direct resistance to cells by altering cell physiology whereas the improved survival from Eleutherococcus is via an indirect action on the whole organism.

The independent application of Eleutherococcus extract (given orally and prophylactically, 5 g/kg) and a chemical radioprotector (adeturone) demonstrated a favourable effect on rats subjected to radiation injury. This favourable effect was only demonstrated on the course of the recovery processes. The two agents mutually potentiated their effects and provided a high degree of protection. This was probably due to an increase in the natural radiation resistance and to the capacity for adaptation during the acute phase of the radiation stress.[29]

Eleutherococcus was found to inhibit spontaneous malignant tumours and tumours induced by a number of carcinogens.[10] Evidence was obtained of a decreased transplantability of tumours in mice and inhibition of metastases occurred in some cases.[10] A decreased incidence of lung cancer in mice was observed when Eleutherococcus was given for several weeks with or after the administration of a carcinogenic agent.[30] Further in vitro research found that components of Eleutherococcus exerted an antiproliferative action upon murine cancer cells.[31] The effect of some cytotoxic drugs was also potentiated by Eleutherococcus, thereby reducing the amount of drug needed.[31] Eleutherococcus lowered the occurrence of chromosomal mutations and increased the survival rate of plants exposed to mutagens.[32]

Immune effects

A preparation of Eleutherococcus increased the in vitro phagocytosis of *Candida albicans* by granulocytes and monocytes from healthy donors by 30–45%. There was no effect observed on intracellular killing of bacteria or yeasts and the preparation did not induce in vitro transformation of lymphocytes.[33]

Resistance to bacterial infection is increased in mice and rabbits by prior dosing with Eleutherococcus. However, simultaneous administration with the infecting organism increased the severity of the disease.[34] This work and clinical experience in Russia support the notion that use of Eleutherococcus should be discontinued during acute infections.[35] Antiviral immunity is also stimulated in vivo and in vitro by prior administration of Eleutherococcus.[36]

Normalizing actions

In terms of a normalizing action, animal experiments have shown that Eleutherococcus impedes both hypertrophy and atrophy of the adrenal and thyroid glands and reduces blood sugar level in hyperglycaemia and increases it in hypoglycaemia. A normalizing action was also obtained in both leucopaenia and leucocytosis.[10]

Cardiovascular effects

Rats fed Eleutherococcus for 2 months displayed a heightened protective activity of their anticoagulant system to administered coagulant drugs[37] and rats recovering from heart damage demonstrated increased repair of heart muscle.[38] Eleutherococcus was found to increase the number of mitochondria in rat cardiac muscle, resulting in greater oxygen metabolism[39] and increased conversion of fat into glycogen for energy.[38] Eleutherococcus countered the effects of cerebral ischaemia in rats.[40]

Other activity

Eleutherococcus displayed a marked antidiabetic effect in diabetic rats by increasing insulin and lowering glucagon.[41] Despite this hypoglycaemic effect in animals, Eleutherococcus has no such effect in diabetes patients.[42] The eleutherosides had an insulin-like activity in diabetic rats[43] and the eleutherans are hypoglycaemic.[9]

In terms of anabolic effects, Eleutherococcus has stimulated weight gain in growing rabbits, improved egg weight and yield in hens and increased reproductive capacity in bulls.[44] When Eleutherococcus was fed to rats it showed protein anabolic effects, as demonstrated by a weight gain and an increase in organ and muscle weight.[45] It is claimed to have a gonadotrophic effect in young male mice, with 1 g of root (by intraperitoneal injection) being equivalent to 6 mg of testosterone (by intramuscular injection).[46] But components of an Eleutherococcus extract have only demonstrated a modest affinity for steroid receptor sites in an in vitro study.[47]

An antitoxic effect has been demonstrated in vivo by the simultaneous administration of drugs or toxins with Eleutherococcus.[48]

Comparison with panax

Panax ginseng is a powerful herb. The steroidal nature of its active constituents gives it a wide range of pharmacological effects, from the individual cell to hormonal control mechanisms.[49] It is unlikely that Eleutherococcus has such far-reaching effects but it is safer and cheaper than panax. According to Brekhman, the use of Eleutherococcus has the following advantages.[25,39]

- Unlike Panax, it rarely causes excitation or a stress-like syndrome in patients.
- It has a more general effect on immunity than Panax.
- It causes a more profound increase in stamina than Panax.

PHARMACOKINETICS

No data available.

CLINICAL TRIALS

Effect on healthy or stressed individuals

Studies on individuals having no pathology have demonstrated an increased capacity to withstand adverse environmental and working conditions. In uncontrolled trials Eleutherococcus has improved the performance and stamina of explorers, sailors, deep sea divers, mine and mountain rescue workers, truck drivers, pilots, factory workers and even cosmonauts.[50] Mental and physical output are increased; for example, proof-readers are quicker and make fewer errors and labourers have improved work capacity.[51] An uncontrolled study of the effect of Eleutherococcus on heat stress in healthy people illustrated how it can help the body function more efficiently. Eleutherococcus caused faster activation and greater intensity of perspiration.[52]

Eleutherococcus is widely used in Russia by track and field athletes, gymnasts and weight lifters due to its actions of increasing endurance and concentration.[53,54] As it has only mild stimulant and anabolic effects, its use is not prohibited. In one study, long-distance runners improved their times by an average of 9%.[55] A Japanese placebo-controlled, double-blind study demonstrated that Eleutherococcus improved maximal work capacity by 23.3% in male athletes compared to a 7.5% increase in the placebo group.[56] This was partly due to improved oxygen metabolism, a finding supported by the discovery that Eleutherococcus increases the number of mitochondria in rat cardiac muscle.[39] In another comparative study on athletes, Eleutherococcus also improved the strength of larger muscles but its effect was weaker than Panax.[57]

Twenty highly trained distance runners randomly assigned in matched pairs participated in an 8-week double-blind study during which they completed five trials of a 10-minute treadmill run at their 10-kilometre race pace and a maximal treadmill test. Following a baseline trial, subjects consumed Eleutherococcus extract or placebo daily for 6 weeks. Data from the measured parameters (including heart rate, respiratory parameters, serum lactate) did not support an ergogenic effect of Eleutherococcus supplementation for submaximal and maximal aerobic exercise tasks.[58]

When Eleutherococcus is taken on a long-term basis, the incidence of acute infections and absenteeism is dramatically reduced.[59,60] In a double-blind study of 1000 workers in a Siberian factory who received Eleutherococcus daily for 30 days, a 40% reduction in lost work days and a 50% reduction in general illness over a 1-year period was observed.[60] A placebo-controlled, double-blind German study demonstrated a strong enhancement of immune function.[43] Populations of both natural killer cells and especially T-helper cells were significantly increased in healthy volunteers, confirming that Eleutherococcus can be considered a non-specific immunostimulant.[61]

Effect on unwell individuals

Administration of Eleutherococcus has a beneficial effect on a wide range of functional and pathological disorders. It has been used in both China and Russia to treat diseases of the heart, kidneys and nervous system. It is likely that Eleutherococcus usually exerts its effects by improving the health of the patient rather than by any direct effect on the pathological process.

The results of a postmarketing surveillance study of 160 patients taking an Eleutherococcus preparation demonstrated a beneficial effect on antibiotic-induced diarrhoea during convalescence. Analysis of a subset of 45 patients with long-term diarrhoea also demonstrated an obvious benefit. Eleutherococcus can be recommended as adjuvant treatment in convalescence after antibiotic therapy to prevent or to clear gastrointestinal complications.[62]

Eleutherococcus has been shown to stimulate the immunological reactivity of patients with cancer. An uncontrolled study of patients given Eleutherococcus while undergoing antitumour treatment demonstrated enhanced non-specific immunity.[63] Eleutherococcus given to cancer patients also minimized the side effects from radiation, chemotherapy and surgery and improved healing and well-being. Eleutherococcus somewhat alleviates the debilitating effects of protracted disease and survival time in patients with terminal disease is lengthened.[64]

Atherosclerotic patients and those with rheumatic heart lesions show an improvement in cardiovascular function and general well-being. Patients with chronic bronchitis, pneumoconiosis and pneumonia show improved well-being and lung capacity. Blood pressure is lowered in hypertensive patients and raised in those with low blood pressure.[65] Hypotensive children demonstrated a significant rise of blood pressure and peripheral resistance when given Eleutherococcus.[66] Children with dysentery responded faster to medical treatment when Eleutherococcus was added.[67] Patients complaining of mild health disturbances including exhaustion, irritability, insomnia and mild depression responded well to a course of Eleutherococcus.[68] All these above results were for uncontrolled trials or case observation studies.

TOXICOLOGY

The acute oral toxicity is very low. The LD_{50} of Eleutherococcus root in mice is 31 g/kg.[69] The LD_{50} of the liquid extract in rats was found to be 10 ml/kg.[45] No toxic manifestations or deaths were observed when Eleutherococcus was fed to rats over their whole lifetime at many times the normal human dose.[69] Rats receiving 10 mg/kg of eleutherosides each day for 2 months showed no evidence of toxic effects.[70] An absence of teratogenicity has been demonstrated in several animal species.[69] Eleutherococcus did not effect spontaneous mutations in the fruit fly and reduced the mutagenic effect of N-nitrosomorpholine.[71]

CONTRAINDICATIONS

In accordance with Russian experiences, Eleutherococcus should not be taken during the acute phase of infections (although it has been used in dysentery in conjunction with antibiotics). Some medical scientists and regulatory bodies[4,72] consider that Eleutherococcus is contraindicated in hypertension (such as in excess of 180/90 mmHg) but it has also been used to treat hypertension.[65]

SPECIAL WARNINGS AND PRECAUTIONS

None required.

INTERACTIONS

None known. The case described below under Side effects was not conclusive as to whether Eleutherococcus caused a real increase in serum digoxin levels, as opposed to an interference with the test method used.

USE IN PREGNANCY AND LACTATION

No adverse effects expected.

EFFECTS ON ABILITY TO DRIVE AND USE MACHINES

No negative influence is expected.

SIDE EFFECTS

'Ginseng abuse syndrome' has been described in the USA, but this study had many flaws.[73] Most notably, it did not differentiate between panax and Eleutherococcus. It is likely that the side effects described, such as insomnia, diarrhoea and hypertension, were due to very high doses of Panax.

Russian studies on Eleutherococcus have noted a general absence of side effects. However, care should be exercised with patients with cardiovascular disorders since insomnia, palpitations, tachycardia and hypertension have been reported in a few cases. Side effects are more likely if normal doses are exceeded.[74]

A case of neonatal androgenization was reported in Canada in 1990.[75] The case was attributed to the mother's use of 'pure Siberian ginseng'. Further follow-up research revealed that the product in question did not contain Eleutherococcus but instead contained *Periploca sepium*.[76,77] A pharmacological study of Eleutherococcus given to rats observed no androgenicity.[78]

A case of apparent elevated serum digoxin levels attributed to consumption of 'Siberian ginseng' has been reported. A 74-year-old man was found to have elevated serum digoxin, which remained high after digoxin therapy was discontinued. The patient was taking a 'Siberian ginseng' product. Testing of serum digoxin levels was undertaken with and without consumption of the product, which indicated it was responsible for the apparent elevation. The capsules were analysed and did not contain any digoxin or digitoxin.[79] The Eleutherococcus contained in the product was not authenticated.

OVERDOSE

Not known.

CURRENT REGULATORY STATUS IN SELECTED COUNTRIES

Eleutherococcus is official in the *Pharmacopoeia of the People's Republic of China* (English edition, 1997). A draft monograph of Eleutherococcus is being prepared and will appear in a future supplement or edition of the *United States Pharmacopeia-National Formulary*.

Eleutherococcus is covered by a positive Commission E monograph and can be used as a tonic to counter exhaustion, to increase stamina, to enhance performance and concentration and to assist convalescence.

Eleutherococcus is not on the UK General Sale List (although 'ginseng' is listed, which probably refers to *Panax ginseng* (Korean ginseng)).

Eleutherococcus does not have GRAS status. However, it is freely available as a 'dietary supplement' in the USA under DSHEA legislation (1994 Dietary Supplement Health and Education Act). Ginseng* has been present as an ingredient in products offered OTC for use as an aphrodisiac. The FDA, however, advises that: 'based on evidence currently available, any OTC drug product containing ingredients for use as an aphrodisiac cannot be generally recognized as safe and effective'.

Eleutherococcus is not included in Part 4 of Schedule 4 of the Therapeutic Goods Act Regulations of Australia.

*The listing in the Code of Federal Regulations (Part 310–New Drugs) lists `ginseng' in addition to Korean ginseng and so is likely to refer to Eleutherococcus.

References

1. Hu SY. The role of botany in Chinese medicinal materials research. In: Chang HM, Yeung HW, Tso WW et al (eds) Advances in Chinese medicinal materials research. World Scientific, Singapore, 1985, pp 28–31.
2. Bensky D, Gamble A. Chinese herbal medicine materia medica. Eastland Press, Seattle, 1986, pp 235–236.
3. Chang HM, But PP. Pharmacology and applications of Chinese materia medica, vol 1. World Scientific, Singapore, 1987, pp 725–735.
4. German Federal Minister of Justice. German Commission E for human medicine monograph, Bundes-Anzeiger (German Federal Gazette), no. 11, dated 17.01.1991.
5. British Herbal Medicine Association. British herbal compendium, vol 1. BHMA, Bournemouth, 1992, pp 89–91.
6. Halstead BW, Hood LL. *Eleutherococcus senticosus*. Siberian ginseng: an introduction to the concept of adaptogenic medicine. Oriental Healing Arts Institute, USA, 1984, pp 2, 71–73.
7. Farnsworth NR, Kinghorn AD, Soefarto DD et al. Siberian ginseng (*Eleutherococcus senticosus*): current status as an adaptogen. In: Farnsworth NR et al (eds) Economic and medicinal plant research, vol 1. Academic Press, London, 1985, p 157.
8. Segiet-Kujawa E, Kaloga M. J Nat Prod 1991; 54 (4): 1044–1048.
9. Hikino H, Takahashi M, Otake K et al. J Nat Prod 1986; 49 (2): 293–297.
10. Brekhman II, Dardymov IV. Ann Rev Pharmacol 1969; 9: 419–430.
11. Wagner H, Proksch A, Riess-Maurer I et al. Arzneim Forsch 1984; 34 (6): 659–661.
12. Nishibe S, Kinoshita H, Takeda H et al. Chem Pharm Bull 1990; 38 (6): 1763–1765.
13. Wagner H, Heur YH, Obermeier A et al. Planta Med 1982; 44 (4): 193–198.
14. Fulder S. The root of being: ginseng and the pharmacology of harmony. Hutchinson, London, 1980, p 137.
15. Golotin VG, Gonenko VA, Zimina VV et al. Vopr Med Khim 1989; 35 (1): 35–37.
16. Farnsworth NR, Kinghorn AD, Soefarto DD et al. Siberian ginseng (*Eleutherococcus senticosus*): current status as an adaptogen. In: Farnsworth NR et al (eds) Economic and medicinal plant research, vol 1. Academic Press, London, 1985, p 202.
17. Fulder S. The root of being: ginseng and the pharmacology of harmony. Hutchinson, London, 1980, pp 161, 255.
18. Chubarev VN, Rubtsova ER, Filatova IV et al. Farmakol Toksikol 1989; 52 (2): 55–59.
19. Saito H, Nishiyama N, Kamegaya T et al. In: Chang HM, Yeung HW, Tso WW et al (eds) Advances in Chinese medicinal materials research. World Scientific, Singapore, 1985, pp 687–688.
20. Streuer M, Jansen G, Winterhoff H et al. International Congress on Phytotherapy, Munich, September 10–13, 1992.
21. Winterhoff H, Gumbinger HG, Vahlensieck U et al. Pharm Pharmacol Lett 1993; 3: 95–98.
22. Lewis W, Zenger VE, Lynch RG. J Ethnopharmacol 1983; 8 (2): 209–214.
23. Abramova ZI, Chernyi ZK, Natalenko VP et al. Lek Sredstva Dal'nego Vostoka 1972; 11: 106–108.
24. Bezdetko GN, Brekhman II, Dardymov IV et al. Vopr Med Khim 1973; 19 (3): 245–248.
25. Medon PJ, Ferguson PW, Watson CF. J Ethnopharmacol 1984; 10 (2): 235–241.
26. Minkova M, Pnatev T, Topalova S et al. Radiobiol-Radiother 1982; 23 (6): 675–678.
27. Miyanomae T, Frindel E. Exp Hematol 1988; 16 (9): 801–806.
28. Ben-Hur E, Fulder S. Am J Chin Med 1981; 9 (1): 48–56.
29. Minkova M, Pantev T. Acta Physiol Pharmacol Bulg 1987; 13 (4): 66–70.
30. Dzhioev FK. Vopr Onkol 1965; 11 (9): T651–T653.
31. Hacker B, Medon PJ. J Pharm Sci 1984; 73 (2): 270–272.

32. Strel'chuk SI. Tsitol Genet 1987; 21 (2): 136–139, 142.
33. Wildfeuer A, Mayerhofer D. Arzneim-Forsch 1994; 44 (3): 361–366.
34. Farnsworth NR, Kinghorn AD, Soefarto DD et al. Siberian ginseng (*Eleutherococcus senticosus*): current status as an adaptogen. In: Farnsworth NR et al (eds) Economic and medicinal plant research, vol 1. Academic Press, London, 1985, p 197.
35. Baranov AI. J Ethnopharmacol 1982; 6 (3): 339–353.
36. Farnsworth NR, Kinghorn AD, Soefarto DD et al. Siberian ginseng (*Eleutherococcus senticosus*): current status as an adaptogen. In: Farnsworth NR et al (eds) Economic and medicinal plant research, vol 1. Academic Press, London, 1985, p 197, 203.
37. Bazaz'ian GG, Liapina LA, Pastorova VE et al. Fiziol Zh SSSR 1987; 73 (10): 1390–1395.
38. Afanasjeva TN, Lebkova NP. Biull Eksp Biol Med 1987; 103 (2): 212–215.
39. Afanesjeva TN, Krivchik AA, Murtasova TP. Proceedings of the 2nd International Symposium on Eleutherococcus, Moscow, 1985.
40. Leonova EV, Bregman IG. Zdravookhr Beloruss 1979; 3: 13–16.
41. Molokovskii DS, Davydov VV, Tiulenev VV. Probl Endokrinol (Mosk) 1989; 35 (6): 82–87.
42. Farnsworth NR, Kinghorn AD, Soefarto DD et al. Siberian ginseng (*Eleutherococcus senticosus*): current status as an adaptogen. In: Farnsworth NR et al (eds) Economic and medicinal plant research, vol 1. Academic Press, London, 1985, p 183.
43. Dardymov IV, Khasina EI, Bezdetko GN. Rastit Resur 1978; 14 (1): 86–89.
44. Farnsworth NR, Kinghorn AD, Soefarto DD et al. Siberian ginseng (*Eleutherococcus senticosus*): current status as an adaptogen. In: Farnsworth NR et al (eds) Economic and medicinal plant research, vol 1. Academic Press, London, 1985, pp 195, 201.
45. Kaemmerer K, Fink J. Prakt Tierarzt 1980; 61 (9): 748, 750–752, 754, 759–760.
46. Farnsworth NR, Kinghorn AD, Soefarto DD et al. Siberian ginseng (*Eleutherococcus senticosus*): current status as an adaptogen. In: Farnsworth NR et al (eds) Economic and medicinal plant research, vol 1. Academic Press, London, 1985, pp 196–197.
47. Pearce PT, Zois I, Wynne KN et al. Endocrinol Japon 1982; 29 (5): 567–573.
48. Farnsworth NR, Kinghorn AD, Soefarto DD et al. Siberian ginseng (*Eleutherococcus senticosus*): current status as an adaptogen. In: Farnsworth NR et al (eds) Economic and medicinal plant research, vol 1. Academic Press, London, 1985, pp 166–167.
49. Fulder S. The root of being: ginseng and the pharmacology of harmony. Hutchinson, London, 1980, pp 166–171.
50. Fulder S. The root of being: ginseng and the pharmacology of harmony. Hutchinson, London, 1980, pp 189, 192, 246–248, 255.
51. Farnsworth NR, Kinghorn AD, Soefarto DD et al. Siberian ginseng (*Eleutherococcus senticosus*): current status as an adaptogen. In: Farnsworth NR et al (eds) Economic and medicinal plant research, vol 1. Academic Press, London, 1985, pp 167, 171, 172.
52. Novozhilov GN, Silchenko KI. Fiziol Chel 1985; 11 (2): 303–306.
53. Fulder S. The root of being: ginseng and the pharmacology of harmony. Hutchinson, London, 1980, p 249.
54. Farnsworth NR, Kinghorn AD, Soefarto DD et al. Siberian ginseng (*Eleutherococcus senticosus*): current status as an adaptogen. In: Farnsworth NR et al (eds) Economic and medicinal plant research, vol 1. Academic Press, London, 1985, p 173.
55. Fulder S. The root of being: ginseng and the pharmacology of harmony. Hutchinson, London, 1980, p 137.
56. Asano K, Takahashi T, Miyashita M et al. Planta Med 1986; 52 (3): 175–177.
57. McNaughton L, Egan G, Caelli G. Int Clin Nutr Rev 1989; 9 (1): 32–35.
58. Dowling EA, Redondo DR, Branch JD et al. Med Sci Sports Exerc 1996; 28 (4): 482–489.
59. Fulder S. The root of being: ginseng and the pharmacology of harmony. Hutchinson, London, 1980, p 189.
60. Farnsworth NR, Kinghorn AD, Soefarto DD et al. Siberian ginseng (*Eleutherococcus senticosus*): current status as an adaptogen. In: Farnsworth NR et al (eds) Economic and medicinal plant research, vol 1. Academic Press, London, 1985, p 178.
61. Bohn B, Nebe CT, Birr C. Arzneim Forsch 1987; 37 (10): 1193–1196.
62. Meyer-Wegener J, Paulus M. Med Welt 1997; 48 (11): 493–496.
63. Kupin VI, Polevaia EB. Vopr Onkol 1986; 32 (7): 21–26.
64. Fulder S. The root of being: ginseng and the pharmacology of harmony. Hutchinson, London, 1980, pp 201–202.
65. Farnsworth NR, Kinghorn AD, Soefarto DD et al. Siberian ginseng (*Eleutherococcus senticosus*): current status as an adaptogen. In: Farnsworth NR et al (eds) Economic and medicinal plant research, vol 1. Academic Press, London, 1985, pp 179–191.
66. Kaloeva ZD. Farmakol Toksikol 1986; 49 (5): 73.
67. Vereshchagin IA. Antibiotiki 1978; 23 (7): 633–636.
68. Farnsworth NR, Kinghorn AD, Soefarto DD et al. Siberian ginseng (*Eleutherococcus senticosus*): current status as an adaptogen. In: Farnsworth NR et al (eds) Economic and medicinal plant research, vol 1. Academic Press, London, 1985, pp 185–186.
69. Farnsworth NR, Kinghorn AD, Soefarto DD et al. Siberian ginseng (*Eleutherococcus senticosus*): current status as an adaptogen. In: Farnsworth NR et al (eds) Economic and medicinal plant research, vol 1. Academic Press, London, 1985, pp 164–166.
70. Dardymov IV, Suprunov NI, Sokolenko LA. Lek Sredstva Dal'nego Vostoka 1972; 11: 66–69.
71. Sakharova TA Revazova YA, Barenboim GM et al. Khim-Farm Zh 1985; 19: 311–312.
72. Dalinger OI. Central nervous stimulants. Tomsk, 1986, pp 112–114. Cited in De Smet PAGM, Keller K, Hansel R et al (eds) Adverse effects of herbal drugs, vol 2. Springer-Verlag, Berlin, 1993, pp 163–164.
73. Siegel RK. JAMA 1979; 241 (15): 1614–1615.
74. Farnsworth NR, Kinghorn AD, Soefarto DD et al. Siberian ginseng (*Eleutherococcus senticosus*): current status as an adaptogen. In: Farnsworth NR et al (eds) Economic and medicinal plant research, vol 1. Academic Press, London, 1985, pp 179, 180–182, 187, 193, 195.
75. Koren G, Randor S, Martin S et al. JAMA 1990; 264 (22): 2866.
76. Awang DVC. JAMA 1991; 266 (3): 363.
77. Awang DVC. JAMA 1991; 265 (14): 1828.
78. Waller DP, Martin AM, Farnsworth NR et al. JAMA 1992; 267 (17): 2329.
79. MacRae S. Can Med Assoc J 1996; 155: 293–295.

St John's wort (*Hypericum perforatum* L.)

SYNONYMS

Hypericum, hardhay (Engl), Hyperici herba (Lat), Johanniskraut, Sonnenwendkraut, Hartheu (Ger), herb de millepertuis (Fr), iperico (Ital), prikbladet perikon (Dan).

WHAT IS IT?

The dried aerial parts of *Hypericum perforatum*, gathered during the flowering period or shortly before, are used medicinally. The generic name of the herb derives from the Greek meaning to 'overcome an apparition' and in earlier times homes would have a plant hanging over the door to ward off evil spirits. This species of hypericum (*H. perforatum*) is referred to as perforate St John's wort due to the perforated appearance of the leaves when they are held up to the light. *H. perforatum* is not a weed in its native Europe, Asia and North Africa but has become a weed in most temperate regions of the world. Hypericum and other species of the genus have been used as a remedy since ancient times particularly to treat ulcers, burns, wounds, abdominal pains and bacterial diseases. Recently it has received attention in clinical trials for the treatment of depression and viral diseases.

EFFECTS

Mild antidepressant activity; useful for wound healing; antiviral activity with application to disorders caused by enveloped viruses.

TRADITIONAL VIEW

Hypericum was considered primarily for the nervous system, particularly for nervous afflictions (excitability, menopausal neurosis, hysteria) and disorders of the spine, spinal injuries, neuralgia, sciatica and muscular rheumatism. It was also used for its supposed diuretic and astringent properties and to treat urinary problems, diarrhoea, dysentery, parasitic infestations, jaundice, haemorrhages, menorrhagia and bed wetting. Hypericum ointment and infused oil were used on a wide range of wounds including ulcers, swellings, bruises and even on tumours.[1,2] In Greece the herb is used externally for the treatment of shingles.[3]

SUMMARY ACTIONS

Antiviral, nervine, antidepressant, vulnerary, antiseptic.

CAN BE USED FOR

INDICATIONS SUPPORTED BY CLINICAL TRIALS

Treatment of mild to moderate depression, particularly when side effects from standard antidepressant drugs become intolerable to the patient; adjunct to standard drug treatment in severe depression; treatment of anxiety; adjunct to light therapy for seasonal affective disorder; psychological symptoms of menopause; aerobic endurance in athletes.

TRADITIONAL THERAPEUTIC USES

Physiological afflictions of the nervous system: spinal injuries, neuralgia, sciatica; muscular rheumatism; mild psychological disorders: excitability, menopausal anxiety and nervousness. Hypericum ointment and infused oil for the treatment of wounds, bruises and shingles.

MAY ALSO BE USED FOR

EXTRAPOLATIONS FROM PHARMACOLOGICAL STUDIES

Treatment and prevention of acute and chronic infections caused by enveloped viruses, e.g. cold sores, herpes genitalis, chicken pox, shingles, glandular fever, cytomegalovirus infection and viral hepatitis; wound healing; conditions requiring increased nocturnal melatonin plasma levels (e.g. circadian rhythm-associated sleep disorders); alcoholism; may also have potential as an anticancer treatment.

OTHER APPLICATIONS

Inclusion in skin care products, particularly for sensitive skin.[4]

PREPARATIONS

Dried or fresh herb for infusion, liquid extract and tablets for internal use.

Infused oil of hypericum is made by mixing the flowers in a good-quality fixed oil (such as olive oil) in a well-sealed vessel in the presence of sunlight over several weeks. The action of the sunlight produces a red oil containing hypericin derivatives, hyperforin, xanthones, flavonoids and the breakdown products of hyperforin.

DOSAGE

- 2–5 g of dried herb per day or the equivalent of 1.0–2.7 mg of total hypericin (TH) per day.
- Hypericum tablets (1.5 g, standardized to contain 0.9 mg TH): 2–3 tablets per day.
- The volume of liquid extract prescribed depends upon the level of TH in the extract; typical doses are 3–6 ml of 1:2 liquid extract per day, 7.5–15 ml of 1:5 tincture per day.

Doses at the higher end of this range have been utilized in the treatment of depression, HIV infection and other viral infections. For the short-term treatment of acute viral infections, even higher doses may be necessary.

DURATION OF USE

No restriction but at least 4 weeks of treatment is required to assess the antidepressant effect. (See the Special warnings section.)

SUMMARY ASSESSMENT OF SAFETY

A scientific investigation found that use of hypericum extract is safer for patients with preexisting cardiac dysfunction or elderly patients than tricyclic antidepressants. Adverse effects are rare from the use of hypericum at normal dosages. Avoidance of excessive exposure to sunlight or artificial UVA light is advisable in patients taking high doses. Hypericum should be used cautiously in patients with known photosensitivity. Practitioners should avoid dispensing the sediment from hypericum extracts. (Refer to Side effects section.)

TECHNICAL DATA

BOTANY

Hypericum is a member of the Clusiaceae (alternative name: Guttiferae) family[5,6] and grows to approximate-ly 1 m with opposite and paired branches. The leaves are opposite, sessile, up to 2 cm long, oblong and contain numerous translucent glandular dots which are visible against the light. The yellow flowers contain five petals with many stamens protruding. The fruit is a capsule.[7,8]

KEY CONSTITUENTS

- Naphthodianthrones (0.05–0.6%), including hypericin and pseudohypericin.[9] The upper level of naphthodianthrones is usually much lower than this quoted value, approximately 0.2%.
- Flavonoids, phenolics including hyperforin;[9] procyanidins,[10] essential oil.[11]

Collectively the naphthodianthrones, hypericin (H) and pseudohypericin (PH) are called 'total hypericin' (TH) and are responsible for the red colour of hypericum extracts. The naphthodianthrones show a restricted solubility in almost all solvents, but more than 40% of the amount present is extractable from the crude herb when preparing a tea with water at 60–80°C.[12] This increase in solubility suggests the possible presence of factors in the herb which modify the solubility of the naphthodianthrones. Accordingly, potassium salts of H and PH have been identified as 'soluble' pigments in *Hypericum species*.[13]

PHARMACODYNAMICS

Antiviral and antiretroviral activity

Hypericin and PH have demonstrated activity against several enveloped viruses in vitro, including vesicular stomatitis virus, herpes simplex virus types 1 and 2, parainfluenza virus, vaccinia virus,[14] murine cytomegalovirus[15] and duck hepatitis B virus.[16] These compounds were inactive against non-enveloped (naked) viruses such as human rhinovirus, adenovirus and poliovirus.[14,17] This suggests that the mechanism of viral inactivation is dependent upon the presence of a viral lipid envelope.[17] The antiviral activity was enhanced by exposure to light[15] and is directed at both the virions and virus-infected cells.[18] Hypericin and PH appear to inactivate the viral fusion function via the generation of singlet oxygen upon illumination[19] which could also occur in vivo in the absence of light if driven by chemically generated excited states.[20] Hypericin and PH also interfere with more than one stage in the virus replication cycle (see also below).[21] Both H and PH demonstrated potent activity, in vitro and in vivo (by oral administration or injection),[22,23] against several retroviruses, including HIV.[24] The antiretroviral activity was enhanced by exposure to light.[18,21] The ring structure, the quinone and phenolic groups are necessary for the antiretroviral activity.[24]

The antiretroviral effect is postulated to be achieved in a number of ways:

- by causing photochemical alterations of the capsid, which inhibits the release of reverse transcriptase

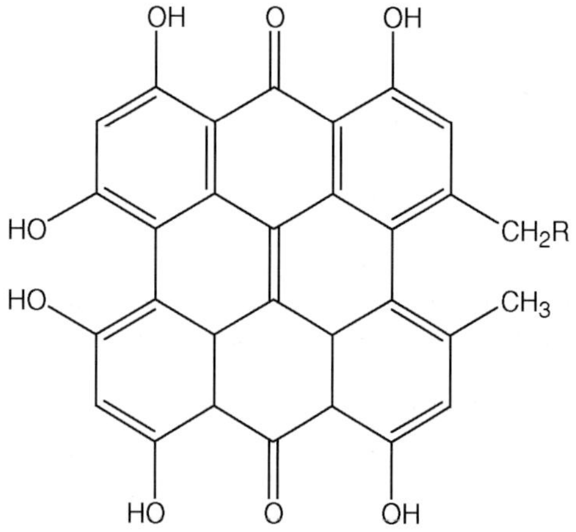

	R
Hypericin	H
Pseudohypericin	OH

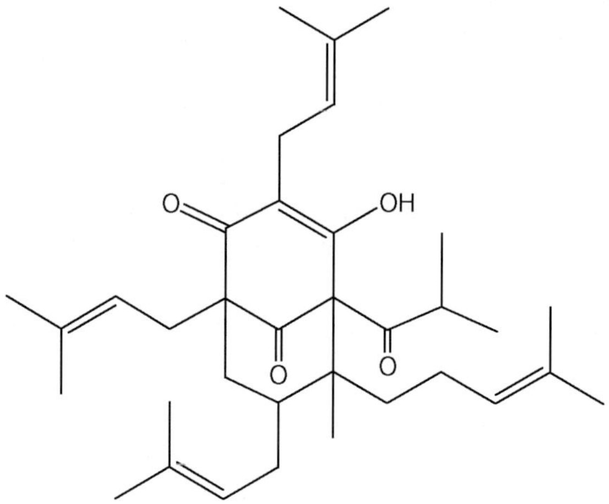

Hyperforin

and prevents reverse transcription of the genome within the target cell;[20]

- by inhibiting intracellular transmission of the HIV-induced cytopathic signal;[25,26]
- by interfering with processing of gag-encoded precursor polyproteins needed for core maturation;[22]
- by impairing the assembly or processing of intact virions;[22]
- by inhibiting the signalling pathway which has an immunosuppressive effect on the host immune system.[27]

The antiretroviral activity is due to a combination of the photodynamic and lipophilic properties of these compounds: H binds cell membranes and crosslinks virus capsid proteins which results in a loss of infectivity and an inability to retrieve the reverse transcriptase activity from the virion.[28]

Antidepressant activity

Information from in vitro studies on key constituents is inconclusive. Hypericum extract and H inhibited dopamine-beta-hydroxylase in vitro.[29] Hypericin also potentiated neurotransmitter binding at the GABA-A, benzodiazepine and serotonin receptors.[30] The non-hypericin fraction of hypericum inhibited monoamine oxidase-A (MAO-A) in vitro, unlike H and the flavanols.[31,32] The xanthones, flavones and flavonols were found to be potent and selective MAO-A inhibitors and the coumarins affected MAO-B in vitro.[32] Amentoflavone demonstrated binding activity at the benzodiazepine receptor in vitro.[33] One group of researchers have suggested, on the basis of their in vitro and in vivo studies, that hyperforin significantly contributes to the antidepressant activity.[34,35] More investigation is required into the role that hyperforin might play in the antidepressant activity of hypericum.

Studies on the whole extract of hypericum have revealed the following results which may reflect on antidepressant activity.

- Inhibition of synaptic uptake of noradrenaline, serotonin and dopamine in vitro and inhibition of GABA reuptake.[36,37,38] It is unusual to find this action on all three uptake systems.[38]
- Downregulation of beta-adrenoceptor density in the frontal cortex after subchronic administration in vivo.[36,38,39] (Note: The downregulation of these receptors in vivo is expected on subchronic administration of antidepressants and is not in contradiction to inhibition of uptake observed in vitro.)
- Upregulation of central serotonergic receptors from cerebral tissue in vivo, which is consistent with effects caused by synthetic antidepressants.[38,40]
- Reduced expression of serotonin receptors in vitro.[41]
- Inhibition of catechol-O-methyltransferase in vitro.[42]

• Suppression of interleukin-6 in blood samples ex vivo.[43] This suppression may assist in deactivating the hypothalamic-pituitary-adrenal axis, leading to inhibition of elevated corticotrophin-releasing factor and other adrenal regulatory hormones. These changes could be linked to antidepressant activity.[44]

• Inhibition of MAO-A and MAO-B activity in vitro,[45] although this inhibition was found to be weak.[38]

• A photosensitizing effect for H, since hypericum treatment has lowered the amount of light necessary to obtain a clinical antidepressant effect.[46]

The relative significance of these in vitro and in vivo results to the mechanism behind the clinical antidepressant activity of hypericum is currently uncertain.

In further work to elaborate the components contributing to antidepressant activity, the antidepressant activity of the clinically proven 80% methanolic extract of hypericum and its various fractions was tested using the forced swimming test and tail suspension test in rats.[47,48] Fraction II (containing flavonoids) and fraction IIIc (containing procyanidins, H and PH) were determined to contribute to the observed in vivo antidepressant activity. Procyanidins in fraction IIIc significantly increased the in vivo effects of H and PH, probably by a solubilizing effect (these compounds otherwise have poor solubility). The effect of solubilized H and PH was antagonized by a dopamine antagonist, suggesting that the dopaminergic system is involved in their action. Hyperforin could not be found in any of the six fractions, presumably because it is unstable. Although this research verifies that H and PH do have experimental antidepressant activity, it should not be interpreted that they are the only compounds with such activity in hypericum.

In a placebo-controlled, two-way crossover trial on 12 healthy volunteers, 6 weeks of hypericum treatment (1.1 mg per day TH equivalent) induced significant differences in EEG patterns. The changes were typical of those induced by antidepressant drugs such as imipramine.[49] In a double-blind, crossover, placebo-controlled study over 4 weeks on 12 older healthy volunteers, hypericum extract (2.7 mg per day TH equivalent) induced an increase in deep sleep during the total sleeping period, as evidenced by EEG and visual analysis. The interference with REM sleep phases which is typical for tricyclic antidepressants and MAO inhibitors did not occur for hypericum. Continuity of sleep, onset of sleep, intermittent wake-up phases and total sleep duration were not improved by hypericum, which implies it does not exert sedative activity.[50]

One hundred and sixty patients suffering from depression completed a randomized, double-blind, multicentre study investigating the electrocardiographic (ECG) effects of high-dose hypericum treatment (1800 mg extract, 5.4 mg TH) compared to imipramine. Analysis of conduction intervals and pathological findings indicated that, for the treatment of patients with a preexisting conductive dysfunction or elderly patients, high-dose hypericum extract is safer with regard to cardiac function than tricyclic antidepressants.[51]

Anticancer activity

Hypericin has produced a potent antitumour activity in vitro against several tumour cells. However, it did not show any toxic effect on normal cells at much higher concentrations. Based on additional experiments it was concluded that H directly inhibits EGF-receptor and PTK activity.[52] Epidermal growth factor (EGF) is a cellular plasma membrane receptor which appears to be involved in the loss of inhibitory constraint on cell growth, a factor in tumour formation. Phosphorylation of proteins on tyrosine residues is a key biochemical reaction that mediates a large variety of cellular signals, including control of the cell cycle and cell differentiation. Enhanced protein tyrosine kinase (PTK) activity is also involved in the transformation of normal cells into tumour cells.

It is premature to conclude that H or hypericum is an effective antiproliferative agent against tumour cells. However, this research looks promising from at least a pharmacokinetic perspective. Concentrations of about 0.3 μM were effective against human colon and stomach cancer cell lines and mouse leukaemia cells. Pharmacokinetic experiments on hypericum extract show that a dose containing 11.25 mg of TH gives a maximum plasma concentration 4 hours later of about 0.3 μM.[53] (Refer to the Pharmacokinetics section below.)

In vitro studies demonstrated a large difference in sensitivity for tumour cell lines towards photo-activated H. Hypericin also demonstrated antitumour activity in vivo after intraperitoneal injection.[54]

An antimutagenic activity was demonstrated by hypericum extract on DNA repair in *Escherichia coli*. Hypericum also reduced the activity of UV-induced beta-galactosidase, indicating that the antimutagenic activity may be due to suppression of error-prone repair.[55]

Other activity

Hypericum extract demonstrated bactericidal activity in vitro against a number of Gram-positive and Gram negative bacteria, including *Staphylococcus aureus*,

Proteus vulgaris, *Escherichia coli* and *Pseudomonas aeruginosa*.[56]

A dry aqueous alcohol extract of hypericum (26.5 mg/kg, oral) induced a marked sedation in vivo compared with diazepam controls. None of the isolated fractions from this extract exhibited the same sedative activity as the extract.[57]

Oral administration of hypericum extracts dose dependently and significantly reduced alcohol intake in two genetic animal models of human alcoholism. Similar results were seen after rats were deprived of alcohol for 20 hours and the extract was administered 30 minutes prior to the return of alcohol. Compared to the control, hypericum extract (0.6 mg/kg) significantly prevented the alcohol deprivation-induced rebound in alcohol intake.[58]

Oral administration of hypericum tincture (0.1 ml of 1:10 tincture) demonstrated improved wound healing in rats. This activity was believed to be due to the facilitation of the collagen maturation phase of wound healing, enhanced new skin growth and an influence on epithelial cell proliferation and migration.[59]

In a controlled in vivo skin test, cosmetic ingredients were considered effective (i.e. antiirritant) when their addition to an irritant (croton oil) led to a decrease in the primary cutaneous irritation index (PII) of more than 0.30. Oily extract of hypericum (3% w/w) demonstrated a significant antiirritant effect (PII = 0.54) in an oil/water emulsion.[60]

In an uncontrolled trial with 13 healthy volunteers, a significant increase in nocturnal melatonin plasma concentration was observed after 3 weeks' administration of hypericum extract (0.5 mg per day TH equivalent).[61]

A randomized, double-blind, placebo-controlled crossover study investigated the interaction of hypericum extract with alcohol. Thirty-two volunteers received either hypericum extract (2.7 mg per day TH equivalent) for 7 days or placebo. At the end of the treatment period they underwent several tests following consumption of alcohol. No interaction between hypericum and alcohol with respect to cognitive capabilities was observed.[62]

In a randomized, double-blind trial, the effect of hypericum extract (2.7 mg per day TH equivalent) was compared with maprotiline on resting EEG and evoked potentials in 24 healthy volunteers. Improved cognitive functions were observed, particularly for hypericum treatment.[63]

PHARMACOKINETICS

In a phase I trial of synthetic H, oral bioavailability of H after a single dose was measured at 14.6–30%.[64] Hypericin and PH are well absorbed into the bloodstream after oral doses of hypericum extract. In pharmacokinetic studies, after hypericum administration to volunteers, H showed better total absorption than PH although PH was more quickly absorbed.[65,66] Over 14 days of treatment with a standardized hypericum extract in 13 healthy volunteers, steady-state levels of H and PH in blood plasma were reached after 7 and 4 days respectively. The systemic availability of H and PH in the extract was roughly estimated to be 14% and 21% respectively.[66] In a single-dose, double-blind study, 13 volunteers received placebo or the following dose of standardized hypericum extract: 900 mg (equivalent to 2.81 mg of TH), 1800 mg (equivalent to 5.62 mg of TH) or 3600 mg (equivalent to 11.25 mg of TH). Approximately 4 hours after intake, maximum TH plasma concentrations were 0, 0.028, 0.061 and 0.159 mg/l respectively.[53] Because of their fat-loving nature, H and PH move readily throughout the body and cross the blood–brain barrier.

CLINICAL TRIALS

Antiviral and antiretroviral activity

In the first reported case studies of HIV-positive patients who had been taking hypericum preparations (0.35–1.2 mg TH per day), nine (of 11) patients demonstrated successful treatment as evidenced by symptomatic relief of fatigue, nausea, mild peripheral neuropathies and abatement of swollen lymph glands. Changes in CD4 cell counts and p24 antigen levels were slower to occur. One patient was asymptomatic.[67]

In 1990 an uncontrolled study was carried out investigating 26 HIV-positive patients self-administering over-the-counter hypericum extract (1 mg per day TH equivalent). At the end of 4 months, p24 antigenaemia disappeared in two of six initially positive patients, both of whom were using the antiretroviral drug AZT. In 10 patients who had never taken AZT, the mean CD4 cell count increased 13% after 1 month and maintained this increase for 4 months. In those using AZT and hypericum, CD4 cell counts fell significantly after an initial mild rise. Liver enzyme elevations occurred in five patients, which returned to baseline after 1 month without hypericum.[68]

In an ongoing uncontrolled trial, 16 HIV patients at various stages of the disease process were treated by intravenous injection and oral route with hypericum. Over 40 months of observation, patients showed stable or increasing CD4 cell counts and only two patients encountered an opportunistic infection. None of the known viral complications due to cytomegalovirus, herpes or Epstein–Barr virus were encountered.

There were no cases of toxoplasmosis, neurological symptoms or photosensitivity.[69] A substantial decline in viral load was observed in most of the 18 AIDS patients undergoing a similar treatment regime (intravenous injection and oral hypericum) for 4–6 years. In those patients who experienced an increase in viral load, there was no effect on the clinical outcome of viral cytomegalovirus, herpes or Epstein–Barr virus complications.[70]

Twenty-four HIV-infected patients in Thailand participated in a study to determine the maximum tolerated effective oral dose (MTD) of H which demonstrates antiviral activity with minimal phototoxic effects. The MTD was found to be 0.05 mg/kg.[71] In a toxicological study involving 10 HIV-positive homosexual men, daily dosages of 0.5, 2.0 4.0 and 8.0 mg H were each administered for 12 weeks. No early, marked anti-HIV activity was found.[72] There have also been two phase I/II studies of synthetic H in HIV-infected subjects, investigating phototoxicity, pharmacokinetics and antiviral activity by oral or intravenous administration.[64,73] A consistent change in antiviral endpoints was not seen with intermittent intravenous dosing. Pharmacokinetic data indicated that chronic oral dosing would achieve sustained blood levels in an antiretroviral range.[64]

Antidepressant and antianxiety activity

Many clinical trials have been conducted over the past 17 years, using some form of standardized hypericum extract (equivalent to 0.4–2.7 mg TH per day). There has been a tendency in later years to use higher doses of TH (2.7 mg per day, about 5 g of herb) and recently even 5.4 mg per day.

Many criticisms have been levelled at the trials conducted from 1979 to 1995 including:

- few trials conducted on severe depression;
- relapses occurring within 1 year after cessation of the studies were not registered;
- dose-response studies were not performed with patients;
- in trials comparing standard antidepressant medications, the doses were too low and the number of patients too small;
- drug interactions were not specifically tested;
- special groups of patients (e.g. geriatric patients, those with renal and hepatic insufficiencies) were not tested.[74]

A critical analysis of 23 randomized clinical trials including a total of 1757 outpatients has shown that hypericum extracts are more effective than placebo for the treatment of mild to moderately severe depressive disorders.[75] Fifteen trials[76,77–90] with 1008 patients were placebo controlled and eight[91–98] with 749 patients compared hypericum to standard antidepressant drugs (maprotiline, imipramine, bromazepam, amitriptyline, desipramine). (Of the eight trials comparing hypericum with other antidepressants, six used single preparations and two used a combination of hypericum and valerian.) Three of the trials used hypericum in combination with other plant extracts,[76,97–98] one trial was single blind,[95] two were open[94,96] and the remainder were double blind. Most trials had reasonably good methodology, with 10 trials scoring 80% or more of the possible points in both assessment systems used.[76,77,80,81,84,85,89,92,93,98] The daily dose of TH varied considerably, between 0.4 and 2.7 mg, as did the duration of treatment (2–12 weeks). Hypericum extracts were significantly superior to placebo, with mean scores on the Hamilton Depression Scale 4.4 points better for patients treated with hypericum (in the nine trials providing data for analysis). Results from comparative trials suggest that hypericum may work as well as standard antidepressants, as indicated by the scores on the Hamilton Depression Scale after treatment. In these trials with standard antidepressants, however, the evidence was insufficient to form definite conclusions due to the limited number of patients included in the trials. In the six trials comparing single hypericum preparations with standard antidepressants, side effects occurred in 20% of patients taking hypericum extracts compared to 36% of patients on standard antidepressants. The authors conclude that further studies are required, with the type of depression among study participants better delineated. They also suggested that comparison of studies using different preparations of hypericum is problematic, even when standardized for TH, as the preparations may vary in other substances contributing to the antidepressant effect.[75]

Clinical trials on hypericum which were not included in the above review and metaanalysis are reviewed below.

In a randomized, multicentre, double-blind trial, 209 patients diagnosed with recurrent severe major depression received either hypericum extract (5.4 mg per day TH equivalent) or 150 mg of imipramine over 6 weeks. Both treatments were found to be equally effective in improving symptoms of severe depression but the decrease in depressive symptoms tended to be greater for imipramine. Even at the higher dose hypericum was better tolerated than imipramine, as evidenced by fewer patients reporting adverse effects and fewer dropouts (one dropout versus eight). There were no reports of photosensitivity.[99] This trial is significant because patients had severe depression and the doses of hypericum and imipramine were both relatively high.

In a randomized, multicentre, double-blind trial, 149 patients with mild to moderate depression received hypericum extract (2.7 mg per day TH equivalent) or amitriptyline over 6 weeks. Comparable efficacy was observed between the two treatments for final Hamilton Depression Scores and global clinical impression. The mean rating scales at the end of the trial favoured amitriptyline. A lower incidence of side effects occurred in the hypericum group.[100] In a randomized, double-blind trial, 102 outpatients with mild to moderate depression received either hypericum extract (2.7 mg per day TH equivalent) or placebo. The placebo group also responded favourably when switched to active treatment for 2 weeks. The total Hamilton score in the hypericum treatment group fell significantly ($p<0.001$) further after 4 weeks than in the placebo group.[101]

In a preliminary single-blind trial, 20 patients with seasonal affective disorder (SAD) were randomized to receive hypericum extract (2.7 mg per day TH equivalent) combined with either bright or dim light therapy for 4 weeks. A significant reduction of Hamilton Depression Scores was observed in both light groups, with no significant difference between the two groups. The favourable response in the dim light group suggests hypericum may be an efficient therapy in patients with SAD, as well as in combination with light therapy.[102] In another similar single-blind trial, 4 weeks' treatment with hypericum extract (2.7 mg per day TH equivalent) was associated with a significant reduction in the total Hamilton score. There was no significant additional advantage for bright light treatment over hypericum.[103]

The effectiveness of hypericum treatment was assessed by 663 medical practitioners in a postmarketing surveillance study of 3250 patients with depressive tendencies. Patients received hypericum extract (2.7 mg per day TH equivalent) for 4 weeks. At the end of treatment, of the 3161 patients remaining in the trial, 79% of patients and 82% of doctors assessed the results as between 'better' and 'symptom free' and 13–16% evaluated results as either 'unchanged' or 'worse'. Patients with light or moderate depression responded better to treatment than those with severe depression.[104]

The safety and efficacy of two hypericum extracts (standardized to 0.5% and 5.0% hyperforin respectively) were compared in 147 patients with mild to moderate depression in a randomized, double-blind, placebo-controlled trial.[105] After 6 weeks of treatment, only the group taking the 5.0% hyperforin extract showed a significant reduction for the Hamilton Depression Score when compared to placebo ($p=0.0004$). This study suggests an antidepressant activity for hyperforin, which is not usually present in conventional hypericum extracts.[47]

From the clinical trials performed between 1993 and 1996 and subsequently, it can be concluded that hypericum is a well-tolerated and effective alternative to standard antidepressants in the treatment of mild to moderate depression, particularly when side effects with the drugs become intolerable to the patient. Patients should be treated long enough and with a sufficiently high daily dose of at least the equivalent of 2.7 mg TH from hypericum extracts.[74]

Other activity

An open, multicentre, postmarketing surveillance study investigated the efficacy and tolerance of a combination of hypericum and black cohosh in the treatment of 812 patients for psychological complaints experienced in menopause. Good improvement was observed in 90% of patients, with improved concentration and reduction in hot flushes. The treatment demonstrated an effect after 3 weeks, with 2% of patients experiencing side effects (most frequently gastrointestinal complaints).[106]

In a double-blind placebo-controlled trial, 72 athletes were randomized into three groups: hypericum plus vitamin E, vitamin E and placebo. The daily dose of hypericum used in the above study was around 170 mg of standardized extract, probably corresponding to about 1 g of dried herb. Measurements of endurance capacity and physical comfort were conducted at 0, 3 and 6 weeks. After 6 weeks, the hypericum plus vitamin E group demonstrated a better aerobic endurance capacity ($p=0.006$) compared to little significant change in the other groups.[107] The trial design does not permit the conclusion that hypericum alone enhances physical endurance (it may only act in this way when combined with the vitamin E and minerals). The daily dose of vitamin E used in the trial was 660 mg.

Phase I/II clinical trials of an oral H formulation for glioblastoma and a topical, light-activated formulation for skin diseases such as psoriasis are continuing.[108]

TOXICOLOGY

Hypericum has very low toxicity. Animals given 2 g/kg per day of dried hypericum for up to a year showed no signs of any toxic changes.[109,110]

Hypericism is a state of sensitivity to sunlight following the ingestion of large quantities of hypericum. When plants are eaten by livestock, weakly pigmented parts of the body become affected by a type of dermatitis. This is due to TH, which causes photosensitization without jaundice and there is no liver damage. Sheep, cattle, horses and goats are affected, with goats the most resistant.[6] The disorder depresses the central nervous system and causes increased sensitivity to handling and temperature change.[111] A review of the effect of hypericum on grazing animals notes that hypericum is more phototoxic if ingested at flowering than when young or dry. The minimum phototoxic dose of foliage for cattle and sheep is approximately 1% and 4% of live weight respectively (i.e. 10 and 40 g/kg).[6] Doses of 3 g/kg or more of ground, dried hypericum aerial parts, given by stomach tube, were able to photosensitize 4–6-month-old calves.[112]

Hypericum given to animals (1–1.5 g/kg per day) did not adversely affect the health of the foetus or of the mother. The fertility of adult animals was not affected.[108] Genotoxicity tests showed no mutagenic effects following hypericum administration.[109,110]

CONTRAINDICATIONS

Hypericum is a safe and effective alternative to orthodox antidepressants in the treatment of mild to moderate depression. But it is not suited for the treatment of serious depression with psychotic symptoms, suicidal risk or signs and symptoms that are so severe that they do not allow the patient's family or work involvements to continue. However, in these cases, hypericum may be a valuable adjunct to other therapy such as drug therapy and psychotherapy.

SPECIAL WARNINGS AND PRECAUTIONS

Hypericum is not advisable in cases of known photosensitivity. (Refer to the Side effects section.) It is recommended that patients on higher doses of hypericum (2.7 mg or more of TH equivalent per day) do not spend excessive amounts of time in the full sun, especially in tropical or subtropical climates, and avoid artificial UVA irradiation. However, total avoidance of sunlight is not advisable because the activity of hypericum may be associated with its photosensitizing activity. Avoidance of foods which interact with MAO-inhibiting drugs, such as tyramine-containing foods (cheeses, beer, wine), and drugs such as L-dopa is not necessary. If a significant response in depressive disorders is not apparent after 4–6 weeks, the treatment should be discontinued.

INTERACTIONS

Negative interactions are not expected. In fact, several cases have been reported indicating a favourable interaction of hypericum with orthodox medication in severe depressive states.[83] However, caution should always be exercised in patients consuming orthodox medication. Patients should be monitored for any symptoms suggestive of serotonin syndrome (such as confusion, fever, shivering, sweating, diarrhoea and muscle spasms). Serotonin syndrome is an adverse drug interaction characterized by altered mental status, autonomic dysfunction and neuromuscular abnormalities. It is most frequently caused by the use of selective serotonin reuptake inhibitors (SSRI) and MAO inhibitors, leading to excess serotonin availability in the CNS at the serotonin 1A receptor.

A case of suspected serotonin syndrome has recently been reported. The 50-year-old woman had stopped taking paroxetine 10 days prior to commencing hypericum (600 mg per day). After this short space of time taking hypericum, she restarted the paroxetine to assist her sleep. The following day she experienced lethargy and grogginess. The author postulated that an adverse reaction occurred between the SSRI (paroxetine) and hypericum.[113] However, the evidence for this conclusion is not strong. A yet-to-be-published study describes two patients who developed what appeared to be classic serotonin syndrome. The syndrome developed in one patient who took hypericum alone and was seen in another patient who took hypericum and trazodone (a weak SSRI) 6 days after the patient stopped taking the SSRI. The authors indicate that it is not clear whether the hypericum caused the serotonin syndrome, the trazodone the one patient was taking, or the combined effect.[114]

USE IN PREGNANCY AND LACTATION

No data available. The scientific committee of ESCOP suggests that in accordance with general medical practice, the product should not be used during pregnancy and lactation without professional advice.[115]

EFFECTS ON ABILITY TO DRIVE AND USE MACHINES

No negative influence is expected.

SIDE EFFECTS

General

In HIV-positive patients receiving oral hypericum extracts containing the equivalent of 1 mg H per day, mild reversible liver enzyme elevations were observed which returned to baseline levels after 1 month without hypericum.[68]

In the postmarketing surveillance study of 3250 patients receiving hypericum extract (equivalent to 2.7 mg per day TH) for treatment of depression, 2.4% reported side effects (mainly minor gastrointestinal complaints and allergic reactions such as pruritus). The incidence of side effects with the hypericum preparation was estimated to be 10 times less than that experienced with orthodox antidepressants.[104]

A case of a dynamic ileus associated with the use of hypericum in a 67-year-old woman has been reported. Her symptoms started 2 weeks after taking the extract, with no other identifiable cause, and resolved gradually and completely after its discontinuation.[116]

Hypericism

There have been no reliable reported cases of hypericism in humans taking oral doses of hypericum. The usual therapeutic doses of hypericum extract are about 30–50 times below the dose needed to induce phototoxicity in calves.[117] However, an oral dose of 0.05 mg/kg per day of pure hypericin over 28 days produced mild photosensitivity of a short duration on exposure to sunlight in three out of four HIV patients in a study in Thailand. When the dose was raised to 0.16 mg/kg, two patients developed intolerable symptoms of photosensitivity and the other developed mild symptoms.[71]

In a single-dose study, healthy volunteers received standardized hypericum extract (equivalent to 2.81, 5.62 or 11.25 mg of TH). No evidence of photosensitivity was observed when their skin was irradiated with both UVA and UVB light 4 hours later. Sensitivity to UVA light was increased only after the highest dose of extract. The results of a multiple-dose study using 1800 mg extract (equivalent to 5.62 mg of TH) over 15 days indicated that hypericum extract caused no significant change in UVB photosensitivity but a moderate increase in UVA photosensitivity. It was concluded that patients should reduce artificial UVA irradiation while taking hypericum, but normal doses of hypericum should represent no concern with regard to photosensitivity.[118,53]

Hypersensitivity reactions

There have been reports of an adverse reaction consisting of sensory nerve hypersensitivity occurring in patients consuming tablets and liquid extracts of hypericum in Australia and New Zealand in recent years. Based on the clinical experience of some Australian practitioners, there is evidence to suggest that these patients ingested hypericum preparations from late harvested herb which contained high levels of resinous constituents which would not normally be ingested, e.g. the sediment in a liquid extract. This can be avoided by not dispensing the sediment and by using hypericum harvested before or at the onset of full flowering. The hypersensitivity reaction was not hypericism.[119]

A possibly related case of subacute toxic neuropathy (nerve damage) has been reported. The woman began to experience sharp pains in areas exposed to the sun (face and hands) after 4 weeks' treatment with an over-the-counter preparation of hypericum (500 mg, concentration undefined). Painful sensitivity on her arms and legs occurred after sunbathing. Her symptoms began to improve and eventually disappeared after she stopped using the product.[120]

OVERDOSE

Overdose with hypericum has not been reported. Phototoxicity could be expected to occur. Typical phototoxic symptoms include rash, pruritus and erythema 24 hours after exposure to ultraviolet light.

CURRENT REGULATORY STATUS IN SELECTED COUNTRIES

Hypericum became official in late 1998 in the *United States Pharmacopeia-National Formulary* (USP23–NF18, 1995–June 1999). Hypericum is covered by a positive Commission E monograph and can be used for psychogenic disturbances, depressive states and excitability. Infused oil of hypericum can be used internally for dyspeptic complaints and externally for the treatment of wounds, bruises, myalgia and first-degree burns.

Hypericum is on the UK General Sale List.

Hypericum does not have GRAS status. However, it is freely available as a 'dietary supplement' in the USA under DSHEA legislation (1994 Dietary Supplement Health and Education Act). Hypericum has been present in OTC digestive aid drug products. The FDA, however, advises that: 'based on evidence currently available, there is inadequate data to establish general recognition of the safety and effectiveness of these ingredients for the specified uses'. Hypericum is also being combined with other constituents such as ma huang (Ephedra) and promoted for weight loss. The FDA has issued a warning that this treatment is not safe and/or effective.

Hypericum is not included in Part 4 of Schedule 4 of the Therapeutic Goods Act Regulations of Australia.

References

1. British Herbal Medicine Association's Scientific Committee. British herbal pharmacopoeia. BHMA, Cowling, 1983, p 115.
2. Felter HW, Lloyd JU. King's American dispensatory, 18th edn, 3rd revision, vol 2, 1905. Reprinted by Eclectic Medical Publications, Portland, 1983, pp 1038–1039.
3. Axarlis S, Mentis A, Demetzos C et al. Phytother Res 1998; 12: 507–511.
4. Smeh NJ. Creating your own cosmetics – naturally. Alliance Publishing Company, Garrisonville, 1995, p 83.
5. Mabberley DJ. The plant book, 2nd edn. Cambridge University Press, Cambridge, 1997, pp 319–320, 356.
6. Campbell MH, Delfosse ES. J Aust Institute Agric Sci 1984; 50 (2): 63–73.
7. Launert EL. The Hamlyn guide to edible and medicinal plants of Britain and Northern Europe. Hamlyn, London, 1981, p 40.
8. Chiej R. The Macdonald encyclopedia of medicinal plants. Macdonald, London, 1984, entry no. 157.
9. Wagner H, Bladt S. Plant drug analysis: a thin layer chromatography atlas, 2nd edn. Springer-Verlag, Berlin, 1996, p 58.
10. Melzer R, Fricke U, Holzl J. Arzneim Forsch 1991; 41 (5): 481–483.
11. Franchomme P, Penoel D. L'aromathérapie exactement: encyclopédie de l'utilisation thérapeutique des huiles essentielles. Roger Jollois Editeur, Limoges, 1990, p 358.
12. Niesel S, Schilcher H. Arch Pharm 1990; 323: 755.
13. Falk H, Schmitzberger W. Monatshefte Chem 1992; 123: 731–739.
14. Andersen DO, Weber ND, Wood SG et al. Antiviral Res 1991; 16 (2): 185–196.
15. Lopez-Bazzocchi I, Hudson JB, Towers GHN. Photochem Photobiol 1991; 54 (1): 95–98.
16. Moraleda G, Wu TT, Jilbert AR et al. Antiviral Res 1993; 20: 235–247.
17. Tang J, Colacino JM, Larsen SH et al. Antiviral Res 1990; 13 (6): 313–325.
18. Hudson JB, Harris L, Towers GHN. Antiviral Res 1993; 20 (2): 173–178.
19. Lenard J, Rabson A, Vanderoef R. Proc Natl Acad Sci USA 1993; 90 (1): 158–162.
20. Degar S, Prince AM, Pascual D et al. AIDS Res Hum Retroviruses 1992; 8 (11): 1929–1936.
21. Carpenter S, Kraus GA. Photochem Photobiol 1991; 53 (2): 169–174.
22. Lavie G, Valentine F, Levin B et al. Proc Natl Acad Sci USA 1989; 86 (15): 5963–5967.
23. Meruelo D, Lavie G, Lavie D et al. Proc Natl Acad Sci USA 1988; 85 (14): 5230–5234.
24. Kraus GA, Pratt D, Tossberg J et al. Biochem Biophys Res Commun 1990; 172 (1): 149–153.
25. Takahashi I, Nakanishi S, Kobayashi E et al. Biochem Biophys Res Commun 1989; 165 (3): 1207–1212.
26. De Witte P, Agostinis P, Van Lint J et al. Biochem Pharmacol 1993; 46 (11): 1929–1936.
27. Panossian AG, Gabrielian E, Manvelian V et al. Phytomed 1996; 3 (1): 19–28.
28. Lavie G, Mazur Y, Lavie D et al. Transfusion 1995; 35 (5): 392–400.
29. Obry T. Diploma work. Cited in Scientific Committee of ESCOP. ESCOP monographs: hyperici herba. European Scientific Cooperative on Phytotherapy, Exeter, 1996.
30. Curle P, Kato G, Hiller KO. Unpublished data. Cited in Scientific Committee of ESCOP. ESCOP monographs: hyperici herba. European Scientific Cooperative on Phytotherapy, Exeter, 1996.
31. Holzl J, Demisch L, Gollinik B. Planta Med 1989; 55: 643.
32. Demisch L, Holzl J, Gollinik B et al. Pharmacopsychiatry 1989; 22(5): 194.
33. Nielsen M, Frokjaer S, Braestrup C. Biochem Pharmacol 1988; 37 (17): 3285–3287.
34. Chatterjee SS, Noldner M, Koch E et al. Pharmacopsychiatry; 1998; 31 (suppl 1): 7–15.
35. Dimpfel W, Schober F, Mannel M. Pharmacopsychiatry 1998; 31 (suppl 1): 30–35.
36. Muller WE. 2nd International Congress on Phytomedicine, Munich, September 11–14, 1996.
37. Perovic S, Muller WE. Arzneim-Forsch 1995; 45 (11): 1145–1148.
38. Muller WE, Rolli M, Schafer C et al. Pharmacopsychiatry 1997; 30 (suppl): 102–107.
39. Muller WE Singer A, Wonnemann M et al. Pharmacopsychiatry 1998; 31 (suppl): 16–21
40. Teufel-Mayer R, Gleitz J. Pharmacopsychiatry 1997; 30 (suppl): 113–116.
41. Muller WEG, Rossol R. Nervenheilkunde 1993; 12: 357–358.
42. Thiede HM, Walper A. Nervenheilkunde 1993; 12: 346–348.
43. Thiele B, Brink I, Ploch M. Nervenheilkunde 1993; 12: 353–356.
44. Nemeroff CB. Sci Am 1998; 278 (6): 42–49.
45. Cott JM. 2nd International Congress on Phytomedicine, Munich, September 11–14, 1996.
46. Harrer G. Therapiewoche 1991; 41 (47): 3092–3098.
47. Butterweck V, Petereit F, Winterhoff H et al. Planta Med 1998; 64: 291–294.
48. Butterweck V, Wall A, Lieflander-Wulf U et al. Pharmacopsychiatry 1997; 30 (suppl 2): 117–124.
49. Johnson D, Ksciuk H, Woelk H et al. TW Neurologie Psychiatrie 1992; 6: 436–444.
50. Schulz H, Jobert M. Nervenheilkunde 1993; 12: 323–327.
51. Czekalla J, Gastpar M, Hubner WD et al. Pharmacopsychiatry 1997; 30 (suppl): 86–88.
52. Kil KS, Yum YN, Seo SH et al. Arch Pharm Res 1996; 19 (6): 490–496.
53. Brockmoller J, Reum T, Bauer S et al. Pharmacopsychiatry 1997; 30 (suppl): 94–101.
54. Vandenbogaerde A, De Witte P. Anticancer Res 1995; 15 (5A): 1757–1758.
55. Vukovic-Gacic B, Simic D. Basic Life Sci 1993; 61: 269–277.
56. Barbagallo C, Chisari G. Fitoterapia 1987; 58 (3): 175–177.
57. Birzu M, Carnat A, Privat AM et al. Phytother Res 1997; 11: 395–397.
58. Rezvani AH, Yang Y, Overstreet D et al. Alcohol Clin Exp Res 1988; 22 (3, suppl): 121A.
59. Gurumadhva Rao S, Laxminarayana Udupa A, Saraswathi Udupa L et al. Fitoterapia 1991; 62 (6): 508–510.
60. Guillot JP Martini MC, Giauffret JY et al. Int J Cosmet Sci 1983; 5: 255–265.
61. Demisch L, Sielaff T, Nispel J et al. AGNP-Symposium, 1991. Cited in Scientific Committee of ESCOP. ESCOP monographs: hyperici herba. European Scientific Cooperative on Phytotherapy, Exeter, 1996.
62. Schmidt U, Harrer G, Kuhn U et al. Nervenheilkunde 1993; 12: 314–319.
63. Johnson D, Ksciuk H, Woelk H et al. Nervenheilkunde 1993; 12: 328–330.
64. McAuliffe V, Gulick R, Hochster H et al. 1st National Conference on Human Retroviruses and Related Infections, December 12–16, 1993, p 159.
65. Staffeldt P, Kerb R, Brockmöller J et al. Nervenheilkunde 1993; 12: 331–338.
66. Kerb R, Brockmöller J, Staffeldt B et al. Antimicrob Agents Chemother 1996; 40 (9): 2087–2093.
67. James JS. AIDS Treatment News 1989; 74: 1–6.
68. Cooper WC, James J. International Conference on AIDS, June 20–23, 1990; 6 (2): 369 (abstract no. 2063).
69. Steinbeck-Klose A, Wernet P. International Conference on AIDS June 6–11, 1993; 9 (1): 470 (abstract no. PO-B26–2012).
70. Vonsover A, Steinbeck KA, Rudich C et al. International Conference on AIDS July 7–12, 1996; 11 (1): 120 (abstract no. Mo-B-1377).
71. Pitisuttithum P, Migasena S, Suntharasamai P et al. International Conference on AIDS July 7–12, 1996; 11 (1): 285 (abstract no. Tu-B-2121).

72. Furner V, Bek M, Gold J. International Conference on AIDS June 16–21, 1991; 7 (2): 199 (abstract no. W-B-2071).
73. National Institute of Allergy and Infectious Diseases, AIDS Clinical Trial Group. Protocol ID number: NIAID ACTG 258, available from AIDSLINE database.
74. Reuter HD. Phytotherapy – Herbal medicine in the twenty-first century. Proceedings of the Symposium presented by the College of Practitioners of Phytotherapy, London, 17–18 May 1997. The School of Phytotherapy, East Sussex, 1997.
75. Linde K, Ramirez G, Mulrow CD et al. Br Med J 1996; 313 (7052): 253–258.
76. Ditzler K, Gressner B, Schatten WFH et al Complement Ther Med 1994; 2: 5–13
77. Quandt J, Schmidt U, Schenk N. Der Allgemeinarzt 1993; 2: 97–102.
78. Schmidt U, Sommer H. Fortschr Med 1993; 111 (19): 339–342.
79. Lehrl S, Willemsen A, Papp R et al. Nervenheilkunde 1993; 12: 281–284.
80. Hansgen KD, Vesper J, Ploch M. Nervenheilkunde 1993; 12: 285–289.
81. Harrer G, Sommer H. Phytomed 1994; 1: 3–8.
82. Hoffmann J, Kuhl ED. Z Allg Med 1979; 55: 776–782.
83. Schlich DF, Braukmann F, Schenk N. Psycho 1987; 13: 440–447.
84. Halama P. Nervenheilkunde 1991; 10: 250–253.
85. Hubner WD, Lande S, Podzuweit H. Nervenheilkunde 1993; 12: 278–280.
86. Harrer G, Schmidt U, Kuhn U. TW Neurologie Psychiatrie 1991; 5: 710–716.
87. Osterheider M, Schmidtke A, Beckmann H. Fortschr Neurol Psychiatr 1992; 60 (suppl 2): 210–211.
88. Schmidt U, Schenk N, Schwarz J et al. Psycho 1989; 15: 665–671.
89. Konig CD. Thesis, University of Basel, 1993. Cited in Linde K, Ramirez G, Mulrow CD et al. Br Med J 1996; 313 (7052): 253–258.
90. Reh C, Laux P, Schenk N. Therapiewoche 1992; 42: 1576–1581.
91. Bergmann R, Nübner J, Demling J et al. TW Neurologie Psychiatrie 1993; 7: 235–240.
92. Harrer G, Hübner WD, Podzuweit H. Nervenheilkunde 1993; 12: 297–301.
93. Vorbach EU, Hübner WD, Arnoldt KH et al. Nervenheilkunde 1993; 12: 290–296.
94. Kugler J Weidenhammer W, Schmidt A et al. Z Allg Med 1990; 66: 21–29.
95. Werth W. Der Kassenarzt 1989; 15: 64–68.
96. Warnecke G. Z Allg Med 1986; 62: 1111–1113.
97. Steger W. Z Allg Med 1985; 61: 914–918.
98. Kniebel R, Burchard HM. Z Allg Med 1988; 64 (23): 689–696.
99. Vorbach EU, Arnoldt KH, Hubner WD. Pharmacopsychiatry 1997; 30 (suppl): 81–85.
100. Wheatley D. 2nd International Congress on Phytomedicine, Munich, September 11–14, 1996.
101. Hansgen KD, Vesper J. Munch Med Wochenschr 1996; 138 (3): 29–33.
102. Martinez B, Kasper S, Ruhrmann B et al. Nervenheilkunde 1993; 12: 302–307.
103. Kasper S. Pharmacopsychiatry 1997; 30 (suppl): 89–93.
104. Woelk H, Burkard G, Grünwald J. Nervenheilkunde 1993; 12: 308–313.
105. Laakmann G, Schüle C, Baghai T et al. Pharmacopsychiatry 1998; 31 (suppl): 54–59.
106. Gerhard I, Liske E, Wustenberg P. 6th Phytotherapy Conference, Berlin, October 5–7, 1995.
107. Hottenrott K, Sommer HM, Lehrl S et al. Deut Zeit Sportzmed 1997; 48 (1): 22–27.
108. Scrip 1998; 2301: 16. Information available from Pharmaprojects, PJB Publications Ltd, Richmond, Surrey, UK or Pharmaprojects Online database.
109. Okpanyi SN, Lidzba H, Scholl BG et al. Arzneim Forsch 1990; 40 (8): 851–855.
110. Horsley CH. J Pharmacol 1934; 50: 310–322.
111. Southwell IA, Campbell MH. Phytochem 1991; 30: 475–478.
112. Araya OS, Ford EJH. J Comp Pathol 1981; 91 (1): 135–142.
113. Gordon JB. Am Fam Phys 1998; 57 (5): 950, 953.
114. Demott K. Clin Psychiatry News 1998; 26 (3): 28.
115. Scientific Committee of ESCOP. ESCOP monographs: hyperici herba. European Scientific Cooperative on Phytotherapy, Exeter, 1996.
116. Tran TL. Curr Clin Strategies 1997; 125 (16): 1022–1087.
117. Seigers CP, Biel S, Wilhelm KP. Nervenheilkunde 1993; 12: 320–322.
118. Roots I, Reum T, Brocknoller J et al. 2nd International Congress on Phytomedicine, Munich, September 11–14, 1996.
119. Baillie N. Modern Phytotherapist 1997; 3 (2): 24–26.
120. Bove GM. Lancet 1998; 352 (9134): 1121–1122.

St Mary's thistle (*Silybum marianum* (L.) Gaertn.)

SYNONYMS

Carduus marianus L. (botanical synonym), milk thistle (Engl), Silybi mariae fructus, Cardui mariae fructus (Lat), Mariendistelfrüchte, Marienkörner (Ger), chardon-Marie (Fr), carduo mariano (Ital), marietidsel (Dan).

WHAT IS IT?

St Mary's thistle is indigenous to the Mediterranean region but has been introduced to most areas of Europe, North and South America and is considered a weed in Australia. The stalk and young leaves have been eaten as a salad vegetable (Culpeper recommends the boiled leaf as a blood cleanser). Although historical references indicate extensive use of St Mary's thistle, even going back 2000 years, its use was revitalized in Germany in the mid-19th century and again in modern practice in the 1930s. Its main constituent, silymarin, has been extensively investigated, particularly as a hepatoprotective and antioxidant. The leaf of St Mary's thistle is also used medicinally but this monograph discusses the fruit (seed).

EFFECTS

Scavenges free radicals, increases intracellular concentration of glutathione; stabilizes hepatocyte membrane against injury and regulates its permeability, assists in cellular regeneration, increases the proliferation of Kupffer cells.

TRADITIONAL VIEW

The seeds of St Mary's thistle were used in Germany for curing jaundice, hepatic and biliary derangements, hepatitis and haemorrhoids and as a demulcent in catarrh and pleurisy.[1,2] External application of the decoction was recommended for some types of cancer. Dioscorides recommended the seeds as a remedy for snakebite. Culpeper suggested infusion of the fresh root and seeds for breaking and expelling gallstones and to treat dropsy (taken internally and applied externally to the liver).[2]

SUMMARY ACTIONS

Hepatoprotective, hepatic trophorestorative, antioxidant, choleretic.

CAN BE USED FOR

INDICATIONS SUPPORTED BY CLINICAL TRIALS

Clinical indications supported by trials using standardized St Mary's thistle extract (70–80% silymarin): non-alcoholic and alcoholic liver damage/disease, including abnormal liver function, diabetes secondary to cirrhosis, fatty liver, exposure to chemical pollutants (drugs, halogenated hydrocarbons, solvents, paints, glues, anaesthesia); treatment of death cap mushroom poisoning. Mixed results have been obtained for treatment of hepatitis, where it should mainly be prescribed for its hepatoprotective properties.

TRADITIONAL THERAPEUTIC USES

Liver and gallbladder problems.

MAY ALSO BE USED FOR

EXTRAPOLATIONS FROM PHARMACOLOGICAL STUDIES

As a prophylactic for conditions caused by oxidative stress; liver problems associated with pregnancy, oral contraceptive use or environmental pollution; to prevent gallstone formation; may assist in cholestasis and the complications of diabetes (such as diabetic neuropathy); may be beneficial as an antiallergic and antiinflammatory agent. Topically, silymarin may be protective against chemical carcinogen- and UVB radiation-induced skin tumours.

PREPARATIONS

Dried seed as a decoction, liquid extract or tablet for internal use.

DOSAGE

- 4–9 g per day of seed.
- 4–9 ml per day of 1:1 liquid extract.
- 1–2 tablets containing 200 mg of extract (standardized to 140 mg silymarin) taken 1–2 times per day.

Higher doses, especially of the tablets, should be used in more severe cases of liver damage. The absorption of silymarin is enhanced by lecithin and simultaneous dosing with a lecithin supplement is recommended.

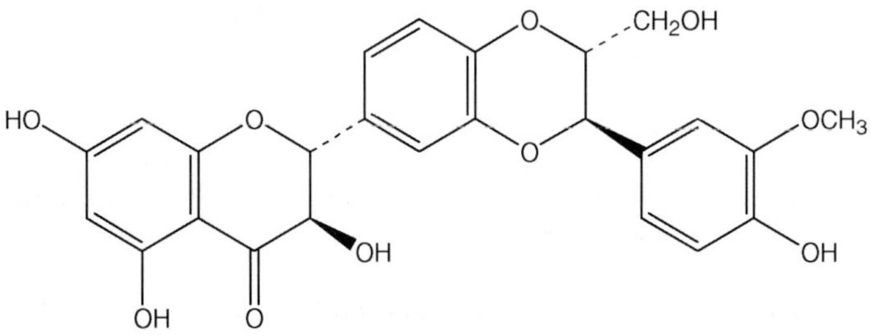

Silybin

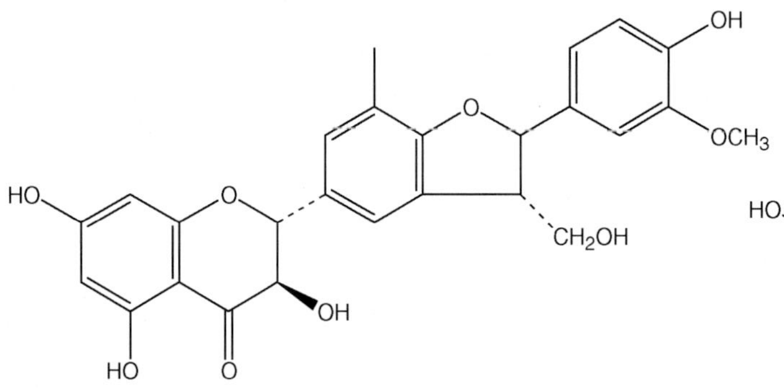

Silychristin

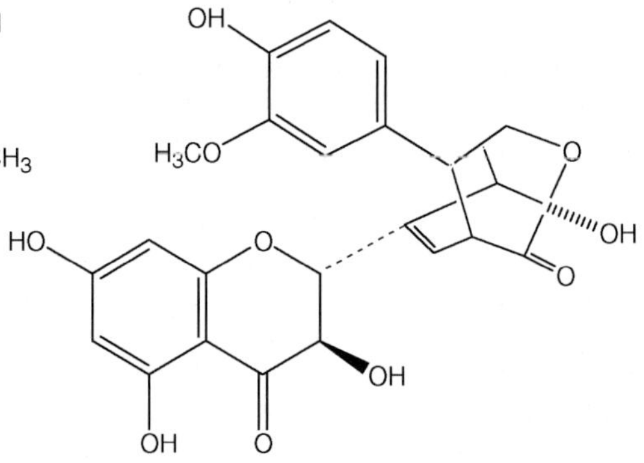

Silydianin

DURATION OF USE

No restriction on long-term use.

SUMMARY ASSESSMENT OF SAFETY

St Mary's thistle is an extremely safe herb.

TECHNICAL DATA

BOTANY

Silybum marianum is a member of the Compositae (daisy) family and in the same tribe as *Cynara scolymus*.[3] It is an annual to biennial herb with a 35–125 cm stem. The leaves are dark green, oblong, pinnatifid with spiny margins. White veins give the leaves a diffusely mottled appearance. The slightly fragrant, hermaphrodite flower heads are also spiny, deep violet in colour, 1–2.5 cm in diameter and sit above an involucre containing rows of spiny bracts. The fruit is an achene, 6–7 mm in length and transversely wrinkled, dark in colour, grey-flecked with a yellow ring near the apex. Attached to the achene is a long white pappus.[4,5]

KEY CONSTITUENTS

- Flavanolignans (1.5–3%): silybin, silychristin, silydianin and 2,3-dehydro derivatives. These flavanolignans are collectively known as silymarin.[6]
- Fixed oil (20–30%), flavonoids, taxifolin, sterols.[7]

Silybin is also called silibinin (particularly in European literature). The flavanolignans are often incorrectly classified as flavonoids. The fixed oil can give liquid extracts a milky colour or may sometimes separate in liquid preparations.

PHARMACODYNAMICS

Antioxidant activity

Silybin demonstrated free radical scavenger and antioxidant activities in vitro when complexed with molecules which increase its solubility.[8] Silybin and silydianin exerted an inhibitory effect on superoxide radical production, peak chemiluminescence and hydrogen peroxide production in stimulated human polymorphonuclear neutrophils in vitro.[9] Oxidative stress induced by a high glucose concentration in human mesangial cell cultures was counteracted by silybin.[10] Silybin increased the activity of both superoxide dismutase and glutathione peroxidase in human erythrocytes in vitro. This may explain the protective effect against free radicals and the stabilizing effect on the red blood cell membrane, as demonstrated by an increase in the time to full haemolysis.[11] Silybin dihemisuccinate sodium salt demonstrated an inhibitory effect in vitro on radiation-induced deactivation of enzymes and peroxidation of membrane lipids in rat liver microsomes.[12] Silybin inhibited linoleate peroxidation in vitro.[13]

Silybin is a potent inhibitor of glutathione S-transferase isoenzymes in vitro and displays a high degree of isoenzyme selectivity.[14] Intraperitoneal administration of silymarin in rats increased the redox state and the total glutathione content of the liver, intestine and stomach, without affecting levels in the kidney, lung and spleen.[15] Although a noticeable effect is observed, the effect of silymarin on lipid peroxidation processes was less marked in patients with chronic diffuse liver diseases than in experiments in vitro.[16]

Effects on detoxification mechanisms

Oral administration of silymarin (100 mg/kg per day) to rats resulted in a significant increase of the activity of the mixed function oxidation system (cytochrome P-450; aminopyrine demethylation, p-nitroanisole demethylation). However, an experimentally induced reduction in the activity of the mixed function oxidation system and glucose-6-phosphatase could not be prevented by pretreatment with silymarin. In human volunteers, treatment with silymarin (210 mg per day for 28 days) had no influence on the metabolism of aminopyrine and phenylbutazone.[17] Oral silymarin (150 mg/kg per day) markedly reversed the alterations in aspirin metabolism and pharmacokinetics observed in portal vein-ligated rats.[18]

Hepatoprotective activity

The pharmacological literature on the hepatoprotective activity of silymarin and silybin is extensive. The following is a selection from publications on this topic. The mechanisms behind the hepatoprotective action of silymarin probably involve the following:[19]

- antioxidant activity by scavenging free radicals and by increasing the intracellular concentration of glutathione;
- a regulatory action on cellular membrane permeability and an increase in its stability against xenobiotic injury;
- activity at the nuclear level: enhancing the synthesis of ribosomal RNA and proteins and thereby cellular regeneration; a possible steroid-like behaviour on the control of DNA expression.

Flavanolignans and other constituents of St Mary's thistle inhibited carbon tetrachloride- and galactosamine-induced cytotoxicity in vitro.[20] Prior intraperitoneal administration of silymarin protected against the effects of carbon tetrachloride in mice, firstly by decreasing its metabolic activation and by acting as an antioxidant.[21] Silymarin and isolated silybin have both shown protective activity against acute administration of liver toxins such as carbon tetrachloride,[22] galactosamine,[23] ethanol,[24] paracetamol,[25] lanthanides and FV3 virus in animal models.[26] Similar protective activity has also been demonstrated against chronic administration of carbon tetrachloride,[27] heavy metals,[28] thioacetamide[29] and several drugs.[30]

Silymarin has shown both prophylactic and curative activities against the toxin of the death cap mushroom (*Amanita phalloides*).[31] It interrupts the enterohepatic recirculation of amanitins, inhibits the binding of alpha-amanitin to hepatocyte membranes, competes with amatoxin for transmembrane transport and inhibits the penetration of amanitin into liver cells.[32,33] Intravenous pretreatment with silybin in animal experiments abolished the morphological changes induced by the toxin and decreased the activities of serum enzymes.[34]

Oral administration of silybin (100 mg/kg) protected against iron-induced hepatic toxicity in rats via an antioxidant mechanism.[35] Oral silymarin (50 mg/kg) ameliorated hepatic collagen accumulation in early and advanced biliary fibrosis secondary to bile duct obliteration in rats.[36] Oral doses of silymarin (5 mg/kg) demonstrated significant hepatoprotective activity against *Plasmodium berghei*-induced hepatic damage in rats. It had no effect on parasitaemia.[37] Oral silymarin (140 mg/kg per day) given to mice over 7 and 14 days after total body gamma irradiation alleviated nucleic acid changes in the liver, spleen and bone marrow.[38]

Although relatively high concentrations of silybin are necessary to diminish free radical formation by activated Kupffer cells, significant inhibition of the 5-lipoxygenase pathway occurs at silybin concentrations which can be achieved in vivo. Selective inhibition of leukotriene formation by Kupffer cells could at least partly account for the hepatoprotective properties of silybin.[39]

Silymarin elicits differential effects on the rate of glucuronidation and contents of UDP-glucuronic acid in isolated rat hepatocytes and in rat liver after administration by intraperitoneal injection.[40] An increase in nuclear RNA synthesis was observed in rat liver as a result of intraperitoneal administration of silybin in the animals. This may explain the acceleration of liver cell regeneration observed clinically with the use of silybin.[41] Silymarin protected against histological changes in the livers of pregnant women and those taking oral contraceptives.[42]

Other gastrointestinal activity

Compared to controls, silybin increased the proliferative activity of Kupffer cells in rats subjected to partial hepatectomy. Phagocytic and bactericidal activities were not modified.[43] Silybin demonstrated anticholestatic activity against paracetamol- and ethynyloestradiol-induced cholestasis by countering the reduction in bile salt output and bile flow.[44]

Oral silymarin demonstrated an anticholesterolaemic effect in rats fed a high-cholesterol diet. The effect was similar to the hypocholesterolaemic drug probucol. In addition, silymarin caused an increase in LDL-cholesterol, a decrease in liver cholesterol content and partially prevented the decrease in liver of reduced glutathione. Silybin was not as effective as silymarin.[45]

Silybin administered at a dose of 100 mg/kg by intraperitoneal injection for 7 days to rats significantly reduced biliary cholesterol and phospholipid concentrations compared to controls. Bile flow, biliary total bile salt concentration and total liver cholesterol content were unchanged. In gallstone patients and in cholecystectomized patients, oral administration of silymarin (420 mg/day for 30 days) reduced biliary cholesterol concentration and bile saturation index compared to placebo treatment.[46]

Antitumour activity

Silybin inhibited the growth of human ovarian and breast cancer cell lines in vitro. It decreased the percentage of cells in the S and G2-M phases of the cell cycle with a concomitant increase in cells in the G0-G1 phases. Silybin also demonstrated synergistic activity with cisplatin and doxorubicin.[47]

Topical application of silymarin prior to carcinogen application resulted in protection against tumour formation in mouse skin. Silymarin inhibited the carcinogen-caused induction of TNF-alpha mRNA expression.[48,49] Topical application of silymarin also reduced tumour incidence, tumour multiplicity and tumour volume per mouse in UVB-induced tumour initiation, promotion and complete carcinogenesis.[50] A sunscreen containing silymarin applied to the skin of mice prior to UVB exposure prevented the formation of pyrimidine dimers.[51]

Antiinflammatory activity

Silybin inhibited arachidonic acid metabolites and arachidonic acid-induced chemiluminescence of human platelets in vitro.[52,53] Silybin, silydianin and silychristin inhibited the formation of prostaglandins in vitro and non-competitively inhibited lipoxygenase from soybeans in vitro.[54] Oral administration of silymarin resulted in antiinflammatory activity in carrageenan-induced rat paw oedema. Topical application of silymarin was more effective than intraperitoneal injection in mouse ear inflammation. Silymarin produced a dose-dependent inhibition of leucocyte accumulation in inflammatory exudates after carrageenan injection and reduced the number of neutrophils. However, it was unable to inhibit phospholipase A_2 in vitro.[55]

Other activity

Silymarin demonstrated potent inhibition of cyclic AMP phosphodiesterase in vitro.[56]

Treatment of diabetic rats with silybin did not affect hyperglycaemia but prevented the inhibition of protein mono-ADP-ribosylation. Silybin treatment was associated with the prevention of substance P-like immunoreactivity loss in the sciatic nerve, which is typical of diabetic neuropathy. Silybin also prevented the increase in ADP-ribosylation of proteins in sciatic nerve Schwann cells. This latter effect is likely to be indirect and secondary to the improvement of diabetic neuropathy.[57,58,59]

The effect of silymarin on corticosteroid secretion was investigated on isolated adrenal cells from an aldosterone-producing adenoma, atrophied adrenal tissues surrounding the adenoma and hyperplastic adrenal tissue from Cushing's syndrome patients. The observed dose-dependent effect of silybin on corticosteroid secretion may be attributed to corresponding changes in the activities of cytochrome P-450 enzymes and the stimulation of ACTH-induced corticosteroidogenesis, which could result from the antioxidant activity of silybin.[60]

Silymarin inhibited microsomal beta-glucuronidase activity in vitro. Silymarin and silybin inhibited beta-glucuronidase of intestinal bacteria and of the faeces of healthy humans and humans with colon cancer. Oral administration of silymarin and silybin protected against the increase in beta-glucuronidase activity in rats treated with carbon tetrachloride.[61]

Silybin enhanced the motility of neutrophils inactivated by formyl-tripeptide, calcium ionophore, lymphokine or human serum and was effective in enhancing spontaneous motility of leucocytes obtained from healthy volunteers 2 hours after administration.[62]

Silybin dose-dependently inhibited f-met peptide and anti-IgE-induced histamine release from human basophils. Further in vitro results suggest the antiallergic activity of silybin may be ascribed to a membrane-stabilizing activity, possibly related to an interference with calcium influx.[63]

Pretreatment with silymarin prevented postischaemic mucosal injury in rats. The inhibitory activity of silymarin on neutrophil function may contribute significantly to its gastroprotective action.[64]

Silybin demonstrated protective effects in rats when administered by intravenous injection one hour prior to cisplatin (an anticancer drug with kidney side effects).[65] In the same model, silybin given alone had no effect on renal function. Administration of silybin did not inhibit the antitumour activity of the drug.[66]

PHARMACOKINETICS

A phase I crossover study using three silymarin products indicated that silybin bioavailability varies with product preparation.[67] Approximately 20–50% of silymarin is absorbed after oral administration, with approximately 80% excreted via the bile.[68]

The flavanolignans preferentially accumulate in the liver and bile. Six volunteers given 560 mg silymarin (240 mg silybin) registered low maximum serum concentrations (0.2–0.6 μg/ml) and low renal excretion (1–2% of the silybin dose over 24 hours). However, bile collected from cholecystectomized patients given 140 mg silymarin (60 mg silybin) was found to contain 11–47 μg/ml, a value approximately 100 times higher than in the serum, despite the lower administered dose.[69] Another study of similar patients showed that after repeated intake of silymarin, a steady state of silybin elimination was reached by the second day at the latest.[70]

A study conducted in 14 cholecystectomized patients indicated that in general there was no relationship between silymarin elimination and bile output. However, in two patients, one with pancreatitis and one with liver metastasis, reduced silybin elimination was linked to a decrease in bile output.[71]

Oral pharmacokinetic studies in rats using silymarin and a silybin-phosphatidylcholine complex indicated lower plasma silybin levels and lower biliary excretion for silymarin alone. The relative bioavailability of the complex was 10 times higher than silymarin.[72] This trend in bioavailability was also observed in healthy human volunteers.[73]

The plasma concentrations of unconjugated and conjugated silybin after intake of a single oral dose of a silybin-phosphatidylcholine complex were evaluated in 12 healthy volunteers. It was concluded that silybin undergoes extensive conversion to conjugated derivatives which are retained in the circulation at relatively high concentrations.[74] An earlier study using the same complex in 14 patients indicated that extrahepatic biliary obstruction is associated with a reduced clearance of conjugated silybin, probably due to impaired excretion of the conjugate in bile.[75]

CLINICAL TRIALS

For many of the clinical trials reviewed in this monograph, patients with a range of liver diseases were grouped together for treatment. These trials have been included in the non-alcoholic liver damage section, whereas trials conducted on patients with only cirrhosis or hepatitis are outlined in those respective sections. The outcomes of many trials have not been consistent, especially those concerned with cirrhosis, hepatitis and alcoholic liver disease (which may have been exacerbated by continuing consumption of alcohol).

Non-alcoholic liver damage

In an uncontrolled study on 2000 patients suffering from toxic liver damage of differing aetiologies, serum levels of hepatic enzymes were considerably reduced.[76] Symptoms such as nausea, discomfort and skin itching were also improved in 83% of patients. Sixty-seven outpatients with toxic-metabolic liver damage, chronic persistent hepatitis and cholangitis with pericholangitis who were treated with silymarin experienced significant reductions in serum transaminases and bromthalein retention. On the basis of liver biopsies, patients with chronic persistent hepatitis were deemed to be cured after 3 months of treatment.[77]

Thirty of the 49 workers with abnormal liver function and/or haematological values as a result of long-term exposure to organic solvent vapours (toluene and/or xylene) were treated orally with silymarin in an uncontrolled study. Liver function tests and platelet counts significantly improved, with leucocytosis and relative lymphocytosis showing a tendency toward improvement.[78]

In a double-blind, placebo-controlled clinical trial, silymarin improved the biochemical, functional and morphological alterations of the liver in 97 patients with slight acute and subacute liver disease who were treated over 4 weeks.[79] In a randomized, double-blind, placebo-controlled clinical study, the efficacy of oral silymarin (800 mg per day) in preventing psychotropic drug-induced hepatic damage was evaluated in 90 patients over a 90-day treatment period. The results indicated that silymarin reduced the lipoperoxidative hepatic damage which occurs during treatment with butyrophenones or phenothiazines.[80]

Alcoholic liver disease

In an open, controlled study, 60 insulin-dependent diabetics with alcoholic cirrhosis received either silymarin (600 mg per day) plus standard therapy or standard therapy alone over a 12-month period. In comparison with baseline values, treatment with silymarin reduced the lipoperoxidation of cell membranes and insulin resistance and significantly decreased insulin overproduction and the need for exogenous insulin administration. This response was not observed for the untreated group.[81] Significant antioxidant activity was verified in a double-blind clinical trial involving 36 patients with alcoholic liver disease.[82]

In a double-blind, placebo-controlled study, patients with cirrhosis were treated with 420 mg of silymarin per day for 6 months (three tablets each containing 140 mg). Serum levels of hepatic enzymes and bilirubin were significantly reduced compared to placebo. These improvements were accompanied by positive histological changes in the livers of patients receiving silymarin.[83] Seventy-two patients with alcoholic liver disease began participation in a randomized, double-blind, placebo-controlled trial and received silymarin (280 mg/day) or placebo tablets. Twelve patients subsequently dropped out of the trial and 10 patients died during the follow-up period (15 months). In those who survived, laboratory values and their changes did not differ between silymarin and placebo treatment. Twenty-two patients were positive for alcohol ingestion during follow-up. Those who abstained from alcohol had a significant fall in gamma-glutamyl transferase but without a significant difference between the two groups.[84]

In a double-blind, placebo-controlled clinical trial, patients with chronic alcoholic liver disease received 6 months' treatment with silymarin (420 mg per day) or placebo. The measured antioxidant and lipid peroxidation parameters were markedly improved in the silymarin group compared to placebo.[85] One hundred and sixteen patients with histologically proven alcoholic hepatitis (58 with cirrhosis) received either silymarin (420 mg per day) or placebo for 3 months. For those who remained in treatment, significant improvement was observed in both groups. Silymarin was not clinically superior to placebo. The rate of abstinence from alcohol was about 50% in both groups.[86]

In a surveillance study, St Mary's thistle extract (200–400 mg per day corresponding to 140–280 mg of silymarin) was administered to 108 patients with alcohol hepatopathies over a 5-week period. Eighty-five percent of patients responded to treatment with reductions in transaminases and procollagen-III-peptide (a fibrosis activity marker).[87]

Cirrhosis

In an open trial in which 11 patients with cirrhosis were treated initially with placebo (14 days) followed by silymarin, improvements in histological findings including regression of inflammatory changes and of lesions were observed. Alkaline phosphatase, serum GOT (glutamic-oxaloacetic transaminase), bilirubin and alpha-globulin decreased, while serum albumin and triglycerides increased.[88]

A randomized, double-blind clinical trial carried out over 4 years showed a significantly higher survival rate from alcoholic cirrhosis for the group of patients treated with silymarin (420 mg per day, $p<0.05$). Treatment of non-alcoholic cirrhosis was not as successful.[89]

In a 4-year, double-blind, randomized study on 170 patients with cirrhosis of different aetiologies, it was demonstrated that long-term treatment up to 2 years with silymarin (420 mg per day) significantly reduced mortality ($p=0.036$).[90] This effect was more pronounced in patients with alcoholic cirrhosis. In a prospective crossover study, the cytoprotective effects of either UDCA (ursodeoxycholic acid, 600 mg per day) or silymarin (420 mg per day) were investigated in 27 patients with active cirrhosis. This was followed by an open trial investigating the effects of a combination therapy (UDCA plus silymarin) versus no therapy or UDCA alone. The entire treatment period spanned 25 months, including a 1-month washout period between single treatments. Both UDCA and silymarin decreased serum transaminase levels, whereas only UDCA significantly diminished serum gamma-glutamyltranspeptidase. Both substances did not influence the functional liver mass when given alone or in combination. Combination therapy did not appear to be more effective than either substance given alone.[91]

Treatment with both silymarin and amino-imidazole-carboxamide phosphate in 60 patients with compensated alcoholic cirrhosis of the liver in a 1 month, double-blind, placebo-controlled clinical trial demonstrated hepatoprotective activity, which was accompanied by favourable changes in the parameters of cellular immunoreactivity.[92]

Hepatitis

In an uncontrolled trial, 29 patients with acute progressive hepatitis, active chronic hepatitis or cirrhosis without liver failure were treated with 210 mg of silymarin per day for a period of 3 months. All patients showed an improvement in their general health and laboratory tests showed a trend towards normal values. Serum bilirubin returned to normal in jaundiced patients.[93] Seventy-two patients with similar conditions including fatty liver demonstrated improvement in enzyme levels after silymarin treatment. Treatment duration varied from 6 months for fatty liver and hepatitis (420 mg) to up to 4 years for cirrhosis (630 mg). Clearcut results in enzyme levels were not achieved for the cirrhosis patients but the progress of the disease was slowed.[94]

In two double-blind, placebo-controlled clinical trials of 12 and 24 patients with chronic hepatitis treated for 3 months to 1 year, laboratory findings did not reveal any significant differences between silymarin (420 mg per day) and placebo. However, histological changes were improved in some of those treated with silymarin, including significant improvement in the mesenchymal intralobular reaction ($p<0.05$). The authors postulated that silymarin may hinder the development of immunological reactions by occupying receptors on the liver cell membrane.[95]

In a randomized, double-blind clinical trial, silymarin demonstrated favourable results in the treatment of 180 patients with chronic persistent hepatitis, chronic active hepatitis and hepatic cirrhosis. The trial lasted for 40 days and no side effects were observed.[96] In a double-blind, placebo-controlled clinical trial conducted at two medical centres, 57 patients with acute viral hepatitis received either silymarin (210 mg per day) or placebo for 3 weeks. Significant differences between bilirubin and GOT values in the placebo and silymarin groups were observed (higher regression after silymarin treatment). A definite trend in the regression of GPT (glutamic-pyruvic transaminase) values in favour of silymarin was also observed. However, the development of immunity was not influenced by silymarin.[97] Similar but significant ($p<0.05$) results for GPT were observed in a double-blind, placebo-controlled trial comprising 77 acute viral hepatitis patients.[98] In a prospective, open, controlled study of 151 acute viral hepatitis patients, silymarin treatment did not demonstrate efficacy (as determined by laboratory findings) compared to no treatment.[99]

In a double-blind trial on chronic persistent hepatitis, silybin treatment (silybin complexed with phosphatidylcholine) for 3 months decreased liver enzymes.[100] Silybin complex reduced the parameters related to hepatocellular necrosis in a short-term, double-blind study on chronic active hepatitis.[101]

Poisoning

A review of 205 cases of clinical poisoning with the death cap mushroom (*Amanita phalloides*) in the period 1971–1980 found the combination of penicillin with silybin to be associated with increased survival.[102] There are many reports of successful treatment of mushroom poisoning.[103–106] Treatment usually involves intravenous administration of silybin, alone or in combination with penicillin and/or other drugs. There are no side effects from parenteral silybin administration, while parenteral penicillin can have significant adverse effects. The clinical picture appears to be markedly mitigated by the early initiation of silybin therapy. A review of 18 cases (1980–1981) found a close relationship between the severity of the intoxication and the time elapsed before commencement of silybin therapy.[107] In a review of 87 patients with signs of poisoning with mushrooms and a long period of incubation, a significant reduction of serum transaminases and prothrombin time was found in those on competitive inhibition with silybin or penicillin, as compared to patients only on plasmapheresis.[108] Intravenous infusion of silybin, in combination with normal management techniques, induced a marked reduction in mortality in a multicentre study on 252 cases of intoxication by *Amanita phalloides*.[109]

Silymarin administered during the pre- and postoperative period prevented the increase of hepatic enzymes in the serum induced by the toxic effect of general anaesthesia.[76] Silymarin also improved liver function in patients who had been exposed for many years to halogenated hydrocarbons.[29] Treatment with silymarin (420 mg per day) in patients with occupational toxic hepatopathy caused by various toxic substances (mostly solvents, paints and glues) resulted in slight variations in some parameters compared to those treated with placebo. The therapeutic effect of silymarin is more evident when the exposure period to toxins is shorter.[110] Improvement in biochemical parameters was observed in 19 patients on psychotropic drugs after 6 months of silymarin treatment.[111]

Other conditions

In an open trial, 14 outpatients with type II hyperlipidaemia were treated with silymarin (420 mg per day) for 3 months, followed by a 2-month placebo period and silymarin treatment for another month. Total cholesterol and HDL-cholesterol levels slightly decreased and apolipoprotein levels were somewhat decreased compared to baseline values. A relative increase in the proportion of cholesterol in the HDL fraction was suggested by the significant decrease of apolipoprotein A-I and A-II values.[112]

Treatment with silybin (231 mg per day for 4 weeks) in 14 non-insulin dependent diabetics resulted in significant reduction of red blood cell sorbitol compared to baseline levels. However, silybin treatment had no effect on fasting blood glucose. This suggests that silybin may be an aldose reductase inhibitor and could be valuable in the prophylaxis and treatment of diabetic complications.[113]

A case of spontaneous regression of hepatocellular carcinoma has been reported. In June 1991, 11 months after being diagnosed with inoperable carcinoma of both lobes, the man presented to the hospital. All laboratory parameters were normal except for one liver enzyme and the liver was clear of the earlier signs of carcinoma. The man claimed to have stopped drinking alcohol and smoking and had been taking silymarin (450 mg per day) for 10 months and glibenclamide (a hypoglycaemic drug).[114]

Silymarin alleviated pruritus associated with intrahepatic cholestasis of pregnancy. However, it did not assist with the biochemical alterations associated with this condition.[115,116]

TOXICOLOGY

The acute toxicology of silymarin is very low. Oral doses of 20 g/kg in mice and 1 g/kg in dogs resulted in no mortality or any signs of adverse effects.[117] Long-term studies (100 mg/kg/day for 16–22 weeks) also failed to demonstrate toxicity or teratogenic effects.[117]

Silymarin is capable of inducing DNA damage (measured as strand breaks) and inhibiting human cell growth. Toxicity was only seen at high micromolar concentrations (levels which are unlikely to be achieved in humans). Neither cytotoxicity nor genotoxicity was associated with the antioxidant enzyme capacity of the test cells.[118]

CONTRAINDICATIONS

None known.

SPECIAL WARNINGS AND PRECAUTIONS

None required.

INTERACTIONS

None known.

USE IN PREGNANCY AND LACTATION

No adverse effects expected.

EFFECTS ON ABILITY TO DRIVE AND USE MACHINES

No negative influence is expected.

SIDE EFFECTS

Drug monitoring studies evaluating more than 3500 patients using silymarin up to 1995 indicate that adverse effects were seen in 1% of patients and consisted mainly of mild gastrointestinal complaints.[119,120] A mild laxative effect is occasionally observed with St Mary's thistle preparations.[26]

A case of anaphylactic shock due to crude St Mary's thistle has been reported in a patient with immediate-type allergy to kiwi fruit. St Mary's thistle tea caused facial oedema, swelling of the oral mucosa, marked respiratory distress, bronchospasm and decreased blood pressure in a 54-year-old man. He exhibited a marked immediate-type reaction to an extract of St Mary's thistle seed in the skin prick test.[121]

OVERDOSE

Not known.

CURRENT REGULATORY STATUS IN SELECTED COUNTRIES

St Mary's thistle became official in mid 1999 in the *United States Pharmacopeia-National Formulary*

(USP23–NF18, 1995–June 1999).

St Mary's thistle is covered by a positive Commission E monograph and has the following applications:

- crude drug: dyspeptic disorders;
- preparations: for toxic liver damage; as supportive treatment in chronic inflammatory liver conditions and liver cirrhosis.

St Mary's thistle is not on the UK General Sale List.

St Mary's thistle does not have GRAS status. However, it is freely available as a 'dietary supplement' in the USA under DSHEA legislation (1994 Dietary Supplement Health and Education Act).

St Mary's thistle is not included in Part 4 of Schedule 4 of the Therapeutic Goods Act Regulations of Australia.

References

1. Madaus G. Lehrbuch der biologischen Heilmettel, Band I. Georg Olms Verlag, Hildesheim, 1976, pp 830–836.
2. Grieve M. A modern herbal, vol 2. Dover Publications, New York, 1971, p 797.
3. Mabberley DJ. The plant book, 2nd edn. Cambridge University Press, Cambridge, 1997, pp 175, 663.
4. Evans WC. Trease and Evans' pharmacognosy, 14th edn. WB Saunders, London, 1996, p 435.
5. Launert EL. The Hamlyn guide to edible and medicinal plants of Britain and Northern Europe. Hamlyn, London, 1981, p 200.
6. Wagner H, Bladt S. Plant drug analysis: a thin layer chromatography atlas, 2nd edn. Springer-Verlag, Berlin, 1996, p 204.
7. Bisset NG (ed). Herbal drugs and phytopharmaceuticals Medpharm Scientific Publishers, Stuttgart, 1994, pp 121–123.
8. Basaga H, Poli G, Tekkaya C et al. Cell Biochem Funct 1997; 15 (1): 27–33.
9. Ignatowicz E, Szaefer H, Zielinska M et al. Acta Biochim Pol 1997; 44 (1): 127–129.
10. Wenzel S, Stolte H, Soose M. J Pharmacol Exp Ther 1996; 279 (3): 1520–1526.
11. Altorjay I, Dalmi L, Sari B et al. Acta Physiol Hung 1992; 80 (1–4): 375–380.
12. Gyorgy I, Antus S, Blazovics A et al. Int J Radiat Biol 1992; 61 (5): 603–609.
13. Valenzuela A, Guerra R, Videla LA. Planta Med 1986; 6: 438–440.
14. Bartholomaeus AR, Bolton R, Ahokas JT. Xenobiotica 1994; 24 (1): 17–24.
15. Valenzuela A, Aspillaga M, Vial S et al. Planta Med 1989; 55: 420–422.
16. Loginov AS, Matiushin BN, Sukhareva GV et al. Ter Arkh 1988; 60 (8): 74–77.
17. Leber HW, Knauff S. Arzneim Forsch 1976; 26 (8): 1603–1605.
18. Favari L, Soto C, Mourelle M. Biopharm Drug Dispos 1997; 18 (1): 53–64.
19. Valenzuela A, Garrido A. Biol Res 1994; 27 (2): 105–112.
20. Hikino H, Kiso Y, Wagner H et al. Planta Med 1984; 50 (3): 248–250.
21. Letteron R, Labbe G, Degott C et al. Biochem Pharmacol 1990; 39 (12): 2027–2034.
22. Vogel G, Trost W, Braatz R et al. Arzneim Forsch 1975; 25 (1): 82–89.
23. Schriewer H, Lohmann J, Rauen HM et al. Arzneim Forsch 1975; 25 (10): 1582–1585.
24. Valenzuela A, Lagos C, Schmidt K et al. Biochem Pharmacol 1985; 34 (12): 2209–2212.
25. Campos R, Garrido A, Guerra R et al. Planta Med 1989; 55: 417–419.
26. German Federal Minister of Justice. German Commission E for human medicine monograph, Bundes-Anzeiger (German Federal Gazette), no. 50, dated 13.03.1986.
27. Mourelle M, Muriel P, Favari L et al. Fundam Clin Pharmacol 1989; 3: 183–191.
28. Barbarino F, Neumann E, Deaciuc I et al. Med Interne 1981; 19 (1): 347–357.
29. Leng-Peschlow E, Strenge-Hesse A. Z Phytother 1991; 12: 162–174.
30. Martines G, Copponi V, Cagnetta G et al. Arch Sci Med (Torino) 1980; 137 (3): 367–386.
31. Choppin J, Desplaces A. Arzneim Forsch 1978; 28 (1): 636–641.
32. Floersheim GL, Eberhard M, Tschumi P et al. Toxicol Appl Pharmacol 1978; 46: 455–462.
33. Kroncke KD, Fricker G, Meier PJ et al. J Biol Chem 1986; 261 (27): 12562–12567.
34. Tuchweber B, Sieck R, Trost W. Toxicol Appl Pharmacol 1979; 51 (2): 265–275.
35. Pietrangelo A, Borella F, Casalgrandi G et al. Gastroenterol 1995; 109 (6): 1941–1949.
36. Boigk G, Stroedter L, Herbst H et al. Hepatology 1997; 26 (3): 643–649.
37. Chander R, Kapoor NK, Dhawan BN. Ind J Med Res [B] Biomed Res Infect Dis 1989; 90: 472–477.
38. Hakova H, Misurova E. Radiats Biol Radioecol 1996; 36 (3): 365–370.
39. Dehmlow C, Erhard J, De Groot H. Hepatology 1996; 23 (4): 749–754.
40. Chrungoo VJ, Reen RK, Singh K et al. Ind J Exp Biol 1997; 35 (3): 256–263.
41. Sonnenbichler J, Zetl I. Hoppe Seylers Z Physiol Chem 1984; 365 (5): 555–566.
42. Martines G, Piva M, Copponi V et al. Arch Sci Med 1979; 136 (3): 443–454.
43. Magliulo E, Scevola D, Carosi GP. Arzneim Forsch 1979; 29 (7): 1024–1028.
44. Shukla B, Visen PK, Patnaik GK et al. Planta Med 1991; 57 (1): 29–33.
45. Krecman V, Skottova N, Walterova D et al. Planta Med 1998; 64: 138–142.
46. Nassuato G, Iemmolo RM, Strazzabosco M et al. J Hepatol 1991; 12 (3): 290–295.
47. Scambia G, De Vincenzo R, Ranelletti FO et al. Eur J Cancer 1996; 32A (5): 877–882.

48. Zi X, Mukhtar H, Agarwal R. Biochem Biophys Res Commun 1997; 239 (1): 334–339.
49. Agarwal R, Katiyar SK, Lundgren DW et al. Carcinogen 1994; 15 (6): 1099–1103.
50. Katiyar SK, Korman NJ, Mukhtar H et al. Natl Cancer Inst 1997; 89 (8): 556–566.
51. Chatterjee ML, Agarwal R, Mukhtar H. Biochem Biophys Res Commun 1996; 229 (2): 590–595.
52. Dehmlow C, Murawski N, De Groot H. Life Sci 1996; 58 (18): 1591–1600.
53. Worner P. Thromb Haemost 1981; 46 (3): 584–589.
54. Fiebrich F, Koch H. Experientia 1979; 35 (12): 1548–1560.
55. Del La Puerta R, Martinez E, Bravo L et al. J Pharm Pharmacol 1996; 48 (9): 968–970.
56. Koch HP, Bachner J, Loffler E. Meth Find Exp Clin Pharmacol 1985; 7 (8): 409–413.
57. Gorio A, Donadoni ML, Finco C et al. Adv Exp Med Biol 1997; 419: 289–295.
58. Gorio A, Donadoni ML, Finco C et al. Eur J Pharmacol 1996; 311 (1): 21–28.
59. Donadoni MI, Gavezzotti R, Borella F et al. J Pharmacol Exp Ther 1995; 274 (1): 570–576.
60. Racz K, Feher J, Csomos G et al. J Endocrinol 1990; 124 (2): 341–345.
61. Kim DH, Jin YH, Park JB et al. Biol Pharm Bull 1994; 17 (3): 443–445.
62. Kalmar L, Kadar J, Somogyi A et al. Agents Actions 1990; 29 (3–4): 239–246.
63. Miadonna A, Tedeschi A, Leggieri E et al. Br J Clin Pharmacol 1987; 24 (6): 747–752.
64. Alarcon De La Lastra AC, Martin MJ, Motilva V et al. Planta Med 1995; 61 (2): 116–119.
65. Gaedeke J, Fels LM, Bokemeyer C et al. Nephrol Dial Transplant 1996; 11 (1): 55–62.
66. Bokemeyer C, Gels LM, Dunn T et al. Br J Cancer 1996; 74 (12): 2036–2041.
67. Schulz HU, Schurer M, Krumbiegel G et al. Arzneim Forsch 1995; 45 (1): 61–64.
68. Mennicke WH. Dtsch Apoth Ztg 1975; 115 (33): 1205–1206.
69. Lorenz D, Lucker PW, Mennicke WH et al. Meth Find Exp Clin Pharmacol 1984; 6 (10): 655–661.
70. Lorenz D, Mennicke WH, Behrendt W. Planta Med 1982; 45 (4): 216–223.
71. Lorenz D, Mennicke WH. Meth Find Exp Clin Pharmacol 1981; 3 (suppl 1): S103–S106.
72. Morazzoni P, Montalbetti A, Malandrino S et al. Eur J Drug Metab Pharmacokinet 1993; 18 (3): 289–297.
73. Barzaghi N, Crema F, Gatti G et al. Eur J Drug Metab Pharmacokinet 1990; 15 (4): 333–338.
74. Gatti G, Perucca E. Int J Clin Pharmacol Ther 1994; 32 (11): 614–617.
75. Schandalik R, Perucca E. Drugs Exp Clin Res 1994; 20 (1): 37–42.
76. Fintelmann V. Med Klin 1973; 68 (24): 809–815.
77. Poser G. Arzneim Forsch 1971; 21 (8): 1209–1212.
78. Szilard S, Szentgyorgyi D, Demeter I. Acta Med Hung 1988; 45 (2): 249–256.
79. Salmi HA, Sarna S. Scand J Gastroenterol 1982; 17 (4): 517–521.
80. Palasciano G, Portincasa P, Palmier V et al. Curr Ther Res Clin Exp 1994; 55 (5): 537–545.
81. Velussi M, Cernigoi AM, De Monte A et al. J Hepatol 1997; 26 (4): 871–879.
82. Feher J, Vereckei A. Z Gastroenterol 1991; 29: 67.
83. Feher J, Deak G, Muzes G et al. Orv Hetil 1989; 130 (51): 2723–2727.
84. Bunout D, Hirsch S, Petermann M et al. Rev Med Chil 1992; 120 (12): 1370–1375.
85. Muzes G, Deak G, Lang I et al. Orv Hetil 1990; 131 (16): 863–866.
86. Trinchet JC, Coste T, Levy VG et al. Gastroenterol Clin Biol 1989; 13 (2): 120–124.
87. Held C. Therapiewoche 1993; 43 (39): 2002–2006.
88. Reutter FW, Haase W. Schweiz Rundsch Med Prax 1975; 64 (36): 1145–1151.
89. Benda L, Dittrich H, Ferenzi P et al. Wien Klin Wochenschr 1980; 92 (19): 678–683.
90. Ferenci P, Dragosics B, Dittrich H et al. J Hepatol 1989; 9 (1): 105–113.
91. Lirussi F, Nassuato G, Orlando R et al. Med Sci Res 1995; 23 (1): 31–33.
92. Lang I, Nekam K, Deak G et al. Ital J Gastroenterol 1990; 22 (5): 283–287.
93. Brodanova M, Filip J. Prak Arzt 1976; 30 (346): 354–367.
94. Ravanelli DV, Haase W. Prak Arzt 1976; 30 (355): 1592–1612.
95. Kiesewetter E, Leodolter I, Thaler H. Leber Magen Darm 1977; 7 (5): 318–323.
96. Tanasescu C, Petrea S, Baldescu R et al. Med Interne 1988; 26 (4): 311–322.
97. Magliulo E, Gagliardi B, Fiori GP. Med Klin 1978; 73 (28–29): 1060–1065.
98. Plomteux G, Albert A, Heusghem C. IRCS Med Sci 1977; 5: 259.
99. Bode JC, Schmidt U, Durr HK. Med Klin 1977; 72 (12): 513–518.
100. Marcelli R Bizzoni P, Conte D et al. Eur Bull Drug Res 1992; 1(3): 131–135.
101. Buzzelli G, Moscarella S, Giusti A et al. Int J Clin Pharmacol Ther Toxicol 1993; 31 (9): 456–460.
102. Floersheim GL, Weber O, Tschumi P et al. Schweiz Med Wochenschr 1982; 112 (34): 1164–1177.
103. Serne EH, Toorians AWFT, Gietema JA et al. Netherlands J Ned 1996; 49: 19–23.
104. Mikos B, Biro E. Orv Hetil 1993; 134 (17): 907–910.
105. Hofer JF, Egermann G, Mach K et al. Wien Klin Wochenschr 1983; 95 (7): 240–243.
106. Carducci R, Armellino MF, Volpe C et al. Minerva Anestesiol 1996; 62 (5): 187–193.
107. Hruby K, Fuhrmann N, Csomos G et al. Wien Klin Wochenschr 1983; 95 (7): 225–231.
108. Gasparovic V, Puljevic D, Radonic R et al. Lijec Vjesn 1991; 113 (1–2): 16–20.
109. Hruby K, Csomós G. 1st IGSC, Amsterdam 1989.
110. Boari C, Montanari FM, Galletti GP et al. Minerva Med 1981; 72 (40): 2679–2688.
111. Saba P, Galeone F, Salvadorini F et al. Gazz Med Ital 1976; 135: 236–251.
112. Somogyi A, Ecsedi GG, Blazovics A et al. Acta Med Hung 1989; 46 (4): 289–295.
113. Zhang JQ, Mao XM, Zhou YP. Chung Kuo Chung Hsi I Chieh Ho Tsa Chih 1993; 13 (12): 725–726.
114. Grossmann M, Hoermann R, Weiss M et al. Am J Gastroenterol 1995; 90 (9): 1500–1503.
115. Reyes H, Simon FR. Semin Liver Dis 1993; 13 (3): 289–301.
116. Reyes H. Gastroenterol Clin North Am 1992; 21 (4): 905–921.
117. Hahn G, Lehmann HD, Kurten M et al. Arzneim Forsch 1968; 18: 698–704.
118. Duthie SJ, Johnson W, Dobson VL. Mutat Res 1997; 390 (1–2): 141–151.
119. Albrecht M, Frerick H, Kuhn H et al. Z Klin Med 1992; 47: 87–92.
120. Grungreiff K, Albrecht M, Strenge-Hesse A. Med Welt 1995; 46: 222–227.
121. Geier J, Fuchs T, Wahl R. Allergolog 1990; 13 (10): 387–388.

Thyme
(*Thymus vulgaris* L.)

SYNONYMS

Common or garden thyme (Engl), Thymi herba, Folia thymi (Lat), Gartenthymian, Thymianblätter (Ger), thym (Fr), timo (Ital), almindelig timian (Dan).

WHAT IS IT?

The leaf and flowers of thyme have been used extensively in cooking, particularly in meat dishes and as a flavouring ingredient in teas and liqueurs. The dried flowers have been used in the same way as lavender, to preserve linen from insects. Thyme oil is used in perfumery, cosmetics, aromatherapy and recently in pest control as a preservative for agricultural commodities such as grains.

The *European Pharmacopoeia* allows the use of whole leaf and flowers of *Thymus zygis* (Spanish thyme) as well as *Thymus vulgaris*.[1]

EFFECTS

Spasmolytic, antiseptic and expectorant for respiratory conditions; antimicrobial in topical application for conditions of the skin and mucous membranes.

TRADITIONAL VIEW

Traditionally thyme has been considered a major antispasmodic cough remedy, particularly when administered in the form of cough syrups. Infusion of thyme, sweetened with honey or sugar, would be prescribed for whooping cough, sore throats and catarrh. Thyme tea was used as a carminative for colic, to treat dyspepsia and to control fever in common colds. Thyme oil was used as a rubifacient and counterirritant in rheumatism and neuralgic pain.[2,3] Eclectic physicians also considered thyme to be an emmenagogue and tonic and prescribed the tea for hysteria, dysmenorrhoea and convalescence after exhausting illness.[3] Thyme was also used for diarrhoea and enuresis in children and as a gargle for tonsillitis.[4]

SUMMARY ACTIONS

Expectorant, spasmolytic, antibacterial, antifungal, antioxidant; rubifacient and antimicrobial in external preparations.

CAN BE USED FOR

INDICATIONS SUPPORTED BY CLINICAL TRIALS

Indications supported by trials using thyme: productive cough.

TRADITIONAL THERAPEUTIC USES

Bronchitis, whooping cough, asthma and catarrh or inflammation of the upper respiratory tract; gastrointestinal disorders including dyspepsia, colic, flatulence and diarrhoea, especially in children; dysmenorrhoea; as an adjunct in convalescence; topically for tonsillitis.

MAY ALSO BE USED FOR

EXTRAPOLATIONS FROM PHARMACOLOGICAL STUDIES

Spasmodic conditions of the gastrointestinal tract; adjunct in treatment of peptic ulcer; possibly as a hypolipidaemic and antioxidant. Topically for fungal and bacterial skin disorders and as a mouthwash to reduce oral bacteria.

OTHER APPLICATIONS

As a flavouring in teas and cough preparations, especially for children,[5,6] steeped in boiling water for inhalation.[7] Thyme oil can be used in toothpastes, soaps, detergents, creams, lotions and perfumes[5] and as an antiseptic agent in lotions, ointments, mouthwashes and ear drops.[8] It can also be used as a component in chest rubs[7] and for healing preparations for oily skin and damaged skin; for hair and scalp treatments including for preventative hair loss; in bath preparations[9] and in massage oils to ease muscle pains and arthritis.[9,10]

PREPARATIONS

As with all essential oil-containing herbs, use of the fresh plant or carefully dried herb is advised. Keep covered if infusing the herb to retain the essential oil.

Liquid extract or essential oil for internal use. Infusion, essential oil or extract for topical use.

DOSAGE

2–6 ml of 1:2 liquid extract per day; 5–15 ml of 1:5 tincture per day. A 5% infusion can be used as a gargle or mouthwash.

DURATION OF USE

No problems known with long-term use.

SUMMARY ASSESSMENT OF SAFETY

No adverse effects are expected from ingestion of thyme.

TECHNICAL DATA

BOTANY

Thymus vulgaris, a member of the Labiatae (mint) family, is a cultivated ornamental indigenous from the western Mediterranean to southern Italy.[11] It is an evergreen subshrub growing up to 25 cm, with a very branched stem. The sessile leaves vary from elliptic to linear or diamond-shaped towards the apex. The flowers are united in spikes at the top of the branches and have a tube-like calyx and tubular corolla with a three lobed lower lip. The fruit consists of a smooth, dark-coloured nutlet and the roots are robust. The whole plant has an aromatic fragrance.[12]

KEY CONSTITUENTS

- Essential oil (1.0–2.5%) containing monoterpenes including thymol (30–70%), carvacrol (70%), thymol methyl ether (1.5–2.5%).[13]
- Flavonoids, including methylated flavones;[14] phenolic glycosides, aliphatic alcohols.[15]
- Biphenyl compounds;[16,17] phenolic acids, including rosmarinic acid.[18]

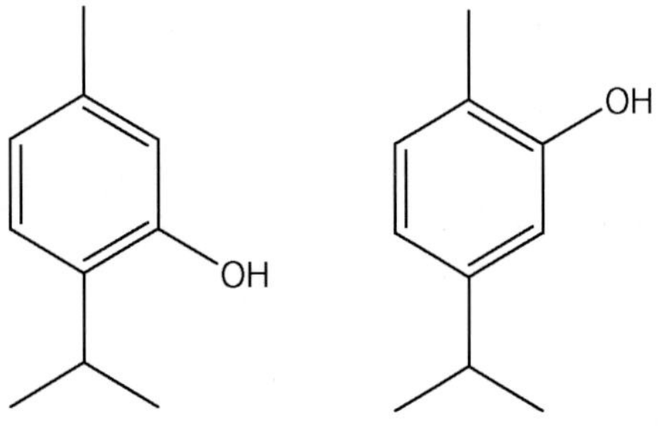

OH

OH

Thymol **Carvacrol**

Spanish thyme has similar essential oil content and composition to that of common thyme but a higher amount of carvacrol and less thymol methyl ether (0.3%).[13]

PHARMACODYNAMICS

Spasmolytic activity

Extracts of dried thyme inhibited agents which stimulate smooth muscle and also demonstrated a spasmolytic effect on various isolated smooth muscles. The relaxing effect of bradykinin was also potentiated.[19] The phenol (thymol and carvacrol) concentration of these and other thyme extracts used in such studies was found to be very low and could not have been responsible for the spasmolytic activity. However, thymol and carvacrol in sufficient dose do have tracheal relaxant activity.[20] Essential oil of thyme also demonstrated a relaxant effect on tracheal smooth muscle and inhibited the phasic contractions of ileal longitudinal muscle. The relaxant effect was higher on tracheal muscle than on the ileal.[21]

Thyme extracts and flavonoids from thyme demonstrated spasmolytic activity on the smooth muscle from ileum, trachea and vas deferens in vitro. Spasm caused by specific receptor agonists (acetylcholine, histamine, L-noradrenaline) as well as non-specific agents was inhibited. The spasmolytic activity may be due to inhibition of calcium ion flux by the flavonoids.[14] In an earlier study, the spasmolytic activity of thymol and carvacrol on isolated ileum and trachea was found to be significantly less potent than flavonoids.[22]

Antibacterial activity

The antibacterial and antifungal activity of thymol is well recognized and no attempt has been made to review this subject comprehensively. Brief exposure to a low concentration of thymol rapidly killed cariogenic and periodontopathogenic bacteria.[23] Thymol has also demonstrated antibacterial activity against other oral bacteria (*Porphyromonas gingivalis, Selenomonas artemidis, Streptococcus sobrinus*). The principal mode of action appears to be membrane perforation, resulting in rapid efflux of intracellular constituents.[24] Thymol, carvacrol, cinnamaldehyde and eugenol showed inhibitory activity on seven oral bacteria. A synergistic effect was observed with certain combinations (such as eugenol and thymol, eugenol and carvacrol, thymol and carvacrol).[25] Thymol and carvacrol are found together in oil of thyme.

Components of thyme oil were effective against seven standard strains of Gram-positive and Gram-negative bacteria.[26] Essential oil of thyme demonstrated antimicrobial and fungicidal activity in vitro.[27]

Thyme oil and thymol decreased the growth of *Salmonella typhimurium*, especially under anaerobic conditions. It is believed that the phenolic compounds of thyme exert antibacterial activity by complexing with the bacterial membrane proteins.[28]

Oil of thyme has demonstrated antibacterial activity against *Sarcina spp* and *Staphylococcus spp*.[29]

A broad spectrum of activity was observed for thymol and carvacrol against bacteria involved in upper respiratory tract infections. A synergistic effect for combination of thymol and carvacrol was also observed.[30] Aqueous and ethanolic extracts of thyme demonstrated significant inhibition of *Helicobacter pylori* in vitro.[31]

Fungicidal activity

Thymol and carvacrol have demonstrated fungitoxic activity towards *Cryptococcus neoformans* in vitro.[32] They also demonstrated strong antifungal activity towards fungal strains known to contaminate food, including *Penicillium spp*. From the range of substances tested, a free hydroxyl group in connection with an alkyl substituent appeared to render the antifungal activity.[33]

Thyme oil (200 ppm) was a highly effective inhibitory agent against eight different species of dermatophytic fungi in vitro[34] and stopped mycelial growth of *Aspergillus parasiticus* at a concentration of 0.1%. Aflatoxin synthesis was also inhibited.[35] Thymol (250 ppm) was highly effective in inhibiting *Aspergillus flavus* growth and aflatoxin production in vitro.[36]

Thyme oil inhibited the growth of several pathogenic fungi, including *Rhizoctonia solani, Pythium ultimum* var. *ultimum, Fusarium solani* and *Colletotrichum lindemuthianum*. The fungicidal activity was attributable to thymol and may be due to degeneration of the fungal hyphae.[37] Thyme oil was fungitoxic to the spores of *Aspergillus flavus, A. niger* and *A. ochraceus* in stored grain.[38] Thyme completely inhibited aflatoxin production on lentil seeds during 8 weeks of incubation.[39]

Antioxidant activity

Rosmarinic acid has demonstrated antioxidant activity in vitro: inhibition of lipid peroxidation, decreased production of the superoxide anion radical[40] and inhibition of the external oxidative effects of polymorphonuclear granulocytes.[41] A biphenyl compound (3,4,3′,4′-tetrahydroxy-5,5′-diisopropyl-2,2′-dimethylbiphenyl) and a flavonoid (eriodictyol) isolated from thyme demonstrated antioxidant activity in vitro by inhibiting superoxide anion production and lipid peroxidation. The biphenyl compound was extremely potent and also protected red blood cells against oxidative haemolysis.[42]

Thymol produced dose-dependent inhibition of endothelial cell-mediated oxidation of low-density lipoprotein.[43] Thymol, carvacrol and p-cymene-2,3-diol isolated from thyme oil demonstrated antioxidant activity in vitro. p-Cymene-2,3-diol exhibited the strongest activity which was greater than alpha-tocopherol.[44] Thymol and carvacrol demonstrated the following antioxidant activities in vitro: decreased peroxidation of phospholipid liposomes and scavenging of peroxyl radicals.[45] A methanol extract of thyme demonstrated strong hydroxyl radical-scavenging activity in vitro.[46]

Antimutagenic activity

Luteolin, a flavonoid isolated from thyme, demonstrated antimutagenic activity against a dietary carcinogen formed during cooking.[47] Extract of thyme demonstrated antimutagenesis with modulating effects on DNA repair in *Escherichia coli*. The antimutagenic activity was a consequence of the stimulation of error-free repair (and not due to suppression of error-prone repair).[48]

Antiallergic and antiinflammatory activity

Rosmarinic acid inhibited immunohaemolysis of erythrocytes in vitro, which was due to inhibition of the classic complement pathway (C3-convertase). Oral administration of rosmarinic acid (1–100 mg/kg) inhibited passive cutaneous anaphylaxis in the rat.[49] In a study of phenolic compounds, thymol inhibited neutrophil chemotaxis in vitro. A positive correlation was observed between superoxide anion generation in neutrophils and inhibition of neutrophil chemotaxis by phenolic compounds. A free phenolic hydroxyl group is essential for both these antiinflammatory activities.[50] Thyme oil inhibited prostaglandin biosynthesis in vitro.[51]

Thyme inhibited immediate allergic reaction via the inhibition of beta-hexosaminidase release from rat basophilic leukaemia cells.[52]

Other activity

Thyme leaf tea had an inhibiting effect on the normal transport velocity of isolated ciliated oesophageal epithelium.[53] This suggests a decrease in expectorant activity, which contrasts with very early work by Gordonoff on thymol and thyme.[54] In addition, the test method in question only demonstrates a partial mechanism of expectoration and an aqueous extract (tea) was used rather than a liquid extract.[55]

Dietary administration (720 μg, every second day) of essential oils (thyme, clove, nutmeg or pepper) to ageing mice had a marked effect on fatty acid distribution. The proportions of polyunsaturated fatty acids within phospholipids were almost restored to levels observed in young mice. The saturated fatty acid to polyunsaturated fatty acid (PUFA) ration decreased from 2.28 to 1.20 for animals treated with thyme oil. Although antioxidant activity was demonstrated in vitro by the oils, it was not responsible for the favourable effect on the PUFA content of tissue.[56]

Biphenyl compounds isolated from thyme demonstrated deodorant activity against methyl mercaptan. The activity was stronger than that of rosmanol, carnosol and sodium copper chlorophylline.[16,17]

PHARMACOKINETICS

A study of the metabolism of thymol and carvacrol in rats indicates that urinary excretion of metabolites is rapid, with only small amounts excreted after 24 hours. Although large amounts of both compounds were excreted unchanged (or as conjugates of glucuronide and sulphate), extensive oxidation of the methyl and isopropyl groups also occurred.[57]

CLINICAL TRIALS

Oral treatment with thymol, in daily doses of 1–4 g in two cycles of 64 and 169 days with a 35-day interval, resolved Kaposi's sarcoma in a 20-year-old woman. Heartburn was observed as a side effect.[58] Oral administration of thymol resolved a case of dermatomyositis[59] and a case of progressive scleroderma.[60]

Note: Large doses of thymol were used in these case studies and these results could not be expected from normal usage of thyme.

In conjunction with maintaining a continuous state of dryness, thymol was successfully used in the treatment of paronychia and onycholysis.[61] (See also the section on Side effects.)

In a double-blind, randomized study, 60 patients with productive cough received either syrup of thyme or bromhexine for a period of 5 days. There was no significant difference between the two groups based on self-reported symptom relief. Both groups made similar gains. A non-statistically significant improvement was observed in the recovery rate of non-smokers compared to smokers in both groups.[62]

Vulval lichen sclerosis in two sisters was successfully treated with a cream containing thyme extract. There were no side effects.[63]

TOXICOLOGY

The LD_{50} of the essential oil is 2.84 g/kg in rats.[64] Oral doses (0.5–3.0 g/kg) of concentrated thyme extract (equivalent to 4.3–26.0 g/kg of thyme) produced decreased locomotor activity and slight slowing down of respiration in mice. An increase in liver and testes weight was observed after chronic administration for 3 months (100 mg/kg equivalent to 0.9 g/kg dried plant per day). Spermatotoxic activity was not demonstrated.[65] Thyme oil had no mutagenic or DNA-damaging activity in the Ames or *Bacillus subtilis* rec-assay.[66] Thymol was not mutagenic in the Ames assay.[67]

CONTRAINDICATIONS

None known.

SPECIAL WARNINGS AND PRECAUTIONS

None required.

INTERACTIONS

None known.

USE IN PREGNANCY AND LACTATION

No data available.

EFFECTS ON ABILITY TO DRIVE AND USE MACHINES

None known.

SIDE EFFECTS

In a group of 100 patients with leg ulcers, 5% gave a positive reaction in patch testing to thyme oil.[68] Allergic contact dermatitis caused by thymol in Listerine for the treatment of paronychia has been reported.[69] Thyme can cause occupational asthma which has been confirmed by inhalation challenges.[70]

OVERDOSE

No toxic effects reported.

CURRENT REGULATORY STATUS IN SELECTED COUNTRIES

Thyme is official in the *European Pharmacopoeia* (1997) and the *British Pharmacopoeia* (1998).

Thyme is covered by a positive Commission E monograph and has the following applications:

- symptoms of bronchitis and whooping cough;
- catarrh of the upper respiratory tract.

Thyme is on the UK General Sale List.

Thyme and thyme oil have GRAS status. It is also freely available as a 'dietary supplement' in the USA under DSHEA legislation (1994 Dietary Supplement Health and Education Act).

Thyme is not included in Part 4 of Schedule 4 of the Therapeutic Goods Act Regulations of Australia.

References

1. European pharmacopoeia, 3rd edn. European Department for the Quality of Medicines within the Council of Europe, Strasbourg, 1996, pp 1638–1639.
2. Grieve M. A modern herbal, vol 2. Dover Publications, New York, 1971, pp 808–813.
3. Felter HW, Lloyd JU. King's American dispensatory, 18th edn, 3rd revision, vol 2, 1905. Reprinted by Eclectic Medical Publications, Portland, 1983, pp 1939–1940.
4. British Herbal Medicine Association's Scientific Committee. British herbal pharmacopoeia. BHMA, Cowling, 1983, pp 212–213.
5. Leung AY, Foster S. Encyclopedia of common natural ingredients used in food, drugs and cosmetics, 2nd edn. John Wiley, New York, 1996, pp 492–495.
6. Schilcher H. Phytotherapy in paediatrics. Medpharm Scientific Publishers, Stuttgart, 1997, p 39.
7. Weiss RF. Herbal medicine. Beaconsfield Publishers, Beaconsfield, 1988, pp 216–217.
8. Tyler VE, Brady LR, Robbers JE. Pharmacognosy, 9th edn. Lea and Febiger, Philadelphia, 1988, pp 127–129.
9. Smeh NJ. Creating your own cosmetics – naturally. Alliance Publishing Company, Garrisonville, 1995, p 95.
10. Pharmaceutical Society of Great Britain. British pharmaceutical codex 1934. Pharmaceutical Press, London, 1934, pp 748–749.
11. Mabberley DJ. The plant book, 2nd edn. Cambridge University Press, Cambridge, 1997, pp 713–714.
12. Chiej R. The Macdonald encyclopedia of medicinal plants. Macdonald, London, 1984, entry no. 309.
13. Wagner H, Bladt S. Plant drug analysis: a thin layer chromatography atlas, 2nd edn. Springer-Verlag, Berlin, 1996, p 155.
14. Van Den Broucke CO, Lemli JA. Pharm Weekbl Sci 1983; 5 (1): 9–14.
15. Scientific Committee of ESCOP. ESCOP monographs: thymi herba. European Scientific Cooperative on Phytotherapy, Exeter, 1996.
16. Nakatani N, Miura K, Inagaki T. Agric Biol Chem 1989; 53 (5): 1375–1382.
17. Miura K, Inagaki T, Nakatani N. Chem Pharm Bull 1989; 37 (7): 1816–1819.
18. Lamaison JL, Petitjean-Freytet C, Carnat A. Ann Pharm Franc 1990; 46 (2): 103–108.
19. Jensen KB, Dyrud OK. Acta Pharmacol Toxicol 1962; 19: 345–355.
20. Van Den Broucke CO, Lemli JA. Planta Med 1981; 41: 129–135.
21. Reiter M, Brandt W. Arzneim Forsch 1985; 35 (1A): 408–414.
22. Van Den Broucke CO. New pharmacologically important flavonoids of Thymus vulgaris. In: Margaris N, Koedam A, Vokou D (eds) Aromatic plants: basic and applied aspects, Martinus Nijhoff, The Hague, 1982, pp 271–276.
23. Shapiro S, Meier A, Guggenheim B. Oral Microbiol Immunol 1994; 9 (4): 202–208.
24. Shapiro S, Guggenheim B. Oral Microbiol Immunol 1995; 10 (4): 241–246.
25. Didry N, Dubreuil L, Pinkas M. Pharm Acta Helv 1994; 69 (1): 25–28.
26. Agnihotri S, Vaidya AD. Indian J Exp Biol 1996; 34 (7): 712–715.
27. Panizzi L, Flamini G, Cioni PL et al. J Ethnopharmacol 1993; 39 (3): 167–170.
28. Juven BJ, Kanner J, Schved F et al. J Appl Bacteriol 1994; 76 (6): 626–631.
29. Vampa G, Albasini A, Provvisionato A et al. Plantes Med Phytother 1988; 22 (3): 195–202.
30. Didry N, Dubreuil L, Pinkas M. Pharmazie 1993; 48 (4): 301–304.
31. Tabak M, Armon R, Potasman I et al. J Appl Bacteriol 1996; 80 (6): 667–672.
32. Viollon C, Chaumont JP. Mycopathologia 1994; 128 (3): 151–153.
33. Pauli A, Knobloch K. Z Lebensm Unters Forsch 1987; 185 (1): 10–13.
34. El-Kady IA, El-Maraghy SSM, Mostafa ME. Qatar Uni Sci J 1993; 13 (1): 63–69.
35. Tantaoui-Elaraki A, Beraoud LJ. Environ Pathol Toxicol Oncol 1994; 13 (1): 67–72.
36. Mahmoud AL. Lett Appl Microbiol 1994; 19 (2): 110–113.
37. Zambonelli A, D'Aulerio AZ, Bianchi A et al. J Phytopathol 1996; 144 (9–10): 491–494.
38. Paster N, Menasherov M, Ravid U et al. J Food Protect 1995; 58 (1): 81–85.
39. El-Maraghy SSM. Folia Microbiol 1995; 40 (5): 490–492.
40. Huang YS, Zhang JT. Yao Hsueh Hsueh Pao 1992; 27 (2): 96–100.
41. Van Kessel KP, Kalter ES, Verhoef J. Agents Actions 1986; 17 (3–4): 375–376.
42. Haraguchi H, Saito T, Ishikawa H et al. Planta Med 1996; 62 (3): 217–221.
43. Pearson DA, Frankel EN, Aeschbach R et al. J Agric Food Chem 1997; 45 (3): 578–582.
44. Schwarz K, Ernst H, Ternes W. J Sci Food Agric 1996; 70 (2): 217–223.
45. Aeschbach R, Loliger J, Scott BC et al. Food Chem Toxicol 1994; 32 (1): 31–36.
46. Chung SK, Osawa T, Kawakishi S. Biosci Biotech Biochem 1997; 61 (1): 118–123.
47. Samejima K, Kanazawa K, Ashida H et al. J Agric Food Chem 1995; 43 (2): 410–414.
48. Vukovic-Gacic B, Simic D. Basic Life Sci 1993; 61: 269–277.
49. Englberger W, Hadding U, Etschenberg E et al. Int J Immunopharmacol 1988; 10 (6): 729–737.
50. Azuma Y, Ozasa N, Ueda Y et al. J Dent Res 1986; 65 (1): 53–56.
51. Wagner H, Wierer M, Bauer R. Planta Med 1986; 52: 184–187.
52. Tanaka Y, Konishi Y, Takagaki Y et al. J Food Hygien Soc Jap 1997; 38 (1): 7–11.
53. Muller-Limmroth W, Frohlich HH. Fortschr Med 1980; 98 (3): 95–101.
54. Gordonoff T, Janett F. Zeit Ges Exp Med 1931; 79: 486–494.
55. Schilcher H. Effects and side-effect of essential oils. In: Baerheim Svendsen A, Scheffer JJC (eds) Essential oils and aromatic plants. Martinus Nijhoff, Dordrecht, 1985, p 217–230.
56. Deans SG, Noble RC, Penzes L et al. Age 1993; 16: 71–74.
57. Austgulen LT, Solheim E, Scheline RR. Pharmacol Toxicol 1987; 61 (2): 98–102.
58. Buccellato G. Giorn Ital Derm 1964; 105: 419–430.
59. Buccellato G. Giorn Ital Derm 1965; 106: 89–94.
60. Buccellato G. Giorn Ital Derm 1965; 106: 373–376.
61. Wilson JW. Arch Dermat 1965; 92: 726–730.
62. Knols G, Stal PC, Van Ree JW. Huisart Wetens 1994; 37 (9): 392–394.
63. Hagedorn M. Z Hautkr 1989; 64 (9): 810: 813–814.
64. Von Skramlik E. Pharmazie 1959; 14: 435–445.
65. Qureshi S, Shah AH, Al-Yahya MA et al. Fitotherapia 1991; 62 (4): 319–323.

66. Zani F, Massimo G, Benvenuti S et al. Planta Med 1991; 57 (3): 237–241.
67. Azizan A, Blevins RD. Arch Environ Contam Toxicol 1995; 28 (2): 248–258.
68. Le Roy R, Grosshans E, Fourssereau J. Derm Beruf Umwelt 1981; 29 (6): 168–170.
69. Fischer AA. Cutis 1989; 43 (6): 531–532.
70. Lemiere C, Cartier A, Lehrer S et al. Allergy 1996; 51 (9): 647–649.

Turmeric (*Curcuma longa* L.)

SYNONYMS

Curcuma domestica Val. (botanical synonym), Indian saffron (Engl), Kurkumawurzelstock, Gelbwurzel (Ger), rhizome de curcuma, safran des Indes (Fr), gurkemeje (Dan), jianghuang (Chin), shati (Sanskrit).

WHAT IS IT?

The rhizome of *Curcuma longa* L. (turmeric) has been used as a medicine, spice and colouring agent for thousands of years. A native of India and South-East Asia, it is now cultivated in many countries but India still accounts for a large percentage of current world production. Turmeric was listed in an Assyrian herbal dating from about 600 BC and was also mentioned by Dioscorides.

EFFECTS

Antiinflammatory (curcumin is a dual inhibitor of arachidonic acid metabolism); antioxidant (particularly by reducing lipid peroxidation); favourably influences cardiovascular function; antimicrobial (particularly by topical application); inhibits carcinogenesis and tumour promotion.

TRADITIONAL VIEW

In India, turmeric is regarded as a stomachic, tonic and blood purifier[1] which is used for poor digestion, fevers, skin conditions, vomiting in pregnancy and liver disorders. Externally, it is used for conjunctivitis, skin infections, cancer, sprains, arthritis, haemorrhoids and eczema.[1,2] Indian women apply it to the skin to reduce hair growth.[3]

In China different uses are attributed to the 'rhizome' and 'tuber'. Turmeric 'rhizome' is said to be a *Blood* and *Qi* (vital energy) stimulant with analgesic properties. It is used to treat chest and abdominal pain and distension, jaundice, frozen shoulder, amenorrhoea due to blood stasis and postpartum abdominal pain due to stasis. It is also used for wounds and injuries.[4] The 'tuber' has similar properties but is used in hot conditions as it is more cooling and has been used to treat viral hepatitis.[5]

In Western herbal medicine, turmeric was regarded as an aromatic digestive stimulant and as a cure for jaundice.[6]

SUMMARY ACTIONS

Antiinflammatory, antiplatelet, antioxidant, hypolipidaemic, choleretic, antimicrobial, carminative, depurative.

CAN BE USED FOR

INDICATIONS SUPPORTED BY CLINICAL TRIALS

Rheumatoid arthritis (curcumin), osteoarthritis (in combination); dyspepsia; topical treatment of cancerous lesions (in an uncontrolled trial).

TRADITIONAL THERAPEUTIC USES

Topically for skin disorders; internal use for poor digestion and liver function.

MAY ALSO BE USED FOR

EXTRAPOLATIONS FROM PHARMACOLOGICAL STUDIES

Inflammatory conditions such as asthma, infections, eczema, psoriasis; long-term prevention and treatment of cardiovascular disease, adjunct in the treatment of hyperlipidaemia; prevention of cancer and adjunct to cancer treatment; to improve gastric and hepatic function; as an antioxidant. Topically for inflammations, skin diseases and skin infections.

PREPARATIONS

Dried root as a decoction, liquid extract; oleoresin or essential oil for internal or external use. The powdered root is also used externally.

DOSAGE

Turmeric should be taken as the powdered rhizome or the 1:1 liquid extract prepared using 45% ethanol or higher. The dose for the liquid extract is 5–14 ml per day which is best taken in 4–5 equal doses throughout the day. A heaped teaspoon of powdered turmeric (about 4 g) can be mixed with water to a slurry and drunk 1–2 times daily. A teaspoon of lecithin can be added to improve absorption. Taking turmeric as a powder may be more desirable for antiinflammatory effects, since aqueous extracts devoid of essential oil

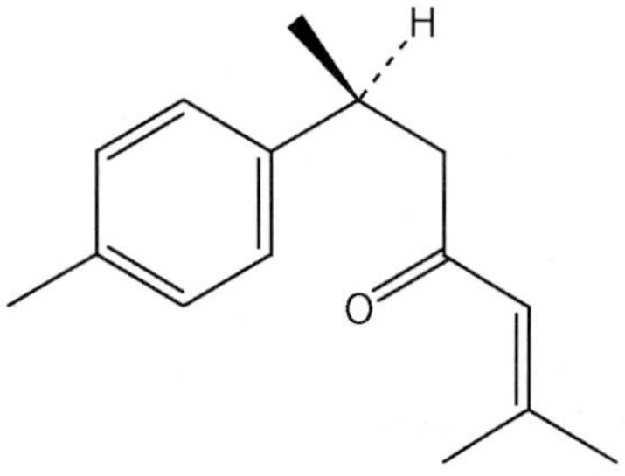

ar-Turmerone

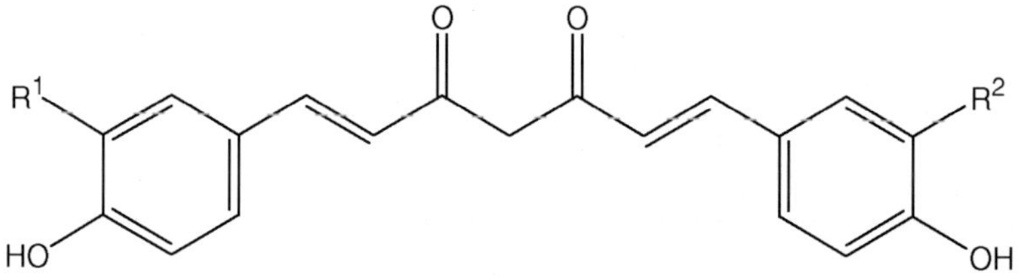

	R^1	R^2
Curcumin	OCH_3	OCH_3
Desmethoxycurcumin	OCH_3	H
Bisdesmethoxycurcumin	H	H

Diarylheptanoids

or curcumin also show significant activity. Turmeric extracts should be stored in dark glass away from direct sunlight due to the decomposition of curcumin on exposure to light.

DURATION OF USE

May be taken in the long term within the recommended dosage.

SUMMARY ASSESSMENT OF SAFETY

No adverse effects from ingestion of turmeric are expected when consumed within the recommended dosage.

TECHNICAL DATA

BOTANY

Turmeric, a member of the Zingiberaceae (ginger) family, is a perennial herb growing up to 1 m high with large tufted leaves. The leaf blade is long and tapers to the base. Pale yellow flowers containing three petals appear close to ground level. The rhizome is oblong or cylindrical and often short-branched. The external colour of the rhizome is brown and internally ranges from yellow to yellow orange.[7,8] The rhizome consists of two parts: an egg-shaped primary rhizome and several cylindrical and branched secondary rhizomes growing from the primary rhizome. These two parts were once differentiated in the Western trade as *C. rotunda* and *C. longa*.[9] In traditional Chinese medicine this differentiation is retained, the primary rhizome being called the 'tuber' and the secondary rhizome, the 'rhizome'.[5]

KEY CONSTITUENTS

- Essential oil (3–5%), containing sesquiterpene ketones (65% including *ar*-turmerone), zingiberene (25%), phellandrene, sabinene, cineole, borneol.[10]
- Yellow pigments (3–6%) known as diarylheptanoids, including curcumin and methoxylated curcumins.[10,11]

PHARMACODYNAMICS

The clinical relevance of in vitro pharmacological studies on curcumin (or where it was administered by injection) is uncertain, especially in the context of oral (but not topical) use of turmeric. This is because curcumin appears to undergo rapid biotransformation during and after gastrointestinal absorption (see also the Pharmacokinetics section). The biotransformation products of curcumin need to be identified and studied, since oral doses of curcumin do appear to exert significant pharmacological activity in several experimental and clinical models.

Antiinflammatory activity of curcumin

The antiinflammatory activity of curcumin was first reported in 1971.[12] In an extension of this work,[13] it was reported that oral doses of curcumin possess significant antiinflammatory action in both acute and chronic animal models. Curcumin was as potent as phenylbutazone and almost as potent as cortisone in the acute test (carrageenan oedema) but only about half as potent as phenylbutazone in chronic tests.

Slaked lime is traditionally mixed with powdered turmeric for topical application as an antiinflammatory agent.[14] This process probably increases the water-solubility of curcumin through salt formation. The antiinflammatory action of sodium curcuminate was investigated in rats as an experimental model of this traditional use.[15] Sodium curcuminate exhibited considerably higher antiinflammatory activity than either curcumin or hydrocortisone in acute and chronic tests. This was confirmed in a later study, which also found that curcumin and sodium curcuminate were more potent than phenylbutazone in acute and chronic models.[16] However, curcumin was only one-tenth as active as ibuprofen in reducing subacute inflammation.[17]

NSAIDs such as phenylbutazone can cause gastric ulceration. Curcumin was found to have a lower ulcerogenic index (0.60) than a nearly equivalent active dose of phenylbutazone (1.70).[13] However, curcumin given orally for 6 consecutive days to rats caused gastric ulceration at a dose of 100 mg/kg but not at a dose of 50 mg/kg.[18] In contrast, lower doses of curcumin in guinea pigs protected against gastric ulceration from phenylbutazone[19] but not histamine.[20] Ulceration caused by high doses of curcumin is associated with a marked reduction in mucin secretion.[18]

The mode of action of curcumin is not fully understood. Curcumin potently inhibited leukotriene production from intact neutrophils and at higher concentrations also inhibited prostaglandin production from bovine seminal vesicles.[21] Curcumin also inhibited the production of leukotrienes and prostaglandins from mouse epidermal microsomes.[22] Thus curcumin is a dual inhibitor of arachidonic acid (AA) metabolism in that it inhibits both the enzymes 5-lipoxygenase and cyclooxygenase. Dual inhibitors of AA metabolism are attracting interest as antiinflammatory agents since they prevent the potentially damaging effects of increased leukotriene production which can result from the use of only cyclooxygenase inhibitors such as aspirin. Moreover, leukotrienes may play an important role in some inflammatory processes. Curcumin is probably only a mild inhibitor of cyclooxygenase in vivo since, unlike aspirin and phenylbutazone, it lacks analgesic and antipyretic activities.[13] Even the more potent sodium curcuminate does not demonstrate analgesic and antipyretic effects.[16]

Curcumin inhibited the 5-lipoxygenase activity in rat peritoneal neutrophils as well as the 12-lipoxygenase and the cyclooxygenase activities in human platelets. In a cell-free peroxidation system, curcumin exerted strong antioxidant activity. Hence its effects on these dioxygenases are probably due to its reducing (antioxidant) capacity.[23]

Curcumin may also possess an indirect antiinflammatory activity via the adrenal cortex although results are conflicting. Curcumin was less effective in adrenalectomized rats,[13] whereas sodium curcuminate maintained its activity.[16] A single dose of sodium curcuminate did not alter plasma cortisol levels[16] but prolonged doses of curcumin doubled plasma cortisol.[17] It is possible that curcumin and sodium curcuminate may be acting via different mechanisms.

Curcumin was more potent than ibuprofen as a stabilizer of liver lysosomal membranes and was also active as an uncoupler of oxidative phosphorylation.[17] Recently it was found that curcumin inhibits aggregation, degranulation and superoxide generation from neutrophils in vitro.[24] It was concluded that at least part of the antiinflammatory action of curcumin is mediated via inhibition of neutrophil function.

Antiinflammatory activity of turmeric extracts and essential oil

Injected doses of the petroleum ether extract of turmeric, and two fractions isolated from it, demonstrated significant antiinflammatory activity when compared to hydrocortisone and phenylbutazone in acute and chronic tests.[25] Successive extraction of turmeric with petroleum ether followed by 50% alcohol and then water gave yields of 2%, 9% and 10% respectively.[26] These fractions, representing 21% by weight of the components of turmeric, were then compared for antiinflammatory activity. In both acute and chronic tests the aqueous extract was significantly more active and was often more active than reference drugs such as hydrocortisone and oxyphenbutazone. Unfortunately no fraction was chemically characterized and doses were administered by intraperitoneal injection, both factors which make the relevance of these findings to the action of oral doses of turmeric difficult to interpret.

Topical application of aqueous extracts of turmeric delayed corneal wound healing in rabbits indicative of 'cortisone-like' antiinflammatory activity.[27] An aqueous-alcoholic extract was inactive but this corresponded to a much lower dose of turmeric. Since curcumin is relatively insoluble in water this local 'cortisone-like' effect must be due to other components of turmeric.

A diethyl ether extract of turmeric inhibited platelet aggregation and altered eicosanoid biosynthesis in human platelets (see below).[28] This research suggests that turmeric may have antiinflammatory activity partly due to its inhibition of AA uptake and release from membrane phospholipids.

Oral doses of the essential oil of turmeric were studied in adjuvant arthritis in rats.[29] Significant antiinflammatory activity was found in this long-term test at doses of 0.1 ml/kg. The essential oil also has antihistaminic properties,[30] which may explain the antiinflammatory effect observed in a short-term test.[29]

Antiplatelet activity

Agents which cause a relative inhibition of platelet aggregation may be useful in the prevention and treatment of cardiovascular degeneration. Sodium curcuminate had no effect on in vitro platelet aggregation stimulated by ADP, epinephrine or collagen.[16] However, curcumin inhibited ADP-, collagen- and epinephrine-induced platelet aggregation in vitro and ex vivo with about the same activity as aspirin.[31] Unlike aspirin, curcumin did not decrease prostacyclin synthesis in rat thoracic aorta. The suggestion that curcumin selectively inhibits thromboxane production was supported by a contemporary publication.[32] In this study curcumin was found to inhibit thromboxane production from platelets in vitro and ex vivo. Also, it was found that increasing doses of curcumin progressively protected against collagen- or epinephrine-induced thrombosis in mice, whereas increasing doses of aspirin beyond a certain level afforded decreased protection. This again suggests a thromboxane-inhibiting but prostacyclin-sparing activity for curcumin.

A recent study found that curcumin inhibited platelet aggregation induced by arachidonate, adrenalin and collagen. Curcumin inhibited thromboxane B_2 production from exogenous radiolabelled arachidonate in washed platelets with a concomitant increase in the formation of 12-lipoxygenase products. It inhibited the incorporation of arachidonate into platelet phospholipids and inhibited the liberation of free arachidonic acid.[33]

A diethyl ether extract of turmeric inhibited AA- but not ADP- and collagen-induced platelet aggregation in vitro and also inhibited thromboxane production from exogenous AA in washed platelets.[28] The turmeric extract also inhibited incorporation of AA into platelet phospholipids and AA release under appropriate stimulation. The chemical content of the diethyl ether extract was not investigated. The author noted that a low incidence of cardiovascular disease is observed in the regions where spices such as turmeric are regularly consumed. Chinese research found that turmeric extract and curcumin enhanced fibrinolytic activity and inhibited platelet aggregation but the essential oil was devoid of these activities.[4]

Antioxidant activity

Curcumin inhibited in vitro lipid peroxide formation in liver homogenates from oedemic mice.[12] Curcumin is also an in vitro inhibitor of lipid peroxidation in brain tissue.[34] Lipid peroxidation induced by air on linoleic acid was inhibited by curcumin and related diarylheptanoids extracted from turmeric.[35] These natural curcuminoids also inhibited haemolysis and lipid peroxidation of mouse erythrocytes induced by hydrogen peroxide but were not as active as vitamin E.[36] Curcumin has a weaker scavenging effect than vitamin C on active oxygen radicals generated by polymorphonuclear leucocytes but is stronger than vitamin E.[37] However, curcumin had the strongest scavenging effect on hydroxyl radicals.

Curcumin was as effective as the antioxidant BHA in inhibiting lipid peroxidation.[38] Curcumin protected DNA against single-strand breaks induced by singlet oxygen. The observed antioxidant activity was both time and dose dependent. The protective ability of curcumin was higher than that of lipoate, alpha-tocopherol and beta-carotene.[39] Curcumin reduced experimentally generated nitrite in vitro. This nitric oxide-scavenging activity was also exhibited by other curcuminoids.[40]

An aqueous extract of turmeric was also found to be an effective inhibitor of oxidation. This unidentified water-soluble antioxidant from turmeric extended 80% protection to DNA against peroxidative injury and has potential as an antipromoter. The active component may have been an antioxidant protein, which has recently been isolated.[41] However, this constituent probably does not account for the in vivo antioxidant activity of turmeric since it would not be present in ethanolic extracts and is probably not absorbed after oral doses.

The efficacy of curcumin in preventing cataract formation was tested ex vivo in a rat model. Lenses from curcumin-treated rats were much more resistant to oxidant-induced opacification than were lenses from control animals.[42] Oral administration of curcumin reduced iron-induced hepatic damage in rats by lowering lipid peroxidation.[43] Dietary turmeric (1%) lowered lipid peroxidation in rats compared to controls by enhancing the activities of antioxidant enzymes (superoxide dismutase, catalase, glutathione peroxidase).[44]

Curcumin completely inhibited the superoxide anion hydrogen peroxide and nitrite radical production ex vivo by rat peritoneal macrophages. Capsaicin and curcumin were fed to rats on a diet containing 8% by weight of coconut oil, olive oil, peanut oil or cod liver oil for 8 weeks. Macrophages isolated from these animals produced lower levels of reactive oxygen species (ROS) compared to the macrophages from the control groups fed the oil alone.[45] Turmeric ethanolic extract administered orally to mice (4 mg/kg/day) for 4 weeks resulted in a decrease in levels of both plasma and liver lipid peroxides, compared to controls.[46] Turmeric extract (equivalent to 20 mg curcumin/day) for 45 days dramatically decreased blood lipid peroxide levels in an uncontrolled study on 18 healthy males.[47]

Hypolipidaemic activity

Toxicity studies on rats to establish the safety of turmeric extracts as a colouring agent also found that liver levels of total cholesterol were somewhat lower than normal.[48] A subsequent study revealed that turmeric extract and curcumin counteracted the increase in liver cholesterol in rats induced by cholesterol feeding.[49]

Dietary levels of curcumin as low as 0.1% significantly reduced the rises in serum and liver cholesterol in rats fed cholesterol but did not lower serum cholesterol in rats fed a normal diet.[50] It was also found that curcumin increased faecal excretion of bile acids and cholesterol in both the normal and hypercholesterolaemic rats and counteracted the rise in body and liver weights caused by cholesterol intake. These findings would suggest that turmeric might raise the ratio of HDL-cholesterol to total cholesterol and this was verified in a subsequent study on hyperlipidaemic rats.[51] Triglyceride levels were also significantly lower with turmeric treatment. Turmeric and curcumin had no effect on cholesterol levels of plasma, liver or egg yolk in hens fed a diet containing cholesterol.[52]

The activity of hepatic cholesterol-7-alpha-hydrolase (the rate-limiting enzyme of bile acid biosynthesis) was significantly elevated in rats fed curcumin. Serum and liver microsomal cholesterol contents were also significantly higher. However, the simultaneous stimulation of cholesterol synthesis by curcumin suggests that this may not be the mechanism for its hypocholesterolaemic action, which may be solely due to interference with exogenous cholesterol absorption.[53]

In experimentally induced diabetic rats maintained on a 0.5% curcumin-containing diet for 8 weeks, blood cholesterol was lowered significantly, exclusively from the LDL-VLDL fraction. Significant decreases in blood triglyceride and phospholipids were also observed. Hepatic cholesterol-7-alpha-hydroxylase activity was markedly higher, suggesting a higher rate of cholesterol catabolism.[54]

Effects on the digestive tract

Early research demonstrated that the essential oil of turmeric[55] and curcumin[56] increased bile secretion. Detailed studies found that while injections of curcumin and essential oil increase bile secretion, the aqueous extract was inactive. Curcumin and the essential oil were each about half as active as sodium deoxycholate administered the same way.[57] Investigations of sodium curcuminate found a stimulation of bile flow although the concentration of solids in the bile was somewhat decreased.[58] At higher doses total excretion of bile salts, bilirubin and cholesterol was enhanced. Such a finding is consistent with animal feeding experiments with curcumin, which also found increased bile acid and cholesterol excretion.[50]

Mice with preestablished cholesterol gallstones were fed a diet containing curcumin (0.5%) for 5 or 10 weeks. After 5 weeks, a regression of gallstones occurred in 45% and after 10 weeks in 80% compared to controls. Biliary cholesterol decreased and phospholipids and bile acids increased over the duration of feeding.[41] Feeding a lithogenic diet supplemented with 0.5% curcumin for 10 weeks reduced the incidence of gallstone formation to 26% when compared to mice fed the lithogenic diet alone. Biliary cholesterol concentration, lithogenic index and the cholesterol/phospholipid ratio of bile were also reduced.[59]

A test meal of 0.5 g/kg of turmeric in rabbits did not show any change in the volume or acid and pepsin content of gastric secretions but the mucin content was considerably increased, suggestive of a mucus stimulatory effect.[60] This contrasts with studies on high doses of curcumin which found ulceration associated with a marked decrease in mucin secretion.[18] Oral doses of 0.5 g/kg of an ethanolic extract of turmeric produced significant protection against ulceration caused by stress, pyloric ligation, indomethacin and reserpine in rats.[61] Turmeric extract increased gastric wall mucus production and also enhanced its cytoprotective quality.

After finding a protective effect for turmeric extract against carbon tetrachloride-induced hepatotoxicity in mice, the various constituents of turmeric were examined for in vitro hepatoprotective activity.[62] Curcumin and related diarylheptanoids (curcuminoids) exhibited considerable intrinsic activity; that is, activity was not due to their metabolites.

Antimicrobial activity

An alcoholic extract of turmeric, its essential oil and curcumin inhibited the growth of Gram-positive bacteria in vitro.[63] However, the antibacterial activity of turmeric is much weaker than conventional antibiotics.[64] The essential oil of turmeric has significant antifungal activity at dilutions of 1 in 500.[65]

An interesting recent discovery is that low concentrations of curcumin are highly toxic to Salmonella in the presence of visible light.[66] This phototoxic effect was thought to be due to unstable intermediates, probably radicals formed during the irradiation. Since an *E. coli* strain with DNA repair capacity was largely resistant to curcumin phototoxicity, this implies that light in combination with curcumin is genotoxic and may be mutagenic. The authors concluded that the observed phototoxicity makes curcumin a potential photosensitizing drug which may be useful in the phototherapy of psoriasis, cancer and bacterial and viral infections.

This study was confirmed by other workers who found that curcumin is more phototoxic to Gram-positive bacteria compared to Gram-negative bacteria.[67] Oxygen is required for the phototoxicity of curcumin and results were suggestive that hydrogen peroxide might be the toxic intermediate.

Turmeric oil (the hexane extract of the rhizome) at dilutions of 1:40 to 1:320 inhibited 15 isolates of dermatophytes and at dilutions of 1:40 to 1:80 inhibited four isolates of pathogenic fungi in vitro (curcumin was inactive). Six isolates of yeasts were insensitive to turmeric oil and curcumin. Turmeric oil (diluted to 1:80) applied topically on the 7th day following dermatophytosis induction with *Trichophyton rubrum* in guinea pigs resulted in improvement within 2–5 days after application and the lesion disappeared at days 6–7.[68]

Cancer prevention

Turmeric and curcumin possess antimutagenic and antipromotion activities which are probably related to the antioxidant and antiinflammatory properties of curcumin. Curcumin showed a dose-dependent decrease in the in vitro mutagenicities of cayenne extract and capsaicin.[69] This was comparable to the effect of known antioxidants such as vitamin E. In the presence of liver homogenate, curcumin also inhibited the in vitro mutagenicity of tobacco smoke condensates, tobacco and benzo (alpha) pyrene (BAP) in a dose-dependent manner.[70] However, it did not inhibit the mutagenicity of sodium azide and streptozocin, which occurs in the absence of liver homogenate. These results indicate that curcumin may alter the metabolism of those carcinogens which require hepatic microsomal activation.

Curcumin and aqueous extract of turmeric protected against DNA damage in human lymphocytes induced by fuel smoke condensate.[71] However, curcumin had no effect on the frequency of mitotic irregularities in virus-transformed cells[72] and curcumin feeding did not inhibit BAP-induced nuclear damage to murine intestinal cells in vivo.[73] In contrast, turmeric at 1% in the diet of mice reduced BAP-induced stomach tumours and also reduced the incidence of spontaneous mammary tumours.[74] A dose-dependent decrease in binding of benzo(alpha)pyrene metabolites to calf thymus DNA was observed in the presence of turmeric, curcumins and aqueous turmeric extract but not in the presence of curcumin-free aqueous turmeric extract. Further studies using mouse liver microsomes indicated that three curcuminoids inhibited benzo(alpha)pyrene-DNA adduct formation.[75]

Topically applied curcumin potently inhibited DNA synthesis and tumour promotion induced by 12–0-tetradecanoylphorbol-13-acetate (TPA) in mouse skin.[76] This effect parallels the inhibitory effect of curcumin on TPA-induced epidermal inflammation and also on epidermal lipoxygenase and cyclooxygenase activities.[22] In other words, the inhibitory effect of curcumin on tumour promotion is related to its antiinflammatory activity. Repeated applications of turmeric or curcumin in the promotion phase produced a significant reduction in mouse skin papillomas induced by DMBA followed by croton oil promotion.[77]

It has been demonstrated that turmeric increases the activity of the carcinogen-detoxifying enzyme glutathione-S-transferase in the stomach, liver and oesophagus of mice.[78] Glutathione levels were also significantly elevated and the in vivo mutagenic effect of BAP in mouse bone marrow cells was suppressed. Curcumin may be responsible for this activity.[79]

Curcuminoids and turmeric caused dose-dependent inhibition of nitrosomethylurea formation in vitro.[80] Nitrosamines can be formed in cured meats through the reaction of secondary amines with nitrites added during manufacturing and are potent carcinogens.

Curcumin and genistein (a component of soybean) were able to inhibit the growth of oestrogen-positive human breast cells induced individually or by a mixture of pesticides or oestradiol. When curcumin and genistein were added together to the cells, a synergistic effect resulting in a total inhibition of cell induction was observed. It was concluded that inclusion of turmeric and soybeans in the diet may assist in the prevention of breast cancer.[81]

Recently several in vitro and in vivo studies have confirmed that curcuminoids inhibit cancer at initiation, promotion and progression stages of development.[82] Curcumin is a potent inhibitor of TPA-induced ornithine decarboxylase activity and arachidonic acid-induced inflammation and topically inhibits

TPA-induced tumour promotion in mouse skin. Structurally related compounds such as chlorogenic acid are less potent inhibitors.[83] Three curcuminoids from turmeric demonstrated potent inhibition of mutagenesis in vitro and in croton oil-induced tumour promotion. Compared to 90% of control animals, 10% of curcumin III-, 20% of curcumin II- and 40% of curcumin I-treated animals developed papillomas.[84]

Dietary administration of curcumin to rats significantly inhibited the incidence of colon adenocarcinomas and the multiplicity of invasive and non-invasive tumours. It also significantly suppressed the colon tumour volume by more than 57% compared to the control diet. The chemopreventive action may at least in part be related to the modulation of arachidonic acid metabolism.[85] Oral administration of turmeric to mice from 2 months of age caused a suppression of mammary tumour virus-related reverse transcriptase activity and preneoplastic changes in mammary glands. Feeding turmeric from 6 months of age resulted in a 100% inhibition of mammary tumours.[86]

Catechin in drinking water and dietary turmeric significantly inhibited the tumour burden and tumour incidence in two tumour models: experimentally induced forestomach tumour in mice and oral mucosal tumour in golden hamsters. Chemoprevention utilizing both catechin and dietary turmeric inhibited both the gross tumour yield and burden more effectively in both tumour models than treatment with the individual components.[87] Oral administration of curcumin via diet inhibited carcinogen-induced forestomach tumorigenesis, duodenal tumorigenesis and colon tumorigenesis in mice. Curcumin inhibited the number of tumours per mouse, the percentage of mice with tumours and also reduced tumour size. Administration of curcumin during the initiation period resulted in a larger decrease in colon tumour incidence compared to administration during the postinitiation period.[88] Turmeric (2% or 5%) in the diet significantly inhibited benzo(alpha)pyrene-induced forestomach tumours in mice and this was dose and time dependent. The 2% diet significantly suppressed skin tumours in mice. The 5% turmeric diet for 7 consecutive days resulted in a 38% decrease in the hepatic cytochrome B-5 and cytochrome P-450 levels. Glutathione content was increased by 12% and glutathione-S-transferase activity was enhanced by 32% in the liver.[89]

Antitumour activity

A turmeric extract prepared with 50% ethanol inhibited the cell growth of normal mammalian cells and was cytotoxic to lymphoma cells at a concentration of 0.4 mg/ml.[90] The active constituent was found to be curcumin which was cytotoxic to lymphoma cells at a concentration of 4 μg/ml. Injections of both turmeric extract and curcumin reduced the development of tumours and enhanced survival in mice injected with lymphoma cells.[90] Sodium curcuminate was devoid of cytotoxic activity in vitro.[91] Earlier work reported that a turmeric extract exhibited cytotoxicity to mammalian cells in vitro by arresting mitosis and altering chromosome morphology.[92] The recently observed cytotoxicity of high concentrations of curcumin to rat hepatocytes was attributed to curcumin's antioxidant capacity and its ability to conjugate with glutathione.[93]

Curcumin III was more active than curcumin I and II as a cytotoxic agent in vitro and in the inhibition of Ehrlich ascites tumour in mice by intraperitoneal infection.[94] Curcumin inhibited the proliferation and cell cycle progression of human umbilical vein endothelial cells. It demonstrated a unique mode of action by effectively blocking the cell cycle progression during the S-phase by inhibiting the activity of thymidine kinase enzyme.[95] Curcumin therefore is a potential angiogenesis inhibitor in vitro.

Other activity

Curcumin inhibited human immunodeficiency virus type-1 integrase in vitro[96] and is a modest inhibitor of the HIV-1 and HIV-2 proteases.[97]

Turmeric (4 g/kg) and curcumin (0.4 g/kg) induced significant increases in hepatic levels of glutathione-S-transferase and acid soluble sulphydryl after 14 or 21 days' treatment in lactating mice and translactationally exposed mouse pups. Cytochrome B-5 and cytochrome P-450 levels were significantly elevated in the mice and their pups.[98]

Curcumin inhibited lipopolysaccharide-induced production of tumour necrosis factor (TNF) and interleukin-1-beta by a human monocytic macrophage cell line. It also inhibited lipopolysaccharide-induced activation of nuclear factor kappa B and reduced the biological activity of TNF in a fibroblast lytic assay.[99] Curcuminoids (I–IV) were ineffective as nematocidal agents when applied independently but the activity increased markedly when mixed, suggesting a synergistic action.[100]

In human peripheral blood mononuclear cells, curcumin dose dependently inhibited the responses to phytohaemagglutinin and mixed lymphocyte reaction. It dose dependently inhibited the proliferation of rabbit vascular smooth muscle cells stimulated by foetal calf serum. Curcumin had a greater inhibitory effect on platelet-derived growth factor-stimulated proliferation than on serum-stimulated proliferation. The characteristics of the curcumin molecule itself were necessary for the activity. Curcumin may therefore be beneficial in the prevention of the pathological changes of atherosclerosis and restenosis.[101]

PHARMACOKINETICS

The uptake, distribution and excretion of curcumin was studied in rats.[102] When administered orally in a single dose, 65–85% of curcumin passes through the gastrointestinal tract unchanged and was found in the faeces, while traces appeared in the urine. Only a small amount of curcumin was found in the bile, liver, kidneys and body fat. After intravenous injection curcumin is actively transported into bile but the majority is rapidly metabolized by the liver.

The poor bioavailability of curcumin was confirmed in a subsequent study on rats, which found that 38% of the administered 400 mg dose remained unchanged in the digestive tract.[103] Only traces were found in body tissues and no curcumin was detected in urine. A subsequent in vitro study suggested that curcumin undergoes transformation to a less polar, colourless compound during absorption from the intestine.[104] This was confirmed using radiolabelled curcumin.[105] While significant levels of radioactivity were absorbed, only traces of curcumin could be measured in body tissues.

When curcumin was given alone in a dose of 2 g/kg to rats, only moderate serum concentrations were achieved over a 4-hour period.[106] Concomitant administration of piperine at 20 mg/kg increased bioavailability by 154%. Administration of 20 mg of piperine to 10 healthy volunteers increased the relative bioavailability of curcumin by 20 times. However, the absolute bioavailability of curcumin under these conditions was still less than 10% and the elimination half-life was relatively rapid at 0.41 ± 0.17 h.

CLINICAL TRIALS

Antiinflammatory activity

In a short-term, double-blind trial on rheumatoid arthritis patients, curcumin (120 mg per day) was compared with phenylbutazone. A significant symptom improvement occurred with curcumin but phenylbutazone gave greater improvement, probably because it also has analgesic activity.[107] When postoperative inflammation was used as a model for evaluating antiinflammatory activity, curcumin (1200 mg per day) was found to have greater activity than phenylbutazone or placebo in a double-blind clinical trial.[108] In both the above trials, use of curcumin was devoid of significant side effects.

In a double-blind, placebo-controlled crossover trial, 42 osteoarthritis patients received either a herb/mineral preparation or placebo for 3 months. After a 15-day wash-out period the patients were transferred to the other treatment for a further 3-month period. The preparation consisted of turmeric, *Withania somnifera, Boswellia serrata* and a zinc complex. Treatment with the herb/mineral preparation produced a significant drop in severity of pain ($p<0.001$) and disability score ($p<0.05$). Radiological assessment did not show any significant changes in either group. Side effects did not necessitate withdrawal of treatment.[109]

Hypolipidaemic activity

An uncontrolled clinical trial on 16 patients in China found that 12 weeks of turmeric extract (equivalent to about 50 g/day of turmeric) lowered plasma cholesterol levels by 49 mg/dl (1.3 mmol/l) and triglycerides by 62 mg/dl.[4] The therapeutic effect was at least equal to clofibrate. Another study on 90 subjects found cholesterol and triglyceride levels were reduced by turmeric in almost all cases.[4] It was found in both studies that use of turmeric somewhat ameliorated the symptoms of angina pectoris.

Anticancer or preventative activity

In an open study, 58 patients with submucous fibrosis received one of the following treatments each day for 3 months: turmeric essential oil (600 mg) mixed with turmeric extract (3 g), turmeric oleoresin (600 mg) mixed with turmeric extract (3 g) or turmeric extract (3 g). Thirty-nine patients completed the treatment and results were compared to 32 healthy subjects who served as a control. All three treatments normalized the number of micronucleated cells both in exfoliated oral mucosal cells and in circulating lymphocytes. Turmeric oleoresin was more effective in reducing the number of micronuclei in oral mucosal cells ($p<0.001$) than the other two treatments. The decrease in micronuclei in circulating lymphocytes was comparable in all three groups.[110]

Turmeric given in doses of 1.5 g/day for 30 days to 16 chronic smokers significantly reduced the urinary excretion of mutagens in an uncontrolled trial. In six non-smokers who served as controls, there was no change in the urinary excretion of mutagens after 30 days. Turmeric had no significant effect on serum aspartate aminotransferase and alanine aminotransferase, blood glucose, creatinine and lipid profile.[111]

In an uncontrolled trial, a 50% ethanol extract of turmeric and an ointment containing curcumin produced symptomatic relief in patients with external cancerous lesions which had failed to respond to conventional treatments.[112] There was a reduction in the odour of the lesions in 90% of cases and also reduction in itching and exudation. In a small number of patients (10%) the thickness of the lesion was reduced.

Digestive tract

The safety and efficacy of turmeric for the treatment of undiagnosed dyspepsia were tested in a three-way, randomized, double-blind, placebo-controlled trial over 7 days.[113] Forty-one patients were in the placebo group, 36 received a herbal formula for flatulence and 39 received 2 g of turmeric powder per day. An 87% favourable outcome was recorded for the turmeric group which was significantly different to the 53% improvement for the placebo group ($p=0.003$). Mild side effects were observed with similar frequency in all three groups.

The effect of turmeric (1000 mg/day) was compared with an antacid formulation in 50 patients over 6 weeks in an open study of the treatment of gastric ulcer.[114] The antacid formula was significantly superior to turmeric in inducing ulcer healing ($p<0.05$). In a joint Vietnam-Sweden prospective, double-blind, two-centre study, turmeric in a dosage of 6 g daily, as suggested in the *Vietnamese Pharmacopoeia*, was compared with placebo in 118 patients suffering from duodenal ulcer.[115] Follow-up endoscopy and/or radiography were performed after 28 ± 4 days and 56 ± 4 days. Turmeric was not superior to placebo in healing duodenal ulcer after either 4 or 8 weeks of treatment. After 8 weeks the ulcer-healing rate of turmeric was 27% while placebo had healed 29%. Both treatments were well tolerated.

HIV/AIDS

Following pharmacological research which suggested that curcumin might weakly inhibit the LTR (long terminal repeat) of HIV-1, a clinical study was conducted. Eighteen HIV-positive patients took an average of 2 g curcumin a day for an average of 127 days.[116] There was a significant increase in CD4 ($p=0.029$) and CD8 ($p=0.009$) lymphocyte counts. A follow-up phase I/II open study using doses of 2.7 g and 4.8 g of curcumin per day failed to show any benefit on viral loads or CD4 count in HIV-positive individuals.[117] It was suggested that the poor bioavailability of curcumin may have been a factor behind this negative result.[118]

Other conditions

A paste consisting of turmeric and neem (*Azadirachta indica*) used in the treatment of scabies in 814 patients resulted in cure in 97% within 3–15 days of treatment. No toxic or adverse reactions were observed.[119]

TOXICOLOGY

Acute and subacute toxicity

The oral LD_{50} in rats of the petroleum ether extract of turmeric was 12.2 g/kg.[25] No toxic effects were observed when this extract was fed to rats at levels of 1 and 2 g/kg for 4 weeks. Rats, guinea pigs and monkeys given 2.5 g/kg of turmeric or 300 mg/kg of the ethanolic extract showed no signs of toxicity and no change in organ weights.[120]

No toxic effects were observed when oral doses of curcumin were given to mice up to 2 g/kg[13] and rats up to 5 g/kg.[102] Sodium curcuminate was not toxic to rats at 3 g/kg in an acute study and at 50 mg/kg/day in a study of 6 weeks' duration.[15]

The acute and chronic toxicity of a 20:1 turmeric ethanolic extract was studied in mice. Acute dosages of extract, given over 24 hours, were 0.5, 1.0 and 3 g/kg body weight and the chronic dosage, given over 90 days, was 100 mg/kg per day. There was no significant body weight gain after chronic treatment. Significant gains in heart and lung weights after chronic treatment were observed. There was a significant fall in the white blood cell and red blood cell levels and there were gains in weight of sexual organs and increased sperm motility but no spermatotoxic effects. No significant mortality or toxic effects were observed after acute doses.[121]

Chronic toxicity and mutagenicity

Turmeric oleoresin (which consists mainly of curcuminoids and essential oil) was fed for 102–109 days to pigs at doses of 60, 296 and 1551 mg/kg. Thyroid enlargement, pericholangitis and epithelial changes in the kidney and bladder were observed in the two higher dose groups. Liver and thyroid weight were increased at all dose levels. The highest dosage group also showed a reduction in weight gain.[122] Turmeric extract and turmeric powder caused hepatotoxicity when fed to mice for 14 days or longer.[123,124] The mouse is probably a susceptible species for turmeric-induced toxicity.

Turmeric extract in direct contact with mammalian cells in vitro caused cytotoxic effects such as chromosomal separation and breakage and mitotic arrest.[92]

Turmeric also caused chromosomal breakage in onion root tip cells.[125] However, turmeric, turmeric oleoresin and curcumin were not mutagenic in vitro in the Ames test[69,126] or in vivo.[127,128] Absence of mutagenicity in vitro was also reported for turmeric extract following activation with caecal microorganisms.[129] Curcumin and the synthetic dye tartrazine were compared for their chromosome-damaging effects on bone marrow cells of mice in vitro. Tartrazine was found to be more clastogenic than curcumin.[130]

Turmeric ethanolic extract was administered to mice (4 mg/kg per day) in their food for 4 weeks while a control group was fed a standard diet. Blood and liver samples taken after treatment indicated that turmeric did not result in any toxic effects on the physiological, behavioural and biochemical parameters measured.[46] Turmeric extracts show antifertility effects at high doses in rats and rabbits.[131]

CONTRAINDICATIONS

There are no contraindications for turmeric other than allergic reaction, which is probably rare. According to the Commission E, turmeric is contraindicated where there is obstruction of the biliary tract and should be used only after seeking professional advice if gallstones are present.[132]

SPECIAL WARNINGS AND PRECAUTIONS

High doses should not be given to patients taking antiplatelet or anticoagulant drugs and care should be exercised with women who wish to conceive or patients complaining of hair loss. Patients applying topical doses should be cautioned against excessive exposure to sunlight.

INTERACTIONS

High doses should not be given to patients taking antiplatelet or anticoagulant drugs.

USE IN PREGNANCY AND LACTATION

No adverse effects expected at the recommended dosage.

EFFECTS ON ABILITY TO DRIVE AND USE MACHINES

None known.

SIDE EFFECTS

Turmeric at 10% of diet caused some hair loss in rats and may have this effect in humans.[133] A case of allergic contact dermatitis to turmeric in a spice shop worker was reported.[3] The authors concluded that turmeric is probably a weak sensitizer and is not a common cause of allergic contact dermatitis.

OVERDOSE

Not known.

CURRENT REGULATORY STATUS IN SELECTED COUNTRIES

Turmeric is official in the *Pharmacopoeia of the People's Republic of China* (English Edition, 1997). It was official in the second edition of the *Indian Pharmacopoeia* (1966) but was not included in the third edition (1985).

Turmeric is covered by a positive Commission E monograph and can be used for the treatment of dyspeptic conditions.

Turmeric is not on the UK General Sale List.

Turmeric and turmeric oleoresin have GRAS status. It is also freely available as a 'dietary supplement' in the USA under DSHEA legislation (1994 Dietary Supplement Health and Education Act).

Turmeric is not included in Part 4 of Schedule 4 of the Therapeutic Goods Act Regulations of Australia.

References

1. Chopra RN, Chopra IC, Handa KL et al. Chopra's indigenous drugs of India, 2nd edn, 1958. Reprinted by Academic Publishers, Calcutta, 1982, pp 325–327.
2. Nadkarni KM, Nadkarni AK. Indian materia medica, vol 1. Popular Prakashan Private, Bombay, 1976, pp 414–418.
3. Goh CL, Ng SK. Contact Derm 1987; 17 (3): 186.
4. Chang HM, But PP. Pharmacology and applications of Chinese materia medica, vol 2. World Scientific Singapore, 1987, pp 936–939.
5. Bensky D, Gamble A. Chinese herbal medicine materia medica. Eastland Press Seattle, 1986, pp 390–391.
6. Grieve M. A modern herbal, vol 2. Dover Publications, New York, 1971, pp 822–823.
7. Kapoor LD. Handbook of Ayurvedic medicinal plants. Boca Raton, CRC Press, 1990, pp 149–150.
8. Bisset NG (ed). Herbal drugs and phytopharmaceuticals Medpharm Scientific Publishers Stuttgart: 1994, pp 173–175.
9. Govindarajan VS. Crit Rev Food Sci Nutr 1980; 12 (3): 199–301.
10. Wagner H, Bladt S. Plant drug analysis: a thin layer chromatography atlas, 2nd edn. Springer-Verlag, Berlin 1996; p 159.
11. Food and Agriculture Organisation of the United Nations. Specifications for identity and purity of certain food additives. Emulsifiers, enzyme preparations, flavouring agents, food colours, thickening agents, miscellaneous food additives. 35th session of JECFA, Rome 1989. FAO Food and Nutrition Papers 1990; 49: 75–78.

12. Srimal RC, Khanna NM, Dhawan BN. Indian J Pharmacol 1971; 3: 10.
13. Srimal RC, Dhawan BN. J Pharm Pharmacol 1973; 25 (6): 447–452.
14. Nadkarni KM, Nadkarni AK. Indian materia medica, vol 1. Popular Prakashan Private, Bombay, 1976; p 417.
15. Ghatak N, Basu N. Indian J Exp Biol 1972; 10 (3): 235–236.
16. Mukhopadhyay A, Basu N, Ghatak N et al. Agents Actions 1982; 12 (4): 508–515.
17. Srivastava R, Srimal RC. Indian J Med Res 1985; 81: 215–223.
18. Gupta B, Kulshrestha VK, Srivastava RK et al. Indian J Med Res 1980; 71: 806–814.
19. Sinha M, Mukherjee BP, Mukherjee B et al. Indian J Pharmacol 1974; 6: 87–90.
20. Bhatia A, Singh GB, Khanna NM. Indian J Exp Biol 1964; 2: 158–160.
21. Flynn DL, Rafferty MF. Prostagland Leukot Med 1986; 22 (3): 357–360.
22. Huang MT, Lysz T, Ferraro T, Abidi TF et al. Cancer Res 1991; 51: 1813–1819.
23. Ammon HP, Safayhi H, Mack T et al. J Ethnopharmacol 1993; 38 (2–3): 113–119.
24. Srivastava R. Agents Actions 1989; 28 (3–4): 298–303.
25. Arora RB, Basu N, Kapoor V et al. Indian J Med Res 1971; 59 (8): 1289–1295.
26. Yegnanarayan R, Saraf AP, Balwani JH. Indian J Med Res 1976; 64 (4): 601–608.
27. Mehra KS, Mikuni I, Gupta V et al. Tokai J Exp Clin Med 1984; 9 (1): 27–31.
28. Srivastava KC. Prostagland Leukot Essent Fatty Acids 1989; 37 (1): 57–64.
29. Chandra D, Gupta SS. Indian J Med Res 1972; 60: 138–142.
30. Gupta SS, Modh PR. Indian J Pharmacol 1969; 1: 22–25.
31. Srivastava R, Puru V, Srima RC et al. Arzneim Forsch 1986; 36: 715–717.
32. Srivastava R, Dikshit M, Srimal RC et al. Thromb Res 1985; 40: 413–417.
33. Srivastava KC, Bordia A, Verma SK. Prostagland Leukot Essent Fatty Acids 1995; 52 (4): 223–227.
34. Sharma OP. Biochem Pharmacol 1976; 25: 1811–1812.
35. Toda S, Miyase T, Arichi H et al. Chem Pharm Bull 1985; 33: 1725–1728.
36. Toda S, Ohnishi M, Kimura M et al. J Ethnopharmacol 1988; 23: 105–108.
37. Zhao BL, Li XJ, He RG et al. Cell Biophys 1989; 14: 175–185.
38. Shalini VK, Srinivas L. Mol Cell Biochem 1987; 77: 3–10.
39. Subramanian M, Sreejayan, Rao MN et al. Mutat Res 1994; 311 (2): 249–255.
40. Sreejayan, Rao MN. J Pharm Pharmacol 1997; 49 (1): 105–107.
41. Selvam R, Subramanian L, Gayathri R et al. J Ethnopharmacol 1995; 47 (2): 59–67.
42. Awasthi S, Srivatava SK, Piper JT et al. Am J Clin Nutr 1996; 64 (5): 761–766.
43. Reddy AC, Lokesh BR. Toxicology 1996; 107 (1): 39–45.
44. Reddy AC, Lokesh BR. Food Chem Toxicol 1994; 32 (3): 279–283.
45. Joe B, Lokesh BR. Biochim Biophys Acta 1994; 1224 (2): 255–263.
46. Miquel J, Martinez M, Diez A et al. Age 1995; 18 (4): 171–174.
47. Ramirez-Bosca A, Soler A, Gutierrez J et al. Age 1995; 18: 167–169.
48. Bhuvaneswaran C, Kapur OP, Sriramachari S et al. Food Sci 1963; 12: 182–185.
49. Srinivasan M, Aiyar AS, Kapur OP et al. Indian J Exp Biol 1964; 2: 104–106.
50. Rao SD, Sekhara CN, Satyanarayana MN et al. J Nutr 1970; 100: 1307–1316.
51. Dixit VP, Jain P, Joshi SC. Indian J Physiol Pharmacol 1988; 32: 299–304.
52. Keshavarz K. Poult Sci 1976; 55: 1077–1083.
53. Srinivasan K, Sambaiah K. Int J Vitam Nutr Res 1991; 61 (4): 364–369.
54. Babu PS, Srinivasan K. Mol Cell Biochem 1997; 166 (1–2): 169–175.
55. Grabe F. Arch Exp Pathol Pharmacol 1935; 176: 673–676.
56. Jentzsch K, Gonda T, Holler H. Pharm Acta Helv 1959; 34: 181–188.
57. Ramprasad C, Sirsi M. J Sci Industr Res 1956; 15C: 262–265.
58. Ramprasad C, Sirsi M. J Sci Industr Res 1957; 16C: 108–110.
59. Hussain MS, Chandrasekhara N. Indian J Med Res 1992; 96: 288–291.
60. Mukerji B, Zaidi SH, Singh GB. J Sci Industr Res 1961; 20C: 25–28.
61. Rafatullah S, Tariq M, Al-Yahya MA et al. J Ethnopharmacol 1990; 29: 25–34.
62. Kiso Y, Suzuki Y, Watanabe N et al. Planta Med 1983; 49: 185–187.
63. Lutomski J, Kedzia B, Debska W. Planta Med 1974; 26: 9–19.
64. Basu AP. Indian J Pharm 1971; 33: 131.
65. Banerjee A, Nigam SS. J Res Indian Med Yoga Homoeopathy 1978; 13: 63–70.
66. Tonnessen HH, De Vries H, Karlsen J et al. J Pharmaceut Sci 1987; 76: 371–373.
67. Dahl TA, McGowan WM, Shard MA et al. Arch Microbiol 1989; 151: 183–185.
68. Apisariyakul A, Vanittanakom N, Buddhasukh D. J Ethnopharmacol 1995; 49 (3): 163–169.
69. Nagabhushan M, Bhide SV. Nutr Cancer 1986; 8 (3): 201–210.
70. Nagabhushan M, Amonkar AJ, Bhide SV. Food Chem Toxicol 1987; 25: 545–547.
71. Shalini VK, Srinivas L. Mol Cell Biochem 1990; 95: 21–30.
72. Stich HF, Tsang SS, Palcic B. Mutat Res 1990; 241: 387–393.
73. Wargovich MJ, Eng VW, Newmark HL. Food Chem Toxicol 1985; 23: 47–49.
74. Nagabhushan M, Bhide SV. J Nutr Growth Cancer 1987; 4 (2): 83–90.
75. Deshpande SS, Maru GB. Cancer Lett 1995; 96 (1): 71–80.
76. Huang M, Smart RC, Wong C et al. Cancer Res 1988; 48: 5941–5946.
77. Soudamini KK, Kuttan R. J Ethnopharmacol 1989; 27: 227–233.
78. Aruna K, Sivaramakrishnan VM. Indian J Exp Biol 1990; 28: 1008–1011.
79. Susan M, Rao MN. Arzneim Forsch 1992; 42 (7): 962–964.
80. Nagabhushan M, Nair UJ, Amonkar AJ et al. Mutat Res 1988; 202 (1): 163–169.
81. Verma SP, Salamone E, Goldin B. Biochem Biophys Res Commun 1997; 233 (3): 692–696.
82. Nagabhushan M, Bhide SV. J Am Coll Nutr 1992; 11 (2): 192–198.
83. Conney AH, Lysz T, Ferraro T et al. Adv Enzyme Regul 1991; 31: 385–396.
84. Anto RJ, George J, Babu KV et al. Mutat Res 1996; 370 (2): 127–131.
85. Rao CV, Rivenson A, Simi B et al. Cancer Res 1995; 55 (2): 259–266.
86. Bhide SV, Azuine MA, Lahiri M et al. Breast Cancer Res Treat 1994; 30 (3): 233–242.
87. Azuine MA, Bhide SV. J Ethnopharmacol 1994; 44 (3): 211–217.
88. Huang MT, Lou YR, Ma W et al. Cancer Res 1994; 54 (22): 5841–5847.
89. Azuine MA, Bhide SV. Nutr Cancer 1992; 17 (1): 77–83.
90. Kuttan R, Bhanumathy P, Nirmala K et al. Cancer Lett 1985; 29: 197–202.
91. Soudamini KK, Kuttan R. 1988. Indian J Pharmacol 1988; 20: 95–101.
92. Goodpasture CE, Arrighi FE. Food Cosmet Toxicol 1976; 14: 9–14.
93. Donatus IA, Vermeulen S, Vermeulen NPE. Biochem Pharmacol 1990; 39: 1869–1875.
94. Ruby AJ, Kuttan G, Babu KD et al. Cancer Lett 1995; 94 (1): 79–83.
95. Singh AK, Sidhu GS, Deepa T et al. Cancer Lett 1996; 107 (1): 109–115.
96. Mazumder A, Raghavan K, Weinstein J et al. Biochem Pharmacol 1995; 49 (8): 1165–1170.
97. Sui Z, Salto R, Li J et al. Bioorg Med Chem 1993; 1 (6): 415–422.
98. Singh A, Singh SP, Bamezai R. Cancer Lett 1995; 96 (1): 87–93.
99. Chan MM. Biochem Pharmacol 1995; 49 (11): 1551–1556.

100. Kiuchi F, Goto Y, Sugimoto N et al. Chem Pharm Bull 1993; 41 (9): 1640–1643.
101. Huang HC, Jan TR, Yeh SF. Eur J Pharmacol 1992; 221 (2–3): 381–384.
102. Wahlström B, Blennow G. Acta Pharmacol Toxicol (Copenh) 1978; 43: 86–92.
103. Ravindranath V, Chandrasekhara N. Toxicology 1980; 16: 259–265.
104. Ravindranath V, Chandrasekhara N. Toxicology 1981; 20: 251–257.
105. Ravindranath V, Chandrasekhara N. Toxicology 1982; 22: 337–344.
106. Shoba G, Joy D, Joseph T et al. Planta Med 1998; 64: 353–356.
107. Deodhar SD, Sethi R, Srimal RC. Indian J Med Res 1980; 71: 632–634.
108. Satoskar RR, Shah SJ, Shenoy SG. Int J Clin Pharmacol 1986; 24: 651–654.
109. Kulkarni RR, Patki PS, Jog VP et al. J Ethnopharmacol 1991; 22 (1–2): 91–95.
110. Hastak K, Lubri N, Jakhi SD et al. Cancer Lett 1997; 116 (2): 265–269.
111. Polasa K, Raghuram TC, Krishna TP et al. Mutagenesis 1992; 7 (2): 107–109.
112. Kuttan R, Sudheeran PC, Joseph CD. Tumori 1987; 73: 29–31.
113. Thamlikitkul MD, Bunyapraphatsara N, Dechatiwongse T et al. J Med Assoc Thai 1989; 72 (11): 613–620.
114. Kositchaiwat C, Kositchaiwat S, Havanondha J. J Med Assoc Thai 1993; 76 (11): 601–605.
115. Van Dau N, Ngoc Ham N, Huy Khac D et al. Phytomed 1998; 5 (1): 29–34.
116. Copeland R, Baker D, Wilson H. Proceedings Int Conf AIDS 1994; 10 (2): 216.
117. Hellinger JA, Cohen CJ, Dugan ME et al. 3rd Conf Retro Opportun Infect 1996 Jan 28-Feb 1, p 78.
118. Gilden D, Smart T. GMHC Treat Issues 1996; 10 (2): 9.
119. Charles V, Charles SX. Trop Geogr Med 1992; 44 (1–2): 178–181.
120. Shankar TNB, Shantha NV, Ramesh HP et al. Indian J Exp Biol 1980; 18: 73–75.
121. Qureshi S, Shah AH, Ageel AM. Planta Med 1992; 58 (2): 124–127.
122. Billie N, Larsen JC, Hansen EV et al. Food Chem Toxicol 1985; 23: 967–973.
123. Deshpande SS, Lalitha VS, Ingle AD et al. Toxicol Lett 1998; 95 (3): 183–193.
124. Kandarkar SV, Sawant SS, Ingle AD et al. Indian J Exp Biol 1998; 36 (7): 675–679.
125. Abraham S, Abraham SK, Radhamony G. Cytologia 1976; 41: 591–595.
126. Jensen NJ. Mutat Res 1982; 105: 393–396.
127. Vijayalaxmi. Mutat Res 1980; 79: 125–132.
128. Abraham SK, Kesavan PC. Mutat Res 1984; 136: 85–88.
129. Shah RG, Netrawali MS. Bull Environ Contam Toxicol 1988; 40 (3): 350–357.
130. Giri AK, Das SK, Talukder G et al. Cytobios 1990; 62: 111–117.
131. Garg SK. Planta Med 1974; 26: 225–227.
132. German Federal Minister of Justice. German Commission E for human medicine monograph, Bundes-Anzeiger (German Federal Gazette), no. 223, dated 30.11.1985: no 164, dated 01.09.1990.
133. Patil TN, Srinivasan M. Indian J Exp Biol 1971; 9 (2): 167–169.

Valerian
(*Valeriana officinalis* L.)

SYNONYMS

European valerian, all heal (Engl), Valerianae radix (Lat), Baldrianwurzel, Katzenwurzel, Balderbrackenwurzel (Ger), racine de valériane (Fr), valeriana, amantilla (Ital), baldrion (Dan).

WHAT IS IT?

In many herbal traditions species of Valeriana have enjoyed a long history of use as mild sedatives. Scientific studies have verified the sedative effect but the exact biochemical mechanism and active components are not fully understood. Although the root and rhizome of *Valeriana officinalis* L. is favoured by the European tradition as a safe and gentle sedative, recent research has demonstrated that other species of Valeriana are also active; in particular, Mexican valerian (*Valeriana edulis* Nutt. ex Torr & Gray, or *V. mexicana* DC) is rich in active constituents. Indian valerian (*V. wallichii* DC or *V. jatamansi* Jones) is also used in herbal medicine. Japanese valerian (*V. fauriei* Briq.) is substantially different from all of these species and will not be considered here. Surprisingly, valerian and its oil have also been utilized in perfumery (valerian root has a strong and characteristic odour).

EFFECTS

Improves sleep latency and sleep quality, lowers periods of wakefulness, increases slow-wave sleep (consolidates non-REM sleep); reduces anxiety; relaxes smooth muscle.

TRADITIONAL VIEW

Valerian has been used in traditional medicine since Dioscorides and Galen. It was used after this time for certain kinds of epilepsy. Valerian was considered to have a remarkable influence on the cerebrospinal system, in particular as a sedative in conditions of nervous unrest, stress and neuralgia. It was used to promote sleep, particularly by the civilian population in Britain during World War II. In Europe, oil of valerian was a popular remedy for cholera.[1,2] The eclectics referred to it as a cerebral stimulant used in chorea, hysteria (with mental depression, despondency) and low forms of fever where a nervous stimulant is required. (The activity here is suggested as aiding cerebral circulation.) It was used to relieve irritability and pain and favour rest and sleep and was considered useful in nervous headache.[3] Both *V. officinalis* and *V. wallichii* have been used in Ayurvedic traditional medicine for hysteria, neurosis and epilepsy. Reference has also been made to extensive use to treat shell shock after World War I. Indian valerian was also regarded as a carminative and antispasmodic.[4]

SUMMARY ACTIONS

Anxiolytic, mild sedative, hypnotic, spasmolytic.

CAN BE USED FOR

INDICATIONS SUPPORTED BY CLINICAL TRIALS

Insomnia, restlessness, nervous tension; may be useful for the treatment of depression or anxiety, especially in combination with other herbs, specifically *Hypericum perforatum*.

TRADITIONAL THERAPEUTIC USES

To promote sleep and as an anxiolytic for nervous unrest, stress, neuralgia, shell shock; epilepsy; to relieve digestive and other spasms of smooth muscle.

MAY ALSO BE USED FOR

EXTRAPOLATIONS FROM PHARMACOLOGICAL STUDIES

Alleviation of the symptoms of benzodiazepine withdrawal.

PREPARATIONS

Root/rhizome as a decoction; liquid extract and tablets for internal use.

DOSAGE

- 3–9 g dried root/rhizome per day.
- 2–6 ml of 1:2 liquid extract per day, 5–15 ml of 1:5 tincture per day.

The Commission E recommends that valerian root may be used for external application, for example as a bath additive, probably as a sedative and to promote sleep.

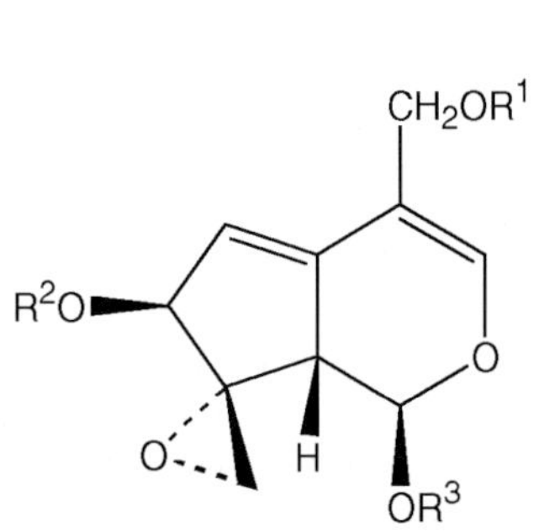

	R^1	R^2	R^3
Valtrate	acetyl	isovaleryl	isovaleryl
Isovaltrate	isovaleryl	acetyl	isovaleryl

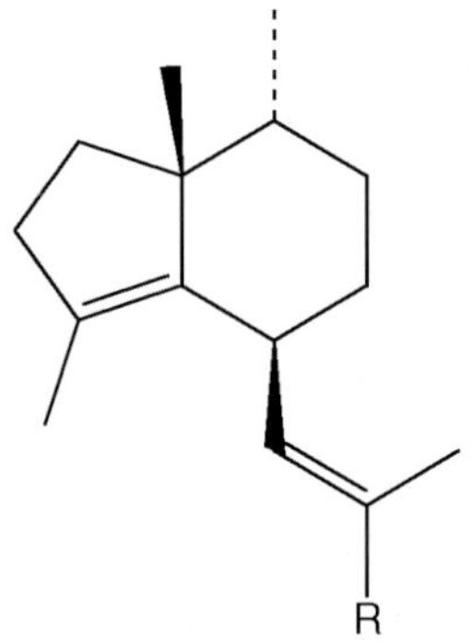

	R
Valerenal	CHO
Valerenic acid	COOH

isovaleryl = $(CH_3)_2CH\text{-}CH_2\text{-}CO\text{-}$

DURATION OF USE

May be used in the long term.

SUMMARY ASSESSMENT OF SAFETY

No adverse effects from ingestion of valerian are expected when consumed within the recommended dosage.

TECHNICAL DATA

BOTANY

Valeriana officinalis, a member of the Valerianaceae family, is a herbaceous plant growing to about 1 m. *Valeriana officinalis* is a collective term and includes subspecies and varieties. Polypoidy occurs in the species, ranging from diploid to octoploid types. The leaves are opposite, pinnate and mostly sessile, although the basal ones are petiolate and the leaflets are sometimes irregularly toothed. The flowers are hermaphrodite, arranged in a terminal cymose inflorescence with a many-toothed calyx and a pink, five-lobed corolla. The fruit is one-seeded with a leathery persistent calyx. It has a short, unbranched rhizome, rarely with stolons and rootlets with hollow centres.[5,6,7]

KEY CONSTITUENTS

The *European Pharmacopoeia* defines valerian root as from *Valeriana officinalis* and containing not less than 5 ml/kg of essential oil.[8]

Valeriana officinalis (European valerian):

- Iridoids (0.5–2%), known as valepotriates (valeriana-epoxy-triesters): including valtrate, isovaltrate, didrovaltrate, acevaltrate.[9]
- Essential oil (0.35–1%), containing monoterpenes (mainly borneol, bornyl acetate), sesquiterpenes (beta-bisabolene, valerenal (fresh root) and carboxylic compounds (esters of valerianic/isovaleric acid).[9]
- Non-volatile cyclopentane sesquiterpenes known as valerenic acid and its derivatives;[9] amino acids,[10] lignans.[11]

Valeriana edulis (Mexican valerian) contains 3–8% iridoids (and a larger valtrate/isovaltrate content); *Valeriana wallichii* (Indian valerian) contains 3–6% iridoids.[9] Valerenic acid and acetoxyvalerenic acid are unique to *V. officinalis*.[12] Studies in The Netherlands indicate there is seasonal variation in the content of these compounds in valerian roots.[13]

Valepotriates are unstable compounds; they are thermolabile and decompose under acid or alkaline conditions or in alcoholic solutions.[14] The baldrinals which form in dried valerian root or its extracts can further decompose into inactive products. The characteristic odour of dried valerian is due to isovaleric acid released on decomposition of the valepotriates.[15]

PHARMACODYNAMICS

Some valepotriates have shown pronounced cytotoxicity in vitro[16] and this caused concern over the safety of valerian. However, subsequent research indicated that the valepotriates were not cytotoxic when given orally; the unstable valepotriates do not survive the acidity of the stomach and form safe decomposition products.[17]

Sedative activity

Valeriana officinalis contains several groups of compounds which are responsible for its sedative activity. While much early research concentrated on the effects of the essential oil,[18,19] it is generally believed that this makes only a minor contribution to its activity (about one-third).[20] Research on valerian in the 1950s demonstrated that the essential oil was not primarily responsible for the sedative activity.[21] This led to the search for other compounds and the valepotriates were discovered about 10 years later.[22] Attention then focused on the valepotriates[15] and later their decomposition products.[23] Recently, attention has focused on valerenic acid and its derivatives as important sedative components unique to European valerian.[24] These compounds may explain the activity of aqueous extract of valerian noted in clinical trials.

When the valepotriates were studied and compared to chlorpromazine (an antipsychotic drug), it was shown that their sedative effect was weaker but, unlike chlorpromazine, they actually improved coordination.[25] Tests of the valepotriates on cats showed no decrease in reactivity but decreases in anxiety and aggression.[25] Whereas diazepam (Valium) increases the toxicity of alcohol, no such effect occurred with the valepotriates.[26]

Intraperitoneal administration of valerenic acid (50–100 mg/kg) demonstrated aspecific central depressant properties in tests conducted on mice and compared to diazepam, chlorpromazine and pentobarbital. A decrease in motility and prolongation of pentobarbital-induced sleeping time were observed. Other isolated sesquiterpenoid compounds such as valerenolic acid and valeranone did not cause impairment of performance. The activity resembled central nervous depression rather than muscle relaxation or a neuroleptic effect.[27]

A study found that valerian in doses of 12.0 mg/kg reversed the anxiogenic effect of acute diazepam withdrawal in dependent rats, whereas doses of 6.0 mg/kg failed to reverse these withdrawal symptoms.[28] Later studies on valerian revealed pronounced sedative properties in mice, by reducing motility and increasing sleeping time. Direct comparison with diazepam and chlorpromazine revealed a moderate sedative activity for valerian.[29]

The sedative effects of valepotriates on humans were confirmed a number of times in German research conducted in the late 1960s.[30,31]

Interaction with neurological receptors

Much scientific research on agents with sedative activity examines potential interaction with receptors mediating sedation. Most of this information in relation to valerian or its components is presented below, although conflicting results are apparent.

Aqueous and hydroalcoholic extracts of valerian displaced bound muscimol from synaptic membranes. The effect is probably only due to their amino acid content, especially gamma-aminobutyric acid (GABA). This therefore does not explain the sedative effect of valerian.[32] An aqueous extract of valerian induced the release of radiolabelled GABA in rat brain synaptosomes. The release was Na^+ dependent, Ca^{2+} independent and sensitive to certain transport inhibitors, suggesting the reversal of the GABA carrier. The increase in GABA release appears to be independent of Na^+-K^+-ATPase activity and membrane potential.[10,33,34] Further in vitro work has shown that the amount of GABA present in aqueous extracts of valerian is sufficient to account for this release from synaptosomes, since valerian extract increased the release of radiolabelled GABA by the same mechanism as exogenous GABA.[10] A comparison of three different valerian extracts on the release of GABA in rat brain synaptosomes found the aqueous and aqueous-alcoholic extracts stimulated the release but the ethanolic extract did not. GABA was absent from the ethanolic extract and present in the other extracts.[35]

An in vitro study of the interaction of valerian extracts and isolated constituents with receptors in rat brain has indicated that the interaction of unknown constituents present in the aqueous extract with GABA-A receptors could represent the basis for the sedative effect of valerian. Aqueous extract, hydroalcoholic extract and the aqueous fraction derived from hydroalcoholic extract showed affinity for the GABA-A receptor, which was not correlated with sesquiterpene or valepotriate content. The lipophilic fraction of the hydroalcoholic extract and dihydrovaltrate showed affinity for the barbiturate receptor and to a lesser extent for the peripheral benzodiazepine receptor. For the hydroalcoholic extract, valepotriates may contribute to the sedative effect due to the interaction with the allosteric sites of GABA receptors controlling chloride anion influx.[36]

Earlier work found that aqueous and hydroalcoholic extracts of valerian did not interact with benzodiazepine receptors. However, a hydroalcoholic extract (but not the aqueous extract) demonstrated a dose-dependent inhibition of the binding to adenosine receptors, indicating a sedative effect.[37] Lignans isolated from valerian roots were shown to act on µ-opiate and 5-HT_{1A} receptors. One of these, (+)-1-hydroxypinoresinol, had a particular affinity for the 5-HT_{1A} receptor.[11]

The ability of various extracts of valerian or valerenic acid to displace radiolabelled melatonin from its receptor sites in the human cerebellum has been assessed. Valerenic acid and aqueous preparations of valerian failed to displace melatonin; however, the ethanolic extract was able to displace melatonin completely in a dose-dependent manner. Valerian in this study showed no significant affinity for the GABA-A receptor.[38] The significance of this finding will only become clear with further studies. The active component has not yet been identified and it is not known whether it acts as an agonist or antagonist for the melatonin receptor. Valerenic acid has some structural similarities with melatonin but it was found to be inactive. Perhaps the valerenic acid derivatives are the active compounds in this model.

Other activity

Intraperitoneal administration of valerian root extract or valerenic acid demonstrated anticonvulsant activity against picrotoxin (but not pentetrazol and harman).[39] The effect of valerian on activation, performance and mood of healthy volunteers under social stress conditions was investigated in a double-blind, placebo-controlled procedure. Undefined valerian extract (100 mg) influenced subjective feelings of somatic arousal, despite high physiological activation during a call-up procedure in which subjects were asked to solve mental arithmetic problems. No sedative effects were demonstrated, which suggested that valerian has thymoleptic activity.[40]

PHARMACOKINETICS

There is very little information on the pharmacokinetics of valerian or its constituents. The main decomposition products of valtrate and isovaltrate include the metabolites baldrinal and homobaldrinal, whereas the decomposition products of dihydrovaltrate do not include baldrinal-like metabolites.[41] Human digestion has the same decomposing effect. This is not an inherent problem since the initial decomposition products of valepotriates are active as sedatives and are probably the active products in the human system.[23] Oral, intravenous and intraduodenal administration of radiolabelled didrovaltrate in mice demonstrated that it is absorbed to a small extent in the unchanged form.[42]

CLINICAL TRIALS

Sleep quality

In a large, uncontrolled, multicentre trial involving over 11 000 patients, treatment with aqueous valerian extract (45 mg per day (5–6:1)) was rated as successful in treating difficulty in falling asleep (72%), discontinuous sleep (76%) and restlessness and tension (72%).[43]

In an early double-blind, placebo-controlled trial, improvement in symptoms was observed for sleep-disturbed elderly patients treated with aqueous dried valerian extract (300 mg per day (5–6:1)) taken for 30 days.[44] Improvements in sleep latency time and sleep quality were observed in 80 elderly patients treated with 270 mg per day of the same extract for 14 days.[45] In a double-blind, placebo-controlled, crossover trial, valerian demonstrated a significant subjective effect on poor sleep ($p<0.001$) in 27 subjects compared to placebo over two consecutive nights. Forty-four percent reported perfect sleep and 89% reported improved sleep. The test preparation contained standardized valerian extract (equivalent to 400 mg of root) and other herbal extracts (hops and lemon balm) which were also present in the placebo tablet, effectively measuring the action of the valerian only.[46]

Swiss researchers studied the effects of an aqueous extract of valerian on sleep in 128 volunteers who tested three sets of tablets taken over three non-consecutive nights: freeze-dried aqueous valerian extract (400 mg, approximately 3:1), a proprietary OTC preparation containing an equivalent amount of valerian extract and a hops extract (200 mg, extract ratio unknown), and placebo. The valerian extract did not contain valepotriates or essential oil but presumably contained valepotriate decomposition products and valerenic acid. Based on a subjective assessment by patients, they found that valerian improved sleep latency ($p<0.05$) and sleep quality without increasing sleepiness the next morning, compared to placebo. Further analysis of results indicated that the group of subjects who rated themselves as good sleepers were largely unaffected by valerian but the poor or irregular sleepers reported a significant improvement ($p<0.05$). Interestingly, valerian did not increase the frequency of 'more sleepy than usual (the next morning)' responses.[47,48,49]

Schulz and co-workers conducted a pilot study of crossover design, with objective and subjective assessment of sleep variables in 14 elderly poor sleepers. Polysomnography was conducted on three nights at 1-week intervals to obtain baseline, a reading 1 hour after tablet consumption and a reading after 1 week of treatment. Eight subjects received valerian (135 mg dried aqueous ethanol extract (5–6:1), three times per day) and six subjects received placebo. Results indicated that valerian had selective effects on non-REM sleep (particularly an increase in slow-wave sleep (SWS)), while REM sleep was unaltered. Despite various shortcomings in the trial design, the authors were confident of the consolidation of non-REM sleep under the acute and repeated administration of the valerian preparation. Valerian seems to induce an increase of SWS in those who have low baseline values and reduced stage 1 sleep. The increase in SWS indicates a different mode of action between valerian and benzodiazepine-type hypnotics.[50]

In a later trial, the efficacy and tolerance of a valerian tablet was evaluated against placebo in the treatment of insomnia. This randomized, double-blind study was conducted on 121 patients with diagnosed insomnia not due to organic causes. Patients were studied over 4 weeks and the daily dosage of aqueous ethanol valerian extract was 600 mg (equivalent to about 2400 mg of dried root and rhizome) taken in the evening. Practitioners rated sleep improvement higher following valerian therapy than after placebo. Patients also preferred valerian and at the 28-day mark there was a significant improvement in the feeling of being rested after sleep for the valerian treatment. Sleep quality also improved significantly in the valerian group. In both the valerian and the placebo group, the rate of side effects was 3.3% and the drop-out rate was also 3.3% for both groups.[51,52] Note that the dosage used was reasonably high and that the paradoxical stimulation which valerian can induce in some patients was not observed at this high dose.

Many trials have measured objective parameters (especially electroencephalograph traces (EEG)) in volunteers or poor sleepers provided with single doses of valerian, often compared to placebo or orthodox drugs. These trials are outlined below. Whilst objective measurements such as these provide valuable information, it should be considered that subjective experience may be a more realistic assessment of sleep quality.[48,49]

A double-blind, placebo-controlled study on eight poor sleepers combined an objective measurement of sleep latency with subjective assessment. Dried aqueous valerian extract corresponding to 1.3 g of root taken 1 hour before retiring reduced the average time taken to fall asleep from 15.8 to 9.0 minutes. Subjects also reported significant improvements in sleep quality and depth without increased sleepiness the next morning. The authors commented that results for valerian compared favourably with those from studies of conventional sleeping pills. Higher doses of valerian 1 hour before retiring were not as beneficial as the 1.3 g dose.[53]

No significant decrease in objective measures of time to fall asleep was observed in 10 volunteers who slept for four nights in a sleep laboratory, although the pattern of results suggested a more rapid onset of stable sleep. On two of the nights volunteers received placebo, on the other two nights dried aqueous valerian extract was given (400 mg, approximately 3:1).[48,49] These subjects were, however, predominantly good sleepers and it is probable that normal sleep latencies were too short for valerian to produce a detectable improvement.

Dosages of 60 mg and 120 mg of a valerian preparation showed a decrease of sleep stage 4 and a slight reduction of REM sleep in healthy volunteers. In contrast, there was an increase in sleep stages 1, 2 and 3. Changes of the beta-intensity of the EEG during REM sleep showed a stronger hypnotic effect for the higher dosage.[54]

The sedative and tranquillizing potential of a number of herbal extracts, including 1200 mg of a dried ethanolic extract of valerian (3–7:1), were tested using EEG in two randomized, double-blind, placebo-controlled trials each comprising 12 sleep-disturbed subjects. Diazepam (10 mg) was utilized as a test substance for comparison. In contrast to diazepam, most of the herbal extracts demonstrated an increase in the relative capacity of the theta wavelengths and did not increase beta-wave frequency. Valerian displayed an increase in delta and theta frequencies and a decrease in beta frequency. In contrast to placebo, most of the herbal extracts (as with diazepam) induced an increase in subjectively evaluated sleepiness.[55] The developmental duration of the effects of dried aqueous ethanolic extract of valerian (3–7:1) following individual (1200 mg) and repeated (600 mg) 14-day administration was evaluated using EEG in a double-blind, placebo-controlled crossover trial on 16 healthy subjects. The absence of an output increase in alpha-1 and beta-2 activity after individual administration compared to placebo, the increase in the output of theta activity and the output alterations in the alpha band after repeated administration supported a sedative effect for valerian. The effect began 1 hour after administration and persisted over the 3 hours during which it was measured. Valerian tended to normalize the sleep profile, lowered periods of wakefulness and increased the efficiency of the sleep period.[56]

The effect of aqueous valerian extract on sleep was investigated in two groups of healthy, young subjects, some of whom slept at home (subjective assessment) and the others in a sleep laboratory (objective assessment). In the home study, both doses of valerian extract (450 mg, 900 mg) reduced perceived sleep latency and wake time after sleep onset. A dose-dependent effect was suggested by the results. In the sleep laboratory where the higher dose was used, no significant differences from placebo were obtained. However, the direction of the changes corresponded to those observed under home conditions.[57] It has been suggested that the lack of significant changes in the objective sleep parameters may have been due to the selection of subjects: young subjects with normal sleep quality, rather than those with disturbed sleep.[50]

Residual sedative effects were examined in a controlled study of 20 healthy volunteers, assigned to four groups receiving the following medication in single dose: tablets of valerian and hops, valerian syrup, flunitrazepam or placebo. Objectively measurable impairment of performance on the morning after medication occurred only in the flunitrazepam group. Fifty percent of volunteers in the flunitrazepam group reported mild side effects compared with 10% from the other groups. Subjective perception of sleep quality was improved in all three medication groups compared to placebo. A very slight impairment of vigilance after taking valerian syrup was statistically significant, as was a retardation in the processing of complex information for the valerian tablets. It was suggested that herbal remedies offer a viable alternative to benzodiazepines with regard to impairment of vigilance on the morning after ingestion.[58]

Valerian has also been combined with other herbal extracts including *Melissa officinalis* (lemon balm), passionflower and hops for the treatment of sleep disorders. The combination of valerian extract (240 mg) and hops extract (400 mg) reduced the noise-induced disturbance of sleep stage patterns (slow-wave sleep and REM) in sleep-disturbed subjects compared to baseline values. The authors recommend that the initial treatment of severe insomnia with strong sleeping pills should be followed by a period of herbal sleeping pill use before discontinuation of therapy.[59]

The effect of a herbal preparation (dried aqueous ethanol extracts of valerian (160 mg, no valepotriates detected; 4.5:1) and lemon balm (80 mg, 5.5:1)) on objective parameters was compared to an orthodox sedative (triazolam) and placebo in 20 volunteers consisting of good and poor sleepers. The herbal preparation induced a significant increase in sleep efficiency in stages 3 and 4 ($p<0.05$). It was apparent that poor sleepers benefited more from treatment as indicated by the significant increase in delta sleep. There was no shortening of sleep latency or wake time, which was observed in the Schulz pilot study. Rebound effects were not observed for either the herbal preparation or triazolam.[60]

A randomized, double-blind, placebo-controlled, multicentre trial investigated the use of the same herbal preparation in 68 ambulatory patients with light insomnia. Those in the test group received two tablets, each containing dried aqueous ethanol extracts of valerian (160 mg, 4.5:1) and lemon balm (80 mg. 5.5:1) twice per day for a period of 3 weeks. Improvement in the primary test criteria (sleep quality, daily condition, initiative, change in condition) occurred after 2 weeks in the treatment group. The valerian and lemon balm combination also improved accompanying indicators such as time to fall asleep, total duration of sleep, concentration and performance ability. There were no hangover, withdrawal or rebound phenomena in the treated group.[61]

Other conditions

A number of clinical trials have investigated the use of combined valerian and *Hypericum perforatum* (St John's wort) preparation for the treatment of depression or anxiety. Some of these trials are outlined below. A combination of valerian root and St John's wort was shown to have equivalent benefits to the drug amitriptyline (Tryptanol) in a randomized, controlled, double-blind study. One hundred and forty-seven outpatients aged between 20 and 65 were given a daily dose of 450–900 mg of valerian and St John's wort concentrates (equivalent to 0.45–0.9 mg total hypericin) or 75–150 mg of amitriptyline over 6 weeks. Benefit was observed for 82% of patients in the herbal group compared to 77% in the amitriptyline group. The total Hamilton Depression Score was reduced from 24.2 to 8.4 after 6 weeks with herbal treatment and from 24.3 to 8.9 after the drug. Statistical analysis showed that the herbal treatment was equivalent in benefit to amitriptyline but without the high frequency of side effects caused by this drug such as dry mouth and lethargy.[62] In an earlier double-blind trial, this herbal combination demonstrated significant improvement compared to the antidepressant desipramine as assessed by physicians after 6 weeks of treatment ($p=0.0004$).[63]

The same combination (0.3–0.6 mg/day total hypericin equivalent) was also shown to be significantly more effective than diazepam (Valium) after 2 weeks of treatment in 100 patients suffering from moderate anxiety in an earlier, double-blind study. Fewer side effects were observed in the herbal treatment group (4%), compared to diazepam treatment (14%).[64] A comparable reduction in symptoms of fear and depressive mood was observed for a valerian-St John's wort combination in comparison to amitriptyline. This double-blind, multicentre trial treated 162 patients diagnosed with fear and depression.[65] In a drug monitoring study which included 5682 patients, only 1.1% of patients reported side effects with the valerian-St John's wort combination. The incidence of side effects was even less than the probability of spontaneous adverse events observed with placebo in clinical trials.[66]

The proven benefits of herbal products as alternatives are particularly relevant given the results of a study which found that, in almost half the patients seeking advice for anxiety, panic and phobias, the cause was benzodiazepines or alcohol. One researcher concluded that when symptoms persist following a distressing event, it is often the case that benzodiazepines or alcohol are sustaining them.[67]

A double-blind, placebo-controlled, three-way crossover trial investigated a valerian and St John's wort extract combination and St John's wort extract for their effects on safety-related performance in 12 volunteers tested over 10 days. The two herbal products were shown to be harmless and comparable to placebo with respect to safety regarding performance and well-being. The effects after simultaneous intake of alcohol were not greater than those of alcohol on its own.[68]

TOXICOLOGY

No acute toxicity was found for valtrate, didrovaltrate and acevaltrate in mice after oral administration up to 4.6 g/kg.[25] A study of prolonged administration (30 days) of valepotriates observed that oral doses were innocuous to pregnant rats and their offspring. However, some toxic effects were observed when the valepotriates were administered by the intraperitoneal route.[69]

Valepotriates developed mutagenic activity only in the presence of S9 mix in the salmonella/microsome test and the SOS-chromotest. Baldrinal and homobaldrinal showed mutagenic effects in both tests with and without metabolic activation.[41] The cytotoxic potential of valerian constituents and valerian tinctures was investigated in two human in vitro cancer cell lines. Valepotriates of the diene type (valtrate, isovaltrate, acevaltrate) demonstrated the highest toxicity. In comparison, valepotriates of the monoene type were two- to threefold less toxic. The decomposition products baldrinal and homobaldrinal were 10–30 times less toxic. Valerenic acids also showed low toxicity. A clear relationship between valepotriate content and toxicity was established for fresh tinctures (*V. officinalis, V. edulis* ssp *procera, V. wallichii*; all 1:5). Significant reduction in cytotoxicity was observed for the same tinctures which had been stored at room temperature for 2 months. These stored tinctures had lower concentrations of valepotriates, which had decomposed.[70]

CONTRAINDICATIONS

None known.

SPECIAL WARNINGS AND PRECAUTIONS

None required.

INTERACTIONS

Although there are no reports to date, valerian may increase the effects of CNS depressants or alcohol when taken together, according to the *US Pharmacopeia*.[71] Despite this warning, early animal studies indicated that valepotriates do not add to the depressant effect of alcohol.[26] A human study confirmed that simultaneous intake of alcohol with valerian/St John's wort combination did not increase the effects of the herbal product[68] and a mixture of valepotriates (valtrate, acevaltrate and didrovaltrate (200–400 mg)) combined with ethanol did not cause a reduction of efficiency.[72]

USE IN PREGNANCY AND LACTATION

No adverse effects expected.

EFFECTS ON ABILITY TO DRIVE AND USE MACHINES

No adverse effect is expected. Evidence from clinical trials indicates that valerian does not cause excessive sedation.

SIDE EFFECTS

In some individuals, valerian can aggravate a sensation of tiredness or drowsiness, particularly in higher doses, but this is usually more a case of an increased awareness of the body's needs rather than a negative depressant effect. A few individuals find valerian stimulating and should avoid its use.

OVERDOSE

The following side effects have been reported when too much is taken: blurred vision, change in heartbeat, excitability, headache, nausea, restlessness, uneasiness.[71] Traditional texts also refer to large doses causing headache, stupor, mental excitement, visual illusions, giddiness, restlessness, agitation and even spasmodic movements.[1,3] In the first reported case of valerian overdose, the patient who had consumed 20 times the recommended therapeutic dose presented with mild symptoms, all of which resolved within 24 hours. The authors described the overdose as benign.[73]

CURRENT REGULATORY STATUS IN SELECTED COUNTRIES

European valerian is official in the *European Pharmacopoeia* (1997), the *British Pharmacopoeia* (1998) and the *United States Pharmacopeia-National Formulary* (USP23–NF18, 1995–June 1999).

Indian valerian was official in the second edition of the *Indian Pharmacopoeia* (1966) but was not included in the third edition (1985).

Valerian is covered by a positive Commission E monograph and has the following applications: restlessness, sleeping disorders based on nervous conditions.

Valerian is on the UK General Sale List.

Valerian does not have GRAS status. However, it is freely available as a 'dietary supplement' in the USA under DSHEA legislation (1994) Dietary Supplement Health and Education Act).

Valerian is not included in Part 4 of Schedule 4 of the Therapeutic Goods Act Regulations of Australia.

References

1. Grieve M. A modern herbal, vol 2. Dover Publications, New York, 1971, pp 824–829.
2. Culpeper's Complete herbal and English physician, 1826. Reprinted by Harvey Sales, 1981, pp 188–189.
3. Felter HW, Lloyd JU. King's American dispensatory, 18th edn, 3rd revision, vol 2, 1905. Reprinted by Eclectic Medical Publications, Portland, 1983, pp 2041–2043.
4. Chopra RN, Chopra IC, Handa KL et al. Chopra's indigenous drugs of India, 2nd edn, 1958. Reprinted by Academic Publishers, Calcutta, 1982, pp 253–255.
5. Chiej R. The Macdonald encyclopedia of medicinal plants. Macdonald, London, 1984, entry no. 323.
6. Launert EL. The Hamlyn guide to edible and medicinal plants of Britain and Northern Europe. Hamlyn, London, 1981, pp 180–181.
7. Evans WC. Trease and Evans' pharmacognosy, 14th edn. WB Saunders, London, 1996, p 323.
8. European pharmacopoeia, 3rd edn. European Department for the Quality of Medicines within the Council of Europe, Strasbourg, 1996, pp 1702–1703.
9. Wagner H, Bladt S. Plant drug analysis: a thin layer chromatography atlas, 2nd edn. Springer-Verlag, Berlin, 1996, pp 342–344.
10. Santos MS, Ferreira F, Faro C et al. Planta Med 1994; 60 (5): 475–476.
11. Bodesheim U, Holzl J. Pharmazie 1997; 52 (5): 386–391.
12. Hansel R, Schultz J. Dtsch Apoth Ztg 1982; 122: 215–219.
13. Bos R, Woerdenbag JH, Scheffer JJC. Planta Med 1993; 59 (7 suppl): A698.
14. De Smet PAGM, Keller K, Hansel R et al (eds). Adverse effects of herbal drugs, vol 3. Springer-Verlag, Berlin, 1997, p 166.
15. Houghton PJ. J Ethnopharmacol 1988; 22: 121–143.
16. Bounthanh C, Bergmann C, Beck JP et al. Planta Med 1981; 41: 21–28.
17. Braun R, Dittmar W, Hubner E et al. Planta Med 1984; 50: 1–4.
18. Hendriks H, Geertsma HJ, Malingre TM. Pharm Weekbl 1981; 116 (43): 1316.
19. Hendriks H, Bos R, Woerdenbag HJ et al. Planta Med 1985; 51: 28–31.
20. Wagner H, Bladt S. Plant drug analysis. Springer-Verlag, New York, 1984, p 264.
21. Gstirmer F, Kleinbauer E. Pharmazie 1958; 13: 415–420.
22. Thies PW, Funke S. Tetrahedron Lett 1966; 11: 1155–1162.
23. Wagner H, Jurcic K, Schaette R. Planta Med 1980; 39: 358–365.
24. Hansel R, Schultz J. Dtsch Apoth Ztg 1982; 122: 215–219.
25. Von Eickstedt KW, Rahman S. Arzneim Forsch 1969; 19: 316–319.
26. Von Eickstedt KW. Arzneim Forsch 1969; 19: 995–997.
27. Hendriks H, Bos R, Woerdenbag HJ et al. Planta Med 1985; 51: 28–31.
28. Andreatini R, Leite JR. Eur J Pharmacol 1994; 260 (2–3): 233–235.
29. Leuschner J, Muller J, Rudmann M. Arzneim Forsch 1993; 43 (6): 638–641.
30. Dziuba K. Med Welt 1968; 35: 1866–1868.
31. Jauch H. Med Klin 1969; 64 (10): 437–439.
32. Cavadas C, Araujo I, Cotrim MD et al. Arzneim Forsch 1995; 45 (7): 753–755.
33. Santos MS, Ferreira F, Cunha AP et al. Arch Int Pharmacodyn Ther 1994; 327 (2): 220–231.
34. Santos MS, Ferreira F, Cunha AP et al. Planta Med 1994; 60 (3): 278–279.
35. Ferreira F, Santos MS, Faro C et al. Rev Port Farm 1996; 46 (2): 74–77.
36. Mennini T, Bernasconi P, Bombardelli E et al. Fitoterapia 1993; 64 (4): 291–300.
37. Balduini W, Cattabeni F. Med Sci Res 1989; 17 (15): 639–640.
38. Fauteck JD. 2nd International Congress on Phytomedicine, Munich, September 11–14, 1996.
39. Hiller KO, Zetler G. Phytother Res 1996; 10 (2): 145–151.
40. Kohnen R, Oswald WD. Pharmacopsychiatry 1988; 21: 447–448.
41. Von Der Hude W, Scheutwinkel-Reich M, Braun R. Mutat Res 1986; 169 (1–2): 23–27.
42. Wagner H, Jurcic K. Planta Med 1980; 38: 366–376.
43. Schmidt-Voigt J. Therapiewoche 1986; 36: 663–667.
44. Jansen W. Therapiewoche 1977; 27 (14): 2779–2786.
45. Kamm-Kohl AV, Jansen W, Brockman P. Med Welt 1984; 35: 1450–1454.
46. Lindahl O, Lindwall L. Pharmacol Biochem Behav 1989; 32: 1065–1066.
47. Leathwood PD, Chauffard F, Heck E et al. Pharmacol Biochem Behav 1982; 17: 65–71.
48. Leathwood PD, Chauffard F. J Psychiatr Res 1982/1983; 17 (2): 115–122.
49. Leathwood PD, Chauffard F, Munoz-Bos R. Sleep 1982. 6th European Congress on Sleep Research, Zurich, 1982, pp 402–405.
50. Schulz H, Stolz C, Muller J. Pharmacopsychiatry 1994; 27 (4): 147–151.
51. Vorbach EU, Arnold KH. 6th Phytotherapy Conference, Berlin, October 5–7, 1995.
52. Vorbach EU, Gortelmeyer R, Bruning J. Psychopharmakotherapie 1996; 3: 109–115.
53. Leathwood PD, Chauffard F. Planta Med 1985; 51: 144–148.
54. Gessner B, Klasser M. EEG EMG Z Elektroenzephalogr Verw Geb 1984; 15 (1): 45–51.

55. Schulz H, Jobert M. 6th Phytotherapy Conference, Berlin, October 5–7, 1995.
56. Donath F, Roots I. 6th Phytotherapy Conference, Berlin, October 5–7, 1995.
57. Balderer G, Borbely AA. Psychopharmacol 1985; 87 (4): 406–409.
58. Gerhard U, Linnenbrink N, Georghiadou C et al. Schweiz Rundsch Med Prax 1996; 85 (15): 473–481.
59. Muller-Limmroth W, Ehrenstein W. Med Klin 1977; 72: 1119–1125.
60. Dressing H, Riemann D, Low H et al. Therapiewoche 1992; 42 (12): 726–736.
61. Dressing H, Kohler S, Muller WE. Psychopharmakother 1996; 3 (3): 123–130.
62. Hiller KO, Rahlfs V. Forschende Komplementärmedizin 1995; 2: 123–132.
63. Steger W. Z Allg Med 1985; 61: 914–918.
64. Panijel M. Therapiewoche 1985; 35 (41): 4659–4668.
65. Kniebel R, Burchard JM. Z Allg Med 1988; 64: 689–696.
66. Quandt J. Therapiewoche 1994; 44: 292–299.
67. Cohen SI. J Roy Soc Med 1995; 88: 73–77.
68. Herberg KW. Therapiewoche 1994; 44 (12): 704–713.
69. Tufik S, Fujita K, De Seabra ML et al. J Ethnopharmacol 1994; 41 (1–2): 39–44.
70. Bos R, Hendriks H, Scheffer JJC et al. Phytomed 1998; 5 (3): 219–225.
71. USP Drug Information, US Pharmacopeia Patient Leaflet, Valerian (Oral). The United States Pharmacopeial Convention, Rockville, 1998.
72. Mayer B, Springer E. Arzneim Forsch 1974; 24: 2066–2070
73. Willey LB, Mady SP, Cobaugh DJ et al. Vet Hum Toxicol 1995; 37 (4): 364–365.

Witchhazel
(*Hamamelis virginiana* L.)

SYNONYMS

Hamamelis (Engl), Hamamelidis folium, Hamamelidis cortex (Lat), virginische Zaubernuβ, Hamamelis, Hexenhasel (Ger), noisietier de la sorcière, hamamélis (Fr), amamelide (Ital), troldnød (Dan).

WHAT IS IT?

Witchhazel is an American shrub that was used by the Native Americans as a poultice for the treatment of painful swellings and tumours. Pond's Extract of Witchhazel was once a very popular general household remedy for burns, scalds, insect bites and inflammatory conditions of the skin. The name Hamamelis was adopted from a Greek word to indicate its resemblance to an apple tree. The parts normally used therapeutically are the leaves and bark, which have similar properties. The distilled twigs of witchhazel (hamamelis water) is still a popular topical remedy.

EFFECTS

Improves vascular tone; astringent and antiinflammatory to mucosa; protects against oxidative stress and ultraviolet radiation when used topically; haemostyptic.

TRADITIONAL VIEW

Witchhazel was used to treat vascular disorders including haemorrhoids, varicose veins, phlebitis, haemorrhages and other conditions associated with poor venous tone or congestion. Other uses included reproductive disorders, such as dysmenorrhoea, menorrhagia and metrorrhagia; acute and chronic diarrhoea in children and adults; renal complaints associated with poor venous tone including haematuria; irritation of the bladder; muscular soreness; aching and bruised sensation whether from cold, exposure, bruises, strains or physical exertion and as a gargle for chronic pharyngitis and inflammation of the gums.[1]

SUMMARY ACTIONS

Astringent, antiinflammatory, haemostyptic.

CAN BE USED FOR

INDICATIONS SUPPORTED BY CLINICAL TRIALS

Topical use for haemorrhoids; topically for mild abrasions and skin inflammation. In combination with Hydrastis for the treatment of varicose veins.

TRADITIONAL THERAPEUTIC USES

Haemorrhoids, varicose veins (topical use as well); diarrhoea, mucous colitis; topical use for bruises and localized inflamed swellings.

MAY ALSO BE USED FOR

EXTRAPOLATIONS FROM PHARMACOLOGICAL STUDIES

The dual inhibition of leukotriene and PAF production in vitro suggests potential therapeutic benefits in the treatment of disorders such as asthma, ulcerative colitis and Crohn's disease. However, these findings need to be confirmed in vivo.

OTHER APPLICATIONS

Use in antiageing or antiwrinkle skin preparations[2] and also as a skin toner.[3]

PREPARATIONS

Dried bark and leaves as a decoction, liquid extract, tablets and suppositories for internal use. Decoction, extract and distilled extract for topical use.

DOSAGE

- 2 g of the dried leaf or bark three times per day or as an infusion.
- 7–14 ml per day of 1:2 liquid extract of leaf.
- Hamamelis water BPC for local application.
- 0.1–1 g in suppositories applied 1–3 times daily.

DURATION OF USE

May be taken long term for external applications. Caution should be exercised with long-term oral intake due to the presence of tannins.

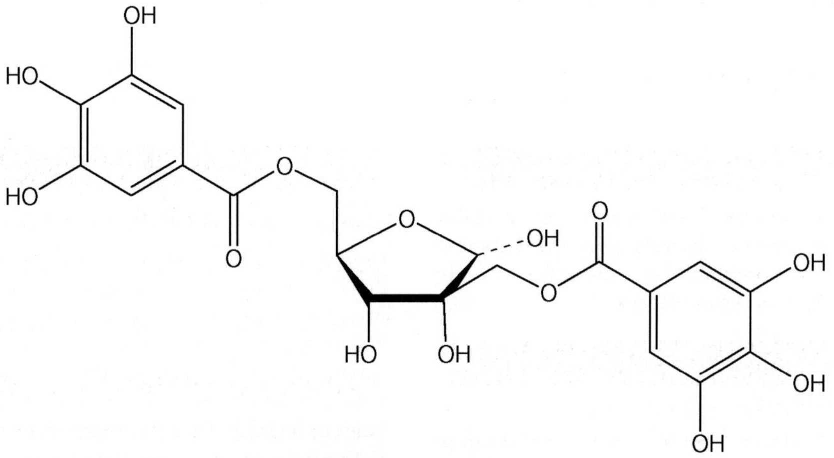

Hamamelitannin

SUMMARY ASSESSMENT OF SAFETY

No significant adverse effects from the ingestion of witchhazel are expected. It may cause irritation of the stomach in a small number of susceptible individuals and topical application can cause contact allergy in rare cases.

TECHNICAL DATA

BOTANY

Hamamelis virginiana L., a member of the Hamamelidaceae family, is a deciduous shrub that grows to approximately 2 m in height and is native to North America. The shrub consists of several crooked branching trunks 10–15 cm in diameter and up to 2 m in height, with a smooth grey bark. The alternate, ovoid, glabrous leaves have crenate margins, are 7–12 cm long and about 7 cm in width on short petioles. The yellow flowers consist of four sepals, four petals, four stamens and two styles and are grouped in two or three axillary glomerules with short peduncles. The fruit is a dehiscent, woody, bilocular capsule containing two dark-coloured glossy edible seeds which are ejected up to 4 m away when ripe. The medicinally useful parts of the plant are gathered in spring.[4,5]

KEY CONSTITUENTS

- A mixture of tannins (3–10%), including hamamelitannin, condensed catechins, gallotannins and procyanidins.[6]
- Essential oil, flavonoids.[6]

The bark contains significantly higher levels of phenylpropanoids and sesquiterpenoids in the volatile fractions compared to the leaves, which contain higher amounts of monoterpenoids.[7] The bark is richer in hydrolysable tannins and the leaves mainly contain condensed tannins.

PHARMACODYNAMICS

Antiinflammatory effects

Hamamelitannin and galloylated proanthocyanidins isolated from witchhazel bark were found to be potent inhibitors of 5-lipoxygenase in vitro. The procyanidins also inhibited lyso-PAF:acetyl-CoA acetyltransferase and thus inhibit the production of PAF. These results demonstrate a dual inhibitory activity in vitro against inflammatory mediators by the procyanidins present in witchhazel.[8]

Oral administration of aqueous ethanolic extract of witchhazel leaf (200 mg/kg) significantly inhibited the chronic phase of adjuvant arthritis-induced rat paw swelling. It was inactive against the acute phase and against carrageenan-induced rat paw oedema.[9] A witchhazel bark concentrate displayed radical scavenging properties, inhibited alpha-glucosidase and human leucocyte elastase in vitro and exhibited strong antiinflammatory effects in the croton oil ear oedema test in the mouse. The extract contained mainly oligomeric to polymeric procyanidins.[10]

The antiinflammatory effect of an aftersun lotion containing 10% witchhazel distillate, the vehicle and the prior aftersun lotion were tested in 20 healthy volunteers using a modified UVB erythema test as a model of inflammation. Test areas on the back were treated with the lotions for 48 hours following irradiation and compared with an untreated, irradiated control area. Erythema suppression ranged from 20% to 27% at 7 and 48 hours respectively for the witchhazel-treated areas. A suppression of 11–15% was recorded in the fields treated with the vehicle and prior aftersun lotion. Witchhazel led to a highly significant reduction in erythema when compared to the prior aftersun lotion (p=0.00039), the vehicle (p=0.00001) or untreated, irradiated skin (p=0.00001).[11]

Antioxidant activity

Hamamelitannin demonstrated in vitro antioxidant activity and protected murine skin fibroblasts from damage induced by UVB irradiation. It protected murine fibroblasts against external active oxygen radicals generated by UVB irradiation by associating with the cell surface through its sugar moiety.[12] Further tests indicated that hamamelitannin has higher protective activity against cell damage induced by superoxide anions than gallic acid (its functional moiety).[13]

In earlier work, hamamelitannin increased the survival rate of fibroblasts compared with controls. Hamamelitannin inhibited superoxide anion radicals at a much lower concentration than ascorbic acid. Further test results supported the superoxide scavenging activity of hamamelitannin.[14] Witchhazel extract demonstrated strong active oxygen-scavenging activity and protected against cell damage induced by active oxygen. The authors recommended witchhazel as a potential antiageing or antiwrinkle material for the skin.[2]

Vasoconstrictive activity

Vasoconstrictive activity has been demonstrated by intravenous administration of witchhazel leaf preparations in isolated rabbit arteries.[15,16] The activity was not blocked by alpha-or beta-sympatholytic agents.[16] Topical application of a witchhazel leaf extract produced a significant reduction in skin temperature in 30 volunteers. The lowered skin temperature was interpreted as a vasoconstrictive activity.[17]

Other activity

A witchhazel concentrate exhibited significant antiviral activity against herpes simplex virus type 1 in vitro.[10]

PHARMACOKINETICS

No data available.

CLINICAL TRIALS

Haemorrhoids and venous tone

In an uncontrolled study, 50 patients with painful skin lesions in the anogenital area were treated with a salve containing witchhazel bark distillate (5%), zinc oxide and vitamins A and D. After a week the healing process was completed in 40 patients.[18] In an uncontrolled trial on 75 patients with itching, painful and bleeding haemorrhoids, application of a salve containing witchhazel bark resulted in a majority of patients becoming free from symptoms after 3 weeks of treatment.[19] A comparison of this witchhazel bark salve with two other salves (one containing corticosteroids) was undertaken in a double-blind trial on 90 patients with grade 1 haemorrhoids. Several patients receiving the witchhazel salve had also received sclerotherapy. All three preparations demonstrated similar efficacy, except that the witchhazel was superior with regard to relief of symptoms: greater reduction in itching and soreness, less frequent bleeding.[20]

In a similar double-blind clinical trial, 90 patients with first-degree haemorrhoids were treated with witchhazel bark ointment and two ointments containing synthetic agents, one of which additionally contained a corticosteroid. Treatment was of 21 days' duration, with follow-up examinations on the third, 14th and 21st day of treatment. Four typical symptoms (pruritus, bleeding, burning sensation, sore sensation) were evaluated by both physician and patient. All three ointments proved highly effective. No major differences were found between the three treatment groups but in the case of some of the test parameters (itch), a positive tendency in favour of the witchhazel ointment was observed.[21]

The therapeutic effect of witchhazel on venous tone was studied in patients with varicose veins in an open trial. Four groups were each given different medications and studied by plethysmography for the next 5 hours. In the untreated controls, venous tone decreased during rest. A reference drug had no effect and the increase in venous tone induced by the ingestion of a high dose of hamamelis-hydrastis mixture was equivalent to that induced by 150 mg of oligomeric procyanidins.[22]

Dermatological conditions

Application of witchhazel leaf cream twice daily for 2 weeks in an uncontrolled study resulted in complete healing or considerable improvement in 37 patients with various forms of eczema or atopic neurodermatitis.[23]

Thirty-six patients with endogenous eczema and 80 patients with toxic degenerative eczema were treated in a double-blind, placebo-controlled trial with either witchhazel salve (25% water distillate from leaf and twigs) or a control preparation. The witchhazel salve was superior to placebo in the treatment of atopic dermatitis but of no benefit in the treatment of primary irritant contact dermatitis.[24] Twenty-two patients with atopic dermatitis were treated with a standardized witchhazel salve on one arm and a non-steroidal antiinflammatory cream (containing bufexamac) on the other over a 3-week period. Both treatments showed a clear improvement in the symptoms investigated: redness, scaling, lichenification, pruritus, infiltration. The salve contained 25 g of water distillate (from 4 g of fresh leaf and twigs) per 100 g of salve, which was also standardized for hamamelis ketone (0.75 mg).[25]

Hamamelis distillate cream (5.35 g hamamelis distillate containing 0.64 mg ketone/100 g) was compared to 0.5% hydrocortisone cream and an unmedicated cream base in a double-blind, randomized trial on 72 patients with moderately severe atopic eczema over a period of 14 days. All treatment regimes significantly reduced itching, erythema and scaling after 1 week. The hydrocortisone cream proved superior to the hamamelis distillate, which was no more effective than the unmedicated base.[26] In a previous study by the same authors, creams containing various concentrations of hamamelis distillate (containing 0.64–2.56 mg hamamelis ketone/100 g) were compared to a chamomile cream and a 1% hydrocortisone cream on human volunteers who had erythema induced by UV irradiation and cellophane tape stripping of the horny layer. A mild antiinflammatory effect was demonstrated for the hamamelis cream, especially if incorporated into a phospholipid base. Although less active than hydrocortisone cream, hamamelis cream was superior to the unmedicated cream base.[27] The antiinflammatory activity described here could, at least in part, be due to a vasoconstrictor activity.[28]

A mild antiinflammatory effect for standardized witchhazel salve (25 g distillate from 4 g fresh leaf and twigs, 0.75 mg of ketone, all per 100 g), compared to its neutral ointment base, was demonstrated by instrumental testing and transcutaneous oxygen measurement in 22 healthy subjects and five patients with dermatosis.[29]

Analgesic activity

A randomized open study of 300 mothers examined the effectiveness of hamamelis water, ice or Epifoam in achieving analgesia for episiotomy associated with forceps delivery. All three agents were equally effective at achieving analgesia on the first day. Approximately one-third of the mothers derived no benefit from any of the treatments.[30]

TOXICOLOGY

A methanol extract and a tincture of witchhazel bark showed dose-dependent inhibition of mutagenicity in the Ames assay. Tannin-free samples did not display any activity. Fractionation yielded two active fractions, both of which contained oligomeric procyanidins. The antimutagenic effect increased with an increasing degree of polymerization in the procyanidins.[31] In a study of 18 substances for mutagenic potential in vitro, witchhazel was not identified as a mutagen.[32]

CONTRAINDICATIONS

None known.

SPECIAL WARNINGS AND PRECAUTIONS

Care should be exercised with long-term oral use due to the presence of tannins.

INTERACTIONS

Tannins inhibit absorption of minerals and B vitamins.

USE IN PREGNANCY AND LACTATION

No adverse effects expected.

EFFECTS ON ABILITY TO DRIVE AND USE MACHINES

No adverse effects expected.

SIDE EFFECTS

Irritation of the stomach may occur in susceptible patients after oral doses.[6] Contact dermatitis caused by the topical use of witchhazel has been reported in rare cases.[33] In a study of 1032 consecutively tested patients, four were found to react to an ointment containing a 25% extract of witchhazel. Two of these patients had reacted positively to the wool fat in the ointment base.[34]

OVERDOSE

No effects known.

CURRENT REGULATORY STATUS IN SELECTED COUNTRIES

Witchhazel leaf is official in the *European Pharmacopoeia* (1997) and distillate made from witchhazel twig is official in the *United States Pharmacopeia-National Formulary* (USP23–NF18, 1995–June 1999).

Witchhazel leaf and bark are covered by positive Commission E monographs and both have the following applications: mild damage to the skin; local inflammation of the skin and mucous membranes, haemorrhoids and varicose veins.

Witchhazel is not on the UK General Sale List.

Witchhazel does not have GRAS status. However, it is freely available as a 'dietary supplement' in the USA under DSHEA legislation (1994 Dietary Supplement Health and Education Act). Witchhazel has been defined as an astringent active ingredient in OTC skin protectant drug products for relief of minor skin irritations due to insect bites, minor cuts, minor scrapes and in OTC anorectal drug products. These OTC products, in a form suitable for topical administration, are generally recognized as safe and effective if they meet the requirements outlined in the Code of Federal Regulations. The FDA, however, advises 'that based on evidence currently available, there is inadequate data to establish general recognition of the safety and effectiveness of these ingredients for the specified uses'.

Witchhazel is not included in Part 4 of Schedule 4 of the Therapeutic Goods Act Regulations of Australia.

References

1. Felter HW, Lloyd JU. King's American dispensatory, 18th edn, 3rd revision, vol 2, 1905. Reprinted by Eclectic Medical Publications, Portland, 1983, pp 974–976.
2. Masaki H, Sakaki S, Atsumi T et al. Biol Pharm Bull 1995; 18 (1): 162–166.
3. Smeh NJ. Creating your own cosmetics – naturally. Alliance Publishing Company, Garrisonville, 1995, p 142.
4. Grieve M. A modern herbal, vol 2. Dover Publications, New York, 1971, p 851.
5. Chiej R. The Macdonald encyclopedia of medicinal plants. Macdonald, London, 1984, entry no. 148.
6. Bisset NG (ed). Herbal drugs and phytopharmaceuticals Medpharm Scientific Publishers, Stuttgart, 1994, pp 245–247.
7. Engel R, Gutmann M, Hartisch C et al. Planta Med 1998; 64: 251–258.
8. Hartisch C, Kolodziej H, Von Bruchhausen F. Planta Med 1997; 63: 106–110.
9. Duwiejua M, Zeitlin IJ, Waterman PG et al. J Pharm Pharmacol 1994; 46 (4): 286–290.
10. Erdelmeier CA, Cinatl J Jr, Rabenau H et al. Planta Med 1996; 62 (3): 241–245.
11. Hughes-Formella BJ, Bohnsack K, Rippke F et al. Dermatology 1998; 196: 316–322.
12. Masaki H, Atsumi T, Sakurai H. J Dermatol Sci 1995; 10 (1): 25–34.
13. Masaki H, Atsumi T, Sakurai H. Biol Pharm Bull 1995; 18 (1): 59–63.
14. Masaki H, Atsumi T, Sakurai H. Free Radic Res Commun 1993; 19 (5): 333–340.
15. Bernard P, Balansard P, Balansard G et al. J Pharm Belg 1972; 27 (4): 505–512.
16. Balansard P, Faure F, Balansard G et al. Therapie 1972; 27 (5): 793–799.
17. Diemunsch AM, Mathis C. STP Pharma 1987; 3: 111–114.
18. Seeberger J. Z Allg Med 1979; 55 (29): 1667–1668.
19. Moosmann EB. Fortschr Med 1991; 109 (116): 5–6.
20. Moosmann EB. Fortschr Med 1991; 109 (116): 7–8.
21. Knoch HG, Klug W, Hübner WD. Fortschr Med 1992; 110 (8): 69–74.
22. Royer RJ, Schmidt CL. Sem Hop 1981; 57 (47–48): 2009–2013.
23. Wokalek H. Deut Dermatol 1995; 5: 498–506.
24. Pfister R. Fortschr Med 1981; 99 (31–32): 1264–1268.
25. Swoboda M, Meurer J. Z Phytother 1991; 12: 114–117.
26. Korting HC, Schafer-Korting M, Klovekorn W et al. Eur J Clin Pharmacol 1995; 48 (6): 461–465.
27. Korting HC, Schafer-Korting M, Hart H et al. Eur J Clin Pharmacol 1993; 44 (4): 315–318.
28. Hormann HP, Korting HC. Phytomed 1994; 1 (2): 161–171.
29. Sorkin B. Phys Med Rehabil 1980; 21 (1): 53–57.
30. Moore W, James DK. J Obst Gynecol 1989; 10 (1): 35–39.
31. Dauer A, Metzner P, Schimmer O. Planta Med 1998; 64: 324–327.
32. McGregor DB, Brown A, Cattanach P et al. Environ Mol Mutagen 1988; 11 (1): 91–118.
33. Granlund H. Contact Derm 1994; 31: 195.
34. Bruynzeel DP, Van Ketel WG, Young E et al. Contact Derm 1992; 27 (4): 278–279.

Withania
(*Withania somnifera* (L.) Dunal)

SYNONYMS

Winter cherry, Indian ginseng (Engl), ashwagandha (Sanskrit), blærebæger (Dan).

WHAT IS IT?

Withania somnifera is an important herb from the Ayurvedic medical system used for the treatment of debility, emaciation, impotence and premature ageing. Not surprisingly, it has been dubbed the 'Indian ginseng'. Its Indian name, ashwagandha, is said to refer to the 'smell and strength of a horse' and alludes to its reputed aphrodisiac properties. Modern research on Withania has stressed its antitumour and adaptogenic actions, reinforcing its comparison with *Panax ginseng*. However, Withania occupies an important place in the herbal materia medica because, while it is not as potent as panax, it lacks the stimulating effects of the latter. In fact, it has a mild sedative action as indicated by its specific name '*somnifera*'. It is therefore ideally suited to the treatment of overactive but debilitated patients, in whom panax would tend to aggravate the overstimulation. Many parts of the plant have been used in traditional medicine, including the leaves, bark and root. Except where specified in this monograph, 'Withania' refers to use of the root.

EFFECTS

Adaptogen (helping to conserve adaptation energy as defined in Selye's general adaptation syndrome); tonic (helping to boost levels of adaptation energy); modulates the immune system; glucocorticoid-like antiinflammatory and antiproliferative activity; potentially cytotoxic and radiosensitizing.

TRADITIONAL VIEW

In Ayurveda, the roots have aphrodisiac, tonic, depurative and anthelmintic properties, besides being useful in vata and kapha conditions and for inflammations, psoriasis, bronchitis, asthma, ulcers, scabies, wasting in children, insomnia and senile debility.[1] Withania is reported as a 'medharasayan' or promoter of learning and memory retrieval.[2] In Unani, the roots have tonic, aphrodisiac and emmenagogue properties and are used in asthma, inflammation, leucoderma, bronchitis, lumbago, arthritis and to promote conception.[1] In the Middle East, Withania root is used as a sedative and hypnotic and is also taken for rheumatic pains.[3]

SUMMARY ACTIONS

Tonic, adaptogen, mild sedative, antiinflammatory, immune modulator, antianaemic, antitumour (in high doses).

CAN BE USED FOR

INDICATIONS SUPPORTED BY CLINICAL TRIALS

Growth promotion in children and antianaemic activity; improvement in conditions associated with ageing; improvement in stamina of athletes (uncontrolled trial).

TRADITIONAL THERAPEUTIC USES

Asthma, bronchitis; psoriasis, arthritis, rheumatic pains; insomnia; senile dementia; promotion of conception.

In India, Withania is given with pungent or heating herbs such as ginger and long pepper to increase its tonic effects.

MAY ALSO BE USED FOR

EXTRAPOLATIONS FROM PHARMACOLOGICAL STUDIES

Debility and nervous exhaustion, especially due to stress; convalescence after acute illness or extreme stress, impotence due to devitalization; chronic diseases, especially those marked by inflammation (e.g. connective tissue diseases); as a general tonic for disease prevention; may be useful for depressed white blood cell count, especially if caused by cytotoxic drugs; possibly as prophylactic against cancer (the leaves, being richer in withaferin A, are a better prospect for cancer therapy).

PREPARATIONS

Dried root as a decoction, liquid extract or tablet for internal use.

DOSAGE

- 3–6 g per day of dried root by decoction.
- 6–12 ml of 1:2 liquid extract per day.

Withanolides

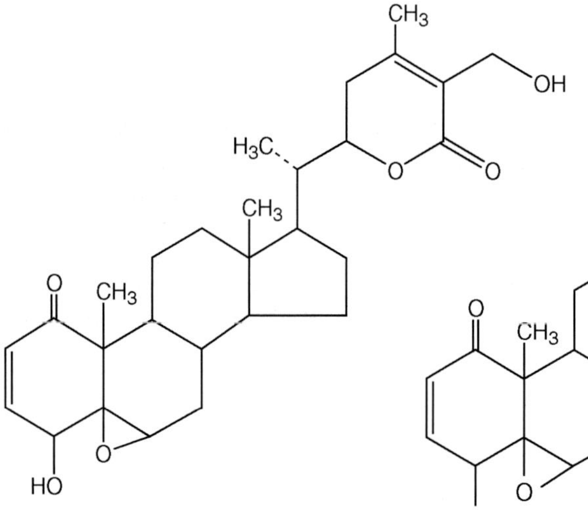

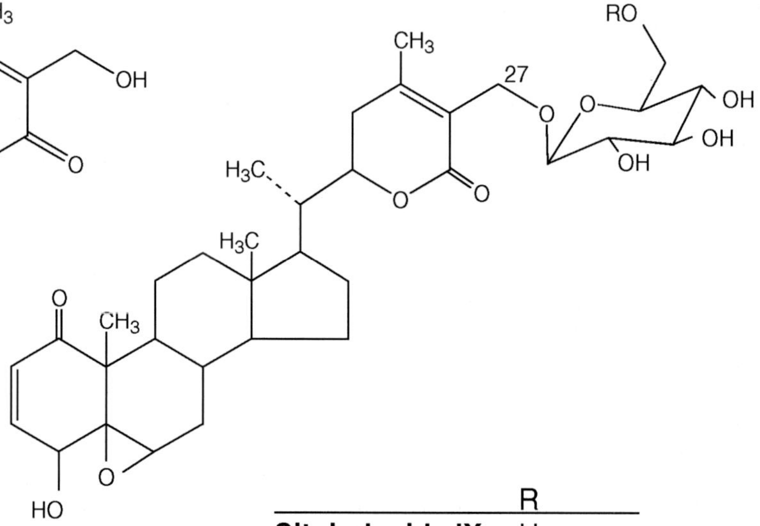

	R
Sitoindoside IX	H
Sitoindoside X	palmitoyl

Withania combines well with a low dose of *Panax ginseng*.

DURATION OF USE

No problems known with long-term use.

SUMMARY ASSESSMENT OF SAFETY

No adverse effects from ingestion of Withania are expected.

TECHNICAL DATA

BOTANY

Withania somnifera, a member of the Solanaceae (nightshade) family, is a small to medium perennial shrub which grows 1–1.5 m in height. It has ovate hair-like branches with simple, alternate leaves, up to 10 cm long. The small, greenish-yellow flowers (approximately 1 cm) are borne together in short axillary clusters. The red fruit (6 mm in diameter) is smooth, spherical and enclosed in the inflated and membranous calyx. The root is long and tuberous.[4]

KEY CONSTITUENTS

- Steroidal compounds, including lactones (withaferin A, sitoindoside IX, X (carbon-27-glycowithanolides)) and acylsteryl glucosides (sitoindosides VII, VIII).[5]
- Alkaloids: tropane-type (tropine, pseudotropine), other alkaloids (including isopelletierine, anaferine).[6]

Withania is also said to be rich in iron.[7]

PHARMACODYNAMICS

Adaptogens increase the ability of an organism to cope with stress. They therefore help to conserve energy, whereas a tonic boosts energy reserves and promotes health in a non-specific manner. In experimental models, adaptogenic effects can be assessed by subjecting an animal to stress, while tonic effects might be assessed by the long-term influence of a substance on the development, health and offspring of a test animal. The antiinflammatory and immunomodulating properties of Withania root are likely to be mild. However, it is possible that significant glucocorticoid-like tonic and

		Day 0	Day 3
Control	Total count	7800	4390
	Neutrophils	3960	1440
Withania	Total count	11 180	8030
	Neutrophils	7020	5060

adaptogenic effects may result from the complex of the many steroidal withanolides which are found in the root. Traditional use emphasizes the tonic properties of Withania root.

Adaptogenic and tonic activity

At an oral dose of 200 mg/kg in rats, Withania countered many of the biochemical changes of cold stress and immobilization stress such as rises in blood sugar, lactic acid, urea and creatinine. It did not, however, counteract the decrease in thymus, liver and kidney weights but did somewhat counteract the increase in adrenal weight.[8] Oral pretreatment with Withania (5, 10 and 20 mg/kg) for 3, 7 and 14 days resulted in protection against stress-induced stomach ulcers in rats.[9] The body weight loss induced by adjuvant arthritis was corrected by 1000 mg/kg Withania given orally over 15 days. Some of the inflammation and bony degenerative changes were also decreased.[10]

Several herbs including Withania were evaluated for their protective effects against cyclophosphamide neutropaenia in mice. The dosage used was 100 mg/kg, given for 15 days prior to a single dose of cyclophosphamide and then for 7 days after. Results are tabulated above.

Withania significantly increased white blood cell and neutrophil counts both before and after treatment with cyclophosphamide (day 3 gave the lowest counts). There were no deaths in the Withania group compared with 10% mortality in other groups.[11]

Young rats were fed Withania or *Asparagus racemosa* at oral doses of 100 mg/g for 8 months and observed for body weight, general condition, number of pregnancies and health of progeny. Weight gain for Withania-treated rats was 227% compared to 159% for *Asparagus racemosa* and 145% for controls. Animals were alert and in good health. While there was no difference in number and size of pregnancies, average body weight of offspring was 70 g for Withania compared to 45 g for controls. This study was followed up with a second short-term study over 4 weeks at 250 mg/g on adult rats. No weight gain was seen, which indicates that Withania's anabolic effect was only exerted in the growth phase. However, other interesting effects in this short-term study were noted. Body temperature was reduced by 1.7°C and liver weight increased for the Withania group. Plasma cortisol was also significantly lower and adrenal weight reduced following Withania treatment.[12] This may reflect on the 'steroid-like' activity of Withania constituents.

A recent pharmacological comparison of Withania and *Panax ginseng* demonstrated that Withania had similar potency to Panax in terms of adaptogenic, tonic and anabolic effects. Significant increases in swimming time were shown by both Withania and panax (100 mg/kg per day, oral administration for 7 days) compared with the control group. Following oral administration of aqueous suspensions at 1 g/kg for 7 days, the increase in body weight seen in the Withania-treated group was greater than that for animals treated with Panax. Gain in wet weight of the levator ani muscle was significant in both Withania ($p<0.01$) and panax groups ($p<0.001$).[13]

Seeds of Withania (100 mg/kg) administered by intraperitoneal injection showed a sparing effect on stress-induced adrenal cortisol and ascorbic acid depletion and on adrenal weight increase. They also showed protective effects against aspirin- and stress-induced ulcers. An anabolic effect at oral doses of 100 mg/kg was also demonstrated.[14]

Sitoindosides protected rats against stress-induced stomach ulcers. Sitoindosides IX and X (50–200 mg/kg) by oral administration produced significant antistress activity in mice and rats and augmented learning acquisition and memory retention in both young and old rats.[15] Aqueous methanolic extract of Withania and a combination of sitoindosides VII, VIII and withaferin A also exhibited significant antistress activity. An antidepressant effect was observed after intraperitoneal administration of sitoindosides VII and VIII to mice subjected to the swimming test.[16]

Acetylcholinesterase activity and levels of neurotransmitter receptor subtypes were investigated in brain slices from rats injected intraperitoneally with a mixture of sitoindosides VII–X and withaferin A (40 mg/kg per day, 7 days). An increase in cortical muscarinic acetylcholine receptor capacity was observed. GABA-A and benzodiazepine receptor binding and glutamate receptor subtypes were not affected. The increase in cortical muscarinic acetylcholine receptor capacity might partly explain the cognition-enhancing and memory-improving effects of Withania observed in animals and humans.[17] The dopaminergic (DA) system in the brain has been implicated in stress.[18] The effect of Withania on the DA system was studied in rats stressed by immobilization. DA receptor population in the corpus striatum was significantly increased after stress and this was prevented by pretreatment with Withania.[19] Withania extract significantly increased the total white blood cell count in normal mice and reduced leucopaenia induced by a sublethal dose of gamma radiation. Treatment increased the bone marrow cellularity significantly and normalized the ratio of normochromatic and polychromatic erythrocytes in mice after radiation exposure.[20]

Immune function

Sitoindosides IX and X (100–400 μg/mouse) produced significant mobilization and activation of peritoneal macrophages, phagocytosis and increased activity of the lysosomal enzymes secreted by activated macrophages. Withaferin A demonstrated immunosuppressive effects, in contrast to immunostimulating activity found for Withania extracts.[15] A steroidal withanolide isolated from roots of *Withania somnifera*[21] demonstrated immunomodulating activity by inhibiting proliferation of murine spleen cell cultures.[22]

Withania alcoholic extract significantly inhibited the experimentally induced suppression of chemotactic activity and production of interleukin-1 and tumour necrosis factor-alpha (TNF-alpha) by macrophages obtained from carcinogen-treated mice ($p<0.005$). Withania was co-administered (100 mg/kg per day) by oral administration with the carcinogen for 17 weeks. TNF-alpha and chemotactic activity was also higher than controls but not significantly.[23]

A significant modulation of immune reactivity by Withania was observed in mice with myelosuppression induced by three different immunosuppressive drugs. In addition, significant increases in haemoglobin concentration ($p<0.01$), red blood cell count ($p<0.01$), white blood cell count ($p<0.05$), platelet count ($p<0.01$) and body weight ($p<0.05$) were observed in Withania-treated mice compared to untreated controls. In an immunostimulatory model, treatment with Withania was accompanied by significant increases in haemolytic antibody responses.[24]

Antitumour activity

The compound withaferin A exhibited cytotoxic activity and radiosensitizing activity even at subtoxic doses in vivo. Pilot clinical studies have demonstrated the effectiveness of its oral administration and lack of systemic toxicity even after repeated administration. Preclinical studies on Withania extract suggest that it may also act as a chemopreventive against tumour induction. However, clinical trials are required to determine the usefulness of this Withania extract in cancer prevention or therapy.[25]

Withaferin A produced a mitotic arrest in the metaphase of dividing Ehrlich ascites carcinoma cells.[26] It also caused disappearance of Ehrlich ascites tumours in mice and the treated mice were resistant to rechallenge with the ascitic tumour cells. Such a response was explained as combined effect of withaferin A and an immune response.[27]

A study of the in vitro mode of action of withaferin A and withanolide D postulated that the cell death of sarcoma-180 tumour cultures was due to inhibition of RNA synthesis.[28] (Several chemotypes of Withania exist; withaferin A is the major withanolide found in leaves of one chemotype and withanolide D is the major one found in another.[29])

Withaferin A produced mitotic arrest in the metaphase of dividing normal human lymphocytes stimulated by phytohaemagglutinin. The membrane system of cells at interphase was also damaged.[30] However, the mechanism of action of the antitumour and radiosensitizing properties of withaferin A cannot be explained wholly on the basis of effects on the cell cycle or macromolecular synthesis.[25,31] Mouse sarcoma-180 solid and ascites tumour cells treated in vitro and in vivo with withaferin A were also affected in a similar way to the above study.[32]

Both withaferin A and withanolide E exhibited specific immunosuppressive effects on human B and T-lymphocytes in vitro. These results are indicative that the steroidal lactone withanolides have antiinflammatory and immunosuppressive effects similar to glucocorticoid drugs, although they were found to have a stronger and more direct action on lymphocytes than hydrocortisone. Intraperitoneal administration of withanolide E was also active against several animal tumour systems. Withaferin A and withanolide D predominate in the leaves of *Withania somnifera* and it is mainly the leaves of Withania which were traditionally used to treat cancerous growths.[33]

Repeated intraperitoneal administration of withaferin A demonstrated significant antitumour activity and radiosensitizing effects on mouse Ehrlich ascites carcinoma in vivo. Different dose fractions were administered with or without gamma irradiation and lifespan and tumour-free survival were studied up to 120 days.[25] In an earlier trial, the ED_{50} of withaferin A for 120-day survival was determined at 33 mg/kg[34] (which is comparable to the LD_{50} value obtained from the above in vitro study). Withaferin A treatment before irradiation synergistically increased survival, even in advanced tumours. A dose of 30 mg/kg appeared to be optimum for combination with radiation.[34] A total dose of 40 mg/kg per day (given as eight fractions of 5 mg/kg) or a total dose of 60 mg/kg per day (given as eight fractions of 7.5 mg/kg) 24 hours after initiation of the tumour process produced 20% tumour cure and tumour-free survival at 120 days. The same total doses of 40 and 60 mg/kg split into two (given as two fractions of 20 mg/kg and two fractions of 30 mg/kg respectively) resulted in 70% and 80% tumour-free survivors respectively at 120 days.[35] This indicates that the dose per fraction rather than the cumulative dose is more important in determining the antitumour efficacy.[25]

Intraperitoneal administration of withaferin A (30 mg/kg per day, 5 days) to mice subjected to gamma radiation resulted in enhanced bone marrow stem cell survival. The treatment increased the survival from 50% of normal after irradiation to more than 80% of normal. Withaferin A was less cytotoxic than the reference antineoplastic drug cyclophosphamide.[36]

Withania root extract was administered by intraperitoneal injection (200–1000 mg/kg per day for 15 days) to mice inoculated with sarcoma cells. Doses of 400 mg/kg and above produced complete regression of tumour after initial growth. The percentage of complete response increased with increasing herb dose, although some mortality was observed at the 1000 mg/kg level. Daily doses of 500–750 mg/kg produced a good response.[37]

A study investigating the effects of Withania, gamma radiation and hyperthermia on sarcoma in mice found that Withania (500 mg/kg per day for 10 days, intraperitoneal administration) produced an 18% rate of complete response. Although the radiation and heat treatments had a greater individual effect on the tumours, Withania increased the effect of these treatments on tumour regression and growth delay when administered concomitantly. The study concluded that Withania had a tumour inhibitory effect and acted as a radiosensitizer.[38] Withania given at 200 mg/kg (whole plant) orally to mice significantly decreased mortality from urethane-induced lung cancers. It countered the decrease in body weight due to the tumours and also decreased their incidence, number and size.[39]

Antiinflammatory activity

Intraperitoneal administration of withaferin A suppressed secondary lesions of adjuvant-induced arthritis in rats and strongly inhibited the graft-versus-host reaction in chicks. The similarity in structure and action with glucocorticoids suggests a complex influence on inflammation and immune response as well as the antiproliferative activity.[40] The effect of Withania on experimentally induced granuloma in rats was compared to cortisone and phenylbutazone. Withania was the most effective treatment in decreasing the glycosaminoglycan content of the granuloma.[41]

Alpha-2-macroglobulin is a liver-synthesized plasma protein which increases markedly during inflammation. Withania was found to be more effective at decreasing this protein during inflammation when compared to standard antiinflammatory drugs.[42] An antiinflammatory effect on granuloma tissue formation in rats was observed using an extract of the aerial parts of Withania. The effect was comparable to that achieved by 5 mg/kg hydrocortisone and was believed to be due to the presence of withaferin A.[43]

CNS activity

One interesting property of Withania root is its activity on the central nervous system. Despite the fact that it is a tonic herb, it has demonstrated sedative and antiepileptic effects but is also a cognition enhancer (confirming traditional use). These effects may be partly modulated by alkaloids (note that these are not to be confused with particular tropane alkaloids found in stramonium and belladonna which can cause marked side effects). Withania may also have some value in opiate addiction.

In high doses, alkaloids from Withania exhibited prolonged hypotensive, bradycardic and respiratory stimulant actions and had a depressant effect on higher cerebral centres.[44] Sedative effects have also been demonstrated.[45] The complex of alkaloids from Withania was only twice as active as the total extract from the root,[44,45] indicating the presence of other components with synergistic or contributive activity.

An in vitro study found that a methanolic extract of Withania contains a component which interacts with the GABA-A receptor and enhances the binding of flunitrazepam (a benzodiazepine drug) to this receptor.[46] This indicates a possible sedative activity and is similar to a postulated action for some steroid hormones.

Oral administration of Withania extract (100 mg/kg) per se did not produce analgesia and did not block morphine-induced analgesia (as measured by tailflick latency). However, repeated administration of withania (at the above dosage) for 9 days attenuated the development of tolerance to morphine-induced analgesia ($p<0.01$). Withania also suppressed morphine withdrawal jumps which are a sign of the development of opiate dependence (as assessed by naloxone precipitation of withdrawal on day 10 of testing).[47]

Pretreatment with sitoindosides VII–X and withaferin A (10–150 mg/kg, intraperitoneal administration) at all doses significantly reversed morphine-induced inhibition of gastrointestinal tract transit ($p<0.05$)

and inhibited development of tolerance to morphine-induced analgesia ($p<0.05$). The treatment per se did not influence intestinal motility nor produce any perceptible analgesic effect. The author suggested that Withania may be useful in the treatment of morphine withdrawal syndromes and the attendant physical dependence on morphine, including immunodepression.[48]

Pretreatment with Withania root extract (100 mg/kg) by oral administration offered significant protection ($p<0.05$) in an experimental epilepsy model in mice. The effect was comparable to diazepam (1 mg/kg). The protective action of Withania appears to involve GABAergic mediation.[49] In an earlier study using electrical stimulation in rats, pretreatment with Withania extract (100 mg/kg) after the establishment of epilepsy resulted in a significant reduction in the severity of motor seizures, as evident from the amplitude and frequency of wave patterns. EEG recordings taken 2 hours after the stimulus showed a normal wave pattern.[50] In vitro and in vivo studies indicate that the anticonvulsant action of Withania extract is mediated via GABAergic mechanism, primarily through the barbiturate site on the nerve cell membrane.[51]

A Withania extract, consisting of equimolar amounts of sitoindosides VII–X and withaferin A, was investigated in an Alzheimer's disease model in rats. Oral administration of the extract (50 mg/kg) significantly reversed the experimentally induced cognitive deficit and the reduction in cholinergic markers after 2 weeks of treatment.[2]

Other activity

Withaferin A has demonstrated antimicrobial activity against Gram-positive bacteria and certain pathogenic fungi.[52] A methanol extract of Withania showed potent inhibition of plaque formation by herpes simplex virus type 1 in cultured cells (without cytotoxicity) at a concentration of 100 μg/ml. This in vitro activity was not demonstrated in vivo (cutaneous HSV-1 infection in mice) but a methanol extract of Withania branches was administered, rather than root.[53]

Withania alkaloids are spasmolytic for intestinal, uterine, bronchial and arterial smooth muscle, with a similar mode of action to papaverine.[45]

Intraperitoneal administration of a mixture of sitoindosides VII–X and withaferin A at doses of 10 and 20 mg/kg per day for 3 weeks to rats induced a dose-related increase in superoxide dismutase, catalase and glutathione peroxidase activities in frontal cortex and striatum. These effects were generally significant on days 14 and 21 and activity was comparable to the test antioxidant deprenyl (2 mg/kg per day).[54]

Simultaneous oral administration of 100 mg/kg of Withania extract with endotoxins prevented the rise in lipid peroxidation in rabbits and mice.[55]

PHARMACOKINETICS

No data available.

CLINICAL TRIALS

A double-blind clinical trial compared the effect of milk fortified with Withania against placebo (lactose powder in milk) in 58 children aged 8–12 years. The dose of Withania was 2 g per day over a period of 60 days. For the Withania-treated children there was a significant increase in mean corpuscular hamoglobin and serum albumin. Blood haemoglobin, serum iron, body weight and strength of hand grip also showed increases which were not statistically significant. There were no significant changes or tendency to change for any of these parameters in the control group. The authors concluded that Withania is a growth promoter with antianaemic activity in children.[7]

The effect of Withania on parameters of ageing was studied in 101 healthy male patients aged 50–59 years under double-blind conditions. Subjects were given 3 g of Withania root or 3 g of starch per day for 1 year. Compared to the placebo control group, Withania caused a significant increase in haemoglobin ($p<0.001$) and red blood cell count ($p<0.02$) and also significantly increased seated stature ($p<0.05$) and hair melanin content (less greying, $p<0.1$) It countered the decrease in nail calcium ($p<0.05$) and also decreased serum cholesterol ($p<0.1$) and erythrocyte sedimentation rate ($p<0.02$). About 71% of subjects receiving Withania reported improvement in sexual performance.[56]

Withania (1 g per day) was administered to trainee mountaineers over 29 days in an uncontrolled trial which included a 5200 m altitude gain through trekking and 6 days' training at that height, including a climb to 6400 m and subsequent descent. Psychological and physiological parameters were tested at various altitudes. Withania improved sleep patterns, responsiveness, alertness and state of awareness together with physical capabilities.[57]

TOXICOLOGY

A single intraperitoneal injection of 1100 mg/kg of Withania extract in mice did not produce any deaths within 24 hours but dosages beyond this level resulted in mortality (100% mortality with a 1500 mg/kg dose).

The acute LD_{50} within 24 hours was 1260 mg/kg. Subacute toxicity studies with repeated intraperitoneal injections of Withania extract at a dose of 100 mg/kg for 30 days in rats did not result in any mortality. An increase in haemoglobin level and a non-significant increase in red blood cell count were observed. Also significant reductions in the weights of spleen, thymus and adrenals were observed in male rats at the end of the experiment. Levels of DNA, RNA, proteins and alkaline and acid phosphates within the liver were normal but the acid phosphatase content of peripheral blood showed a significant increase from controls.[58]

CONTRAINDICATIONS

None known.

SPECIAL WARNINGS AND PRECAUTIONS

None required.

INTERACTIONS

None known.

USE IN PREGNANCY AND LACTATION

No adverse effects expected.

EFFECTS ON ABILITY TO DRIVE AND USE MACHINES

No negative influence is expected at the recommended dosage.

SIDE EFFECTS

Side effects from ingestion of Withania have not been reported.

OVERDOSE

Not known.

CURRENT REGULATORY STATUS IN SELECTED COUNTRIES

Withania was official in the second edition of the *Indian Pharmacopoeia* (1966) but was not included in the third edition (1985).

Withania is not covered by a Commission E monograph and is not on the UK General Sale List.

Withania does not have GRAS status. However, it is freely available as a 'dietary supplement' in the USA under DSHEA legislation (1994 Dietary Supplement Health and Education Act).

Withania is not included in Part 4 of Schedule 4 of the Therapeutic Goods Act Regulations of Australia.

References

1. Thakur RS, Puri HS, Husain A. Major medicinal plants of India. Central Institute of Medicinal and Aromatic Plants, Lucknow, 1989, pp 531–535.
2. Bhattacharya SK, Kumar A, Ghosal S. Phytother Res 1995; 9 (2): 110–113.
3. Miller AG, Morris M. Plants of Dhofar. The Office of the Adviser for Conservation of the Environment, Diwan of Royal Court Sultanate of Oman, 1988, p 274.
4. Kapoor LD. CRC handbook of Ayurvedic medicinal plants. CRC Press, Boca Raton, 1990, pp 337–338.
5. Wagner H, Norr H, Winterhoff H. Phytomed 1994; 1: 63–76.
6. Atal CK, Gupta OP, Raghunathan K et al. Pharmacognosy and phytochemistry of *Withania somnifera* (Linn) Dunal (Ashwagandha). Central Council for Research in Indian Medicine and Homoeopathy, New Delhi, 1975, pp 47–53.
7. Venkataraghavan S, Seshadri C, Sundaresan TP et al. J Res Ayu Sid 1980; 1: 370–385.
8. Dadkar VN, Ranadive NU, Dhar HL. Ind J Clin Biochem 1987; 2: 101–108.
9. Roy U, Mukhopadhyay S, Poddar MK et al. International seminar – traditional medicine, Calcutta, November 7–9, 1992, p 141.
10. Begum VH, Sadique J. Indian J Exp Biol 1988; 26 (11): 877–882.
11. Thatte UM, Chhabria SN, Karandikar SM et al. J Postgrad Med 1987; 33 (4): 185–188.
12. Sharma S, Dahanukar S, Karandikar SM. Indian Drugs 1986; 23 (3): 133–139.
13. Grandhi A, Mujumdar AM, Patwardhan B. J Ethnopharmacol 1994; 44 (3): 131–135.
14. Singh N, Nath R, Lata A et al. Int J Crude Drug Res 1982; 20 (1): 29–35.
15. Ghosal S, Lah J, Srivastava R et al. Phytother Res 1989; 3 (5): 201–206.
16. Bhattacharya SK, Goel RK, Kaur R et al. Phytother Res 1987; 1 (1): 32–37.
17. Schliebs R, Liebmann A, Bhattacharya SK et al. Neurochem Int 1997; 30 (2): 181–190.
18. Roth KA, Mefford IM, Barchas JD. Brain Res 1982; 239 (2): 417–424.
19. Saksena AK, Singh SP, Dixit KS et al. Planta Med 1989; 55: 95.
20. Kuttan G. Indian J Exp Biol 1996; 34 (9): 854–856.
21. Menssen HG, Stapel G. Planta Med 1973; 24 (1): 8–12.
22. Bähr V, Hänsel R. Planta Med 1982; 44 (1): 32–33.
23. Dhuley JN. J Ethnopharmacol 1997; 58 (1): 15–20.
24. Ziauddin M, Phansalkar N, Patki P et al. J Ethnopharmacol 1996; 50 (2): 69–76.
25. Devi PU. Indian J Exp Biol 1996; 34 (10): 927–932.
26. Shohat B, Gitter S, Lavie D. Int J Cancer 1970; 5 (2): 244–252.
27. Shohat B, Joshua H. Int J Cancer 1971; 8 (3): 487–496.
28. Chowdhury K, Neogy RK. Biochem Pharmacol 1975; 24: 919–920.
29. Chakraborti SK, De BK, Bandyopadhyay T. Experientia 1974; 30 (8): 852–853.
30. Shohat B, Ben-Bassat M, Shaltiel A et al. Cancer Lett 1976; 2 (2): 63–70.
31. Devi PU, Akagi K, Ostapenko V et al. Int J Radiat Biol 1996; 69 (2): 193–197.
32. Shohat B, Shaltiel A, Ben-Bassat M et al. Cancer Lett 1976; 2 (2): 71–77.

33. Shohat B, Kirson I, Lavie D. Biomed 1978; 28 (1): 18–24.
34. Devi PU, Sharada AC, Solomon FE. Cancer Lett 1995; 95 (1–2): 189–193.
35. Sharada AC, Solomon FE, Devi PU et al. Acta Oncol 1996; 35 (1): 95–100.
36. Ganasoundari A, Zare SM, Devi PU. Br J Radiol 1997; 70 (834): 599–602.
37. Devi PU, Sharada AC, Solomon FE et al. Indian J Exp Biol 1992; 30 (3): 169–172.
38. Devi PU, Sharada AC, Solomon FE. Indian J Exp Biol 1993; 31 (7): 607–611.
39. Singh N, Singh SP, Nath R et al. Int J Crude Drug Res 1986; 24 (2): 90–100.
40. Fugner A. Arzneim Forsch 1973; 23 (7): 932–935.
41. Begum VH, Sadique J. Biochem Med Metab Biol 1987; 38 (3): 272–277.
42. Anbalagan K, Sadique J. Int J Crude Drug Res 1985; 23 (4): 177–183.
43. Al-Hindawi MK, Al-Khafaji SH, Abdul-Nabi MH. J Ethnopharmacol 1992; 37 (2): 113–116.
44. Malhotra CL, Das PK, Dhalla NS et al. Indian J Med Res 1961; 49: 448–460.
45. Malhotra CL, Mehta VL, Prasad K et al. Indian J Physiol Pharmacol 1965; 9: 9–15.
46. Mehta AK, Binkley P, Gandhi SS et al. Indian J Med Res 1991; 94: 312–315.
47. Kulkarni SK, Ninan I. J Ethnopharmacol 1997; 57 (3): 213–217.
48. Ramarao P, Rao KT, Srivastava RS et al. Phytother Res 1995; 9 (1): 66–68.
49. Kulkarni SK, George B. Phytother Res 1996; 10 (5): 447–449.
50. Kulkarni SK, George B, Nayar U. Indian Drugs 1995; 32 (1): 37–49.
51. Kulkarni SK, Sharma A, Verma A et al. Indian Drugs 1993; 30 (7): 305–312.
52. Das Gupta IR, Sethi PD, Sarma KB et al. Indian J Pharm 1970; 32: 70.
53. Hattori M, Nakabayashi T, Lim YA et al. Phytother Res 1995; 9 (4): 270–276.
54. Bhattacharya SK, Satyan KS, Ghosal S. Indian J Exp Biol 1997; 35 (3): 236–239.
55. Dhuley JN. J Ethnopharmacol 1998; 60 (2): 173–178.
56. Kuppurajan K, Rajagopalan SS, Sitaraman R et al. J Res Ayu Sid 1980; 1: 247–258.
57. Roy AS, Acharya SB, De AK et al. International seminar – traditional medicine, Calcutta, November 7–9, 1992, p 161.
58. Sharada AC, Soloman FE, Devi PU. Int J Pharmacog 1993; 31 (3): 205–212.

Actions index

Conditions index

General index